Comprehensive Evaluation and Treatment: Provides a step-wise approach to the evaluation and treatment of coma, seizures, shock, and other common complications of poisoning and to the proper use of gastric decontamination and dialysis procedures.

Emergency Treatment

Specific Poisons and Drugs: Diagnosis and Treatment: Alphabetical listing of specific drugs and poisons, including the pathophysiology, toxic dose and level, clinical presentation, diagnosis, and specific treatment associated with each substance.

Common Poisons & Drugs

Therapeutic Drugs and Antidotes: Descriptions of therapeutic drugs and antidotes discussed in the two preceding sections, including their pharmacology, indications, adverse effects, drug interactions, recommended dosage, and formulations.

Antidotes & Drug Therapy

Environmental and Occupational Toxicology: Approach to hazardous materials incidents; evaluation of occupational exposures; and the toxic effects, physical properties, and workplace exposure limits fo over 500 common industrial chemicals.

Industrial Chemicals

Index: Includes generic drug and chemical ...d numerous brand name drugs and commercial products

Index

seventh edition

POISONING & DRUG OVERDOSE

Edited by

Kent R. Olson, MD, FACEP, FACMT, FAACT
Clinical Professor of Medicine and Pharmacy,
University of California, San Francisco;
Co-Medical Director, California Poison Control System,
San Francisco Division (retired)

Associate Editors

Ilene B. Anderson, PharmD
Clinical Professor of Pharmacy, University of California, San Francisco;
Senior Toxicology Management Specialist,
California Poison Control System,
San Francisco Division

Neal L. Benowitz, MD
Professor of Medicine
and Chief, Division of Clinical Pharmacology and Toxicology,
University of California, San Francisco;
Associate Medical Director,
California Poison Control System,
San Francisco Division

Paul D. Blanc, MD, MSPH
Professor of Medicine and Chief, Division of Occupational and Environmental Medicine,
University of California, San Francisco

Richard F. Clark, MD, FACEP
Professor of Medicine,
University of California, San Diego;
Director, Division of Medical Toxicology and Medical Director,
California Poison Control System,
San Diego Division

Thomas E. Kearney, PharmD, ABAT
Professor of Clinical Pharmacy, and
Associate Dean for Academic Affairs
University of California, San Francisco;
Clinical Consultant
California Poison Control System,
San Francisco Division

Susan Y. Kim-Katz, Pha ID
Clinical Professor of P macy,
University of Calif ia, San Francisco;
Senior Toxico Management Specialist,
California P Control System,
San Fra Division

Alan H. B. Wu, PhD cine,
Professor of Laborat Francisco;
University of Califo Laboratory
Chief, Clinical C Hospital
San Francisc

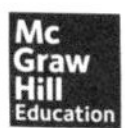

New York Chicago San ul Lisbon London Madrid Mexico City
Milan New Delhi Sa Singapore Sydney Toronto

Poisoning & Drug Overdose, Seventh Edition

1 2 3 4 5 6 7 8 9 LCR 22 21 20 19 18 17

ISBN 978-0-07-183979-2
MHID 0-07-183979-8
ISSN 1048-8847

Notice

Medicine is an ever-changing science. As new research and clinical experience broaden our knowledge, changes in treatment and drug therapy are required. The authors and the publisher of this work have checked with sources believed to be reliable in their efforts to provide information that is complete and generally in accord with the standards accepted at the time of publication. However, in view of the possibility of human error or changes in medical sciences, neither the authors nor the publisher nor any other party who has been involved in the preparation or publication of this work warrants that the information contained herein is in every respect accurate or complete, and they disclaim all responsibility for any errors or omissions or for the results obtained from use of the information contained in this work. Readers are encouraged to confirm the information contained herein with other sources. For example and in particular, readers are advised to check the product information sheet included in the package of each drug they plan to administer to be certain that the information contained in this work is accurate and that changes have not been made in the recommended dose or in the contraindications for administration. This recommendation is of particular importance in connection with new or infrequently used drugs.

This book was se[illegible] Helvetica LT Std by Aptara, Inc.
The editors were Bria[illegible] Belval and Christie Naglieri.
The production supervis[illegible] was Richard Ruzycka.
Project management was [illegible]vided by Indu Jawwad, Aptara, Inc.
The index was prepared by [illegible]hy Pitcoff.
Cover image credit: Astrid & [illegible]s-Frieder Michler/Science Source.
LSC Communications was prin[illegible]d binder.

This book is printed on acid-free pa[illegible]

McGraw-Hill Education books are ava[illegible]t special quantity discounts to use as premiums and sales promotions or for us[illegible]porate training programs. To contact [illegible] representation, please visit the Contact [illegible]s at www.mhprofessional.com.

seventh edition

POISONING & DRUG OVERDOSE

Edited by

Kent R. Olson, MD, FACEP, FACMT, FAACT
Clinical Professor of Medicine and Pharmacy,
University of California, San Francisco;
Co-Medical Director, California Poison Control System,
San Francisco Division (retired)

Associate Editors

Ilene B. Anderson, PharmD
Clinical Professor of Pharmacy, University of California, San Francisco;
Senior Toxicology Management Specialist,
California Poison Control System,
San Francisco Division

Neal L. Benowitz, MD
Professor of Medicine
and Chief, Division of Clinical Pharmacology and Toxicology,
University of California, San Francisco;
Associate Medical Director,
California Poison Control System,
San Francisco Division

Paul D. Blanc, MD, MSPH
Professor of Medicine and Chief, Division of Occupational and Environmental Medicine,
University of California, San Francisco

Richard F. Clark, MD, FACEP
Professor of Medicine,
University of California, San Diego;
Director, Division of Medical Toxicology and Medical Director,
California Poison Control System,
San Diego Division

Thomas E. Kearney, PharmD, ABAT
Professor of Clinical Pharmacy, and
Associate Dean for Academic Affairs
University of California, San Francisco;
Clinical Consultant
California Poison Control System,
San Francisco Division

Susan Y. Kim-Katz, PharmD
Clinical Professor of Pharmacy,
University of California, San Francisco;
Senior Toxicology Management Specialist,
California Poison Control System,
San Francisco Division

Alan H. B. Wu, PhD
Professor of Laboratory Medicine,
University of California, San Francisco;
Chief, Clinical Chemistry Laboratory
San Francisco General Hospital

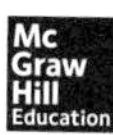

New York Chicago San Francisco Lisbon London Madrid Mexico City
Milan New Delhi San Juan Seoul Singapore Sydney Toronto

Poisoning & Drug Overdose, Seventh Edition

1 2 3 4 5 6 7 8 9 LCR 22 21 20 19 18 17

ISBN 978-0-07-183979-2
MHID 0-07-183979-8
ISSN 1048-8847

Notice

Medicine is an ever-changing science. As new research and clinical experience broaden our knowledge, changes in treatment and drug therapy are required. The authors and the publisher of this work have checked with sources believed to be reliable in their efforts to provide information that is complete and generally in accord with the standards accepted at the time of publication. However, in view of the possibility of human error or changes in medical sciences, neither the authors nor the publisher nor any other party who has been involved in the preparation or publication of this work warrants that the information contained herein is in every respect accurate or complete, and they disclaim all responsibility for any errors or omissions or for the results obtained from use of the information contained in this work. Readers are encouraged to confirm the information contained herein with other sources. For example and in particular, readers are advised to check the product information sheet included in the package of each drug they plan to administer to be certain that the information contained in this work is accurate and that changes have not been made in the recommended dose or in the contraindications for administration. This recommendation is of particular importance in connection with new or infrequently used drugs.

This book was set in Helvetica LT Std by Aptara, Inc.
The editors were Brian Belval and Christie Naglieri.
The production supervisor was Richard Ruzycka.
Project management was provided by Indu Jawwad, Aptara, Inc.
The index was prepared by Kathy Pitcoff.
Cover image credit: Astrid & Hanns-Frieder Michler/Science Source.
LSC Communications was printer and binder.

This book is printed on acid-free paper.

Contents

Authors

Suad Abdullah Saif Al Abri, MD, ABEM, OBEM
Medical Toxicology Fellow, California Poison Control System, San Francisco Division, University of California, San Francisco; Consultant Emergency Physician and Medical Toxicologist, Emergency Department, Sultan Qaboos University Hospital, Muscat, Oman

Timothy E. Albertson, MD, MPH, PhD
Professor of Medicine, Medical Pharmacology and Toxicology, University of California Medical Center, Davis; Medical Director, California Poison Control System, Sacramento Division

Ilene B. Anderson, PharmD
Clinical Professor of Pharmacy, University of California, San Francisco; Senior Toxicology Management Specialist, California Poison Control System, San Francisco Division

Gilberto Araya-Rodriguez, Licenciado en Farmacia (Costa Rica)
Volunteer, California Poison Control System, San Francisco Division, San Francisco, California

Ann Arens, MD
Medical Toxicology Fellow, Department of Medicine, University of California, San Francisco, California; Medical Toxicologist, Minnesota Poison Control System; Assistant Professor, Department of Emergency Medicine, University of Minnesota

Patil Armenian, MD
Associate Professor, Assistant Research Director, Department of Emergency Medicine, University of California, San Francisco-Fresno

John R. Balmes, MD
Professor of Medicine, University of California, San Francisco; Division of Environmental Health Sciences, School of Public Health, University of California, Berkeley

Neal L. Benowitz, MD
Professor of Medicine and Chief, Division of Clinical Pharmacology, Medicine and Bioengineering & Therapeutic Sciences, Zuckerberg San Francisco General Hospital/ University of California, San Francisco

Kathleen Birnbaum, PharmD
Toxicology Management Specialist, California Poison Control System, San Diego Division

Paul D. Blanc, MD, MSPH
Professor of Medicine, Division of Occupational and Environmental Medicine, University of California, San Francisco and the Veteran Affairs Medical Center, San Francisco

Stephen C. Born, MD, MPH
Clinical Professor Emeritus, Division of Occupational and Environmental Medicine, University of California, San Francisco

F. Lee Cantrell, PharmD
Managing Director, California Poison Control System, San Diego Division; Professor of Clinical Pharmacy, University of California, San Francisco; Clinical Professor of Pharmacy and Medicine, University of California, San Diego

James Chenoweth, MD, MAS
Assistant Professor, Director of Toxicology Research, Department of Emergency Medicine, University of California, Davis

Richard F. Clark, MD
Medical Director, San Diego Division, California Poison Control System; Director, Division of Medical Toxicology, University of California, San Diego Medical Center

Michael A. Darracq, MD, MPH
Associate Professor of Clinical Emergency Medicine, University of California, San Francisco-Fresno

G. Patrick Daubert, MD, FACEP
Division of Emergency Medicine, Kaiser Permanente, South Sacramento Medical Center, Sacramento, California

Timur S. Durrani, MD, MPH, MBA
Medical Director, Occupational Health Services, Zuckerberg San Francisco General Hospital; Assistant Medical Director, San Francisco Division, California Poison Control System; Principal Investigator, UCSF Pediatric Environmental Health Specialty Unit; Assistant Clinical Professor of Medicine, University of California San Francisco

Jo Ellen Dyer, PharmD
Clinical Professor of Pharmacy, University of California, San Francisco; Senior Toxicology Management Specialist, California Poison Control System, San Francisco Division

Gary W. Everson, PharmD
Toxicology Management Specialist, California Poison Control System, Fresno/Madera Division

Jeffrey Fay, PharmD
Assistant Clinical Professor of Pharmacy, University of California, San Francisco; Toxicology Management Specialist, California Poison Control System, Fresno/Madera Division

Jonathan B. Ford, MD
Assistant Professor, Emergency Medicine, University of California, Davis

Thomas J. Ferguson, MD, PhD
Associate Clinical Professor, Departments of Internal Medicine and Public Health, University of California, Davis

Frederick Fung, MD, MS
Clinical Professor of Occupational Medicine, University of California, Irvine; Medical Director, Occupational Medicine Department and Toxicology Services, Sharp Rees-Stealy Medical Group, San Diego, California

Fabian Garza, PharmD
Assistant Clinical Professor of Pharmacy, University of California, San Francisco; Toxicology Management Specialist, California Poison Control System, Fresno/Madera Division

Curtis Geier, PharmD
Emergency Medicine Clinical Pharmacist, Zuckerberg San Francisco General Hospital, San Francisco, California, Assistant Clinical Professor of Pharmacy, University of California, San Francisco

Richard J. Geller, MD, MPH
Associate Clinical Professor of Emergency Medicine, University of California, San Francisco; Medical and Managing Director, California Poison Control System, Fresno/Madera Division

Nasim Ghafouri, PharmD
Toxicology Management Specialist, California Poison Control System, San Diego Division

Joyce Go, PharmD
Emergency Medicine Clinical Pharmacist, Department of Pharmacy, Zuckerberg San Francisco General Hospital and Trauma Center, San Francisco, California

Joanne M. Goralka, PharmD
Department of Clinical Pharmacy, University of California, San Francisco; Toxicology Management Specialist, California Poison Control System, Sacramento Division

Hallam Gugelmann, MD, MPH
Attending Physician in Emergency Medicine, CPMC St. Luke's Hospital; Assistant Medical Director, California Poison Control System, San Francisco Division

Sandra A. Hayashi, PharmD
Assistant Clinical Professor, University of California, San Francisco; Toxicology Management Specialist, California Poison Control System, San Francisco Division

Patricia Hess Hiatt, BS
Operations Manager (retired), San Francisco Division, California Poison Control System

Raymond Y. Ho, PharmD
Managing Director, California Poison Control System, San Francisco Division

Leslie M. Israel, DO, MPH
Medical Director, Occupational Health Services, Los Angeles Department of Water and Power, Los Angeles, California

Sam Jackson, MD, MBA
Chief Medical Officer, Alkahest, Inc., San Carlos, California

Thomas E. Kearney, PharmD, DABAT
Professor of Clinical Pharmacy and Associate Dean for Academic Affairs, University of California, San Francisco; Clinical Consultant, California Poison Control System, San Francisco Division

Paul Khasigian, PharmD
Toxicology Management Specialist, California Poison Control System, Fresno/Madera Division

Susan Kim-Katz, PharmD
Professor of Clinical Pharmacy, University of California, San Francisco; Senior Toxicology Management Specialist, California Poison Control System, San Francisco Division

Richard Ko, PharmD, PhD
Pharmaceutical Consultant, Herbal Synergy, Pinole, California

Michael J. Kosnett, MD, MPH, FACMT
Associate Clinical Professor, Division of Clinical Pharmacology & Toxicology, Department of Medicine, University of Colorado School of Medicine Denver, Colorado

Allyson Kreshak, MD, FACMT, FACEP
Assistant Clinical Professor, Department of Emergency Medicine, University of California San Diego

Chi-Leung Lai, PharmD
Assistant Clinical Professor of Pharmacy, University of California, San Francisco; Assistant Clinical Professor of Medicine, University of California, Davis; Toxicology Management Specialist, California Poison Control System, Sacramento Division

Darren H. Lew, PharmD
Toxicology Management Specialist, California Poison Control System, Fresno/Madera Division

Justin C. Lewis, PharmD, DABAT
Managing Director, California Poison Control System, Sacramento Division

Kai Li, MD
Medical Toxicology Fellow, Department of Emergency Medicine, University of California, San Francisco

Derrick Lung, MD, MPH
Assistant Clinical Professor, Division of Clinical Pharmacology and Toxicology, Department of Medicine, University of California, San Francisco

Binh T. Ly, MD, FACMT, FACEP
Professor and Vice Chair (Education), Department of Emergency Medicine (Medical Toxicology), University of California, San Diego

Conan MacDougall, PharmD, MAS
Professor of Clinical Pharmacy, University of California San Francisco

Tanya M. Mamantov, MD, MPH
Medical Toxicology Attending Physician, Zuckerberg San Francisco General Hospital and California Poison Control System, San Francisco Division

Beth H. Manning, PharmD
Assistant Clinical Professor of Pharmacy, University of California, San Francisco; Toxicology Management Specialist, California Poison Control System, San Francisco Division

Kathryn H. Meier, PharmD
Assistant Clinical Professor of Pharmacy, University of California, San Francisco; Toxicology Management Specialist, California Poison Control System, San Francisco Division

Alicia B. Minns, MD
Assistant Clinical Professor of Emergency Medicine, Department of Emergency Medicine, University of California, San Diego

Eileen Morentz
Poison Information Provider, California Poison Control System, San Francisco Division

Stephen W. Munday, MD, MPH, MS
Chair, Department of Occupational Medicine, Sharp Rees Stealy Medical Group, San Diego; California Poison Control System, San Diego Division

Sean Patrick Nordt, MD, PharmD, DABAT, FAACT, FAAEM, FACMT
Associate Professor of Clinical Emergency Medicine, Keck School of Medicine, University of Southern California

Charles W. O'Connell, MD
Clinical Professor of Emergency Medicine, Division of Medical Toxicology, University of California, San Diego

Steven R. Offerman, MD
Assistant Professor, Department of Emergency Medicine, University of California, Davis; Division of Emergency Medicine, Kaiser Permanente, South Sacramento Medical Center, Sacramento, California

Kent R. Olson, MD, FACEP, FACMT, FAACT
Clinical Professor of Medicine and Pharmacy, University of California, San Francisco; Co-Medical Director, California Poison Control System, San Francisco Division, San Francisco (retired)

Michael A. O'Malley, MD, MPH
Associate Clinical Professor, Public Health Sciences, University of California, Davis

Annamariam Pajouhi, PharmD
Assistant Clinical Professor of Pharmacy, University of California, San Francisco; Toxicology Management Specialist, California Poison Control System, Sacramento Division

Mariam Qozi, PharmD
Toxicology Management Specialist, California Poison Control System, San Diego Division

Joshua B. Radke
Medical Toxicology Fellow, Department of Emergency Medicine, University of California, Davis

Cyrus Rangan, MD
Assistant Medical Director, California Poison Control System; Director, Toxics Epidemiology Program, Los Angeles County Department of Health Services; Attending Staff, Children's Hospital, Los Angeles, California

Daniel J. Repplinger, MD
Assistant Clinical Professor, Department of Emergency Medicine, University of California, San Francisco; Zuckerberg San Francisco General Hospital, San Francisco, California

Freda M. Rowley, PharmD
Assistant Clinical Professor of Pharmacy, University of California, San Francisco; Toxicology Management Specialist, California Poison Control System, San Francisco Division

Thomas R. Sands, PharmD
Assistant Clinical Professor of Pharmacy, University of California, San Francisco; Associate Clinical Professor, School of Medicine, University of California, Davis; Toxicology Management Specialist, California Poison Control System, Sacramento Division (retired)

Aaron Schneir, MD
Professor of Emergency Medicine, Division of Medical Toxicology, Department of Emergency Medicine, University of California, San Diego

Jay Schrader, CPhT
Poison Information Provider, California Poison Control System, San Francisco Division

Dennis Shusterman, MD, MPH
Professor of Clinical Medicine, Emeritus, Division of Occupational and Environmental Medicine, University of California, San Francisco

Craig Smollin, MD
Medical Director, California Poison Control System, San Francisco Division; Associate Professor of Emergency Medicine, University of California, San Francisco

Jeffrey R. Suchard, MD
Professor of Clinical Emergency Medicine and Pharmacology, Department of Emergency Medicine, University of California, Irvine

Mark E. Sutter, MD
Associate Professor of Emergency Medicine, University of California, Davis

R. Steven Tharratt, MD, MPVM
Clinical Professor of Medicine, Division of Pulmonary, Critical Care & Sleep Medicine, University of California, Davis

Ben T. Tsutaoka, PharmD
Assistant Clinical Professor of Pharmacy, University of California, San Francisco; Toxicology Management Specialist, California Poison Control System, San Francisco Division

Janna H. Villano, MD
Clinical Faculty, Emergency Medicine, University of California, San Diego

Kathy Vo, MD
Medical Toxicology Fellow, California Poison Control System, San Francisco Division, University of California, San Francisco; Assistant Clinical Professor of Emergency Medicine, University of California, San Francisco

Rais Vohra, MD
Assistant Professor of Emergency Medicine, University of California, San Francisco-Fresno

Michael J. Walsh, PharmD
Assistant Clinical Professor of Pharmacy, University of California, San Francisco; Toxicology Management Specialist, California Poison Control System, Sacramento Division

R. David West, PharmD
Toxicology Management Specialist, California Poison Control System, Fresno/Madera Division

Michael Young, DO, FACEP, FACMT
Associate Director, Division of Toxicology, Kaiser Permanente, San Diego, California

Preface

Poisoning & Drug Overdose provides practical advice for the diagnosis and management of poisoning and drug overdose and concise information about common industrial chemicals.

The manual is divided into four sections and an index, each identified by a black tab in the right margin. **Section I** leads the reader through initial emergency management, including treatment of coma, hypotension, and other common complications; physical and laboratory diagnosis; and methods of decontamination and enhanced elimination of poisons. **Section II** provides detailed information for approximately 150 common drugs and poisons. **Section III** describes the use and side effects of approximately 60 antidotes and therapeutic drugs. **Section IV** describes the medical management of chemical spills and occupational chemical exposures and includes a table of over 500 chemicals. The **Index** is comprehensive and extensively cross-referenced.

The manual is designed to allow the reader to move quickly from section to section, obtaining the needed information from each. For example, in managing a patient with isoniazid intoxication, the reader will find specific information about isoniazid toxicity in **Section II,** practical advice for gut decontamination and management of complications such as seizures in **Section I,** and detailed information about dosing and side effects for the antidote pyridoxine in **Section III.**

ACKNOWLEDGMENTS

The success of the first and second editions of this manual would not have been possible without the combined efforts of the staff, faculty, and fellows of the San Francisco Bay Area Regional Poison Control Center, to whom I am deeply indebted. From its inception, this book has been a project by and for our poison center; as a result, all royalties from its sale have gone to our center's operating fund and not to any individual editor or author.

In January 1997, four independent poison control centers joined their talents to become the California Poison Control System, administered by the University of California, San Francisco. With the third, fourth, fifth, and sixth editions, the manual became a project of our statewide system, bringing in new authors and editors.

On behalf of the authors and editors of the seventh edition, my sincere thanks go to all those who contributed to one or more of the first six editions:

Timothy E. Albertson, MD, PhD
Judith A. Alsop, PharmD
Ilene Brewer Anderson, PharmD
Patil Armenian, MD
Margaret Atterbury, MD
Georgeanne M. Backman
John Balmes, MD
Shireen Banerji, PharmD
James David Barry, MD
Charles E. Becker, MD
Neal L. Benowitz, MD
Bruce Bernard, MD
David P. Betten, MD
Kathleen Birnbaum, PharmD
Paul D. Blanc, MD, MSPH
Stephen Born, MD
Christopher R. Brown, MD
Randall G. Browning, MD, MPH
James F. Buchanan, PharmD
Alan Buchwald, MD
Cindy Burkhardt, PharmD
Chris Camillieri, DO
F. Lee Cantrell, PharmD
Terry Carlson, PharmD
Shaun D. Carstairs, MD
Gregory Cham, MD
Chulathida Chomchai, MD
Summon Chomchai, MD
Richard F. Clark, MD
Matthew D. Cook, MD

G. Patrick Daubert, MD
Delia Dempsey, MD
Charlene Doss
Chris Dutra, MD
Jo Ellen Dyer, PharmD
Brent R. Ekins, PharmD
Andrew Erdman, MD
Gary Everson, PharmD
Jeffrey Fay, PharmD
Thomas J. Ferguson, MD, PhD
Donna E. Foliart, MD, MPH
Frederick Fung, MD
Mark J. Galbo, MS
Fabian Garza, PharmD
Richard J. Geller, MD, MPH
Robert L. Goldberg, MD
Joanna Goralka, PharmD
Colin S. Goto, MD
Gail M. Gullickson, MD
Christine A. Haller, MD
Jennifer Hannum, MD
Sandra Hayashi, PharmD
Patricia H. Hiatt, BS
Raymond Ho, PharmD
B. Zane Horowitz, MD
Yao-min Hung, MD
David L. Irons, PharmD
Leslie M. Israel, DO, MPH
Sam Jackson, MD, MBA
Thanjira Jiranankatan, MD
Gerald Joe, PharmD
Jeffrey R. Jones, MPH, CIH
Paul A. Khasigian, PharmD
Thomas E. Kearney, PharmD
Kathryn H. Keller, PharmD
Michael T. Kelley, MD
Susan Y. Kim-Katz, PharmD
Lada Kokan, MD
Michael J. Kosnett, MD
Allyson Kreshak, MD
Amy Kunihiro, MD
Grant D. Lackey, PharmD
Chi-Leung Lai, PharmD
Rita Lam, PharmD
Shelly Lam, PharmD
John P. Lamb, PharmD
Belle L. Lee, PharmD
Darrem Lew, PharmD
Diane Liu, MD, MPH
Jon Lorett, PharmD
Derrick Lung, MD, MPH
Binh T. Ly, MD
Richard Lynton, MD
Tatiana M. Mamantov, MD
Beth H. Manning, PharmD
Anthony S. Manoguerra, PharmD
Kathy Marquardt, PharmD
Michael J. Matteucci, MD
Timothy D. McCarthy, PharmD
Howard E. McKinney, PharmD
Kathryn H. Meier, PharmD
Michael A. Miller, MD
Alicia Minns, MD
S. Todd Mitchell, MD
Eileen Morentz
Walter H. Mullen, PharmD
Stephen W. Munday, MD, MPH, MS
Nancy G. Murphy, MD
Frank J. Mycroft, PhD, MPH
Joshua Nogar, MD
Sean Patrick Nordt, MD, PharmD
Steve Offerman, MD
Kent R. Olson, MD
Michael O'Malley, MD, MPH
Gary Joseph Ordog, MD
John D. Osterloh, MD
Kelly P. Owen, MD
Gary Pasternak, MD
Manish Patel, MD
Paul D. Pearigen, MD
Cyrus Rangan, MD
Brett A. Roth, MD
Freda M. Rowley, PharmD
Thomas R. Sands, PharmD
Aaron Schnier, MD
Jay Schrader, CPhT
Kerry Schwarz, PharmD
Dennis J. Shusterman, MD, MPH
Craig Smollin, MD
Karl A. Sporer, MD
Jeffrey R. Suchard, MD
Mark E. Sutter, MD
Winnie W. Tai, PharmD
David A. Tanen, MD
S. Alan Tani, PharmD
John H. Tegzes, VMD
R. Steven Tharratt, MD
Josef G. Thundiyil, MD, MPH
Christian Tomaszewski, MD
Ben T. Tsutaoka, PharmD
Mary Tweig, MD
Rais Vohra, MD
Peter H. Wald, MD, MPH
Michael J. Walsh, PharmD
Jonathan Wasserberger, MD
Janet S. Weiss, MD
R. David West, PharmD
Timothy J. Wiegand, MD
Saralyn R. Williams, MD
Joyce Wong, PharmD

Olga F. Woo, PharmD
Alan H. B. Wu, PhD
Lisa Wu, MD
Evan T. Wythe, MD
Peter Yip, MD
Shoshana Zevin, MD

We are also grateful for the numerous comments and suggestions received from colleagues, students, and the editorial staff at McGraw-Hill, which helped us to improve the manual with each edition.

Kent R. Olson, MD

San Francisco, California
September 2017

SECTION I. Comprehensive Evaluation and Treatment

▶ EMERGENCY EVALUATION AND TREATMENT

Kent R. Olson, MD and Rais Vohra, MD

Even though they may not appear to be acutely ill, all poisoned patients should be treated as if they have a potentially life-threatening intoxication. Figure I-1 provides a checklist of emergency evaluation and treatment procedures. More detailed information on the diagnosis and treatment for each emergency step is referenced by page and presented immediately after the checklist. For immediate expert advice on diagnosis and management of poisoning, call a regional **poison control center** (in the United States, **toll-free 1-800-222-1222**).

When treating suspected poisoning cases, **quickly review the checklist** to determine the scope of appropriate interventions and **begin needed life-saving treatment.** If further information is required for any step, turn to the cited pages for a detailed discussion of each topic. Although the checklist is presented in a **sequential format,** many steps may be performed **simultaneously** (eg, airway management, naloxone and dextrose administration, and gastric lavage).

AIRWAY

I. **Assessment.** The most common factor contributing to death from drug overdose or poisoning is loss of airway-protective reflexes with subsequent airway obstruction caused by the flaccid tongue, pulmonary aspiration of gastric contents, or respiratory arrest. All poisoned patients should be suspected of having a potentially compromised airway.
   A. **Patients who are awake** and talking are likely to have intact airway reflexes but should be monitored closely because worsening intoxication can result in rapid loss of airway control.
   B. **In a lethargic or obtunded patient,** the response to stimulation of the nasopharynx (eg, does the patient react to placement of a nasal airway?) or the presence of a spontaneous cough reflex may provide an indirect indication of the patient's ability to protect the airway. If there is any doubt, it is best to perform endotracheal intubation (see below).

II. **Treatment.** Optimize the airway position and perform endotracheal intubation if necessary. Early use of naloxone (p 584) or flumazenil (p 556) may awaken a patient intoxicated with opioids or benzodiazepines, respectively, and obviate the need for endotracheal intubation. (***Note:*** Flumazenil is ***not*** recommended except in very select circumstances, as its use may precipitate seizures.)
   A. **Position the patient and clear the airway**.
      1. **Optimize the airway position** to force the flaccid tongue forward and maximize the airway opening. The following techniques are useful. ***Caution:*** Do ***not*** perform neck manipulation if you suspect a neck injury.
         a. Place the neck and head in the **"sniffing" position**, with the neck flexed forward and the head extended.
         b. Apply the "**jaw thrust**" maneuver to create forward movement of the tongue without flexing or extending the neck. Pull the jaw forward by placing the fingers of each hand on the angle of the mandible just below the ears. (This motion also causes a painful stimulus to the angle of the jaw, the response to which reflects the patient's depth of coma.)
         c. Place the patient in a **head-down**, **left-sided position** that allows the tongue to fall forward and secretions or vomitus to drain out of the mouth.

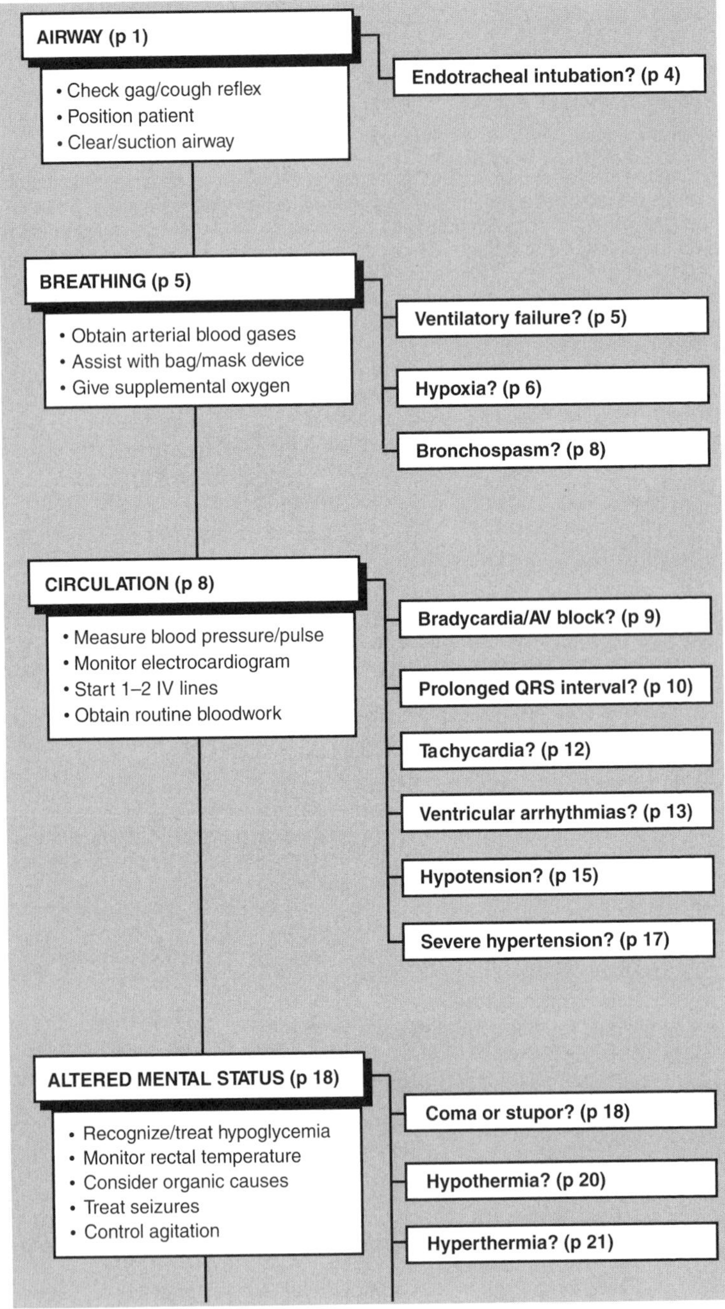

FIGURE I–1. Checklist of emergency evaluation and treatment procedures.

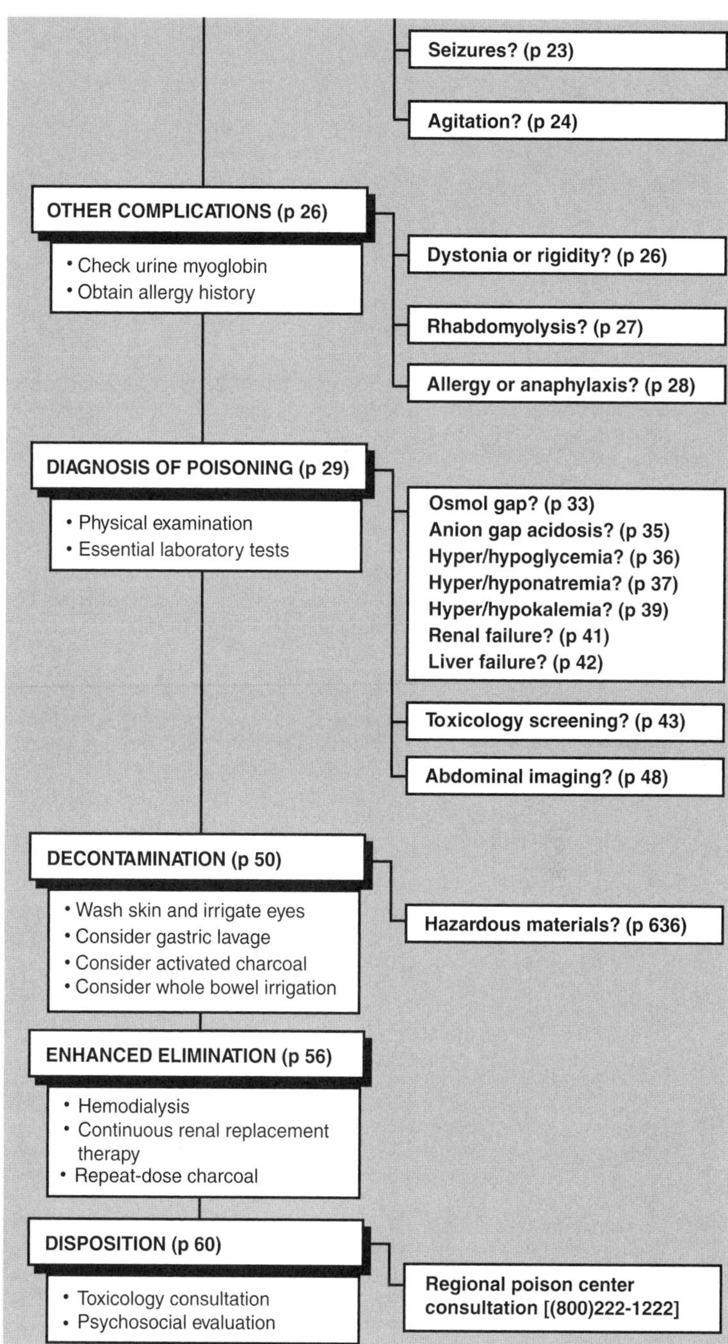
Seizures? (p 23)
Agitation? (p 24)
OTHER COMPLICATIONS (p 26)
• Check urine myoglobin
• Obtain allergy history
Dystonia or rigidity? (p 26)
Rhabdomyolysis? (p 27)
Allergy or anaphylaxis? (p 28)
DIAGNOSIS OF POISONING (p 29)
• Physical examination
• Essential laboratory tests
Osmol gap? (p 33)
Anion gap acidosis? (p 35)
Hyper/hypoglycemia? (p 36)
Hyper/hyponatremia? (p 37)
Hyper/hypokalemia? (p 39)
Renal failure? (p 41)
Liver failure? (p 42)
Toxicology screening? (p 43)
Abdominal imaging? (p 48)
DECONTAMINATION (p 50)
• Wash skin and irrigate eyes
• Consider gastric lavage
• Consider activated charcoal
• Consider whole bowel irrigation
Hazardous materials? (p 636)
ENHANCED ELIMINATION (p 56)
• Hemodialysis
• Continuous renal replacement therapy
• Repeat-dose charcoal
DISPOSITION (p 60)
• Toxicology consultation
• Psychosocial evaluation
Regional poison center consultation [(800)222-1222]

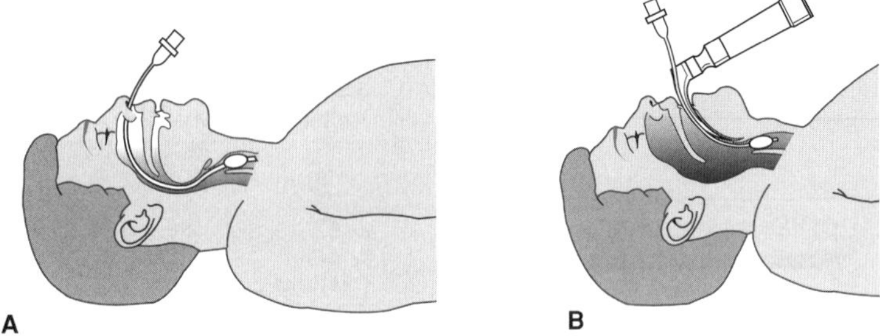

FIGURE I–2. Two routes for endotracheal intubation. **A:** Nasotracheal intubation. **B:** Orotracheal intubation.

2. If the airway is still not patent, examine the oropharynx and **remove any obstruction or secretions** by suction, by a sweep with the finger, or with Magill forceps.
3. The airway can also be maintained with **artificial oropharyngeal or nasopharyngeal airway devices**. These devices are placed in the mouth or nose to lift the tongue and push it forward. They are only temporary measures. A patient who can tolerate an artificial airway without complaint probably needs an endotracheal tube.

B. Perform endotracheal intubation if personnel trained in the procedure are available. Intubation of the trachea provides the most reliable protection of the airway, preventing obstruction and reducing the risk for pulmonary aspiration of gastric contents as well as allowing mechanically assisted ventilation. However, it is not a simple procedure and *should be attempted only by those with training and experience.* Complications include vomiting with pulmonary aspiration; local trauma to the oropharynx, nasopharynx, and larynx; inadvertent intubation of the esophagus or a mainstem bronchus; worsening acidosis due to apnea; and failure to intubate the patient after respiratory arrest has been induced by a neuromuscular blocker. There are two routes for endotracheal intubation: nasotracheal and orotracheal.

1. **Nasotracheal intubation.** In nasotracheal intubation, a soft, flexible tube is passed through the nose and into the trachea by using a "blind" technique (Figure I–2A).
   a. **Advantages**
      (1) It may be performed in a conscious or semiconscious patient without the need for neuromuscular paralysis.
      (2) Once placed, it is usually better tolerated than an orotracheal tube.
   b. **Disadvantages**
      (1) Perforation of the nasal mucosa with epistaxis.
      (2) Stimulation of vomiting in an obtunded patient.
      (3) Patient must be breathing spontaneously.
      (4) Anatomically more difficult in infants because of their anterior epiglottis.
2. **Orotracheal intubation.** In orotracheal intubation, the tube is passed through the patient's mouth into the trachea under direct vision (Figure I–2B), with the aid of a video laryngoscope device, or with the aid of a long, flexible stylet (bougie).
   a. **Technique**
   b. **Advantages**
      (1) Performed under direct or video-assisted visualization, making accidental esophageal intubation less likely than with nasotracheal intubation.
      (2) Insignificant risk for bleeding.
      (3) Patient need not be breathing spontaneously.
      (4) Higher success rate than that achieved via the nasotracheal route.

c. Disadvantages

(1) Frequently requires neuromuscular paralysis, creating a risk for respiratory acidosis, or fatal respiratory arrest if intubation is unsuccessful.

(2) Requires neck manipulation, which may cause spinal cord injury if the patient has also had neck trauma.

3. Cricothyrotomy or tracheotomy may be necessary in the rare patient whose larynx is damaged or distorted making endotracheal intubation through the pharynx impossible.

C. Extraglottic airway devices. The role of newer advanced airway equipment, such as the laryngeal mask airway (LMA), in patients with poisoning or drug overdose is not known; although these devices are easier to insert than endotracheal tubes, especially in some patients with "difficult" airways, they do not provide adequate protection against pulmonary aspiration of gastric contents, and they cannot be used in patients with laryngeal edema, injury, or laryngospasm.

BREATHING

Along with airway problems, breathing difficulties are the major cause of morbidity and death in patients with poisoning or drug overdose. Patients may have one or more of the following complications: ventilatory failure, hypoxia, and bronchospasm.

I. Ventilatory failure

A. Assessment. Normal ventilation, or gas exchange, requires a number of interdependent physiological processes. Ventilatory failure can have multiple causes, including failure of the ventilatory muscles, central depression of respiratory drive, and severe pneumonia or pulmonary edema. Examples of drugs and toxins that cause ventilatory failure, and the causative mechanisms, are listed in Table I–1.

B. Complications. Ventilatory failure is the most common cause of death in poisoned patients.

1. Hypoxia may result in brain damage, cardiac dysrhythmias, and cardiac arrest.

2. Hypercarbia results in acidosis, which may contribute to worsening systemic toxicity and dysrhythmias, especially in patients with salicylate toxicity or tricyclic antidepressant overdoses.

C. Differential diagnosis. Rule out the following:

1. Bacterial or viral pneumonia.

2. Viral encephalitis or myelitis (eg, polio).

3. Traumatic or ischemic spinal cord or central nervous system (CNS) injury.

4. Tetanus, causing rigidity of chest wall muscles.

5. Pneumothorax.

TABLE I–1. SELECTED DRUGS AND TOXINS CAUSING VENTILATORY FAILURE[a]

Paralysis of ventilatory muscles	Depression of central respiratory drive
Botulinum toxin (botulism)	Antihistamines
Neuromuscular blockers	Barbiturates
Nicotine	Clonidine and other sympatholytic agents
Organophosphates and carbamates	Ethanol and alcohols
Saxitoxin ("red tide")	Gamma-hydroxybutyrate (GHB)
Snakebite (elapids and some vipers)	Opioids
Strychnine and tetanus (muscle rigidity)	Phenothiazines and other antipsychotics
Tetrodotoxin	Sedative-hypnotics
Warfare nerve gases	Tricyclic antidepressants

[a]Adapted in part, with permission, from Olson KR, Pentel PR, Kelly MT. Physical assessment and differential diagnosis of the poisoned patient. *Med Toxicol.* 1987;2:52.

D. Treatment. Obtain measurements of the arterial blood gases. Quickly estimate the adequacy of ventilation from the P_{CO_2} level; obtundation with an elevated or rising P_{CO_2} (eg, >60 mm Hg) indicates a need for assisted ventilation. Do ***not*** wait until the patient is apneic or until the P_{CO_2} is above 60 mmHg to begin assisted ventilation.

1. Assist breathing manually with a bag-valve-mask device or bag-valve endotracheal tube device until the mechanical ventilator is ready for use.
2. If not already accomplished, **perform endotracheal intubation**.
3. **Program the mechanical ventilator** for tidal volume (usually 15 mL/kg), rate (usually 12–15 breaths/min), and oxygen concentration (usually 30–35% to start). Monitor the patient's response to the ventilator settings frequently by obtaining arterial blood gas values. ***Note:*** In salicylate-poisoned patients with severe acidosis and marked compensatory tachypnea, the ventilator should be programmed to match the patient's high minute ventilation. Otherwise, any rise in the patient's P_{CO_2} and consequent fall in blood pH can dramatically increase tissue levels of salicylate, with disastrous consequences.
   a. If the patient has some spontaneous ventilation, the machine can be set to allow the patient to breathe spontaneously with only intermittent mandatory ventilation (usually 10–12 breaths/min).
   b. If the endotracheal tube has been placed only for airway protection, the patient can be left to breathe entirely spontaneously with blow-by oxygen mist (T-piece).
4. Although often used as respiratory care adjuncts, noninvasive ventilation techniques such as Bilevel Positive Airway Pressure (BiPAP) have not been adequately evaluated in patients with acute respiratory failure due to intoxication.

II. Hypoxia

A. Assessment. Physical examination is insensitive but the presence of cyanosis, pallor, respiratory distress, or shock are indications of tissue hypoxia. Pulse oximeter monitoring, arterial blood gas measurement, and co-oximetry testing are the most helpful diagnostic tests for hypoxia. Examples of drugs or toxins causing hypoxia are listed in Table I–2. Hypoxia can be caused by the following conditions:

1. **Insufficient oxygen** in ambient air (eg, displacement of oxygen by inert gases).

TABLE I–2. SELECTED CAUSES OF HYPOXIA[a]

Inert gases	**Pneumonia or noncardiogenic pulmonary edema**
Carbon dioxide	Aspiration of gastric contents
Methane and propane	Aspiration of hydrocarbons
Nitrogen	Chlorine and other irritant gases
Cardiogenic pulmonary edema	Cocaine
Beta receptor antagonists	Ethchlorvynol (IV and oral)
Calcium channel blockers (eg, verapamil)	Ethylene glycol
Stimulant cardiomyopathy	Hydrogen sulfide
Quinidine, procainamide, and disopyramide	Mercury vapor
Tricyclic antidepressants	Metal fumes ("metal fumes fever")
Cellular hypoxia	Nitrogen dioxide
Carbon monoxide	Opioids
Cyanide	Paraquat
Hydrogen sulfide	Phosgene
Methemoglobinemia	Salicylates
Sulfhemoglobinemia	Sedative-hypnotic drugs
	Smoke inhalation

[a]See also Table I–1.

2. **Disruption of oxygen absorption** by the lung (eg, resulting from pneumonia or pulmonary edema).
   a. **Pneumonia.** The most common cause of pneumonia in overdosed patients is pulmonary aspiration of gastric contents. Pneumonia may also be caused by the IV injection of foreign material or bacteria, aspiration of hydrocarbons or petroleum distillates, or inhalation of irritant gases.
   b. **Pulmonary edema.** All agents that cause chemical pneumonitis (eg, irritant gases and hydrocarbons) can also cause pulmonary edema, due to alteration of permeability in pulmonary capillaries. In noncardiogenic pulmonary edema, the pulmonary capillary wedge pressure (reflecting filling pressure in the left ventricle) is usually normal or low. In contrast, **cardiogenic** pulmonary edema caused by cardiac depressant drugs is characterized by low cardiac output with elevated pulmonary wedge pressure.
3. **Cellular hypoxia**, which may be present despite a normal arterial blood gas value.
   a. **Carbon monoxide** poisoning (p 182) and **methemoglobinemia** (p 317) may severely limit oxygen binding to hemoglobin (and therefore the oxygen-carrying capacity of blood) without altering the PO_2 because routine blood gas determination measures dissolved oxygen in the plasma but does not measure actual oxygen content. In such cases, only the direct measurement of oxygen saturation with a co-oximeter (not its calculation from the PO_2) will reveal decreased oxyhemoglobin saturation. ***Note:*** Conventional pulse oximetry gives falsely normal or inaccurate results and is not reliable. A newer pulse oximetry device (the Masimo pulse co-oximeter) can estimate carboxyhemoglobin and methemoglobin concentrations, but its accuracy and sensitivity are uncertain.
   b. **Cyanide** poisoning (p 208) and **hydrogen sulfide** poisoning (p 271) interfere with cellular oxygen utilization, resulting in decreased oxygen uptake by the tissues, and may cause abnormally high venous oxygen saturation.

B. **Complications.** Significant or sustained hypoxia may result in brain damage and cardiac dysrhythmias.

C. **Differential diagnosis.** Rule out the following:
1. Erroneous sampling (eg, inadvertently measuring venous blood gases rather than arterial blood gases).
2. Bacterial or viral pneumonia.
3. Pulmonary contusion caused by trauma.
4. Cardiac pump failure.

D. **Treatment**
1. **Provide supplemental oxygen** as indicated, based on arterial PO_2. Intubation and assisted ventilation may be required.
   a. If carbon monoxide poisoning is suspected, give 100% oxygen and consider hyperbaric oxygen (p 599).
   b. See also treatment guides for cyanide (p 208), hydrogen sulfide (p 271), and methemoglobinemia (p 317).
2. **Treat pneumonia.** Obtain sputum samples and initiate appropriate antibiotic therapy when there is evidence of infection.
3. **Treat pulmonary edema.**
   a. Avoid excessive fluid administration. Assessment of volume status by ultrasound or pulmonary artery cannulation and wedge pressure measurements may be necessary to guide fluid therapy.
   b. Administer supplemental oxygen to maintain a PO_2 of at least 60–70 mm Hg. Endotracheal intubation and the use of positive end-expiratory pressure (PEEP) ventilation may be necessary to maintain adequate oxygenation.

TABLE I–3. SELECTED DRUGS AND TOXINS CAUSING BRONCHOSPASM

Beta receptor antagonists	Isocyanates
Brevetoxin	Nickel carbonyl
Chlorine and other irritant gases	Nitrogen oxides
Drugs causing allergic reactions	Organophosphates and other anticholinesterases
Formaldehyde	Particulate dusts
Glutaraldehyde	Smoke inhalation
Hydrocarbon aspiration	Sulfites (eg, in foods)

III. Bronchospasm

A. Assessment. Wheezes, tachypnea, inability to speak full sentences, and a prolonged expiratory phase are all signs of bronchospasm (***Note:*** in severe cases, air exchange may be so compromised that no wheezes are heard). Examples of drugs and toxins that cause bronchospasm are listed in Table I–3. Bronchospasm may result from the following:

1. **Direct irritant injury** from the inhalation of gases or pulmonary aspiration of petroleum distillates or stomach contents.
2. **Pharmacologic effects** of toxins (eg, organophosphate or carbamate insecticides or beta-adrenergic antagonists).
3. **Hypersensitivity** or allergic reactions.

B. Complications. Severe bronchospasm may result in hypoxia and ventilatory failure. Exposure to high concentrations of irritant gases can lead to asthma (reactive airway dysfunction syndrome [RADS]).

C. Differential diagnosis. Rule out the following:

1. Asthma or other pre-existing bronchospastic disorders.
2. Stridor caused by upper airway injury and edema (progressive airway edema may result in acute airway obstruction).
3. Airway obstruction by a foreign body.
4. Congestive heart failure can cause fine crackles and wheezes ("cardiac asthma") due to the presence of excess pulmonary interstitial fluid.

D. Treatment

1. Administer supplemental oxygen. Assist ventilation and perform endotracheal intubation if needed.
2. Remove the patient from the source of exposure to any irritant gas or other offending agent.
3. Immediately discontinue any beta-adrenergic antagonist treatment.
4. Administer bronchodilators:
   - **a.** Aerosolized $beta_2$ receptor stimulant (eg, albuterol [2.5–5 mg] in nebulizer). Repeat as needed or give 5–15 mg as a continuous nebulizer treatment over 1 hour (children: 0.3–0.5 mg/kg/h).
   - **b.** Aerosolized ipratropium bromide, 0.5 mg every 4–6 hours, especially if excessive cholinergic stimulation is suspected.
   - **c.** For reactive airways, consider inhaled or oral steroids.
5. For patients with bronchospasm and bronchorrhea caused by organophosphate, carbamate, or other cholinesterase inhibitor poisoning, give atropine (p 512) IV. Ipratropium bromide (see Item 4.b above) may also be helpful.

CIRCULATION

I. General assessment and initial treatment

A. Check blood pressure and pulse rate and rhythm. Perform cardiopulmonary resuscitation (CPR) if there is no pulse and perform advanced cardiac life support (ACLS) for dysrhythmias and shock. ***Note:*** Some ACLS drugs may be ineffective or dangerous in patients with drug- or poison-induced cardiac disorders.

For example, type Ia antiarrhythmic drugs are contraindicated in patients with tricyclic antidepressant or other sodium channel–blocker overdose.

B. **Obtain a 12-lead ECG and begin continuous electrocardiographic (ECG) monitoring.** Dysrhythmias may complicate a variety of drug overdoses, and all patients with potentially cardiotoxic drug poisoning should be monitored in the emergency department or an intensive care unit for at least 6 hours after the ingestion.

C. **Secure venous access.** Antecubital or forearm veins are usually easy to cannulate. Alternative sites include femoral, subclavian, internal jugular, and other central veins. Access to central veins is technically more difficult but allows measurement of the central venous pressure and placement of a pacemaker or pulmonary artery lines. **Intraosseous** (IO) access may also be used in urgent situations.

D. **Draw blood** for routine studies (p 33).

E. **Begin IV infusion** of normal saline (NS), 5% dextrose in NS (D_5NS), 5% dextrose in half NS (D_5W 0.45% sodium chloride), or 5% dextrose in water (D_5W) at a keep-open rate; for children, use 5% dextrose in quarter NS (D_5W 0.25% sodium chloride). If the patient is hypotensive (p 15), NS or another isotonic crystalloid solution is preferred.

F. In seriously ill patients (eg, those who are hypotensive, obtunded, convulsing, or comatose), **place a Foley catheter** in the bladder, obtain urine for routine and toxicologic testing, and measure hourly urine output.

II. **Bradycardia and atrioventricular (AV) block**

A. **Assessment.** Examples of drugs and toxins causing bradycardia or AV block and their mechanisms are listed in Table I–4.

1. Bradycardia and AV block are common features of intoxication with calcium antagonists (p 172) and drugs that depress sympathetic tone (eg, clonidine, beta blockers) or increase parasympathetic tone (eg, digoxin). These conditions may also result from severe intoxication with sodium channel–blocking drugs (eg, tricyclic antidepressants, quinidine, and other types Ia and Ic antiarrhythmic agents).
2. Bradycardia or AV block may also be a reflex response (baroreceptor reflex) to hypertension induced by alpha-adrenergic agents such as phenylpropanolamine and phenylephrine.
3. In children, bradycardia is commonly caused by respiratory compromise and usually responds to ventilation and oxygenation.

B. **Complications.** Bradycardia and AV block frequently cause hypotension, which may progress to asystolic cardiac arrest.

C. **Differential diagnosis.** Rule out the following:

1. Hypothermia.

TABLE I–4. SELECTED DRUGS AND TOXINS CAUSING BRADYCARDIA OR ATRIOVENTRICULAR BLOCK[a]

Cholinergic or vagotonic agents	**Sympatholytic agents**
Digitalis glycosides	Beta receptor antagonists
Organophosphates and carbamates	Clonidine
Physostigmine, neostigmine	Opioids
Membrane-depressant drugs	**Other**
Propranolol	Calcium antagonists
Encainide and flecainide	Carbamazepine
Quinidine and other Type Ia antidysrhythmics	Lithium
Tricyclic antidepressants	Phenylpropanolamine and other alpha-adrenergic agonists
	Propoxyphene

[a]Adapted in part, with permission, from Olson KR, et al. *Med Toxicol.* 1987;2:71.

TABLE I–5. SELECTED DRUGS AND TOXINS CAUSING QRS INTERVAL PROLONGATION[a]

Bupropion	Lamotrigine
Chloroquine and related agents	Phenothiazines (thioridazine)
Cocaine (high-dose)	Propoxyphene
Digitalis glycosides (complete heart block)	Propranolol
Diphenhydramine (high-dose)	Quinidine and other Type Ia antidysrhythmics
Encainide and flecainide	Tricyclic antidepressants
Hyperkalemia	Venlafaxine

[a]Adapted in part, with permission, from Olson KR, et al. *Med Toxicol.* 1987;2:71.

2. Myocardial ischemia or infarction.
3. Electrolyte abnormality (eg, hyperkalemia).
4. Metabolic disturbance (eg, hypothyroidism).
5. Physiologic origin, resulting from a baroreceptor response to hypertension, an intrinsically slow pulse rate (common in athletes), or an acute vasovagal reaction.
6. Cushing reflex (caused by severe intracranial hypertension).

D. Treatment. Do ***not*** treat bradycardia or AV block unless the patient is symptomatic (eg, exhibits signs of syncope or hypotension). ***Note:*** Bradycardia or even AV block may be a protective baroreceptor reflex to lower the blood pressure in a patient with severe hypertension (see Item VII below).

1. Maintain an open airway and assist ventilation (pp 1–6) if necessary. Administer supplemental oxygen.
2. Rewarm hypothermic patients. A sinus bradycardia of 40–50 beats/min is common when the body temperature is 32–35°C (90–95°F) and will usually return to normal with warming.
3. Administer atropine, 0.01–0.03 mg/kg IV (p 512). If this is not successful, use isoproterenol, 1–10 mcg/min IV (p 568), titrated to the desired rate, or use an emergency transcutaneous or transvenous pacemaker.
4. Use the following specific antidotes if appropriate:
   - **a.** For beta receptor antagonist overdose, give glucagon (p 559).
   - **b.** For digoxin, digitalis, or other cardiac glycoside intoxication, use Fab antibody fragments (p 542).
   - **c.** For tricyclic antidepressant or membrane-depressant drug overdose, administer sodium bicarbonate (p 520).
   - **d.** For calcium antagonist overdose, give calcium (p 526), hyperinsulin-euglycemia therapy (p 564), or lipid emulsion (p 574).

III. QRS interval prolongation

A. Assessment. Normal QRS interval is 80–100 msec. Examples of drugs and toxins causing QRS interval prolongation are listed in Table I–5.

1. QRS interval prolongation of greater than 100 msec in the limb leads (Figure I–3) is common in poisoning by tricyclic antidepressants (p 107) or other membrane-depressant drugs (eg, quinidine [p 398], flecainide [p 88], chloroquine [p 194], and propranolol [p 158]). Rightward axis deviation of the terminal 40 msec of the ECG, which is easily recognized as a late R wave in the aVR lead, may precede QRS widening in patients with tricyclic antidepressant intoxication (Figure I–4).
2. QRS interval prolongation may also result from a ventricular escape rhythm in a patient with complete heart block (eg, from digitalis, calcium antagonist poisoning, or intrinsic cardiac disease).

B. Complications. QRS interval prolongation in patients with tricyclic antidepressant or similar drug poisoning is often accompanied by hypotension, AV block, and seizures. Widening of QRS beyond 160 msec is associated with an increased likelihood of ventricular arrhythmias (ventricular tachycardia, bigeminy, idioventricular rhythm) and shock.

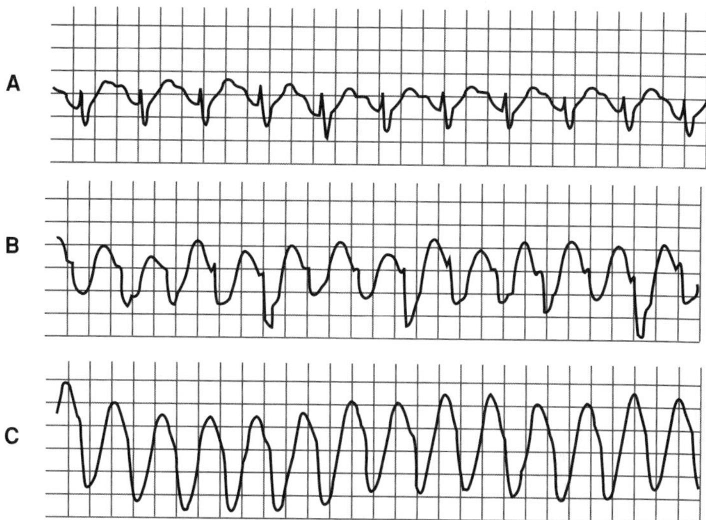

FIGURE I–3. Widened QRS interval caused by tricyclic antidepressant overdose. **A:** Delayed intraventricular conduction results in prolonged QRS interval (0.18 s). **B** and **C:** Supraventricular tachycardia with progressive widening of QRS complexes mimics ventricular tachycardia. (Modified and reproduced, with permission, from Benowitz NL, Goldschlager N. Cardiac disturbances in the toxicologic patient. In: Haddad LM, Winchester JF, eds. *Clinical Management of Poisoning and Drug Overdose.* 3rd ed., p 94. WB Saunders; 1998. © Elsevier.)

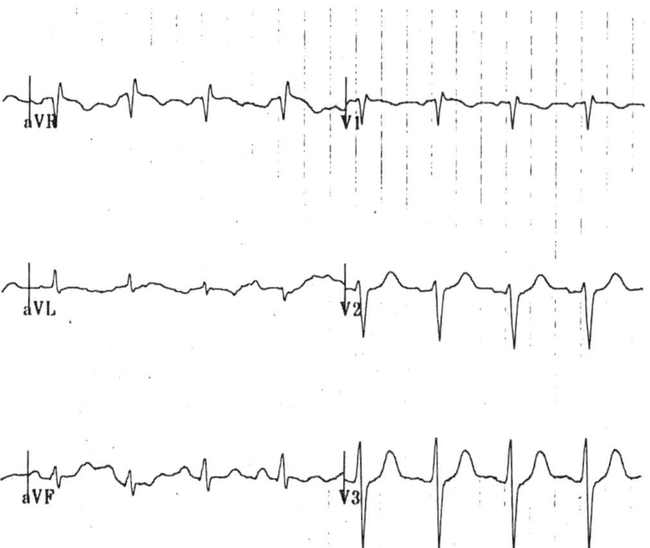

FIGURE I–4. Right axis deviation of the terminal 40 msec, easily recognized as a late R wave in aVR.

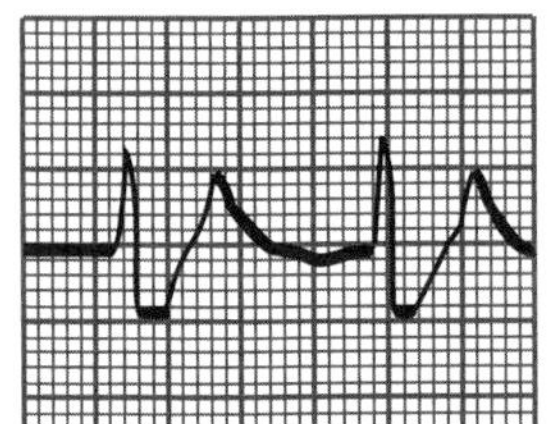

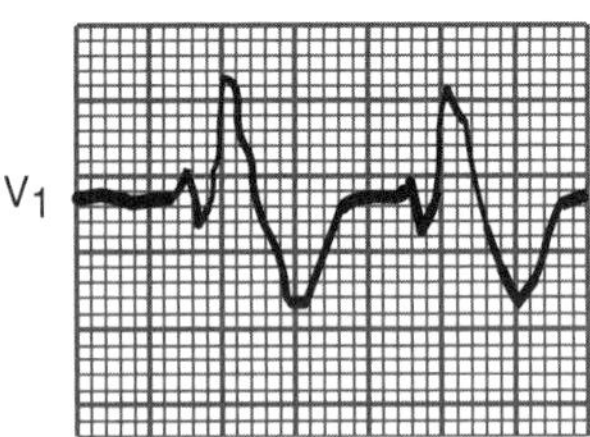

FIGURE I–5. Electrocardiogram of a patient with hyperkalemia. (Modified and reproduced, with permission, from Goldschlager N, Goldman MJ. Effect of drugs and electrolytes on the electrocardiogram. In: Goldschlager N, Goldman MJ, eds. *Electrocardiography: Essentials of Interpretation,* p 199. Appleton & Lange; 1984.)

C. **Differential diagnosis.** Rule out the following:
   1. Intrinsic conduction system disease (bundle branch block or complete heart block). Check an old ECG if available.
   2. Brugada syndrome.
   3. **Hyperkalemia** with critical cardiac toxicity may appear as a "sine wave" pattern with markedly wide QRS complexes. These are usually preceded by peaked T waves (Figure I–5).
   4. **Hypothermia** with a core temperature of less than 32°C (90°F) often causes an extraterminal QRS deflection (J wave or Osborne wave), resulting in a widened QRS appearance (Figure I–6).

D. **Treatment**
   1. For tricyclic antidepressant or other sodium channel–blocking drug overdose, give sodium bicarbonate, 1- to 2-mEq/kg IV bolus (p 520); repeat as needed.
   2. Maintain the airway and assist ventilation if necessary (pp 1–4). Administer supplemental oxygen.
   3. Treat hyperkalemia (p 39) and hypothermia (p 20) if they occur.
   4. Treat AV block with atropine (p 512), isoproterenol (p 568), and a pacemaker if necessary.

IV. **Tachycardia**

A. **Assessment.** Examples of drugs and toxins causing tachycardia and their mechanisms are listed in Table I–6.
   1. Sinus tachycardia and supraventricular tachycardia are often caused by excessive sympathetic stimulation or inhibition of parasympathetic tone. Sinus tachycardia may also be a reflex response to hypotension or hypoxia.
   2. Sinus tachycardia and supraventricular tachycardia accompanied by QRS interval prolongation (eg, with tricyclic antidepressant poisoning) may have the appearance of ventricular tachycardia (see Figure I–3).

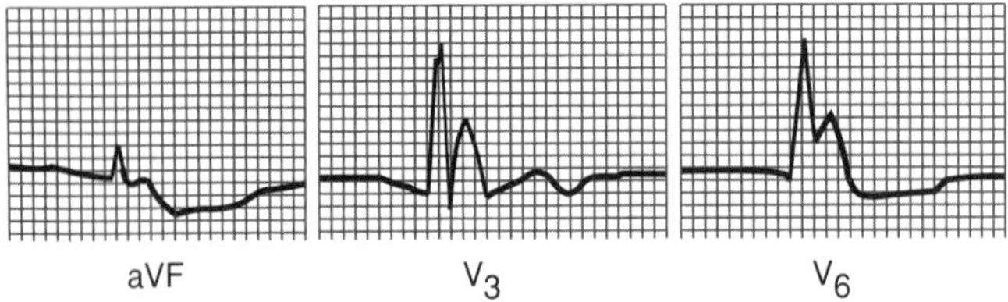

FIGURE I–6. Electrocardiogram of a patient with hypothermia, showing prominent J waves. (Modified and reproduced, with permission, from Goldschlager N, Goldman MJ. Miscellaneous abnormal electrocardiogram patterns. In: Goldschlager N, Goldman MJ, eds. *Electrocardiography: Essentials of Interpretation,* p 227. Appleton & Lange; 1984.)

TABLE I–6. SELECTED DRUGS AND TOXINS CAUSING TACHYCARDIA[a]

Sympathomimetic agents	**Anticholinergic agents**
Amphetamines and derivatives	*Amanita muscaria* mushrooms
Caffeine	Antihistamines
Cocaine	Atropine and other anticholinergics
Ephedrine and pseudoephedrine	Phenothiazines
Phencyclidine (PCP)	Plants (many [p 375])
Theophylline	Tricyclic antidepressants
Agents causing cellular hypoxia	**Other**
Carbon monoxide	Ethanol or sedative-hypnotic drug withdrawal
Cyanide	
Hydrogen sulfide	Vasodilators (reflex tachycardia)
Oxidizing agents (methemoglobinemia)	Thyroid hormone

[a]Adapted, with permission, from Olson KR, et al. *Med Toxicol,* 1987;2:71.

B. Complications. Simple sinus tachycardia (heart rate <140 beats/min) is rarely of hemodynamic consequence; children and healthy adults easily tolerate rates of up to 160–180 beats/min. However, sustained rapid rates may result in hypotension, chest pain, myocardial ischemia, or syncope.

C. Differential diagnosis. Rule out the following:

1. Occult blood loss (eg, from gastrointestinal bleeding or trauma).
2. Fluid loss (eg, third spacing, gastroenteritis).
3. Hypoxia.
4. Fever and infection.
5. Myocardial infarction.
6. Anxiety.
7. Intrinsic conduction system disease (eg, Wolff–Parkinson–White syndrome) causing tachydysrhythmia.

D. Treatment. If tachycardia is not associated with hypotension or chest pain, observation and sedation with benzodiazepines (especially for stimulant intoxication) are usually adequate.

1. Sympathomimetic-induced tachycardia resulting in ischemia or rate-related hypotension: give a short-acting, titratable beta blocker such as esmolol, 0.025–0.1 mg/kg/min IV (p 552). ***Note:*** If tachycardia is accompanied by hypertension, add a vasodilator (see Item VII.D.2 below).
2. Anticholinergic-induced tachycardia may respond to physostigmine (p 609) or neostigmine, but tachycardia alone is rarely an indication for use of these drugs. Moreover, in patients with tricyclic antidepressant overdose, additive depression of conduction by these drugs may result in severe bradycardia, heart block, or asystole.

V. Ventricular dysrhythmias

A. Assessment. Examples of drugs and toxins causing ventricular dysrhythmias are listed in Table I–7.

1. Ventricular irritability is commonly associated with excessive sympathetic stimulation (eg, from cocaine or amphetamines). Patients intoxicated by chlorinated, fluorinated, or other hydrocarbons may have heightened myocardial sensitivity to the arrhythmogenic effects of catecholamines.
2. Ventricular tachycardia may also be a manifestation of intoxication by a tricyclic antidepressant or another sodium channel–blocking drug, although with these drugs true ventricular tachycardia may be difficult to distinguish from sinus or supraventricular tachycardia accompanied by QRS interval prolongation (see Figure I–3).
3. Agents that cause **QT interval prolongation** (QTc >0.43 seconds in men, >0.45 seconds in women) may produce torsade de pointes. **Torsade de pointes** is a polymorphous ventricular tachycardia in which the axis

TABLE I–7. SELECTED DRUGS AND TOXINS CAUSING VENTRICULAR ARRHYTHMIAS[a]

Ventricular tachycardia or fibrillation	
Amphetamines and other sympathomimetic agents	Cocaine
Aromatic hydrocarbon solvents	Digitalis glycosides
Barium	Fluoride/hydrofluoric acid
Caffeine and theophylline	Phenothiazines
Chloral hydrate	Theophylline
Chlorinated or fluorinated hydrocarbon solvents	Tricyclic antidepressants
QT prolongation with well-documented risk for torsade de pointes[b]	
Amiodarone	Ibutilide
Arsenic trioxide	Levomethadyl
Astemizole	Mesoridazine
Azithromycin	Metoclopramide
Bepridil	Methadone
Chloroquine	Pentamidine
Chlorpromazine	Pimozide
Cisapride	Probucol
Clarithromycin	Procainamide
Disopyramide	Organophosphate insecticides
Dofetilide	Quinidine
Domperidone	Sotalol
Droperidol	Sparfloxacin
Erythromycin	Terfenadine
Halofantrine	Thallium
Haloperidol	Thioridazine

[a]Olson KR. et al. *Med Toxicol.* 1987;2:71; and Arizona Center for Education and Research on Therapeutics: Drugs With Risk of Torsades de Pointes. http://www.torsades.org. Accessed March 3, 2010.
[b]Torsade de pointes can deteriorate into ventricular fibrillation and cardiac arrest.

appears to rotate continuously (Figure I–7). Torsade de pointes may also be caused by hypokalemia, hypocalcemia, or hypomagnesemia.

B. Complications. Ventricular tachycardia in patients with a pulse may be associated with hypotension or may deteriorate into pulseless ventricular tachycardia or ventricular fibrillation.

C. Differential diagnosis. Rule out the following possible causes of ventricular premature beats, ventricular tachycardia, or ventricular fibrillation:

1. Hypoxemia.
2. Hypokalemia.

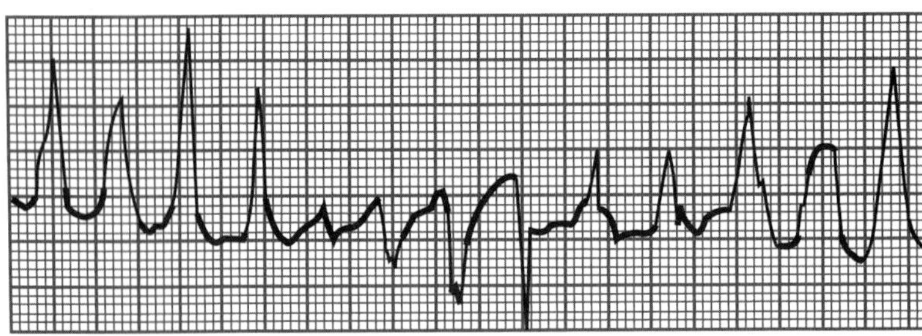

FIGURE I–7. Polymorphic ventricular tachycardia (torsade de pointes). (Modified and reproduced, with permission, from Goldschlager N, Goldman MJ. Effect of drugs and electrolytes on the electrocardiogram. In: Goldschlager N, Goldman MJ, eds. *Electrocardiography: Essentials of Interpretation,* p 197. Appleton & Lange; 1984.)

3. Metabolic acidosis.
4. Myocardial ischemia or infarction.
5. Electrolyte disturbances (eg, hypocalcemia or hypomagnesemia) or congenital disorders that may cause QT prolongation and torsade de pointes.
6. Brugada syndrome.

D. Treatment. Perform CPR if necessary and follow standard ACLS guidelines for the management of dysrhythmias, with the exception that type Ia antiarrhythmic drugs should ***not*** be used, especially if tricyclic antidepressant or sodium channel–blocking drug overdose is suspected.

1. Maintain an open airway and assist ventilation if necessary (pp 1–7). Administer supplemental oxygen.
2. Correct acid–base and electrolyte disturbances.
3. For suspected myocardial sensitivity caused by chloral hydrate or halogenated or aromatic hydrocarbons, use esmolol, 0.025–0.1 mg/kg/min IV (p 552), or propranolol, 0.5–3 mg IV (p 617).
4. **For ventricular dysrhythmias due to tricyclic antidepressant or other sodium channel–blocking drug overdose**, administer sodium bicarbonate, 1–2 mEq/kg IV (p 520) in repeated boluses until the dysrhythmia is interrupted and QRS interval narrows to less than 160 msec or the serum pH exceeds 7.7.
5. **For polymorphic ventricular tachycardia (torsade de pointes),** do the following:
   a. Administer IV magnesium sulfate, 1–2 g in adults, over 20–30 minutes (p 577).
   b. Use overdrive pacing or isoproterenol, 1–10 mcg/min IV (p 568), to increase the heart rate (this makes repolarization more homogeneous and abolishes the dysrhythmia).
   c. As with other types of ventricular dysrhythmias, immediate defibrillation is warranted if the patient is unstable or pulseless.

VI. Hypotension

A. Assessment. Examples of drugs and toxins causing hypotension and their mechanisms are listed in Table I–8.

1. Physiologic derangements resulting in hypotension include volume loss because of vomiting, diarrhea, or bleeding; apparent volume depletion caused by venodilation, arteriolar dilation, depression of cardiac contractility, and dysrhythmias that interfere with cardiac output; and hypothermia.
2. **Check the pulse rate.** Volume loss, venodilation, and arteriolar dilation are likely to result in hypotension with reflex tachycardia. In contrast, hypotension accompanied by bradycardia should suggest intoxication by sympatholytic agents, membrane-depressant drugs, calcium antagonists, or cardiac glycosides, or the presence of hypothermia.

B. Complications. Severe or prolonged hypotension can cause acute renal tubular necrosis, brain damage, hepatic necrosis, and cardiac ischemia. Metabolic acidosis is a common finding.

C. Differential diagnosis. Rule out the following:

1. Hypothermia, which results in a decreased metabolic rate and lowered blood pressure demands.
2. Hyperthermia, which causes arteriolar dilation and venodilation and direct myocardial depression.
3. Fluid loss caused by gastroenteritis.
4. Blood loss (eg, from trauma or gastrointestinal bleeding).
5. Myocardial infarction.
6. Sepsis.
7. Spinal cord injury.

D. Treatment. Fortunately, hypotension usually responds readily to empiric therapy with IV fluids and low doses of vasoactive drugs (eg, dopamine, norepinephrine). When hypotension does not resolve after simple measures,

TABLE I–8. SELECTED DRUGS AND TOXINS CAUSING HYPOTENSION[a]

HYPOTENSION WITH RELATIVE BRADYCARDIA	HYPOTENSION WITH TACHYCARDIA
Sympatholytic agents	**Fluid loss or third spacing**
Beta receptor antagonists	Amatoxin-containing mushrooms
Bretylium	Arsenic
Clonidine and methyldopa	Colchicine
Hypothermia	Copper sulfate
Opioids	Hyperthermia
Reserpine	Iron
Tetrahydrozoline and oxymetazoline	Rattlesnake envenomation
Membrane-depressant drugs	Sedative-hypnotic agents
Encainide and flecainide	**Peripheral venous or arteriolar dilation**
Quinidine, procainamide, and disopyramide	Alpha antagonists (doxazosin, prazosin, terazosin)
Propoxyphene	$Beta_2$ receptor agonists (eg, albuterol)
Propranolol	Caffeine
Tricyclic antidepressants	Calcium antagonists (nifedipine, amlodipine, nicardipine)
Others	Hydralazine
Barbiturates	Hyperthermia
Calcium antagonists (verapamil, diltiazem)	Minoxidil
Cyanide	Nitrites
Fluoride	Sodium nitroprusside
Hydrogen sulfide	Phenothiazines
Organophosphates and carbamates	Quetiapine
Sedative-hypnotic agents	Theophylline
Tilmicosin	Tricyclic antidepressants

[a]Adapted in part, with permission, from Olson KR, et al. *Med Toxicol.* 1987;2:57.

a systematic approach should be followed to determine the cause of hypotension and select the appropriate treatment.

1. Maintain an open airway and assist ventilation if necessary (pp 1–7). Administer supplemental oxygen.
2. Treat cardiac dysrhythmias that may contribute to hypotension (heart rate <40–50 beats/min or >180–200 beats/min [pp 9–15]).
3. Hypotension associated with hypothermia often will not be relieved unless the patient is rewarmed. A systolic blood pressure of 80–90 mm Hg is expected when the body temperature is 32°C (90°F).
4. Give an IV fluid challenge with NS, 10–20 mL/kg, or another crystalloid solution.
5. Administer **dopamine**, 5–15 mcg/kg/min (p 545). Note that dopamine (an indirect vasopressor) may be ineffective in some patients with depleted catecholamines (eg, from disulfiram [p 226] or tricyclic antidepressant [p 107] overdose) or in patients in whom alpha-adrenergic receptors may be blocked (tricyclic antidepressants, phenothiazines). In such cases, a direct-acting vasopressor such as **norepinephrine**, 0.1 mcg/kg/min IV (p 595), or **phenylephrine** (p 606) may be more effective.
6. Consider specific antidotes for some toxins:
   a. Sodium bicarbonate (p 520) for tricyclic antidepressant or other sodium channel–blocking drug overdose.
   b. Glucagon (p 559) for beta receptor antagonist overdose.
   c. Calcium (p 526) for calcium antagonist overdose.
   d. Propranolol (p 617) or esmolol (p 552) for theophylline, caffeine, or albuterol or other beta agonist overdose (which cause peripheral vasodilation mediated through $beta_2$ receptors).

7. Other treatments:
   a. Severe hypotension due to calcium antagonist or beta blocker poisoning may respond to hyperinsulin-euglycemia therapy (p 564).
   b. Lipid emulsion (p 574) may be useful for severe cardiotoxicity due to lipid-soluble drugs (eg, bupivacaine, verapamil, bupropion).
   c. If adrenal insufficiency is suspected, administer corticosteroids (eg, hydrocortisone, 100 mg IV every 8 hours).
8. If empiric measures to restore the blood pressure are unsuccessful, assess volume status and cardiac contractility with bedside ultrasound, or insert a central venous pressure (CVP) monitor or pulmonary artery catheter. Although invasive, CVP monitoring can help to determine whether further IV fluids are needed and to measure the cardiac output (CO) and calculate the systemic vascular resistance (SVR):

$$SVR = \frac{80\ (MAP - CVP)}{CO}$$

   Select further therapy on the basis of the following:
   a. If the central venous pressure or pulmonary artery wedge pressure remains low, give more IV fluids.
   b. If the cardiac output is low, give more dopamine or dobutamine.
   c. If the systemic vascular resistance is low, administer norepinephrine, 4–8 mcg/min (p 595), or phenylephrine (p 606).
9. Patients refractory to medical interventions may benefit from **extracorporeal membrane oxygenation** (ECMO, or "heart–lung bypass"), which helps to perfuse the vital organs until the toxin can be eliminated or metabolized.

VII. Hypertension

A. Assessment. Hypertension is frequently overlooked in drug-intoxicated patients and often goes untreated. Many young people have normal blood pressures in the range of 90/60–100/70 mm Hg; in such a person, an abrupt elevation to 170/100 mm Hg is much more significant (and potentially catastrophic) than the same blood pressure elevation in an older person with chronic hypertension. Examples of drugs and toxins causing hypertension are listed in Table I–9. Hypertension may be caused by a variety of mechanisms:

1. Amphetamines and other related drugs cause hypertension and tachycardia through generalized sympathetic stimulation.
2. Selective alpha-adrenergic agents cause hypertension with reflex (baroreceptor-mediated) bradycardia or even AV block.
3. Anticholinergic agents cause mild hypertension with tachycardia.
4. Substances that stimulate nicotinic cholinergic receptors (eg, organophosphates) may initially cause tachycardia and hypertension, followed later by bradycardia and hypotension.
5. Withdrawal from sedative-hypnotic drugs, ethanol, opioids, or clonidine can cause hypertension and tachycardia.

B. Complications. Severe hypertension can result in intracranial hemorrhage, aortic dissection, myocardial infarction, renal injury, and congestive heart failure.

C. Differential diagnosis. Rule out the following:

1. Idiopathic hypertension (which is common in the general population). However, without a prior history of hypertension, it should not be initially assumed to be the cause of the elevated blood pressure.
2. Pheochromocytoma or other paraganglionic tumors that secrete epinephrine, norepinephrine, or both are rare but potentially lethal. They typically cause paroxysmal attacks of hypertension, headache, perspiration, and palpitations.
3. Increased intracranial pressure caused by spontaneous hemorrhage, trauma, or other causes. This may result in hypertension with reflex bradycardia (Cushing reflex).

TABLE I–9. SELECTED DRUGS AND TOXINS CAUSING HYPERTENSION[a]

HYPERTENSION WITH TACHYCARDIA

Generalized sympathomimetic agents
- Amphetamines and derivatives
- Cocaine
- Ephedrine and pseudoephedrine
- Epinephrine
- Levodopa
- LSD (lysergic acid diethylamide)
- Marijuana
- Monoamine oxidase inhibitors
- Synthetic cathinones and cannabinoids

Anticholinergic agents[b]
- Antihistamines
- Atropine and other anticholinergics
- Tricyclic antidepressants

Others
- Ethanol and sedative-hypnotic drug withdrawal
- Nicotine (early stage)
- Organophosphates (early stage)

HYPERTENSION WITH BRADYCARDIA OR ATRIOVENTRICULAR BLOCK
- Clonidine, tetrahydrozoline, and oxymetazoline[c]
- Ergot derivatives
- Methoxamine
- Norepinephrine
- Phenylephrine
- Phenylpropanolamine

[a]Adapted in part, with permission, from Olson KR, et al. *Med Toxicol.* 1987;2:56.
[b]Hypertension is usually mild and associated with therapeutic or slightly supratherapeutic levels. Overdose may cause hypotension, especially with tricyclics.
[c]Hypertension is often transient and followed by hypotension.

D. Treatment. Rapid lowering of the blood pressure is desirable as long as it does not result in hypotension, which can potentially cause an ischemic cerebral infarction in older patients with cerebrovascular disease. For a patient with chronic hypertension, lowering the diastolic pressure to 100 mm Hg is acceptable. However, for a young person whose normal diastolic blood pressure is 60 mm Hg, the diastolic pressure should be lowered to 80 mm Hg.

1. **For hypertension with little or no tachycardia**, vasodilator treatment is recommended. Use phentolamine, 0.02–0.1 mg/kg IV (p 605), or nitroprusside, 2–10 mcg/kg/min IV (p 593).
2. **For hypertension with tachycardia**, add a beta blocker to the vasodilator treatment in Item 1 above. Give esmolol, 0.025–0.1 mg/kg/min IV (p 552), or labetalol, 0.2–0.3 mg/kg IV (p 571). ***Caution:*** Do not use beta blockers without a vasodilator to treat hypertensive crisis; beta receptor antagonists may paradoxically worsen hypertension because any alpha-mediated vasoconstriction is unopposed when $beta_2$-mediated vasodilation is blocked. Although labetalol has some alpha-adrenergic receptor blocker activity, it may be insufficient to overcome unopposed alpha effects.
3. **If hypertension is accompanied by a focally abnormal neurologic examination** (eg, hemiparesis), perform computed tomography (CT) as quickly as possible. In a patient with a cerebrovascular accident, hypertension should generally not be treated unless specific complications of the elevated pressure (eg, heart failure or cardiac ischemia) are present. Consult a neurologist or neurosurgeon.

ALTERED MENTAL STATUS

I. Coma and stupor

A. Assessment. A decreased level of consciousness is the most common serious complication of drug overdose or poisoning. Examples of commonly encountered drugs and toxins that cause coma are listed in Table I–10. ***Note:*** this is not an exhaustive list because almost any toxin has the potential to depress mental function.

TABLE I–10. SELECTED DRUGS AND TOXINS CAUSING COMA OR STUPOR[a]

General central nervous system depressants	**Cellular hypoxia**
Anticholinergics	Carbon monoxide
Antihistamines	Cyanide
Baclofen	Hydrogen sulfide
Barbiturates	Methemoglobinemia
Benzodiazepines	Sodium azide
Carbamazepine	**Other or unknown mechanisms**
Ethanol and other alcohols	Acetaminophen (massive ingestion)
GHB (gamma hydroxybutyrate)	Bromide
Phenothiazines and other antipsychotic drugs	Diquat
Sedative-hypnotic agents	Disulfiram
Tricyclic and other antidepressants	Hypoglycemic agents
Valproic acid	Ifosfamide
Sympatholytic agents	Lead
Clonidine, tetrahydrozoline, and oxymetazoline	Lithium
Methyldopa	Nonsteroidal anti-inflammatory drugs (NSAIDs)
Opioids	Phencyclidine (PCP)
	Salicylates

[a]Adapted in part, with permission, from Olson KR, et al. *Med Toxicol.* 1987;2:61.

1. Coma is most often a result of global depression of the brain's reticular activating system, caused by anticholinergic agents, sympatholytic drugs, generalized CNS depressants, or toxins that result in cellular hypoxia.
2. Coma sometimes represents a postictal phenomenon after a drug- or toxin-induced seizure.
3. Coma may also be caused by brain injury associated with infarction or intracranial bleeding. Brain injury is suggested by the presence of focal neurologic deficits and is confirmed by CT or MRI.

B. Complications. Coma frequently is accompanied by respiratory depression, which is a major cause of death. Other conditions that may accompany or complicate coma include hypotension (p 15), hypothermia (p 20), hyperthermia (p 21), and rhabdomyolysis (p 27).

C. Differential diagnosis. Rule out the following:

1. Head trauma or other causes of intracranial bleeding.
2. Vital signs abnormalities which contribute to cerebral hypoperfusion, such as hypotension or hypoxia.
3. Abnormal levels of blood glucose, sodium, or other electrolytes. **Hypoglycemia is a common cause of altered mental status.**
4. Hypothyroidism.
5. Liver or renal failure.
6. Environmental hyperthermia or hypothermia.
7. Serious CNS infections such as encephalitis and meningitis or systemic processes such as sepsis.

D. Treatment

1. Maintain the airway and assist ventilation if necessary (pp 1–7). Administer supplemental oxygen.
2. Consider administration of dextrose, thiamine, naloxone, and possibly flumazenil.
   a. **Dextrose.** All patients with depressed consciousness should receive concentrated dextrose (p 562) unless hypoglycemia is ruled out with an immediate bedside glucose determination. Use a secure vein and avoid

extravasation; concentrated dextrose is highly irritating to tissues. Initial doses include the following:

(1) Adults: 50% dextrose, 50 mL (25 g) IV.

(2) Children: 25% dextrose, 2 mL/kg IV.

b. Thiamine. Thiamine is given to prevent or treat Wernicke syndrome resulting from thiamine deficiency in alcoholic patients and others with suspected vitamin deficiencies. It is not given routinely to children. Give thiamine, 100 mg, in the IV solution or IM (p 628). It can also be given orally if the patient is awake.

c. Naloxone. All patients with respiratory depression should receive naloxone (p 584); if a patient is already intubated and is being artificially ventilated, naloxone is not immediately necessary and can be considered a diagnostic rather than a therapeutic drug. ***Caution:*** naloxone may precipitate abrupt opioid withdrawal or unmask stimulant-mediated hypertension, tachycardia, or psychosis in patients with amphetamine or cocaine intoxication. In addition, acute pulmonary edema is sometimes temporally associated with abrupt naloxone reversal of opioid intoxication.

(1) Give naloxone, 0.2–0.4 mg IV (may also be given IM or through an intraosseous line, or intranasally).

(2) If there is no response within 1–2 minutes, give naloxone, 2 mg IV.

(3) If there is still no response and opioid overdose is highly suspected by the history or clinical presentation (pinpoint pupils, apnea, or hypotension), give naloxone, up to 10–20 mg IV.

d. Consider **flumazenil** if benzodiazepines are the only suspected cause of coma and there are no contraindications (p 556). ***Caution:*** The use of flumazenil can precipitate seizures in patients who are dependent on benzodiazepines or who have co-ingested a convulsant drug or poison.

3. Treat hypothermia or hyperthermia if present.

4. If there is any question of CNS trauma or cerebrovascular accident, perform a CT scan of the head.

5. If meningitis or encephalitis is suspected, perform a lumbar puncture and treat with appropriate antibiotics.

II. Hypothermia

A. Assessment. Hypothermia may mimic or complicate drug overdose and should be suspected in every comatose patient. Examples of drugs and toxins that cause hypothermia are listed in Table I–11.

1. Hypothermia is usually caused by exposure to low ambient temperatures in a patient with blunted thermoregulatory response mechanisms. Drugs and toxins may induce hypothermia by causing vasodilation, inhibiting the shivering response, decreasing metabolic activity, or causing loss of consciousness in a cold environment.

2. A patient whose temperature is lower than 30°C (86°F) may appear to be dead, with a barely detectable pulse or blood pressure and without reflexes. The ECG may reveal an abnormal terminal deflection (J wave or Osborne wave [see Figure I–6]).

B. Complications. Because there is a generalized reduction of metabolic activity and less demand for blood flow, hypothermia is commonly accompanied by hypotension and bradycardia.

TABLE I–11. SELECTED DRUGS AND TOXINS ASSOCIATED WITH HYPOTHERMIA[a]

Barbiturates	Phenothiazines
Ethanol and other alcohols	Sedative-hypnotic agents
Hypoglycemic agents	Tricyclic antidepressants
Opioids	Vasodilators

[a]Adapted in part, with permission, from Olson KR, et al. *Med Toxicol.* 1987;2:60.

1. Mild hypotension (systolic blood pressure of 70–90 mm Hg) in a patient with hypothermia should not be treated aggressively; excessive IV fluids may cause fluid overload and further lowering of the temperature.
2. Severe hypothermia (temperature <28–30°C) may cause intractable ventricular fibrillation and cardiac arrest. This may occur abruptly, such as when the patient is moved or rewarmed too quickly or when CPR is performed.

C. Differential diagnosis. Rule out the following:

1. Sepsis.
2. Hypoglycemia.
3. Hypothyroidism.
4. Adrenal insufficiency.
5. Thiamine deficiency.

D. Treatment

1. Maintain the airway and assist ventilation if necessary (pp 1–4). Administer supplemental oxygen.
2. Because the pulse rate may be profoundly slow and weak, perform careful cardiac evaluation before assuming that the patient is in cardiac arrest. Bedside ultrasound can also help rapidly confirm cardiac activity.
3. Unless the patient is in cardiac arrest (asystole or ventricular fibrillation), rewarm slowly (with blankets, warmed IV fluids, and inhalation of warmed mist) to prevent rewarming dysrhythmias.
4. For patients in cardiac arrest, usual antiarrhythmic agents and direct current countershock are frequently ineffective until the core temperature is above 30–32°C (86–90°F). Perform CPR and initiate active internal rewarming (eg, pleural or peritoneal lavage with warmed fluids; extracorporeal bypass; endovascular rewarming catheters).
5. Open cardiac massage, with direct warm irrigation of the ventricle, or a partial cardiopulmonary bypass may be necessary in hypothermic patients in cardiac arrest who are unresponsive to the aforementioned treatment.
6. If the patient is hypoglycemic, give dextrose (p 562) and thiamine (p 628).
7. If adrenal insufficiency is suspected, draw blood for a serum cortisol level and administer 100 mg of hydrocortisone IV.
8. Consider severe hypothyroidism (myxedema coma) as a cause of hypothermia if the patient has a history of thyroid dysfunction or a surgical neck scar.

III. Hyperthermia

A. Assessment. Hyperthermia (temperature >40°C or 104°F) is a potentially catastrophic complication of intoxication by a variety of drugs and toxins (Table I–12). It can be caused by excessive heat generation resulting from sustained seizures, rigidity, or other muscular hyperactivity; an increased metabolic rate; impaired dissipation of heat secondary to impaired sweating (eg, anticholinergic agents); or hypothalamic disorders.

1. **Neuroleptic malignant syndrome (NMS)** is a hyperthermic disorder related to use of antipsychotic agents. Often developing over days to weeks before diagnosis, NMS is characterized by hyperthermia, generalized muscle rigidity (often so severe as to be called "lead pipe" rigidity), metabolic acidosis, rhabdomyolysis, dehydration, and confusion. This may also occur after sudden withdrawal of dopaminergic agents (eg, carbidopa/levodopa, bromocriptine) in patients being treated for Parkinson disease.
2. **Malignant hyperthermia** is an inherited disorder of muscle relaxation that manifests as severe hyperthermia, metabolic acidosis, and rigidity minutes after the administration of certain anesthetic agents (most commonly succinylcholine and inhaled anesthetics). Typical findings include masseter (jaw) spasm, chest wall rigidity, and failure to ventilate. Hyperthermia is often a preterminal event.
3. **Serotonin syndrome** occurs primarily in patients taking combinations of antidepressants and other agents which enhance serotonin pathways in the brain.

TABLE I–12. SELECTED DRUGS AND TOXINS ASSOCIATED WITH HYPERTHERMIA[a]

Excessive muscular hyperactivity, rigidity, or seizures	Impaired heat dissipation or disrupted thermoregulation
Amoxapine	Amoxapine
Amphetamines and derivatives (including MDMA)	Anticholinergic agents
Cocaine	Antihistamines (eg, diphenhydramine)
Lithium	Phenothiazines and other antipsychotic agents
LSD (lysergic acid diethylamide)	Tricyclic antidepressants
Maprotiline	**Other**
Monoamine oxidase inhibitors	Exertional heatstroke
Phencyclidine (PCP)	Malignant hyperthermia
Tricyclic antidepressants	Metal fume fever
Increased metabolic rate	Neuroleptic malignant syndrome (NMS)
Dinitrophenol and pentachlorophenol	Serotonin syndrome
Salicylates	Withdrawal from carbidopa/levodopa or bromocriptine
Thyroid hormone	Withdrawal from ethanol or sedative-hypnotic drugs

[a]Adapted, with permission, from Olson KR, et al. *Med Toxicol.* 1987;2:59.

Common triggers include selective serotonin reuptake inhibitors (SSRIs) and monoamine oxidase (MAO) inhibitors as well as lithium, cocaine, and methylenedioxymethamphetamine (MDMA). Serotonin syndrome typically manifests within 24 hours of an overdose or medication dose change, and it is characterized by confusion, muscle rigidity, and myoclonus (especially of the lower extremities), diaphoresis, autonomic instability, and hyperthermia.

B. Complications. Untreated, severe hyperthermia is likely to result in hypotension, rhabdomyolysis, coagulopathy, cardiac and renal failure, brain injury, and death. Survivors often have permanent neurologic sequelae.

C. Differential diagnosis. Rule out the following:

1. Sedative-hypnotic drug or ethanol withdrawal (delirium tremens).
2. Exertional or environmental heat stroke.
3. Thyrotoxicosis.
4. Meningitis or encephalitis.
5. Other serious infections.

D. Treatment. Immediate rapid cooling is essential to prevent death or serious brain damage.

1. Maintain the airway and assist ventilation if necessary (pp 1–7). Administer supplemental oxygen.
2. Administer glucose-containing IV fluids and give a concentrated glucose bolus (p 562) if the patient is hypoglycemic.
3. Rapidly gain control of seizures (p 23), agitation (p 24), or muscular rigidity (p 26).
4. Begin external cooling with tepid (lukewarm) sponging and fanning. This evaporative method is the most efficient method of external cooling.
5. Shivering often occurs with rapid external cooling, and it may generate even more heat. Use a benzodiazepine such as diazepam, 0.1–0.2 mg/kg IV, or lorazepam, 0.05–0.1 mg/kg IV, or midazolam, 0.05–0.1 mg/kg IV or IM (p 516), or use neuromuscular paralysis (see below).
6. The most rapidly effective and reliable means of lowering the temperature is neuromuscular paralysis. Administer a nondepolarizing agent (p 586) such as vecuronium, 0.1 mg/kg IV. ***Caution:*** The patient will stop breathing; be prepared to ventilate and intubate endotracheally.
7. **Malignant hyperthermia.** If muscle rigidity persists despite administration of neuromuscular blockers, a defect at the muscle cell level (ie, malignant

hyperthermia) should be suspected. **Give dantrolene**, 1–10 mg/kg IV (p 537) immediately.

8. **Neuroleptic malignant syndrome (NMS).** Withdrawal of the offending agent, initiation of cooling measures, and rehydration with IV fluids are the mainstays of treatment. For severe cases, consider bromocriptine (p 524).
9. **Serotonin syndrome.** As with NMS, withdrawal of the offending agent or agents, initiation of cooling measures and rehydration with IV fluids are the mainstays of treatment. Benzodiazepines are useful for control of agitation. Anecdotal case reports suggest benefit with cyproheptadine (Periactin), 12 mg orally (PO) initially, followed by 4 mg every hour for 3–4 doses (p 537). Chlorpromazine has also been used; it can be given intravenously (25–50 mg) and titrated to effect, but is a vasodilator and can cause hypotension so patients should be volume-loaded.

IV. Seizures

A. Assessment. Seizures are a major cause of morbidity and mortality from drug overdose or poisoning. Seizures may be single and brief or multiple and sustained and may result from a variety of mechanisms (Table I–13).

1. Generalized seizures usually result in loss of consciousness, often accompanied by tongue biting and fecal and urinary incontinence.
2. Other causes of muscular hyperactivity or rigidity (p 26) may be mistaken for seizures, especially if the patient is also unconscious.

TABLE I–13. SELECTED DRUGS AND TOXINS CAUSING SEIZURES[a]

Adrenergic-sympathomimetic agents	**Antidepressants and antipsychotics**
Amphetamines and derivatives (including MDMA)	Amoxapine
Caffeine and theophylline	Bupropion
Cocaine	Haloperidol and droperidol
Ephedrine	Loxapine, clozapine, and olanzapine
Phencyclidine (PCP)	Phenothiazines
Phenylpropanolamine	Serotonin reuptake inhibitors
Synthetic cathinones ("bath salts") and cannabinoids	Tricyclic antidepressants
	Venlafaxine
Others	
Antihistamines (diphenhydramine, hydroxyzine)	Lamotrigine
Boric acid	Lead and other heavy metals
Camphor	Lidocaine and other local anesthetics
Carbamazepine	Lithium
Cellular hypoxia (eg, carbon monoxide, cyanide, hydrogen sulfide)	Mefenamic acid
Chlorinated hydrocarbons	Meperidine (normeperidine metabolite)
Cholinergic agents (carbamates, nicotine, organophosphates)	Metaldehyde
Cicutoxin (water hemlock) and other plant toxins	Methanol
Citrate	Methyl bromide
DEET (diethyltoluamide) (rare)	Phenols
Ethylene glycol	Phenylbutazone
Fipronil	Piroxicam
Fluoride	Propranolol
Foscarnet	Salicylates
GHB (gamma hydroxybutyrate)	Strychnine (opisthotonus and rigidity)
Isoniazid (INH)	Tetramine (rodenticide)
	Tiagabine
	Tramadol
	Withdrawal from ethanol or sedative-hypnotic drugs

[a]Adapted in part, with permission, from Olson KR, et al. *Med Toxicol.* 1987;2:63.

B. Complications

1. Any seizure can cause airway compromise, resulting in apnea or pulmonary aspiration.
2. Multiple or prolonged seizures may cause severe metabolic acidosis, hyperthermia, rhabdomyolysis, and brain damage.

C. Differential diagnosis. Rule out the following:

1. Any serious metabolic disturbance (eg, hypoglycemia, hyponatremia, hypocalcemia, or hypoxia).
2. Head trauma with intracranial injury.
3. Idiopathic epilepsy.
4. Withdrawal from alcohol or a sedative-hypnotic drug.
5. Exertional or environmental hyperthermia.
6. CNS infection such as meningitis or encephalitis.
7. Febrile seizures in children.

D. Treatment

1. Maintain an open airway and assist ventilation if necessary (pp 1–7). Administer supplemental oxygen.
2. Administer naloxone (p 584) if seizures are thought to be caused by hypoxia resulting from opioid-associated respiratory depression.
3. Check for hypoglycemia and administer dextrose and thiamine as for coma (p 19).
4. Use one or more of the following anticonvulsants. ***Caution:*** Anticonvulsants can cause hypotension, cardiac arrest, or respiratory arrest if administered too rapidly.
   a. Diazepam, 0.1–0.2 mg/kg IV (p 516).
   b. Lorazepam, 0.05–0.1 mg/kg IV (p 516).
   c. Midazolam, 0.1–0.2 mg/kg IM (useful when IV access is difficult) or 0.05–0.1 mg/kg IV (p 516).
   d. Phenobarbital, 10–15 mg/kg IV; slow infusion over 15–20 minutes (p 604).
   e. Pentobarbital, 5–6 mg/kg IV; slow infusion over 8–10 minutes, then continuous infusion at 0.5–3 mg/kg/h titrated to effect (p 602).
   f. Propofol, 1–2 mg/kg IV (p 613), infused in increments IV every 10–20 seconds until desired effect, followed by continuous infusion 1.2–12 mg/kg/h.
   g. Phenytoin is ineffective for convulsions caused by drug-induced seizures and is not recommended in the setting of drug overdose.
5. Immediately check the rectal or tympanic **temperature** and cool the patient rapidly (p 21) if the temperature is above 40°C (104°F). The most rapid and reliably effective method of temperature control is neuromuscular paralysis with vecuronium, 0.1 mg/kg IV (p 586) or another nondepolarizing neuromuscular blocker. ***Caution:*** If paralysis is used, the patient must be intubated and ventilated; in addition, monitor the electroencephalogram for continued brain seizure activity because peripheral muscular convulsions are no longer visible.
6. Use the following specific antidotes if available:
   a. Pyridoxine (p 621) for seizures due to isoniazid (INH; p 281) or monomethylhydrazine-containing mushrooms (see p 330).
   b. Pralidoxime (2-PAM; p 613) or atropine (p 512) or both for organophosphate or carbamate insecticides (p 353).

V. Agitation, delirium, or psychosis

A. Assessment. Agitation, delirium, or psychosis may be caused by a variety of drugs and toxins (Table I–14). In addition, such symptoms may result from a functional thought disorder or metabolic encephalopathy caused by medical illness.

1. Functional psychosis or stimulant-induced agitation and psychosis are usually associated with an intact sensorium, and hallucinations are predominantly auditory.

TABLE I–14. SELECTED DRUGS AND TOXINS CAUSING AGITATION, DELIRIUM, OR CONFUSION[a]

Predominant confusion or delirium	Predominant agitation or psychosis
Amantadine	Amphetamines and derivatives
Anticholinergic agents	Caffeine and theophylline
Antihistamines	Cocaine
Bromide	Cycloserine
Carbon monoxide	Dextromethorphan
Cimetidine	LSD (lysergic acid diethylamide)
Disulfiram	Marijuana
Lead and other heavy metals	Mercury
Levodopa	Phencyclidine (PCP)
Lidocaine and other local anesthetics	Procaine
Lithium	Serotonin reuptake inhibitors (SSRIs)
Salicylates	Steroids (eg, prednisone)
Withdrawal from ethanol or sedative-hypnotic drugs	Synthetic cathinones and cannabinoids

[a]Adapted in part, with permission, from Olson KR, et al. *Med Toxicol.* 1987;2:62.

2. With metabolic encephalopathy or drug-induced delirium, there is usually alteration of the sensorium (manifested by confusion or disorientation). Hallucinations, when they occur, are predominantly visual. Anticholinergic delirium is often accompanied by tachycardia, dilated pupils, flushing, dry skin and mucous membranes, decreased peristalsis, and urinary retention.

B. Complications. Agitation, especially if accompanied by hyperkinetic behavior and struggling, may result in hyperthermia (p 21) and rhabdomyolysis (p 27).

C. Differential diagnosis. Rule out the following:

1. Serious metabolic disturbance (hypoxia, hypoglycemia, or hyponatremia).
2. Alcohol or sedative-hypnotic drug withdrawal.
3. Thyrotoxicosis.
4. CNS infection such as meningitis or encephalitis.
5. Exertion-induced or environmental hyperthermia.

D. Treatment. Sometimes, the patient can be calmed with reassuring words and reduction of noise, light, and physical stimulation. If this is not quickly effective, rapidly gain control of the patient to determine the rectal or tympanic temperature and begin rapid cooling and other treatment if needed.

1. Maintain an open airway and assist ventilation if necessary (pp 1–7). Administer supplemental oxygen.
2. Treat hypoglycemia (p 36), hyperthermia (p 21), hypoxia (p 6), or other metabolic disturbances.
3. Administer one of the following benzodiazepines (p 516):
 a. Midazolam, 0.05–0.1 mg/kg IV over 1 minute, or 0.1–0.2 mg/kg IM.
 c. Lorazepam, 0.05–0.1 mg/kg IV over 1 minute.
 d. Diazepam, 0.1–0.2 mg/kg IV over 1 minute.
4. Consider use of an antipsychotic agent (p 503):
 a. Ziprasidone, 10–20 mg IM, or olanzapine, 5–10 mg IM.
 b. An older antipsychotic drug that is often used for agitation is haloperidol, 0.1–0.2 mg/kg IM or IV over 1 minute. ***Note:*** Do not give haloperidol *decanoate* salt intravenously; it is a long-acting preparation designed for depot use every 4 weeks.
 c. ***Caution:*** Haloperidol and other antipsychotic agents can cause prolongation of the QT interval and polymorphic ventricular tachycardia (torsade de pointes). Avoid or use with great caution in patients with preexisting QT prolongation or with toxicity from agents known to prolong the QT interval. Haloperidol can also induce an acute dystonic reaction (see below).

5. For agitated patients not responding adequately to benzodiazepines or antipsychotics, consider **dexmedetomidine** (p 540) or **ketamine** (p 569).
6. For anticholinergic-induced agitated delirium, consider use of **physostigmine**, 0.5–1 mg IV (p 609). ***Caution:*** Do not use in patients with tricyclic antidepressant or other sodium channel–blocker overdose if there is evidence of a cardiac conduction disturbance (eg, prolonged QRS interval).
7. If **hyperthermia** occurs as a result of excessive muscular hyperactivity, skeletal muscle paralysis is indicated. Use vecuronium, 0.1 mg/kg IV (p 586), or another nondepolarizing neuromuscular blocker. ***Caution:*** Be prepared to ventilate and endotracheally intubate the patient after muscle paralysis.

OTHER COMPLICATIONS

I. Dystonia, dyskinesia, and rigidity

A. Assessment. Examples of drugs and toxins causing abnormal movements or rigidity are listed in Table I–15.

1. **Dystonic reactions** are common with therapeutic or toxic doses of many antipsychotic agents and with some antiemetics. The mechanism triggering these reactions is thought to be related to central dopamine blockade. Dystonias usually consist of forced, involuntary, and often painful muscle contractions resulting in neck rotation (torticollis), tongue protrusion, jaw extension, or trismus. Other extrapyramidal or parkinsonian movement disorders (eg, pill rolling, bradykinesia, and masked facies) may also be seen. **Akathisia** is a sensation of inner restlessness.
2. In contrast, **dyskinesias** are usually rapid, repetitive body movements that may involve small, localized muscle groups (eg, tongue darting, focal myoclonus) or may consist of generalized hyperkinetic activity. The cause is not dopamine blockade but, more commonly, increased central dopamine activity or blockade of central cholinergic effects.
3. **Rigidity** may also be seen with a number of toxins and may be caused by CNS effects or spinal cord stimulation. Neuroleptic malignant syndrome and serotonin syndrome (p 21) are characterized by rigidity, hyperthermia, metabolic acidosis, and an altered mental status. Rigidity seen with

TABLE I–15. SELECTED DRUGS AND TOXINS CAUSING DYSTONIAS, DYSKINESIAS, AND RIGIDITY[a]

Dystonia and/or akathisia	Dyskinesias
Haloperidol and droperidol	Amphetamines
Metoclopramide	Anticholinergic agents
Phenothiazines (prochlorperazine)	Antihistamines
Ziprasidone and other atypical antipsychotic agents	Bismuth
Rigidity	Caffeine
Black widow spider bite	Carbamazepine
Lithium	Carisoprodol
Malignant hyperthermia	Cocaine
Manganese	GHB (gamma hydroxybutyrate)
Methaqualone	Ketamine
Monoamine oxidase inhibitors	Levodopa
Neuroleptic malignant syndrome	Lithium
Phencyclidine (PCP)	Phencyclidine (PCP)
Strychnine	Serotonin reuptake inhibitors (SSRIs)
Tetanus	Tricyclic antidepressants

[a]Adapted in part, with permission, from Olson KR, et al. *Med Toxicol.* 1987;2:64.

malignant hyperthermia (p 21) is caused by a defect at the muscle cell level and may not reverse with neuromuscular blockade.

B. Complications. Sustained muscular rigidity or hyperactivity may result in rhabdomyolysis (p 27), hyperthermia (p 21), ventilatory failure (p 5), or metabolic acidosis (p 35).

C. Differential diagnosis. Rule out the following:

1. Catatonic rigidity caused by functional thought disorder.
2. Tetanus.
3. Cerebrovascular accident.
4. Postanoxic encephalopathy.
5. Idiopathic parkinsonism.

D. Treatment

1. Maintain the airway and assist ventilation if necessary (pp 1–7). Administer supplemental oxygen.
2. Check the rectal or tympanic temperature and treat hyperthermia (p 21) rapidly if the temperature is above 40°C (102.2°F).
3. **Dystonia.** Administer an anticholinergic agent such as diphenhydramine (p 544), 0.5–1 mg/kg IM or IV, or benztropine (p 519), 1–4 mg IM, in adults. Follow this treatment with oral therapy for 2–3 days.
4. **Dyskinesia.** Do not treat with anticholinergic agents. Instead, administer a sedative such as diazepam, 0.1–0.2 mg/kg IV, or lorazepam, 0.05–0.1 mg/kg IV or IM, or midazolam, 0.05–0.1 mg/kg IV or 0.1–0.2 mg/kg IM (p 516).
5. **Rigidity.** Do not treat with anticholinergic agents. Instead, administer a sedative (see Item 4 directly above) or provide specific pharmacologic therapy as follows:
   a. Dantrolene (p 537) for malignant hyperthermia.
   b. Bromocriptine (p 524) for neuroleptic malignant syndrome.
   c. Benzodiazepines or *Latrodectus* antivenom (p 508) for a black widow spider bite (p 426).

II. Rhabdomyolysis

A. Assessment. Muscle cell necrosis is a common complication of poisoning. Examples of drugs and toxins that cause rhabdomyolysis are listed in Table I–16.

1. Causes of rhabdomyolysis include prolonged immobilization on a hard surface, excessive seizures or muscular hyperactivity, hyperthermia, hypoxia, and direct cytotoxic effects of the drug or toxin (eg, carbon monoxide, colchicine, hemlock, *Tricholoma* and *Russula* mushrooms, and some snake venoms).
2. The diagnosis is made by finding Hematest-positive urine with few or no intact red blood cells or an elevated serum creatine kinase (CK) level. Serum aminotransferase levels are usually elevated, AST more than ALT.

B. Complications. Myoglobin released by damaged muscle cells may precipitate in the kidneys, causing acute tubular necrosis and renal failure. This is more likely when the serum CK level exceeds several thousand IU/L and if the patient is dehydrated. With severe rhabdomyolysis, hyperkalemia, hyperphosphatemia, hyperuricemia, and hypocalcemia may also occur.

C. Differential diagnosis. Hemolysis leading to hemoglobinuria may also produce Hematest-positive urine.

D. Treatment

1. Aggressively restore volume in dehydrated patients. Then establish a steady urine flow rate (3–5 mL/kg/h) with IV fluids. For massive rhabdomyolysis accompanied by oliguria, also consider a bolus of **mannitol**, 0.5 g/kg IV (p 578).
2. Some clinicians alkalinize the urine by adding 100 mEq of sodium bicarbonate to each liter of 5% dextrose. The rationale for this treatment is that acidic urine promotes the deposition of myoglobin in the renal tubules, possibly exacerbating the acute kidney injury.

TABLE I–16. SELECTED DRUGS AND TOXINS ASSOCIATED WITH RHABDOMYOLYSIS

Excessive muscular hyperactivity, rigidity, or seizures	Other or unknown mechanisms
Amphetamines and derivatives	Carbon monoxide
Antihistamines and anticholinergics	Chlorophenoxy herbicides
Cholinesterase inhibitors (fasciculations)	Colchicine
Clozapine and olanzapine	Ethanol
Cocaine	Ethylene glycol
Lithium	Gemfibrozil
Monoamine oxidase inhibitors	Haff disease (unknown toxin found in Baltic fish, buffalo fish)
Phencyclidine (PCP)	Hemlock
Seizures caused by a variety of agents	Hyperthermia caused by a variety of agents
Strychnine	Hypokalemia
Tetanus	Mushrooms (some *Amanita, Russula, Tricholoma* species)
Tricyclic antidepressants	Paraphenylenediamine (hair dye)
	Prolonged immobility (eg, coma due to central nervous system depressant drug overdose)
	"Statin" cholesterol drugs (eg, cerivastatin)
	Trauma

3. Provide intensive supportive care, including hemodialysis if needed, for acute renal failure. Kidney function is usually regained in 2–3 weeks.

III. Anaphylactic and anaphylactoid reactions

A. Assessment. Examples of drugs and toxins that cause anaphylactic or anaphylactoid reactions are listed in Table I–17. These reactions are characterized by bronchospasm and increased vascular permeability that may lead to laryngeal edema, skin rash, and hypotension.

1. Anaphylaxis occurs when a patient with antigen-specific immunoglobulin E (IgE) bound to the surface of mast cells and basophils is exposed to the antigen, triggering the release of histamine and various other vasoactive compounds.

2. Anaphylactoid reactions are also caused by release of active compounds from mast cells but do not involve prior sensitization or mediation through IgE.

B. Complications. Severe anaphylactic or anaphylactoid reactions can result in laryngeal obstruction, respiratory arrest, hypotension, and death.

C. Differential diagnosis. Rule out the following:

1. Bronchospasm or laryngeal edema from irritant gas exposure.

2. Nonallergic pharmacologic effects of the drug or toxin.

3. Vasovagal syncope or hyperventilation.

TABLE I–17. EXAMPLES OF DRUGS AND TOXINS CAUSING ANAPHYLACTIC OR ANAPHYLACTOID REACTIONS

Anaphylactic reactions (IgE-mediated)	Anaphylactoid reactions (not IgE-mediated)
Antisera (antivenins)	Acetylcysteine (when given IV)
Foods (nuts, fish, shellfish)	Blood products
Hymenoptera and other insect stings	Iodinated contrast media
Immunotherapy allergen extracts	Opioids (eg, morphine)
Penicillins and other antibiotics	Scombroid
Vaccines	Tubocurarine
Other or unclassified	
Exercise	
Sulfites	
Tartrazine dye	

D. Treatment

1. Maintain the airway and assist ventilation if necessary (pp 1–7). Endotracheal intubation may be needed if laryngeal swelling is severe. Administer supplemental oxygen.
2. Treat hypotension with IV crystalloid fluids (eg, normal saline) and place the patient in a supine position.
3. Administer epinephrine (p 551) as follows:
   a. For mild-to-moderate reactions, administer 0.3–0.5 mg subcutaneously (SC; children: 0.01 mg/kg to a maximum of 0.5 mg).
   b. For severe reactions, administer a 0.05- to 0.1-mg IV bolus every 5 minutes, or give an infusion starting at a rate of 1–4 mcg/min and titrating upward as needed.
4. Administer diphenhydramine (p 544), 0.5–1 mg/kg IV over 1 minute. Follow with oral therapy for 2–3 days. A histamine2 (H2) blocker such as ranitidine (p 532), 150 mg IV every 12 hours, is also helpful.
5. Administer a corticosteroid such as hydrocortisone, 200–300 mg IV, or methylprednisolone, 40–80 mg IV.
6. Bronchodilator therapy (nebulized $beta_2$ agonists or anticholinergics) may help bronchospasm.

DIAGNOSIS OF POISONING

The diagnosis and treatment of poisoning often must proceed rapidly without the results of extensive toxicologic screening. Fortunately, in most cases the correct diagnosis can be made by using carefully collected data from the history, a directed physical examination, and commonly available laboratory tests.

I. History. Although frequently unreliable or incomplete, the history of ingestion may be very useful if carefully obtained.

A. Ask the patient about all drugs taken, including nonprescription drugs, herbal medicines, and vitamins.

B. Ask family members, friends, and paramedical personnel about any prescriptions or over-the-counter medications known to be used by the patient or others in the house.

C. Obtain any available drugs or drug paraphernalia for later testing, but handle them very carefully to avoid poisoning by skin contact or an inadvertent needle stick with potential for hepatitis B or human immunodeficiency virus (HIV) transmission.

D. Check with the pharmacy on the label of any medications found with the patient to determine whether other prescription drugs have been obtained there.

E. Check the patient's cell phone for a better estimate of the time of ingestion, as patients sometimes text their contacts or loved ones just minutes before or after an ingestion.

II. Physical examination

A. General findings. Perform serial examinations because findings in intoxicated patients invariably change over time. A carefully directed examination may uncover one of the common autonomic syndromes or "toxidromes" (see Table I–18). ***Note:*** patients may not manifest a classic toxidrome, especially in the presence of opposing effects from multiple medications or underlying medical conditions.

1. **Alpha-adrenergic syndrome.** Hypertension with reflex bradycardia is characteristic. The pupils are usually dilated (eg, phenylpropanolamine and phenylephrine).
2. **Beta-adrenergic syndrome.** $Beta_2$-mediated vasodilation may cause hypotension. Tachycardia is common (eg, albuterol, metaproterenol, theophylline, and caffeine).

TABLE I–18. AUTONOMIC SYNDROMES[a,b]

	Blood Pressure	Pulse Rate	Pupil Size	Sweating	Peristalsis
Alpha-adrenergic	+	−	+	+	−
Beta-adrenergic	±	+	±	±	±
Mixed adrenergic	+	+	+	+	−
Sympatholytic	−	−	--	−	−
Nicotinic	+	+	±	+	+
Muscarinic	−	--	--	+	+
Mixed cholinergic	±	±	--	+	+
Anticholinergic (antimuscarinic)	±	+	+	--	--

[a]Key to symbols: +, increased; ++, markedly increased; −, decreased; --, markedly decreased; ±, mixed effect, no effect, or unpredictable.
[b]Adapted, with permission, from Olson KR, et al. *Med Toxicol.* 1987;2:54.

3. **Mixed alpha- and beta-adrenergic syndrome.** Hypertension is accompanied by tachycardia. The pupils are dilated. The skin is sweaty, although mucous membranes are dry (eg, cocaine and amphetamines).
4. **Sympatholytic syndrome.** Blood pressure and pulse rate are both decreased. (Exceptions: Peripheral alpha receptor antagonists may cause hypotension with reflex tachycardia; $alpha_2$ agonists may cause peripheral vasoconstriction with transient hypertension.) The pupils are small, often of pinpoint size. Peristalsis is often decreased (eg, centrally acting $alpha_2$ agonists [clonidine and methyldopa], opioids, and phenothiazines).
5. **Nicotinic cholinergic syndrome.** Stimulation of nicotinic receptors at autonomic ganglia and neuromuscular junctions activates both parasympathetic and sympathetic systems, with unpredictable or biphasic results. Initial tachycardia may be followed by bradycardia, and muscle fasciculations may be followed by paralysis. (eg, nicotine and the depolarizing neuromuscular blocker succinylcholine, which act on nicotinic receptors in skeletal muscle).
6. **Muscarinic cholinergic syndrome.** Muscarinic receptors are located at effector organs of the parasympathetic system and in general mediate secretory functions. Stimulation causes bradycardia, miosis, sweating, hyperperistalsis, bronchorrhea, wheezing, excessive salivation, and urinary incontinence (eg, bethanechol).
7. **Mixed cholinergic syndrome.** When both nicotinic and muscarinic receptors are stimulated, mixed effects may be seen. The pupils are usually miotic (of pinpoint size). The skin is sweaty, and peristaltic activity is increased. Fasciculations are a manifestation of nicotinic stimulation of the neuromuscular junction and may progress to muscle weakness or paralysis (eg, organophosphate and carbamate insecticides and physostigmine).
8. **Anticholinergic (antimuscarinic) syndrome.** Tachycardia with mild hypertension is common. The pupils are widely dilated. The skin is flushed, hot, and dry. Peristalsis is decreased, and urinary retention is common. Patients may have myoclonic jerking or choreoathetoid movements. Agitated delirium is common, and hyperthermia may occur (eg, atropine, scopolamine, benztropine, antihistamines, and antidepressants; all of these drugs are primarily antimuscarinic).

B. **Eye findings**
   1. **Pupil size** is affected by a number of drugs that act on the autonomic nervous system. Table I–19 lists common causes of miosis and mydriasis.

TABLE I–19. SELECTED CAUSES OF PUPIL SIZE CHANGES[a]

CONSTRICTED PUPILS (MIOSIS)	DILATED PUPILS (MYDRIASIS)
Sympatholytic agents	**Sympathomimetic agents**
Clonidine	Amphetamines and derivatives
Opioids	Cocaine
Phenothiazines	Dopamine
Tetrahydrozoline and oxymetazoline	LSD (lysergic acid diethylamide)
Valproic acid	Monoamine oxidase inhibitors
Cholinergic agents	Nicotine[b]
Carbamate insecticides	**Anticholinergic agents**
Nicotine[b]	Antihistamines
Organophosphates	Atropine and other anticholinergics
Physostigmine	Carbamazepine
Pilocarpine	Glutethimide
Others	Tricyclic antidepressants
Heatstroke	**Retinal toxins (fixed, dilated pupils)**
Pontine infarct	Methanol
Subarachnoid hemorrhage	Quinine

[a]Adapted in part, with permission, from Olson KR, et al. *Med Toxicol.* 1987;2:66.
[b]Nicotine can cause the pupils to be dilated (rare) or constricted (common).

2. Horizontal-gaze **nystagmus** is common with a variety of drugs and toxins, including barbiturates, ethanol, carbamazepine, phenytoin, and scorpion envenomation. Phencyclidine (PCP) may cause horizontal, vertical, and even rotatory nystagmus.
3. **Hippus or pupillary athetosis** refers to rhythmically dilating and contracting pupil size, and can be caused by aconitine, some hallucinogens, or seizure activity.
4. **Cranial neuropathy** involving the eyes can indicate a lesion of the brain matter (eg, ischemic stroke), cranial nerves (eg, cerebral edema impinging on cranial nerve VI, causing an abducens palsy), or ocular muscles (eg, botulism presenting with ptosis or disconjugate gaze).
5. Problems with **visual acuity** or **papilledema** fundoscopic testing suggest retinal toxins such as methanol (formic acid) or chloroquine and related antimalarials.
6. Corneal injury can be caused by irritant or corrosive substances.
7. Chronic digoxin toxicity can cause xanthopsia (the illusion of seeing yellow halos around objects).
8. Hallucinations or illusions can result from mind-altering recreational substances. Synesthesis ("seeing sounds and hearing colors") is typical of serotonergic hallucinogens such as LSD.

C. **Neuropathy.** A variety of drugs and poisons can cause sensory or motor neuropathy, usually after chronic repeated exposure (Table I–20). Some agents (eg, arsenic and thallium) can cause neuropathy after a single large exposure.

D. **Abdominal findings.** Peristaltic activity is commonly affected by drugs and toxins (see Table I–18).

1. Ileus may also be caused by **mechanical factors** such as injury to the gastrointestinal tract with perforation and peritonitis or mechanical obstruction by a swallowed foreign body.
2. Abdominal distension and ileus may also be a manifestation of acute **bowel infarction,** a rare but catastrophic complication that results from prolonged hypotension or mesenteric artery vasospasm (caused, eg, by ergot, cocaine, or amphetamines). Radiographs or CT scans may reveal air in the intestinal wall, biliary tree, or hepatic vein. The serum phosphorus

TABLE I–20. SELECTED CAUSES OF NEUROPATHY

Cause	Comments
Acrylamide	Sensory and motor distal axonal neuropathy
Antineoplastic agents	Vincristine most strongly associated (p 114)
Antiretroviral agents	Nucleoside reverse transcriptase inhibitors (p 134)
Arsenic	Sensory-predominant mixed axonal neuropathy (p 140)
Buckthorn (*K humboldtiana*)	Livestock and human demyelinating neuropathy (p 379)
Carbon disulfide	Sensory and motor distal axonal neuropathy (p 181)
Dimethylaminopropionitrile	Urogenital and distal sensory neuropathy
Disulfiram	Sensory and motor distal axonal neuropathy (p 226)
Ethanol	Sensory and motor distal axonal neuropathy (p 231)
n-Hexane	Sensory and motor distal axonal neuropathy (p 718)
Isoniazid (INH)	Preventable with coadministration of pyridoxine (p 281)
Lead	Motor-predominant mixed axonal neuropathy (p 286)
Mercury	Organic mercury compounds (p 305)
Methyl *n*-butyl ketone	Acts like *n*-hexane via 2,5-hexanedione metabolite
Nitrofurantoin	Sensory and motor distal axonal neuropathy
Nitrous oxide	Sensory axonal neuropathy with loss of proprioception (p 343)
Organophosphate insecticides	Specific agents only (eg, triorthocresyl phosphate)
Pyridoxine (vitamin B_6)	Sensory neuropathy with chronic excessive dosing (p 621)
Selenium	Polyneuritis (p 416)
Thallium	Sensory and motor distal axonal neuropathy (p 433)
Tick paralysis	Ascending flaccid paralysis after bites by several tick species

and alkaline phosphatase levels are often elevated, as are nonspecific indicators of systemic stress such white blood cell count and lactic acid.

3. Vomiting, especially with hematemesis, may indicate the ingestion of a corrosive substance.
4. Diarrhea can result from GI irritation by a variety of toxins, withdrawal from opioids, or cholinergic excess (eg, organophosphate or carbamate poisoning).

E. Skin findings

1. **Sweating** or the absence of sweating may provide a clue to one of the autonomic syndromes (see Table I–18).
2. **Flushed red skin** may be caused by carbon monoxide poisoning, boric acid toxicity, chemical burns from corrosives or hydrocarbons, or anticholinergic agents. It may also result from vasodilation (eg, phenothiazines or disulfiram–ethanol interaction).
3. **Pale coloration** with diaphoresis is frequently caused by acute anemia or sympathomimetic agents. Severe localized pallor should suggest possible arterial vasospasm, such as that caused by ergot (p 229) or some amphetamines (p 81). Jaundice or uremia can also blanch the skin tone.
4. **Cyanosis** may indicate hypoxia, sulfhemoglobinemia, or methemoglobinemia (p 317).

F. Odors. A number of toxins may have characteristic odors (Table I–21). However, the odor may be subtle and may be obscured by the smell of vomit or by other ambient odors. In addition, the ability to smell an odor may vary; for example, only about 50% of the general population can smell the "bitter almond" odor of cyanide. Thus, the absence of an odor does not guarantee the absence of the toxin.

G. Urine.

1. **Color**
   a. **Red-pink or orange** urine may be seen with pyridium, rifampin, or treatment with deferoxamine or hydroxocobalamin.
   b. **Violet or blue** urine can be caused by methylene blue or methocarbamol.

TABLE I–21. SOME COMMON ODORS CAUSED BY TOXINS AND DRUGS[a]

Odor	Drug or Toxin
Acetone	Acetone, isopropyl alcohol
Acrid or pearlike	Chloral hydrate, paraldehyde
Bitter almonds	Cyanide
Carrots	Cicutoxin (water hemlock)
Disinfectant	Phenol, pine oil-based cleaners, turpentine
Garlic	Arsenic (arsine), organophosphates, selenium, thallium
Hay (freshly mown)	Phosgene
Mothballs	Naphthalene, paradichlorobenzene, camphor
New Shower Curtains	Ethchlorvynol
Rotten eggs	Hydrogen sulfide, stibine, mercaptans, old sulfa drugs
Wintergreen	Methyl salicylate

[a]Adapted in part, with permission, from Olson KR, et al. *Med Toxicol.* 1987;2:67.

c. **Brown or black** urine can indicate the presence of phenol, myoglobin (eg, rhabdomyolysis), and the plant-based laxative cascara.

d. Fluorescence under ultraviolet light (Wood lamp) suggests presence of fluorescein, which is found in most antifreeze products. However, other substances in the urine can also be fluorescent.

2. Crystals of calcium oxalate may be seen in the urine of patients with ethylene glycol poisoning (p 234).

III. **Essential clinical laboratory tests.** Simple, readily available clinical laboratory tests may provide important clues to the diagnosis of poisoning and may guide the investigation toward specific toxicology testing. When the diagnosis is obvious, broad laboratory testing may not be necessary.

A. **Routine tests.** The following tests may be useful for screening of the overdose patient with an uncertain diagnosis. ***Note:*** Each test comes with limitations which are important to keep in mind when selecting a diagnostic strategy. Like physical examination findings, laboratory values in poisoned patients are dynamic and serial assessment is often warranted in high risk or critically ill patients.

a. Serum glucose (rapid bedside device).
b. ECG.
c. Serum acetaminophen level.
d. Electrolytes for determination of the sodium, potassium, bicarbonate, and anion gap.
e. Blood alcohol (ethanol) level.
f. Measured serum osmolality and calculation of the osmol gap.
g. Complete blood cell count or hemogram.
h. Hepatic aminotransferases (AST, ALT) and synthetic hepatic function (eg, bilirubin and coagulation) tests.
i. Blood urea nitrogen (BUN) and creatinine for evaluation of renal function.
j. Urinalysis to check for crystalluria, hemoglobinuria, or myoglobinuria.
k. Pregnancy test (females of childbearing age).
l. Creatine kinase to check for rhabdomyolysis.

B. **Serum osmolality and osmol gap.** Under normal circumstances, the measured serum osmolality is approximately 290 mOsm/L and can be calculated from the results of the sodium, glucose, and blood urea nitrogen (BUN) tests. The difference between the calculated osmolality and the osmolality measured in the laboratory is the osmol gap (Table I–22). ***Note:*** Clinical studies suggest that the normal osmol gap may vary from –14 to +10 mOsm/L. Thus, small osmol gaps may be difficult to interpret.

1. **Causes of an elevated osmol gap** (see Table I–22)

a. The osmol gap may be increased in the presence of low–molecular-weight substances such as ethanol, other alcohols, and glycols, any of

TABLE I–22. CAUSES OF ELEVATED OSMOL GAP[a]

Acetone	Mannitol
Dimethyl sulfoxide (DMSO)	Metaldehyde
Ethanol	Methanol
Ethyl ether	Osmotic contrast dyes
Ethylene glycol and other low–molecular-weight glycols	Propylene glycol
Glycerol	Renal failure without dialysis
Isopropyl alcohol	Severe alcoholic ketoacidosis, diabetic ketoacidosis, or lactic acidosis
Magnesium	

[a]Osmol gap = measured – calculated osmolality. Normal = 0 ± 5–10 (see text). Calculated osmolality = 2[Na] + [glucose]/18 + [BUN]/2.8. Na (serum sodium) in mEq/L; glucose and BUN (blood urea nitrogen) in mg/dL. ***Note:*** The osmolality may be measured as falsely normal if a vaporization point osmometer is used instead of the freezing point device because volatile alcohols will be boiled off.

which can contribute to the measured but not the calculated osmolality. Table I–23 describes how to estimate alcohol and glycol levels by using the osmol gap.

b. An osmol gap accompanied by, or immediately preceding, a worsening anion gap acidosis should immediately suggest poisoning by methanol (p 314) or ethylene glycol (p 234).

2. Differential diagnosis

a. Combined osmol and anion gap elevation may also be seen with severe alcoholic ketoacidosis or diabetic ketoacidosis, owing to the accumulation of unmeasured anions (beta-hydroxybutyrate) and osmotically active substances (acetone, glycerol, and amino acids).

b. Patients with chronic renal failure who are not undergoing hemodialysis may have an elevated osmol gap owing to the accumulation of low–molecular-weight solutes.

c. False elevation of the osmol gap may be caused by the use of an inappropriate sample tube (lavender top, ethylenediaminetetraacetic acid [EDTA]; gray top, fluoride-oxalate; blue top, citrate; see Table I–33).

d. A falsely elevated osmol gap may also occur in patients with severe hyperlipidemia or hyperglobulinemia with resulting pseudohyponatremia.

3. Pitfalls and limitations of the osmol gap

a. Measurements of the osmolality, sodium, BUN, and glucose must be done on the same serum specimen; otherwise, the gap may be falsely low or high.

TABLE I–23. ESTIMATION OF ALCOHOL AND GLYCOL LEVELS FROM THE OSMOL GAP[a]

Alcohol or Glycol	Molecular Weight (mg/mmol)	Conversion Factor[b]
Acetone	58	5.8
Ethanol	46	4.6[c]
Ethylene glycol	62	6.2
Glycerol	92	9.2
Isopropyl alcohol	60	6
Mannitol	182	18.2
Methanol	32	3.2
Propylene glycol	76	7.6

[a]Adapted, with permission, from Ho MT, Saunders CE, eds. *Current Emergency Diagnosis & Treatment.* 3rd ed. Appleton & Lange; 1990.
[b]To obtain estimated serum level (in mg/dL), multiply osmol gap by conversion factor.
[c]One clinical study (Purssell RA, et al, *Ann Emerg Med.* 2001;38:653) found that a conversion factor of 3.7 was more accurate for estimating the contribution of ethanol to the osmol gap.

b. Serum osmolality should be measured using a freezing point–depression osmometer. A falsely normal osmol gap despite the presence of volatile alcohols may result from using a heat-of-vaporization method to measure osmolality because the alcohols will boil off before the serum boiling point is reached.

4. **Treatment** depends on the cause. If ethylene glycol (p 234) or methanol (p 314) poisoning is suspected, antidotal therapy (eg, fomepizole [p 558] or ethanol [p 553]) and hemodialysis may be indicated.

C. **Anion gap metabolic acidosis.** The normal anion gap of 8–12 mEq/L accounts for unmeasured anions (eg, phosphate, sulfate, and anionic proteins) in the plasma. Metabolic acidosis is usually associated with an elevated anion gap.

1. **Causes of elevated anion gap** (Table I–24)

a. An elevated anion gap acidosis is commonly caused by an accumulation of lactic acid but may also be caused by other unmeasured acid anions, such as formate (eg, methanol poisoning), glycolate or oxalate (eg, ethylene glycol poisoning), beta-hydroxybutyrate (in patients with ketoacidosis), and 5-oxoproline.

b. In any patient with an elevated anion gap, also check the osmol gap; a combination of elevated anion and osmol gaps suggests poisoning by methanol or ethylene glycol. ***Note:*** Combined osmol and anion gap elevation may also be seen with severe alcoholic ketoacidosis and diabetic ketoacidosis.

c. A **narrow anion gap** may occur with an overdose by bromide or nitrate, both of which can increase the serum chloride level measured by some laboratory instruments. Also, high concentrations of lithium, calcium, or magnesium can narrow the anion gap owing to relative lowering of the serum sodium concentration or the presence of their salts (chloride, carbonate). Finally, severe hypoalbuminemia may reduce the anion gap.

2. **Differential diagnosis.** Rule out the following:

a. Common causes of lactic acidosis such as hypoxia and ischemia.

b. False depression of the serum bicarbonate and P_{CO_2} measurements, which can occur from incomplete filling of the red-topped Vacutainer blood collection tube.

c. False depression of the P_{CO_2} and calculated bicarbonate measurements, which can result from excess heparin when arterial blood gases are

TABLE I–24. SELECTED DRUGS AND TOXINS CAUSING ELEVATED ANION GAP ACIDOSIS[a]

Lactic acidosis	Other than lactic acidosis
Acetaminophen (levels >600 mg/L)	Alcoholic ketoacidosis (beta-hydroxybutyrate)
Antiretroviral drugs	Benzyl alcohol
Beta-adrenergic receptor agonists	Diabetic ketoacidosis
Caffeine and Theophylline	Ethylene glycol (glycolic and other acids)
Carbon monoxide	Exogenous organic and mineral acids
Cyanide	Formaldehyde (formic acid)
Hydrogen sulfide	Ibuprofen (propionic acid)
Iron	Metaldehyde
Isoniazid (INH)	Methanol (formic acid)
Metformin and phenformin	5-Oxoprolinuria and other organic acidurias
Propofol (high dose, children)	Salicylates (salicylic acid)
Propylene glycol	Starvation ketosis
Seizures, shock, or hypoxia	Valproic acid
Sodium azide	

[a]Anion gap = [Na] − [Cl] − [HCO_3] = 8–12 mEq/L. Adapted in part, with permission, from Olson KR, et al. *Med Toxicol.* 1987;2:73.

obtained (0.25 mL of heparin in 2 mL of blood falsely lowers the P_{CO_2} by about 8 mm Hg and bicarbonate by about 5 mEq/L).

d. False elevation of the serum lactate owing to anaerobic glycolysis in the blood sample tube before separation and testing.

e. The presence of a second, nongap acidosis (eg, respiratory acidosis due to hypoventilation) can exacerbate the clinical effects of the metabolic acidosis. In a pure metabolic acidosis, the expected P_{CO_2} in a blood gas sample should be 1.5 times the serum bicarbonate level (±6–10); a value outside this range suggests a second acid–base abnormality.

3. Treatment

a. Treat the underlying cause of the acidosis.

(1) Treat seizures (p 23) with anticonvulsants or neuromuscular paralysis.

(2) Treat hypoxia (p 6) and hypotension (p 15) if they occur.

(3) Treat methanol (p 314) or ethylene glycol (p 234) poisoning with fomepizole (or ethanol) and hemodialysis.

(4) Treat salicylate intoxication (p 410) with alkaline diuresis and hemodialysis.

b. Treatment of the acidemia itself is not generally necessary unless the pH is less than 7–7.1. In fact, mild acidosis may be beneficial by promoting oxygen release to tissues. However, acidemia may be harmful in poisoning by tricyclic antidepressants or salicylates.

(1) In a tricyclic antidepressant overdose (p 107), acidemia enhances cardiotoxicity. Maintain the serum pH at 7.45–7.5 with boluses of sodium bicarbonate. ***Note:*** although some sources recommend continuous bicarbonate infusions for TCA overdose, we prefer to give intermittent 1–2 mEq/kg boluses only as needed for QRS prolongation, which may help avoid excessive alkalemia.

(2) In salicylate intoxication (p 410), acidemia enhances salicylate entry into the brain and must be prevented. Alkalinization with a continuous infusion of sodium bicarbonate prevents academia and promotes salicylate elimination in the urine. A bolus prior to rapid sequence intubation may help blunt the effect of transient respiratory acidosis due to neuromuscular paralysis.

D. Hyperglycemia and hypoglycemia. A variety of drugs and disease states can cause alterations in the serum glucose level (Table I–25). A patient's blood glucose level can be altered by the nutritional state, endogenous insulin levels, and endocrine and liver function and by the presence of various drugs or

TABLE I–25. SELECTED CAUSES OF ALTERATIONS IN SERUM GLUCOSE

Hyperglycemia	Hypoglycemia
$Beta_2$-adrenergic receptor agonists	Ackee or lychee fruit (unripe)
Caffeine intoxication	Endocrine disorders (hypopituitarism, Addison disease, myxedema)
Corticosteroids	Ethanol intoxication (especially pediatric)
Dextrose administration	Fasting
Diabetes mellitus	Hepatic failure
Diazoxide	Insulin
Excessive circulating epinephrine	Oral sulfonylurea hypoglycemic agents
Glucagon	Pentamidine
Iron poisoning	Propranolol intoxication
Theophylline intoxication	Renal failure
Thiazide diuretics	Salicylate intoxication
Vacor	Streptozocin
	Valproic acid intoxication

toxins. If insulin administration is suspected as the cause of the hypoglycemia, obtain serum levels of insulin and C-peptide; a low C-peptide level in the presence of a high insulin level suggests an exogenous source.

1. **Hyperglycemia,** especially if severe (>500 mg/dL [28 mmol/L]) or sustained, may result in dehydration and electrolyte imbalance caused by the osmotic effect of excess glucose in the urine; in addition, the shifting of water from the brain into plasma may result in hyperosmolar coma. More commonly, hyperglycemia in poisoning or drug overdose cases is mild and transient. Significant or sustained hyperglycemia should be treated if it is not resolving spontaneously or if the patient is symptomatic.
   - **a.** If the patient has altered mental status, maintain an open airway, assist ventilation if necessary, and administer supplemental oxygen (pp 1–7).
   - **b.** Replace fluid deficits with IV normal saline or another isotonic crystalloid solution. Monitor serum potassium levels, which may fall sharply as the blood glucose is corrected, and give supplemental potassium as needed.
   - **c.** Correct acid–base and electrolyte disturbances.
   - **d.** Administer regular insulin, 5–10 U IV initially, followed by infusion of 5–10 U/h, while monitoring the effects on the serum glucose level (children: administer 0.1 U/kg initially and 0.1 U/kg/h [p 564]).
2. **Hypoglycemia,** if severe (serum glucose <40 mg/dL [2.2 mmol/L]) and sustained, can rapidly cause permanent brain injury. For this reason, whenever hypoglycemia is suspected as a cause of seizures, coma, or altered mental status, immediate empiric treatment with dextrose is indicated.
   - **a.** If the patient has altered mental status, maintain an open airway, assist ventilation if necessary, and administer supplemental oxygen (pp 1–7).
   - **b.** Perform rapid bedside blood glucose testing: hypoglycemia is considered a "supplemental vital sign" for patients with altered mental status.
   - **c.** If the blood glucose is low (<60–70 mg/dL [3.3–3.9 mmol/L]) or if bedside testing is not available, administer concentrated 50% dextrose, 50 mL IV (25 g). In children, give 25% dextrose, 2 mL/kg (p 562). In small infants, some clinicians use 10% dextrose.
   - **d.** In malnourished or alcoholic patients, also give thiamine, 100 mg IM or IV, to treat or prevent acute Wernicke syndrome. Thiamine (p 628) can also be given orally if the patient is awake.
   - **e.** For hypoglycemia caused by oral sulfonylurea drug overdose (p 217), consider antidotal therapy with octreotide (p 596) to prevent recurrence of hypoglycemic episodes.

E. Hypernatremia and hyponatremia. Sodium disorders occur infrequently in poisoned patients (see Table I–26). More commonly they are associated with

TABLE I–26. SELECTED DRUGS AND TOXINS ASSOCIATED WITH ALTERED SERUM SODIUM

Hypernatremia	Hyponatremia
Cathartic abuse	Beer potomania
Lactulose therapy	Cerebral salt wasting syndrome (eg, after trauma)
Lithium therapy (nephrogenic diabetes insipidus)	Diuretics
Mannitol	Iatrogenic (IV fluid therapy)
Severe gastroenteritis (many poisons)	Syndrome of inappropriate ADH (SIADH):
Sodium or salt overdose	Amitriptyline
Valproic acid (divalproex sodium)	Carbamazepine and oxcarbazepine
	Chlorpropamide
	Clofibrate
	MDMA (ecstasy)
	Oxytocin
	Phenothiazines

underlying disease states. Antidiuretic hormone (ADH) is responsible for concentrating the urine and preventing excess water loss.

1. **Hypernatremia** (serum sodium >145 mEq/L) may be caused by excessive sodium intake, excessive free water loss, or impaired renal concentrating ability.
   a. **Dehydration with normal kidney function.** Excessive sweating, hyperventilation, diarrhea, or osmotic diuresis (eg, hyperglycemia or mannitol administration) may cause disproportional water loss. The urine osmolality is usually greater than 400 mOsm/kg, and the antidiuretic hormone (ADH) function is normal.
   b. **Impaired renal concentrating ability.** Excess free water is lost in the urine, and urine osmolality is usually less than 250 mOsm/L. This may be caused by hypothalamic dysfunction with reduced ADH production (diabetes insipidus [DI]) or impaired kidney response to ADH (nephrogenic DI). Nephrogenic DI has been associated with long-term lithium therapy as well as acute overdose.
2. **Treatment of hypernatremia.** Treatment depends on the cause, but in most cases, the patient is hypovolemic and needs fluids. ***Caution:*** Do ***not*** reduce the serum sodium level too quickly because osmotic imbalance may cause excessive fluid shift into brain cells, resulting in cerebral edema. The correction should take place over 24–36 hours; the serum sodium should be lowered about 1 mEq/L/h. Note: if the disturbance occurred rapidly (eg, acute salt ingestion), then speedier correction is appropriate.
   a. **Hypovolemia.** Administer NS (0.9% sodium chloride) to restore volume, then switch to half NS in dextrose (D_5W 0.45% sodium chloride).
   b. **Volume overload.** Treat with a combination of sodium-free or low-sodium fluid (eg, 5% dextrose or D_5W 0.25% sodium chloride) and a loop diuretic such as furosemide, 0.5–1 mg/kg IV.
   c. **Lithium-induced nephrogenic DI.** Administer fluids (see Item 2.a above). Discontinue lithium therapy. Partial improvement may be seen with oral administration of indomethacin, 50 mg 3 times a day, and hydrochlorothiazide, 50–100 mg/d. (***Note:*** However, thiazides may also impair renal lithium clearance.)
3. **Hyponatremia** (serum sodium <130 mEq/L) is a common electrolyte abnormality and may result from a variety of mechanisms. Severe hyponatremia (serum sodium <110–120 mEq/L) can result in seizures and altered mental status.
   a. **Pseudohyponatremia** may result from a shift of water from the extracellular space (eg, hyperglycemia). Plasma sodium falls by about 1.6 mEq/L for each 100-mg/dL (5.6-mmol/L) rise in glucose. Reduced relative blood water volume (eg, hyperlipidemia or hyperproteinemia) may also produce pseudohyponatremia if older (flame emission) detector devices are used, but this is unlikely with current direct measurement electrodes.
   b. **Hyponatremia with hypovolemia** may be caused by excessive volume loss (sodium and water) that is partially replaced by free water. To maintain intravascular volume, the body secretes ADH, which causes water retention. A urine sodium level of less than 10 mEq/L suggests that the kidney is appropriately attempting to compensate for volume losses. An elevated urine sodium level (>20 mEq/L) implies renal salt wasting, which can be caused by diuretics, adrenal insufficiency, or nephropathy. A syndrome of salt wasting has been reported in some patients with head trauma ("cerebral salt wasting syndrome").
   c. **Hyponatremia with volume overload** occurs in conditions such as congestive heart failure and cirrhosis. Although the total body sodium is increased, baroreceptors sense an inadequate circulating volume and stimulate the release of ADH. The urine sodium level is normally less than 10 mEq/L unless the patient has been on diuretics.

d. **Hyponatremia with normal volume** occurs in a variety of situations. Measurement of serum and urine osmolalities may help determine the diagnosis.

(1) **Syndrome of inappropriate ADH secretion (SIADH).** ADH is secreted independently of volume or osmolality. Causes include malignancies, pulmonary disease, severe head injury, and some drugs (see Table I–26). The serum osmolality is low, but the urine osmolality is inappropriately increased (>300 mOsm/L). The serum BUN is usually low (<10 mg/dL [3.6 mmol/L]).

(2) **Psychogenic polydipsia,** or compulsive water drinking (generally >10 L/d), causes reduced serum sodium because of the excessive free water intake and because the kidney excretes sodium to maintain euvolemia. The urine sodium level may be elevated, but urine osmolality is appropriately low because the kidney is attempting to excrete the excess water and ADH secretion is suppressed.

(3) **Beer potomania** may result from chronic daily excessive beer drinking (>4 L/d) without intake of adequate solutes and electrolytes, a process which degrades the normal electrolyte gradient needed for free water excretion from the kidney. It usually occurs in patients with cirrhosis who already have elevated ADH levels.

(4) Other causes of euvolemic hyponatremia include hypothyroidism, postoperative state, and idiosyncratic reactions to diuretics (generally thiazides).

4. **Treatment of hyponatremia.** Treatment depends on the cause, the patient's volume status, and, most importantly, the patient's clinical condition. ***Caution:*** Avoid overly rapid correction of the sodium because brain damage (central pontine myelinolysis) may occur if the sodium is increased by more than 25 mEq/L in the first 24 hours, unless the disorder occurred rapidly (eg, acute water ingestion), in which case speedier correction is appropriate. Obtain frequent measurements of the serum and urine sodium levels and adjust the rate of infusion as needed to increase the serum sodium by no more than 1–1.5 mEq/h. Arrange consultation with a nephrologist as soon as possible. **For patients with profound hyponatremia** (serum sodium <110 mEq/L) accompanied by coma or seizures, administer hypertonic (3% sodium chloride) saline, 100–200 mL.

a. **Hyponatremia with hypovolemia.** Replace lost volume with NS (0.9% sodium chloride). If adrenal insufficiency is suspected, give hydrocortisone, 100 mg every 6–8 hours. Hypertonic saline (3% sodium chloride) is rarely indicated.

b. **Hyponatremia with volume overload.** Restrict water (0.5–1 L/d) and treat the underlying condition (eg, congestive heart failure). If diuretics are given, do ***not*** allow excessive free water intake. Hypertonic saline is dangerous in these patients; if it is used, also administer furosemide, 0.5–1 mg/kg IV. Consider hemodialysis to reduce volume and restore the sodium level.

c. **Hyponatremia with normal volume.** Asymptomatic patients may be treated conservatively with water restriction (0.5–1 L/d). Psychogenic compulsive water drinkers may have to be restrained or separated from all sources of water, including washbasins and toilets. Demeclocycline (a tetracycline antibiotic that can produce nephrogenic DI), 300–600 mg twice a day, can be used to treat mild chronic SIADH; the onset of action may require a week. For patients with coma or seizures, give hypertonic (3%) saline, 100–200 mL, along with furosemide, 0.5–1 mg/kg.

F. **Hyperkalemia and hypokalemia.** A variety of drugs and toxins can cause serious alterations in the serum potassium level (Table I–27). Potassium levels are dependent on potassium intake and release (eg, from muscles), diuretic use, proper functioning of the ATPase pump, serum pH, and beta-adrenergic

TABLE I–27. SELECTED DRUGS AND TOXINS AND OTHER CAUSES OF ALTERED SERUM POTASSIUM[a]

Hyperkalemia	Hypokalemia
Acidosis	Alkalosis
Adrenal insufficiency (chronic steroid use)	Barium
Angiotensin-converting enzyme (ACE) inhibitors	Beta-adrenergic drugs
Beta receptor antagonists	Caffeine
Digitalis glycosides	Cesium
Fluoride	Chloroquine
Lithium	Diuretics (chronic)
Potassium	Epinephrine
Renal failure	Hypomagnesemia
Rhabdomyolysis	Salicylate poisoning (with dehydration)
	Theophylline
	Toluene (chronic)

[a]Adapted in part, with permission, from Olson KR, et al. *Med Toxicol.* 1987;2:73.

activity. Changes in serum potassium levels do not always reflect overall body gain or loss but may be caused by intracellular shifts (eg, acidosis drives potassium out of cells, while beta-adrenergic stimulation drives it into cells).

1. **Hyperkalemia** (serum potassium >5 mEq/L) produces muscle weakness and interferes with normal cardiac conduction. Peaked T waves and prolonged PR intervals are the earliest signs of cardiotoxicity. Critical hyperkalemia produces widened QRS intervals, AV block, ventricular fibrillation, and cardiac arrest (see Figure I–5).
   a. Hyperkalemia caused by **fluoride intoxication** (p 240) is usually accompanied by hypocalcemia.
   b. **Digoxin or other cardiac glycoside intoxication** associated with hyperkalemia is an indication for administration of digoxin-specific Fab antibodies (p 542).
2. **Treatment of hyperkalemia.** A potassium level higher than 6 mEq/L is a medical emergency; a level higher than 7 mEq/L is critical.
   a. Monitor the ECG. QRS prolongation indicates critical cardiac poisoning.
   b. Administer 10% calcium chloride, 5–10 mL, or 10% calcium gluconate, 10–20 mL (p 526), if there are signs of critical cardiac toxicity such as wide QRS complexes, absent P waves, and bradycardia.
   c. Glucose plus insulin promotes intracellular movement of potassium. Give 50% dextrose, 50 mL (25% dextrose, 2 mL/kg in children), plus regular insulin, 0.1 U/kg IV.
   d. Inhaled beta$_2$-adrenergic agonists such as albuterol also enhance potassium entry into cells and can provide a rapid supplemental method of lowering serum potassium levels.
   e. Hemodialysis rapidly lowers serum potassium levels.
   f. Hyperkalemia due to cardiac glycoside toxicity (see p 222) usually rapidly improves with administration of digoxin-specific antibodies (see p 542).
   g. Sodium bicarbonate, 1–2 mEq/kg IV (p 520), may drive potassium into cells and lower the serum level, but this effect takes up to 60 minutes and clinical studies show equivocal results.
   h. Sodium polystyrene sulfonate (SPS; Kayexalate), 0.3–0.6 g/kg orally in 2 mL of 70% sorbitol per kilogram, is commonly recommended as a potassium-binding resin that can enhance enteric elimination over several hours. However, recent evidence suggests that it is not very effective, and colonic necrosis has been reported in patients with ileus, constipation, gastric ulceration, or other high-risk conditions. Use with caution, if at all.

3. **Hypokalemia** (serum potassium <3.5 mEq/L) may cause muscle weakness, hyporeflexia, and ileus. Rhabdomyolysis may occur. The ECG shows flattened T waves and prominent U waves. In severe hypokalemia, AV block, ventricular dysrhythmias, and cardiac arrest may occur.
   a. With **theophylline, caffeine, or beta$_2$ agonist** intoxication, an intracellular shift of potassium may produce a very low serum potassium level with normal total body stores. Patients usually do not have serious symptoms or ECG signs of hypokalemia, and aggressive potassium therapy is not required.
   b. With **barium** poisoning (p 152), profound hypokalemia may lead to respiratory muscle weakness and cardiac and respiratory arrest; therefore, intensive potassium therapy is necessary. Up to 420 mEq has been given in 24 hours.
   c. Hypokalemia resulting from **diuretic therapy** may contribute to ventricular dysrhythmias, especially those associated with chronic digitalis glycoside poisoning.
4. **Treatment of hypokalemia.** Mild hypokalemia (potassium, 3–3.5 mEq/L) is usually not associated with serious symptoms.
   a. Administer potassium chloride orally or IV. See p 611 for recommended doses and infusion rates.
   b. Monitor serum potassium and the ECG for signs of hyperkalemia from excessive potassium therapy.
   c. If hypokalemia is caused by diuretic therapy, malnutrition, or gastrointestinal fluid losses, measure and replace other ions, including sodium, chloride, and especially magnesium (which protects against renal potassium wasting).

G. **Renal failure.** Examples of drugs and toxins that cause renal failure are listed in Table I–28. Acute kidney injury may be caused by a direct nephrotoxic action of the poison or acute massive tubular precipitation of myoglobin (rhabdomyolysis), hemoglobin (hemolysis), or calcium oxalate crystals (ethylene glycol). Acute kidney injury may also be secondary to shock caused by blood or fluid loss or cardiovascular collapse.
1. **Assessment.** Renal failure is characterized by a progressive rise in the serum creatinine and blood urea nitrogen (BUN) levels, usually accompanied by oliguria or anuria.
   a. The serum creatinine concentration usually rises about 1–1.5 mg/dL per day (88–132 micromol/L/d) after total anuric renal failure.

TABLE I–28. EXAMPLES OF DRUGS AND TOXINS AND OTHER CAUSES OF ACUTE RENAL FAILURE

Direct nephrotoxic effect
- Acetaminophen
- Acyclovir (chronic, high-dose treatment)
- *Amanita phalloides* mushrooms
- *Amanita smithiana* mushrooms
- Analgesics (eg, ibuprofen, phenacetin)
- Antibiotics (eg, aminoglycosides)
- Bromates
- Chlorates
- Chlorinated hydrocarbons
- *Cortinarius* species mushrooms
- Cyclosporine
- Ethylenediaminetetraacetic acid (EDTA)
- Ethylene glycol (glycolate, oxalate)
- Foscarnet
- Heavy metals (eg, mercury) salts
- Indinavir

Hemolysis
- Arsine
- Naphthalene
- Oxidizing agents (especially in patients with glucose-6-phosphate dehydrogenase [G6PD] deficiency)

Rhabdomyolysis (see also TABLE I-16)
- Amphetamines and cocaine
- Coma with prolonged immobility
- Hyperthermia
- Phencyclidine (PCP)
- Status epilepticus
- Strychnine

b. A more abrupt rise should suggest rapid muscle breakdown (rhabdomyolysis), which increases the creatine load and also results in elevated serum CK levels that may interfere with a determination of the serum creatinine level.

c. Oliguria may be seen before renal failure occurs, especially with hypovolemia, hypotension, or heart failure. In this case, the BUN level is usually elevated out of proportion to the serum creatinine level.

d. **False elevation of the creatinine** level can be caused by nitromethane, isopropyl alcohol, and ketoacidosis owing to interference with the usual colorimetric laboratory (Jaffe) method. The BUN remains normal, which may help to distinguish false from real elevation of the creatinine.

2. **Complications.** The earliest complication of acute renal failure is hyperkalemia (p 39); this may be more pronounced if the cause of the renal failure is rhabdomyolysis or hemolysis, both of which release large amounts of intracellular potassium into the circulation. Later complications include metabolic acidosis, delirium, and coma.

3. **Treatment**

a. Prevent renal failure, if possible, by administering specific treatment (eg, acetylcysteine for acetaminophen overdose [although of uncertain benefit for this complication], British anti-Lewisite [BAL; dimercaprol] chelation for mercury poisoning, and IV fluids for rhabdomyolysis or shock).

b. Monitor the serum potassium level frequently and treat hyperkalemia (p 39) if it occurs.

c. Do ***not*** give supplemental potassium, and avoid cathartics or other medications containing magnesium, phosphate, or sodium, which can build up in uremic patients.

d. Initiate hemodialysis as needed.

H. **Hepatic failure.** A variety of drugs and toxins may cause hepatic injury (Table I–29). Mechanisms of toxicity include direct hepatocellular damage (eg, *Amanita phalloides* and related mushrooms [p 333]), metabolic creation of a hepatotoxic intermediate (eg, acetaminophen [p 73] or carbon tetrachloride [p 184]), and hepatic veno-occlusive disease (eg, pyrrolizidine alkaloids; see "Plants," p 375).

1. **Assessment.** Laboratory and clinical evidence of hepatitis often does not become apparent until 24–36 hours after exposure to the poison. Then aminotransferase (AST, ALT) levels rise sharply and may fall to normal over the next 3–5 days. If hepatic damage is severe, measurements of hepatic function (eg, bilirubin and prothrombin time) will continue to worsen after 2–3 days, even as aminotransferase levels are returning to normal. Metabolic acidosis and hypoglycemia usually indicate a poor prognosis.

TABLE I–29. EXAMPLES OF DRUGS AND TOXINS CAUSING HEPATIC DAMAGE

Acetaminophen	Kava
Amanita phalloides and similar mushrooms	Niacin (sustained-release formulation)
Arsenic	2-Nitropropane
Carbon tetrachloride and other chlorinated hydrocarbons	Pennyroyal oil
Copper	Phenol
Dimethylformamide	Phosphorus
Ethanol	Polychlorinated biphenyls (PCBs)
Green tea extracts	Pyrrolizidine alkaloids (see "Plants" [p 375])
Gyromitra mushrooms	Thallium
Halothane	Troglitazone (removed from US market)
Iron	Valproic acid

2. **Complications**
   a. Abnormal hepatic function may result in excessive bleeding owing to insufficient production of vitamin K–dependent coagulation factors.
   b. Fulminant hepatic failure often leads to acute kidney injury, respiratory failure, coma and death, usually within 5–7 days.
3. **Treatment**
   a. Prevent hepatic injury if possible by administering specific treatment (eg, acetylcysteine for acetaminophen overdose).
   b. Obtain baseline and daily electrolytes, aminotransferase, bilirubin, glucose levels, and prothrombin time. In addition to direct tests of hepatic function, acidosis and renal dysfunction indicate a poor prognosis.
   c. Provide intensive supportive care for hepatic failure and encephalopathy (eg, glucose for hypoglycemia, fresh-frozen plasma or clotting factor concentrates for coagulopathy, or lactulose for encephalopathy).
   d. Extracorporeal liver assist devices have been used to augment hepatic function ("hepatic dialysis") in experimental studies and small clinical trials. However, these are not widely available, and routine use is not currently recommended.
   e. Liver transplant may be the only effective treatment once massive hepatic necrosis has resulted in severe encephalopathy and metabolic derangements.

IV. Toxicology screening.[1] To maximize the utility of the toxicology laboratory, it is necessary to understand what the laboratory can and cannot do and how knowledge of the results will affect the patient. Comprehensive blood and urine screening is of little practical value in the initial care of the poisoned patient, mainly because of the delay in obtaining results. However, specific toxicologic analyses and quantitative levels of certain drugs may be extremely helpful. Before ordering any tests, always ask these two questions: (1) How will the result of the test alter the approach to treatment? and (2) Can the result of the test be returned in time to affect therapy positively?

A. Limitations of toxicology screens. Owing to long turnaround time (1–5 days), lack of availability, reliability factors, and the low risk for serious morbidity with supportive clinical management, toxicology screening is estimated to affect management in fewer than 15% of all cases of poisoning or drug overdose.

1. Although immunoassays for urine drug testing are widely available and inexpensive, and have fast turnaround times, some assays suffer from poor sensitivity for some members of a drug class (eg, benzodiazepines), whereas other assays produce false-positive results to structural analogs and drugs that are themselves not part of a targeted drug class (eg, amphetamine screens). In many other cases, there are no immunoassays available at all (eg, most of the newer antipsychotic drugs).
2. Comprehensive toxicology screens or panels may look specifically for 200–300 drugs among more than 10,000 possible drugs or toxins (or 6 million chemicals). However, the drugs listed in Tables I–30 and I–31 account for more than 80% of overdoses.
3. Comprehensive screening performed by mass spectrometry (GC-MS or LC-MS/MS) have high specificity and sensitivity but results are usually not available in real time. Some drugs that are present in therapeutic amounts may be detected on the screen even though they are causing no clinical symptoms (clinical false positives).
4. Because many agents are neither sought nor detected during a toxicology screening (Table I–32), a negative result does not always rule out poisoning;

[1]By Alan Wu, PhD.

TABLE I–30. DRUGS COMMONLY INCLUDED IN A COMPREHENSIVE URINE SCREEN[a]

Alcohols	**Sedative-hypnotic drugs**
Acetone	Barbiturates[c]
Ethanol	Benzodiazepines[c]
Isopropyl alcohol	Carisoprodol
Methanol	Chloral hydrate
Analgesics	Ethchlorvynol
Acetaminophen	Glutethimide
Salicylates	Meprobamate
Anticonvulsants	**Stimulants**
Carbamazepine	Amphetamines[c]
Phenobarbital	Caffeine
Phenytoin	Cocaine and benzoylecgonine
Primidone	Phencyclidine (PCP)
Antihistamines	Strychnine
Benztropine	**Tricyclic antidepressants**
Chlorpheniramine	Amitriptyline
Diphenhydramine	Desipramine
Pyrilamine	Doxepin
Trihexyphenidyl	Imipramine
Opioids	Nortriptyline
Codeine	Protriptyline
Dextromethorphan	**Cardiac drugs**
Fentanyl	Diltiazem
Hydrocodone	Lidocaine
Meperidine	Procainamide
Methadone	Propranolol
Morphine and 6-acetylmorphine	Quinidine and quinine
Oxycodone[b]	Verapamil
Pentazocine	**Oral hypoglycemic drugs**
Propoxyphene	Glipizide
Phenothiazines	Glyburide
Chlorpromazine	**Newer antipsychotic drugs**
Prochlorperazine	Bupropion
Promethazine	Quetiapine
Thioridazine	
Trifluoperazine	

[a]Newer drugs in any category may not be included in screening.
[b]Depends on the order of testing.
[c]Not all drugs in this class are detected.

the negative predictive value of the screen is only about 70%. In contrast, a positive result has a predictive value of about 90%.

5. The specificity of toxicologic tests is dependent on the method and the laboratory. The presence of other drugs, drug metabolites, disease states, or incorrect sampling may cause erroneous results (Table I–33).

B. Adulteration of urine may be attempted by persons undergoing enforced drug testing to evade drug detection. Methods used include ingestion of water or diuretics to dilute the urine, and addition of substances to the urine (eg, acids, baking soda, bleach, metal salts, nitrite salts, glutaraldehyde, or pyridinium chlorochromate) to inactivate, either chemically or biologically, the initial screening immunoassay to produce a negative test. Adulteration is variably successful depending on the agent used and the type of immunoassay. Laboratories that routinely perform urine testing for drug surveillance programs

TABLE I–31. DRUGS COMMONLY INCLUDED IN A HOSPITAL URINE "DRUGS OF ABUSE" PANEL[a]

Drug	Detection Time Window for Recreational Doses	Comments
Amphetamines	2 days	Often misses MDA or MDMA. Many false positives (see Table I-33)
Barbiturates	Less than 2 days for most drugs, up to 1 week for phenobarbital	
Benzodiazepines	2–7 days (varies with specific drug and duration of use)	May not detect triazolam, lorazepam, alprazolam, other newer drugs
Cocaine	2 days	Detects metabolite benzoylecgonine
Ethanol	Less than 1 day	
Marijuana (tetrahydro-cannabinol [THC])	2–5 days after single use (longer for chronic use)	
Opioids	2–3 days	Synthetic opioids (meperidine, methadone, propoxyphene, oxycodone) are often not detected. Separate testing for methadone and oxycodone is sometimes offered
Phencyclidine (PCP)	Up to 7 days	See Table I-33

[a]Laboratories often perform only some of these tests, depending on what their emergency department requests and local patterns of drug use in the community. Also, positive results are usually not confirmed with a second, more specific test; thus, false positives may be reported.

often have methods to test for some of the adulterants as well as assay indicators that suggest possible adulterations.

C. Uses for toxicology screens

1. Comprehensive screening of urine and blood should be carried out whenever the diagnosis of brain death is being considered to rule out the presence of common depressant drugs that might result in a temporary loss

TABLE I–32. DRUGS AND TOXINS NOT COMMONLY INCLUDED IN EMERGENCY TOXICOLOGIC SCREENING PANELS[a]

Anesthetic gases	Ethylene glycol
Antiarrhythmic agents	Fluoride
Antibiotics	Formate (formic acid, from methanol poisoning)
Antidepressants (newer)	Hypoglycemic agents
Antihypertensives	Isoniazid (INH)
Antipsychotic agents (newer)	Lithium (available as a quantitative TDM assay)
Benzodiazepines (newer)	LSD (lysergic acid diethylamide)
Beta receptor antagonists (other than propranolol)	MAO inhibitors
Borate	Noxious gases
Bromide	Plant, fungal, and microbiologic toxins
Calcium antagonists (newer)	Pressors (eg, dopamine)
Colchicine	Solvents and hydrocarbons
Cyanide	Theophylline
Digitalis glycosides	Valproic acid (available as a quantitative TDM assay)
Diuretics	Vasodilators
Ergot alkaloids	

[a]Many of these are available as separate specific tests.

TABLE I–33. INTERFERENCES IN TOXICOLOGIC BLOOD OR URINE TESTS

Drug or Toxin	Method[a]	Causes of Falsely Increased Level
Acetaminophen	SC[b]	Salicylate, salicylamide, methyl salicylate (each will increase acetaminophen level by 10% of their level in mg/L); bilirubin; phenols; renal failure (each 1-mg/dL increase in creatinine can increase acetaminophen level by 30 mg/L).
	GC, IA	Phenacetin (banned by the FDA in 1983).
Amitriptyline	HPLC, GC	Cyclobenzaprine.
Amphetamines (urine)	GC[c]	Other volatile stimulant amines (misidentified). GC mass spectrometry poorly distinguishes *d*-methamphetamine from *l*-methamphetamine (found in Vicks inhaler).
	IA[c]	All assays are reactive to methamphetamine and amphetamine as well as drugs that are metabolized to amphetamines (benzphetamine, clobenzorex, famprofazone, fenproporex, selegiline). The polyclonal assay is sensitive to cross-reacting sympathomimetic amines (ephedrine, fenfluramine, isometheptene, MDA, MDMA, *phentermine,* phenmetrazine, phenylpropanolamine, pseudoephedrine, and other *amphetamine* analogs); cross-reacting nonstimulant drugs (aripiprazole, bupropion, chlorpromazine, labetalol, ranitidine, sertraline, trazodone, trimethobenzamide), and dimethylamylamine (DMAA). The monoclonal assay is reactive to *d*-amphetamine and *d*-methamphetamine; in addition, many have some reactivity toward MDA and MDMA. Variable cross-reactivities for designer amines found in "bath salts."
Benzodiazepines	IA	Efavirenz (depending on the immunoassay); oxaprozin. Note that some benzodiazepine assays give false-negative results for drugs that do not metabolize to oxazepam or nordiazepam (eg, lorazepam, alprazolam, others).
Chloride	SC, EC	Bromide (variable interference).
Creatinine	SC[b]	Ketoacidosis (acetoacetate may increase creatinine up to 2–3 mg/dL in non-rate methods); isopropyl alcohol (acetone); nitromethane (up to 100-fold increase in measured creatinine with use of Jaffe reaction); cephalosporins; creatine (eg, with rhabdomyolysis).
	EZ	Creatine, lidocaine metabolite, 5-fluorouracil, nitromethane "fuel"
Cyanide	SC	Thiosulfate
Digoxin	IA	Endogenous digoxin-like immunoreactive factor in newborns and in patients with hypervolemic states (cirrhosis, heart failure, uremia, pregnancy) and renal failure (up to 0.5 ng/mL); plant or animal glycosides bufotoxins; Chan Su; oleander); after digoxin antibody (Fab) administration (with tests that measure total serum digoxin); presence of heterophile or human antimouse antibodies (up to 45.6 ng/mL reported in one case).
	MEIA	Falsely lowered serum digoxin concentrations during therapy with spironolactone, canrenone.
Ethanol	SC[b]	Other alcohols, ketones (by oxidation methods).
	EZ	Isopropyl alcohol; patients with elevated lactate and LDH.

(*continued*)

TABLE I–33. INTERFERENCES IN TOXICOLOGIC BLOOD OR URINE TESTS (CONTINUED)

Drug or Toxin	Method[a]	Causes of Falsely Increased Level
Ethylene glycol	EZ	Other glycols, elevated triglycerides, 2,3-butanediol (observed in some patients with diabetic or starvation ketoacidosis). Note: the presence of glycerol or propylene glycol interferes with some ethylene glycol enzymatic assays.
	GC	Propylene glycol (may also decrease the ethylene glycol level).
Glucose	Any method	Glucose level may fall by up to 30 mg/dL/h when transport to laboratory is delayed. (This does not occur if specimen is collected in gray-top tube.)
Iron	SC	Deferoxamine causes 15% lowering of total iron-binding capacity (TIBC). Lavender-top Vacutainer tube contains EDTA, which lowers total iron.
Isopropanol	GC	Skin disinfectant containing isopropyl alcohol used before venipuncture (highly variable, usually trivial, but up to 40 mg/dL).
Ketones	SC	Acetylcysteine, valproic acid, captopril, levodopa. Note: Acetest method is primarily sensitive to acetoacetic acid, which may be low in patients with alcoholic ketoacidosis. An assay specific for beta-hydroxybutyric acid is a more reliable marker for early evaluation of acidosis and ketosis.
Lactate	EZ	Ethylene glycol (some point-of-care assays).
Lithium	SC, ISE	Green-top Vacutainer specimen tube (may contain lithium heparin) can cause marked elevation (up to 6–8 mEq/L).
	SC	Procainamide, quinidine can produce 5–15% elevation.
Methadone (urine)	IA	Diphenhydramine, disopyramide, doxylamine, verapamil.
Methemoglobin	SC	Sulfhemoglobin (cross-positive ~10% by co-oximeter); methylene blue (2-mg/kg dose gives transiently false-positive 15% methemoglobin level); hyperlipidemia (triglyceride level of 6,000 mg/dL may give false methemoglobin of 28.6%).
		Falsely decreased level with in vitro spontaneous reduction to hemoglobin in Vacutainer tube (~10%/h). Analyze within 1 hour.
Morphine/codeine (urine)	IA[c]	Cross-reacting opioids: hydrocodone, hydromorphone, monoacetylmorphine, tapentadol, tramadol; morphine from poppy seed ingestion. Also rifampicin and ofloxacin and other quinolones in different IAs. Note: Methadone, oxycodone, fentanyl and many other opioids are often not detected by routine opiate screen, may require separate specific immunoassays.
Osmolality	Osm	Lavender-top (EDTA) Vacutainer specimen tube (15 mOsm/L); gray-top (fluoride-oxalate) tube (150 mOsm/L); blue-top (citrate) tube 10 mOsm/L); green-top (lithium heparin) tube (theoretically, up to 6–8 mOsm/L).
		Falsely normal if vapor pressure method used (alcohols are volatilized).
Phencyclidine (urine)	IA[c]	Many false positives reported: chlorpromazine, dextromethorphan, diphenhydramine, doxylamine, ibuprofen, imipramine, ketamine, meperidine, methadone, thioridazine, tramadol, venlafaxine.

(continued)

TABLE I–33. INTERFERENCES IN TOXICOLOGIC BLOOD OR URINE TESTS (CONTINUED)

Drug or Toxin	Method[a]	Causes of Falsely Increased Level
Salicylate	SC	Phenothiazines (urine), diflunisal, ketosis,[c] salicylamide, accumulated salicylate metabolites in patients with renal failure (~10% increase).
	EZ	Acetaminophen (slight salicylate elevation).
	IA, SC	Diflunisal.
	SC	Decreased or altered salicylate level: bilirubin, phenylketones.
Tetrahydrocannabinol (THC, marijuana)	IA	Pantoprazole, efavirenz, riboflavin, promethazine, nonsteroidal anti-inflammatory drugs (depending on the immunoassay). Largely negative for synthetic cannabinoids.
Tricyclic antidepressants	IA	Carbamazepine, cyclobenzaprine, dextromethorphan, diphenhydramine, quetiapine.

[a]EC, electrochemical; EZ, enzymatic; GC, gas chromatography (interferences primarily with older methods); HPLC, high-pressure liquid chromatography; IA, immunoassay; ISE, ion selective electrode; MEIA, microparticle enzymatic immunoassay; SC, spectrochemical; TLC, thin-layer chromatography.
[b]Uncommon methodology, no longer performed in most clinical laboratories.
[c]More common with urine test. Confirmation by a second test is required. Note: Urine testing is sometimes affected by intentional adulteration to avoid drug detection (see text).
For more information on drugs of abuse testing errors, the reader is referred to: Saitman et al. False–positive interferences of common urine drug screen immunoassays: a review. *J Anal Toxicol* 2014;38:387–396.

of brain activity and mimic brain death. Toxicology screens may be used to confirm clinical impressions during hospitalization and can be inserted in the permanent medicolegal record. This may be important if homicide, assault, or child abuse is suspected.

2. **Selective screens** (eg, for "drugs of abuse") with rapid turnaround times are often used to confirm clinical impressions and may aid in disposition of the patient. Positive results may need to be verified by confirmatory testing with a second method, depending on the circumstances.

D. Approach to toxicology testing

1. Communicate clinical suspicions to the laboratory.
2. Obtain blood and urine specimens on admission in unusual cases and have the laboratory store them temporarily. If the patient recovers rapidly, they can be discarded.
3. Urine is usually the best sample for broad qualitative screening. Compared with urine, blood testing has a narrow window of detection, depending on the half-life of the drug. When the drug is present in the blood, quantitation may help evaluate impairment of the subject by the drug.
4. Decide if a specific quantitative blood level may assist in management decisions (eg, use of an antidote or dialysis; Table I–34). Quantitative levels are helpful only if there is a predictable correlation between the serum level and toxic effects.
5. A regional poison control center (1-800-222-1222) or toxicology consultant may provide assistance in considering certain drug etiologies and in selecting specific tests.

V. Imaging studies may reveal important aspects of toxic exposures.

A. Radiographs can detect radiopaque foreign bodies (such as broken needles at subcutaneous injection sites), ingested tablets, drug-filled condoms or packets, and some ingested or injected liquids (eg, chloral hydrate, arsenic).

1. The radiograph is useful only if positive; recent studies suggest that few types of tablets are predictably visible (Table I–35).

TABLE I–34. SPECIFIC QUANTITATIVE LEVELS AND POTENTIAL INTERVENTIONS[a]

Drug or Toxin	Potential Intervention
Acetaminophen	Acetylcysteine
Carbamazepine	Repeat-dose charcoal, hemoperfusion
Carboxyhemoglobin	100% oxygen
Digoxin	Digoxin-specific antibodies
Ethanol	Low level indicates search for other toxins
Ethylene glycol	Ethanol or fomepizole therapy, hemodialysis
Iron	Deferoxamine chelation
Lithium	Hemodialysis
Methanol	Ethanol or fomepizole therapy, hemodialysis
Methemoglobin	Methylene blue
Salicylate	Alkalinization, hemodialysis
Theophylline	Repeat-dose charcoal, hemoperfusion
Valproic acid	Hemodialysis, repeat-dose charcoal

[a]For specific guidance, see individual chapters in Section II.

2. Do ***not*** attempt to determine the radiopacity of a tablet by placing it directly on the x-ray plate. This often produces a false-positive result because of an air contrast effect.

B. **Ultrasound** of soft tissues can detect the depth and spread of subcutaneous edema following high-pressure hydrocarbon injection injuries or cytotoxic snakebites.

TABLE I–35. RADIOPAQUE DRUGS AND POISONS[a]

Usually visible
Bismuth subsalicylate (Pepto-Bismol)
Calcium carbonate (Tums)
Iron tablets
Lead and lead-containing paint
Metallic foreign bodies (eg, coins, disc batteries, magnets)
Potassium tablets
Sometimes/weakly visible
Acetazolamide
Arsenic
Brompheniramine and dexbrompheniramine
Busulfan
Chloral hydrate
Drug-filled condoms, balloons, or other packets
Enteric-coated or sustained-release preparations (highly variable)
Meclizine
Mothballs (paradichlorobenzene)
Perphenazine with amitriptyline
Phosphorus/phosphides
Prochlorperazine
Sodium chloride
Thiamine
Tranylcypromine
Trifluoperazine
Trimeprazine
Zinc sulfate

[a]Savitt DL, Hawkins HH, Roberts JR. The radiopacity of ingested medications. *Ann Emerg Med.* 1987;16:331.

C. Computerized tomography (CT) scans and **magnetic resonance imaging (MRI)** are increasingly used.

1. CT and MRI can identify intracranial complications of poisoning, such as basal ganglia infarcts (carbon monoxide; cyanide) or hemorrhage (methanol), cerebral edema, anoxic/ischemic injury, leukoencephalopathy (toluene or vaporized heroin) or gas emboli (concentrated hydrogen peroxide).
2. Abdominal imaging with CT/MRI has also been used to detect ingested drug packets, pipes, vials, or other paraphernalia, although the sensitivity is uncertain.
3. CT scans of the chest and abdomen can be used to evaluate the extent of injury from corrosive chemicals, as an adjunct to endoscopic assessment.

DECONTAMINATION

I. Surface decontamination

A. Skin. Corrosive agents rapidly injure the skin and must be removed immediately. In addition, many toxins are readily absorbed through the skin, and systemic absorption can be prevented only by rapid action. Table II–21 (p 187) lists several corrosive chemical agents that can have systemic toxicity, and many of them are readily absorbed through the skin.

1. Be careful not to expose yourself or other care providers to potentially contaminating substances. Wear protective gear (gloves, gown, and goggles) and wash exposed areas promptly. Contact a regional poison control center for information about the hazards of the chemicals involved; in the majority of cases, health care providers are not at significant personal risk for secondary contamination, and simple measures such as emergency department gowns and plain examination gloves, and a well-ventilated room, provide sufficient protection. For radiation and other hazardous materials incidents, see also Section IV (p 636).
2. Remove contaminated clothing and flush exposed areas with copious quantities of tepid (lukewarm) water or saline. Wash carefully behind ears, under nails, and in skin folds. Use soap and shampoo for oily substances.
3. There is rarely a need for chemical neutralization of a substance spilled on the skin. In fact, the heat generated by chemical neutralization can potentially create worse injury. Some of the few exceptions to this rule are listed in Table I–36.
4. Some medications can cause tissue necrosis due to extravasation (eg, chemotherapeutic agents, concentrated potassium, dextrose, or calcium solutions, phenytoin, IV contrast dye). Stop the infusion immediately and apply a warm towel to facilitate systemic absorption by vasodilation. More specific therapies, such as local injection of hyaluronidase (which transiently increases absorptive capacity of subcutaneous tissues) or neutralizing agents may be indicated depending on the agent.

TABLE I–36. SOME TOPICAL AGENTS FOR CHEMICAL EXPOSURES TO THE SKIN[a]

Chemical Corrosive Agent	Topical Treatment
Hydrofluoric acid	Calcium soaks
Oxalic acid	Calcium soaks
Phenol	Mineral oil or other oil; isopropyl alcohol; polyethylene glycol
Phosphorus (white)	Copper sulfate 1% (colors embedded granules blue, facilitates mechanical removal)
Potassium permanganate	Dilute oxalic acid (can remove dermal staining)

[a]Edelman PA: Chemical and electrical burns. In: Achauer BM, ed. *Management of the Burned Patient,* pp 183–202. Appleton & Lange; 1987.

B. Eyes. The cornea is especially sensitive to corrosive agents and hydrocarbon solvents that may rapidly damage the corneal surface and lead to permanent scarring.

1. Act quickly to prevent serious damage. Remove any contact lenses. If available, instill local anesthetic drops in the eye to facilitate irrigation. Flush exposed eyes with copious quantities of fluids (lactated ringer's solution is closest in composition to tear fluid so it is preferred, but saline or even tap water can be used if these are more readily available).
2. Apply Morgan's lenses (ocular irrigation device) after placing the victim in a supine position. Connect the tubing to lactated ringer's solution (preferred) or normal saline, and irrigate 1 L of fluid. If Morgan's lenses are not available, nasal cannula tubing can be repurposed to direct a stream of water into the medial aspect of the eye. Tape the nasal cannula to the bridge of the nose and connect the tubing to IV fluid bags. Reassure the patient and check frequently to ensure that each prong drips fluid into the medial canthus.
3. If the offending substance is an acid or a base, check the pH of the victim's tears after irrigation and continue irrigation if the pH remains abnormal.
4. Do not instill neutralizing solution in an attempt to normalize the pH; there is no evidence that such treatment works, and it may further damage the eye.
5. After irrigation is complete, check the conjunctival and corneal surfaces carefully for evidence of full-thickness injury. Check visual acuity, and perform a fluorescein examination of the eye with a Wood lamp to reveal corneal injury.
6. Patients with serious conjunctival or corneal injury should be referred to an ophthalmologist immediately.

C. Inhalation. Agents that injure the pulmonary system may be acutely irritating gases or fumes and may have good or poor warning properties (p 255).

1. Be careful not to expose yourself or other care providers to toxic gases or fumes without adequate respiratory protection (p 641).
2. Remove the victim from exposure and give supplemental humidified oxygen, if available. Assist ventilation if necessary (pp 1–7).
3. Observe closely for evidence of upper respiratory tract edema, which is heralded by a hoarse voice and stridor and may progress rapidly to complete airway obstruction. Endotracheally intubate patients who show evidence of progressive airway compromise.
4. Also observe for late-onset noncardiogenic pulmonary edema resulting from more slowly acting toxins (eg, nitrogen oxide, phosgene), which may take several hours to appear. Early signs and symptoms include dyspnea, hypoxemia, and tachypnea (p 255).

II. Gastrointestinal decontamination. There remains controversy about the role of gastric emptying and activated charcoal to decontaminate the gastrointestinal tract in the management of ingested poisons. There is little support in the medical literature for gut-emptying procedures, and studies have shown that after a delay of 60 minutes or more, only a small proportion of the ingested dose is removed by induced emesis or gastric lavage. Moreover, studies suggest that in the typical overdosed patient, simple oral administration of activated charcoal without prior gut emptying is probably just as effective as the traditional sequence of gut emptying followed by charcoal. For many overdose patients who have ingested a small dose, a relatively nontoxic substance, or a drug that is rapidly absorbed, it is even questionable whether activated charcoal makes a difference in outcome.

However, there are some circumstances in which aggressive gut decontamination may potentially be life-saving and is advised, even after more than 1–2 hours. Examples include ingestion of highly toxic drugs (eg, calcium antagonists, colchicine), ingestion of drugs not adsorbed to charcoal (eg, iron, lithium), ingestion of massive amounts of a drug (eg, 150–200 aspirin tablets), and ingestion of sustained-release or enteric-coated products.

A. Emesis. Syrup of ipecac-induced emesis is no longer recommended in the home, prehospital, or emergency settings. Adverse effects of ipecac include persistent vomiting with the potential for esophageal tear or rupture, electrolyte derangements, dehydration, and cardiomyopathy from repeated daily use (eg, by bulimic patients). Other emetics such as manual digital stimulation, copper sulfate, salt water, sodium bicarbonate, mustard water, apomorphine, and potassium permanganate are unsafe and should not be used.

B. Gastric lavage. Gastric lavage is only occasionally done in hospital emergency departments. There is little clinical evidence to support its routine use. Gastric lavage may be effective for recently ingested liquid substances. However, it does not reliably remove undissolved pills or pill fragments (especially sustained-release or enteric-coated products). In addition, the procedure may delay the administration of activated charcoal and may hasten the movement of drugs and poisons into the small intestine, especially if the patient is supine or in the right decubitus position. Gastric lavage is not necessary for small-to-moderate ingestions of most substances if activated charcoal can be given promptly.

1. Indications

a. To remove ingested liquid and solid drugs and poisons when the patient has taken a massive overdose or has ingested a particularly toxic substance. Lavage is more likely to be effective if initiated within 30–60 minutes of the ingestion, before gastric emptying has occurred.

b. A nasogastric tube may be needed in order to administer activated charcoal and whole-bowel irrigation to patients unwilling or unable to swallow them.

c. To dilute and remove corrosive liquids from the stomach and to empty the stomach in preparation for endoscopy.

2. Contraindications

a. Obtunded, comatose, or convulsing patients. Because it may disturb the normal physiology of the esophagus and airway protective mechanisms, gastric lavage must be used with caution in obtunded patients whose airway reflexes are dulled. In such cases, endotracheal intubation with a cuffed endotracheal tube should be performed first to protect the airway.

b. Ingestion of sustained-release or enteric-coated tablets. (Owing to the size of most tablets, lavage is unlikely to return intact tablets, even through a 40F orogastric hose.) In such cases, whole-bowel irrigation (see below) is preferable.

c. Use of gastric lavage after ingestion of a corrosive substance is controversial; some gastroenterologists recommend that insertion of a gastric tube and aspiration of gastric contents be performed as soon as possible after liquid caustic ingestion to remove corrosive material from the stomach and to prepare for endoscopy.

3. Adverse effects

a. Perforation of the esophagus or stomach.

b. Bleeding from mucosal trauma during passage of the tube.

c. Inadvertent tracheal intubation.

d. Vomiting resulting in pulmonary aspiration of gastric contents in an obtunded patient without airway protection.

4. Technique

a. If the patient is deeply obtunded, first protect the airway by intubating the trachea with a cuffed endotracheal tube.

b. Place the patient in the left lateral decubitus position. This helps prevent ingested material from being pushed into the duodenum during lavage.

c. Insert a large gastric tube through the mouth or nose and into the stomach (36–40F [catheter size] in adults; a smaller tube will suffice for removal of liquid poisons or if simple administration of charcoal is all that is intended). Check tube position with air insufflation while listening with a stethoscope positioned on the patient's stomach. If time permits, a rapid portable x-ray can also help confirm placement.

d. Withdraw as much of the stomach contents as possible. If the ingested poison is a toxic chemical that may contaminate hospital personnel (eg, cyanide, organophosphate insecticide), take steps to isolate it immediately (eg, use a self-contained wall suction unit).

e. Administer activated charcoal, 60–100 g (1 g/kg; see Item II.C below), down the tube before starting lavage to begin adsorption of material that may enter the intestine during the lavage procedure.

f. Instill tepid (lukewarm) water or saline, 200- to 300-mL aliquots, and remove by gravity or active suction. Use repeated aliquots for a total of 2 L or until the return is free of pills or toxic material. ***Caution:*** Use of excessive volumes of lavage fluid or plain tap water can result in hypothermia or electrolyte imbalance in infants and small children.

C. Activated charcoal is a highly adsorbent powdered material made from a distillation of wood pulp. Owing to its very large surface area, it is highly effective in adsorbing most toxins when given in a ratio of approximately 10:1 (charcoal to toxin). Only a few toxins are poorly adsorbed to charcoal (Table I–37), and in some cases this requires a higher ratio (eg, for cyanide a ratio of about 100:1 is necessary). Studies in volunteers taking nontoxic doses of various substances suggest that activated charcoal given alone without prior gastric emptying is as effective as or even more effective than emesis and lavage procedures in reducing drug absorption. However, there are no well-designed prospective randomized clinical studies demonstrating its effectiveness in poisoned patients, and there is a risk of vomiting and subsequent aspiration of gastric contents. As a result, some toxicologists advise against its routine use.

1. Indications

a. Used after ingestion to limit drug absorption from the gastrointestinal tract if it can be given safely and in a reasonable time period after the ingestion.

b. Charcoal is often given even if the offending substance may not be well adsorbed to charcoal in case other substances have been co-ingested.

c. Repeated oral doses of activated charcoal may enhance the elimination of some drugs from the bloodstream (p 59).

2. Contraindications. Ileus without distension is not a contraindication to a single dose of charcoal, but further doses should be withheld. Charcoal should not be given to a drowsy patient unless the airway is adequately protected.

3. Adverse effects

a. Constipation or intestinal impaction and charcoal bezoar are potential complications, especially if multiple doses of charcoal are given and the patient is not adequately hydrated.

TABLE I–37. DRUGS AND TOXINS POORLY ADSORBED BY ACTIVATED CHARCOAL[a]

Alkali	Hydrocarbons
Cyanide[b]	Inorganic salts (variable)
Ethanol and other alcohols	Iron
Ethylene glycol	Lithium
Fluoride	Mineral acids
Heavy metals (variable)	Potassium

[a]Few studies have been performed to determine the in vivo adsorption of these and other toxins to activated charcoal. Adsorption may also depend on the specific type and concentration of charcoal.

[b]Charcoal should still be given because usual doses of charcoal (60–100 g) will adsorb usual lethal ingested doses of cyanide (200–300 mg).

TABLE I–38. GUIDELINES FOR ADMINISTRATION OF ACTIVATED CHARCOAL

General

The risk of the poisoning justifies the risk of charcoal administration. Activated charcoal can be administered within 60 minutes of the ingestion.[a]

Prehospital

The patient is alert and cooperative.

Activated charcoal without sorbitol is readily available.

Administration of charcoal will not delay transport to a health care facility.

Hospital

The patient is alert and cooperative, or the activated charcoal will be given via gastric tube (assuming the airway is intact or protected).

[a]The time after ingestion during which charcoal remains an effective decontamination modality has not been established with certainty in clinical trials. For drugs with slow or erratic intestinal absorption, or for those with anticholinergic or opioid effects or other pharmacologic effects that may delay gastric emptying into the small intestine, or for drugs in a modified-release formulation, or after massive ingestions that may produce a tablet mass or bezoar, it is appropriate to administer charcoal more than 60 minutes after ingestion, or even several hours after ingestion.

b. Distension of the stomach with a potential risk for pulmonary aspiration, especially in a drowsy patient.

c. Many commercially available charcoal products contain charcoal and the cathartic sorbitol in a premixed suspension. Even single doses of sorbitol often cause stomach cramps and vomiting, and repeated doses may cause serious fluid shifts to the intestine, diarrhea, dehydration, and hypernatremia, especially in young children and elderly persons.

d. May bind coadministered acetylcysteine (not clinically significant).

4. Technique. (See Table I–38 for guidelines on prehospital and hospital use.)

a. Give activated charcoal aqueous suspension (without sorbitol), 60–100 g (1 g/kg), orally or by gastric tube.

b. One or two additional doses of activated charcoal may be given at 1- or 2-hour intervals to ensure adequate gut decontamination, particularly after large ingestions. In rare cases, as many as 8 or 10 repeated doses may be needed to achieve the desired 10:1 ratio of charcoal to poison (eg, after an ingestion of 200 aspirin tablets); in such circumstances, the doses should be given over a period of several hours.

c. Although charcoal has a neutral taste, some patients refuse to drink it because of its gritty texture and black appearance. Covering the lid and adding charcoal to juice or milk can help facilitate administration.

D. Cathartics. Controversy remains over the use of cathartics to hasten elimination of toxins from the gastrointestinal tract. Some toxicologists still use cathartics routinely when giving activated charcoal, even though few data exist to support their efficacy.

1. Indications

a. To enhance gastrointestinal transit of the charcoal–toxin complex, decreasing the likelihood of desorption of toxin or the development of a "charcoal bezoar."

b. To hasten the passage of iron tablets and other ingestions not adsorbed by charcoal.

2. Contraindications

a. Ileus or intestinal obstruction.

b. Sodium- or magnesium-containing cathartics should not be used in patients with fluid overload or renal insufficiency, respectively.

c. There is no role for oil-based cathartics (previously recommended for hydrocarbon poisoning).

3. Adverse effects

a. Severe fluid loss, hypernatremia, and hyperosmolarity may result from overuse or repeated doses of cathartics; deaths have occurred in very young, elderly, or frail patients.

b. Hypermagnesemia may occur in patients with renal insufficiency who are given magnesium-based cathartics.

c. Abdominal cramping and vomiting may occur, especially with sorbitol.

d. Colonic intestinal necrosis has been associated with sorbitol–sodium polystyrene sulfonate (Kayexalate) combinations used to treat hyperkalemia.

4. Technique

a. Administer the cathartic of choice (10% magnesium citrate, 3–4 mL/kg, or 70% sorbitol, 1 mL/kg) along with activated charcoal or mixed together as a slurry. Avoid using commercially available combination products containing charcoal plus sorbitol because they have a larger-than-desirable amount of sorbitol (eg, 96 g of sorbitol/50 g of charcoal).

b. Repeat with one-half the original dose if there is no charcoal stool after 6–8 hours.

E. Whole-bowel irrigation. Whole-bowel irrigation has become an accepted method for the elimination of some drugs and poisons from the gut. The technique makes use of a surgical bowel-cleansing solution containing a nonabsorbable polyethylene glycol in a balanced electrolyte solution that is formulated to pass through the intestinal tract without being absorbed. This solution is given at high flow rates to wash intestinal contents out by sheer volume.

1. Indications

a. Large ingestions of iron, lithium, or other drugs poorly adsorbed to activated charcoal.

b. Large ingestions of sustained-release or enteric-coated tablets containing valproic acid (eg, Depakote), theophylline (eg, Theo-Dur), aspirin (eg, Ecotrin), verapamil (eg, Calan SR), diltiazem (eg, Cardizem CD), or other dangerous drugs.

c. Ingestion of foreign bodies or drug-filled packets or condoms. Although controversy persists about the optimal gut decontamination for "body stuffers" (persons who hastily ingest drug-containing packets to hide incriminating evidence), prudent management involves several hours of whole-bowel irrigation accompanied by activated charcoal. Follow-up imaging studies may be indicated to search for retained packets if the amount of drug or its packaging is of concern.

2. Contraindications

a. Ileus or intestinal obstruction.

b. Obtunded, comatose, or convulsing patient unless the airway is protected.

3. Adverse effects

a. Nausea, diarrhea, and bloating.

b. Regurgitation and pulmonary aspiration.

c. Activated charcoal may not be as effective when given with whole-bowel irrigation.

4. Technique

a. Administer bowel preparation solution (eg, CoLyte or GoLytely), 2 L/h by gastric tube (children: 500 mL/h or 35 mL/kg/h), until rectal effluent is clear or a total of 10–15 L have been passed. Continued treatment may occasionally be needed (eg, if an x-ray demonstrates the presence of iron tablets remaining in the GI tract).

b. Some toxicologists recommend the administration of activated charcoal 25–50 g every 2–3 hours while whole-bowel irrigation is proceeding, if the ingested drug is adsorbed by charcoal.

c. Be prepared for a large-volume stool within 1–2 hours. Pass a rectal tube or, preferably, have the patient sit on a commode.

TABLE I–39. SELECTED ORAL BINDING AGENTS

Drug or Toxin	Binding Agent(s)
Calcium	Cellulose sodium phosphate
Chlorinated hydrocarbons	Cholestyramine resin
Digitoxin[a]	Cholestyramine resin
Heavy metals (arsenic, mercury)	Demulcents (egg white, milk)
Iron	Sodium bicarbonate
Iodine	Starchy food or milk; sodium thiosulfate
Lithium	Sodium polystyrene sulfonate (Kayexalate)[b]
Paraquat[a]	Fuller's earth, Bentonite
Potassium	Sodium polystyrene sulfonate (Kayexalate)[b]
Thallium, ^{137}Cesium	Prussian blue

[a]Activated charcoal is also very effective.
[b]Uncertain effectiveness; may cause gut necrosis.

d. Stop administration after 8–10 L (children: 150–200 mL/kg) if no rectal effluent has appeared.

F. Other oral binding agents. Other binding agents may be given in certain circumstances to trap toxins in the gut, although activated charcoal is the most widely used effective adsorbent. Table I–39 lists some alternative binding agents and the toxin(s) for which they may be useful. Most have not been proven beneficial in well-designed studies, while some have been associated with potential harm (eg, Kayexalate and bowel necrosis).

G. Surgical removal. Occasionally, drug-filled packets or condoms, intact tablets, or tablet concretions persist despite aggressive gastric lavage or whole-gut lavage, and surgical or endoscopic removal may be necessary. Consult a regional poison control center or a medical toxicologist for advice.

ENHANCED ELIMINATION

Measures to enhance elimination of drugs and toxins have been overemphasized in the past. Although a desirable goal, rapid elimination of most drugs and toxins is frequently not practical and may be unsafe. A logical understanding of pharmacokinetics as it applies to toxicology (toxicokinetics) is necessary for the appropriate use of enhanced removal procedures.

I. Assessment. Three critical questions must be answered:

A. Does the patient need enhanced removal? Ask the following questions: How is the patient doing? Will supportive care enable the patient to recover fully? Is there an antidote or another specific drug that might be used? Important indications for enhanced drug removal include the following:

1. Obviously severe or critical intoxication with a deteriorating condition despite maximal supportive care (eg, phenobarbital overdose with intractable hypotension).
2. The normal or usual route of elimination is impaired (eg, lithium overdose in a patient with renal failure).
3. The patient has ingested a known lethal dose or has a lethal blood level (eg, theophylline or methanol).
4. The patient has underlying medical problems that could increase the hazards of prolonged coma or other complications (eg, severe chronic obstructive pulmonary disease or congestive heart failure).

B. Is the drug or toxin accessible to the removal procedure? For a drug to be accessible to removal by extracorporeal procedures, it should be located

TABLE I–40. VOLUME OF DISTRIBUTION OF SOME DRUGS AND POISONS

Large Vd (>5–10 L/kg)	Small Vd (<1 L/kg)
Antidepressants	Alcohols
Digoxin	Carbamazepine
Lindane	Lithium
Opioids	Phenobarbital
Phencyclidine (PCP)	Salicylate
Phenothiazines	Theophylline

primarily within the bloodstream or in the extracellular fluid. If it is extensively distributed to tissues, it is not likely to be easily removed.

1. **The volume of distribution (Vd)** is a numeric concept that provides an indication of the accessibility of the drug:

$$\begin{aligned} Vd &= \text{apparent volume into which the drug is distributed} \\ &= (\text{amount of drug in the body})/(\text{plasma concentration}) \\ &= (\text{mg/kg})/(\text{mg/L}) = \text{L/kg} \end{aligned}$$

Thus, a drug with a very large Vd has a relatively low plasma concentration compared to total body stores. In contrast, a drug with a small Vd is potentially quite accessible by extracorporeal removal procedures. Table I-40 lists some common volumes of distribution.

2. **Protein binding.** Highly protein-bound drugs have low free drug concentrations and are difficult to remove by dialysis.

C. **Will the method work?** Does the removal procedure efficiently extract the toxin from the blood?

1. The **clearance (CL)** is the rate at which a given volume of fluid can be "cleared" of the substance.

   a. The CL may be calculated from the extraction ratio across the dialysis machine or hemoperfusion column, multiplied by the blood flow rate through the following system:

$$CL = \text{extraction ratio} \times \text{blood flow rate}$$

   b. A crude urinary CL measurement may be useful for estimating the effectiveness of fluid therapy for enhancing renal elimination of substances not secreted or absorbed by the renal tubule (eg, lithium):

$$\text{Renal CL} = \text{urine flow rate} \times \frac{\text{urine drug level}}{\text{serum drug level}}$$

Note: The units of clearance are milliliters per minute. Clearance is not the same as elimination rate (milligrams per minute). If the blood concentration is small, the actual amount of drug removed is also small.

2. **Total CL** is the sum of all sources of clearance (eg, renal excretion plus hepatic metabolism plus respiratory and skin excretion plus dialysis). If the contribution of dialysis is small compared with the total clearance rate, the procedure will contribute little to the overall elimination rate (Table I–41).

3. The **half-life** ($T_{1/2}$) depends on the volume of distribution and the clearance:

$$T_{1/2} = \frac{0.693 \times Vd}{CL}$$

where the unit of measurement of Vd is liters (L) and that of CL is liters per hour (L/h). For many substances, half-life is prolonged in overdose because elimination mechanisms become saturated.

TABLE I–41. ELIMINATION OF SELECTED DRUGS AND TOXINS[a]

Drug or Toxin	Volume of Distribution (L/kg)	Usual Body Clearance (mL/min)	Reported Clearance by: Dialysis (mL/min)	Reported Clearance by: Hemoperfusion[b] (mL/min)
Acetaminophen	0.8–1	400	120–150	125–300
Amitriptyline	6–10	500–800	NHD[c]	240[d]
Bromide	0.7	5	100	N/A[c]
Carbamazepine	1.4–3	60–90	59–100[e]	80–130
Digitoxin	1.5	4	10–26	N/A[c]
Digoxin	5–10	150–200	NHD[c]	90–140
Ethanol	0.7	100–300	100–200	NHP[c]
Ethchlorvynol	2–4	120–140	20–80	150–300[d]
Ethylene glycol	0.6–0.8	200	100–200	NHP[c]
Glutethimide	2.7	200	70	300[d]
Isopropyl alcohol	0.7	30	100–200	NHP[c]
Lithium	0.7–1.4	25–30	50–150	NHP[c]
Meprobamate	0.75	60	60	85–150
Metformin	80 L[f]	491–652[g]	68–170	56[h]
Methanol	0.7	40–60	100–200	NHP[c]
Formic acid (methanol metabolite)		198–248		
Methaqualone	2.4–6.4	130–175	23	150–270
Methotrexate	0.5–1	50–100	N/A[c]	54
Nadolol	2	135	46–102	N/A[c]
Nortriptyline	15–27	500–1000	24–34	216[d]
Paraquat	2.8	30–200	10	50–155
Pentobarbital	0.65–1	27–36	23–55	200–300
Phenobarbital	0.5–1	2–15	144–188[i]	100–300
Phenytoin	0.5–0.8	15–30	NHD	76–189
Procainamide	1.5–2.5	650	70	75
N-acetylprocainamide (NAPA)	1.4	220	48	75
Salicylate	0.1–0.3	30	35–80	57–116
Theophylline	0.5	80–120	30–50	60–225
Thiocyanate (cyanide metabolite)			83–102	
Trichloroethanol (chloral hydrate)	0.6–1.6	25	68–162	119–200
Valproic acid	0.1–0.5	10	23	55

[a]Adapted in part, with permission, from Pond SM: Diuresis, dialysis, and hemoperfusion: indications and benefits. *Emerg Med Clin North Am.* 1984;2:29; and Cutler RE, et al. Extracorporeal removal of drugs and poisons by hemodialysis and hemoperfusion. *Ann Rev Pharmacol Toxicol.* 1987;27:169.
[b]Hemoperfusion data are mainly for charcoal hemoperfusion.
[c]N/A, not available; NHD, not hemodialyzable; NHP, not hemoperfusable.
[d]Data are for XAD-4 resin hemoperfusion.
[e]Lower clearances (14–59 mL/min) reported with older dialysis equipment; newer high-flux dialysis may produce clearances of 59 mL/min up to estimated 100 mL/min (based on case reports).
[f]Literature reports of metformin Vd vary widely.
[g]Metformin clearance is markedly reduced in patients with renal insufficiency (108–130 mL/min).
[h]Clearance by continuous venovenous hemofiltration (CVVH).
[i]Lower clearances of 60–75 mL/min reported with older dialysis equipment; newer high-flux dialysis may produce clearances of 144–188 mL/min (Palmer BF. *Am J Kid Dis.* 2000;36:640).

II. Methods available for enhanced elimination

A. Urinary manipulation. These methods require that the kidney be a significant contributor to total clearance.

1. Forced diuresis may increase the glomerular filtration rate, and ion trapping by urinary pH manipulation may enhance the elimination of polar drugs.

2. Alkalinization is commonly used for salicylate overdose, but "forced" diuresis (producing urine volumes of up to 1 L/h) is generally not used because of the risk for fluid overload.

B. **Hemodialysis.** Blood is taken from a large vein (usually a femoral vein) with a double-lumen catheter and pumped through an extracorporeal blood purification system. The patient must be given anticoagulant medication to prevent clotting of blood in the dialyzer. Drugs and toxins flow passively across the semipermeable membrane down a concentration gradient into a dialysate (electrolyte and buffer) solution. Fluid and electrolyte abnormalities can be corrected concurrently.

1. Flow rates of up to 300–500 mL/min can be achieved, and clearance rates may reach 200–300 mL/min or more. Removal of drug is dependent on the flow rate—insufficient flow (ie, due to clotting) will reduce clearance proportionately.
2. Characteristics of the drug or toxin that enhance its extractability include small size (molecular weight <500 daltons), water solubility, and low protein binding.
3. ***Note:*** Smaller, portable dialysis units that use a resin column or filter to recycle a smaller volume of dialysate ("mini-dialysis") do not efficiently remove drugs or poisons and should not be used.

C. **Hemoperfusion.** With the use of equipment and vascular access similar to that for hemodialysis, the blood is pumped directly through a column containing an adsorbent material (either charcoal or Amberlite resin). Because the drug or toxin is in direct contact with the adsorbent material, drug size, water solubility, and protein binding are less important limiting factors. Systemic anticoagulation is required, often in higher doses than are used for hemodialysis, and thrombocytopenia is a common complication. At the present time, few dialysis centers have the equipment for hemoperfusion, and the procedure is rarely carried out.

D. **Peritoneal dialysis.** Dialysate fluid is infused into the peritoneal cavity through a transcutaneous catheter and drained off, and the procedure is repeated with fresh dialysate. The gut wall and peritoneal lining serve as the semipermeable membrane.

1. Peritoneal dialysis is easier to perform than hemodialysis or hemoperfusion and does not require anticoagulation, but it is only about 10–15% as effective owing to poor extraction ratios and slower flow rates (clearance rates, 10–15 mL/min).
2. However, peritoneal dialysis can be performed continuously, 24 hours a day; a 24-hour peritoneal dialysis with dialysate exchange every 1–2 hours is approximately equal to 4 hours of hemodialysis.
3. Peritoneal dialysis is rarely used in the treatment of acute poisoning.

E. **Continuous renal replacement therapy** (eg, continuous arteriovenous hemofiltration [CAVH], continuous venovenous hemofiltration [CVVH], continuous arteriovenous hemodiafiltration [CAVHDF], or continuous venovenous hemodiafiltration [CVVHDF]) has been suggested as an alternative to conventional hemodialysis when the need for rapid removal of the drug is less urgent. Like peritoneal dialysis, these procedures are associated with lower clearance rates but have the advantage of being minimally invasive, with no significant impact on hemodynamics, and can be carried out "continuously" for many hours. However, their role in the management of acute poisoning remains uncertain.

F. **Repeat-dose activated charcoal.** Repeated doses of activated charcoal (20–30 g or 0.5–1 g/kg every 2–3 hours) are given orally or via gastric tube. The presence of a slurry of activated charcoal throughout several meters of the intestinal lumen reduces blood concentrations by interrupting enterohepatic or enteroenteric recirculation of the drug or toxin, a mode of action quite

TABLE I–42. SOME DRUGS REMOVED BY REPEAT-DOSE ACTIVATED CHARCOAL[a]

Caffeine	Phenobarbital
Carbamazepine	Phenylbutazone
Chlordecone	Phenytoin
Dapsone	Salicylate
Digitoxin	Theophylline
Nadolol	

[a]*Note:* Based on volunteer studies. There are few data on clinical benefit in drug overdose.

distinct from the simple adsorption of ingested but unabsorbed tablets. This technique is easy and noninvasive and has been shown to shorten the half-life of phenobarbital, theophylline, and several other drugs (Table I–42). However, it has not been proven in clinical trials to alter patient outcome. ***Caution:*** Repeat-dose charcoal may cause serious fluid and electrolyte disturbance secondary to large-volume diarrhea, especially if premixed charcoal–sorbitol suspensions are used. Also, it should not be used in patients with ileus or obstruction.

G. A number of extracorporeal methods have been used to enhance elimination or support vital organs while a toxin is eliminated, but the level of evidence for their use is limited to case reports and small case series. These modalities include exchange transfusion, plasmapheresis, cerebrospinal fluid (CSF) exchange for intrathecal overdoses, and extracorporeal membrane oxygenation (ECMO).

DISPOSITION OF THE PATIENT

I. Emergency department discharge or intensive care unit admission?

A. All patients with potentially serious overdose should be observed for at least 6–8 hours before discharge or transfer to a nonmedical (eg, psychiatric) facility. If signs or symptoms of intoxication develop during this time, admission for further observation and treatment is required. ***Caution:*** Beware of delayed complications from the slow absorption of medications (eg, from a tablet concretion or bezoar or sustained-release or enteric-coated preparations). In these circumstances, a longer period of observation is warranted. If specific drug levels are determined, obtain repeated serum levels to be certain that they are decreasing as expected.

B. Most patients admitted for poisoning or drug overdose will need observation in an intensive care unit, although this depends on the potential for serious cardiorespiratory complications. Any patient with suicidal intent must be kept under close observation.

II. Regional poison control center consultation: 1-800-222-1222. Consult with a regional poison control center to determine the need for further observation or admission, administration of antidotes or therapeutic drugs, selection of appropriate laboratory tests, or decisions about extracorporeal removal. An experienced clinical toxicologist is usually available for immediate consultation. A single toll-free number is in effect nationwide and will automatically connect the caller to the regional poison control center.

III. Psychosocial evaluation

A. Psychiatric consultation for suicide risk. All patients with intentional poisoning or drug overdose should undergo a psychiatric evaluation for suicidal intent.

1. It is not appropriate to discharge a potentially suicidal patient from the emergency department without a careful psychiatric evaluation. Most states have provisions for the physician to place an emergency psychiatric hold, forcing involuntary patients to remain under psychiatric observation for up to 72 hours.

2. Patients calling from home after an intentional ingestion should always be referred to an emergency department for medical and psychiatric evaluation.

B. **Child abuse** (see also below) or **sexual abuse**

1. Children should be evaluated for the possibility that the ingestion was not accidental. Sometimes parents or other adults intentionally give children sedatives or tranquilizers to control their behavior.
2. Accidental poisonings may also warrant social services referral. Occasionally, children get into stimulants or other abused drugs that are left around the home. Repeated ingestions suggest overly casual or negligent parental behavior.
3. Intentional overdose in a child or adolescent should raise the possibility of physical or sexual abuse. Teenage girls may have overdosed because of unwanted pregnancy.

IV. **Overdose in the pregnant patient**

A. In general, it is prudent to check for pregnancy in any young woman with drug overdose or poisoning. Unwanted pregnancy may be a cause for intentional overdose, or special concerns may be raised about treatment of the pregnant patient.

B. Gastric lavage, whole-bowel irrigation and oral activated charcoal can be performed in all trimesters, but be aware of the higher risk of pulmonary aspiration or GI tract perforation as a result of upward displacement by the uterine fundus.

C. Some toxins are known to be teratogenic or mutagenic (see below and Table I–45, p 66). However, adverse effects on the fetus are generally associated with chronic, repeated use as opposed to acute, single exposure.

▶ SPECIAL CONSIDERATIONS IN PEDIATRIC PATIENTS

Cyrus Rangan, MD

The majority of calls to poison control centers involve children younger than 5 years. Fortunately, children account for a minority of serious **poisonings** requiring emergency hospital treatment. Most common childhood ingestions involve nontoxic substances or nontoxic doses of potentially toxic drugs or products (p 347). Table I–43 lists important causes of serious or fatal childhood poisoning, which include iron supplements (p 277); tricyclic antidepressants (p 107); cardiovascular medications such as digitalis (p 222), beta receptor antagonists (p 158), or calcium antagonists (p 172); methyl salicylate (p 410); and hydrocarbons (p 266).

I. **High-risk populations.** Two age groups are commonly involved in pediatric poisonings: children between 1 and 5 years and adolescents.

A. **Ingestions in toddlers and young children** usually result from oral and tactile exploration. Unintentional exposures in children younger than 6 months or between the ages of 5 and adolescence are relatively rare. In young infants, consider the possibility of intentional administration by an older child or adult. In school-aged children, suspect abuse or neglect.

B. **In adolescents and young adults,** overdoses often are the result of suicidal or other self-harm intent, but may also occur in the settings of drug abuse, bullying, underlying mental health conditions, or experimentation. Common underlying reasons for adolescent suicide attempts include pregnancy; sexual, physical, or mental abuse; school failure; conflict with peers; conflict with homosexual orientation; a sudden or severe loss; and alcoholism or illicit drug use. Any adolescent with intentional poisoning must undergo psychiatric evaluation and follow-up.

TABLE I–43. EXAMPLES OF POTENT PEDIATRIC POISONS[a]

Drug or Poison	Potentially Fatal Dose in a 10-kg Toddler
Antiarrhythmics	
Flecainide	One or two 150-mg tablets
Quinidine	Two 300-mg tablets
Antipsychotics	
Chlorpromazine	One or two 200-mg tablets
Thioridazine	One 200-mg tablet
Benzocaine	2 mL of a 10% gel
Calcium channel blockers	
Nifedipine	One or two 90-mg tablets
Verapamil	One or two 240-mg tablets
Camphor	5 mL of 20% oil
Chloroquine	One 500-mg tablet
Diphenoxylate/atropine (Lomotil)	Five 2.5-mg tablets
Hydrocarbons (eg, kerosene)	One swallow (if aspirated)
Hypoglycemic sulfonylureas	One 5-mg glyburide tablet
Iron	Ten adult-strength tablets
Lindane	Two teaspoons (10 mL)
Methyl salicylate	<5 mL of oil of wintergreen
Opioids	
Codeine	Three 60-mg tablets
Hydrocodone	One 5-mg tablet
Methadone	One 40-mg tablet
Morphine	One 200-mg tablet
Selenious acid (gun bluing)	One swallow
Theophylline	One 500-mg tablet
Tricyclic antidepressants	
Desipramine	Two 75-mg tablets
Imipramine	One 150-mg tablet

[a]Bar-Oz B, Levichek Z, Koren G. Medications that can be fatal for a toddler with one tablet or teaspoon-ful: a 2004 update. *Paediatric Drugs.* 2004;6(2):123–126; Koren G. Medications which can kill a toddler with one teaspoon or tablet. *Clin Toxicol.* 1993;31(3):407; Osterhoudt K. *Toxtalk* 1997;8(7); Litovitz T, Manoguerra A. Comparison of pediatric poisoning hazards: an analysis of 3.8 million exposure incidents. *Pediatrics.* 1992;89(6):999.

II. Poisoning prevention. Young children with unintentional exposures are at higher risk for subsequent exposures compared to the general population. After an incident, prevention strategies must be reviewed. If the family does not understand or comply with the advice, or if a child presents with a subsequent poisoning, consider a home evaluation for child-proofing by a public health nurse, child protective services official, or other health care professional.

A. Enhance child safety in the home, day care setting, and any households the child commonly visits (eg, grandparents and other relatives). Store all medicines, chemicals, and cleaning products out of the reach of children or in locked cabinets. All products should remain in their original containers, and must never be stored in food or drink containers, or in the same cabinets as food. Children commonly find medications and other products on bedside tables, kitchen counters, and in visitors' purses or backpacks.

B. **Use child-resistant containers** to store prescription and nonprescription medications. It should be understood that child-resistant containers are not child-proof; they only lessen the time it takes a determined child to get into the container. Children should never be allowed to play with medication containers.

C. **Medication errors** are a preventable cause of severe injury or death in children, especially those younger than 1 year. These errors are commonly associated with concentrated drugs in small volumes (<1-mL intended dosages); 10-fold dosing errors secondary to mislabeling or misinterpreted directions; unintentional repeated dosing secondary to multiple caregivers administering the same medication; and unintentional use of more than one product with the same ingredients (ie, a child with fever and cough is given acetaminophen for fever as well as a combination cough medicine that also contains acetaminophen). In one study, the leading causes of death due to medication errors in children were the following: acetaminophen, cough and cold preparations (especially those containing opiates), fosphenytoin, metoclopramide, viscous lidocaine, diphenoxylate/atropine, morphine, digoxin, and sodium phenyl butyrate.

III. **Child abuse.** Consider the possibility that the child was intentionally given the drug or toxin, or that the exposure occurred as a result of neglect. Most states require all health care professionals to report suspected cases of child abuse or neglect, making it a ***legal obligation to report any suspicious incident, rather than a discretionary decision.*** Parents or guardians should be informed in a straightforward, nonjudgmental manner that a report is being made under this legal obligation. Reports of suspected abuse should be made before the child is released, so that local law enforcement or child protection services can decide whether it is safe to release the child to the parents or guardians. In unclear situations, the child can be admitted for observation to allow time for officials to evaluate the social circumstances fully. The following should alert medical personnel to the possibility of abuse or neglect:

A. Medical, social, of family history that does not make sense or seems inconsistent with the presentation; a recount from a caregiver that changes upon re-questioning; or different caregivers providing differing or conflicting accounts of the incident.

B. The child is nonambulatory, or with very limited access to the poison (eg, a child younger than 6 months, or a child with physical/cognitive disabilities). Carefully review how the child gained access to the drug or toxin.

C. The child is older than 4–5 years. Accidental ingestions are relatively rare in older children; ingestion may be a signal of abuse or neglect.

D. The drug ingested was a tranquilizer (eg, haloperidol, chlorpromazine), a drug of abuse (eg, cocaine, heroin), a sedative (eg, diazepam, carisoprodol), or ethanol. On occasion, parents may be simultaneously intoxicated.

E. There is a long interval between the time of ingestion and the time the child presents for medical evaluation.

F. There are signs of physical or sexual abuse or neglect: multiple or unusual bruises; a broken bone or burns; a very dirty, unkempt child; or a child with a flat affect or indifferent or inappropriate behavior.

G. A history of repeated episodes of possible or documented poisonings, or a history of prior abuse.

H. Munchausen syndrome by proxy: Drugs or toxins are given to the child to simulate or promote illness. Many perpetrators are mothers with a medical background. This is a rare diagnosis.

IV. **Clinical evaluation.** Physical and laboratory evaluation is essentially the same as for adults. However, normal vital signs vary with age (Table I–44).

A. **Heart rate.** Newborns may have normal heart rates as high as 190 beats/min, and 2-year-olds up to 120 beats/min. Abnormal tachycardia or bradycardia

TABLE I–44. PEDIATRIC VITAL SIGNS[a]

Age	Respiratory Rate (breaths/min)	Heart Rate (beats/min)	Blood Pressure (mm Hg)			
			Lower Limit	Average	Upper Limit	Severe
Newborn	30–80	110–190	52/25	50–55[b]	95/72	110/85
1 mo	30–50	100–170	64/30	85/50	105/68	120/85
6 mo	30–50	100–170	60/40	90/55	110/72	125/85
1 y	20–40	100–160	66/40	90/55	110/72	125/88
2 y	20–30	100–160	74/40	90/55	110/72	125/88
4 y	20–25	80–130	79/45	95/55	112/75	128/88
8 y	15–25	70–110	85/48	100/60	118/75	135/92
12 y	15–20	60–100	95/50	108/65	125/84	142/95

[a]Dieckmann RA, Coulter K. Pediatric emergencies. In: Saunders CE, Ho MT, eds: *Current Emergency Diagnosis & Treatment.* 4th ed, p 811. Appleton & Lange; 1992; Gundy JH: The pediatric physical exam. In: Hoekelman RA, et al., eds. *Primary Pediatric Care,* p 68. Mosby; 1987; Hoffman JIE. Systemic arterial hypertension. In: Rudolph AM, et al., eds. *Rudolph's Pediatrics.* 19th ed, p 1438. Appleton & Lange, 1991; Liebman J, Freed MD. Cardiovascular system. In: Behrman RE, Kleigman R, eds: *Nelson's Essentials of Pediatrics,* p 447. WB Saunders; 1990; Lum GM. Kidney and urinary tract. In: Hathaway WE, et al., eds. *Current Pediatric Diagnosis & Treatment.* 10th ed, p 624. Appleton & Lange; 1991.

[b]Mean arterial pressure range on the first day of life.

suggests the possibility of hypoxemia in addition to the numerous drugs and poisons that affect heart rate and rhythm (see Tables I–4 [p 9] through I–7 [p 14]).

B. Blood pressure is a very important vital sign in a poisoned child. The blood pressure cuff must be of the proper size; cuffs that are too small can falsely elevate blood pressure. Blood pressures of infants are difficult to obtain by auscultation, and may more easily be obtained by Doppler in some cases.

1. Many children tend to have blood pressures lower than that of adults. However, low blood pressure in the context of a poisoning should be regarded as normal only if the child is alert and active, behaves appropriately, and has normal peripheral perfusion.
2. Idiopathic or essential hypertension is rare in children. Elevated blood pressure should be assumed to indicate an acute condition, although the systolic blood pressure can be transiently elevated if the child is vigorously crying or screaming. Unless a child's baseline blood pressure is known, values at the upper limit of normal should be assumed to be elevated. The decision to treat elevated blood pressure is based on the clinical scenario and the toxin involved.

V. Neonates present specific challenges, including unique pharmacokinetics and potentially severe withdrawal from prenatal drug exposure.

A. Neonatal pharmacokinetics. Newborns (birth–1 month) and infants (1–12 months) are unique from a toxicological and pharmacological perspective. Drug absorption, distribution, metabolism, protein binding, and elimination may be significantly different from those in older children and adults. Incorrect dosing, trans-placental passage proximate to the time of birth, breast-feeding, dermal absorption, and intentional poisoning are potential routes of toxic exposure. Enhanced skin absorption and reduced drug elimination may lead to significant toxicity after relatively mild exposure.

1. **Skin absorption.** Neonates have a very high ratio of surface area to body weight, which predisposes them to poisoning via percutaneous absorption (eg, hexachlorophene, boric acid, or alcohols).

2. **Elimination** of many drugs (eg, acetaminophen, many antibiotics, caffeine, lidocaine, morphine, phenytoin, and theophylline) is prolonged in neonates. For example, the half-life of caffeine is approximately 3 hours in adults but may be greater than 100 hours in newborns.

B. **Neonatal drug withdrawal** may occur in infants with chronic prenatal exposure to illicit or therapeutic drugs. The onset is usually within 72 hours of birth, but postnatal onset as late as 14 days has been reported. Signs usually commence in the nursery, and patients should not be discharged until clinically stable. However, with early discharge from nurseries being encouraged in many health care settings, an infant's first presentation of withdrawal may be to an emergency department or other outpatient setting. Initial presentation may include nonspecific signs such as mild colic or poor feeding, or may include severe findings such as withdrawal seizures or excessive diarrhea.

1. **Opioids** (especially methadone and heroin) are the most common cause of serious neonatal drug withdrawal symptoms. Other drugs for which a withdrawal syndrome has been reported include phencyclidine (PCP), cocaine, amphetamines, tricyclic antidepressants, phenothiazines, benzodiazepines, barbiturates, ethanol, clonidine, diphenhydramine, lithium, meprobamate, and theophylline. A careful drug history from the mother should include exposures to illicit drugs, alcohol, and prescription and over-the-counter medications, and whether she is breast-feeding.

2. **The manifestations of neonatal opioid withdrawal** include inability to sleep, irritability, tremulousness, inconsolability, high-pitched incessant cry, hypertonia, hyperreflexia, sneezing and yawning, lacrimation, disorganized suck, poor feeding, vomiting, diarrhea, tachypnea or respiratory distress, tachycardia, autonomic dysfunction, sweating, fevers, and seizures. Morbidity and mortality from untreated opioid withdrawal can be significant, may be associated with weight loss, metabolic acidosis, respiratory alkalosis, dehydration, electrolyte imbalance, and seizures. Withdrawal is a diagnosis of exclusion; other diagnostic considerations include sepsis, hypoglycemia, hypocalcemia, and hypoxia, hyperbilirubinemia, hypomagnesemia, hyperthyroidism, and intracranial hemorrhage. Seizures do not usually occur as the only clinical manifestation of opioid withdrawal.

3. **Treatment of neonatal opioid withdrawal** is largely supportive, and includes swaddling, rocking, a quiet room, frequent small feedings with a high-calorie formula, and intravenous fluids or parental nutrition as necessary. A variety of drugs have been used, including morphine, paregoric, tincture of opium, diazepam, lorazepam, chlorpromazine, and phenobarbital. Abstinence-scoring systems may yield objective findings to evaluate and to treat opioid withdrawal. The scoring and treatment of a neonate in withdrawal should be supervised by a neonatologist or pediatric provider experienced with neonatal withdrawal.

VI. **Pregnancy and drugs or chemicals.** The etiology of congenital abnormalities and adverse pregnancy outcomes is multi-factorial; only approximately 1–5% of all defects may be attributable to prescription medications, chemicals, hyperthermia, ionizing radiation, and other reproductive toxins and teratogens.

A. Adverse effects of drugs and chemicals in pregnancy are dose- and time-dependent. Pregnancy termination is not indicated simply based on exposure to a contraindicated drug. Risks must be carefully considered and evaluated by the patient and health care provider. Although some exposures are associated with well-documented teratogenicity (eg, valproic acid), the majority of drug-exposed fetuses incur little or no adverse effect with close medical monitoring and supervision.

B. The adverse effects of the drug or chemical on pregnancy or the fetus may include prevention of implantation (eg, nonsteroidal anti-inflammatory drugs [NSAIDs]), fetal death (eg, intra-amniotic methylene blue), malformations

TABLE I–45. DRUGS AND CHEMICALS THAT POSE A RISK TO THE FETUS OR PREGNANCY

Drug Name	FDA[a] Category	Recommendation or Comments[b]
Amantadine	C	Contraindicated (first trimester)
Aminoglutethimide (anticonvulsant)	D	No data
Aminopterin	X	Contraindicated (any trimester)
Amiodarone	D	Risk (third trimester)
Amphetamine	C	Risk (third trimester)
Androgenic hormones	X	Contraindicated (any trimester)
Angiotensin-converting enzyme (ACE) inhibitors	C/D	Risk (second and third trimesters)
Angiotensin II receptor antagonists	C/D	Risk (second and third trimesters)
Antidepressants	C	Risk (third trimester)
Antineoplastic cytotoxic agents	C/D/X	Look up individual drugs. Only category X drugs are given in table. Recommendations vary widely.
Azathioprine	D	Risk (third trimester)
Barbiturates	C or D	Recommendation by drug varies from Probably Compatible to Risk (first and third trimesters)
Benzodiazepines	D/X	Recommendation varies by agent from Low Risk (animal data) to Contraindicated (any trimester). Look up individual agents.
Benzphetamine	X	Contraindicated (any trimester)
Beta-adrenergic blockers	C/D	Risk (second and third trimesters)
Bexarotene	X	Contraindicated (any trimester)
Blue cohosh (herb)	C	Risk (third trimester)—used to stimulate labor
Bromides, anticonvulsant	D	Risk (third trimester)
Carbamazepine	D	Compatible: benefits >> risks
Carbarsone, 29% arsenic	D	Contraindicated (any trimester)
Carbimazole	D	Risk (third trimester); use propylthiouracil (PTH)
Chenodiol	X	Contraindicated (any trimester)
Ciguatoxin		Contraindicated (any trimester)
Clarithromycin	C	High risk (animal data)
Clomiphene (fertility agent)	X	Contraindicated (any trimester)
Clonazepam, anticonvulsant	D	Low risk (animal data)
Cocaine, systemic use	C/X	Contraindicated (any trimester; topical use okay)
Colchicine	D	Risk (animal data)
Corticosteroids	C/D	Recommendation varies from compatible, to benefits >> risks, to risk in third trimester. Look up individual agents.
Coumarin derivatives	D/X	Contraindicated (any trimester)
Diazoxide	C	Risk (third trimester)
Dihydroergotamine	X	Contraindicated (any trimester)
Diuretics	B or C/D	Compatible but do not use for gestational hypertension (Category D)
"Ecstasy" (methylenedioxy-methamphetamine, MDMA)	C	Contraindicated (any trimester)
Edrophonium	C	Risk (third trimester)
Electricity	D	Risk (third trimester); stillbirth associated with relatively mild shocks
Epinephrine	C	Risk (third trimester)
Ergotamine	X	Contraindicated (any trimester)

(continued)

TABLE I–45. DRUGS AND CHEMICALS THAT POSE A RISK TO THE FETUS OR PREGNANCY (CONTINUED)

Drug Name	FDA[a] Category	Recommendation or Comments[b]
Erythromycin (estolate salt)		Hepatic toxicity in pregnant women. Other salts are compatible
Estrogenic hormones	X	Contraindicated (any trimester)
Ethanol	D/X	Contraindicated (any trimester)
Ethotoin	D	Compatible (benefits >> risks)
Fenfluramine	C	Contraindicated (any trimester)
Fluconazole ≥ 400 mg/d	C	Risk (third trimester)
Flucytosine	C	Contraindicated (first trimester)
Fluorouracil	D/X	Contraindicated (first trimester)
Fluphenazine	C	Risk (third trimester)
HMG Co-A[c] reductase inhibitors: all drugs in this class	X	Contraindicated (any trimester)
Iodide ^{125}I and ^{131}I (radiopharmaceuticals)	X	Contraindicated (any trimester)—ablates fetal Thyroid
Iodine and iodide-containing compounds, including topicals, expectorants, and diagnostic agents	D/X	Varies from contraindicated (any trimester) to risk (second and third trimesters). Fetal and neonatal goiter and hypothyroidism
Kanamycin	D	Risk (third trimester)
Leflunomide	X	Contraindicated (any trimester)
Lenalidomide (potent thalidomide analog)	X	Contraindicated (any trimester)
Leuprolide	X	Contraindicated (any trimester)
Lithium	D	Risk (third trimester)
LSD (lysergic acid diethylamide)	C	Contraindicated (any trimester)
Marijuana	X	Contraindicated (any trimester)
Measles vaccine (live attenuated)	C	Contraindicated (any trimester)—avoid from 1–2 months before pregnancy until after delivery
Menadiol, menadione, vitamin K_3	C	Risk (third trimester)
Mephobarbital, anticonvulsant	D	Compatible: benefits >> risks
Meprobamate	D	Contraindicated (first trimester)
Metaraminol	C	Risk (second and third trimesters)
Methaqualone	D	No data
Methimazole	D	Risk (third trimester); use propylthiouracil (PTH)
Methotrexate	X	Contraindicated (any trimester)
Methylene blue, intra-amniotic	C/D	Contraindicated (second and third trimesters)
Methylergonovine maleate, ergot derivative	C	Contraindicated (any trimester)
Mifepristone, RU 486	X	Contraindicated (any trimester)
Misoprostol (oral)	X	Contraindicated (any trimester)
Misoprostol: low dose for cervical ripening	X	Low risk (human data)
Mumps vaccine (live attenuated)	C	Contraindicated (any trimester)
Naloxone	B	Compatible
Narcotic agonist analgesics	B or C/D	Risk (third trimester): Category D—risk associated with prolonged use or high doses at term
Narcotic agonist-antagonist analgesics	B or C/D	Risk (third trimester)
Narcotic antagonists (except naloxone)	D	Risk (third trimester) or no data; use naloxone.

(*continued*)

TABLE I–45. DRUGS AND CHEMICALS THAT POSE A RISK TO THE FETUS OR PREGNANCY (CONTINUED)

Drug Name	FDA[a] Category	Recommendation or Comments[b]
Nonsteroidal anti-inflammatory drugs (NSAIDs, full-dose aspirin)	B or C/D	Risk (first and third trimesters)
Norepinephrine	D	Risk (third trimester)
Oral antidiabetic agents	C	Insulin is the preferred agent for management of diabetes during pregnancy. Oral antidiabetic agents cross placenta—risk for severe hypoglycemia in newborn
p-Aminosalicylic acid	C	Risk (third trimester)
Paramethadione	D	Contraindicated (first trimester)
Penicillamine	D	Risk (third trimester)
Phencyclidine	X	Contraindicated (any trimester)
Phensuximide	D	Risk (third trimester)
Phentermine	C	Contraindicated (any trimester)
Phenylephrine	C	Risk (third trimester)
Phenytoin	D	Compatible: benefits >> risks
Plicamycin, mithramycin	X	Contraindicated (first trimester)
Podofilox, podophyllum	C	Contraindicated (any trimester)
Primidone	D	Risk (third trimester)
Progestogenic hormones	D or X	Contraindicated (any trimester)
Quinine, antimalarial	D/X	Risk (third trimester)
Quinolone antibiotics	C	Arthropathy in immature animals
Retinoid agents	X	Contraindicated (any trimester)
Ribavirin, antiviral	X	Contraindicated (any trimester)
Rubella vaccine (live attenuated)	C/D	Contraindicated (any trimester)—avoid from 1–2 months before pregnancy until after delivery
Smallpox vaccine (live attenuated)	X	Epidemic: compatible (benefits >> risks); otherwise risk (third trimester)
Streptomycin	D	Risk (third trimester)
Sulfonamides	C/D	Risk (third trimester)
Tacrolimus	C	Risk (third trimester)
Tamoxifen	D	Contraindicated (any trimester)
Terpin hydrate	D	Contraindicated (any trimester) owing to ethanol content
Tetracyclines, all	D	Contraindicated (second and third trimesters)
Thalidomide and analogs	X	Contraindicated (any trimester)
Tramadol	C	Risk (third trimester)
Tretinoin: topical doses	C	Low risk (human data)
Triamterene	C/D	Risk (any trimester)—weak folic acid antagonist, and Category D for gestational hypertension use
Trimethadione	D	Contraindicated (first trimester)
Trimethaphan	C	Contraindicated (any trimester)
Trimethoprim	C	Risk (third trimester)
Valproic acid	D	Risk (third trimester)
Varicella vaccine (live attenuated)	C	Contraindicated (any trimester)—avoid from 1–2 months before pregnancy until after delivery
Venezuelan equine encephalitis vaccine, VEE TC-84 (live attenuated)	X	Contraindicated (any trimester)—avoid from 1–2 months before pregnancy until after delivery
Vidarabine, antiviral	C	Teratogenic in animals

(continued)

TABLE I–45. DRUGS AND CHEMICALS THAT POSE A RISK TO THE FETUS OR PREGNANCY (CONTINUED)

Drug Name	FDA[a] Category	Recommendation or Comments[b]
Vitamin A	A/X	Contraindicated (any trimester) in doses greater than FDA RDA[c]
Vitamin D	A/D	Compatible except for doses greater than FDA RDA[c]
Vitamin K_3, menadiol, menadione	C	Risk (third trimester)
Voriconazole	D	Teratogenic in animals
Warfarin	D/X	Contraindicated (any trimester)
Yellow fever vaccine (live attenuated)	D	Epidemic: compatible (benefits >> risks). Otherwise avoid from 1–2 months before pregnancy until after delivery
Zonisamide, anticonvulsant	C	Teratogenic in animals

[a]FDA categories (see also p 498): A = controlled study has shown no risk; B = no evidence of risk in humans; C = risk cannot be ruled out; D = positive evidence of risk; X = contraindicated in pregnancy. Note: in November 2016 the FDA removed the categories A, B, C, D and X to be replaced by more explanatory labeling.
[b]Data from Briggs GG, Freeman RK, Yaffe SJ. *Drugs in Pregnancy and Lactation: A Reference Guide to Fetal and Neonatal Risk.* 8th ed. Lippincott Williams & Wilkins; 2008. All recommendations are based on human data. Animal data are cited only if human data are unavailable and animal data show serious toxicity in multiple species. Risk: Human data suggest risk; exposure during pregnancy should be avoided unless the benefits of the drug outweigh the risks. Contraindicated: Human exposure data indicate that the drug should not be used in pregnancy. Numbers in parentheses indicate times during pregnancy when the drug is contraindicated or poses risk: All: any time during pregnancy.
[c]HMG Co-A, hepatic hydroxymethylglutaryl coenzyme A; RDA, recommended daily allowance.

(eg, thalidomide), postnatal adverse physiologic effects (eg, oral hypoglycemics), and adverse outcomes that may manifest years after birth (eg, diethylstilbestrol).

Certain drugs with a very long half-life (eg, ribavirin, retinoids) may require cessation of exposure for several months before conception.

C. For clinical assistance in determining the risk posed to a pregnancy by a specific exposure, contact **Motherisk** (*www.motherisk.org*, 1-877-439-2744 toll-free, or 416-813-6780). Motherisk is an evidence-based information and phone consultation service based in Toronto, Canada devoted to the study of the safety or risk of drugs, chemicals, and disease during pregnancy and lactation.

D. Breastfeeding. Some drugs can enter breast milk and cause intoxication in the infant. A number of variables determine whether the drug may pose a risk, including its size, lipid solubility, and oral bioavailability. A useful information resource is **LactMed** (https://toxnet.nlm.nih.gov/newtoxnet/lactmed.htm).

E. Table I–45 lists the **FDA pregnancy ratings** of drugs and chemicals (see also TABLE III–1). Some drugs have more than one pregnancy category because the category changes with the trimester or because different manufacturers/authorities are not in agreement. Briggs GG, Freeman RK, Yaffe SJ. *Drugs in Pregnancy and Lactation: A Reference Guide to Fetal and Neonatal Risk.* 9th ed. Lippincott Williams & Wilkins; 2011 provide a comprehensive source of material regarding the effects of drugs and chemicals on pregnancy and lactation. This source organizes data for individual drugs into monographs, with evidence-based recommendations regarding usage and risk. Drugs in pregnancy category D or X, and those noted with additional "risk" or "contraindication" by Briggs et al. are included in Table I–45. Drugs that are labeled FDA category D or X and selected anticonvulsants may still be administered during pregnancy with close medical monitoring and supervision, if the benefits to the mother outweigh the risks to the fetus (maternal benefit >> fetal risk).

▶ SPECIAL CONSIDERATIONS IN THE EVALUATION OF DRUG-FACILITATED CRIMES

Jo Ellen Dyer, PharmD

Since 1996, reports of drug-facilitated crimes have been increasing. Drugs may be used to render the victim helpless or unconscious so that the assailant can commit a rape or robbery. The amnestic effects of many of the drugs used often leave little or no recollection of the events, making investigation, and prosecution of the suspect more difficult.

I. **High-risk populations** include single women, men or unsuspecting travelers, new to an area, without companions. Drug administration may occur in a bar, club, or on public transportation when the victim leaves a drink unattended or accepts an opened bottle or drink. In one series of self-reported cases, half the victims reported meeting the assailant in a public place, and more than 70% of the victims knew the assailant (eg, a friend or colleague).

II. **Drugs used.** Contrary to the popular belief that specific "date rape drugs" are involved in these crimes, a variety of drugs with amnestic or central nervous system (CNS) depressant effects can be used to facilitate assault, including opioids, anesthetics, benzodiazepines, other sedative-hypnotic drugs, skeletal muscle relaxants, anticholinergics, hallucinogens, clonidine, aromatic solvents, and of course ethanol (Table I-46).

   A. Note that many of these drugs are also commonly used to "get high" and may have been self-administered by the victim for this purpose.

TABLE I–46. EXAMPLES OF SUBSTANCES DETECTED IN URINE OF DRUG-FACILITATED ASSAULT VICTIMS

Drug	Usual Duration of Detection in Urine[a]
Amphetamines	1–3 days
Barbiturates	2–7 days
Benzodiazepines	2–7 days
Benzoylecgonine	1–2 days
Cannabinoids	2–5 days (single use)
Carisoprodol	1–2 days[b]
Chloral hydrate	1–2 days[b]
Clonidine	1–2 days[b]
Cyclobenzaprine	1–2 days[b]
Diphenhydramine	1–2 days[b]
Ethanol	Less than 1 day
Gamma hydroxybutyrate (GHB)	Less than 1 day[b]
Ketamine	1–2 days[b]
Meprobamate	1–2 days[b]
Opioids	2–3 days
Scopolamine	1–2 days[b]

[a]Estimate of the duration of detection, with the use of methods more sensitive than typical drug screening. Actual detection will depend on individual metabolism, dose, and concentration in specimen. Also, assays vary in sensitivity and specificity depending on the laboratory, so it is important to consult with the laboratory for definitive information.

[b]Specific information not available; duration given is an estimate.

B. Benzodiazepines are often selected for their anterograde amnestic effect, which is related to but distinct from sedation. The strength of the amnestic effects can be predicted to increase with the dose, rapidity of onset, lipophilic character, and slow redistribution from the CNS.

III. Routes of surreptitious drug administration

A. Drink: tablet, ice, liquid in eyedropper.

B. Smoke: applied to a cigarette or joint.

C. Ingestion: brownie, gelatin, fruit, other food.

D. Vaginal syringe: drug in contraceptive gel.

E. Represented as another drug.

IV. **Clinical evaluation.** If the victims present early after the assault, they may still be under the influence of the drug and may appear inappropriately disinhibited or relaxed for the situation. Unfortunately, victims often present many hours, days, or even weeks after the assault, making the collection of physical and biochemical evidence much more difficult. Determining the time course of drug effects with estimation of last memory and first recall may provide useful information to investigators.

A. Use open-ended questions to avoid suggesting symptoms to a victim who may be trying to fill in a lapse in memory.

B. Perform a thorough examination and maintain the legal chain of custody for any specimens obtained.

V. **Laboratory.** Timing of laboratory analysis may be crucial, as elimination rates of commonly used sedative and amnestic drugs vary and some may be extremely short. Immediate collection of toxicology specimens is important to avoid loss of evidence. For a service that deals in assaults or sexual abuse, it is important to confer in advance with the laboratory so that it is clearly understood what type of testing will be performed; the laboratory can then develop a testing strategy (what tests to use, the sequence of tests and confirmations, and the level of sensitivity and specificity). Such a service should ideally be part of law enforcement. Note that most clinical laboratories do not have the ability to document the chain of custody often needed in criminal proceedings.

A. **Blood.** Collect a 10- to 30-mL specimen as soon as possible and within 24 hours of the alleged assault. Have the specimen centrifuged and the plasma or serum frozen for future analysis. Pharmacokinetic evaluation of multiple blood levels may allow estimations of time course, level of consciousness, and amount ingested.

B. **Urine.** Collect a 100-mL specimen if it is within 72 hours of suspected ingestion and freeze for analysis. (***Note:*** Flunitrazepam [Rohypnol] may be detected for up to 96 hours.)

C. **Hair.** Collect four strands of about 100 hairs each from the vertex posterior close to the scalp 4–5 weeks after the offense and mark the root end. Hair analysis may become a useful complement to conventional blood and urine drug analysis. Currently, however, few forensic laboratories perform hair analysis, and legally defensible methods and values are needed for a single drug exposure.

D. **Analysis** (see **Table I-46**). Hospital laboratories doing routine toxicology testing have different testing strategies and levels of detection and may not detect drugs used to facilitate assault. Rapid toxicology screens (eg, "drugs of abuse" screens) *will not detect* all commonly available benzodiazepines or other CNS depressants (eg, ketamine, gamma-hydroxybutyrate, and carisoprodol) that are popular drugs of abuse. It may be necessary to contract for special services through national reference laboratories, state laboratories, or a local medical examiner's office to identify less common drugs used for assault and to detect very low levels of drugs that remain in cases of late presentation.

VI. **Treatment** of the intoxication is based on the clinical effects of the drug(s) involved. The assessment and treatment of effects related to individual drugs are detailed in Section II of this book. In addition, victims often need psychological support and counseling and the involvement of law enforcement authorities. If the assault involves a minor, state law generally mandates reporting to child protection services and law enforcement officials.

GENERAL TEXTBOOKS AND OTHER REFERENCES IN CLINICAL TOXICOLOGY

Brent J, Walace K, Burkhart K, et al. *Critical Care Toxicology: Diagnosis and Management of the Critically Poisoned Patient*. 1st ed. Mosby; 2005.

Dart RC, et al., eds. *Medical Toxicology*. 3rd ed. Lippincott Williams & Wilkins; 2004.

Ford M, ed. *Clinical Toxicology.* WB Saunders, 2000.

Goldfrank LR, et al., eds. *Goldfrank's Toxicologic Emergencies.* 10th ed. McGraw-Hill; 2014.

Haddad LM, Winchester JF, Shannon M, eds. *Clinical Management of Poisoning and Drug Overdose.* 3rd ed. WB Saunders; 1998.

Poisindex [computerized poison information system, available as CD-ROM or mainframe application, updated quarterly]. Micromedex [updated quarterly]. Medical Economics.

SELECTED INTERNET SITES

American Academy of Clinical Toxicology: *http://www.clintox.org*
American Association of Poison Control Centers: *http://www.aapcc.org*
American College of Medical Toxicology: *http://www.acmt.net*
Agency for Toxic Substances and Disease Registry: *http://www.atsdr.cdc.gov*
Animal Poison Control Center: *http://www.aspca.org*
California Poison Control System. www.calpoison.org
Centers for Disease Control: *http://www.cdc.gov*
Food and Drug Administration: *http://www.fda.gov*
National Institute on Drug Abuse: *http://www.nida.nih.gov*
National Pesticide Information Center: *http://www.npic.orst.edu*
PubMed: *http://www.ncbi.nlm.nih.gov*
QT Prolonging Drugs: *http://www.qtdrugs.org*
Substance Abuse and Mental Health Services Administration: *http://workplace.samhsa.gov*
TOXNET databases: *http://toxnet.nlm.nih.gov/index.html*

SECTION II. Specific Poisons and Drugs: Diagnosis and Treatment

▶ ACETAMINOPHEN

Kent R. Olson, MD

Acetaminophen (Anacin-3, Liquiprin, Panadol, Paracetamol, Tempra, Tylenol, and many other brands) is a widely used drug found in many over-the-counter and prescription analgesics and cold remedies. When it is combined with another drug, such as diphenhydramine, codeine, hydrocodone, oxycodone, dextromethorphan, or propoxyphene, the more dramatic acute symptoms caused by the other drug may mask the mild and nonspecific symptoms of early acetaminophen toxicity, resulting in a missed diagnosis or delayed antidotal treatment. Common combination products containing acetaminophen include the following: Darvocet, Excedrin ES, Lorcet, Norco, NyQuil, Percocet, Unisom Dual Relief Formula, Sominex 2, Tylenol with Codeine, Tylenol PM, Tylox, Vicks Formula 44-D, and Vicodin.

I. **Mechanism of toxicity**
   - A. **Hepatic injury.** One of the products of normal metabolism of acetaminophen by cytochrome P450 (CYP) mixed-function oxidase enzymes is highly toxic; normally this reactive metabolite (NAPQI) is detoxified rapidly by glutathione in liver cells. However, in an overdose, production of NAPQI exceeds glutathione capacity and the metabolite reacts directly with hepatic macromolecules, causing liver injury.
   - B. **Renal damage** may occur by the same mechanism, owing to renal CYP metabolism.
   - C. Overdose during **pregnancy** has been associated with fetal death and spontaneous abortion.
   - D. **Very high levels** of acetaminophen can cause lactic acidosis and altered mental status by uncertain mechanisms, probably involving mitochondrial dysfunction.
   - E. **Pharmacokinetics.** Acetaminophen is rapidly absorbed, with peak levels usually reached within 30–120 minutes. (***Note:*** Absorption may be delayed after ingestion of sustained-release products [Tylenol Extended Release, Tylenol Arthritis] or with co-ingestion of opioids or anticholinergics.) Volume of distribution (Vd) is 0.8–1 L/kg. Elimination is mainly by liver conjugation (90%) to nontoxic glucuronides or sulfates; mixed-function oxidase (CYP2E1, CYP1A2) accounts for only about 3–8% but produces a toxic intermediate (see Item A above). The elimination half-life is 1–3 hours after a therapeutic dose but may be greater than 12 hours after an overdose (see also Table II–66, p 462).

II. **Toxic dose**
   - A. **Acute ingestion** of more than 200 mg/kg in children or 6–7 g in adults is potentially hepatotoxic.
     1. Children younger than 10–12 years appear to be less susceptible to hepatotoxicity because of the smaller contribution of CYP to acetaminophen metabolism.
     2. In contrast, the margin of safety may be lower in patients with induced CYP microsomal enzymes because more of the toxic metabolite may be produced. **High-risk patients** include alcoholics and patients taking inducers of CYP2E1, such as isoniazid. Fasting and malnutrition may also increase the risk for hepatotoxicity, presumably by lowering cellular glutathione stores.
   - B. **Chronic toxicity** has been reported after daily consumption of supratherapeutic doses. A consensus guideline from the American Association of Poison Control Centers (AAPCC) recommends medical evaluation if more than 150 mg/kg/d (or 6 g/d) has been ingested for 2 days or longer. One study

reported elevated transaminases in more than one-third of healthy volunteers given doses of 4 g/d for several days.

1. Children have developed toxicity after receiving as little as 100–150 mg/kg/d for 2–8 days. The AAPCC guideline recommends medical evaluation for doses of more than 150 mg/kg/d for 2 days or 100 mg/kg/d for 3 days or more. There is a single case report of hepatotoxicity in an infant receiving 72 mg/kg/d for 10 days.
2. As with acute overdose, the risk for injury from chronic use may be greater in alcoholic patients and persons taking isoniazid and other drugs that induce CYP2E1.

C. **Intravenous acetaminophen** (10 mg/mL) is now available and 10-fold dosing errors have occurred. An acute overdose of more than 150 mg/kg is considered potentially toxic. (One report of hepatotoxicity after 75 mg/kg IV acetaminophen was probably due to other complications leading to ischemic liver injury.)

III. **Clinical presentation.** Clinical manifestations depend on the time after ingestion.

A. **Early** after acute acetaminophen overdose, there are usually no symptoms other than anorexia, nausea, or vomiting. Rarely, a massive overdose may cause altered mental status, hypotension, and metabolic acidosis in the absence of any laboratory evidence of liver damage. Transient prolongation of the prothrombin time/international normalized ratio (PT/INR) in the absence of hepatitis has been noted in the first 24 hours; some, but not all, of these patients go on to develop liver injury.

B. **After 24–48 hours,** when aspartate aminotransferase (AST) and alanine aminotransferase (ALT) begin to rise, hepatic necrosis becomes evident. If acute fulminant hepatic failure occurs, death may ensue. Encephalopathy, metabolic acidosis, and a continuing rise in PT/INR indicate a poor prognosis. Acute renal failure occasionally occurs, with or without concomitant liver failure.

C. **Chronic** excessive use of acetaminophen.

1. Patients often have nausea and vomiting, and may already show evidence of hepatic injury by the time they seek medical care.
2. Glutathione depletion associated with chronic acetaminophen ingestion has also been associated with anion gap metabolic acidosis due to the accumulation of 5-oxoproline.

IV. **Diagnosis.** Prompt diagnosis is possible only if the ingestion is suspected and a serum acetaminophen level is obtained. However, patients may fail to provide the history of acetaminophen ingestion because they are unable (eg, comatose from another ingestion), unwilling, or unaware of its importance. Therefore, many clinicians routinely order acetaminophen levels in all overdose patients regardless of the history of substances ingested.

A. **Specific levels.** ***Note:*** 1 mg/L = 1 mcg/mL = 6.6 mcmol/L.

1. After an acute oral or intravenous overdose, obtain a serum acetaminophen level 4 hours after the overdose and use the nomogram (Figure II–1) to predict the likelihood of toxicity. Do not attempt to interpret a level drawn before 4 hours unless it is "nondetectable." Obtain a second level at 8 hours if the 4-hour value is borderline or if delayed absorption is anticipated.
2. The nomogram should not be used to assess chronic or repeated ingestions.
3. Falsely elevated acetaminophen levels may occur in the presence of high levels of salicylate and other interferents by certain older laboratory methods (see Table I–33, p 46). This problem is rare with currently used analytic methods.

B. **Other useful laboratory studies** include electrolytes (presence of an anion gap), glucose, BUN, creatinine, liver aminotransferases, bilirubin, and PT/INR.

V. **Treatment**

A. **Emergency and supportive measures**

1. **Spontaneous vomiting** may delay the oral administration of antidote or charcoal (see below) and can be treated with metoclopramide (p 581) or a serotonin (5-HT3) receptor antagonist such as ondansetron (p 597).

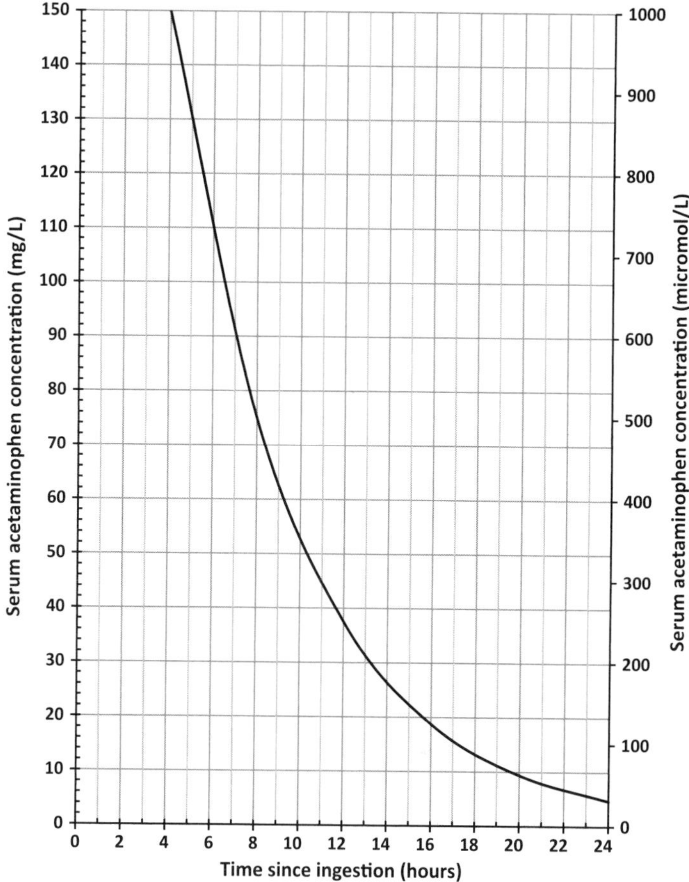

FIGURE II–1. Nomogram for prediction of acetaminophen hepatotoxicity following acute overdosage. Patients with serum levels above the line after acute overdose should receive antidotal treatment. (Adapted, with permission, from Daly FF et al. Guidelines for the management of paracetamol poisoning in Australia and New Zealand–explanation and elaboration. A consensus statement from clinical toxicologists consulting to the Australasian poisons information centres. *Med J Austr.* 2008;188:296. © Copyright The Medical Journal of Australia.)

2. Provide general supportive care for hepatic or renal failure if it occurs. Emergency **liver transplant** may be necessary for fulminant hepatic failure. Encephalopathy, metabolic acidosis, hypoglycemia, and a progressive rise in the prothrombin time are indications of severe liver injury.

B. Specific drugs and antidotes

1. **Acute single** ingestion or intravenous overdose
   a. If the serum level falls above the treatment line on the nomogram or if stat serum levels are not immediately available, initiate antidotal therapy with ***N*-acetylcysteine** (NAC; p 499). The effectiveness of NAC depends on **early treatment**, before the toxic metabolite accumulates; it is of maximal benefit if started within 8–10 hours and of diminishing value

after 12–16 hours; however, treatment should not be withheld even if the delay is 24 hours or more. If vomiting interferes with or threatens to delay oral acetylcysteine administration, give the NAC IV.

b. If the serum level falls below but near the nomogram line, consider giving NAC if the patient is at increased risk for toxicity—for example, if the patient is alcoholic, is taking a drug that induces CYP2E1 activity (eg, isoniazid [INH]), or has taken multiple or subacute overdoses—or if the time of ingestion is uncertain or unreliable.

c. If the serum level falls well below the nomogram line, few clinicians would treat with NAC unless the time of ingestion is very uncertain or the patient is considered to be at particularly high risk.

d. ***Note:*** After ingestion of **extended-release** tablets (eg, Tylenol Extended Release, Tylenol Arthritis Pain), which are designed for prolonged absorption, there may be a delay before the peak acetaminophen level is reached. This can also occur after co-ingestion of drugs that delay gastric emptying, such as opioids and anticholinergics (eg, Tylenol PM). In such circumstances, repeat the serum acetaminophen level at 8 hours and possibly 12 hours. In such cases, it may be prudent to initiate NAC therapy before 8 hours while waiting for subsequent levels.

e. Duration of NAC treatment. The conventional US protocol for the treatment of acetaminophen poisoning calls for 17 doses of oral NAC given over approximately 72 hours. However, for decades successful protocols in the United States, Canada, the United Kingdom, and Europe have used IV NAC for only 20 hours. In uncomplicated cases, give NAC (orally or IV) for 20 hours (or until acetaminophen levels are no longer detectable) and follow hepatic transaminase levels and the PT/INR; if evidence of liver injury develops, continue NAC until liver function tests are improving.

f. Massive ingestion. Although data is lacking, it is recommended to use a higher dose of NAC to treat very large overdoses. The intravenous NAC protocol delivers a total of only 300 mg/kg NAC over 21 hours, compared with the oral regimen which delivers a total of 1,190 mg/kg NAC over 72 hours. See NAC, p 499 for detailed recommendations.

2. Chronic or repeated acetaminophen ingestions: Patients may give a history of several doses taken over 24 hours or more, in which case the nomogram cannot accurately estimate the risk for hepatotoxicity. In such cases, we advise NAC treatment if the amount ingested was more than 200 mg/kg within a 24-hour period, 150 mg/kg/d for 2 days, or 100 mg/kg/d for 3 days or more; if liver enzymes are elevated; if there is detectable acetaminophen in the serum; or if the patient falls within a high-risk group (see above). Treatment may be stopped when acetaminophen is no longer detectable if the liver enzymes and PT/INR are normal.

C. Decontamination (p 50). Administer activated charcoal orally if conditions are appropriate (see Table I–38, p 54). Gastric lavage is not necessary after small-to-moderate ingestions if activated charcoal can be given promptly.

1. Although activated charcoal adsorbs some of the orally administered antidote NAC, this effect is not considered clinically important.

2. Do not administer charcoal if more than 1–2 hours has passed since ingestion unless delayed absorption is suspected (eg, as with Tylenol Extended Release, Tylenol Arthritis Pain, or co-ingestants containing opioids or anticholinergic agents).

D. Enhanced elimination. Hemodialysis effectively removes acetaminophen from the blood but is not generally indicated because antidotal therapy is so effective. Dialysis should be considered for massive ingestions with very high levels (eg, over 900–1,000 mg/L) complicated by severe acidosis, coma and/or hypotension.

▶ ACONITE AND OTHER SODIUM CHANNEL OPENERS

G. Patrick Daubert, MD

Aconitine is probably the best-known of the sodium channel openers and is found in monkshood or wolfsbane (*Aconitum napellus*). Other sodium channel openers include veratridine from false or green hellebore (*Veratrum* genus), grayanotoxins from azalea and rhododendron (*Rhododendron* species), death camas (*Zigadenus*), and mountain laurel (*Kalmia latifolia*).

Aconitine has been found in a number of Chinese herbal remedies, most notably *chuanwu* and *caowu* and the Tibetan medicine *Manquin*. Most cases of acute poisoning result from the ingestion of herbs containing aconitine. Grayanotoxins have largely been reported to cause intoxication in regions where honey is produced from *Rhododendron* species. Veratridine has historically been used in both insecticides and medicinals.

Symptoms of sodium channel opener poisoning include numbness, tingling of the lips and tongue, bradycardia or irregular pulse, gastroenteritis, respiratory failure, and vagus nerve stimulation. The paramount concern in managing acute poisoning is the management of lethal arrhythmias.

I. Mechanism of toxicity

A. These toxins primarily activate voltage-gated sodium channels. They are lipid soluble, which allows them access to the sodium channel–binding site embedded within the plasma membrane, where they preferentially bind to the open state of the sodium channel. They exert their action on nerve and muscle membranes by persistent activation of channel at the resting membrane potential.

B. Sodium channel openers cause early and delayed after-depolarizations in ventricular myocytes, which may be due to increased intracellular calcium and sodium. This may explain the reports of biventricular tachycardia and torsade de pointes in patients with aconitine intoxication.

II. Toxic dose

A. The amount and composition of plant alkaloids are the main factors determining the severity of intoxication, and these vary greatly with different species, the time of harvesting, and the method of processing. The lethal dose of aconitine is 0.1 mg/kg in mice and approximately 2 mg orally in humans.

III. Clinical presentation

A. Poisoning results in a combination of cardiovascular and neurologic toxicity. The onset of symptoms is 3 minutes to 2 hours, but typically within 10–20 minutes. Initial symptoms may include sneezing, diaphoresis, chills, weakness, perioral and limb numbness, and paresthesias, which are followed by vomiting, diarrhea, bradycardia with first-degree heart block or junctional bradycardia, dysrhythmias (including torsade de pointes), hypotension, CNS and respiratory depression, and seizures.

B. Death is usually due to ventricular arrhythmias. A characteristic but uncommon electrocardiographic finding is bidirectional ventricular tachycardia, similar to that seen with digoxin and other cardiac steroids.

C. In a retrospective review of 17 patients who had ingested herbal aconitine, the recovery time was from 1.5 to 2 days in mildly intoxicated patients, whereas patients with cardiovascular complications, including ventricular tachycardia, recovered in 7–9 days.

D. Hyperventilation resulting in respiratory alkalosis may be seen as a consequence of the central effect of aconitine on the medullary center.

IV. Diagnosis of sodium channel opener poisoning should be considered in anyone with the rapid onset of paresthesias, weakness, and ventricular tachycardia.

A. Specific levels. Diagnosis is based on a history of exposure. Routine laboratory testing is unlikely to be helpful. Blood and urine aconitine, veratridine, and grayanotoxins can be obtained by using liquid and gas chromatography with mass spectrometry.

B. Other useful studies include electrocardiogram, electrolytes, and glucose.

V. **Treatment**

A. **Emergency and supportive measures.** Treatment is therapeutically challenging and based primarily on case report data. Patients who have ingested plants with aconitine alkaloids should be admitted to a monitored setting, even if initially asymptomatic.

1. Protect the airway and assist ventilation (pp 1–7) if necessary.
2. Treat bradycardia (p 9), hypotension (p 15), coma (p 18), and seizures (p 23) if they occur.
3. Amiodarone and flecainide are reasonable first-line agents for ventricular tachycardia.
4. Magnesium (p 577) is recommended for prolonged QT interval and torsade de pointes.

B. **Specific drugs and antidotes.** None.

C. **Decontamination**

1. Single-dose activated charcoal (p 50) should be considered in patients who present within 1 hour of ingestion and have an intact or protected airway. Gastric lavage is not necessary after small-to-moderate ingestions if activated charcoal can be given promptly.
2. Whole-bowel irrigation has not been evaluated in the management of *Aconitum* or other sodium channel opener ingestions. Because of the rapid absorption of these diterpene alkaloids, it is not recommended.

D. **Enhanced elimination.** These compounds are rapidly absorbed and metabolized by the body, and extracorporeal methods of elimination would not be expected to enhance their elimination. The molecules are not likely dialyzable because of their high lipophilicity (resulting in large volumes of distribution).

▶ AMANTADINE

Ann Arens, MD

Amantadine (Symmetrel) is an antiviral agent whose dopaminergic properties make it effective in the treatment of Parkinson's disease and for prophylaxis against the parkinsonian side effects of neuroleptic agents. Although amantadine is no longer recommended for the treatment or prophylaxis of influenza because of resistance, it has been studied as a potential treatment for hepatitis C, Huntington's disease, brain injury or encephalopathy, and cocaine dependence. Its effects in acute overdose have been associated with seizures, arrhythmias, and death. Withdrawal from amantadine has also been linked to neuroleptic malignant syndrome.

I. **Mechanism of toxicity**

A. Amantadine is thought to increase dopamine levels in the peripheral and central nervous systems by enhancing the release of dopamine and preventing dopamine reuptake. It also acts as a noncompetitive antagonist at the *N*-methyl-D-aspartate (NMDA) receptor. It blocks potassium and sodium channels in cardiac myocytes, leading to QT prolongation and widened QRS intervals. In addition, it has anticholinergic properties, especially in overdose.

B. **Pharmacokinetics.** Peak absorption 1–4 hours; volume of distribution (Vd) 4–8 L/kg. Eliminated renally with a half-life of 7–37 hours (see also Table II–66, p 462).

II. **Toxic dose.** The toxic dose has not been determined. Because the elimination of amantadine depends almost entirely on kidney function, patients with renal insufficiency may develop intoxication with therapeutic doses. Ingestion of an estimated 800–1,500 mg caused status epilepticus in a 2-year-old child.

III. **Clinical presentation**

A. **Amantadine intoxication** causes agitation, visual hallucinations, nightmares, disorientation, delirium, slurred speech, ataxia, myoclonus, tremor, and sometimes seizures. Anticholinergic manifestations include dry mouth, urinary retention, and mydriasis. Obstructive acute renal failure due to urinary retention has also been reported. Interval changes on the ECG, such as QT prolongation and QRS widening, may be seen. Ventricular arrhythmias, including torsade de pointes (p 13) and premature ventricular contractions, may occur. Amantadine has also been reported to cause heart failure and acute respiratory distress syndrome (ARDS).

B. **Amantadine withdrawal,** either after standard therapeutic use or in the days after an acute overdose, may result in hyperthermia and rigidity (similar to neuroleptic malignant syndrome [p 21]).

IV. **Diagnosis** is based on a history of acute ingestion or is made by noting the aforementioned constellation of symptoms and signs in a patient taking amantadine.

A. **Specific levels** are not readily available. When available, serum amantadine levels above 1.5 mg/L have been associated with toxicity.

B. **Other useful laboratory studies** include electrolytes, BUN, creatinine, creatine kinase (CK), and ECG.

V. **Treatment**

A. **Emergency and supportive measures**

1. Maintain an open airway and assist ventilation if necessary (pp 1–4).
2. Treat coma (p 18), seizures (p 23), arrhythmias (p 13), and hyperthermia (p 21) if they occur.
3. Monitor an asymptomatic patient for at least 8–12 hours after acute ingestion.

B. **Specific drugs and antidotes.** There is no known antidote. Although some of the manifestations of toxicity are caused by the anticholinergic effects of amantadine, physostigmine should not be used if there is evidence of cardiac conduction disturbance (eg, wide QRS).

1. Treat **tachyarrhythmias** with lidocaine or amiodarone (if wide-complex) or beta blockers (if narrow-complex) such as propranolol (p 617) and esmolol (p 552). Use amiodarone with caution in patients with QT prolongation.
2. **Hyperthermia** requires urgent cooling measures (p 21) and may respond to muscle relaxants such as dantrolene (p 537). When hyperthermia occurs in the setting of amantadine withdrawal, some have advocated using amantadine as therapy.

C. **Decontamination.** Administer activated charcoal orally if conditions are appropriate (see Table I–38, p 54). Gastric lavage is not necessary after small-to-moderate ingestions if activated charcoal can be given promptly.

D. **Enhanced elimination.** Amantadine is not effectively removed by dialysis because the volume of distribution is very large (4–8 L/kg). In a patient with no renal function, dialysis may be attempted to remove a portion of the drug.

▶ AMMONIA

R. Steven Tharratt, MD, MPVM

Ammonia is widely used as a refrigerant, a fertilizer, and a household and commercial cleaning agent. Anhydrous ammonia (NH3) is a highly irritating gas that is very water soluble. It is also a key ingredient in the illicit production of methamphetamine. Aqueous solutions of ammonia may be strongly alkaline, depending on the concentration. Solutions for household use are usually 5–10% ammonia, but commercial solutions may be 25–30% or more. The addition of ammonia to chlorine or hypochlorite solutions will produce chloramine gas, an irritant with properties similar to those of chlorine (p 191).

I. **Mechanism of toxicity.** Ammonia gas is highly water soluble and rapidly produces an alkaline corrosive effect on contact with moist tissues, such as those of the eyes and upper respiratory tract. Exposure to aqueous solutions causes corrosive alkaline injury to the eyes, skin, or GI tract (see "Caustic and Corrosive Agents," p 186).

II. **Toxic dose**

A. **Ammonia gas.** The odor of ammonia is detectable at 3–5 ppm, and persons without protective gear will experience respiratory irritation at 50 ppm and usually self-evacuate the area. Eye irritation is common at 100 ppm. The workplace recommended exposure limit (ACGIH TLV-TWA) for anhydrous ammonia gas is 25 ppm as an 8-hour time-weighted average, and the short-term exposure limit (STEL) is 35 ppm. The level considered immediately dangerous to life or health (IDLH) is 300 ppm. The Emergency Response Planning Guidelines (ERPG) suggest that 25 ppm will cause no more than mild, transient health effects for exposures of up to 1 hour.

B. **Aqueous solutions.** Diluted aqueous solutions of ammonia (eg, <5%) rarely cause serious burns but are moderately irritating. More concentrated industrial cleaners (eg, 25–30% ammonia) are much more likely to cause serious corrosive injury.

III. **Clinical presentation.** Clinical manifestations depend on the physical state and route of exposure.

A. **Inhalation of ammonia gas.** Symptoms are rapid in onset owing to the high water solubility of ammonia and include immediate burning of the eyes, nose, and throat, accompanied by coughing. With serious exposure, swelling of the upper airway may rapidly cause airway obstruction, preceded by croupy cough, hoarseness, and stridor. Bronchospasm with wheezing may occur. Massive inhalational exposure may cause noncardiogenic pulmonary edema.

B. **Ingestion of aqueous solutions.** Immediate burning in the mouth and throat is common. With more concentrated solutions, serious esophageal and gastric burns are possible, and victims may have dysphagia, drooling, and severe throat, chest, and abdominal pain. Hematemesis and perforation of the esophagus or stomach may occur. The absence of oral burns does not rule out significant esophageal or gastric injury.

C. **Skin or eye contact with gas or solution.** Serious alkaline corrosive burns may occur. Contact with liquefied ammonia can cause frostbite injury.

IV. **Diagnosis** is based on a history of exposure and description of the typical ammonia smell, accompanied by typical irritative or corrosive effects on the eyes, skin, and upper respiratory or GI tract.

A. **Specific levels.** Blood ammonia levels may be elevated (normal, 8–33 mcmol/L) but are not predictive of toxicity. Testing should be performed on a stat basis because ammonia levels increase after blood collection owing to the breakdown of proteins.

B. **Other useful laboratory studies** may include electrolytes, arterial blood gases or pulse oximetry, and chest radiographs.

V. **Treatment**

A. **Emergency and supportive measures.** Treatment depends on the physical state of the ammonia and the route of exposure.

1. Inhalation of ammonia gas

   a. Observe carefully for signs of progressive upper airway obstruction, and intubate early if necessary (p 4).

   b. Administer humidified supplemental oxygen and bronchodilators for wheezing (p 8). Treat noncardiogenic pulmonary edema (p 7) if it occurs.

   c. Asymptomatic or mildly symptomatic patients may be discharged after a brief observation period.

2. **Ingestion of aqueous solution.** If a solution of 10% or greater has been ingested or if there are any symptoms of corrosive injury (dysphagia, drooling, or pain), perform flexible endoscopy to evaluate for serious esophageal or gastric injury. Obtain chest and abdominal radiographs to look for mediastinal or abdominal free air, which suggests esophageal or GI perforation.

3. **Eye exposure.** After eye irrigation, perform fluorescein examination and refer the patient to an ophthalmologist if there is evidence of corneal injury.

B. **Specific drugs and antidotes.** There is no specific antidote for these or other common caustic burns. The use of corticosteroids in alkaline corrosive ingestions has been proved ineffective and may be harmful in patients with perforation or serious infection.

C. **Decontamination** (p 50)

1. **Inhalation.** Remove immediately from exposure, and give supplemental oxygen if available.
2. **Ingestion**
   a. Immediately give water by mouth to dilute the ammonia. Do ***not*** induce vomiting because this may aggravate corrosive effects. Do ***not*** attempt to neutralize the ammonia (eg, with an acidic solution).
   b. Gastric lavage may be useful to remove liquid caustic in the stomach (in cases of deliberate ingestion of large quantities) and to prepare for endoscopy; use a small, flexible tube and pass it gently to avoid injury to damaged mucosa.
   c. Do ***not*** use activated charcoal; it does not adsorb ammonia, and it may obscure the endoscopist's view.
3. **Skin and eyes.** Remove contaminated clothing and wash exposed skin with water. Irrigate exposed eyes with copious amounts of tepid water or saline (p 51).

D. **Enhanced elimination.** There is no role for dialysis or other enhanced elimination procedures.

▶ AMPHETAMINES

Timothy E. Albertson, MD, MPH, PhD

Dextroamphetamine (Dexedrine) and **methylphenidate** (Ritalin) are used for the treatment of narcolepsy and for attention-deficit disorders in children. **Methamphetamine** ("crank," "speed"), 3,4-**methylenedioxymethamphetamine** (MDMA; "ecstasy"), **paramethoxyamphetamine** (PMA), and several other amphetamine derivatives, as well as a number of prescription drugs, are used as illicit stimulants and hallucinogens (see also "Lysergic Acid Diethylamide [LSD] and Other Hallucinogens," p 297). "Ice" is a high purity, smokable crystalline form of methamphetamine. Methamphetamine precursors such as pseudoephedrine, ephedrine, and other over-the-counter decongestants are discussed on p 394. Several amphetamine-related drugs (benzphetamine, diethylpropion, phendimetrazine, phenmetrazine, and phentermine) are marketed as prescription anorectic medications for use in weight reduction (Table II–1). **Fenfluramine** and **dexfenfluramine** were marketed as anorectic medications but were withdrawn from the market in 1997 because of concerns about cardiopulmonary toxicity with long-term use.

Cathinone (found in the shrub *Catha edulis,* or khat), **methcathinone,** and **mephedrone** (4-methylmethcathinone) are chemically related drugs with amphetamine-like effects. Newer synthetic analogs, such as 3,4-methylenedioxypyrovalerone and various derivatives of methcathinone, are becoming popular drugs of abuse, often sold on the Internet as **"bath salts"** with names such as "Ivory Wave," "Bounce," "Bubbles," "Mad Cow," and "Meow Meow." **Piperazine-like** compounds such as 1-benzyl-piperazine (BZP), 1-(4-methoxyphenyl)-piperazine (pMeOPP), 1-(3-chlorophenyl)-piperazine (mCPP), and 1-(3-trifluoromethylphenyl)-piperazine (TFMPP) are also designer drugs of abuse with stimulant effects.

Atomoxetine is a specific norepinephrine reuptake inhibitor approved as a nonstimulant alternative for the treatment of attention-deficit/hyperactivity disorder (ADHD). **Modafinil** is a nonamphetamine stimulant used in the treatment of narcolepsy, sleep disorders associated with shift work, and sleep apnea.

TABLE II–1. AMPHETAMINEMINE-LIKE PRESCRIPTION DRUGS[a]

Drug	Clinical Indications	Typical Adult Dose (mg)	Half-life (h)[b]
Atomoxetine[c]	Hyperactivity	40–120	3–4
Benzphetamine	Anorectant	25–50	6–12
Dexfenfluramine (withdrawn from US market in 1997)	Anorectant	15	17–20
Dextroamphetamine	Narcolepsy, hyperactivity (children)	5–15	10–12
Diethylpropion	Anorectant	25, 75 (sustained-release)	2.5–6
Fenfluramine (withdrawn from US market in 1997)	Anorectant	20–40	10–30
Mazindol	Anorectant	1–2	10
Methamphetamine	Narcolepsy, hyperactivity (children)	5–15	4–15
Methylphenidate	Hyperactivity (children)	5–20	2–7
Modafinil[c]	Narcolepsy, shift work sleepdisorder, sleep apnea	100–600	15
Pemoline	Narcolepsy, hyperactivity (children)	18.7–75	9–14
Phendimetrazine	Anorectant	35, 105 (sustained-release)	5–12.5
Phenmetrazine	Anorectant	25, 75 (sustained-release)	8
Phentermine	Anorectant	8, 30 (sustained release)	7–24

[a]See also Table II–35 ("Hallucinogens"), p 298.
[b]Half-life variable, dependent on urine pH.
[c]Not an amphetamine, but has some stimulant properties.

I. **Mechanism of toxicity**
   A. **Amphetamine and related drugs** activate the sympathetic nervous system via CNS stimulation, peripheral release of catecholamines, inhibition of neuronal reuptake of catecholamines, and inhibition of monoamine oxidase. Amphetamines, particularly MDMA, PMA, fenfluramine, and dexfenfluramine, also cause serotonin release and block neuronal serotonin uptake. The various drugs in this group have different profiles of catecholamine and serotonin action, resulting in different levels of CNS and peripheral stimulation.
   B. **Modafinil** is a nonamphetamine stimulant. Its mechanism of action is unclear, but extracellular CNS levels of dopamine, norepinephrine, serotonin, histamine, and glutamate are increased while gamma aminobutyric acid (GABA) is decreased. **Atomoxetine** is a specific norepinephrine reuptake inhibitor.
   C. **Piperazine-like** compounds have stimulant properties and enhance the release of catecholamines particularly dopamine and serotonin.
   D. **Pharmacokinetics.** All these drugs are well absorbed orally and have large volumes of distribution (Vd = 3–33 L/kg), except for pemoline (Vd = 0.2–0.6 L/kg), and they are generally extensively metabolized by the liver. Excretion of most amphetamines is highly dependent on urine pH, with amphetamines eliminated more rapidly in an acidic urine (see also Table II–66, p 462). There is limited pharmacokinetic data for piperazine-like compounds.

II. **Toxic dose.** These drugs generally have a low therapeutic index, with toxicity at levels only slightly above usual doses. However, a high degree of tolerance can develop after repeated use. Acute ingestion of more than 1 mg/kg of dextroamphetamine (or an equivalent dose of other drugs; see Table II–1) should be considered potentially life-threatening.

III. Clinical presentation

A. Acute CNS effects of intoxication of amphetamines include euphoria, talkativeness, anorexia, anxiety, restlessness, agitation, psychosis, seizures, and coma. Intracranial hemorrhage may occur owing to hypertension or cerebral vasculitis.

B. Acute peripheral manifestations include sweating, tremor, muscle fasciculations and rigidity, bruxism, tachycardia, hypertension, acute myocardial ischemia, and infarction (even with normal coronary arteries). Inadvertent intra-arterial injection may cause vasospasm resulting in gangrene; this has also occurred with oral use of DOB (2,5-dimethoxy-4-bromoamphetamine; see "Lysergic Acid Diethylamide [LSD] and Other Hallucinogens," p 297).

C. Death may be caused by ventricular arrhythmia, status epilepticus, intracranial hemorrhage, or hyperthermia. **Hyperthermia** frequently results from seizures and muscular hyperactivity and may cause brain damage, rhabdomyolysis, and myoglobinuric renal failure (p 21).

D. Acute modafinil and atomoxetine overdoses are generally mild to moderate in severity. Overdoses of modafinil up to 8 g are generally well tolerated with neurological complaints of anxiety, agitation, headaches, dizziness, insomnia, tremors, and dystonia. Similarly, overdoses of atomoxetine are usually mild and present with drowsiness, agitation, hyperactivity, GI upset, tremor, hyperreflexia, tachycardia, hypertension, and seizures.

E. Acute exposures to piperazine-like compounds including BZP, pMeOPP, mCPP, and TFMPP result in palpitations, agitation, anxiety, confusion, dizziness, insomnia, headache, hallucinations, depression, paranoia, tremor, mydriasis, urinary retention, nausea, and vomiting. Seizures have also been reported along with multi-organ failure. Symptoms have persisted for up to 24 hours after ingestion. Consistent with sympathomimetic effects, patients often present with tachycardia and hypertension.

F. Chronic effects of amphetamine abuse include weight loss, cardiomyopathy, pulmonary hypertension, dental changes, stereotypic behavior (eg, picking at the skin), paranoia, and paranoid psychosis. Psychiatric disturbances may persist for days or weeks. After cessation of habitual use, patients may experience fatigue, hypersomnia, hyperphagia, and depression lasting several days.

G. Prolonged use (usually 3 months or longer) of fenfluramine or dexfenfluramine in combination with phentermine ("fen-phen") has been associated with an increased risk for pulmonary hypertension and fibrotic valvular heart disease (primarily aortic, mitral, and tricuspid regurgitation). The pathology of the valvular disease is identical to that seen with carcinoid syndrome.

H. Illicit manufacture of methamphetamine can expose the "chemist" and his or her family to various toxic chemicals, including corrosive agents, solvents, and heavy metals.

IV. Diagnosis is usually based on a history of amphetamine use and clinical features of sympathomimetic drug intoxication.

A. Specific levels. Amphetamines and many related drugs can be detected in blood, urine and gastric samples, providing confirmation of exposure. However, quantitative serum levels do not closely correlate with the severity of clinical effects and are not generally available. Amphetamine derivatives and adrenergic amines may cross-react in immunoassays (see Table I–33, p 46), and distinguishing the specific drug requires confirmatory testing (eg, with thin-layer chromatography, gas chromatography [GC], or GC/mass spectrometry). Selegiline (a drug used in Parkinson disease) is metabolized to *l*-amphetamine and *l*-methamphetamine, and Clobenzorex (an anorectic drug sold in Mexico) is metabolized to amphetamine; these drugs can produce a positive result for amphetamines on urine and blood tested with immunoassays (unless a specific monoclonal antibody amphetamine assay is used) or GC/mass spectrometry (unless a special chiral derivative or column is used). Amphetamine, methamphetamine, and MDMA can be screened for by using hair and liquid chromatography—mass spectrometry.

B. Other useful laboratory studies include electrolytes, glucose, BUN and creatinine, creatine kinase (CK), urinalysis, urine dipstick test for occult hemoglobin (positive in patients with rhabdomyolysis with myoglobinuria), ECG and ECG monitoring, and CT scan of the head (if hemorrhage is suspected). Echocardiography and right heart catheterization may be useful for detecting valvular disease or pulmonary hypertension.

V. Treatment

A. Emergency and supportive measures

1. Maintain an open airway and assist ventilation if necessary (pp 1–7).
2. Treat agitation (p 24), seizures (p 23), coma (p 18), and hyperthermia (p 21) if they occur.
3. Continuously monitor the temperature, other vital signs, and the ECG for a minimum of 6 hours.

B. Specific drugs and antidotes. There is no specific antidote.

1. **Agitation.** Benzodiazepines (p 516) are usually satisfactory, although antipsychotic agents (p 503) may be added as needed.
2. **Hypertension** (p 17) is best treated with sedation and, if this is not effective, a parenteral vasodilator such as phentolamine (p 605) or nitroprusside (p 593).
3. Treat **tachyarrhythmias** (p 12) with propranolol (p 617) or esmolol (p 552). ***Note:*** Paradoxical hypertension is postulated to occur due to unopposed alpha-adrenergic effects when $beta_2$-mediated vasodilation is blocked; be prepared to give a vasodilator (see Item B.2 above) if needed.
4. Treat **arterial vasospasm** as described for ergots (p 229).

C. Decontamination. Administer activated charcoal orally if conditions are appropriate (see Table I–38, p 54). Gastric lavage is not necessary after small-to-moderate ingestions if activated charcoal can be given promptly. Consider whole-bowel irrigation (p 55) and repeated doses of charcoal after ingestion of drug-filled packets ("body stuffers").

D. Enhanced elimination. Dialysis and hemoperfusion are not effective. Repeat-dose charcoal has not been studied. Renal elimination of dextroamphetamine may be enhanced by acidification of the urine, but this is not recommended because of the risk for aggravating the nephrotoxicity of myoglobinuria.

► ANESTHETICS, LOCAL

Neal L. Benowitz, MD

Local anesthetics are used widely to provide anesthesia via local subcutaneous (SC) injection; topical application to skin and mucous membranes; and epidural, spinal, and regional nerve blocks. In addition, lidocaine (p 573) is used IV as an antiarrhythmic agent, and cocaine (p 201) is a popular drug of abuse. Commonly used agents are divided into two chemical groups: ester-linked and amide-linked (Table II–2).

Toxicity from local anesthetics (other than cocaine) is usually caused by therapeutic overdose (ie, excessive doses for local nerve blocks), inadvertent acceleration of IV infusions (lidocaine), or accidental injection of products meant for dilution (eg, 20% lidocaine) instead of those formulated for direct administration (2% solution). Acute injection of lidocaine has also been used as a method of homicide. To prolong the duration of effect, local anesthetics are often administered together with epinephrine, which can also cause toxicity.

I. Mechanism of toxicity

A. Local anesthetics bind to sodium channels in nerve fibers, blocking the sodium current responsible for nerve conduction and thereby increasing the threshold

TABLE II–2. LOCAL ANESTHETICS

Anesthetic	Usual Half-life	Maximum Adult Single Dose[a] (mg)
Ester-linked		
Benzocaine[b]		N/A
Benzonatate[c]		200
Butacaine[b]		N/A
Butamben[b]		N/A
Chloroprocaine	1.5–6 min	800
Cocaine[b]	1–2.5 h	N/A
Hexylcaine[b]		N/A
Procaine	7–8 min	600
Proparacaine[b]		N/A
Propoxycaine		75
Tetracaine	5–10 min	15
Amide-linked		
Articaine	1–2 h	500
Bupivacaine	2–5 h	400
Dibucaine		10
Etidocaine	1.5 h	400
Levobupivacaine	1–3 h	300
Lidocaine	1.2 h	300
Lidocaine with epinephrine	2 h	500
Mepivacaine		400
Prilocaine		600
Ropivacaine		225
Other (neither ester- nor amide-linked)		
Dyclonine[b]		N/A
Pramoxine[b]		N/A

[a]Maximum single dose for subcutaneous infiltration. N/A, not applicable.
[b]Used only for topical anesthesia.
[c]Given orally as an antitussive.

for conduction and reversibly slowing or blocking impulse generation. In therapeutic concentrations, this results in local anesthesia. In high concentrations, such actions may result in CNS and cardiovascular toxicity.

B. Bupivacaine is more cardiotoxic than other local anesthetics, with a very narrow toxic-to-therapeutic ratio and with numerous reports of rapid cardiovascular collapse and sometimes death. In addition to causing sodium channel blockade, bupivacaine inhibits carnitine acyltransferase, which is essential for fatty acid transport, resulting in mitochondrial dysfunction that is thought to contribute to cardiotoxicity.

C. In addition, some local anesthetics (eg, benzocaine, prilocaine, lidocaine) can cause methemoglobinemia (p 317).

D. Pharmacokinetics. With local subcutaneous injection, peak blood levels are reached in 10–60 minutes, depending on the vascularity of the tissue and whether a vasoconstrictor such as epinephrine has been added. **Ester-type**

drugs are hydrolyzed rapidly by plasma cholinesterase and have short half-lives. **Amide-type** drugs are metabolized by the liver, have a longer duration of effect, and may accumulate after repeated doses in patients with hepatic insufficiency. For other kinetic values, see Table II–66, p 462.

II. Toxic dose. Systemic toxicity occurs when brain levels exceed a certain threshold. Toxic levels can be achieved with a single large subcutaneous injection, with rapid IV injection of a smaller dose, inadvertent intravascular injection, or by accumulation of drug with repeated doses. The recommended maximum single subcutaneous doses of the common agents are listed in Table II–2. With IV regional anesthesia, doses as low as 1.4 mg/kg for lidocaine and 1.3 mg/kg for bupivacaine have caused seizures, and doses as low as 2.5 mg/kg for lidocaine and 1.6 mg/kg for bupivacaine have caused cardiac arrest.

III. Clinical presentation

A. Toxicity due to **local anesthetic effects** includes prolonged anesthesia and, rarely, permanent sensory or motor deficits. Spinal anesthesia may block nerves to the muscles of respiration, causing respiratory arrest, or may cause sympathetic blockade, resulting in hypotension.

B. Toxicity resulting from **systemic absorption** of local anesthetics most commonly affects the CNS and the cardiovascular system. For some anesthetics such as lidocaine and mepivacaine, CNS toxicity precedes cardiovascular toxicity, while the reverse is seen with bupivacaine.

1. Neurological toxicity includes headache, confusion, tinnitus, perioral paresthesias, slurred speech, muscle twitching, agitation, convulsions, coma, and respiratory arrest.

2. Cardiotoxic effects include hypotension, sinus arrest, widening of the QRS complex, bradycardia, atrioventricular block, ventricular tachycardia/fibrillation, and asystole. Cardiac arrest due to bupivacaine is often refractory to usual treatment.

3. Epinephrine toxicity may include palpitations, headache, tachycardia, hypertension, and ventricular arrhythmias.

C. Methemoglobinemia (see also p 317) may occur after exposure to benzocaine, prilocaine, or lidocaine.

D. Allergic reactions (bronchospasm, hives, and shock) are uncommon and occur almost exclusively with ester-linked local anesthetics. Methylparaben, which is used as a preservative in some multidose vials, may be the cause of some reported hypersensitivity reactions.

E. Features of toxicity caused by **cocaine** are discussed on p 201.

IV. Diagnosis is based on a history of local anesthetic use and typical clinical features. Abrupt onset of confusion, slurred speech, or convulsions in a patient receiving lidocaine infusion for arrhythmias should suggest lidocaine toxicity.

A. Specific levels. Serum levels of some local anesthetics may confirm their role in producing suspected toxic effects, but these levels must be obtained promptly because they fall rapidly.

1. Serum concentrations of lidocaine greater than 6–10 mg/L are considered toxic.

2. Lidocaine is often detected in comprehensive urine toxicology screening as a result of use either as a local anesthetic (eg, for minor procedures in the emergency department) or as a cutting agent for drugs of abuse.

B. Other useful laboratory studies include electrolytes, glucose, BUN and creatinine, ECG monitoring, arterial blood gases or pulse oximetry, and methemoglobin level (benzocaine).

V. Treatment

A. Emergency and supportive measures

1. Maintain an open airway and assist ventilation if necessary (pp 1–7).

2. Treat coma (p 18), seizures (p 23), hypotension (p 15), arrhythmias (p 13), and anaphylaxis (p 28) if they occur. Low-dose epinephrine is preferred for pressor support. Extracorporeal circulatory assistance (eg, balloon pump or partial cardiopulmonary bypass) has been used for the short-term support of patients after acute massive overdose with 20% lidocaine solution or inadvertent intravascular administration of bupivacaine.

3. Monitor vital signs and ECG for at least 6 hours.

B. **Specific drugs and antidotes. Intravenous lipid emulsion** (Intralipid) therapy (p 574) may augment the return of spontaneous circulation after cardiac arrest caused by bupivacaine, levobupivacaine, ropivacaine, or mepivacaine. Administer a 1.5-mL/kg bolus of Intralipid 20%, repeated up to two times if necessary, followed by an infusion of 0.25–0.50 mL/kg/min for 30–60 minutes.

C. **Decontamination**

1. **Parenteral exposure.** Decontamination is not feasible.
2. **Ingestion**. Administer activated charcoal orally if conditions are appropriate (see Table I–38, p 54). Gastric lavage is not necessary after small-to-moderate ingestions if activated charcoal can be given promptly.

D. **Enhanced elimination.** The role of extracorporeal elimination is limited. Lidocaine has a moderate volume of distribution, but at therapeutic levels a large percentage (40–80%) is protein bound making hemodialysis relatively ineffective. Dialysis might be considered after a massive overdose or when metabolic elimination is impaired because of circulatory collapse or severe liver disease.

▶ ANGIOTENSIN BLOCKERS AND ACE INHIBITORS

Sandra A. Hayashi, PharmD

The angiotensin-converting enzyme (ACE) inhibitors and angiotensin receptor (AR) blockers are widely used for the treatment of patients with hypertension or heart failure and patients who have had a myocardial infarction. Currently, at least 10 ACE inhibitors and 7 AR blockers are marketed in the United States.

I. **Mechanism of toxicity**

A. ACE inhibitors reduce vasoconstriction and aldosterone activity by blocking the enzyme that converts angiotensin I to angiotensin II. AR blockers directly inhibit the action of angiotensin II.

B. All the ACE inhibitors except captopril and lisinopril are prodrugs that must be metabolized to their active moieties (eg, enalapril is converted to enalaprilat) following oral administration.

C. Angioedema and cough associated with ACE inhibitors are thought to be mediated by bradykinin, which normally is broken down by angiotensin-converting enzyme. However, it has also been rarely reported with AR blockers, which do not alter bradykinin elimination.

D. Rare cases of acute liver injury (hepatocellular and/or cholestatic) have been associated with both ACE inhibitors and AR blockers, by unclear mechanisms.

E. **Pharmacokinetics** (see also Table II–66). The volume of distribution (Vd) of ACE inhibitors is fairly small (eg, 0.7 L/kg for captopril). The parent drugs are rapidly converted to their active metabolites, with half-lives of 0.75–1.5 hours. The active metabolites have elimination half-lives of 5.9–35 hours. The AR blockers have half-lives of 5–24 hours; losartan has an active metabolite.

II. **Toxic dose.** Only mild toxicity has resulted from most reported overdoses of up to 7.5 g of captopril, 440 mg of enalapril (serum level 2.8 mg/L at 15 hours), and 420 mg of lisinopril. A 75-year-old man was found dead after ingesting approximately 1,125 mg of captopril. A 45-year-old woman recovered without sequelae after intentional ingestion of 160 mg of candesartan cilexetil along with several other drugs. A 2.5-year-old girl ingested 2 mg/kg of perindopril and experienced an asymptomatic transient drop in blood pressure to 65/45 mm Hg approximately 4 hours later. A 14-month-old boy ingested 15 mg/kg of irbesartan and reportedly became unsteady on his feet within 1 hour of ingestion and had mild hypotension, but he was acting normally 3 hours later and was discharged home.

III. Clinical presentation

A. Hypotension, usually **responsive** to fluid therapy, has been reported with acute overdose. Bradycardia may also occur.

B. Hyperkalemia has been reported with therapeutic use, especially in patients with renal insufficiency and those taking nonsteroidal anti-inflammatory drugs.

C. Bradykinin-mediated effects in patients taking therapeutic doses of ACE **inhibitors** include dry **cough** (generally mild but often persistent and annoying) and **acute angioedema**, usually involving the tongue, lips, and face, which may lead to life-threatening airway obstruction.

IV. Diagnosis is based on a history of exposure.

A. Specific levels. Blood levels are not readily available and do not correlate with clinical effects.

B. Other useful laboratory studies include electrolytes, glucose, BUN, and creatinine.

V. Treatment

A. Emergency and supportive measures. Monitor blood pressure and heart rate for 6 hours after ingestion. If symptomatic or significant hypotension develops, observe for at least 24 hours.

1. If hypotension occurs, treat it with supine positioning and IV fluids (p 15). Vasopressors are rarely necessary.
2. Treat angioedema with usual measures (eg, diphenhydramine, corticosteroids) and discontinue the ACE inhibitor. Switching to an AR blocker may not be appropriate as angioedema has also been reported with these agents.
3. Treat hyperkalemia (p 39) if it occurs.

B. Specific drugs and antidotes. No specific antidote is available.

C. Decontamination (p 50). Administer activated charcoal orally if conditions are appropriate (see Table I–38, p 54). Gastric lavage is not necessary after small-to-moderate ingestions if activated charcoal can be given promptly.

D. Enhanced elimination. Hemodialysis may effectively remove these drugs but is not likely to be indicated clinically.

▶ ANTIARRHYTHMIC DRUGS

Alicia B. Minns, MD

Because of their actions on the heart, antiarrhythmic drugs are extremely toxic, and overdoses are often life-threatening. Several classes of antiarrhythmic drugs are discussed elsewhere in Section II: type Ia drugs (quinidine, disopyramide, and procainamide, p 398); type II drugs (beta blockers, p 158); type IV drugs (calcium antagonists, p 172); and the older type Ib drugs (lidocaine, p 84, and phenytoin, p 369). This section describes toxicity caused by type Ib (tocainide and mexiletine); type Ic (flecainide, encainide, propafenone, and moricizine); and type III (bretylium, amiodarone, dronedarone, and dofetilide) antiarrhythmic drugs. Sotalol, which also has type III antiarrhythmic actions, is discussed in the section on beta-adrenergic blockers (p 158).

I. Mechanism of toxicity

A. Type I drugs in general act by inhibiting the fast sodium channel responsible for initial cardiac cell depolarization and impulse conduction. Type Ia and type Ic (which also block potassium channels) slow depolarization and conduction in normal cardiac tissue, and even at normal therapeutic doses the QT (types Ia and Ic) and QRS intervals (type Ic) are prolonged. Type Ib drugs slow depolarization primarily in ischemic tissue and have little effect on normal tissue or on the ECG. In overdose, all type I drugs have the potential to markedly depress myocardial automaticity, conduction, and contractility.

B. **Type II and type IV drugs** act by blocking beta-adrenergic receptors (type II) or calcium channels (type IV). Their actions are discussed elsewhere (type II, p 158; type IV, p 172).

C. **Type III drugs** act primarily by blocking potassium channels to prolong the duration of the action potential and the effective refractory period, resulting in QT-interval prolongation at therapeutic doses.

1. IV administration of **bretylium** initially causes release of catecholamines from nerve endings, followed by inhibition of catecholamine release.
2. **Amiodarone** is also a noncompetitive beta-adrenergic blocker and has sodium and calcium channel–blocking effects, which may explain its tendency to cause bradyarrhythmias. Amiodarone may also release iodine, and chronic use has resulted in altered thyroid function (both hyper- and hypothyroidism).
3. **Dronedarone** is an analog of amiodarone but does not contain iodine and does not affect thyroid function. It exhibits properties of all four antiarrhythmic classes.
4. **Dofetilide** is used to maintain sinus rhythm in patients with atrial fibrillation. It is associated with QT prolongation and a risk for torsade de pointes, as discussed further in the following text.

D. **Relevant pharmacokinetics.** All the drugs discussed in this section are widely distributed to body tissues. Most are extensively metabolized, but significant fractions of tocainide (40%), flecainide (40%), dofetilide (80%), and bretylium (>90%) are excreted unchanged by the kidneys (see also Table II–66, p 462).

II. **Toxic dose.** In general, these drugs have a narrow therapeutic index, and severe toxicity may occur slightly above or sometimes even within the therapeutic range, especially if two or more antiarrhythmic drugs are taken together.

A. Ingestion of **twice the daily therapeutic dose** should be considered potentially life-threatening (usual therapeutic doses are given in Table II–3).

B. An exception to this rule of thumb is amiodarone, which is **distributed** so extensively to tissues that even massive single overdoses produce little or no toxicity (toxicity usually occurs only after accumulation during chronic amiodarone dosing).

III. **Clinical presentation**

A. **Tocainide and mexiletine**

1. **Side effects** with therapeutic use may include dizziness, paresthesias, tremor, ataxia, and GI disturbance (nausea, vomiting, heartburn). A hypersensitivity syndrome (fever, rash, eosinophilia) has been described with mexiletine, and most commonly affects Japanese males.
2. **Overdose** may cause sedation, confusion, coma, seizures, respiratory arrest, and cardiac toxicity (sinus arrest, atrioventricular [AV] block, asystole, and hypotension). As with lidocaine, the QRS and QT intervals are usually normal, although they may be prolonged after massive overdose.

B. **Flecainide, propafenone, and moricizine**

1. **Side effects** with therapeutic use include dizziness, blurred vision, headache, and GI upset. Ventricular arrhythmias (monomorphic or polymorphic ventricular tachycardia; see p 13) and sudden death may occur at therapeutic levels, especially in persons receiving high doses and those with reduced ventricular function. Propafenone has been associated with cholestatic hepatitis.
2. **Overdose** causes hypotension, seizures, bradycardia, sinoatrial and AV nodal block, and asystole. The QRS and QT intervals are prolonged, and ventricular arrhythmias may occur. Flecainide may slow atrial fibrillation and convert it to atrial flutter with rapid conduction.

C. **Bretylium** is no longer widely used and has been removed from advanced cardiac life support (ACLS) guidelines.

TABLE II–3. ANTIARRHYTHMIC DRUGS

Class	Drug	Usual Half-life (h)	Therapeutic Daily Dose (mg)	Therapeutic Serum Levels (mg/L)	Major Toxicity[a]
Ia	Quinidine and related drugs (p 398)				
Ib	Tocainide[d]	11–15	1,200–2,400	4–10	S,B,H
	Mexiletine	10–12	300–1,200	0.8–2	S,B,H
	Lidocaine (p 84)				
	Phenytoin (p 369)				
Ic	Flecainide	14–15	200–600	0.2–1	B,V,H
	Encainide[b,d]	2–11	75–300		S,B,V,H
	Propafenone[b]	2–10[c]	450–900	0.5–1	S,B,V,H
	Moricizine[d]	1.5–3.5	600–900	0.02–0.18	B,V,H
II	Beta blockers (p 158)				
III	Amiodarone	50 days	200–600	1.0–2.5	B,V,H
	Bretylium	5–14	5–10 mg/kg (IV loading dose)	1–3	H
	Dofetilide	10	0.125–1		B,V
	Dronedarone	13–19	800		B
	Ibutilide	2–12	N/A		B,V,H
	Sotalol (p 158)				
IV	Calcium antagonists (p 172)				
Miscellaneous	Adenosine	<10 seconds	N/A		S,B,V,H

[a]Major toxicity: B, bradyarrhythmias; H, hypotension; S, seizures; V, ventricular arrhythmias.
[b]Active metabolite may contribute to toxicity; level not established.
[c]Genetically slow metabolizers may have half-lives of 10–32 hours. Also, metabolism is nonlinear, so half-lives may be longer in patients with overdose.
[d]Encainide, morizicine, and tocainide are no longer sold in the United States.
This table was updated with assistance from Elizabeth Birdsall, PharmD.

1. The major toxic **side effect** of bretylium is hypotension caused by inhibition of catecholamine release. Orthostatic hypotension may persist for several hours.
2. After **rapid IV injection**, transient hypertension, nausea, and vomiting may occur.

D. Amiodarone, dronedarone, and dofetilide

1. **Acute overdose** in a person not already on amiodarone is not expected to cause toxicity. Bradyarrhythmias, hypotension, and asystole have been observed during IV loading. Acute hepatitis and acute pneumonitis have rarely been associated with IV loading doses given over several days. Few overdoses of dofetilide have been reported but would be expected to produce QT-interval prolongation and torsade de pointes, as this is the major dose-related toxicity.
2. With **chronic use, amiodarone** may cause ventricular arrhythmias (monomorphic or polymorphic ventricular tachycardia; see p 13) or bradyarrhythmias (sinus arrest, AV block). The most important life-threatening toxicity from amiodarone is pulmonary toxicity (hypersensitivity pneumonitis or interstitial/

alveolar pneumonitis), which has a fatality rate of 10%. Amiodarone may also cause hepatitis, photosensitivity dermatitis, corneal deposits, hypothyroidism or hyperthyroidism, tremor, ataxia, and peripheral neuropathy. Mild elevation in liver enzymes is common; severe liver toxicity is rare. Chronic **dronedarone** use doubles the risk of death in patients with symptomatic heart failure. It is also contraindicated in patients with permanent atrial fibrillation. **Dofetilide** has been associated with QT prolongation and torsade de pointes, particularly in people whose renal function has deteriorated or who are taking other QT-prolonging drugs, and with the development of hypokalemia and/or hypomagnesemia.

IV. Diagnosis is usually based on a history of antiarrhythmic drug use and typical cardiac and ECG findings. Syncope in any patient taking these drugs should suggest possible drug-induced arrhythmia.

A. Specific levels. Serum levels are available for most type Ia and type Ib drugs (see Table II–3); however, because toxicity is immediately life-threatening, measurement of drug levels is used primarily for therapeutic drug monitoring or to confirm the diagnosis rather than to determine emergency treatment. The following antiarrhythmic drugs may be detected in *comprehensive* urine toxicology screening: diltiazem, flecainide, lidocaine, metoprolol, phenytoin, propranolol, quinidine, and verapamil.

B. Other useful laboratory studies include electrolytes, glucose, BUN and creatinine, liver enzymes, thyroid panel (chronic amiodarone), and ECG monitoring.

V. Treatment

A. Emergency and supportive measures

1. Maintain an open airway and assist ventilation if necessary (pp 1–7).
2. Treat coma (p 18), seizures (p 23), hypotension (p 15), and arrhythmias (pp 9–14) if they occur. ***Note:*** Type Ia antiarrhythmic agents should not be used to treat cardiotoxicity caused by type Ia, type Ic, or type III drug.
3. Continuously monitor vital signs and ECG for a minimum of 6 hours after exposure, and admit the patient for 24 hours of intensive monitoring if there is evidence of toxicity.

B. Specific drugs and antidotes. In patients with intoxication by type Ia or type Ic drug, QRS prolongation, bradyarrhythmias, and hypotension may respond to **sodium bicarbonate**, 1–2 mEq/kg IV (p 520). The sodium bicarbonate reverses cardiac-depressant effects caused by inhibition of the fast sodium channel. Torsade de pointes should be treated with IV magnesium, repletion of potassium, and, if necessary, overdrive cardiac pacing.

C. Decontamination (p 50). Administer activated charcoal orally if conditions are appropriate (see Table I–38, p 54). Gastric lavage is not necessary after small-to-moderate ingestions if activated charcoal can be given promptly.

D. Enhanced elimination. Owing to extensive tissue binding with resulting large volumes of distribution, dialysis and hemoperfusion are not likely to be effective for most of these agents. Hemodialysis may be of benefit for tocainide or flecainide overdose in patients with renal failure, but prolonged and repeated dialysis would be necessary. No data are available on the effectiveness of repeat-dose charcoal.

► ANTIBACTERIAL AGENTS

Conan MacDougall, PharmD, MAS

The antibacterial group of drugs has proliferated immensely since the first clinical use of sulfonamide in 1936 and the mass production of penicillin in 1941. In general, harmful effects have resulted from allergic reactions or inadvertent intravenous overdose. Serious toxicity from a single acute ingestion is rare. Table II–4 lists common and newer antibacterial agents that have been associated with significant toxic effects.

TABLE II–4. ANTIBACTERIAL DRUGS

Drug	Half-life[a]	Toxic Dose or Serum Level	Toxicity
Aminoglycosides			
Amikacin	2–3 h	Varies	Toxic to vestibular and cochlear cells; nephrotoxicity causing proximal tubular damage and acute tubular necrosis; competitive neuromuscular blockade if given rapidly IV with other neuromuscular-blocking drugs. Threshold for toxic effects varies with the drug, dosage schedule, treatment duration, and sampling time.
Gentamicin	2 h	Varies	
Kanamycin	2–3 h	>30 mg/L	
Neomycin		0.5–1 g/d	
Streptomycin	2.5 h	>40–50 mg/L	
Tobramycin	2–2.5 h	Varies	
Antimycobacterials			Used for treatment of tuberculosis and other mycobacterial infections
Bedaquiline	4–5 mo	Unknown	QT prolongation, hepatotoxicity
Ethambutol	4 h	Chronic; 15 mg/kg/d and up	Optic neuritis, red-green color blindness, peripheral neuropathy. Risk of ocular adverse effects increases with dose: 1% at 15 mg/kg/d, 5% at 25 mg/kg/d, 18% at 35 mg/kg/d.
Ethionamide	1.92 ± 0.27 h	GI intolerance acute; other effects chronic	Severe nausea/vomiting, hepatitis, hypothyroidism, hypoglycemia, photosensitivity, neurotoxic effects
Isoniazid (INH)	0.5–4 h	1–2 g orally	Convulsions, metabolic acidosis, hypotension, acute hepatic failure; hepatotoxicity and peripheral neuropathy with chronic use
Pyrazinamide	9–10 h	40–50 mg/kg/d for prolonged period	Hepatotoxicity, hyperuricemia
Rifampin, rifabutin, rifapentine	1.5–5 h, 36 h, 13 h	100 mg/kg/d (fatal exposures at 14–60 g)	All patients will develop harmless red discoloration of urine, sweat, and tears. With acute exposure, abdominal pain, vomiting and diarrhea (may be red), facial edema, pruritus. Severe toxicity includes acute hepatic failure, seizures, cardiac arrest. Antibiotics of rifamycin class are inducers of hepatic cytochrome P450 enzymes, especially CYP3A4.
Bacitracin		Unknown	Minimal enteric systemic absorption; if administered parenterally or absorbed via breaks in skin, ototoxicity and nephrotoxicity
Carbapenems			Hypersensitivity reactions; seizures associated with renal dysfunction and high doses
Doripenem	1 h	Chronic	
Ertapenem	4 h (2.5 h in ages 3 mo–12 y)	Chronic	

(*continued*)

TABLE II–4. ANTIBACTERIAL DRUGS (CONTINUED)

Drug	Half-life[a]	Toxic Dose or Serum Level	Toxicity
Imipenems/ cilastatin	1 h	Acute: >1 g every 6 h; Chronic	Highest seizure risk for imipenem
Meropenem	1 h	Chronic	
Cephalosporins			Hypersensitivity reactions; convulsions reported in patients with renal insufficiency and excessive doses
Cefazolin Cephalothin	90–120 min	Unknown	Coagulopathy associated with cefazolin
Cefaclor	0.6–0.9 h	Chronic	Neutropenia
Cefoperazone Cefamandole Cefotetan Moxalactam Cefmetazole	102–156 min 30–60 min 3–4.6 h 114–150 min 72 min	3–4 mg/L	One case of symptomatic hepatitis. All these antibiotics have the N-methylthiotetrazole side chain, which may inhibit aldehyde dehydrogenase to cause a disulfiram-like interaction with ethanol (p 226) and coagulopathy (inhibition of vitamin K production).
Ceftriaxone	4.3–4.6 h; extensive excretion in bile	IV bolus over <3–5 min	Pseudolithiasis ("gallbladder sludge"). Should be administered IV over 30 min
Cefepime	2 h	Chronic	Encephalopathy, nonconvulsive status epilepticus associated with high doses, renal dysfunction.
Chloramphenicol	4 h	>40 mg/L	Leukopenia, reticulocytopenia, circulatory collapse ("gray baby" syndrome)
Clindamycin, lincomycin,	2.4–3 h, 4.4–6.4 h	Unknown	Hypotension and cardiopulmonary arrest after rapid intravenous administration
Daptomycin	8–9 h	Chronic	May cause muscle pain, weakness, or asymptomatic elevation of the CK level. Rare cases of rhabdomyolysis, dosage-related.
Fidaxomicin	12 h	Unknown	Minimal systemic absorption; nausea/vomiting/abdominal pain possible
Folate antagonists			Bone marrow suppression
Pyrimethamine	2–6 h	Acute ≥300 mg; Chronic	Seizures, hypersensitivity reactions, folic acid deficiency
Trimethoprim	8–11 h	Unknown	Methemoglobinemia, hyperkalemia
Fosfomycin	12 h	Unknown	Low serum concentrations with oral administration; nausea, vomiting. Ototoxicity and taste disturbances in overdoses
Glycopeptides			
Dalbavancin	346 h	Unknown	Highly protein bound; administered once weekly. No experience in overdose; possible hepatotoxicity, bleeding risk.

(continued)

TABLE II–4. ANTIBACTERIAL DRUGS (CONTINUED)

Drug	Half-life[a]	Toxic Dose or Serum Level	Toxicity
Oritavancin	245 h	Unknown	Highly protein bound; administered once weekly. P450 drug interactions. Interferes with coagulation lab tests (aPTT, INR).
Telavancin	8 ± 1.5 h	Chronic	Nephrotoxic; may cause QTc prolongation, foamy urine, "red man" syndrome; interferes with coagulation tests.
Vancomycin	4–6 h	>80 mg/L acute; >25 mg/L chronic	Nephrotoxic at high doses. Hypotension, skin rash/flushing ("red man" syndrome) associated with rapid IV administration. Possible ototoxicity.
Gramicidin		Unknown	Topical/ophthalmic agent. Hemolysis if systemically absorbed.
Linezolid, tedizolid	4.5–5.5 h, 12 h	Duration-related (>2 wk)	Thrombocytopenia, anemia; lactic acidosis (rare); peripheral neuropathy and optic neuritis with prolonged use. Linezolid is an inhibitor of monoamine oxidase (p 326); serotonin syndrome reported when combined with antidepressants.
Macrolides			Can prolong the QT interval and lead to torsade de pointes (atypical ventricular tachycardia). Inhibitors of CYP enzymes.
Azithromycin	68 h	Chronic	Least likely of the macrolides to induce torsade in animal studies and least potent P450 inhibitor.
Clarithromycin	3–4 h	Chronic	
Dirithromycin	44 (16–55) h	Chronic	Hepatotoxicity
Erythromycin	1.4 h	Unknown	Abdominal pain; idiosyncratic hepatotoxicity with estolate salt. Administration of more than 4 g/d may cause tinnitus, ototoxicity.
Tilmicosin (veterinary drug)	Death may occur within 1 h	Minimum toxic dose unknown, but 1–1.5 mL (300–450 mg) caused serious symptoms	Cardiotoxic: tachycardia, decreased contractility, cardiac arrest
Nitrofurantoin	20 min	Unknown	Nausea/vomiting with acute overdose; hemolysis in G6PD-deficient patients is possible. Pulmonary hypersensitivity reactions with long-term use.
Nitroimidazoles			Seizures with acute overdose; peripheral neuropathy with chronic use; disulfiram-like reactions with ethanol (p 226)
Metronidazole	6–14 h	5 g/d	

(continued)

TABLE II–4. ANTIBACTERIAL DRUGS (CONTINUED)

Drug	Half-life[a]	Toxic Dose or Serum Level	Toxicity
Tinidazole	12–14 h	Chronic	
Penicillins			Hypersensitivity reactions; seizures with single high dose or chronic excessive doses in patients with renal dysfunction
Ampicillin, amoxicillin	1.5 h 1.3 h	Unknown	Acute renal failure caused by crystal deposition
Methicillin	30 min	Unknown	Interstitial nephritis, leukopenia
Nafcillin	1.0 h	Unknown	Neutropenia
Penicillin G	30 min	10 million units/d IV (6 g), or CSF >5 mg/L	Administration of long-acting IM salt formulations (benzathine, procaine) via IV route associated with cardiovascular collapse and death.
Penicillins, anti-pseudomonal			
Carbenicillin	1.0–1.5 h	>300 mg/kg/d or >250 mg/L	Bleeding disorders due to impaired platelet function; hypokalemia (formulations have high sodium content). Risk for toxicity higher in patients with renal insufficiency.
Mezlocillin	0.8–1.1 h	>300 mg/kg/d	
Piperacillin/ tazobactam	0.6–1.2 h	>300 mg/kg/d	
Ticarcillin	1.0–1.2 h	>275 mg/kg/d	
Polymyxins			Nephrotoxicity and noncompetitive neuromuscular blockade
Polymyxin B	4.3–6 h	30,000 units/ kg/d	
Polymyxin E (colistin)	2–3 h	250 mg IM in a 10-month-old caused acute renal failure	
Quinolones			Tendonitis and tendon rupture (higher risk with increased age, corticosteroid use, renal dysfunction) Potentially irreversible peripheral neuropathy. Some agents can prolong the QT interval. Headache, dizzinesss, seizures. Acute liver injury. Dysglycemia in susceptible populations.
Ciprofloxacin	4 h	Acute 7.5 g	Crystalluria associated with doses above daily maximum and with alkaline urine. Inhibits CYP1A2 – interactions with theophylline and caffeine.
Gatifloxacin	7–14 h	Hypoglycemia or hyperglycemia within 6 and 5 days of therapy, respectively	Case reports of induced cholestatic hepatitis and hallucinations. Hypoglycemia or hyperglycemia. Oral and parenteral products withdrawn from US market.
Gemifloxacin	7 h	Chronic	Encephalopathy
Levofloxacin	6–8 h	Chronic	Hepatotoxicity, vision impairment, pseudotumor cerebri, autoimmune hemolytic anemia; interactions with herbal and natural supplements may cause cardiotoxicity.

(continued)

TABLE II–4. ANTIBACTERIAL DRUGS (CONTINUED)

Drug	Half-life[a]	Toxic Dose or Serum Level	Toxicity
Lomefloxacin	8 h	Chronic	Phototoxicity, seizures
Moxifloxacin	12 h	Chronic	Highest QT prolongation of quinolones available in the United States.
Nalidixic acid	1.1–2.5 h	50 mg/kg/d	Metabolic acidosis; intracranial hypertension
Norfloxacin	3–4 h	Chronic	Crystalluria associated with doses above daily maximum and with alkaline urine
Ofloxacin	7.86 ± 1.81 h	Chronic	Psychotoxicity
Sparfloxacin	16–30 h	Chronic	Associated with prolonged QT interval and torsade de pointes. Photosensitivity (use at least SPF 15 in sun-exposed areas).
Sulfonamides and Sulfones			Hypersensitivity reactions, including severe rash; frequently co-administered with folate antagonists
Dapsone	10–50 h	As little as 100 mg in an 18-month-old	Methemoglobinemia (see p 211), sulfhemoglobinemia, hemolysis; metabolic acidosis; hallucinations, confusion; hepatitis
Sulfamethoxazole		Unknown	Acute renal failure caused by crystal deposition
Tetracyclines			Use of tetracyclines may discolor/damage developing teeth, avoid in pregnancy and children <8 y. Risk of fetal harm in pregnancy.
Demeclocycline	10–17 h	Chronic	Nephrogenic diabetes insipidus
Doxycycline	12–20 h	Chronic	Rare esophageal ulceration
Minocycline	11–26 h	Chronic	Vestibular symptoms
Tetracycline	6–12 h	>1 g/d in infants	Benign intracranial hypertension. Degradation products (eg, expired prescriptions) are nephrotoxic, may cause Fanconi-like syndrome. Some products contain sulfites
		>4 g/d in pregnancy or >15 mg/L	Acute fatty liver
Tigecycline	37–67 h	Chronic	Nausea and vomiting common.

[a]Normal renal function.

I. Mechanism of toxicity. The precise mechanisms underlying toxic effects vary with the agent and are not well understood.

A. In some cases, toxicity is caused by an extension of **pharmacologic** effects, whereas in other cases, **allergic** or **idiosyncratic** reactions are responsible (especially penicillins, cephalosporins, and sulfonamides).

B. Some IV preparations may contain **preservatives** such as benzyl alcohol or large amounts of potassium or sodium.

C. **Drug interactions** may increase toxic effects by inhibiting metabolism of the antibacterial; **macrolides** are frequently implicated in drug–drug interactions.

D. **Prolonged QT interval** and **torsade de pointes** (atypical ventricular tachycardia) have emerged as serious effects of **macrolides** or **quinolones** when they are used alone or interact with other medications.

II. **Toxic dose.** The toxic dose is highly variable, depending on the agent. Life-threatening allergic reactions may occur after even subtherapeutic doses in hypersensitive individuals.

III. **Clinical presentation.** After acute oral overdose, most agents cause only nausea, vomiting, and diarrhea. Specific features of toxicity are described in Table II–4.

IV. **Diagnosis** is usually based on the history of exposure.

A. **Specific levels.** Serum levels for antibacterials are typically only rapidly available for **aminoglycosides** and **vancomycin;** there is a relatively predictable concentration–toxicity relationship for these agents.

B. **Other useful laboratory studies** include CBC, electrolytes, glucose, BUN and creatinine, liver function tests, urinalysis, ECG (including QT interval), and methemoglobin level (for patients with dapsone overdose).

V. **Treatment**

A. **Emergency and supportive measures**

1. Maintain an open airway and assist ventilation if necessary (pp 1–7).
2. Treat coma (p 18), seizures (p 23), hypotension (p 15), anaphylaxis (p 28), and hemolysis (see "Rhabdomyolysis," p 27) if they occur.
3. Replace fluid losses resulting from gastroenteritis with IV crystalloids.
4. Maintain steady urine flow with fluids to alleviate crystalluria from overdoses of **sulfonamides, ampicillin**, or **amoxicillin**.

B. **Specific drugs and antidotes**

1. **Trimethoprim** or **pyrimethamine** poisoning: Administer **leucovorin** (folinic acid [p 572]). Folic acid is not effective.
2. **Dapsone** overdose (see also p 211): Administer **methylene blue** (p 579) for symptomatic methemoglobinemia.
3. Treat **isoniazid** (INH) overdose (see also p 281) with **pyridoxine** (p 621).

C. **Decontamination** (p 50). Administer activated charcoal orally if conditions are appropriate (see Table I–38, p 54). Gastric lavage is not necessary after small-to-moderate ingestions if activated charcoal can be given promptly.

D. **Enhanced elimination.** Most antibacterials are excreted unchanged in the urine, so maintenance of adequate urine flow is important. The role of forced diuresis is unclear. Hemodialysis is not usually indicated, except perhaps in patients with renal dysfunction and a high level of a toxic agent.

1. Charcoal hemoperfusion effectively removes **chloramphenicol** and is indicated after a severe overdose with a high serum level and metabolic acidosis.
2. **Dapsone** undergoes enterohepatic recirculation and is eliminated more rapidly with repeat-dose activated charcoal (p 59).
3. Hemodialysis may remove **isoniazid** (p 281), but it is rarely indicated due to the short half-life of isoniazid and generally adequate response to treatment with benzodiazepines and pyridoxine.

► ANTICHOLINERGICS

Beth H. Manning, PharmD

Anticholinergic intoxication can occur with a wide variety of prescription and over-the-counter medications and with numerous plants and mushrooms. Common drugs that have anticholinergic activity include antihistamines (p 110), antipsychotics (p 130), antispasmodics, skeletal muscle relaxants (p 419), and tricyclic antidepressants

TABLE II–5. ANTICHOLINERGIC DRUGS[a]

Tertiary Amines	Usual Adult Single Dose (mg)	Quaternary Amines	Usual Adult Single Dose (mg)
Atropine	0.4–1	Anisotropine	50
Benztropine	1–6	Clidinium	2.5–5
Biperiden	2–5	Glycopyrrolate	1
Darifenacin	7.5–15	Hexocyclium	25
Dicyclomine	10–20	Ipratropium bromide	N/A[b]
Flavoxate	100–200	Isopropamide	5
Fesoterodine	4–8	Mepenzolate	25
L-Hyoscyamine	0.15–0.3	Methantheline	50–100
Oxybutynin	5	Methscopolamine	2.5
Oxyphencyclimine	10	Propantheline	7.5–15
Procyclidine	5	Tiotropium	N/A[c]
Scopolamine	0.4–1	Tridihexethyl	25–50
Solifenacin succinate	5–10	Trospium chloride	20
Tolterodine	2–4		
Trihexyphenidyl	6–10		

[a]These drugs act mainly at muscarinic cholinergic receptors and sometimes are more correctly referred to as antimuscarinic drugs.
[b]Not used orally; available as metered-dose inhaler and 0.02% inhalation solution and 0.03% nasal spray.
[c]Supplied as 18-mcg capsules for inhalation.

(p 107). Common combination products containing anticholinergic drugs include Atrohist, Donnagel, Donnatal, Hyland's Teething Tablets, Lomotil, Motofen, Ru-Tuss, Urised, and Urispas. Common anticholinergic medications are described in Table II–5. Plants and mushrooms containing anticholinergic alkaloids include jimsonweed (*Datura stramonium*), deadly nightshade (*Atropa belladonna*), and fly agaric (*Amanita muscaria*).

I. Mechanism of toxicity

A. Anticholinergic agents competitively antagonize the effects of acetylcholine at peripheral muscarinic and central receptors. Exocrine glands, such as those responsible for sweating and salivation, and smooth muscle are mostly affected. The inhibition of muscarinic activity in the heart leads to a rapid heartbeat.

B. Tertiary amines such as atropine are well absorbed centrally, whereas quaternary amines such as glycopyrrolate have a less central effect.

C. Pharmacokinetics. Absorption may be delayed because of the pharmacologic effects of these drugs on GI motility. The duration of toxic effects can be quite prolonged (eg, benztropine intoxication may persist for 2–3 days; see also Table II–66, p 462).

II. Toxic dose. The range of toxicity is highly variable and unpredictable. The potentially lethal dose of atropine has been estimated to be greater than 10 mg in adults. Ingestion of 30–50 jimsonweed seeds has been reported to cause significant toxicity. Doses up to 360 mg of trospium chloride produced increased heart rate and dry mouth but no other significant toxicity in healthy adults.

III. Clinical presentation. The anticholinergic syndrome is characterized by warm, dry, flushed skin; dry mouth; mydriasis; delirium; tachycardia; ileus; and urinary retention. Jerky myoclonic movements and choreoathetosis are common and may lead to rhabdomyolysis. Hyperthermia, coma, and respiratory arrest may occur. Seizures are rare with pure antimuscarinic agents, although they may result from other pharmacologic properties of the drug (eg, tricyclic antidepressants and antihistamines).

IV. **Diagnosis** is based on a history of exposure and the presence of typical features, such as dilated pupils and flushed skin. A trial dose of physostigmine (see below) can be used to confirm the presence of anticholinergic toxicity; rapid reversal of signs and symptoms is consistent with the diagnosis.

A. **Specific levels.** Concentrations in body fluids are not generally available. Common over-the-counter (OTC) agents are usually detectable on comprehensive urine toxicology screening but are not found on hospital drugs of abuse panels.

B. **Other useful laboratory studies** include electrolytes, glucose, creatine kinase (CK), arterial blood gases or pulse oximetry, and ECG monitoring.

V. **Treatment**

A. **Emergency and supportive measures**

1. Maintain an open airway and assist ventilation if needed (pp 1–7).
2. Treat hyperthermia (p 21), coma (p 18), rhabdomyolysis (p 27), and seizures (p 23) if they occur.

B. **Specific drugs and antidotes**

1. A small dose of **physostigmine** (p 609), 0.5–2 mg IV in an adult, can be given to patients with severe toxicity (eg, hyperthermia, severe delirium, or tachycardia). If an initial response is seen, but delirium recurs, a continuous infusion of physostigmine may be useful. ***Caution:*** Physostigmine can cause atrioventricular (AV) block, asystole, and seizures, especially in patients with tricyclic antidepressant overdose.
2. **Neostigmine** (p 609), a peripherally acting cholinesterase inhibitor, may be useful in treating anticholinergic-induced ileus.

C. **Decontamination** (p 50). Administer activated charcoal orally if conditions are appropriate (see Table I–38, p 54). Gastric lavage is not necessary after small-to-moderate ingestions if activated charcoal can be given promptly. Because of slowed GI motility, gut decontamination procedures may be helpful, even in late-presenting patients.

D. **Enhanced elimination.** Hemodialysis, hemoperfusion, peritoneal dialysis, and repeat-dose charcoal are not effective in removing anticholinergic agents.

▶ ANTICOAGULANTS, NEWER

Charles W. O'Connell, MD

The newer target-specific oral anticoagulant medications dabigatran, rivaroxaban, apixaban, and edoxaban have become increasingly popular alternatives to the vitamin K antagonist, warfarin (see p 459), the former mainstay of oral anticoagulation for prevention and treatment of venous thrombus events and stroke risk reduction in atrial fibrillation. These newer drugs inhibit a single target-specific step in coagulation rather than blocking multiple vitamin K–dependent blood factors as done by warfarin.

I. **Mechanism of toxicity**

A. **Dabigatran** is a competitive, direct inhibitor of both bound and free thrombin.

B. The factor Xa inhibitors **rivaroxaban**, **apixaban,** and **edoxaban** affect both free and bound factor Xa.

C. All of these agents also cause some small degree of indirect inhibition of platelet aggregation due to the decreased thrombin activity.

D. The resulting anticoagulation is both the intended benefit of these drugs and also the mechanism of toxicity in the event of adverse bleeding, ranging from minor to life-threatening hemorrhage.

TABLE II–6. NEWER ORAL ANTICOAGULANTS

Drug	Usual Adult Daily Dose (mg/24 h)	Peak Effect (h)	Elimination Half-life (h)	Renal Excretion (%)	Hepatic Metabolism
Dabigatran	150–300	1–3	12–17	80	No
Apixaban	5–10	1–3	8–15	25	Minimal
Edoxaban	30–60	1–3	9–11	50	Yes
Rivaroxaban	15–20	2–4	5–9[a]	35	Yes

[a]Half-life is 11–13 h in the elderly.

E. Overdose during **pregnancy**. FDA pregnancy categories B (apixaban) and C (dabigatran, edoxaban, and rivaroxaban). There is insufficient information regarding overdose in pregnancy for these agents.

F. **Pharmacokinetics.**

1. These agents have a more rapid onset of action and shorter half-lives than warfarin (see Table II–6).
2. They also have the advantage of far fewer food–drug and drug–drug interactions compared to warfarin, although drug concentrations of all these drugs may be increased in the presence of p-glycoprotein (p-gp) inhibitors.
3. Apixaban and rivaroxaban are highly protein bound, 87% and 92–95% respectively, whereas dabigatran protein binding is much less at 35%.
4. Decline in renal function may lead to increased drug concentrations, especially with use of dabigatran.
5. Dabigatran etexilate is a prodrug which is hydrolyzed to form its active moiety; its bioavailability is significantly increased (from 3–7% to 75%) when the pellets are ingested without the capsule shell.

II. **Toxic dose**

A. **Acute ingestion.** Impaired coagulation can occur with any ingestion; however, this does not imply that bleeding will occur. Systemic absorption of rivaroxaban is thought to be self-limited with no further increase in plasma levels with oral doses above 50 mg. Apixaban has been shown to be well tolerated at doses up to 50 mg PO daily for 3–7 days without clinically significant events.

B. **Chronic.** The majority of reported clinically significant bleeding has occurred with chronic ingestion.

III. **Clinical presentation.**

A. **Bleeding** has ranged from minor to life-threatening hemorrhage, including bleeding gums, ecchymoses, hematemesis, hemoptysis, hematochezia, melena, hematuria, menorrhagia, hematoma, or signs and symptoms of intracranial hemorrhage. Bleeding may be occult or may present with lightheadedness, fatigue, anemia, or hemodynamic instability if blood loss is severe or prolonged. Bleeding-associated fatalities have been reported.

B. **Acute ingestion.** There has been little symptomatic toxicity seen with intentional or accidental acute ingestions. In observational case series, low-dose single ingestions of dabigatran, apixaban, and rivaroxaban did not result in clinically significant bleeding. Acute self-harm ingestions in the absence of trauma have resulted in anticoagulation but rarely significant bleeding.

C. **Chronic overmedication.** The majority of adverse and significant bleeding events have been seen with chronic ingestions both with therapeutic use and unintentional overdoses.

IV. **Diagnosis** is based on history and evidence of excessive anticoagulation and/or bleeding.

A. **Specific levels.** Current laboratory diagnostic testing that reliably and accurately assesses the presence and degree of activity of these drugs is not available at most health centers.

1. Drug-specific concentrations are not typically readily available.
2. These drugs can alter common coagulation assays (PTT, PT), but there is an inconsistent relationship between drug effect and assay response. Effects on assays vary based on concentration ranges as well.
   a. A normal PTT excludes excess dabigatran concentrations.
   b. A normal PT excludes significant rivaroxaban concentrations, but is insensitive for apixaban and edoxaban.
   c. The hemoclot assay, a diluted thrombin time assay, has shown some utility in measuring anticoagulant effects in dabigatran concentrations up to 4,000 nanomol/L (1,886 ng/mL). Ecarin based assays have shown utility in correlation with dabigatran as well.
   d. Anti-FXa activity calibrated to the specific FXa inhibitors is the best diagnostic test for the FXa inhibitors, but is not widely available.

B. **Other useful laboratory studies** include BUN, creatinine, CBC, blood type, and cross-match.

V. **Treatment**

A. **Emergency and supportive measures**

1. If significant bleeding occurs, attempt to identify the source of bleeding and provide local control or hemostasis if possible. Give intravenous volume replacement as needed and closely monitor hemodynamics. Obtain immediate neurosurgical consult if intracranial bleeding is suspected.
2. Administer specific antidote as directed.
3. For severe or life-threatening bleeding, use a **specific reversal agent** (see V.B., below) or consider one of the **prothrombin complex concentrates** (PCCs) or **activated PCC** (APCC). For dabigatran, APCC is the preferred agent; for factor Xa inhibitors, a 4-factor PCC is preferred (see p 534). The utility of these concentrates is limited by the stoichiometric ratio needed to overcome the effects of the newer direct anticoagulants.
4. **Fresh-frozen plasma** is likely of limited utility given volume constraints and sheer amount that would be required to overcome drug effect, but may have a role for coagulopathies caused by dilution or DIC.
5. Consider **platelet transfusion** for patients on concurrent antiplatelet agents.
6. **Desmopressin** enhances hemostasis by increasing the release of von Willebrand factor and can be considered as an adjunct. The usual dose is 0.3 mcg/kg IV or subcutaneously, or 150–300 mcg intranasally.
7. Packed red blood cell transfusions should be administered as indicated for blood loss.
8. Take care not to precipitate hemorrhage in severely anticoagulated patients. Proper fall precautions should be taken and invasive procedures should be avoided if possible.

B. **Specific drugs and antidotes.**

1. **Idarucizumab** (Praxbind), an antibody fragment, has been shown to rapidly decrease the plasma concentration of **dabigatran**, decrease ecarin clotting time and plasma-diluted thrombin time, and improve hemostasis.
2. **Andexanet alfa**, a recombinant derivative of factor Xa, acts as a decoy receptor for the reversal of anticoagulation by the **factor Xa inhibitors** (apixaban, edoxaban, and rivaroxaban).

C. **Decontamination.** Administer activated charcoal orally if conditions are appropriate (see Table I–38, p 54). Activated charcoal given 2 and 6 hours after single dose ingestion of apixaban reduced mean apixaban absorption by 50% and 27% in a healthy volunteer study.

D. **Enhanced elimination.**

1. Hemodialysis (HD) can remove **dabigatran**, but the potential complications of placing an HD catheter (mainly bleeding) should be considered. HD has

been shown to remove 62–68% of the dabigatran dose in patients with end-stage renal disease.

2. The other newer anticoagulants are poor candidates for HD due to greater protein binding.

▶ ANTICONVULSANTS, NEWER

Freda M. Rowley, PharmD

Developed for the treatment of partial and generalized seizure disorders, these second- and third-generation anticonvulsants are finding wider use in the treatment of chronic and neuropathic pain syndromes; mood disorders, including bipolar and generalized anxiety disorders ; and migraine headache prophylaxis. Serious adverse effects with the therapeutic use of ezogabine (retinal pigment abnormalities, blue skin discoloration), felbamate (aplastic anemia, hepatic failure) and vigabatrin (permanent visual field deficits) have led to restrictions in their use.

Characteristics of several of these drugs are listed in Table II–7.

I. **Mechanism of toxicity.** Anticonvulsants suppress neuronal excitation by one of four major mechanisms.

A. **Blockade of voltage-gated sodium channels** by lamotrigine, topiramate, zonisamide, and felbamate. Lacosamide selectively enhances slow inactivation of these channels.

B. **Blockade of voltage-gated calcium channels** by gabapentin, levetiracetam, and zonisamide. Pregabalin binds to the alpha-2 delta subunit of L-type calcium channels.

C. **Inhibition of excitatory amines.** Lamotrigine inhibits glutamate release via sodium channel effects on presynaptic membranes. Felbamate is a competitive glutamate antagonist at the *N*-methyl-D-aspartate (NMDA) receptor. Perampanel is a selective noncompetitive antagonist at postsynaptic amino-3-hydroxy-5-methyl-4-isoxazolepropionic acid (AMPA) glutamate receptors.

D. **Gamma-aminobutyric acid (GABA) enhancement.** Tiagabine inhibits GABA transporter GAT-1, preventing reuptake into presynaptic neurons. Vigabatrin inhibits GABA transaminase, blocking GABA metabolism. Gabapentin and pregabalin are GABA analogs that have no known activity at GABA receptors.

E. **Pharmacokinetics** (see Tables II–7 and II–66 [p 462])

II. **Toxic dose varies** with each medication. A 4-year-old boy had a **10**-minute tonic–clonic seizure after the ingestion of 52 mg (3 mg/kg) of **tiagabine.** Ingestion of 91 g of **gabapentin** by an adult resulted in dizziness, slurred speech, and nystagmus that resolved after 11 hours. A 26-year-old man ingested 1,350 mg of **lamotrigine** and presented with nystagmus, ataxia, tachycardia, and a QRS interval of 112 msec, but never developed seizures; his 3-hour lamotrigine level was 17.4 mg/L (therapeutic range, 2.1–15 mg/L). A 56-year-old man became asystolic within 20 minutes after ingestion of 7 g of **lacosamide**; ECG after resuscitation showed QRS 206 msec, and serum lacosamide level was 27.7 mcg/mL (therapeutic range, 6.6–18.3).

III. **Clinical presentation.** See Table II–7.

IV. **Diagnosis** usually is based on the history of ingestion or is suspected in any patient on these medications who presents with altered mental status, ataxia, or seizures.

A. **Specific levels.** Serum levels can be requested from reference laboratories but are not usually available in time to make them useful for emergency management decisions.

B. **Other useful laboratory studies** include electrolytes, glucose, serum creatinine (gabapentin, lacosamide, pregabalin, topiramate), CBC (felbamate), liver aminotransferases (felbamate, lacosamide), bilirubin (felbamate), and ECG monitoring (lamotrigine, lacosamide, ezogabine).

TABLE II–7. ANTICONVULSANT DRUGS (NEWER)

Drug	Usual Elimination Half-life (h)	Usual Daily Dose (mg/d)	Reported Potential Toxic Effects
Ezogabine	7–11	300–1,200	CNS depression, dizziness, ataxia; agitation, aggressive behavior (>2.5 g), hallucinations, seizures; QT prolongation, dysrhythmias
Felbamate	20–23	1,800–4,800	Mild CNS depression, nystagmus, ataxia; tachycardia; nausea and vomiting; delayed (>12 h) crystalluria, hematuria, renal dysfunction
Gabapentin	5–7	900–3,600	Somnolence, dizziness, ataxia, myoclonus, slurred speech, diplopia; tachycardia, hypotension or hypertension; diarrhea
Lacosamide	13	200–600	CNS depression, headache, dizziness, ataxia, nystagmus, nausea and vomiting; QRS widening, AV block, hypotension, tachycardia; transient transaminase elevation
Lamotrigine	22–36	200–500	Lethargy, dizziness, ataxia, stupor, nystagmus, hypertonia, seizures; hypotension, tachycardia, QRS prolongation; nausea and vomiting; hypokalemia; hypersensitivity: fever, rash (Stevens–Johnson syndrome), hepatitis, renal failure
Levetiracetam	6–8	1,000–3,000	Drowsiness, ataxia
Perampanel	52–129	2–12	CNS depression, dizziness, ataxia, vertigo; agitation, euphoria, seizures; hyponatremia, nausea, and vomiting
Pregabalin	6-9	50–600	CNS depression, dizziness, headache, ataxia, agitation, confusion, seizures; nausea and vomiting; hypotension, peripheral edema
Tiagabine	7–9	30–70	Somnolence, confusion, agitation, dizziness, ataxia, tremor, clonus, seizures, status epilepticus
Topiramate	21	200–600	Sedation, confusion, slurred speech, ataxia, tremor, anxiety, agitation, seizures; hypotension; hyperchloremic non–anion gap metabolic acidosis
Vigabatrin	4–8	2,000–4,000	Sedation, confusion, coma, agitation, delirium, psychotic disturbances (hallucinations, delusions, paranoia)
Zonisamide	50–68	100–400	Somnolence, ataxia, agitation; bradycardia, hypotension; respiratory depression

V. Treatment

A. Emergency and supportive measures

1. Maintain an open airway and assist ventilation if necessary (pp 1–7). Administer supplemental oxygen.
2. Treat stupor and coma (p 18) if they occur. Protect the patient from self-injury secondary to ataxia.
3. Treat anticonvulsant-induced seizures using benzodiazepines (p 516).

4. Treat agitation and delirium (p 24) if they occur.
5. Monitor asymptomatic patients for a minimum of 4–6 hours. Admit symptomatic patients for at least 24 hours after lamotrigine, lacosamide, felbamate, topiramate, or zonisamide ingestions.

B. **Specific drugs and antidotes.** There are no specific antidotes. Sodium bicarbonate (p 520) may be useful for lamotrigine-induced QRS-interval prolongation. It also appeared to narrow the QRS in a lacosamide poisoning.

C. **Decontamination** (p 50). Administer activated charcoal orally if conditions are appropriate (see Table I–38, p 54). Gastric lavage is not necessary after small-to-moderate ingestions if activated charcoal can be given promptly.

D. **Enhanced elimination.** Hemodialysis is effective at removing **gabapentin, lacosamide, pregabalin,** and **topiramate,** but clinical manifestations are usually responsive to supportive care, making enhanced removal procedures unnecessary.

▶ ANTIDEPRESSANTS, GENERAL (NONCYCLIC)

Neal L. Benowitz, MD

Many noncyclic antidepressants are available. These can be classified as selective serotonin reuptake inhibitors (SSRIs), including fluoxetine (Prozac), sertraline (Zoloft), citalopram (Celexa), escitalopram (Lexapro), paroxetine (Paxil), and fluvoxamine (Luvox); serotonin-norepinephrine reuptake inhibitors (SNRIs), including venlafaxine (Effexor), desvenlafaxine (Pristiq) duloxetine (Cymbalta), milnacipran (Savella) and levomilnacipran (Fetzima); norepinephrine-dopamine reuptake inhibitors (NDRIs), including bupropion (Wellbutrin); and others, including trazodone (Desyrel) and mirtazapine (Remeron), the latter a tetracyclic antidepressant. Bupropion is also marketed under the brand name Zyban for smoking cessation. In overdose these drugs are generally less toxic than the **tricyclic antidepressants** (p 107) and the **monoamine oxidase (MAO) inhibitors** (p 326), although serious effects, such as seizures, hypotension, cardiac arrhythmias, and serotonin syndrome, occasionally occur. Noncyclic and tricyclic antidepressants are described in Table II–8.

I. **Mechanism of toxicity**

A. **SSRIs** inhibit serotonin reuptake transporters resulting in increased stimulation of serotonin receptors in the brain. **SNRIs** inhibit both serotonin and norepinephrine reuptake transporters and also increase stimulation of CNS norepinephrine receptors. Most agents cause CNS depression. Bupropion is a stimulant that can also cause seizures, presumably related to inhibition of reuptake of dopamine and norepinephrine.

B. Trazodone and mirtazapine produce peripheral alpha-adrenergic blockade, which can result in hypotension and priapism.

C. Serotonin reuptake inhibitors, such as fluoxetine, citalopram, sertraline, paroxetine, fluvoxamine, venlafaxine, and trazodone, may interact with each other, with chronic use of an MAO inhibitor (p 326), or with dextromethorphan (p 215) to produce the "**serotonin syndrome**" (see below and p 21).

D. None of the drugs in this group has significant anticholinergic effects.

E. **Pharmacokinetics.** These drugs have large volumes of distribution (Vd = 12–88 L/kg), except for trazodone (Vd = 1.3 L/kg). Most are eliminated via hepatic metabolism (see also Table II–66, p 462). Fluoxetine and paroxetine are potent inhibitors of the drug-metabolizing cytochrome P450 enzyme CYP2D6, which leads to many potential drug interactions. **Absorption may be delayed with extended-release formulations (eg, Wellbutrin-XL).**

II. **Toxic dose.** The noncyclic antidepressants generally have a wide therapeutic index, with doses in excess of 10 times the usual therapeutic dose tolerated without serious toxicity. Bupropion can cause seizures in some patients with

TABLE II–8. ANTIDEPRESSANTS

	Usual Adult Daily Dose (mg)	Neurotransmitter Effects[a]	Toxicity[b]
Tricyclic antidepressants			
Amitriptyline	75–200	NE, 5-HT	A, H, QRS, Sz
Amoxapine	150–300	NE, DA	A, H, Sz
Clomipramine	100–250	NE, 5-HT	A, H, QRS, Sz
Desipramine	75–200	NE	A, H, Sz
Doxepin	75–300	NE, 5-HT	A, H, QRS, Sz
Imipramine	75–200	NE, 5-HT	A, H, QRS, Sz
Maprotiline	75–300	NE	A, H, QRS, Sz
Nortriptyline	75–150	NE	A, H, QRS, Sz
Protriptyline	20–40	NE	A, H, QRS, Sz
Trimipramine	75–200	NE, 5-HT	A, H, QRS, Sz
Newer, noncyclic drugs			
Bupropion	200–450	DA, NE	Sz
Citalopram	20–40	5-HT	Sz, SS
Desvenlafaxine	50	5-HT, NE	Sz, SS
Duloxetine	30–180	5-HT, NE	Sz, SS
Escitalopram	10–30	5-HT	Sz, SS
Fluoxetine	20–80	5-HT	Sz, SS
Fluvoxamine	50–300	5-HT	Sz, SS
Levomilnacipran	40–120	5-HT, NE	Sz, SS
Milnacipran	100–200	5-HT, NE	Sz, SS
Mirtazapine	15–45	$Alpha_2$	Sz
Nefazodone	100–600	5-HT, $Alpha_2$	H
Paroxetine	20–50	5-HT	Sz, SS
Sertraline	50–200	5-HT	Sz, SS
Trazodone	50–400	5-HT, $Alpha_2$	H, Sz, SS
Venlafaxine	30–600	5-HT, NE	Sz, SS
Monoamine oxidase inhibitors	See p 326		

[a]$Alpha_2$, central $alpha_2$-adrenergic receptor agonist; DA, dopamine reuptake inhibitor; 5-HT, serotonin reuptake inhibitor; NE, norepinephrine reuptake inhibitor.
[b]A, anticholinergic effects; H, hypotension; QRS, QRS prolongation; SS, serotonin syndrome; Sz, seizures.

moderate overdoses or even in therapeutic doses, particularly in people with a history of seizure disorders.

III. Clinical presentation

A. Central nervous system. The usual presentation after SSRI overdose includes ataxia, sedation, and coma. Respiratory depression may occur, especially with co-ingestion of alcohol or other drugs. These agents, particularly bupropion, can cause restlessness, anxiety, and agitation. Tremor and seizures are common with bupropion but occur occasionally after overdose with SSRIs, particularly citalopram, as well as the SNRIs venlafaxine and duloxetine.

B. **Cardiovascular** effects are usually not life-threatening, although trazodone can cause hypotension and orthostatic hypotension, bupropion and SNRIs can cause sinus tachycardia and hypertension, and citalopram and escitalopram can cause sinus bradycardia with hypotension.

1. Severe cardiotoxicity, including QRS-interval prolongation, hypotension, and cardiac arrest, has been reported with overdoses involving bupropion, citalopram, and venlafaxine.
2. Venlafaxine and citalopram also cause QT-interval prolongation, and the FDA has recommended a maximal daily citalopram dose of 40 mg to minimize the risk of torsade de pointes.

C. **Serotonin syndrome** (p 21) is characterized by a triad of clinical features: neuromuscular hyperactivity (hyperreflexia, spontaneous or induced clonus, ocular clonus, rigidity, shivering); autonomic instability (tachycardia, hypertension, diaphoresis, hyperthermia, mydriasis, tremor); and mental status changes (agitation, anxiety, confusion, hypomania).

1. This reaction may be seen when a patient taking an MAO inhibitor (p 326) ingests a serotonin uptake blocker. Because of the long duration of effects of MAO inhibitors and most of the serotonin uptake blockers, this reaction can occur up to several days to weeks after either treatment regimen has been discontinued.
2. The syndrome has also been described in patients taking an overdose of a single SSRI or SNRI, an SSRI with meperidine, fentanyl, amphetamines, and derivatives (eg, methylenedioxymethamphetamine [MDMA]), dextromethorphan, linezolid, lithium, St. John's wort or combinations of various SSRIs and/or SNRIs. The FDA has issued a warning about the risk for serotonin syndrome from the combination of triptans with SSRIs, but causation is still not established.

IV. **Diagnosis.** A noncyclic antidepressant overdose should be suspected in patients with a history of depression who develop lethargy, coma, or seizures. As these agents uncommonly affect cardiac conduction, QRS-interval prolongation should suggest a tricyclic antidepressant overdose (p 107).

A. **Specific levels**. Blood and urine assays are not routinely available and are not useful for emergency management. These drugs are not likely to appear on a rapid "drugs of abuse" screen, and they may or may not appear on comprehensive toxicology screening, depending on the laboratory.

B. **Other useful laboratory studies** include electrolytes, glucose, arterial blood gases or pulse oximetry, and ECG monitoring.

V. **Treatment**

A. Emergency and supportive measures

1. Maintain an open airway and assist ventilation if needed (pp 1–7). Administer supplemental oxygen.
2. Treat coma (p 18), QRS-interval prolongation (p 10), QT prolongation or arrhythmias (p 13), hypotension (p 15), hypertension, and seizures (p 23) if they occur.
3. For mild serotonin syndrome (p 21), benzodiazepines can be used for control of agitation and tremor. Severe serotonin syndrome with hyperthermia requires hospitalization and aggressive cooling measures, which often include neuromuscular paralysis and endotracheal intubation.
4. Because of the potential for delayed onset of seizures, observe patients for 24 hours after sustained-release bupropion or venlafaxine overdose.

B. **Specific drugs and antidotes.** For suspected serotonin syndrome, anecdotal reports and case series claim benefit from cyproheptadine (p 537), 12 mg orally or by nasogastric tube, followed by 4 mg every hour for 3–4 doses. Chlorpromazine, 25–50 mg IV, has also been recommended.

C. **Decontamination** (p 50). Administer activated charcoal orally if conditions are appropriate (see Table I–38, p 54). Gastric lavage is not necessary after small-to-moderate ingestions if activated charcoal can be given promptly.

D. Enhanced elimination. In general, owing to extensive protein binding and large volumes of distribution, dialysis, hemoperfusion, peritoneal dialysis, and repeat-dose charcoal are not effective.

▶ ANTIDEPRESSANTS, TRICYCLIC

Neal L. Benowitz, MD

Tricyclic antidepressants taken in overdose by suicidal patients are a substantial cause of poisoning hospitalizations and deaths. Currently available tricyclic antidepressants are described in Table II–8. Amitriptyline also is marketed in combination with chlordiazepoxide (Limbitrol) or perphenazine (Etrafon or Triavil). **Cyclobenzaprine** (Flexeril), a centrally acting muscle relaxant (p 419), is structurally related to the tricyclic antidepressants but exhibits minimal cardiotoxic and variable CNS effects. **Newer, noncyclic antidepressants** are discussed on p 104. **Monoamine oxidase inhibitors** are discussed on p 326.

I. **Mechanism of toxicity.** Tricyclic antidepressant toxicity affects primarily the cardiovascular and central nervous systems.
   A. **Cardiovascular effects.** Several mechanisms contribute to cardiovascular toxicity:
      1. Anticholinergic effects and inhibition of neuronal reuptake of catecholamines result in tachycardia and mild hypertension.
      2. Peripheral alpha-adrenergic blockade causes vasodilation and contributes to hypotension.
      3. Membrane-depressant (quinidine-like) effects cause myocardial depression and cardiac conduction disturbances by inhibition of the fast sodium channel that initiates the cardiac cell action potential. Metabolic or respiratory acidosis may contribute to cardiotoxicity by further inhibiting the fast sodium channel.
   B. **Central nervous system effects.** These effects result in part from anticholinergic toxicity (eg, sedation and coma), but seizures are probably a result of inhibition of reuptake of norepinephrine or serotonin in the brain or other central effects.
   C. **Pharmacokinetics.** Anticholinergic effects of these drugs may retard gastric emptying, resulting in slow or erratic absorption. Most of these drugs are extensively bound to body tissues and plasma proteins, resulting in very large volumes of distribution and long elimination half-lives (see Tables II–8 and II–66). Tricyclic antidepressants are metabolized primarily by the liver, with only a small fraction excreted unchanged in the urine. Active metabolites may contribute to toxicity; several drugs are metabolized to other well-known tricyclic antidepressants (eg, amitriptyline to nortriptyline, imipramine to desipramine).

II. **Toxic dose.** Most of the tricyclic antidepressants have a narrow therapeutic index, so that doses of less than 10 times the therapeutic daily dose may produce severe intoxication. In general, ingestion of 10–20 mg/kg is potentially life-threatening.

III. **Clinical presentation.** Tricyclic antidepressant poisoning may produce any of three major toxic syndromes: anticholinergic effects, cardiovascular effects, and seizures. Hyponatremia is also common. Depending on the dose and the drug, patients may experience some or all of these toxic effects. Symptoms usually begin within 30–40 minutes of ingestion but may be delayed owing to slow and erratic gut absorption. Patients who are awake initially may abruptly lose consciousness or develop seizures without warning.
   A. **Anticholinergic** effects include sedation, delirium, coma, dilated pupils, dry skin and mucous membranes, diminished sweating, tachycardia, diminished or

absent bowel sounds, and urinary retention. Myoclonic muscle jerking is common with anticholinergic intoxication and may be mistaken for seizure activity.

B. **Cardiovascular** toxicity manifests as abnormal cardiac conduction, arrhythmias, and hypotension.

1. Typical **electrocardiographic findings** include sinus tachycardia with prolongation of the PR, QRS, and QT intervals. A prominent terminal R wave is often seen in lead aVR. Various degrees of atrioventricular (AV) block may be seen. A Brugada pattern (down-sloping ST-segment elevation in V1–V3 in association with a right bundle branch block) has also been reported.
   a. Prolongation of the QRS complex to 0.12 seconds or longer, a terminal R wave of 3 mm or more in aVR, and a terminal R wave/S wave ratio of 0.7 or more in aVR are fairly reliable predictors of serious cardiovascular and neurologic toxicity (except in the case of amoxapine, which causes seizures and coma with no change in the QRS interval).
   b. Sinus tachycardia accompanied by QRS-interval prolongation may resemble ventricular tachycardia (see Figure I–3, p 11). True ventricular tachycardia and fibrillation may also occur.
   c. Atypical or polymorphous ventricular tachycardia (torsade de pointes; see Figure I–7, p 14) associated with QT-interval prolongation may occur with therapeutic dosing but is actually uncommon in overdose.
   d. Development of bradyarrhythmias usually indicates a severely poisoned heart and carries a poor prognosis.
2. **Hypotension** caused by venodilation is common and usually mild. In severe cases, hypotension results from myocardial depression and may be refractory to treatment; some patients die with progressive, intractable cardiogenic shock. Pulmonary edema is also common in severe poisonings.

C. **Seizures** are common with tricyclic antidepressant toxicity and may be recurrent or persistent. The muscular hyperactivity from seizures and myoclonic jerking, combined with diminished sweating, can lead to severe hyperthermia (p 21), resulting in rhabdomyolysis, brain damage, multisystem failure, and death.

D. **Death** from tricyclic antidepressant overdose usually occurs within a few hours of admission and may result from ventricular fibrillation, intractable cardiogenic shock, or status epilepticus with hyperthermia. Sudden death several days after apparent recovery has been reported occasionally, but in all such cases, there was evidence of continuing cardiac toxicity within 24 hours of death.

IV. **Diagnosis.** Tricyclic antidepressant poisoning should be suspected in any patient with lethargy, coma, or seizures accompanied by QRS-interval prolongation or a terminal R wave in aVR of greater than 3 mm.

A. **Specific levels**

1. Plasma levels of some of the tricyclic antidepressants can be measured by clinical laboratories. Therapeutic concentrations are usually less than 0.3 mg/L (300 ng/mL). Total concentrations of parent drug plus metabolite of 1 mg/L (1,000 ng/mL) or greater usually are associated with serious poisoning. Generally, plasma levels are not used in emergency management because the QRS interval and clinical manifestations of overdose are reliable and more readily available indicators of toxicity.
2. Most tricyclics are detectable on comprehensive urine toxicology screening. Some rapid immunologic techniques are available and have sufficiently broad cross-reactivity to detect several tricyclics. However, use of these assays for rapid screening in the hospital laboratory is not recommended because they may miss some important drugs and give false-positive results for other drugs (eg, cyclobenzaprine or diphenhydramine) that are present in therapeutic concentrations. Because diphenhydramine is widely used, it causes many more false-positive than true-positive tricyclic antidepressant results, leading to significant diagnostic ambiguity.

B. Other useful laboratory studies include electrolytes, glucose, BUN, creatinine, creatine kinase (CK), urinalysis for myoglobin, arterial blood gases or oximetry, 12-lead ECG and continuous ECG monitoring, and chest radiography.

V. Treatment

A. Emergency and supportive measures

1. Maintain an open airway and assist ventilation if necessary (pp 1–7). ***Caution:*** Respiratory arrest can occur abruptly and without warning.
2. Treat coma (p 18), seizures (p 23), hyperthermia (p 21), hypotension (p 15), and arrhythmias (pp 13–15) if they occur. ***Note:*** Do **not** use procainamide or other type Ia or Ic antiarrhythmic agents for ventricular tachycardia because these drugs may aggravate cardiotoxicity.
3. Consider cardiac pacing for bradyarrhythmias and high-degree AV block, and overdrive pacing for torsade de pointes.
4. Mechanical support of the circulation (eg, cardiopulmonary bypass) may be useful (based on anecdotal reports) in stabilizing patients with refractory shock, allowing time for the body to eliminate some of the drug.
5. If seizures are not immediately controlled with usual anticonvulsants, paralyze the patient with a neuromuscular blocker (p 586) to prevent hyperthermia, which may induce further seizures, and lactic acidosis, which aggravates cardiotoxicity. ***Note:*** Paralysis abolishes the muscular manifestations of seizures but has no effect on brain seizure activity. After paralysis, electroencephalographic (EEG) monitoring is necessary to determine the efficacy of anticonvulsant therapy.
6. Continuously monitor the temperature, other vital signs, and ECG in asymptomatic patients for a minimum of 6 hours, and admit patients to an intensive care setting for at least 24 hours if there are any signs of toxicity.
7. If the patient is resuscitated after cardiac arrest, therapeutic hypothermia has been suggested to be beneficial in a case report.

B. Specific drugs and antidotes

1. In patients with QRS-interval prolongation or hypotension, administer sodium bicarbonate (p 520), 1–2 mEq/kg IV, and repeat as needed to maintain arterial pH between 7.45 and 7.55. **Sodium bicarbonate** may reverse membrane-depressant effects by increasing extracellular sodium concentrations and by a direct effect of pH on the fast sodium channel. Hypertonic sodium chloride has similar effects in animal studies and some human case reports.
2. When cardiotoxicity persists despite treatment with sodium bicarbonate, the use of **lidocaine** can be considered, although evidence in people is still limited. Lidocaine competes with tricyclic antidepressants for binding at the sodium channel but binds for a shorter period of time and thus may reverse some of sodium channel blockade.
3. For severe tricyclic overdose, particularly with amitriptyline and clomipramine, the use of **intravenous lipid emulsion** therapy has been reported to be beneficial (p 574).
4. Hyperventilation, by inducing a respiratory alkalosis (or reversing respiratory acidosis), may also be of benefit but works only transiently and may provoke seizures.
5. Although **physostigmine** was advocated in the past, it should ***not*** be administered routinely to patients with tricyclic antidepressant poisoning; it may aggravate conduction disturbances, causing asystole; further impair myocardial contractility, worsening hypotension; and contribute to seizures.

C. Decontamination (p 50). Administer activated charcoal orally if conditions are appropriate (see Table I–38, p 54). Gastric lavage is not necessary after small-to-moderate ingestions if activated charcoal can be given promptly, but it should be considered for large ingestions (eg, >20–30 mg/kg).

D. Enhanced elimination. Owing to extensive tissue and protein binding with a resulting large volume of distribution, dialysis and hemoperfusion are not effective. Although repeat-dose charcoal has been reported to accelerate tricyclic antidepressant elimination, the data are not convincing.

▶ ANTIHISTAMINES

Beth Manning, PharmD

Antihistamines (H_1 receptor antagonists) are commonly found in over-the-counter and prescription medications used for motion sickness, control of allergy-related itching, and cough and cold palliation and used as sleep aids (Table II–9). Acute intoxication with antihistamines results in symptoms very similar to those of anticholinergic poisoning. H_2 receptor blockers (cimetidine, ranitidine, and famotidine) inhibit gastric acid secretion but otherwise share no effects with H_1 agents, do not produce significant intoxication, and are not discussed here. Common combination products containing antihistamines include Actifed, Allerest, Contac, Coricidin, Dimetapp, Dristan, Drixoral, Excedrin PM, Nyquil, Nytol, Pamprin, PediaCare, Tavist, Triaminic, Triaminicol, Unisom Dual Relief Formula, and Vicks Pediatric Formula 44.

I. Mechanism of toxicity

A. H_1 blocker antihistamines are structurally related to histamine and antagonize the effects of histamine on H_1 receptor sites. They have anticholinergic effects (except the "nonsedating" agents: cetirizine, desloratadine, fexofenadine, levocetirizine, and loratadine). They may also stimulate or depress the CNS, and some agents (eg, diphenhydramine) have local anesthetic and membrane-depressant effects in large doses.

B. Pharmacokinetics. Drug absorption may be delayed because of the pharmacologic effects of these agents on the GI tract. Volumes of distribution are generally large (3–20 L/kg). Elimination half-lives are highly variable, ranging from 1–4 hours for diphenhydramine to 7–24 hours for many of the others (see also Table II–66, p 462).

II. Toxic dose. The estimated fatal oral dose of diphenhydramine is 20–40 mg/kg. Children are more sensitive to the toxic effects of antihistamines than are adults. Pediatric ingestions of less than 7.5 mg/kg of diphenhydramine are not expected to cause significant toxicity. The nonsedating agents are associated with less toxicity. Up to 300 mg of loratadine is expected to cause only minor effects in pediatric patients.

III. Clinical presentation

A. An overdose results in many symptoms similar to those of anticholinergic poisoning: drowsiness, dilated pupils, flushed dry skin, fever, tachycardia,

TABLE II–9. ANTIHISTAMINES

Drug	Usual Duration of Action (h)	Usual Single Adult Dose (mg)	Sedation
Ethanolamines			
Bromodiphenhydramine	4–6	12.5–25	+++
Carbinoxamine	3–4	4–8	++
Clemastine	10–12	0.67–2.68	++
Dimenhydrinate	4–6	50–100	+++
Diphenhydramine	4–6	25–50	+++
Diphenylpyraline	6–8	5	++

(continued)

TABLE II–9. ANTIHISTAMINES (CONTINUED)

Drug	Usual Duration of Action (h)	Usual Single Adult Dose (mg)	Sedation
Doxylamine	4–6	25	+++
Phenyltoloxamine	6–8	50	+++
Ethylenediamines			
Pyrilamine	4–6	25–50	++
Thenyldiamine	8	10	++
Tripelennamine	4–6	25–50	++
Alkylamines			
Acrivastine	6–8	8	+
Brompheniramine	4–6	4–8	+
Chlorpheniramine	4–6	4–8	+
Dexbrompheniramine	6–8	2–4	+
Dexchlorpheniramine	6–8	2–4	+
Dimethindene	8	1–2	+
Pheniramine	8–12	25–50	+
Pyrrobutamine	8–12	15	+
Triprolidine	4–6	2.5	+
Piperazines			
Buclizine	8	50	
Cetirizine	24	5–10	+/–
Cinnarizine	8	15–30	+
Cyclizine	4–6	25–50	+
Flunarizine	24	5–10	+
Hydroxyzine	20–25	25–50	+++
Levocetirizine	24	5	+
Meclizine	12–24	25–50	+
Phenothiazines			
Methdilazine	6–12	4–8	+++
Promethazine	4–8	25–50	+++
Trimeprazine	6	2.5	+++
Others			
Astemizole[a]	30–60 days	10	+/–
Azatidine	12	1–2	++
Cyproheptadine	8	2–4	+
Desloratadine	24	5	+/–
Fexofenadine	24	60	+/–
Loratadine	>24	10	+/–
Phenindamine	4–6	25	+/–
Terfenadine[a]	12	60	+/–

[a]Withdrawn from the US market because of reports of prolonged-QT syndrome and torsade-type atypical ventricular tachycardia.

delirium, hallucinations, and myoclonic or choreoathetoid movements. Convulsions, rhabdomyolysis, and hyperthermia may occur with a serious overdose, and complications such as renal failure and pancreatitis have been reported.

B. **Massive diphenhydramine** overdoses have been reported to cause QRS widening and myocardial depression, similar to tricyclic antidepressant overdoses (p 107).

C. **QT-interval prolongation** and torsade-type atypical ventricular tachycardia (p 14) have been associated with elevated serum levels of **terfenadine** or **astemizole. (Both of these drugs have been removed from the US market.)** It has also been reported with a large diphenhydramine overdose.

IV. **Diagnosis** is generally based on the history of ingestion and can usually be readily confirmed by the presence of a typical anticholinergic syndrome. Comprehensive urine toxicology screening will detect most common antihistamines.

A. **Specific levels** are not generally available or useful.

B. **Other useful laboratory studies** include electrolytes, glucose, creatine kinase (CK), arterial blood gases or pulse oximetry, and ECG monitoring (diphenhydramine, terfenadine, or astemizole).

V. **Treatment**

A. **Emergency and supportive measures**

1. Maintain an open airway and assist ventilation if necessary (pp 1–7).
2. Treat coma (p 18), seizures (p 23), hyperthermia (p 21), and atypical ventricular tachycardia (p 14) if they occur.
3. Monitor the patient for at least 6–8 hours after ingestion.

B. **Specific drugs and antidotes**. There is no specific antidote for antihistamine overdose. As for anticholinergic poisoning (p 97), **physostigmine** has been used for the treatment of severe delirium or tachycardia. However, because antihistamine overdoses carry a greater risk for seizures and wide-complex tachycardia, physostigmine is not recommended routinely. **Sodium bicarbonate** (p 520), 1–2 mEq/kg IV, may be useful for myocardial depression and QRS-interval prolongation after a massive diphenhydramine overdose.

C. **Decontamination** (p 50). Administer activated charcoal orally if conditions are appropriate (see Table I–38, p 54). Gastric lavage is not necessary after small-to-moderate ingestions if activated charcoal can be given promptly. Because of slowed GI motility, gut decontamination procedures may be helpful, even in late-presenting patients.

D. **Enhanced elimination.** Hemodialysis, hemoperfusion, peritoneal dialysis, and repeat-dose activated charcoal are not effective in removing antihistamines.

▶ ANTIMONY AND STIBINE

Rais Vohra, MD

Antimony (Sb) is a versatile trace element widely used for hardening soft metal alloys; for compounding rubber; as a major flame retardant component (5–20%) in plastics, textiles, and clothing; and as a coloring agent in dyes, varnishes, paints, and glazes. Exposure to antimony dusts and fumes may occur during mining and refining of ores, in glassworking, and from the discharge of firearms. Organic pentavalent antimony compounds (sodium stibogluconate and antimoniate meglumine) are commonly used worldwide as antiparasitic drugs. Foreign or folk remedies may contain antimony potassium tartrate ("tartar emetic" or trivalent antimony), which was widely used in previous centuries as an emetic, purgative, and aversive therapy for alcohol abuse. **Stibine** (antimony hydride, SbH3) is a colorless gas with the odor of rotten eggs that is produced as a by-product when antimony-containing ore or furnace slag is treated with acid.

I. **Mechanism of toxicity.** The mechanism of antimony and stibine toxicity is not known. Because these compounds are chemically related to arsenic and arsine gas, respectively, their modes of action may be similar.

A. **Antimony** compounds probably act by binding to sulfhydryl groups, enhancing oxidative stress, and inactivating key enzymes. Ingested antimonials are corrosive to GI mucosal membranes and demonstrate significant enterohepatic recirculation.

B. **Stibine,** like arsine, may cause hemolysis. It is also an irritant gas.

II. **Toxic dose**

A. An estimated toxic amount of the organic antimony compound tartar emetic (nonelemental antimony) is 0.1–1 g. The lethal oral dose of metallic **antimony** in rats is 100 mg/kg of body weight; the trivalent and pentavalent oxides are less toxic, with LD50 in rats ranging from 3,200 to 4,000 mg/kg of body weight. The recommended workplace limit (ACGIH TLV-TWA) for antimony is 0.5 mg/m^3 as an 8-hour time-weighted average. The air level considered to be immediately dangerous to life or health (IDLH) is 50 mg/m^3.

B. The recommended workplace limit (ACGIH TLV-TWA) for **stibine** is 0.1 ppm as an 8-hour time-weighted average. The air level considered immediately dangerous to life or health (IDLH) is 5 ppm.

III. **Clinical presentation**

A. **Acute ingestion of antimony** causes nausea, vomiting, hemorrhagic gastritis, and diarrhea. Hepatitis, renal insufficiency, and prolongation of the QTc interval may occur. Cardiac dysrhythmias (including torsade de pointes), hyperkalemia, pancreatitis, aplastic crisis, and arthralgias have been associated with the use of antimonial antiprotozoal drugs, such as stibogluconate, for the treatment of parasitic infections.

B. **Acute stibine gas inhalation** causes acute hemolysis, resulting in anemia, jaundice, hemoglobinuria, and renal failure.

C. **Chronic exposure to antimony dusts and fumes** in the workplace is the most common type of exposure and may result in headache, anorexia, respiratory tract and eye irritation, pneumonitis/pneumoconiosis, peptic ulcers, and dermatitis ("antimony spots"). Sudden death presumably resulting from a direct cardiotoxic effect has been reported in workers exposed to antimony trisulfide. Based on evidence of in vitro genotoxicity and limited rodent carcinogenicity testing, antimony trioxide is a suspected carcinogen (IARC 2B).

1. In 2009, the Centers for Disease Control and Prevention (CDC) investigated a cluster of nonspecific neurologic symptoms among firefighters in Florida, concluding that antimony-containing flame retardant uniforms did not cause clinical or laboratory changes consistent with antimony toxicity.
2. A suspected causal link between antimony and the sudden infant death syndrome (SIDS) has been refuted.

IV. **Diagnosis** is based on a history of exposure and typical clinical presentation.

A. **Specific levels.** Urine antimony levels are normally below 2 mcg/L. Serum and whole-blood levels are not reliable and are no longer used. Urine concentrations correlate poorly with workplace exposure, but exposure to air concentrations greater than the TLV-TWA will increase urinary levels. Urinary antimony is increased after firearm discharge exposure. Hair analysis is not recommended because of the risk for external contamination. There is no established toxic antimony level after stibine exposure.

B. **Other useful investigations** include CBC, plasma-free hemoglobin, serum lactate dehydrogenase (LDH), free haptoglobin, electrolytes, BUN, creatinine, urinalysis for free hemoglobin, liver aminotransferases, bilirubin, ammonia, prothrombin time, cardiac injury biomarkers and 12-lead ECG. Chest radiography is recommended for chronic respiratory exposures.

V. **Treatment**

A. **Emergency and supportive measures**

1. **Antimony.** Large-volume IV fluid resuscitation may be necessary for shock caused by gastroenteritis (p 15). Electrolyte abnormalities should be corrected, and intensive supportive care may be necessary for patients with

multiple-organ failure. Perform continuous cardiac monitoring and treat torsade de pointes if it occurs (p 14).

2. **Stibine.** Blood transfusion may be necessary after massive hemolysis. Treat hemoglobinuria with fluids and bicarbonate as for rhabdomyolysis (p 27).

B. **Specific drugs and antidotes.** There is no specific antidote. British anti-lewisite (BAL; dimercaprol), dimercaptosuccinic acid (DMSA), and dimercaptopropanesulfonic acid (DMPS) have been proposed as chelators for antimony, although data in human poisoning are conflicting. Chelation therapy is not expected to be effective for stibine. Case reports have described the use of NAC (N-acetylcysteine, p 499) to facilitate the conjugation of trivalent antimony to glutathione.

C. **Decontamination** (p 50)

1. **Inhalation.** Remove the patient from exposure, and give supplemental oxygen if available. Protect rescuers from exposure.
2. **Ingestion** of antimony salts. Activated charcoal is probably not effective in light of its poor adsorption of antimony. Gastric lavage may be helpful if performed soon after a large ingestion.

D. **Enhanced elimination.** Hemodialysis, hemoperfusion, and forced diuresis are ***not*** effective at removing antimony or stibine. Exchange transfusion may be effective in treating massive hemolysis caused by stibine.

► ANTINEOPLASTIC AGENTS

Susan Kim-Katz, PharmD

Other than iatrogenic errors, relatively few acute overdoses of antineoplastic drugs have been reported. However, because of the inherently cytotoxic nature of most of these agents, an overdose is more likely to be extremely serious. In this chapter, antineoplastic drugs are classified into 12 broad categories and are listed alphabetically in Table II–10. Radiologic agents are not included in this chapter, and arsenic is discussed on p 140.

I. **Mechanism of toxicity.** In general, toxic effects are extensions of the pharmacologic properties of these drugs.

A. **Alkylating agents.** These drugs attack nucleophilic sites on DNA, resulting in alkylation and cross-linking and thus inhibiting replication and transcription. Binding to RNA or protein moieties appears to contribute little to cytotoxic effects.

B. **Antibiotics.** These drugs intercalate within base pairs in DNA, inhibiting DNA-directed RNA synthesis. Another potential mechanism may be the generation of cytotoxic free radicals.

C. **Antimetabolites.** These agents interfere with normal nucleic acid biosynthesis at various stages. Antimetabolites may also be incorporated into nucleic acids in place of corresponding normal nucleotides.

D. **DNA demethylation agents.** Hypermethylation of DNA is a common characteristic of some cancers, particularly myelodysplasias. Hypomethylation can confer direct cytotoxic effects as well as alterations of gene expression that may prevent disease progression.

E. Histone deacetylases (HDACs) catalyze the removal of acetyl groups from lysine residues of proteins. In some cancer cells, HDACs may be overexpressed or be recruited for oncogenic transcription factors. **Histone deacetylase inhibitors** allow for the accumulation of acetylated histones, resulting in cell cycle arrest or apoptosis.

F. **Hormones.** Steroid hormones regulate the synthesis of steroid-specific proteins. The exact mechanism of antineoplastic action is unknown.

G. **Kinase inhibitors.** Mutation of protein kinases can trigger unregulated growth of the cell. Inhibition of kinase activity can result in decreased cellular proliferation, cell cycle arrest, and apoptosis.

TABLE II–10. ANTINEOPLASTIC DRUGS

Drug	Mechanism of Action[a]	Major Site(s) of Toxicity[b]	Comments
Abiraterone acetate	F (antiandrogen)	En+, H+	Risk of excess mineralocorticoid activity, adrenocortical insufficiency, hypophosphatemia. Potent inhibitor of cytochrome P450. Peak level 2 hours after oral dose.
Ado-trastuzumab emtansine	L	C+, G+, H+, M+, N+, P+	Thrombocytopenia common. Reduction in left ventricular ejection fraction seen. Watch for hypokalemia.
Afatinib	G	C+, D++, G++, H+, P+, R+	Diarrhea may be severe. Two adolescents developed nausea, vomiting, asthenia, dizziness, headache, abdominal pain, and elevated amylase after ingesting 360 mg. They recovered with supportive care. Peak level at 2–5 hours after oral dose.
Aldesleukin (interleukin 2)	L	An++, C++, D+, En+, G+, M+, N+, P++, R++	Commonly causes capillary leak syndrome resulting in severe hypotension. Respiratory distress may be life threatening.
Altretamine	A	G+, M+, N+	Reversible peripheral sensory neuropathy. Pyridoxine used to prevent neuropathy during therapy. Unknown if helpful with acute overdose. Peak plasma levels at 0.5–3 hours after oral dose.
Anastrozole	F (aromatase inhibitor)	En+, G±	High risk of osteoporosis. Acute toxic effects unlikely. Peak level within 2 hours.
Arsenic trioxide			See "Arsenic" p 140
Asparaginase	L	An++, En+, G+, H++, N++, R+	A 3yo boy who received a 10-fold overdose developed hyperammonemia, increased levels of glutamic and aspartic acid, and decreased levels of glutamine and asparagine. The laboratory values returned to normal after 1 week. Repeated plasmapheresis was performed on a 48yo with fulminant hepatic failure attributed to asparaginase and recovered fully.
Axitinib	G	C++, D+, En+, G+, H+, M+, N+, P+	Severe hypertension, hemorrhage, thromboembolic events. Doses up to 20 mg twice daily have resulted in dizziness, hypertension, seizures, and fatal hemoptysis. Peak plasma concentration 2.5–4.1 hours after oral dose.
Azacitidine	D	En+, G++, H+, M++, N+, R+	One patient experienced diarrhea, nausea, and vomiting after receiving a single IV dose of approximately 290 mg/m^2, almost 4 times the recommended starting dose.

(*continued*)

TABLE II–10. ANTINEOPLASTIC DRUGS (CONTINUED)

Drug	Mechanism of Action[a]	Major Site(s) of Toxicity[b]	Comments
BCG (intravesical)	L	G+	Attenuated Mycobacterium bovis. Bladder irritation, flulike symptoms common. Risk for sepsis in immunocompromised patients.
Bendamustine	A	An+, D++, G+, M++	Potentially fatal dermatologic reactions. Watch for tumor lysis syndrome. Of 4 patients treated at maximum single dose of 280 mg/m^2, 3 showed ECG changes, including QT prolongation, ST-segment and T-wave deviations, and left anterior fascicular block.
Bevacizumab	I	C++, G+, M+, N+,P+, R+	Severe and fatal hemorrhages, including GI perforation, wound dehiscence, hemoptysis, up to 5 times more frequent than in control groups. Hypertension, at times severe, common.
Bexarotene	L	D+, En+, G+, M+, N+	Serious lipid and thyroid abnormalities, fatal pancreatitis during therapy. Peak level 2–4 hours after oral dose.
Bicalutamide	F (antiandrogen)	En+, H+	Gynecomastia, hot flashes
Bleomycin	B	An++, D++, G+, P++	Pulmonary toxicity (eg, pneumonitis, fibrosis) in about 10% of patients. High concentration of inhaled oxygen may worsen injury. Febrile reaction in 20–25% of patients.
Bortezomib	L	An+, C+, G++, M++, N++	Peripheral neuropathy common. Overdose of twice the recommended dosage was fatal due to hypotension, thrombocytopenia.
Bosutinib	G	An+, D+, G++, H+, M++	Fluid retention may be severe. Time to peak after oral dose is 4–6 hours.
Brentuximab vedotin	L	An+, D+, G+, M++, N++	Peripheral sensory neuropathy common. Fatal Progressive Multifocal Leukoencephalopathy reported.
Busulfan	A	D+, En+, G++, M++, N+, P++	Pulmonary fibrosis, adrenal insufficiency with chronic use. Acute overdose of 2.4 g was fatal in a 10yo, and 140 mg resulted in pancytopenia in a 4yo. A 14yo who received 9 doses of 4 mg/kg every 6 hours developed seizures. Hemodialysis may be effective.
Cabazitaxel	H	A++, G+, M++, N+, R+	Severe hypersensitivity reaction can occur. Hematuria seen during therapy.
Cabozantinib	G	C+, D++, G++, M++, N+	Ingestion of 200 mg daily (twice the therapeutic dose) for 9 days caused memory loss, cognitive disturbance. Risk of GI perforation and fistulas, wound complications. Hand-foot syndrome common. Watch for hypocalcemia. Peak plasma levels at 2–5 hours after oral dose.

(continued)

TABLE II–10. ANTINEOPLASTIC DRUGS (CONTINUED)

Drug	Mechanism of Action[a]	Major Site(s) of Toxicity[b]	Comments
Capecitabine	C	C+, D+, G+, M+	Prodrug, converted to 5-fluorouracil. Hand-foot syndrome common. Hemodialysis may be effective. Peak level 1–1.5 hours after oral dose.
Carboplatin	J	An+, Ex+, G++, H+, M++, R+	Peripheral neuropathy in 4–10% of patients. Deaths from renal, hepatic failure; thrombocytopenia; thrombotic microangiopathic hemolytic anemia. Early dialysis may be effective. Peritoneal dialysis was not effective in one pediatric case.
Carfilzomib	L	An+, C+, G+, H+, M++, P+	Risk of worsening CHF, sudden cardiac death. Thrombocytopenia can be severe.
Carmustine (BCNU)	A	D+, Ex+, G++, H+, M+, P+	Flushing, hypotension, and tachycardia with rapid IV injection
Cetuximab	I	An++, D++, G+, N+, P+	Potentially fatal infusion reaction in 3% of patients. Low Mg^{2+} common.
Chlorambucil	A	D+, G+, H+, M+,N++	Seizures, confusion, coma reported after overdose. Acute overdoses of 0.125–6.8 mg/kg in children caused seizures up to 3–4 hours after ingestion. Bone marrow suppression with >6.5 mg/kg. Peak serum level 0.8 hours after oral dose.
Cisplatin	J	An+, Ex+, G++, H+, M+, N+, P+, R++	Ototoxic, nephrotoxic. A 750-mg acute IV overdose was fatal. A 33yo died 18 days after inadvertently receiving 100 mg/m^2 daily for 4 days. Good hydration essential. Plasmapheresis and plasma exchange may be helpful. Hemodialysis not effective. Amifostine and sodium thiosulfate have been used to reduce cytotoxic effects.
Cladribine	C	An+, D+, M++, N++, R++	Irreversible paraparesis/quadriparesis seen in high doses.
Clofarabine	C	C+, D+, En++, G++, H++, M++	Systemic inflammatory response syndrome, capillary leak possible. Severe hypokalemia, hypophosphatemia common.
Crizotinib	G	G+, H+, M++, N+P+	Life-threatening or fatal pneumonitis seen. QTc prolongation possible. Vision disorders common. Peak level at 4–6 hours after oral dose.
Cyclophosphamide	A	Al++, C+, D+, En+, G++, M++, P+, R+	Severe left ventricular dysfunction, respiratory distress, moderate transaminitis after 16,200 mg over 3 days. Hemodialysis may be effective. Mesna and N-acetylcysteine have been used investigationally to reduce hemorrhagic cystitis.

(*continued*)

TABLE II–10. ANTINEOPLASTIC DRUGS (CONTINUED)

Drug	Mechanism of Action[a]	Major Site(s) of Toxicity[b]	Comments
Cytarabine	C	An+, En+, G++, H+, M+, N++, P++	Cytarabine syndrome: fever, myalgia, bone pain, rash, malaise. Capillary leak syndrome with ARDS in 16% of cases. Cerebellar dysfunction may be severe. Hemodialysis may be effective if initiated very soon after an overdose.
Dabrafenib	G	Al+, An++, D+, En++	Hyperglycemia, hypophosphatemia common. Risk of hemolytic anemia in G6PD deficient patients. QTc prolongation risk. Time to peak 2 hours after oral dose.
Dacarbazine	A	Al+, An+, En+, G++, H+, M+	May produce flulike syndrome. Photosensitivity reported.
Dactinomycin (actinomycin D)	B	Al++, D+, Ex++, G++, M++, N+	A 10-fold overdose in a 1yo child resulted in severe hypotension, pancytopenia, acute renal failure, choreoathetosis. Highly corrosive to soft tissue.
Dasatinib	G	C+, D+, En+, G+, M++, N+, P+	High risk for severe fluid retention, hemorrhage. QT prolongation seen. Peak level 0.5–6 hours after oral dose.
Daunorubicin	B	Al+, An+, C++, Ex++, G+, M++, N+	Congestive cardiomyopathy risk after total cumulative dose >400 mg/m^2. A 3yo died after receiving 17 mg intrathecally. Dexrazoxane may be cardioprotective and beneficial for treatment of extravasation. Plasma exchange may remove liposomal daunorubicin.
Decitabine	D	An+, D+, En+, G+, M++, P+	Electrolyte abnormalities (low Mg^{++}, Na^+, K^+), peripheral edema common.
Degarelix	F (gonadotropin-releasing hormone antagonist)	H+	QTc prolongation possible.
Docetaxel	H	Al+, An++, C+, D+, Ex+, G+, M++, N+, P+	Severe fluid retention and edema in 6–9% of patients. Two patients who received 150–200 mg/m^2 over 1 hour developed severe neutropenia, cutaneous reactions and mild asthenia and paresthesias.
Doxorubicin	B	Al+, An+, C++, D+, Ex++, G++, M++, N+	CHF and cardiomyopathy may occur after total cumulative dose >400 mg/m^2. Arrhythmias after acute overdose. Two patients survived doxorubicin overdoses of 540 mg as a single dose and 300 mg over 2 days. Complications included severe mucositis and bone marrow suppression Hemoperfusion may be effective. Dexrazoxane is given for cardioprotection and extravasation.

(*continued*)

TABLE II–10. ANTINEOPLASTIC DRUGS (CONTINUED)

Drug	Mechanism of Action[a]	Major Site(s) of Toxicity[b]	Comments
Enzalutamide	F (antiandrogen)	En+, N+	Seizures have been reported following doses of 360–600 mg. Peak levels at 0.5–3 hours after oral dose.
Epirubicin	B	Al+, C++, Ex++, G++, M++	Death from multiple-organ failure reported in a 63yo woman after a single dose of 320 mg/m^2. Risk for congestive heart failure increases steeply after cumulative dose of 900 mg/m^2. Acute/early cardiotoxicity manifest as arrhythmias, ECG abnormalities. Dexrazoxane conferred protection from epirubicin-induced cardiotoxicity in several studies.
Eribulin mesylate	H	Al+, An+, G+, M++, N++, P+	Overdose of 4 times the therapeutic dose caused grade 3 neutropenia for 7 days and grade 3 hypersensitivity for 1 day. Watch for QTc prolongation.
Erlotinib	G	D+, G+, H+, P+	Fatal interstitial lung disease reported. Overdoses of 1,000 mg in healthy and up to 1,600 mg in cancer patients tolerated. Peak level 4 hours after oral dose.
Estramustine	A	En ±, G+, H±, M ±	Has weak estrogenic and alkylating activity
Etoposide	H	Al+, An+, Ex+, G+, M++, P+	A 25yo woman mistakenly took 4,900 mg over 25 days. She presented with fatigue, fever, cough, diarrhea, and grade 1–2 myelosuppression. Peak level 1–1.5 hours after oral dose.
Everolimus	G	An+, D+, En+, G+, H+, M+, P+, R+	Hyperglycemia, hyperlipidemia common. Fatal noninfectious pneumonitis seen. Peak level 1–2 hours after oral dose.
Exemestane	F (aromatase inhibitor)	En+, G±, H+, M+	Leukocytosis 1 hour after exemestane 25-mg ingestion in a child. Peak level at 2–4 hours post ingestion.
Floxuridine	C	Al+, G++, M++	Prodrug of 5-fluorouracil.
Fludarabine	C	An+, G+, M++, N++, P+	Blindness, seizures, coma, death at high doses. Peak level 1 hour after oral dose.
5-Fluorouracil	C	Al+, C+, D+, G++, M++, N+	Acute cerebellar syndrome seen. Cardiac arrest, sudden death during therapy. Death has occurred with 1,000 mg. Leucovorin may worsen toxicity. Uridine triacetate is a specific antidote (see text).
Flutamide	F (antiandrogen)	En+, H+	Gynecomastia. Aniline metabolite of flutamide has caused methemoglobinemia (p 317). A single dose of 5 g resulted in no sequelae.
Fulvestrant	F (antiestrogen)	Al ±, D ±, En ±, G ±	Acute toxic effects unlikely

(continued)

TABLE II–10. ANTINEOPLASTIC DRUGS (CONTINUED)

Drug	Mechanism of Action[a]	Major Site(s) of Toxicity[b]	Comments
Gemcitabine	C	An+, D+, G+, H++, M++, P++, R+	Can cause bronchospasm, severe ARDS, potentially fatal hemolytic-uremic syndrome.
Goserelin	F (gonadotropin-releasing hormone inhibitor)	En+	Initial increase in luteinizing hormone, follicle-stimulating hormone
Histrelin	F (gonadotropin-releasing hormone inhibitor)	En+	Initial increase in luteinizing hormone, follicle-stimulating hormone
Hydroxyurea	C	Al+, D+, G+, H+, M++	Leukopenia, anemia more common than thrombocytopenia. A 2yo girl developed only mild myelosuppression after ingesting 612 mg/kg acutely. Peak serum level 1–4 hours after oral dose.
Ibritumomab tiuxetan	I	An++, D+, Ex+, G+, M++, P+	Given with radiolabeled drug. Severe, fatal infusion reactions reported.
Ibrutinib	G	Al+, C+, G+, M++, P+, R+	Severe bleeding events (subdural hematoma, gastrointestinal bleeding, hematuria, and postprocedural bleeding) have occurred. Time to peak 1–2 hours after oral dose.
Idarubicin	B	Al+, C+, Ex++, G++, M++	Congestive heart failure may occur. Severe arrhythmias reported in one case of fatal overdose. One patient died after receiving 135 mg/m^2 (>10 times the therapeutic dose) over 3 days.
Ifosfamide	A	Al++, M++, N++, G++, R++	Hemorrhagic cystitis, somnolence, confusion, hallucinations, status epilepticus, coma seen during therapy. Cumulative dose of 26 g/m^2/cycle has caused irreversible renal failure. Combined hemodialysis and hemoperfusion reduced serum levels by 84%. Coadministration of Mesna decreases incidence and severity of bladder toxicity. N-acetylcystine may mitigate renal toxicity. Methylene blue may protect against and treat encephalopathy.
Imatinib	G	C+, D+, En+, G+, H+, M+, N+	Fluid retention and edema, muscle cramps common. Acute overdose of 6,400 mg by a 21yo caused severe vomiting, transient decrease in neutrophils, and mild transaminitis. A 53yo woman had severe abdominal pain and vomiting after ingesting 16 gm. A 47yo developed severe muscle cramps, CPK of 3,880 u/L after ingestion of 2 g. Ingestion of 400 mg by a 3yo resulted in vomiting, diarrhea, and anorexia. Another 3yo with ingestion of 980 mg developed leukopenia and diarrhea. Peak level 2–4 hours after oral dose.

(continued)

TABLE II–10. ANTINEOPLASTIC DRUGS (CONTINUED)

Drug	Mechanism of Action[a]	Major Site(s) of Toxicity[b]	Comments
Ipilimumab	I	D+, En+, G+, H+, N+	Potentially fatal immune mediated reactions most commonly include enterocolitis, hepatitis, dermatitis, neuropathy and endrocrinopathy (hypothyroidism, adrenal insufficiency).
Irinotecan	K	Al+, An+, G++, H+, M++, P+	Severe diarrhea, may be fatal. Cholinergic syndrome during infusion.
Ixabepilone	H	Al+, G+, M++, N++	Peripheral neuropathy common. One patient who mistakenly received 100 mg/m^2 (2.5 times therapeutic dose) experienced mild myalgia and fatigue one day after infusion, and recovered without further incident.
Lapatinib	G	C+, D+, G+, H+, M+, P+	Left ventricular ejection fraction decrease, QT prolongation seen. Grade 3 diarrhea and vomiting were reported in an adult on day 10 after taking 3,000 mg daily for 10 days. Peak level 4 hours after oral dose.
Letrozole	F (aromatase inhibitor)	En+, G±	No toxicity from 62.5-mg letrozole acute overdose
Leuprolide	F (gonadotropin-releasing hormone analog)	En+	Acute toxic effects unlikely. Initial increase in luteinizing hormone, follicle-stimulating hormone
Levamisole	L	G+, M+, N+	Nicotinic and muscarinic effects at cholinergic receptors. Gastroenteritis, dizziness, headache after 2.5-mg/kg dose. Fatality after ingestion of 15 mg/kg in a 3yo and 32 mg/kg in an adult. Several reports of agranulocytosis from cocaine adulterated with levamisole. Peak level 1.5–2 hours after oral dose.
Lomustine (CCNU)	A	Al+, G++, H+, M+, P+	Two patients developed grade 4 neutropenia and thrombocytopenia approximately 2 weeks after taking 800 mg orally over 4–5 days but recovered. 1,400 mg taken over 1 week was fatal in an adult. Peak level 1–4 hours after oral dose.
Mechlorethamine	A	D+, Ex++, G++, M++, N+	Powerful vesicant. Avoid contact with powder or vapors. Lymphocytopenia may occur within 24 hours. Watch for hyperuricemia.
Medroxyprogesterone	F (progestin)	An ±, En+, G±	Acute toxic effects unlikely. May induce porphyria in susceptible patients.
Megestrol	F (progestin)	An ±, En+, G±	Acute toxic effects unlikely. Potential for adrenal insufficiency with chronic use.

(continued)

TABLE II–10. ANTINEOPLASTIC DRUGS (CONTINUED)

Drug	Mechanism of Action[a]	Major Site(s) of Toxicity[b]	Comments
Melphalan	A	An+, En+, G+, M+, N+, P+	Hyponatremia, SIADH seen during therapy. A 1yo received 140 mg of IV (a 10-fold overdose) and developed pronounced lymphopenia within 24 hours then neutropenia, thrombocytopenia, and diarrhea by day 7. Peak level at 1 hour after oral dose.
6-Mercaptopurine	C	D+, G+, H++, M+	A 22-month-old child who ingested 86 mg/kg had severe neutropenia with nadir at 11 days. A 2yo with a maximum potential ingestion of 400 mg (26 mg/kg) did not develop clinical or laboratory evidence of toxicity. Peak level 1 hour after oral dose.
Methotrexate (p 319)	C	Al+, D+, G++, H+, M++, N+, P+, R+	Folinic acid (leucovorin [p 572]) is a specific antidote. Hemoperfusion questionably effective. Urinary alkalinization and repeat-dose charcoal may be helpful. Peak serum level 1–2 hours after oral dose.
Mitomycin	B	Al+, C+, D+, Ex++, G++, H+, M++, P+, R+	Hemolytic-uremic syndrome reported with therapeutic doses. Pulmonary toxicity at an average cumulative dose of 78 mg. The incidence of renal toxicity significantly increases with total cumulative doses of 120 mg.
Mitotane	L	Al+, D+, En++, G++, N++	Adrenal suppression; glucocorticoid replacement essential during stress.
Mitoxantrone	L	Al+, C+, Ex+, G++, M++, P+	Four patients died of severe leukopenia and infection after overdose. Reversible cardiomyopathy in one overdose case. Hemoperfusion was ineffective.
Nelarabine	D	G+, M++, N++, P+	Paralysis, seizures, coma, Guillain-Barre–like symptoms reported during treatment.
Nilotinib	G	C+, D+, En+, G+, H+, M++	Causes QT prolongation, electrolyte abnormalities. Peak level 3 hours after oral dose.
Nilutamide	F (antiandrogen)	En+, H+, P+	Ingestion of 13 g resulted in no evidence of toxicity
Obinutuzumab	I	An++, En+, H+, M++, R+	Severe infusion reactions. Tumor lysis syndrome 12–24 hours following infusion. May reactivate hepatitis B virus.
Ofatumumab	I	An++, D+, G+, M++, P+	Fatal infections in 17% of treated patients. Risk of serious infusion reactions, including bronchospasms, pulmonary edema. Tumor lysis syndrome. May reactivate hepatitis B virus.
Omacetaxine	L	An+, En+, G+, M++, N+	May induce glucose intolerance.

(continued)

TABLE II–10. ANTINEOPLASTIC DRUGS (CONTINUED)

Drug	Mechanism of Action[a]	Major Site(s) of Toxicity[b]	Comments
Oxaliplatin	J	An+, Ex+, G+,H+, M+, N++, P+	A 64yo woman developed peripheral neuropathy, diarrhea, thrombocytopenia, and neutropenia after receiving 500 mg. A 7yo had severe lower limb pain, respiratory distress, vomiting, diarrhea, severe thrombocytopenia, mild anemia, mild renal failure, and neurological symptoms (ie, nystagmus, lower limb weakness, hyperextension of the right foot) after inadvertently receiving 800 mg instead of 80 mg. An overdose of 500 mg IV resulted in fatality from respiratory failure, bradycardia.
Paclitaxel	H	Al++, An+, C+, G+, M++, N++	Severe hypersensitivity reactions, including death, reported. Hypotension, bradycardia, ECG abnormalities, conduction abnormalities may occur. Fatal myocardial infarction 15 hours into infusion reported.
Panitumumab	I	An+, D++, G+, P+	Severe infusion reaction possible. Watch for electrolyte depletion, especially K^+, Mg^{2+}
Pazopanib	G	C++, En+, G+, H++, M++	Hypertension, hyperglycemia common. Electrolyte depletion. Peak concentration 2–4 hours after oral dose.
Pegaspargase	L	An++, G+, H+, N+	Bleeding diathesis from low fibrinogen and antithrombin III. Incidence of pancreatitis 18% during treatment.
Pemetrexed	C	D+, G+, H+, M+, P+	Folic acid antagonist. Leucovorin may be useful. One report of using thymidine to prevent worsening renal injury. Patients must take daily vitamin B_{12}, folic acid.
Pentostatin	C	An+, C+, D+, G+, H+, M+, N+, P+, R+,	Central nervous system depression, convulsions, coma seen at high doses.
Pertuzumab	I	Al+, An+, C+, D+, G++, M++	Decreased left ventricular ejection fraction in 8–16% of patients.
Ponatinib	G	An+, C+, D+, En+, G+, H++, M++, N+, P+	Arterial and venous thrombosis and occlusion in at least 27% of patients. One patient given estimated 540 mg developed QT prolongation within 2 hours and died 9 days later from pneumonia and sepsis. Another patient who took 165 mg on cycle 1 and 2 experienced fatigue and noncardiac chest pain on day 3. Ingestion of 90 mg/day for 12 days resulted in pneumonia, systemic inflammatory response, atrial fibrillation, and a moderate pericardial effusion. Peak concentration 6 hours after oral dose.

(*continued*)

TABLE II–10. ANTINEOPLASTIC DRUGS (CONTINUED)

Drug	Mechanism of Action[a]	Major Site(s) of Toxicity[b]	Comments
Porfimer	L	D+, G+, P+	Used in conjunction with phototherapy; risk for photosensitivity.
Pralatrexate	C	D+, G++, M+, P+	Mucositis is common and can be severe. Consider leucovorin (p 572) rescue for overdose.
Procarbazine	L	An+, D+, En+, G++, M++, N++	Monoamine oxidase inhibitor activity. Disulfiram-like ethanol interaction. Coma, seizures during therapy.
Rasburicase	C	An++, En+, G+, H+, M+	Hemolysis in G6PD-deficient patients. Methemoglobinemia reported. Risk of fluid overload, hyper- or hypo-phosphatemia.
Regorafenib	G	C+, D++, En++, G+, H++, M+, N+	Hypertension common and can be severe. Risk of hemorrhage. Various electrolyte disturbances. Peak level 4 hours after oral dose.
Rituximab	I	An++, C+, D+,En+, G+, M++, P+, R+	Severe, fatal hypersensitivity reaction possible. Tumor lysis syndrome has caused acute renal failure. Potentially fatal mucocutaneous reactions reported. Electrolyte disturbance.
Romidepsin	E	C+, En++, G+, H+, M++, N+	Risk of supraventricular and ventricular arrhythmias, electrolyte disturbance (especially phosphate).
Ruxolitinib	G	C+, En+, G+, H+, M++	Severe withdrawal syndrome, including septic shock-like symptoms, possible. Up to 200 mg acutely tolerated with minimal symptoms. Peak level at 1–2 hours after oral dose
Sorafenib	G	Al+, C+, D+, G+, M++	Hypertension, hand-foot syndrome common. INR elevation. Risk of hypocalcemia, hypophosphatemia. Peak level 3 hours after oral dose.
Streptozocin	A	En+, Ex+, G++, H+, M+, R++	Destroys pancreatic beta islet cells, may produce acute diabetes mellitus. Niacinamide may be effective in preventing islet cell destruction. Renal toxicity in two-thirds of patients.
Sunitinib	G	C++, D+, En+, G+, H+ M+	Left ventricular dysfunction (21%), hemorrhagic events (30%). Hypertension can be severe. Risk of electrolyte abnormalities, hypothyroidism. No adverse reactions reported with an intentional overdose of 1,500 mg. Peak level 6–12 hours after oral dose.
Tamoxifen	F (antiestrogen)	Al ±, D ±, En ±, G ±, H+	Tremors, hyperreflexia, unsteady gait, QT prolongation with high-dose therapy. Peak levels 3–6 hours after oral dose.

(*continued*)

TABLE II–10. ANTINEOPLASTIC DRUGS (CONTINUED)

Drug	Mechanism of Action[a]	Major Site(s) of Toxicity[b]	Comments
Temozolomide	A	Al+, G+, M++, N+	Overdose of 5,500 mg over 2 days caused pancytopenia between 1 and 4 weeks. Another overdose of 2,000 mg per day for 5 days resulted in death from multiorgan failure, pancytopenia. Peak plasma level at 1 hour after oral dose.
Temsirolimus	G	An+, D+, En+, G+, H+, M++, P+, R+	Hyperglycemia, hyperlipidemia, hypertriglyceridemia common.
Teniposide	H	An+, Ex+, G+, M++	One report of sudden death from hypotension, cardiac arrhythmias. Hypotension from rapid IV. Injection solution contains benzyl alcohol.
6-Thioguanine	C	H+, M+, R+	Reversible myelosuppression after oral dose of 35 mg/kg. Peak level 8 hours after oral dose.
Thiotepa (triethylenethiophosphoramide, TSPA, TESPA)	A	An+, G++, M++	Bone marrow suppression usually very severe.
Topotecan	K	Al+, An+, G+, M++, P+	Severe pancytopenia, especially neutropenia, leukopenia, common. A patient who received double the IV dose developed severe neutropenia 14 days later. Fourfold increase in clearance during hemodialysis in one patient with renal failure. Peak level 1–2 hours after oral dose.
Toremifene	F (antiestrogen)	Al ±, D ±, En ±, G ±	Risk of QTc prolongation, hypercalcemia and tumor flare. Headache and dizziness observed in healthy volunteers with 680 mg daily for 5 days.
Tositumomab	I	An+, En+, G+, M++	Given with radiolabeled iodine complex. May cause hypothyroidism.
Trametinib	G	An++, C+, D++, En++, G+, H+, M++	Watch for electrolyte disturbances (hyponatremia, hypomagnesemia), QTc prolongation. Time to peak 1.5 hours after oral dose.
Trastuzumab	I	An++, C+, G+, H+, N+, P+	Can precipitate congestive heart failure. Severe, fatal hypersensitivity, infusion reactions and pulmonary toxicity reported. Ado-trastuzumab emtansine, a complex of a small molecule cytotoxin bound to trastuzumab, has caused fatal hepatotoxicity.
Tretinoin	L	An+, C+, D+, G+, H+, M+, N+, P+	Retinoic acid syndrome in 25% of patients with acute promyelocytic leukemia: fever, dyspnea, pulmonary infiltrates, and pleural or pericardial effusions. Fatal multiple-organ thrombosis reported. Acute oral overdose of 1,000 mg in a 31yo caused only diarrhea. A 32yo with an overdose of 525 mg had only vomiting. Peak level 1–2 hours after oral dose.

(*continued*)

TABLE II–10. ANTINEOPLASTIC DRUGS (CONTINUED)

Drug	Mechanism of Action[a]	Major Site(s) of Toxicity[b]	Comments
Triptorelin	F (gonadotropin-releasing hormone analog)	En+	Acute toxic effects unlikely. Initial increase in luteinizing hormone, follicle-stimulating hormone
Valrubicin	B	M++	Used intravesically, but highly myelotoxic if systemically absorbed. Conventional and peritoneal dialysis ineffective.
Vandetanib	G	C++, D+, En+, G++, H+, N+	Can cause QTprolongation, severe hypertension, hypocalcemia. Peak level 4–10 hours (median 6) after oral dose.
Vemurafenib	G	Al+, An+, D++, G+, H+	Severe dermatologic reactions, including Stevens–Johnson, seen. QTc prolongation risk. Peak level at 3 hours after oral dose.
Vinblastine	H	Al+, Ex++, G+, M++, N+, P+	Fatal if given intrathecally. An 83yo given 5 mg of IM daily for 6 days developed neutropenia, thrombocytopenia, fever, and pneumonia and died 10 days after initial dose. A 5yo who received 10 times the intended dose developed seizures, coma, myelosuppression and gastrointestinal symptoms (vomiting, adynamic ileus) but recovered. A 12yo had severe musculoskeletal pain, fever, intestinal hypotonia, severe esophagitis, and peripheral neuropathy after receiving almost double the maximum recommended dose. Two plasma exchange transfusions were performed at 4 and 18 hours after the overdose. Patient recovered from the incident.
Vincristine	H	Al+, Ex++, G+, M ±, N++, P+	Fatal if given intrathecally. Delayed (up to 9 days) seizures, coma reported after overdoses. A 13yo inadvertently given 32 mg of vincristine IV developed abdominal distension, fever, hypertension then hypotension, and died 33 hours later. A 7yo given 10 times the intended IV dose developed hypotension, ileus, urinary retention, myelosuppression, hyponatremia and respiratory distress and died 68 hours after the overdose. A 5yo who received 7.5 mg IV exhibited fever, elevated liver enzymes, areflexia, bloody diarrhea, neutropenia, hallucinations and died 9 days after overdose. Exchange transfusion and plasmapheresis have reduced vincristine concentrations after overdoses. Leucovorin, pyridoxine, and glutamic acid (PO or IV) may reduce the incidence of neurotoxicity.

(*continued*)

TABLE II–10. ANTINEOPLASTIC DRUGS (CONTINUED)

Drug	Mechanism of Action[a]	Major Site(s) of Toxicity[b]	Comments
Vinorelbine	H	D+, Ex++, G+, H+, M++, N+, P+	Fatal if given intrathecally. After receiving 10 times the intended dose, a woman developed fever, pulmonary edema, severe mucositis, diarrhea, paralytic ileus, severe cutaneous desquamation, peripheral neuropathy and severe bone marrow suppression but survived.
Vismodegib	L	Al+, G+	Muscle spasms common. Watch for hyponatremia, hypokalemia.
Vorinostat	E	C+, G+, M+, P+	Risk of thromboembolism, hyperglycemia. Can prolong QT. Peak level at a median of 4 hours after oral dose.
Ziv-aflibercept	L	C++, G++, H+, M++, R++	Potentially fatal bleeding events, GI perforation, compromised wound healing. Risk of severe hypertension, proteinuria.

[a]A, alkylating agents; B, antibiotics; C, antimetabolites; D, DNA demethylation agents; E, histone deacetylase inhibitors; F, hormones; G, kinase inhibitors; H, mitotic inhibitors; I, monoclonal antibodies; J, platinum-containing complexes; K, topoisomerase inhibitors; L, miscellaneous.
[b]Al, alopecia; An, anaphylaxis, allergy, or drug fever; C, cardiac; D, dermatologic; En, endocrine and metabolic; Ex, extravasation risk; G, gastrointestinal; H, hepatic; M, myelosuppressive; N, neurologic; P, pulmonary; R, renal; +, mild to moderate severity; ++, severe toxicity; ±, minimal.

H. **Mitotic inhibitors.** These agents act in various ways to inhibit orderly mitosis, thereby arresting cell division.

I. **Monoclonal antibodies** target antigens specific to or overexpressed in cancerous cells. The antibodies may be directly cytotoxic or may be used to deliver radionuclides or cytotoxins to the target cells.

J. **Platinum-**containing complexes produce intra-and/or interstrand platinum-DNA cross-links.

K. **Topoisomerase inhibitors** inhibit topoisomerase I, an enzyme that relieves torsional strain during DNA replication. The cleavable complex normally formed between DNA and topoisomerase I is stabilized by these drugs, resulting in breaks in single-stranded DNA.

L. **Miscellaneous.** The cytotoxic actions of other antineoplastic drugs result from a variety of mechanisms, including blockade of protein synthesis and inhibition of hormone release.

M. **Pharmacokinetics.** Most oral antineoplastic agents are readily absorbed (see Table II–10). As a result of rapid intracellular incorporation and the delayed onset of toxicity, pharmacokinetic values are usually of little utility in managing acute overdose.

II. **Toxic dose.** Because of the highly toxic nature of these agents (except for hormones), exposure to even therapeutic amounts should be considered potentially serious.

III. **Clinical presentation.** The organ systems affected by the various agents are listed in Table II–10. The most common sites of toxicity are the hematopoietic and GI systems.

A. **Leukopenia** is the most common manifestation of bone marrow depression. Thrombocytopenia and anemia may also occur. Death may result from overwhelming infections or hemorrhagic diathesis. With alkylating agents, the lowest blood counts occur 1–4 weeks after exposure, whereas with antibiotics, antimetabolites, and mitotic inhibitors, the lowest blood counts occur 1–2 weeks after exposure.

B. **Gastrointestinal** toxicity is also very common. Nausea, vomiting, and diarrhea often accompany therapeutic administration, and severe ulcerative gastroenteritis and extensive fluid loss may occur. Pretreatment with aprepitant (Emend) and dexamethasone is often used for highly emetogenic regimens.

C. **Systemic inflammatory response syndrome (SIRS) or capillary leak syndrome** due to cytokine release may manifest as tachypnea, tachycardia, hypotension, and pulmonary edema. Cytotoxic agents can also cause **tumor lysis syndrome** (hyperuricemia, hyperkalemia, renal failure) as a consequence of rapid lysis of malignant cells and release of intracellular components.

D. Palmar-plantar erythrodysesthesia (**hand-foot syndrome**), painful erythema of palms of the hands and soles of the feet that can progress to paresthesias, is often associated with capecitabine, cytarabine, docetaxel, doxorubicin, fluorouracil, and sunitinib.

E. **Extravasation** of some antineoplastic drugs at the IV injection site may cause severe local injury, with skin necrosis and sloughing. Drugs that bind to nucleic acids in DNA, such as anthracyclines (eg, daunorubicin, doxorubicin), cause direct local cell death and are more likely to cause severe injury.

IV. **Diagnosis** is usually based on the history. Because some of the most serious toxic effects may be delayed until several days after exposure, early clinical symptoms and signs may not be dramatic.

A. **Specific levels.** Not generally available. For methotrexate, see "Methotrexate" (p 319).

B. **Other useful laboratory studies** include CBC with differential, platelet count, electrolytes, glucose, BUN and creatinine, liver enzymes, and prothrombin time. Electrocardiography may be indicated for cardiotoxic agents, and pulmonary function tests are indicated for agents with known pulmonary toxicity.

C. **Genetic polymorphisms.** Some individuals are genetically predisposed to the hematopoietic and GI effects of irinotecan (eg, UGT1A1 *28/*28 genotype), and thiopurine drugs such as azathioprine and 6-mercaptopurine (eg, TPMT *2, *3A, or *3C genotypes). Tests available through reference laboratories.

V. **Treatment**

A. **Emergency and supportive measures**

1. Maintain an open airway and assist ventilation if necessary (pp 1–7).
2. Treat coma (p 18), seizures (p 23), hypotension (p 15), and arrhythmias (pp 10–15) if they occur.
3. Treat nausea and vomiting with ondansetron (p 597) or metoclopramide (p 581). Consider adding a benzodiazepine (p 516). Treat fluid losses caused by gastroenteritis with IV crystalloid fluids.
4. **Bone marrow depression** should be treated with the assistance of an experienced hematologist or oncologist. Transfusions of packed red blood cells and platelets may be needed for episodes of bleeding. Recombinant erythropoietin may be useful for severe anemia, and hematopoietic colony-stimulating factors may be useful for neutropenia.
5. **Extravasation.** Immediately stop the infusion and withdraw as much fluid as possible by applying negative pressure on the syringe. Elevate the affected limb. Surgical intervention may be necessary. Specific treatment recommendations vary by institutional preferences.

   a. Local injection with **sodium thiosulfate** may be helpful for extravasation from **cisplatin**, **cyclophosphamide, mechlorethamine, and mitomycin**. Mix 4 mL of sodium thiosulfate 10% solution with 6 mL of sterile water for injection, and inject 3–10 mL of the mixture subcutaneously into the extravasation site.

b. Topical application of **dimethyl sulfoxide (DMSO)** 99% (or 50% if readily available) may be beneficial for **carboplatin, cisplatin, dactinomycin, daunorubicin, doxorubicin, epirubicin, idarubicin, mitomycin, and mitoxantrone**. Apply a thin layer with a sterile gauze to the area of infiltration every 2 hours for the first 24 hours then 6–8 hours for 7–14 days (do not cover).

c. Local injection with **hyaluronidase** may help diffuse the drug through the interstitial space and enhance systemic absorption. Reconstitute with normal saline and inject 150–900 units subcutaneously or intradermally. Its use may be of benefit for **carmustine, docetaxel, etoposide, oxaliplatin, paclitaxel, teniposide, vinblastine, vincristine,** and **vinorelbine**. Do not use for doxorubicin or other anthracycline extravasation.

d. Totect (United States) and Savene (Europe), brands of **dexrazoxane**, are approved for the treatment of extravasation from anthracyclines: **daunorubicin**, **doxorubicin**, **epirubicin**, and **idarubicin**. Give an IV infusion of 1,000 mg/m^2 of body surface area (maximum, 2,000 mg) over 1–2 hours, no later than 6 hours after extravasation. Repeat the same dose 24 hours later, then 500 mg/m^2 (maximum 1,000 mg) 48 hours after the first dose. Infuse in a large vein in an area remote from the extravasation. Do not use for local infiltration. Do not use DMSO for patients receiving dexrazoxane.

e. For most chemotherapeutic agents, apply **cool compresses** to the extravasation site for 15 minutes 4 times daily for 2–3 days. Do not use cool compresses for vinca alkaloids (eg, vinblastine, vincristine).

f. Apply **warm compresses**/heating pad intermittently (15–30 minutes 4 times a day) for 1–2 days specifically for **vinblastine**, **vincristine**, and **vinorelbine**. Do not apply heat for anthracyclines.

g. Application of both cool and warm compresses has been recommended for **carboplatin, carmustine, dacarbazine, docetaxel, etoposide, fluorouracil, methotrexate, oxaliplatin**, and **paclitaxel**.

h. There is no justification for injection of hydrocortisone or sodium bicarbonate.

B. **Specific drugs and antidotes.** Very few specific treatments or antidotes are available (see Table II–10).

1. **Amifostine** is approved for reduction of cumulative renal toxicity from cisplatin. It has also been used for cisplatin-induced neurotoxicity, cyclophosphamide-induced granulocytopenia, and radiation and/or chemotherapy-induced mucositis.
2. **Dexrazoxane** protects against doxorubicin-induced cardiotoxicity and may be protective for other anthracyclines (epirubicin, idarubicin, and mitoxantrone).
3. **Mesna** is approved for the prophylaxis of ifosfamide-induced hemorrhagic cystitis and may be beneficial for cyclophosphamide-induced hemorrhagic cystitis.
4. **Palifermin** is used to decrease the incidence and duration of severe oral mucositis in patients with hematologic malignancies who are receiving myelotoxic therapy requiring hematopoietic stem cell support.
5. **Uridine triacetate** is approved for treatment of 5-fluorouracil and capecitabine overdose. Contact Wellstat Therapeutics at 1-844-374-0604.

C. **Decontamination** (p 50). Administer activated charcoal orally if conditions are appropriate (see Table I–38, p 54). Gastric lavage is not necessary after small-to-moderate ingestions if activated charcoal can be given promptly.

D. **Enhanced elimination.** Because of the rapid intracellular incorporation of most of these agents, dialysis and other extracorporeal removal procedures are generally not effective (see Table II–10 for exceptions).

▶ ANTIPSYCHOTIC DRUGS, INCLUDING PHENOTHIAZINES

Justin C. Lewis, PharmD

Phenothiazines, butyrophenones, and other related drugs are used widely to treat psychosis and agitated depression. In addition, some of these drugs (eg, prochlorperazine, promethazine, trimethobenzamide, and droperidol) are used as antiemetic agents. Suicidal overdoses are common, but because of the high toxic-therapeutic ratio, acute overdose seldom results in death. A large number of newer agents that often are

TABLE II–11. ANTIPSYCHOTIC DRUGS

Drug	Type[a]	Usual Adult Daily Dose (mg)	Toxicity[b]
Aripiprazole	O	10–30	A, E, H, Q
Asenapine	O	10–20	E
Chlorpromazine	P	200–800	A, E, H, Q
Chlorprothixene	T	100–200	E
Clozapine	D	100–900	A, H
Droperidol[c]	B	2–10	E, Q
Ethopropazine	P	50–600	A, H
Fluphenazine	P	2.5–40	E, A
Haloperidol	B	1–100	E, Q
Iloperidone	O	12–24	E, H, Q
Loxapine	D	20–100	E
Lurasidone	O	20–120	E,H
Mesoridazine	P	100–400	A, H, Q
Molindone	O	50–225	E
Olanzapine	D	5–20	A, E, H
Paliperidone	O	3–12	E, H, Q
Perphenazine	P	12–64	E
Pimozide	O	1–10	E, Q
Prochlorperazine[c]	P	15–4	E
Promethazine[c,d]	P	12.5–1,500	A, E
Quetiapine	D	300–800	A, E, H, Q
Risperidone	O	2–16	E, H, Q
Thioridazine	P	150–800	A, H, Q
Thiothixene	T	5–60	E
Trifluoperazine	P	4–40	E
Trimethobenzamide[c]	O	600–1,200	A, E
Ziprasidone	O	40–160	A, E, H, Q

[a]B, butyrophenone; D, dibenzodiazepine; P, phenothiazine; O, other ("atypical" antipsychotic); T, thiothixine.
[b]A, anticholinergic effects; E, extrapyramidal reactions; H, hypotension; Q, QT-interval prolongation.
[c]Used primarily as an antiemetic.
[d]Promethazine: Administer IM into deep muscle (preferred route of administration). IV administration is *not* the preferred route; extravasation can cause severe tissue damage.

referred to as "atypical antipsychotics" have been developed. Atypical antipsychotics differ from other neuroleptics in their binding to dopamine receptors and their effects on dopamine-mediated behaviors. Overdose experience with these agents is limited. Table II–11 describes available antipsychotic agents.

I. **Mechanism of toxicity.** A variety of pharmacologic effects are responsible for toxicity, involving primarily the cardiovascular system and CNS.

A. **Cardiovascular system.** Anticholinergic effects may produce tachycardia. Alpha-adrenergic blockade may cause hypotension, especially orthostatic hypotension. With very large overdoses of some agents, quinidine-like membrane-depressant effects on the heart may occur. Many of these agents can cause QT prolongation (p 14).

B. **Central nervous system.** Centrally mediated sedation and anticholinergic effects contribute to CNS depression. Alpha-adrenergic blockade causes small pupils despite anticholinergic effects on other systems. Extrapyramidal dystonic reactions are relatively common with therapeutic doses and probably are caused by central dopamine receptor blockade. The seizure threshold may be lowered by unknown mechanisms. Temperature regulation is also disturbed, resulting in poikilothermia.

C. **Pharmacokinetics.** These drugs have large volumes of distribution (Vd = 10–30 L/kg), and most have long elimination half-lives (eg, chlorpromazine half-life = 18–30 hours). Elimination is largely by hepatic metabolism (see Table II–66, p 462).

II. **Toxic dose.** Extrapyramidal reactions, anticholinergic side effects, and orthostatic hypotension are often seen with therapeutic doses. Tolerance to the sedating effects of the antipsychotics is well described, and patients on chronic therapy may tolerate much larger doses than do other persons.

A. Typical daily doses are given in Table II–11.

B. The toxic dose after acute ingestion is highly variable. Serious CNS depression and hypotension may occur after ingestion of 200–1,000 mg of chlorpromazine in children or of 3–5 g in adults.

III. **Clinical presentation.** Major toxicity is manifested in the cardiovascular system and CNS. Also, anticholinergic intoxication (p 97) may occur as a result of ingestion of benztropine (Cogentin) or other co-administered drugs.

A. **Mild intoxication** causes sedation, small pupils, and orthostatic hypotension. Anticholinergic manifestations include dry mouth, absence of sweating, tachycardia, and urinary retention. Paradoxically, clozapine causes hypersalivation through an unknown mechanism.

B. **Severe intoxication** may cause coma, seizures, and respiratory arrest. The ECG usually shows QT-interval prolongation and occasionally QRS prolongation (particularly with thioridazine [Mellaril]). Hypothermia or hyperthermia may occur. Clozapine can cause a prolonged confusional state and rarely cardiac toxicity. Risperidone, aripiprazole, and quetiapine can cause QT-interval prolongation, but delirium is less severe.

C. **Extrapyramidal** dystonic side effects of therapeutic doses include torticollis, jaw muscle spasm, oculogyric crisis, rigidity, bradykinesia, and pill-rolling tremor. These are more common with the butyrophenones.

D. Patients on chronic antipsychotic medication may develop the **neuroleptic malignant syndrome** (p 21), which is characterized by rigidity, hyperthermia, sweating, lactic acidosis, and rhabdomyolysis.

E. **Clozapine** use has been associated with agranulocytosis.

F. **Promethazine** can cause severe tissue damage after perivascular extravasation or unintentional intra-arterial, intraneural, or perineural injection. IV administration is **not** recommended unless the line is freely flowing and the drug is given slowly.

IV. **Diagnosis** is based on a history of ingestion and findings of sedation, small pupils, hypotension, and QT-interval prolongation. Dystonias in children should always suggest the possibility of antipsychotic exposure, often as a result of intentional administration by parents. Phenothiazines are occasionally visible on plain abdominal radiographs (see Table I–35, p 49).

A. **Specific levels.** Quantitative blood levels are not routinely available and do not help in diagnosis or treatment. Qualitative screening may easily detect phenothiazines in urine or gastric juice, but butyrophenones such as haloperidol are usually not included in toxicologic screens (see Table I–30, p 44).

B. **Other useful laboratory studies** include electrolytes, glucose, BUN, creatinine, creatine kinase (CK), arterial blood gases or oximetry, abdominal radiography (to look for radiopaque pills), and chest radiography.

V. **Treatment**

A. **Emergency and supportive measures**

1. Maintain an open airway and assist ventilation if necessary (pp 1–7). Administer supplemental oxygen.
2. Treat coma (p 18), seizures (p 23), hypotension (p 15), and hyperthermia (p 21) if they occur.
3. Monitor vital signs and ECG for at least 6 hours and admit the patient for at least 24 hours if there are signs of significant intoxication. Children with antipsychotic intoxication should be evaluated for possible intentional abuse.

B. **Specific drugs and antidotes.** There is no specific antidote.

1. **Dystonic reactions.** Give diphenhydramine, 0.5–1 mg/kg IM or IV (p 544), or benztropine (p 519).
2. QRS-interval prolongation. Treat quinidine-like cardiotoxic effects with bicarbonate, 1–2 mEq/kg IV (p 520).
3. **Hypotension** from these dugs probably involves vasodilation caused by alpha1 receptor blockade. Treat with IV fluids and, if needed, a vasoconstrictor such as norepinephrine or phenylephrine. Theoretically, drugs with beta2 activity (eg, epinephrine, isoproterenol) may worsen hypotension.
4. **QT prolongation and torsade** may respond to magnesium infusion or overdrive pacing (p 14).

C. **Decontamination** (p 50). Administer activated charcoal orally if conditions are appropriate (see Table I–38, p 54). Gastric lavage is not necessary after small-to-moderate ingestions if activated charcoal can be given promptly.

D. **Enhanced elimination.** Owing to extensive tissue distribution, these drugs are not effectively removed by dialysis or hemoperfusion. Repeat-dose activated charcoal has not been evaluated.

► ANTISEPTICS AND DISINFECTANTS

Kent R. Olson, MD

Antiseptics are applied to living tissue to kill or prevent the growth of microorganisms. **Disinfectants** are applied to inanimate objects to destroy pathogenic microorganisms. Despite the lack of rigorous evidence that they prevent infection, they are used widely in households, the food industry, and hospitals. This chapter describes toxicity caused by **chlorhexidine, glutaraldehyde, hexylresorcinol, hydrogen peroxide, ichthammol,** and **potassium permanganate.** These agents are often used as dilute solutions that usually cause little or no toxicity. Hexylresorcinol is commonly found in throat lozenges. Ichthammol is found in many topical salves. Descriptions of the toxicity of other antiseptics and disinfectants appear elsewhere in this book, including the following: hypochlorite (p 191), iodine (p 274), isopropyl alcohol (p 282), mercurochrome (p 305), phenol (p 368), and pine oil (p 266).

I. **Mechanism of toxicity**

A. **Chlorhexidine** is commonly found in dental rinses, mouthwashes, skin cleansers, and a variety of cosmetics. Many preparations also contain isopropyl alcohol. Systemic absorption of chlorhexidine salts is minimal. Ingestion of products with a concentration less than 0.12% is not likely to cause more than minor irritation, but higher concentrations have caused corrosive injury.

B. Glutaraldehyde (pH 3–4) is used to disinfect medical equipment, as a tissue preservative, and topically as an antifungal and is found in some x-ray solutions. It is highly irritating to the skin and respiratory tract and has caused allergic contact dermatitis with repeated exposures.

C. Hexylresorcinol is related to phenol but is much less toxic, although alcohol-based solutions have vesicant properties.

D. Hydrogen peroxide is an oxidizing agent, but it is very unstable and readily breaks down to oxygen and water. Generation of oxygen gas in closed-body cavities can potentially cause mechanical distention that results in gastric or intestinal perforation, as well as venous or arterial gas embolization. Hydrogen peroxide is found in many dental products, including mouth rinses and tooth whiteners, skin disinfectants, hair products, and earwax removers, and it has many industrial uses. In veterinary medicine it is used to induce emesis.

E. Ichthammol (ichthyol, ammonium ichthosulfonate) contains about 10% sulfur in the form of organic sulfonates and is keratolytic to tissues.

F. Potassium permanganate is an oxidant, and the crystalline form and concentrated solutions are corrosive owing to the release of potassium hydroxide when potassium permanganate comes in contact with water.

II. Toxic dose

A. Chlorhexidine ingestions of less than 4% are expected to cause irritation, and ingestion of 150 mL of 20% solution caused esophageal damage and hepatic injury.

B. The lethal dose of **glutaraldehyde** is estimated to be 5–50 g/kg. Topical application of 10% solutions can cause dermatitis, and 2% solutions have caused ocular damage.

C. Hexylresorcinol is used in some antihelminthics, in doses of 400 mg (for children age 1–7 years) to 1 g (older children and adults). Most lozenges contain only about 2–4 mg.

D. Hydrogen peroxide for household use is available in 3–5% solutions and causes only mild throat and gastric irritation with ingestion of less than 1 oz. However, gas embolization has occurred with low concentrations used in surgical irrigations. Concentrations above 10% are found in some hair-bleaching solutions and are potentially corrosive. Most reported deaths have been associated with ingestion of undiluted 35% hydrogen peroxide, marketed as "hyperoxygen therapy" in health food stores or "food grade" in industry.

E. Potassium permanganate solutions of greater than 1:5,000 strength may cause corrosive burns.

III. Clinical presentation. Most low-concentration antiseptic ingestions are benign, and mild irritation is self-limited. Spontaneous vomiting and diarrhea may occur, especially after a large-volume ingestion.

A. Exposure to **concentrated** antiseptic solutions may cause corrosive burns on the skin and mucous membranes, and oropharyngeal, esophageal, or gastric injury may occur. Glottic edema has been reported after ingestion of concentrated potassium permanganate.

B. Permanganate may also cause **methemoglobinemia** (p 317).

C. Hydrogen peroxide ingestion may cause gastric distension and, rarely, perforation. Severe corrosive injury and **air emboli** have been reported with ingestion of the concentrated forms and may be caused by the entry of gas through damaged gastric mucosa or oxygen gas liberation within the venous or arterial circulation.

IV. Diagnosis is based on a history of exposure and the presence of mild GI upset or frank corrosive injury. Solutions of potassium permanganate are dark purple, and skin and mucous membranes are often stained brown-black.

A. Specific levels. Drug levels in body fluids are not generally useful or available.

B. **Other useful laboratory studies** include electrolytes, glucose, methemoglobin level (for potassium permanganate exposure), and upright chest radiography (for suspected gastric perforation).

V. **Treatment**

A. **Emergency and supportive measures**

1. In patients who have ingested concentrated solutions, monitor the airway for swelling and intubate if necessary.
2. Consult a gastroenterologist for possible endoscopy after ingestions of corrosive agents such as concentrated hydrogen peroxide and potassium permanganate. Most ingestions are benign, and mild irritation is self-limited.
3. Consider **hyperbaric oxygen** treatment for gas emboli associated with concentrated peroxide ingestion.

B. **Specific drugs and antidotes.** No specific antidotes are available for irritant or corrosive effects. If **methemoglobinemia** occurs, administer methylene blue (p 579).

C. **Decontamination** (p 50)

1. Ingestion of concentrated corrosive agents (see also p 186)
   a. Dilute immediately with water or milk.
   b. Do ***not*** induce vomiting because of the risk for corrosive injury. Perform gastric lavage cautiously.
   c. Activated charcoal and cathartics are probably not effective. Moreover, charcoal may interfere with the endoscopist's view of the esophagus and stomach in cases of suspected corrosive injury.
2. **Eyes and skin.** Irrigate the eyes and skin with copious amounts of tepid water. Remove contaminated clothing.

D. **Enhanced elimination.** Enhanced elimination methods are neither necessary nor effective.

▶ ANTIVIRAL AND ANTIRETROVIRAL AGENTS

Conan MacDougall, PharmD, MAS

Antiviral drugs are used for a variety of infections, including herpesvirus, hepatitis B (HBV) and C (HCV), and influenza. Antiviral drugs that target human immunodeficiency virus (HIV) are referred to as antiretrovirals. A wide variety of antiretroviral agents from different mechanistic classes are now available (Table II–12). Antiretrovirals are typically given in combination to treat HIV infection. New multiple-drug combined formulations have been developed to decrease the number of pills to take per day and increase adherence to treatment regimens. Some antiretrovirals are also active against HBV. The management of HCV has been revolutionized by the development of new anti-HCV agents, usually given in combination.

I. **Mechanism of toxicity.** The mechanism underlying toxic effects varies with the agent and is usually an extension of its pharmacologic effect.

A. **Neurotoxicity** may be the result of inhibition of mitochondrial DNA polymerase and altered mitochondrial cell function.

B. **Hepatic steatosis, severe lactic acidosis**, and **lipodystrophy** may be due to inhibition of DNA polymerase-gamma, which depletes mitochondrial DNA and flavoprotein cofactors, impairing electron transport and causing mitochondrial dysfunction. Mitochondrial RNA formation may also be inhibited.

C. Acyclovir crystal deposition in the tubular lumen leading to an obstructive nephropathy may cause **acute renal failure**. Indinavir is poorly water soluble and can precipitate in the kidney, causing kidney stones and interstitial nephritis.

D. Other serious toxicities that develop after chronic use of many of these agents include bone marrow depression, diabetes mellitus, hepatotoxicity, lactic

TABLE II–12. ANTIVIRAL AND ANTIRETROVIRAL DRUGS

Drug	Half-life	Toxic Dose or Serum Level	Toxicity
Antiherpesvirus drugs			
Acyclovir Valacyclovir (acyclovir prodrug)	2.5–3.3 h	Chronic	High-dose chronic therapy has caused crystalluria and renal failure, leukopenia. Coma, seizures, renal failure after large acute overdoses. Hallucinations and confusion after IV administration, especially in renal impairment.
Cidofovir	2.5 h	16.3 and 17.4 mg/kg (case reports)	No renal dysfunction after treatment with probenecid and IV hydration.
Foscarnet	3.3–4 h	1.14–8 times recommended dose (average, 4 times)	Seizures, renal impairment. One patient had seizures and died after receiving 12.5 g daily for 3 days.
Ganciclovir Valganciclovir (ganciclovir prodrug)	3.5 h (IV) 4 h (oral val-ganciclovir)	Adults: 5–7 g or 25 mg/kg IV	Neutropenia, thrombocytopenia, pancytopenia, increased serum creatinine; 9 mg/kg IV caused a seizure; 10 mg/kg IV daily caused hepatitis. Children: 1 g instead of 31 mg in a 21-month-old had no toxic effect; an 18-month-old received 60 mg/kg IV, was treated with exchange transfusion, and had no effect; a 4-month-old received 500 mg, was treated with peritoneal dialysis, and had no effect; 40 mg in a 2-kg infant caused hepatitis. One adult developed fatal bone marrow suppression after several days of dosing with valganciclovir at a level 10-fold greater than recommended for the patient's renal function.
Penciclovir Famciclovir (penciclovir produg)	2–2.3 h		Extensive intracellular metabolism.
Trifluridine	12–18 minutes (ophthalmic)	15–30 mg/kg IV	Reversible bone marrow toxicity reported after 3–5 courses of IV treatment. Systemic absorption is negligible after ophthalmic instillation. Ingestion of contents of one bottle (7.5 mL, 75 mg) unlikely to cause any adverse effects.
Vidarabine	Rapid deamination to ara-hypoxanthine metabolite, whose half-life is 2.4–3.3 h	Chronic 1–20 mg/kg/d IV for 10–15 d	Nausea, vomiting, diarrhea, dizziness, ataxia, tremor, confusion, hallucinations, psychosis; decreased Hct, Hgb, WBC, platelets; increased AST, ALT, LDH. Poorly absorbed orally; no toxicity expected if one tube (3.5 g, 105 mg) ingested.

(*continued*)

TABLE II–12. ANTIVIRAL AND ANTIRETROVIRAL DRUGS (CONTINUED)

Drug	Half-life	Toxic Dose or Serum Level	Toxicity
Anti-influenza drugs			
Oseltamivir carboxylate	6–10 h	Chronic	Doses up to 1,000 mg resulted only in nausea and vomiting in clinical trials. Delirium, hallucinations, psychosis, seizures reported with therapeutic use; may relate to underlying influenza infection.
Peramivir	20 h	Chronic	No reported overdoses
Zanamivir	2.5–5.1 h	Chronic	Bronchospasm with therapeutic use
Nucleoside (NRTIs) or nucleotide (NtRTIs) reverse transcriptase inhibitors			Lactic acidosis, mitochondrial toxicity, hepatotoxicity.
Abacavir (ABC)	1.54 ± 0.63 h	Chronic	Hypersensitivity syndrome with rash, fever, nausea/vomiting. May progress to life-threatening hypotension and death with continued administration or rechallenge. Perioral paresthesias.
Adefovir	7.5 h	≥60 mg/d	Nephrotoxicity.
Didanosine (ddi)	1.5 ± 0.4 h	Chronic	Diarrhea, pancreatitis, peripheral neuropathy, salt overload with buffered product.
Emtricitabine (FTC)	10 h	Chronic	Lactic acidosis and severe hepatomegaly with steatosis.
Entecavir	128–149 h	Chronic	Headache, nasopharyngitis, cough, pyrexia, upper abdominal pain, fatigue, diarrhea, lactic acidosis, hepatomegaly.
Lamivudine (3TC)	5–7 h	Chronic	Headaches, nausea. Some preparations co-formulated with zidovudine with or without abacavir.
Stavudine (d4T)	1.15 h IV 1.44 h PO	Chronic	Hepatic steatosis, lactic acidosis, peripheral neuropathy.
Telbivudine	15 h	Chronic	Myopathy, peripheral neuropathy.
Tenofovir[a] (TDF)	17 h	Chronic	Diarrhea, flatulence, nausea, vomiting. Some preparations co-formulated with emtricitabine with or without efavirenz or dolutegravir.
Zidovudine (AZT, ZDV)	0.5–1.5 h	Chronic	Anemia, fatigue, headaches, nausea, neutropenia, neuropathy, myopathy.
Nonnucleoside reverse transcriptase inhibitors (NNRTIs)			Hepatotoxicity, rash
Delavirdine (DLV)	5.8 h (range, 2–11 h)	Chronic	Hepatotoxicity, rash.
Efavirenz (EFV)	40–76 h	Chronic	CNS effects: confusion, disengagement, dizziness, hallucinations, insomnia, somnolence, vivid dreams. Some preparations co-formulated with emtricitabine and tenofovir.

(continued)

TABLE II–12. ANTIVIRAL AND ANTIRETROVIRAL DRUGS (CONTINUED)

Drug	Half-life	Toxic Dose or Serum Level	Toxicity
Etravirine (ETR)	40 ± 20 h	Chronic	Severe skin and hypersensitivity reactions.
Nevirapine (NVP)	45 h, single dose; 25–30 h, multiple doses	Chronic	Hepatotoxicity, rash.
Rilpivirine (RPV)	50 h	Chronic	Hepatotoxicity, rash. Co-formulated with emtricitabine, tenofovir.
Protease inhibitors			Dyslipidemias, insulin resistance (diabetes mellitus), hepatotoxicity, lipodystrophy; osteoporosis.
Atazanavir (ATV)	6.5–7.9 h	Chronic	Commonly causes elevated bilirubin, concentration- and dose-dependent prolongation of PR interval.
Darunavir (DRV)	15 h (CYP3A)	Chronic	Hepatotoxic; 3.2-g doses tolerated without adverse effects. Given in combination with ritonavir, which limits its metabolism and boosts drug levels.
Fosamprenavir (FPV)	7.7 h	Chronic	Contains a sulfonamide moiety. Skin rash commonly occurs; onset usually at 11 days, duration of 13 days. One case of Stevens–Johnson syndrome. Spontaneous bleeding may occur in hemophiliacs.
Indinavir (IDV)	1.8 h	Chronic	Hyperbilirubinemia, kidney stones, nausea.
Lopinavir/ritonavir (LPV/r)	5–6 h	Chronic	Diarrhea, nausea, increased cholesterol, triglycerides, and GGT. Solution contains 42.4% alcohol. Pills co-formulated with ritonavir.
Nelfinavir (NFV)	3–5 h	Chronic	Diarrhea, nausea, vomiting.
Ritonavir (RTV)	2–4 h	Chronic	Diarrhea, nausea, vomiting, significant drug interactions.
Saquinavir (SQV)	?	Chronic	Abdominal pain, diarrhea, nausea; fetal harm during first trimester of pregnancy. Possible garlic-drug interaction to lower blood levels.
Tipranavir (TPV)	5.5 h	Chronic	Increased risk for hepatotoxicity in patients with chronic hepatitis B or hepatitis C.
Fusion inhibitor			
Enfuvirtide (T-20)	3.8 ± 0.6 h	Chronic	Increased risk for a bacterial pneumonia to occur; infection at injection site (abscess, cellulitis). Does not inhibit cytochrome P450 enzymes.
Integrase inhibitor			
Dolutegravir (DTG)	14 h	Chronic	Hepatotoxicity, hyperglycemia.
Elvitegravir (EVG/COBI/FTC/TDF)	13 h	Chronic	Diarrhea, nausea. Co-formulated with cobicistat, emtricitabine, tenofovir.

(continued)

TABLE II–12. ANTIVIRAL AND ANTIRETROVIRAL DRUGS (CONTINUED)

Drug	Half-life	Toxic Dose or Serum Level	Toxicity
Raltegravir (RAL)	9 h	Chronic	Hyperglycemia, diarrhea. Rare muscle problems, Stevens–Johnson syndrome.
Chemokine receptor antagonist			
Maraviroc (MVC)	14–18 h	Chronic; postural hypotension observed at 600 mg	Possible hepatic and cardiac toxicity; elevated cholesterol levels.
Anti-Hepatitis C drugs			
Boceprevir	3.4 h	Chronic	Anemia, neutropenia. Dysgeusia, vomiting. Co-administered with ribavirin and interferon.
Dasabuvir	5.5–6 h	Chronic	Hepatotoxicity, pruritis, rash. Usually co-administered with ombitasvir/paritaprevir/ritonavir.
Ledipasvir/ Sofosbuvir	47 h	Chronic	Fatigue, headache.
Ombitasvir/ Paritaprevir/ Ritonavir	Ombitasvir: 21–25h Paritaprevir: 5.5 h	Chronic	Hepatotoxicity, pruritis, rash.
Ribavirin	298 h	Up to 20 g acute ingestion	Hemolytic anemia, neutropenia, thrombocytopenia; suicidal ideation.
Simeprevir	10–13 h	Chronic	Rash, photosensitivity, pruritis.
Sofosbuvir	27 h (active metabolite)	Chronic	Fatigue, headache.
Telaprevir	9–11 h	Chronic	Nausea, vomiting, dysguesia, rash. Co-administered with ribavirin and interferon.

[a]Tenofovir is a nucleotide reverse transcriptase inhibitor (NtRTI).

acidosis, lipodystrophy, lipoatrophy, myopathies and rhabdomyolysis, pancreatitis, peripheral neuropathy, renal failure, and seizures.

E. Antiviral/retroviral drugs that are metabolized mainly via the hepatic cytochrome P450 isoenzyme system may be associated with clinically significant interactions with other drugs and dietary supplements (eg, St. John wort, garlic).

II. Toxic dose. Acute single ingestions are infrequent, and toxicity has been generally mild. Chronic toxicity, however, commonly occurs.

A. Acyclovir. Chronic high-dose therapy has caused crystalluria and renal failure. A patient who had an acute ingestion of 20 g recovered. A 1.5-day-old infant and a 2-year-old child recovered from accidental overdoses involving 100 mg/kg IV 3 times a day for 4 days and 800 mg IV, respectively. A patient with an acute ingestion of 30 g of valacyclovir experienced acute kidney injury with recovery after oral hydration.

B. Atazanavir. Laboratory evidence of hyperbilirubinemia is common and is not dose-dependent. The abnormality is reversible when the drug is discontinued.

C. Cidofovir. Two adults who received overdoses of 16.3 and 17.4 mg/kg, respectively, were treated with IV hydration and probenecid and had no toxic effects.

D. **Efavirenz.** A 33-year-old woman who ingested 54 g developed manic symptoms and recovered after 5 days.

E. **Enfuvirtide.** This drug is given by injection, and patients often develop local injection site reactions (eg, abscess, cellulitis, nodules, and cysts).

F. **Fosamprenavir** is a water-soluble prodrug to amprenavir that commonly causes skin reactions. The drug contains a sulfonamide moiety, and caution should be exercised in patients with an allergy to sulfonamides. Life-threatening Stevens–Johnson syndrome has been reported to the manufacturer.

G. **Foscarnet.** An adult receiving 12.5 g for 3 days developed seizures and died. Adults who received 1.14–8 times (average of 4 times) the recommended doses developed seizures and renal impairment.

H. **Ganciclovir.** All toxic reports have been after IV administration. The doses producing toxic effects after chronic high dosing or inadvertent acute IV overdose have been variable. No toxic effects were noted in two adults who were given 3.5 g and 11 mg/kg, respectively, for seven doses over 3 days. However, single doses of 25 mg/kg and 6 g, or daily doses of 8 mg/kg for 4 days or 3 g for 2 days, resulted in neutropenia, granulocytopenia, pancytopenia, and/or thrombocytopenia. An adult and a 2-kg infant developed hepatitis after 10-mg/kg and 40-mg doses, respectively. An adult developed seizures after a 9-mg/kg dose, and others have had increased serum creatinine levels after 5- to 7-g doses.

I. **Indinavir.** Patients with acute and chronic overdoses, up to 23 times the recommended total daily dose of 2,400 mg, which resulted in interstitial nephritis, kidney stones, or acute renal dysfunction, recovered after IV fluid therapy.

J. **Nevirapine.** An alleged 6-g ingestion in an adult was benign.

K. **Oseltamivir.** Doses up to 1,000 mg resulted only in nausea and vomiting in clinical trials. In a series of reported overdoses, minor effects were reported in 15% of patients with a mean dose of 245 mg and moderate effects reported in 5% with a mean dose of 190 mg.

L. **Ribavirin.** Up to 20-g acute ingestions have not been fatal, but hematopoietic effects are more severe than those associated with therapeutic doses.

M. **Zidovudine.** Acute overdoses have been mild with ingestions of less than 25 g.

III. **Clinical presentation.** Gastrointestinal symptoms are common after therapeutic doses and are more remarkable after an acute overdose. Specific features of toxicity are described in Table II–12. **Lactic acidosis,** often severe and sometimes fatal, has been reported with antiretroviral drugs, particularly nucleoside reverse transcriptase inhibitors (NRTIs).

IV. **Diagnosis** is usually based on the history of exposure. Unexplained mental status changes, neurologic deficits, weight gain, and renal abnormalities occurred after the erroneous administration of acyclovir, particularly in pediatric patients.

A. **Specific levels.** Serum levels are not commonly available for these agents and have not been particularly useful for predicting toxic effects.

B. **Other useful laboratory studies** include CBC, electrolytes, glucose, BUN, creatinine, liver function tests, and urinalysis. Plasma lactate levels and arterial blood gases are recommended if lactic acidosis is suspected.

C. **Genetic polymorphisms.** Individuals who have the HLA-B*5701 genotype are at risk for developing Stevens–Johnson syndrome and toxic epidermal necrolysis with abacavir. The prevalence rate of this mutation is highest among Caucasians and Africans, and is rare among Asians. Testing is available through reference laboratories.

V. **Treatment**

A. Emergency and supportive measures

1. Maintain an open airway and assist ventilation if necessary.
2. Treat coma (p 18), seizures (p 23), hypotension (p 15), torsade de pointes (p 14), rhabdomyolysis (p 27), and anaphylaxis (p 28) if they occur.

3. Replace fluid losses resulting from gastroenteritis with IV crystalloids.
4. Maintain steady urine flow with IV fluids to alleviate crystalluria and reverse renal dysfunction.
5. Treat lactic acidosis with judicious doses of sodium bicarbonate and by withdrawal of the offending drug.

B. **Specific drugs and antidotes.** There are no specific antidotes for these agents. Anecdotal cases of patients with severe lactic acidosis suggest that vitamin deficiency may be a contributor to the development of a life-threatening condition. Riboflavin (50 mg/d) and/or thiamine (100 mg twice a day) may be beneficial if levels are low.

C. **Decontamination** (p 50). Administer activated charcoal orally if conditions are appropriate (see Table I–38, p 54). Gastric lavage is not necessary after small-to-moderate ingestions if activated charcoal can be given promptly.

D. **Enhanced elimination.** The few reported overdoses with these agents have been benign or associated with mild toxicities. Hemodialysis may remove 60% of the total body burden of acyclovir, 50% of ganciclovir, and approximately 30% of emtricitabine over 3–4 hours. Enhanced elimination, however, has yet to be evaluated or employed after acute overdoses.

▶ ARSENIC

Michael J. Kosnett, MD, MPH

Arsenic compounds are found in a select group of industrial, commercial, and pharmaceutical products. Use of arsenic as a wood preservative in industrial applications (eg, marine timbers and utility poles) accounts for two-thirds of domestic consumption, but former widespread use in new lumber sold for residential purposes (eg, decks, fencing, play structures) ended with a voluntary ban effective at the end of 2003. Arsenic-treated lumber used in residential structures and objects created before 2004 has not been officially recalled or removed. Virtually all arsenic in pesticides and herbicides in the United States have been withdrawn or subject to phaseout with the exception of the limited use of monosodium methane arsonate (MSMA) as an herbicide. Until recently phenylarsenic compounds were used as feed additives for poultry and swine, and poultry litter used as a soil amendment sometimes contained low levels of soluble arsenic. Intravenous arsenic trioxide, reintroduced to the US Pharmacopoeia in 2000, is used as a drug for cancer chemotherapy. Inorganic arsenic is used in the production of nonferrous alloys, semiconductors, and certain types of glass. Inorganic arsenic is sometimes found in folk remedies and tonics, particularly from Asian sources. Artesian well water can be contaminated by inorganic arsenic from natural geologic deposits, and elevated levels of arsenic may be encountered in mine tailings and sediments and coal fly ash. Arsine, a hydride gas of arsenic, is discussed on p 144.

I. **Mechanism of toxicity.** Arsenic compounds may be organic or inorganic and may contain arsenic in either a pentavalent (arsenate) or a trivalent (arsenite) form. Once absorbed, arsenicals exert their toxic effects through multiple mechanisms, including inhibition of enzymatic reactions vital to cellular metabolism, induction of oxidative stress, and alteration in gene expression and cell signal transduction. Although arsenite and arsenate undergo in vivo biotransformation to less toxic pentavalent monomethyl and dimethyl forms, there is evidence that the process also forms more toxic trivalent methylated compounds. Thioarsenite compounds, which occur in vivo as minor metabolites, may also contribute to toxicity.

A. **Soluble arsenic compounds,** which are well absorbed after ingestion or inhalation, pose the greatest risk for acute human intoxication.

B. **Inorganic arsenic dusts** (eg, arsenic trioxide) may exert irritant effects on the skin and mucous membranes. Contact dermatitis has also been reported.

Although the skin is a minor route of absorption for most arsenic compounds, systemic toxicity has resulted from industrial accidents involving percutaneous exposure to highly concentrated liquid formulations.

C. The chemical warfare agent **lewisite** (dichloro [2-chlorovinyl] arsine) is a volatile vesicant liquid that causes immediate severe irritation and necrosis to the eyes, skin, and airways (see also p 452).

D. Arsenate and arsenite are **known human carcinogens** by both ingestion and inhalation.

II. **Toxic dose.** The toxicity of arsenic compounds varies considerably with the valence state, chemical composition, and solubility. Humans are generally more sensitive than other animals to the acute and chronic effects of arsenicals.

A. **Inorganic arsenic compounds.** In general, trivalent arsenic (As^{3+}) is 2–10 times more acutely toxic than pentavalent arsenic (As^{5+}). However, overexposure to either form produces a similar pattern of effects, requiring the same clinical approach and management.

1. Acute ingestion of as little as 100–300 mg of a soluble trivalent arsenic compound (eg, sodium arsenite) can be fatal.
2. The lowest observed acute effect level (LOAEL) for acute human toxicity is approximately 0.05 mg/kg, a dose associated with GI distress in some individuals.
3. Death attributable to malignant arrhythmias has been reported after days to weeks of cancer chemotherapy regimens in which arsenic trioxide at a dosage of 0.15 mg/kg/d was administered IV.
4. Repeated ingestion of approximately 0.04 mg/kg/d can result in GI distress and hematologic effects after weeks to months and peripheral neuropathy after 6 months to several years. Lower chronic exposures, approximately 0.01 mg/kg/d, can result in characteristic skin changes (initially spotted pigmentation, followed within years by palmar-plantar hyperkeratosis) after intervals of 5–15 years.
5. The US National Research Council (2001) estimated that chronic ingestion of drinking water containing arsenic at a concentration of 10 mcg/L can be associated with an excess lifetime cancer risk greater than 1 in 1,000. The latency period for development of arsenic-induced cancer is probably a decade or longer.

B. **Organic arsenic.** In general, pentavalent organoarsenic compounds are less toxic than either trivalent organoarsenic compounds or inorganic arsenic compounds. Marine organisms may contain large quantities of arsenobetaine, an organic trimethylated compound that is excreted unchanged in the urine and produces no known toxic effects. Arsenosugars (dimethylarsinoyl riboside derivatives) and arsenolipids are present in some marine and freshwater animals (eg, bivalve mollusks) and marine algae (eg, seaweeds, often used in Asian foods).

III. **Clinical presentation**

A. **Acute exposure** most commonly occurs after accidental, suicidal, or deliberate poisoning by ingestion. A single massive dose produces a constellation of multisystemic signs and symptoms that emerge over the course of hours to weeks.

1. **Gastrointestinal effects.** After a delay of minutes to hours, diffuse capillary damage results in hemorrhagic gastroenteritis. Nausea, vomiting, abdominal pain, and watery diarrhea are common. Although prominent GI symptoms may subside within 24–48 hours, severe multisystemic effects may still ensue.
2. **Cardiovascular effects.** In severe cases, extensive tissue third spacing of fluids combined with fluid loss from gastroenteritis may lead to hypotension, tachycardia, shock, and death. Metabolic acidosis and rhabdomyolysis may be present. After a delay of 1–6 days, there may be a second phase of congestive cardiomyopathy, cardiogenic or noncardiogenic pulmonary edema, and isolated or recurrent cardiac arrhythmias. Prolongation of the QT interval may be associated with torsade de pointes ventricular arrhythmia.

3. **Neurologic effects.** Mental status may be normal, or there may be lethargy, agitation, or delirium. Delirium or obtundation may be delayed by 2–6 days. Generalized seizures may occur but are rare. Symmetric sensorimotor axonal peripheral neuropathy may evolve 1–5 weeks after acute ingestion, beginning with painful distal dysesthesias, particularly in the feet. Ascending weakness and paralysis may ensue, leading in severe cases to quadriplegia and neuromuscular respiratory failure.
4. **Hematologic effects.** Pancytopenia, particularly leukopenia and anemia, characteristically develops within 1–2 weeks after acute ingestion. A relative eosinophilia may be present, and there may be basophilic stippling of red blood cells.
5. **Dermatologic effects.** Findings that occasionally appear after a delay of 1–6 weeks include desquamation (particularly involving the palms and soles), a diffuse maculopapular rash, periorbital edema, and herpes zoster or herpes simplex. Transverse white striae in the nails (Aldrich-Mees lines) may become apparent months after an acute intoxication.

B. **Chronic intoxication** is also associated with multisystemic effects, which may include fatigue and malaise, gastroenteritis, leukopenia and anemia (occasionally megaloblastic), sensory-predominant peripheral neuropathy, hepatic transaminase elevation, noncirrhotic portal hypertension, and peripheral vascular insufficiency. Skin disorders and cancer may occur (see below), and a growing body of epidemiologic evidence links chronic arsenic ingestion with an increased risk for hypertension, cardiovascular mortality, diabetes mellitus, and chronic nonmalignant respiratory disease. Genetic factors affecting the methylation of arsenic, particularly those associated with an elevated percentage of urinary monomethylarsonic acid (MMA), may increase the risk for arsenic-related chronic disease.

1. **Skin lesions,** which emerge gradually over a period of 1–10 years, typically begin with a characteristic pattern of spotted ("raindrop") pigmentation on the torso and extremities, followed after several years by the development of hyperkeratotic changes on the palms and soles. Skin lesions may occur after lower doses than those causing neuropathy or anemia. Arsenic-related skin cancer, which includes squamous cell carcinoma, Bowen disease, and basal cell carcinoma, is characteristically multicentric and occurs in non–sunexposed areas.
2. **Cancer.** Chronic inhalation increases the risk for lung cancer. Chronic ingestion is an established cause of cancer of the lung, bladder, and skin, and epidemiological studies have increasingly linked arsenic to certain types of renal cancer and liver cancer.

IV. **Diagnosis** usually is based on a history of exposure combined with a typical pattern of multisystemic signs and symptoms. Suspect acute arsenic poisoning in a patient with an abrupt onset of abdominal pain, nausea, vomiting, watery diarrhea, and hypotension, particularly when followed by an evolving pattern of delayed cardiac dysfunction, pancytopenia, and peripheral neuropathy. Metabolic acidosis and elevated creatine kinase (CK) may occur early in the course of severe cases. Some arsenic compounds, particularly those of lower solubility, are radiopaque and may be visible on a plain abdominal radiograph.

A. **Specific levels.** In the first 2–3 days after acute symptomatic poisoning, total 24-hour urinary arsenic excretion is typically in excess of several thousand micrograms (spot urine >1,000 mcg/L) and, depending on the severity of poisoning, may not return to background levels (<70 mcg in a 24-hour specimen or <50 mcg/L in a spot urine) for several weeks. Spot urine analyses are usually sufficient for diagnostic purposes.

1. **Ingestion of seafood** (eg, fin fish, shellfish and marine plants such as seaweed), which may contain very large amounts of nontoxic organoarsenicals such as arsenobetaine and arsenosugars, can "falsely" elevate

measurements of *total* urinary arsenic for up to 3 days. Speciation of urinary arsenic by a laboratory capable of reporting the concentration of inorganic arsenic and its primary human metabolites, monomethylarsonic acid (MMA) and dimethylarsinic acid (DMA), may sometimes be helpful; background urine concentration of the sum of urinary inorganic arsenic, MMA, and DMA is usually less than 20 mcg/L in the absence of recent seafood ingestion. (In the 2011–2012 National Health and Nutrition Examination Survey [NHANES] of the US general population, the median and 95% percentile values were 6.15 and 17.2 mcg/L, respectively.) It should be noted that although arsenobetaine is excreted unchanged in the urine, arsenosugars, which are abundant in bivalve mollusks and seaweed, are metabolized in part to DMA as well as recently recognized methylated thioarsenic species. Among terrestrial foods, rice naturally contains relatively high concentrations of arsenic (albeit at concentrations usually <1 ppm).

2. **Blood levels** are highly variable and are rarely of value in the diagnosis of arsenic poisoning or management of patients capable of producing urine. Although whole-blood arsenic, normally less than 5 mcg/L, may be elevated early in acute intoxication, it may decline rapidly to the normal range despite persistent elevated urinary arsenic excretion and continuing symptoms.
3. **Elevated concentrations of arsenic in nails or hair** (normally <1 ppm) may be detectable in certain segmental samples for months after urine levels normalize but should be interpreted cautiously owing to the possibility of external contamination.

B. Other useful laboratory studies include CBC with differential and smear for basophilic stippling, electrolytes, glucose, BUN and creatinine, liver enzymes, creatine kinase (CK), urinalysis, ECG and ECG monitoring (with particular attention to the QT interval), and abdominal and chest radiography.

V. Treatment

A. Emergency and supportive measures

1. Maintain an open airway and assist ventilation if necessary (pp 1–7).
2. Treat coma (p 18), shock (p 15), and arrhythmias (pp 10–15) if they occur. Because of the association of arsenic with prolonged QT intervals, avoid quinidine, procainamide, and other type Ia antiarrhythmic agents. Phenothiazines should not be given as antiemetics or antipsychotics because of their ability to prolong the QT interval and lower the seizure threshold.
3. Treat hypotension and fluid loss with aggressive use of IV crystalloid solutions, along with vasopressor agents if needed, to support blood pressure and optimize urine output.
4. Prolonged in-patient support and observation are indicated for patients with significant acute intoxication because cardiopulmonary and neurologic complications may be delayed for several days. Continuous cardiac monitoring beyond 48 hours is warranted in patients with persistent symptoms or evidence of toxin-related cardiovascular disturbance, including ECG abnormalities, or any degree of congestive heart failure.

B. Specific drugs and antidotes. Treat seriously symptomatic patients with *chelating agents,* which have shown therapeutic benefit in animal models of acute arsenic intoxication when administered promptly (ie, minutes to hours) after exposure. Treatment should not be delayed during the several days often required to obtain specific laboratory confirmation.

1. **Unithiol** (2,3-dimercaptopropanesulfonic acid, DMPS, Dimaval [p 630]), a water-soluble analog of dimercaprol (BAL) that can be administered IV, has the most favorable pharmacologic profile for the treatment of acute arsenic intoxication. Although published experience is sparse, 3–5 mg/kg every 4 hours by slow IV infusion over 20 minutes is a suggested starting dose. In the United States, the drug is available through compounding pharmacists.

2. **Dimercaprol** (BAL, British anti-lewisite, 2,3-dimercaptopropanol [p 514]) is the chelating agent of second choice if unithiol is not immediately available. The starting dose is 3–5 mg/kg by deep IM injection every 4–6 hours. Lewisite burns to the skin and eyes can be treated with topical inunctions of dimercaprol.
3. Once patients are hemodynamically stable and GI symptoms have subsided, parenteral chelation may be changed to oral chelation with either **oral unithiol** or **oral succimer** (DMSA, 2,3-dimercaptosuccinic acid [p 624]). A suggested dose of unithiol is 4–8 mg/kg orally every 6 hours. Alternatively, give succimer, 7.5 mg/kg orally every 6 hours or 10 mg/kg orally every 8 hours.
4. The therapeutic end points of chelation are poorly defined. For chelation instituted to treat symptomatic acute intoxication, one empiric approach would be to continue treatment (initially parenterally, then orally) until total urinary arsenic levels are less than 500 mcg/24 h (or spot urine <300 mcg/L), levels below those associated with overt symptoms in acutely poisoned adults. Alternatively, oral chelation could be continued until total urinary arsenic levels reach background levels (<70 mcg/24 h or spot urine <50 mcg/L). The value of chelation for the treatment of an established neuropathy (or prevention of an incipient neuropathy) has not been proved.

C. **Decontamination** (p 50). Administer activated charcoal orally if conditions are appropriate (see Table I–38, p 54). However, note that animal and in vitro studies suggest that activated charcoal has a relatively poor affinity for inorganic arsenic salts. Consider gastric lavage or whole-bowel irrigation for large ingestions.

D. **Enhanced elimination**. Hemodialysis may be of possible benefit in patients with concomitant renal failure but otherwise contributes minimally to arsenic clearance. There is no known role for diuresis, hemoperfusion, or repeat-dose charcoal.

▶ ARSINE

Michael Kosnett, MD, MPH

Arsine is a colorless hydride gas (AsH_3) formed when arsenic comes in contact with hydrogen or with reducing agents in aqueous solution. Typically, exposure to arsine gas occurs in smelting operations or other industrial settings when arsenic-containing ores, alloys, or metallic objects come in contact with acidic (or occasionally alkaline) solutions and newly formed arsine is liberated. Arsine is also used as a dopant in the microelectronics industry, and it may be accidentally encountered in the recycling of scrap gallium arsenic semiconductors.

I. **Mechanism of toxicity.** Arsine is a potent hemolytic agent. Recent investigations suggest that hemolysis occurs when arsine interacts with oxyheme in hemoglobin to form a reactive intermediate that alters transmembrane ion flux and greatly increases intracellular calcium. ***Note:*** Arsenite and other oxidized forms of arsenic do ***not*** cause hemolysis. Deposition of massive amounts of hemoglobin in the renal tubule can cause acute renal injury. Massive hemolysis also decreases systemic oxygen delivery and creates hypoxic stress, and arsine and/or its reaction products exert direct cytotoxic effects on multiple organs.

II. **Toxic dose.** Arsine is the most toxic form of arsenic. Acute exposure guideline levels (AEGLs) recently developed by the US Environmental Protection Agency and the National Research Council indicate that disabling effects (AEGL-2) may occur after 30 minutes of exposure to ≥0.21 ppm, 1 hour of exposure to ≥0.17 ppm, or 8 hours of exposure to ≥0.02 ppm. Lethal or life-threatening effects (AEGL-3) may occur from 30 minutes of exposure to ≥0.63 ppm, 4 hours of exposure to ≥0.13 ppm, or 8 hours of exposure to ≥0.06 ppm. The level considered by the National Institute for Occupational Safety and Health (NIOSH; 1994) as "immediately dangerous to life or health" (IDLH) is 3 ppm. The odor threshold of 0.5–1.0 ppm provides insufficient warning properties. Exclusive dermal exposure did not result in absorption in a hairless mouse model, suggesting that percutaneous absorption will not pose a risk to first responders or workers with adequate respiratory protection.

III. Clinical presentation

A. Acute effects. Because arsine gas is not acutely irritating, inhalation causes **no immediate symptoms.** Those exposed to high concentrations may sometimes detect a garlic-like odor, but more typically they are unaware of the presence of a significant exposure. In most industrial accidents involving arsine, the hazardous exposure occurred over the course of 30 minutes to a few hours.

B. After a **latent period of 2–24 hours** (depending on the intensity of exposure), massive hemolysis occurs, along with early symptoms that may include malaise, headache, fever or chills, and numbness or coldness in the extremities. There may be concomitant GI complaints of nausea, vomiting, and cramping pain in the abdomen, flank, or low back. In severe exposures, abrupt cardiovascular collapse and death may occur within 1 or 2 hours.

C. Hemoglobinuria imparts a dark, reddish color to the urine, and the skin may develop a copper, bronze, or "jaundiced" discoloration that may be attributable to elevated plasma hemoglobin.

D. Oliguria and **acute renal failure** often occur 1–3 days after exposure and are a major aspect of arsine-related morbidity.

E. A minority of patients may develop agitation and delirium within 1–2 days of presentation.

F. Chronic arsine poisoning, a rarely reported condition, has been associated with headache, weakness, shortness of breath, nausea, vomiting, and anemia.

IV. Diagnosis. Arsine poisoning should be suspected in a patient who presents with the abrupt onset of hemolysis, hemoglobinuria, and progressive oliguria. A consistent work history or another likely source of exposure increases the index of suspicion but is not always apparent.

A. Specific levels. Urine and whole-blood arsenic levels may be elevated but are rarely available in time to assist with prompt diagnosis and management. Whole-blood arsenic concentrations in patients with severe arsine poisoning have ranged from several hundred to several thousand micrograms per liter.

B. Other useful laboratory studies

1. The CBC in the first few hours after acute exposure may be normal or reveal only moderate depression of the hematocrit or hemoglobin. However, within approximately 12–36 hours these values will decline progressively, with hemoglobin levels declining to 5–10 g/100 mL. The peripheral blood smear may reveal erythrocyte fragmentation and abnormal red blood cell forms, including characteristic "ghost cells" in which an enlarged membrane encloses a pale or vacant interior. Leukocytosis is common. Measurement of *plasma or serum* hemoglobin may guide management (see below).
2. Initial urinalysis will typically be heme-positive on dipstick, but with scant formed red blood cells on microscopic examination. Later, as oliguria progresses, an active urine sediment with red blood cells and casts will often emerge. Quantitative measurement of urine hemoglobin may rise to 3 g/L during significant hemolysis and in some instances may exceed 10 g/L.
3. Serum bilirubin may show mild-to-moderate elevations (eg, 2–5 mg/dL) during the first 48 hours, with only a slight rise in liver aminotransferases.
4. Increases in BUN and serum creatinine will reflect acute renal insufficiency.

V. Treatment

A. Emergency and supportive measures

1. Provide vigorous IV **hydration** and, if needed, **osmotic diuresis with mannitol** (p 578) to maintain urine output and reduce the risk for acute hemoglobinuric renal failure.

2. Clinical reports indicate that **prompt exchange transfusion with whole blood** is a key therapeutic intervention and should be initiated for patients with a free serum hemoglobin level of 1.5 g/dL or higher and/or signs of renal insufficiency or early acute tubular necrosis. Because of the time delay needed to obtain matched blood, the possible need for exchange transfusion in significantly exposed patients should be anticipated soon after they present.
3. Hemodialysis may be needed to treat progressive renal failure but is not a substitute for exchange transfusion, which, unlike hemodialysis, removes arsenic-hemoprotein complexes thought to contribute to the ongoing hemolytic state.

B. Specific drugs and antidotes

1. The scant clinical experience with chelation in acute arsine poisoning is inconclusive, but limited animal and in vitro experimental studies suggest it is reasonable to initiate treatment with dimercaprol (BAL, British anti-lewisite [p 514]), a relatively lipid-soluble chelator, in patients who present within 24 hours of exposure. The dose of **dimercaprol** during the first 24 hours is 3–5 mg/kg every 4–6 hours by deep IM injection.
2. After 24 hours, consider chelation with the water-soluble dimercapto chelating agents: oral or parenteral **unithiol** (DMPS [p 630]) or oral **succimer** (DMSA, Chemet [p 624]).
3. Note that the recommendation to use dimercaprol rather than unithiol or succimer during the initial phases of poisoning is unique to arsine and differs from the chelation recommendation for poisoning by other inorganic arsenicals, in which initial use of unithiol is favored.
4. Chelation is of uncertain efficacy and should not substitute for or delay the vigorous supportive measures outlined earlier.

C. Decontamination. Remove the victim from exposure. First responders should use self-contained breathing apparatus (SCBA) to protect themselves from any arsine remaining in the environment.

D. Enhanced elimination. As noted earlier, **prompt exchange transfusion with whole blood** is useful in patients with evidence of significant active hemolysis or evolving renal insufficiency. Whole donor blood may be infused through a central line at the same rate of blood removal through a peripheral vein, or techniques using automated cell separators to exchange both erythrocytes and plasma can be considered.

▶ ASBESTOS

John R. Balmes, MD

Asbestos is the name given to a group of naturally occurring silicates—chrysotile, amosite, crocidolite, tremolite, actinolite, and anthophyllite. Exposure to asbestos is a well-documented cause of pulmonary and pleural fibrosis, lung cancer, and mesothelioma, illnesses that may appear many years after exposure.

I. Mechanism of toxicity. Fiber size, biopersistence, and chemical composition are the key determinants of the toxicity of inhaled asbestos fibers, with longer fibers (>5 μm) less easily cleared from the lungs. Asbestos fibers in the lungs are known to generate reactive oxygen species, and the subsequent cell damage and inflammatory response can lead to fibrosis. Long fibers have been shown to interfere physically with the mitotic spindle and cause chromosomal damage, especially deletions, which likely plays a role in asbestos-induced carcinogenesis. Cigarette smoking enhances the risk for lung cancer in asbestos-exposed individuals.

II. Toxic dose. A safe threshold of exposure to asbestos has not been established. Balancing potential health risks against feasibility of workplace control, the current Occupational Safety & Health Administration (OSHA) federal asbestos standard sets a permissible exposure limit (PEL) of 0.1 fiber per cubic centimeter (fiber/cc) as an 8-hour time-weighted average. No worker should be exposed to concentrations in excess of 1 fiber/cc over a 30-minute period.

III. **Clinical presentation.** After a latent period of 15–20 years, the patient may develop one or more of the following clinical syndromes:
   A. **Asbestosis** is a slowly progressive fibrosing disease of the lungs. Pulmonary impairment resulting from lung restriction and decreased gas exchange is common.
   B. **Pleural plaques** typically involve only the parietal pleura and are usually asymptomatic but provide a marker of asbestos exposure. Rarely, significant lung restriction occurs as a result of severe pleural fibrosis involving both the parietal and visceral surfaces (diffuse pleural thickening).
   C. **Pleural effusions** may occur as early as 5–10 years after the onset of exposure and are often not recognized as asbestos related.
   D. **Lung cancer** is a common cause of death in patients with asbestos exposure, especially in cigarette smokers. **Mesothelioma** is a malignancy that may affect the pleura or the peritoneum. The incidence of **gastrointestinal cancer** may be increased in asbestos-exposed workers.

IV. **Diagnosis** is based on a history of exposure to asbestos (usually at least 15–20 years before the onset of symptoms) and a clinical presentation of one or more of the syndromes described earlier. Chest radiograph typically shows small, irregular, round opacities distributed primarily in the lower lung fields. Pleural plaques, diffuse thickening, or calcification may be present. Pulmonary function tests reveal decreased vital capacity and total lung capacity and impairment of carbon monoxide diffusion.
   A. **Specific tests.** There are no specific blood or urine tests.
   B. **Other useful laboratory studies** include chest imaging, arterial blood gases, and pulmonary function tests.

V. **Treatment**
   A. **Emergency and supportive measures.** Emphasis should be placed on **prevention** of exposure. All asbestos workers should be encouraged to stop smoking and observe workplace control measures stringently.
   B. **Specific drugs and antidotes.** There are none.
   C. **Decontamination** (p 50)
      1. **Inhalation.** Persons exposed to asbestos dust and those assisting victims should wear protective equipment, including appropriate respirators and disposable gowns and caps. Watering down any dried material will help prevent its dispersion into the air as dust.
      2. **Skin exposure.** Asbestos is not absorbed through the skin. However, it may be inhaled from skin and clothes, so removal of clothes and washing the skin are recommended.
      3. **Ingestion.** Asbestos is not known to be harmful by ingestion, so no decontamination is necessary.
   D. **Enhanced elimination.** There is no role for these procedures.

► AZIDE, SODIUM

Jo Ellen Dyer, PharmD

Sodium azide is a highly toxic white crystalline solid. It has come into widespread use in automobile air bags; its explosive decomposition to nitrogen gas provides rapid inflation of the air bag (***Note:*** some newer-generation airbags utilize ammonium nitrate as the explosive chemical). In addition, sodium azide is used in the production of metallic azide explosives and as a preservative in laboratories. It has no current medical uses, but because of its potent vasodilator effects, it has been evaluated as an antihypertensive agent.

I. Mechanism of toxicity

A. The mechanism of azide toxicity is unclear. Like cyanide and hydrogen sulfide, azide inhibits iron-containing respiratory enzymes such as cytochrome oxidase, resulting in cellular asphyxiation. In the CNS, enhanced excitatory transmission occurs. Azide is also a potent direct-acting vasodilator.

B. Although neutral solutions are stable, acidification rapidly converts the azide salt to **hydrazoic acid**, particularly in the presence of solid metals (eg, drain pipes). Hydrazoic acid vapors are pungent and (at high concentrations) explosive. The acute toxicity of hydrazoic acid has been compared with that of hydrogen cyanide and hydrogen sulfide.

II. Toxic dose. Although several grams of azide are found in an automobile airbag, it is completely consumed and converted to nitrogen during the explosive inflation process, and toxicity has not been reported from exposure to spent air bags. However, sodium hydroxide is a by-product of the combustion reaction, and talc or cornstarch used to lubricate the fabric may appear as white dust or smoke after air bag deployment.

A. Inhalation. Irritation symptoms or a pungent odor does not give adequate warning of toxicity. The recommended workplace ceiling limit (ACGIH TLV-C) is 0.29 mg/m^3 for sodium azide and 0.11 ppm for hydrazoic acid. Air concentrations as low as 0.5 ppm may result in mucous membrane irritation, hypotension, and headache. A chemist who intentionally sniffed the vapor above a 1% hydrazoic acid solution became hypotensive, collapsed, and recovered 15 minutes later with residual headache. Workers in a lead azide plant exposed to air concentrations of 0.3–3.9 ppm experienced symptoms of headache, weakness, palpitations, and mild smarting of the eyes and nose, in addition to a drop in blood pressure. Laboratory workers adjacent to a sulfur analyzer that was emitting vapor concentrations of 0.5 ppm experienced symptoms of nasal stuffiness without detecting a pungent odor.

B. Dermal absorption. Industrial workers handling bulk sodium azide experienced headache, nausea, faintness, and hypotension, but it is unclear whether the exposure occurred via dermal absorption or inhalation. An explosion of a metal waste drum containing a 1% sodium azide solution caused burns over a 45% body surface area and led to typical azide toxicity with a time course similar to that of oral ingestion; coma and hypotension developed within 1 hour, followed by refractory metabolic acidosis, shock, and death 14 hours later.

C. Ingestion. Several serious or fatal poisonings occurred as a result of drinking large quantities of laboratory saline or distilled water containing 0.1–0.2% sodium azide as a preservative.

1. Ingestion of several grams can cause death within 1–2 hours.
2. Ingestion of 700 mg resulted in myocardial failure after 72 hours. Ingestion of 150 mg produced shortness of breath, tachycardia, restlessness, nausea, vomiting, and diarrhea within 15 minutes. Later, polydipsia, T-wave changes on ECG, leukocytosis, and numbness occurred, lasting 10 days.
3. Doses of 0.65–3.9 mg/d given for up to 2.5 years have been used experimentally as an antihypertensive. The hypotensive effect occurred within 1 minute. Headache was the only complaint noted in these patients.

III. Clinical presentation

A. Irritation. Exposure to dust or gas may produce reddened conjunctivae and nasal and bronchial irritation that may progress to pulmonary edema.

B. Systemic toxicity. Both inhalation and ingestion are associated with a variety of dose-dependent systemic symptoms. Early in the course, hypotension and tachycardia occur that can evolve to bradycardia, ventricular fibrillation, and myocardial failure. Neurologic symptoms include headache, restlessness, facial flushing, loss of vision, faintness, weakness, hyporeflexia, seizures, coma, and respiratory failure. Nausea, vomiting, diarrhea, diaphoresis, and lactic acidosis also appear during the course.

IV. Diagnosis is based on the history of exposure and clinical presentation.

A. Specific levels. Specific blood or serum levels are not routinely available. A simple qualitative test can be used on powders and solid materials: Azide forms a red precipitate in the presence of ferric chloride (use gloves and respiratory protection when handling the azide).

B. Other useful laboratory studies include electrolytes, glucose, arterial blood gases or pulse oximetry, and ECG.

V. Treatment. ***Caution:*** Cases involving severe azide ingestion are potentially dangerous to health care providers. In the acidic environment of the stomach, azide salts are converted to hydrazoic acid, which is highly volatile. Quickly isolate all vomitus or gastric washings and keep the patient in a well-ventilated area. Wear appropriate respiratory protective gear if available; personnel should be trained to use it. Dispose of azide with care. On contact with heavy metals, including copper or lead found in water pipes, metal azides form that may explode.

A. Emergency and supportive measures

1. Protect the airway and assist ventilation (pp 1–7) if necessary. Insert an IV line and monitor the ECG and vital signs.
2. Treat coma (p 18), hypotension (p 15), seizures (p 23), and arrhythmias (pp 10–15) if they occur.

B. Specific drugs and antidotes. There is no specific antidote.

C. Decontamination (p 50)

1. **Inhalation.** Remove the victim from exposure and give supplemental oxygen if available. Rescuers should wear self-contained breathing apparatus and appropriate chemical-protective clothing.
2. **Skin.** Remove and bag contaminated clothing and wash affected areas copiously with soap and water.
3. **Ingestion.** Administer activated charcoal. (The affinity of charcoal for azide is not known.) Consider gastric lavage if presentation is early after ingestion. See the caution statement above; isolate all vomitus or gastric washings to avoid exposure to volatile hydrazoic acid.

D. Enhanced elimination. There is no role for dialysis or hemoperfusion in acute azide poisoning.

▶ BACLOFEN

Daniel J. Repplinger, MD

Baclofen (Lioresal, Liofen, Gablofen) is a centrally acting muscle relaxant used therapeutically to treat muscle spasticity, often secondary to conditions such as spinal cord injury and multiple sclerosis. It has also been abused for recreational purposes.

I. Mechanism of toxicity

A. As a presynaptic GABA(B) agonist, baclofen is capable of producing CNS and respiratory depression. It is also associated with paradoxical hypertonicity and seizure-like activity. In withdrawal, baclofen may cause seizures, hallucinations, and hyperthermia. Additionally, bradycardia has been reported in up to 30% of ingestions.

B. Pharmacokinetics. Baclofen is rapidly absorbed from the GI tract with possible prolonged absorption in the setting of overdose. Peak absorption occurs within 2 hours of oral ingestion. Toxic effects may be seen within minutes of intrathecal overdose. The apparent volume of distribution is 1–2.5 L/kg. Protein binding is about 30%. Approximately 85% is excreted unchanged in urine while 15% is eliminated in the stool. The usual elimination half-life is 2.5–4 hours in therapeutic dosing, but may be prolonged in overdose (see also Table II–66, p 464).

II. Toxic dose. Toxicity has been reported with ingestions of 200 mg in healthy adults, while intrathecal doses of 1.5 mg have been associated with severe CNS and respiratory depression. Death has occurred with ingestions of 1 g or more. A dose of 120 mg in an infant resulted in respiratory failure.

III. Clinical presentation

A. **Baclofen intoxication** causes nausea, vomiting, confusion, somnolence, lethargy, and occasionally paradoxical hallucinations, agitation, and seizures. More severe toxicity is manifested by coma, respiratory failure, bradycardia, hypotension, flaccidity, mydriasis, and hypothermia. Deep coma can mimic brain death and may persist for several days postingestion. Rhabdomyolysis, status epilepticus, and first-degree AV block are rarely reported events.

B. **Baclofen withdrawal** generally occurs in the setting of abrupt discontinuation of an intrathecal pump but may also occur after cessation of oral dosing. The onset is typically 24–48 hours after the dose reduction. Symptoms include agitation, seizures, tachycardia, hyperthermia, hyper- or hypotension, muscle rigidity, and hallucinations. Severe withdrawal has been reported to cause rhabdomyolysis, multi-organ system failure, and death.

IV. Diagnosis is usually based on a history of ingestion or known history of baclofen pump placement or manipulation as well as the clinical findings mentioned earlier. The differential diagnosis should include intoxication and/or withdrawal from other sedative-hypnotic agents (p 414), gamma hydroxybutyrate (GHB, p 252), or ethanol (p 231).

A. **Specific levels** are not readily available and would not aid in the management of acute overdose, but might be necessary if the patient remains in deep coma and brain death is being considered.

B. **Other useful laboratory studies** include glucose, electrolytes, BUN, creatinine, creatine kinase (CK), telemetry monitoring, and pulse oximetry.

V. Treatment

A. **Emergency and supportive measures**

1. Maintain an open airway and assist ventilation if necessary (pp 1–7).
2. Treat coma (p 18), seizures (p 23), arrhythmias (p 13), hypothermia (p 20), and hyperthermia (p 21) if they occur. Hypotension is usually responsive to supine position and IV fluid resuscitation.
3. Monitor an asymptomatic patient for at least 6 hours after acute ingestion.

B. **Specific drugs and antidotes.** There is no known specific antidote and treatment is supportive. Withdrawal symptoms may respond to benzodiazepines but definitive treatment is re-institution of baclofen followed later by gradually tapering the dose if indicated.

C. **Decontamination.** Administer activated charcoal orally if conditions are appropriate (see Table I–38, p 54). Gastric lavage is not necessary after small-to-moderate ingestions if activated charcoal can be given promptly.

D. **Enhanced elimination.** While most patients do well with supportive care, hemodialysis may be warranted in patients with severe toxicity, particularly those with renal compromise as baclofen is excreted largely by the kidneys.

► BARBITURATES

Timothy E. Albertson, MD, MPH, PhD

Barbiturates have been used as hypnotic and sedative agents, for the induction of anesthesia, and for the treatment of epilepsy and status epilepticus. They have been largely replaced by newer drugs and calls to poison control centers have decreased significantly. They often are divided into four major groups according to their pharmacologic activity and clinical use: **ultra–short-acting, short-acting, intermediate-acting,** and **long-acting** (Table II–13); and *combination products* containing barbiturates include Fiorinal (50 mg butalbital) and Donnatal (16 mg phenobarbital). Veterinary euthanasia products often contain barbiturates such as pentobarbital.

TABLE II–13. BARBITURATES

Drug	Normal Terminal Elimination Half-life (h)	Usual Duration of Effect (h)	Usual Hypnotic Dose, Adult (mg)	Minimum Toxic Level (mg/L)
Ultra–short-acting				
Methohexital	3–5	<0.5	50–120	>5
Thiopental	8–10	<0.5	50–75	>5
Short-acting				
Pentobarbital	15–50	>3–4	50–200	>10
Secobarbital	15–40	>3–4	100–200	>10
Intermediate-acting				
Amobarbital	10–40	>4–6	65–200	>10
Aprobarbital	14–34	>4–6	40–160	>10
Butabarbital	35–50	>4–6	100–200	>10
Butalbital	35		100–200	>7
Long-acting				
Mephobarbital	10–70	>6–12	50–100	>30
Phenobarbital	80–120	>6–12	100–320	>30

I. Mechanism of toxicity

A. All barbiturates cause generalized **depression of neuronal activity** in the brain. Interaction with a barbiturate receptor leads to enhanced gamma-aminobutyric acid (GABA)–mediated chloride currents and results in synaptic inhibition. Hypotension that occurs with large doses is caused by depression of central sympathetic tone as well as by direct depression of cardiac contractility.

B. Pharmacokinetics vary by agent and group (see Table II–13 and Table II–66, p 462).

1. **Ultra–short-acting** barbiturates are highly lipid soluble and rapidly penetrate the brain to induce anesthesia, then are quickly redistributed to other tissues. For this reason, the clinical duration of effect is much shorter than the elimination half-life for these compounds.
2. **Long-acting barbiturates like phenobarbital** are distributed more evenly and have long elimination half-lives, making them useful for once-daily treatment of epilepsy. Primidone (Mysoline) is metabolized to phenobarbital and phenylethylmalonamide (PEMA); although the longer-acting phenobarbital accounts for only about 25% of the metabolites, it has the greatest anticonvulsant activity.

II. Toxic dose. The toxic dose of barbiturates varies widely and depends on the drug, the route and rate of administration, and individual patient tolerance. In general, toxicity is likely when the dose exceeds 5–10 times the hypnotic dose. Chronic users or abusers may have striking tolerance to depressant effects.

A. The potentially fatal **oral dose** of the shorter-acting agents such as pentobarbital is 2–3 g, compared with 6–10 g for phenobarbital.

B. Several deaths were reported in young women undergoing therapeutic abortion after they received rapid **IV injections** of as little as 1–3 mg of methohexital per kilogram.

III. Clinical presentation. The onset of symptoms depends on the drug and the route of administration.

A. Lethargy, slurred speech, nystagmus, and ataxia are common with mild-to-moderate intoxication. With higher doses, hypotension, coma, and respiratory arrest commonly occur. With deep coma, the pupils are usually small or mid-position but as the dose increases the patient may lose all reflex activity and can neurologically appear dead.

B. **Hypothermia** is common in patients with deep coma, especially if the victim has been exposed to a cool environment. Hypotension and bradycardia commonly accompany hypothermia.

IV. **Diagnosis** is usually based on a history of ingestion and should be suspected in any epileptic patient with stupor or coma. Although skin bullae sometimes are seen with barbiturate overdose, they are not specific for barbiturates. Other causes of coma should also be considered (p 18).

A. **Specific levels** of phenobarbital are usually readily available from hospital clinical laboratories; concentrations greater than 60–80 mg/L are usually associated with coma, and those greater than 150–200 mg/L with severe hypotension. For short- and intermediate-acting barbiturates, coma is likely when the serum concentration exceeds 20–30 mg/L. Barbiturates are easily detected in routine urine toxicologic screening.

B. **Other useful laboratory studies** include electrolytes, glucose, BUN, creatinine, arterial blood gases or pulse oximetry, and chest radiography.

V. **Treatment**

A. **Emergency and supportive measures**

1. Protect the airway and assist ventilation (pp 1–7) if necessary.
2. Treat coma (p 18), hypothermia (p 20), and hypotension (p 15) if they occur.

B. **Specific drugs and antidotes.** There is no specific antidote.

C. **Decontamination** (p 50). Administer activated charcoal orally if conditions are appropriate (see Table I–38, p 54). Gastric lavage is not necessary after small-to-moderate ingestions if activated charcoal can be given promptly.

D. **Enhanced elimination (p 56)**

1. **Alkalinization** of the urine (p 59) increases the urinary elimination of phenobarbital (a weak acid) but not other barbiturates. Its value in acute overdose is unproven, and it may potentially contribute to fluid overload and pulmonary edema.
2. **Repeat-dose activated charcoal** has been shown to decrease the half-life of phenobarbital and its metabolites, but data are conflicting regarding its effects on the duration of coma, time on mechanical ventilation, and time to extubation.
3. **Hemodialysis** or hemoperfusion may be necessary for severely intoxicated patients who are not responding to supportive care (ie, with intractable hypotension). Continuous venovenous hemodiafiltration has been reported to accelerate elimination.

► BARIUM

Alicia B. Minns, MD

Barium poisonings are uncommon and usually result from accidental contamination of food sources, suicidal ingestion, or occupational inhalation exposure. Accidental mass poisoning has occurred from the addition of barium carbonate to flour and the contamination of table salt. The incidence of barium poisoning in developing countries is much higher than in developed countries.

Barium is a dense alkaline earth metal that exists in nature as a divalent cation in combination with other elements. The water-soluble barium salts (acetate, chloride, fluoride, hydroxide, nitrate, and sulfide) are highly toxic. The solubility of barium carbonate is low at physiologic pH, but increases considerably as the pH is lowered (such as in the presence of gastric acid). Soluble barium salts are found in depilatories, ceramic glazes, and rodenticides and are used in the manufacture of glass and in dyeing textiles. Barium chlorate is a common ingredient in fireworks, producing a green color on ignition. Barium sulfide and polysulfide may also produce hydrogen sulfide toxicity (p 271). Barium may also enter the air during mining and refining processes, the burning of coal and gas, and the production of barium compounds. The oil and gas industries use barium compounds to make drilling mud, which lubricates the drill while it passes through rocks.

The insoluble salts, such as barium sulfate, are poorly absorbed. However, intravasation from a radiologic study has occurred, where barium sulfate administered under pressure leaked into the peritoneal cavity or portal venous system. Cardiovascular collapse has been reported although it is unclear if this was directly from the barium or from overwhelming sepsis.

I. Mechanism of toxicity

A. Systemic barium poisoning is characterized by profound hypokalemia, leading to respiratory and cardiac arrest. Barium is a competitive blocker of potassium channels, interfering with the efflux of intracellular potassium out of the cell. Barium ions may also have a direct effect on either skeletal muscle or neuromuscular transmission. In the GI tract, barium stimulates acid and histamine secretion and peristalsis.

B. Inhalation of insoluble inorganic barium salts can cause baritosis, a benign pneumoconiosis. One death resulted from barium peroxide inhalation. Detonation of barium styphnate caused severe poisoning from inhalation and dermal absorption.

C. Pharmacokinetics. After ingestion, soluble barium salts are rapidly absorbed by the digestive mucosa. A rapid redistribution phase is followed by a slow decrease in barium levels, with a half-life ranging from 18 hours to 3.6 days. The predominant route of elimination is the feces, with renal elimination accounting for 10–28%. Barium is irreversibly stored in bone.

II. Toxic dose. The minimum oral toxic dose of soluble barium salts is undetermined but may be as low as 200 mg. Lethal doses range from 1 to 30 g for various barium salts because absorption is influenced by gastric pH and foods high in sulfate. Patients have survived ingestions of 129 and 421 g of barium sulfide. The US Environmental Protection agency (EPA) has set an oral reference dose for barium of 0.07 mg/kg/d. A level of 50 mg/m^3 may be immediately dangerous to life and health (IDLH).

III. Clinical presentation. Acute intoxication manifests within 10–60 minutes with severe gastrointestinal symptoms, such as vomiting, epigastric discomfort, and profuse watery diarrhea. This is soon followed by skeletal muscle weakness due to profound hypokalemia, that progresses to flaccid paralysis, areflexia, and respiratory failure. Ventricular arrhythmias, hypophosphatemia, mydriasis, impaired visual accommodation, myoclonus, salivation, hypertension, convulsions, rhabdomyolysis, acute renal failure, and coagulopathy may also occur. Profound lactic acidosis and CNS depression may be present. More often, patients remain conscious even when severely poisoned.

IV. Diagnosis is based on a history of exposure, accompanied by rapidly progressive hypokalemia and muscle weakness. A plain abdominal radiograph may detect radiopaque material, but the sensitivity and specificity of radiography have not been determined for barium ingestions.

A. Specific levels. Serum barium levels are not readily available. They can be measured by a variety of techniques, and levels greater than 0.2 mg/L are considered abnormal.

B. Other useful laboratory studies include electrolytes, BUN, creatinine, phosphorus, arterial blood gases or pulse oximetry, and continuous ECG monitoring. Measure serum potassium levels frequently.

V. Treatment

A. Emergency and supportive measures

1. Maintain an open airway and assist ventilation if necessary (pp 1–7).

2. Treat fluid losses from gastroenteritis with IV crystalloids.
3. Attach a cardiac monitor and observe the patient closely for at least 6–8 hours after ingestion.

B. **Specific drugs and antidotes**. Administer **potassium chloride** (p 611) to treat symptomatic or severe hypokalemia. Large doses of potassium may be necessary (doses as high as 420 mEq over 24 hours have been given). Use potassium phosphate if the patient has hypophosphatemia. Serum potassium levels should be followed closely as rebound hyperkalemia has been reported.

C. **Decontamination** (p 50)
1. Activated charcoal does not bind barium and is not recommended unless other agents are suspected or have been ingested.
2. Consider gastric lavage for a large recent ingestion.
3. **Magnesium sulfate or sodium sulfate** (adults, 30 g; children, 250 mg/kg) should be administered **orally** to precipitate ingested barium as the insoluble sulfate salt. IV magnesium sulfate or sodium sulfate is not advised as it may result in the precipitation of barium in the renal tubules, leading to renal failure.

D. **Enhanced elimination.** Hemodialysis has been associated with rapid clinical improvement and a faster reduction in barium plasma half-life in several case reports. In one case report, continuous venovenous hemodialfiltration (CVVHD) was successfully used, reducing the serum barium half-life by a factor of 3, with resulting complete neurologic recovery within 24 hours. Either method of enhanced elimination should be considered in any severely poisoned patient who does not respond to correction of hypokalemia.

► BENZENE

Timur S. Durrani, MD, MPH, MBA

Benzene, a highly flammable, clear, volatile liquid with an acrid, aromatic odor, is one of the most widely used industrial chemicals. It is a constituent by-product in gasoline, and it is used as an industrial solvent and as a chemical intermediate in the synthesis of a variety of materials. Benzene can be found in dyes, plastics, insecticides, and many other materials and products. Industries with the highest benzene usage include leather production, electronics manufacturing, machinery manufacturing and spray painting. Benzene is generally not present in household products.

I. **Mechanism of toxicity.** Like other hydrocarbons, benzene can cause a chemical pneumonia if it is aspirated. See p 266 for a general discussion of hydrocarbon toxicity.
   A. Once absorbed, benzene causes CNS depression and may sensitize the myocardium to the arrhythmogenic effects of catecholamines.
   B. Benzene is also known for its chronic effects on the hematopoietic system, which are thought to be mediated by a reactive toxic intermediate metabolite.
   C. Benzene is a known human carcinogen (IARC Group 1).

II. **Toxic dose.** Benzene is absorbed rapidly by inhalation and ingestion and, to a limited extent, percutaneously.
   A. Acute ingestion of 2 mL may produce neurotoxicity, and as little as 15 mL has caused death.
   B. The recommended workplace limit (ACGIH TLV-TWA) for benzene **vapor** is 0.5 ppm (1.6 mg/m^3) as an 8-hour time-weighted average. The short-term exposure limit (STEL) is 2.5 ppm. The level considered immediately dangerous to life or health (IDLH) is 500 ppm. A single exposure to 7,500–20,000 ppm can be fatal. Chronic exposure to air concentrations well below the threshold for smell (2 ppm) is associated with hematopoietic toxicity.

C. The US Environmental Protection Agency maximum contaminant level (MCL) in water is 5 ppb.

III. Clinical presentation

A. **Acute exposure** may cause immediate CNS effects, including headache, nausea, dizziness, tremor, convulsions, and coma. Symptoms of CNS toxicity should be apparent immediately after inhalation or within 30–60 minutes after ingestion. Severe inhalation may result in noncardiogenic pulmonary edema. Ventricular arrhythmias may result from increased sensitivity of the myocardium to catecholamines. Benzene can cause chemical burns to the skin with prolonged or massive exposure.

B. After **chronic exposure**, hematologic disorders such as pancytopenia, aplastic anemia, and acute myelogenous leukemia/acute nonlymphocytic leukemia and its variants may occur. Causality is suspected for chronic myelogenous leukemia, chronic lymphocytic leukemia, multiple myeloma, non-Hodgkin lymphoma, and paroxysmal nocturnal hemoglobinuria. There is an unproven association between benzene exposure and acute lymphoblastic leukemia, myelofibrosis, and lymphomas. Chromosomal abnormalities have been reported, although no effects on fertility have been described in women after occupational exposure.

IV. Diagnosis of benzene poisoning is based on a history of exposure and typical clinical findings. With chronic hematologic toxicity, erythrocyte, leukocyte, and thrombocyte counts may first increase and then decrease before the onset of aplastic anemia.

A. **Specific levels. *Note:*** Smoke from one cigarette contains 60–80 mcg of benzene; a typical smoker inhales 1–2 mg of benzene daily. This may confound measurements of low-level benzene exposures.

1. Urine phenol levels may be useful for monitoring workplace benzene exposure (if diet is carefully controlled for phenol products). A spot urine phenol measurement higher than 50 mg/L suggests excessive occupational exposure. Urinary *trans*-muconic acid and *S*-phenylmercapturic acid (SPMA) are more sensitive and specific indicators of low-level benzene exposure but are usually not readily available. SPMA in urine is normally less than 15 mcg/g of creatinine.
2. Benzene can also be measured in expired air for up to 2 days after exposure.
3. Blood levels of benzene or metabolites are not clinically useful except after an acute exposure. Normal levels are less than 0.5 mcg/L.

B. **Other useful laboratory studies** include CBC, electrolytes, BUN, creatinine, liver function tests, ECG monitoring, and chest radiography (if aspiration is suspected).

V. Treatment

A. **Emergency and supportive measures**

1. Maintain an open airway and assist ventilation if necessary (pp 1–7).
2. Treat coma (p 18), seizures (p 23), arrhythmias (pp 10–15), and other complications if they occur.
3. Be cautious with the use of any beta-adrenergic agents (eg, epinephrine, albuterol) because of the possibility of dysrhythmias due to myocardial sensitization.
4. Monitor vital signs and ECG for 12–24 hours after significant exposure.

B. **Specific drugs and antidotes.** There is no specific antidote.

C. **Decontamination** (p 50)

1. **Inhalation.** Immediately move the victim to fresh air and administer oxygen if available.
2. **Skin and eyes.** Remove clothing and wash the skin; irrigate exposed eyes with copious amounts of water or saline.
3. **Ingestion**. Administer activated charcoal orally if conditions are appropriate (see Table I–38, p 54). Consider gastric aspiration with a small flexible

tube if the ingestion was large (eg, >150–200 mL) and occurred within the previous 30–60 minutes.

D. Enhanced elimination. Dialysis and hemoperfusion are not effective.

▶ BENZODIAZEPINES

Ben Tsutaoka, PharmD

The drug class of benzodiazepines includes many compounds that vary widely in potency, duration of effect, the presence or absence of active metabolites, and clinical use (Table II–14). Three nonbenzodiazepines—eszopiclone, zaleplon, and zolpidem—have similar clinical effects and are included here. In general, death from benzodiazepine overdose is rare unless the drugs are combined with other CNS-depressant agents, such as ethanol, opioids, and barbiturates. Newer potent, short-acting agents have been considered the sole cause of death in recent forensic cases.

I. Mechanism of toxicity. Benzodiazepines enhance the action of the inhibitory neurotransmitter gamma-aminobutyric acid (GABA). They also inhibit other neuronal systems by poorly defined mechanisms. The result is generalized depression of spinal reflexes and the reticular activating system. This can cause coma and respiratory arrest.

TABLE II–14. BENZODIAZEPINES

Drug	Half-life (h)	Active Metabolite	Oral Adult Dose (mg)
Alprazolam	6.3–26.9	No	0.25–0.5
Bromazepam	8–30	Yes	3–30
Chlordiazepoxide	18–96[a]	Yes	5–50
Clobazam	10–50	Yes	5–40
Clonazepam	18–50	No	0.5–2
Clorazepate	40–120[a]	Yes	3.75–30
Diazepam	40–120[a]	Yes	5–20
Estazolam	8–28	No	1–2
Eszopiclone[c]	6	No	2–3
Flunitrazepam	9–30	No	1–2
Flurazepam	47–100[a]	Yes	15–30
Lorazepam	10–20	No	2–4
Midazolam	2.2–6.8	Yes	1–5[b]
Oxazepam	5–20	No	15–30
Phenazepam	15–60	Yes	0.5–2
Quazepam	70–75[a]	Yes	7.5–15
Temazepam	3.5–18.4	No	15–30
Triazolam	1.5–5.5	No	0.125–0.5
Zaleplon[c]	1	No	5–20
Zolpidem[c]	1.4–4.5	No	5–10

[a]Half-life of active metabolite, to which effects can be attributed.
[b]IM or IV.
[c]Not a benzodiazepine, but similar mechanism of action and clinical effects, which may be reversed with flumazenil.

A. Respiratory arrest is more likely with newer short-acting benzodiazepines such as triazolam (Halcion), alprazolam (Xanax), and midazolam (Versed). It has also been reported with zolpidem (Ambien).

B. Cardiopulmonary arrest has occurred after rapid injection of diazepam, possibly because of CNS-depressant effects or because of the toxic effects of the diluent propylene glycol.

C. **Pharmacokinetics.** Most of these agents are highly protein bound (80–100%). Time to peak blood level, elimination half-lives, the presence or absence of active metabolites, and other pharmacokinetic values are given in Table II–66 (p 462).

II. **Toxic dose.** In general, the toxic-therapeutic ratio for benzodiazepines is very high. For example, oral overdoses of diazepam have been reported in excess of 15–20 times the therapeutic dose without serious depression of consciousness. However, respiratory arrest has been reported after ingestion of 5 mg of triazolam and after rapid IV injection of diazepam, midazolam, and many other benzodiazepines. Also, ingestion of another drug with CNS-depressant properties (eg, ethanol, barbiturates, opioids) probably will produce additive effects.

III. **Clinical presentation.** Onset of CNS depression may be observed within 30–120 minutes of ingestion, depending on the compound. Lethargy, slurred speech, ataxia, coma, and respiratory arrest may occur. Generally, patients with benzodiazepine-induced coma have hyporeflexia and midposition or small pupils. Hypothermia may occur. Serious complications are more likely when newer short-acting agents are involved or when other depressant drugs have been ingested.

IV. **Diagnosis** usually is based on the history of ingestion or recent injection. The differential diagnosis should include other sedative-hypnotic agents, antidepressants, antipsychotics, and narcotics. Coma and small pupils do not respond to naloxone but will reverse with administration of flumazenil (see below).

A. **Specific levels.** Serum drug levels are often available from commercial toxicology laboratories but are rarely of value in emergency management. Urine and blood qualitative screening may provide rapid confirmation of exposure. Immunoassays are sensitive to the benzodiazepines that metabolize to oxazepam (eg, diazepam, chlordiazepoxide, and temazepam), but may not detect newer benzodiazepines or those in low concentrations.

B. Other useful laboratory studies **include glucose, arterial blood gases, and pulse oximetry**.

V. **Treatment**

A. **Emergency and supportive measures**

1. Protect the airway and assist ventilation if necessary (pp 1–7).
2. Treat coma (p 18), hypotension (p 15), and hypothermia (p 20) if they occur. Hypotension usually responds promptly to supine position and IV fluids.

B. **Specific drugs and antidotes. Flumazenil** (p 556) is a specific benzodiazepine receptor antagonist that can rapidly reverse coma. However, because benzodiazepine overdose by itself is rarely fatal, the role of flumazenil in routine management has not been established. It is administered IV with a starting dose of 0.1–0.2 mg, repeated as needed up to a maximum of 3 mg. It has some important potential drawbacks:

1. It may induce seizures in patients who have co-ingested medications with proconvulsant activity.
2. It may induce acute withdrawal, including seizures and autonomic instability, in patients who are addicted to benzodiazepines.
3. Resedation is common when the drug wears off after 1–2 hours, and repeated dosing or a continuous infusion is often required.

C. **Decontamination** (p 50). Consider activated charcoal if the ingestion occurred within the previous 30 minutes and other conditions are appropriate (see Table I–38, p 54). Gastric lavage is not necessary after small-to-moderate ingestions if activated charcoal can be given promptly.

D. **Enhanced elimination.** There is no role for diuresis, dialysis, or hemoperfusion. Repeat-dose charcoal has not been studied.

▶ BETA-ADRENERGIC BLOCKERS

Neal L. Benowitz, MD

Beta-adrenergic–blocking agents are widely used for the treatment of hypertension, arrhythmias, angina pectoris, heart failure, migraine headaches, and glaucoma. Beta-blocker poisoning is the most common cause of drug-induced cardiogenic shock in the United States. Many patients with beta-blocker overdose will have underlying cardiovascular diseases or will be taking other cardioactive medications, both of which may aggravate beta-blocker overdose. Of particular concern are combined ingestions with calcium blockers or tricyclic antidepressants. A variety of beta blockers are available, with various pharmacologic effects and clinical uses (Table II–15).

I. **Mechanism of toxicity.** Excessive beta-adrenergic blockade is common to overdose with all drugs in this category. Although beta receptor specificity is seen at low doses, it is lost in overdose.

A. **Propranolol, acebutolol,** and other agents with membrane-depressant (quinidine-like) effects further depress myocardial contractility and conduction and may be associated with ventricular tachyarrhythmias. Propranolol is also lipid soluble, which enhances brain penetration and can cause seizures and coma.

B. **Pindolol, acebutolol, and penbutolol,** agents with partial beta agonist activity, may cause tachycardia and hypertension.

TABLE II–15. BETA-ADRENERGIC BLOCKERS

Drug	Usual Daily Adult Dose (mg/24 h)	Cardio-selective	Membrane Depression	Partial Agonist	Normal Half-life (h)
Acebutolol	400–800	+	+	+	3–6
Alprenolol	200–800	0	+	++	2–3
Atenolol	50–100	+	0	0	4–10
Betaxolol[a]	10–20	+	0	0	12–22
Bisoprolol	5–20	+	0	0	8–12
Carteolol	2.5–10	0	0	+	6
Carvedilol[c]	6.25–50	0	0	0	6–10
Esmolol[b]		+	0	0	9 min
Labetalol[c]	200–800	0	+	0	6–8
Levobunolol[a]		0	0	0	5–6
Metoprolol	100–450	+	+/–	0	3–7
Nadolol	80–240	0	0	0	10–24
Nebivolol[e]	5–40	+	0	0	12–19
Oxprenolol	40–480	0	+	++	1–3
Penbutolol	20–40	0	0	+	17–26
Pindolol	5–60	0	+	+++	3–4
Propranolol	40–360	0	++	0	2–6
Sotalol[d]	160–480	0	0	0	7–18
Timolol[a]	20–80	0	0	+/–	2–4

[a]Also available as an ophthalmic preparation.
[b]Intravenous infusion.
[c]Also has alpha-adrenergic–blocking activity.
[d]Class III antiarrhythmic activity.
[e]Also vasodilates by increasing endothelial nitric oxide (NO) release.

C. **Sotalol,** which also has type III antiarrhythmic activity, prolongs the QT interval in a dose-dependent manner and may cause torsade de pointes (p 14) and ventricular fibrillation.

D. **Labetalol** and **carvedilol** have combined nonselective beta- and alpha-adrenergic–blocking actions, and **nebivolol** is a selective $beta_1$ antagonist with vasodilating properties not mediated by alpha blockade. With these drugs, direct vasodilation can contribute to hypotension in overdose.

E. **Pharmacokinetics.** Peak absorption occurs within 1–4 hours but may be much longer with sustained-release preparations. Volumes of distribution are generally large. Elimination of most agents is by hepatic metabolism, although nadolol, atenolol, and carteolol are excreted unchanged in the urine and esmolol is rapidly inactivated by red blood cell esterases (see also Table II–66, p 462).

II. **Toxic dose.** The response to beta-blocker overdose is highly variable, depending on underlying medical disease or other medications. Susceptible patients may have severe or even fatal reactions to therapeutic doses. There are no clear guidelines, but ingestion of only 2–3 times the therapeutic dose (see Table II–15) should be considered potentially life-threatening in all patients.

III. **Clinical presentation.** The pharmacokinetics of beta blockers varies considerably, and duration of poisoning may range from minutes to days.

A. **Cardiac disturbances,** including first-degree heart block, hypotension, and bradycardia, are the most common manifestations of poisoning. High-degree atrioventricular block, intraventricular conduction disturbances, cardiogenic shock, and asystole may occur with severe overdose, especially with membrane-depressant drugs such as propranolol. The ECG usually shows a normal QRS duration with increased PR intervals; QRS widening occurs with massive intoxication. QT prolongation and torsade de pointes can occur with sotalol.

B. **Central nervous system toxicity,** including convulsions, coma, and respiratory arrest, is commonly seen with propranolol and other membrane-depressant and lipid-soluble drugs.

C. **Bronchospasm** is most common in patients with pre-existing asthma or chronic bronchospastic disease.

D. **Hypoglycemia** and **hyperkalemia** may occur.

IV. **Diagnosis** is based on the history of ingestion, accompanied by bradycardia and hypotension. Other drugs that may cause a similar presentation after overdose include sympatholytic and antihypertensive drugs, digitalis, and calcium channel blockers.

A. **Specific levels.** Measurement of beta-blocker serum levels may confirm the diagnosis but does not contribute to emergency management and is not routinely available. Metoprolol, labetalol, and propranolol may be detected in comprehensive urine toxicology screening.

B. **Other useful laboratory studies** include electrolytes, glucose, BUN, creatinine, arterial blood gases, and 12-lead ECG and ECG monitoring.

V. **Treatment**

A. **Emergency and supportive measures**

1. Maintain an open airway and assist ventilation if necessary (pp 1–7).
2. Treat coma (p 18), seizures (p 23), hypotension (p 15), hyperkalemia (p 39), and hypoglycemia (p 36) if they occur.
3. Treat bradycardia with glucagon, as discussed in the following text, and if necessary with atropine, 0.01–0.03 mg/kg IV; isoproterenol (start with 4 mcg/min and increase infusion as needed, see p 568); or cardiac pacing.
4. Treat bronchospasm with nebulized bronchodilators (p 7).
5. Continuously monitor the vital signs and ECG for at least 6 hours after ingestion.

B. **Specific drugs and antidotes**

1. Bradycardia and hypotension resistant to the measures listed above should be treated with **glucagon**, 5- to 10-mg IV bolus, repeated as needed and

followed by an infusion of 1–5 mg/h (p 559). **Epinephrine** (IV infusion started at 1–4 mcg/min and titrated to effect [p 551]) may also be useful. **High-dose insulin** plus glucose therapy (see also p 564) has shown benefit in animal studies and case reports of beta-blocker poisoning. IV lipid emulsion therapy (p 574) was reported helpful for propranolol, atenolol, and nebivolol overdoses in animal studies and/or in a few case reports. Mechanical life support (intra-aortic balloon pump, cardiopulmonary bypass or extracorporeal membrane oxygenation) should be considered for intractable shock.

2. Wide-QRS-complex conduction defects and associated hypotension caused by membrane-depressant poisoning may respond to **sodium bicarbonate**, 1–2 mEq/kg, as given for tricyclic antidepressant overdose (p 520).
3. Torsade de pointes polymorphous ventricular tachycardia associated with QT prolongation resulting from sotalol poisoning can be treated with **isoproterenol** infusion, **magnesium**, or **overdrive pacing** (p 14). Correction of hypokalemia may also be useful.

C. **Decontamination** (p 50). Administer activated charcoal orally if conditions are appropriate (see Table I–38, p 54). Gastric lavage is not necessary after small-to-moderate ingestions if activated charcoal can be given promptly. Consider whole-bowel irrigation for large ingestions involving sustained-release formulations.

D. **Enhanced elimination.** Most beta blockers, especially the more toxic drugs such as propranolol, are highly lipophilic and have a large volume of distribution. For those with a relatively small volume of distribution coupled with a long half-life or low intrinsic clearance (eg, acebutolol, atenolol, nadolol, and sotalol), hemoperfusion, hemodialysis, or repeat-dose charcoal may be effective. Hemodialysis has been shown to be effective for atenolol intoxication, and should be considered particularly when renal function is severely impaired.

► BETA$_2$-ADRENERGIC STIMULANTS

Susan Kim-Katz, PharmD

Beta-adrenergic agonists can be broadly categorized as having beta$_1$ and beta$_2$ receptor activity. This section describes the toxicity of beta$_2$-selective agonists that are commonly available for oral use: albuterol (salbutamol), metaproterenol, and terbutaline (Table II–16). Clenbuterol, a potent beta$_2$ agonist, is not approved for human use in the United States but is abused for its anabolic effects.

I. **Mechanism of toxicity**

A. Stimulation of beta$_2$ receptors results in relaxation of smooth muscles in the bronchi, uterus, and skeletal muscle vessels. At high doses, selectivity for beta$_2$ receptors may be lost, and beta$_1$ effects may be seen.

TABLE II–16. BETA$_2$-SELECTIVE AGONISTS

Drug	Oral Adult Dose (mg/d)	Oral Pediatric Dose (mg/kg/d)	Duration (h)
Albuterol	8–16	0.3–0.8	4–8
Clenbuterol	40–80 mcg	1 mcg/kg per dose	8–12
Metaproterenol	60–80	0.9–2.0	4
Ritodrine[a]	40–120	N/A	4–6
Terbutaline	7.5–20	0.15–0.6	4–8

[a]No longer available as an oral formulation in the United States.
N/A, pediatric dose not available.

B. Pharmacokinetics. These agents are readily absorbed orally or by inhalation. Half-lives and other pharmacokinetic parameters are described in Table II–66 (p 462).

II. Toxic dose. Generally, a single ingestion of more than the total usual daily dose (see Table II–16) may be expected to produce signs and symptoms of toxicity. Pediatric ingestion of less than 1 mg/kg of **albuterol** is not likely to cause serious toxicity. Tonic–clonic seizures were observed 16 hours after ingestion of 4 mg/kg of **albuterol** in a 3-year old. A 22-year-old woman developed acidosis, rhabdomyolysis, and acute renal failure following ingestion of 225 mg of **terbutaline**. Dangerously exaggerated responses to therapeutic doses of **terbutaline** have been reported in pregnant women, presumably as a result of pregnancy-induced hemodynamic changes. Ingestion of 109 mcg of **clenbuterol** in a 31-year-old man resulted in supraventricular tachycardia and atrial fibrillation lasting 3 days, and ingestion of 5,000 mcg by a 23-year-old male resulted in myocardial infarction.

III. Clinical presentation. Overdoses of these drugs affect primarily the cardiovascular system. Most overdoses, especially in children, result in only mild toxicity.

A. Vasodilation results in reduced peripheral vascular resistance and can lead to significant hypotension. The diastolic pressure usually is reduced to a greater extent than is the systolic pressure, resulting in a wide pulse pressure and bounding pulse.

B. Tachycardia is a common reflex response to vasodilation and may also be caused by direct stimulation of $beta_1$ receptors as $beta_2$ selectivity is lost in high doses. Supraventricular tachycardia or ventricular extrasystoles are reported occasionally.

C. Myocardial ischemia and infarction have been reported after IV administration of albuterol and oral abuse of clenbuterol.

D. Agitation and skeletal muscle tremors are common. Rhabdomyolysis is possible. Seizures are rare.

E. Metabolic effects include hypokalemia, hyperglycemia, and lactic acidosis. Delayed hypoglycemia may follow initial hyperglycemia. Hypokalemia is caused by an intracellular shift of potassium rather than true depletion.

IV. Diagnosis is based on the history of ingestion. The findings of tachycardia, hypotension with a wide pulse pressure, tremor, and hypokalemia are strongly suggestive. Theophylline overdose (p 435) may present with similar manifestations.

A. Specific levels are not generally available and do not contribute to emergency management. These drugs are not usually detectable on comprehensive urine toxicology screening.

B. Other useful laboratory studies include electrolytes, glucose, BUN, creatinine, creatine kinase (CK; if excessive muscle activity suggests rhabdomyolysis), lactate, cardiac enzymes, and ECG monitoring.

V. Treatment. Most overdoses are mild and do not require aggressive treatment.

A. Emergency and supportive measures

1. Maintain an open airway and assist ventilation if necessary (pp 1–7).
2. Monitor the vital signs and ECG for about 4–6 hours after ingestion.
3. If seizures and/or altered mental status occur, they are most likely caused by cerebral hypoperfusion and should respond to treatment of hypotension (see below).
4. Treat hypotension initially with boluses of IV crystalloid, 10–30 mL/kg. If this fails to raise the blood pressure, use a beta-adrenergic blocker (see Item B, below).
5. Sinus tachycardia rarely requires treatment, especially in children, unless accompanied by hypotension or ventricular dysrhythmias. If treatment is necessary, use beta-adrenergic blockers (see Item B, below).
6. Hypokalemia does not usually require treatment because it is transient and does not reflect a total body potassium deficit.

B. Specific drugs and antidotes. Hypotension, tachycardia, and ventricular arrhythmias are caused by excessive beta-adrenergic stimulation, and beta blockers are specific antagonists. Give propranolol, 0.01–0.02 mg/kg IV (p 617), or esmolol, 0.025–0.1 mg/kg/min IV (p 552). Use beta blockers cautiously in patients with a prior history of asthma or wheezing.

C. Decontamination (p 50). Administer activated charcoal orally if conditions are appropriate (see Table I–38, p 54). Gastric lavage is not necessary after small-to-moderate ingestions if activated charcoal can be given promptly.

D. Enhanced elimination. There is no role for these procedures.

▶ BORIC ACID, BORATES, AND BORON

Chi-Leung Lai, PharmD

Boric acid and sodium borate have been used for many years in a variety of products as antiseptics and as fungistatic agents in baby talcum powder. Boric acid powder (99%) is still used as a pesticide against ants and cockroaches. In the past, repeated and indiscriminate application of boric acid to broken or abraded skin resulted in many cases of severe poisoning. Epidemics have also occurred after boric acid was added mistakenly to infant formula or used in food preparation. Although chronic toxicity seldom occurs now, acute ingestion by children at home is more common.

Other boron-containing compounds with similar toxicity include boron oxide and orthoboric acid (sassolite).

I. Mechanism of toxicity

A. The mechanism of borate poisoning is unknown. Boric acid is not highly corrosive but is irritating to mucous membranes. It probably acts as a general cellular poison. The organ systems most commonly affected are the skin, GI tract, brain, liver, and kidneys.

B. Pharmacokinetics. The volume of distribution (Vd) is 0.17–0.50 L/kg. Elimination is mainly through the kidneys, and 85–100% of a dose may be found in the urine over 5–7 days. The elimination half-life is 12–27 hours.

II. Toxic dose

A. The **acute** single oral toxic dose is highly variable, but serious poisoning is reported to occur with 1–3 g in newborns, 5 g in infants, and 20 g in adults. A teaspoon of 99% boric acid contains 3–4 g. Most accidental ingestions in children result in minimal or no toxicity.

B. Chronic ingestion or application to abraded skin is much more serious than acute single ingestion. Serious toxicity and death occurred in infants ingesting 5–15 g in formula over several days; serum borate levels were 400–1,600 mg/L.

III. Clinical presentation

A. After oral or dermal absorption, the earliest symptoms are GI, with vomiting and diarrhea. Vomit and stool may have a blue-green color. Significant dehydration and renal failure can occur, with death caused by profound shock.

B. Neurologic symptoms of hyperactivity, agitation, and seizures may occur early.

C. An erythrodermic rash ("boiled-lobster" appearance) is followed by exfoliation after 2–5 days. Alopecia totalis has been reported.

IV. Diagnosis is based on a history of exposure, the presence of gastroenteritis (possibly with blue-green vomit), erythematous rash, acute renal failure, and elevated serum borate levels (although these are not commonly available in clinical laboratories).

A. Specific levels. Serum or blood borate levels are not generally available and may not correlate accurately with the level of intoxication. Analysis of serum for borates can be obtained from National Medical Services (1-866-522-2206) or other large regional commercial laboratories. Normal serum or blood levels vary with diet but are usually less than 7 mg/L. The serum boron level can be estimated by dividing the serum borate by 5.72.

B. Other useful laboratory studies include electrolytes, glucose, BUN, creatinine, and urinalysis.

V. **Treatment**

A. **Emergency and supportive measures**

1. Maintain an open airway and assist ventilation if necessary (pp 1–7).
2. Treat coma (p 18), seizures (p 23), hypotension (p 15), and renal failure (p 41) if they occur.

B. **Specific drugs and antidotes.** There is no specific antidote.

C. **Decontamination** (p 50). Activated charcoal is not very effective. Consider gastric lavage for very large ingestions.

D. **Enhanced elimination**

1. **Hemodialysis** is effective and is indicated after massive ingestions and for supportive care of renal failure. Continuous venovenous hemodialysis has also been reported effective. Peritoneal dialysis has not proved effective in enhancing elimination in infants.
2. One animal study showed increased urinary excretion of boric acid with *N*-acetylcysteine. There are no human case reports of this treatment.

▶ BOTULISM

Ilene B. Anderson, PharmD

German physicians first identified botulism in the late 18th century when patients developed an often fatal disease after eating spoiled sausage. Five distinct clinical syndromes are now recognized: **food-borne botulism, infant botulism, wound botulism, adult intestinal colonization,** and **iatrogenic botulism**. Food-borne botulism, the best-known form, results from ingestion of preformed toxin in improperly preserved home-canned vegetables, fish, or meats. In the last few decades, noncanned foods have also been reported to cause food-borne botulism. Examples include fresh garlic in olive oil, sautéed onions, beef or turkey pot pie, baked potatoes, potato salad, smoked whitefish, turkey loaf, untreated well water, home-fermented tofu, turkey stuffing, and "pruno" (an alcoholic beverage illicitly brewed in prison settings).

I. **Mechanism of toxicity**

A. Botulism is caused by a heat-labile neurotoxin (botulin) produced by the bacterium *Clostridium botulinum.* Different strains of the bacterium produce eight distinct exotoxins: A, B, C, D, E, F, G and H; types A, B, and E are most frequently involved in human disease. Botulin toxin irreversibly binds to cholinergic nerve terminals and prevents acetylcholine release from the axon. Severe muscle weakness results, and death is caused by respiratory failure. Symptoms may be slow in onset but are sometimes rapidly progressive. The toxin does not cross the blood–brain barrier.

B. Botulinum spores are ubiquitous in nature, and except in infants (and in rare situations adults), the ingestion of spores is harmless. However, in an anaerobic environment with a pH of 4.6–7, the spores germinate and produce botulinum toxin. The spores are relatively heat-stable but can be destroyed by pressure cooking at a temperature of at least 120°C (250°F) for 30 minutes. The toxin is heat-labile and can be destroyed by boiling at 100°C (212°F) for 10 minutes or heating at 80°C (176°F) for 20 minutes. Nitrites added to meats and canned foods inhibit the growth of clostridia.

II. **Toxic dose.** Botulin toxin is extremely potent; as little as one taste of botulinum-contaminated food (approximately 0.05 mcg of toxin) may be fatal.

III. **Clinical presentation**

A. Classic **food-borne botulism** occurs after ingestion of preformed toxin in contaminated food. Initial symptoms are nonspecific and may include nausea, vomiting, dry or sore throat, and abdominal discomfort. The onset of neurologic symptoms is typically delayed 12–36 hours but may vary from a few hours to as long as 8 days. The earlier the onset of symptoms, the more severe the illness. Diplopia, ptosis, sluggishly reactive pupils, dysarthria, dysphagia, dysphonia, and other cranial nerve weaknesses occur, followed by progressive symmetric descending paralysis. The patient's mentation remains clear, and there is no sensory loss. Pupils may be either dilated and unreactive or normal. Constipation and ileus resulting from decreased motility may occur. Profound weakness involving the respiratory muscles may cause respiratory failure and death.

B. **Infant botulism,** the most commonly reported type, is caused by ingestion of botulism spores (not preformed toxin) followed by in vivo production of toxin (typically type A or B) in the immature infant gut. Risk factors include age younger than 1 year, breastfeeding, and ingestion of corn syrup or honey (which commonly contains botulism spores). It has also occurred in infants fed chamomile tea. The illness is characterized by hypotonia, constipation, tachycardia, difficulty in feeding, poor head control, and diminished gag, sucking, and swallowing reflexes. It is rarely fatal, and infants usually recover strength within 4–6 weeks.

C. **Wound botulism** occurs when the spores contaminate a wound, germinate in the anaerobic environment, and produce toxin in vivo that then is absorbed systemically, resulting in illness. It occurs most commonly in IV drug abusers who "skin pop" (inject the drug subcutaneously rather than intravenously), particularly those using "black tar" heroin. It has also been reported rarely with open fractures, dental abscesses, lacerations, puncture wounds, gunshot wounds, and sinusitis. The clinical manifestations are similar to those of food-borne botulism, although nausea and vomiting are usually absent and fever may be present. Manifestations of botulism occur after an incubation period of 1–3 weeks.

D. **Adult intestinal colonization botulism** occurs rarely in adults after ingestion of botulism spores (not preformed toxin). As in infant botulism, spores germinate in the intestinal tract, and the toxin is produced in vivo. Conditions predisposing patients to this rare form of botulism include a history of extensive gastrointestinal (GI) surgery, decreased gastric or bile acids, ileus, and prolonged antibiotic therapy altering GI flora.

E. **Iatrogenic botulism** occurs following the injection of botulinum toxin type A (Botox and unlicensed concentrated preparations) for cosmetic purposes or the treatment of blepharospasm, strabismus, spasticity, or axillary hyperhidrosis. Reported complications include muscle weakness, diplopia, asthenia, dysphagia, dyspnea, and stridor. Symptom onset is expected within 1–2 days of exposure and may persist for months.

IV. **Diagnosis** is based on a high index of suspicion in any patient with a dry sore throat, clinical findings of descending cranial nerve palsies, and a history of exposure (eg, ingestion of home-canned food, "skin popping," or treatment with botulinum toxin type A). Electromyography (EMG) testing may reveal small muscle action potentials of uniform amplitude in response to repetitive low-frequency nerve stimulation, whereas high-frequency repetitive nerve stimulation results in muscle action potentials of increasing amplitude. However, EMG findings may change over time and differ among various muscle groups and therefore should not be depended on for diagnosis. The differential diagnosis includes myasthenia gravis, Eaton–Lambert syndrome, the Miller–Fisher variant of Guillain–Barré syndrome, sudden infant death syndrome (SIDS), magnesium intoxication, paralytic shellfish poisoning, and tick-related paralysis (eg, *Dermacentor andersoni*).

A. **Specific levels.** Diagnosis is confirmed by determination of the toxin in serum, stool, gastric aspirate, or a wound. Although these tests are useful for public health investigation, they cannot be used to determine initial treatment because the analysis takes more than 24 hours to perform. Obtain serum, stool, wound pus, vomitus, and gastric contents, and suspect food for toxin analysis by the local or state health department. Microbiological test results may be negative owing to toxin levels below the level of detection or improper sample collection or storage.

B. **Other useful laboratory studies** include electrolytes, blood sugar, arterial blood gases, electromyography, and cerebrospinal fluid (CSF) if CNS infection is suspected.

V. **Treatment**

A. **Emergency and supportive measures**

1. Maintain an open airway and assist ventilation if necessary (pp 1–7). Patients with a vital capacity of less than 30% are likely to require intubation and ventilatory support.
2. Obtain arterial blood gases and observe closely for respiratory weakness; respiratory arrest can occur abruptly.

B. **Specific drugs and antidotes**

1. **Food-borne, wound, adult intestinal colonization, and iatrogenic botulism**

a. **Botulinum antitoxin** (p 522) binds the circulating free toxin and prevents the progression of illness; however, it does not reverse established neurologic manifestations. It is most effective when given within 24 hours of the onset of symptoms.

Contact the local or state health department or the Centers for Disease Control in Atlanta, Georgia, telephone 1-770-488-7100 (24-hour number), to obtain antitoxin. Antitoxin is not stocked by hospital pharmacies.

b. **Guanidine** increases the release of acetylcholine at the nerve terminal but has not been shown to be clinically effective.

c. For **wound botulism**, antibiotic (eg, penicillin) treatment is indicated, along with wound debridement and irrigation. Aminoglycosides should be avoided because they may exacerbate neuromuscular blockade.

2. **Infant botulism**

a. **BabyBIG (Botulism Immune Globulin Intravenous [Human]** [page 522]) is indicated for the treatment of infant botulism caused by toxin type A or B in patients younger than 1 year of age. To inquire about obtaining **BabyBIG**, contact the Centers for Disease Control in Atlanta, Georgia, telephone 1-770-488-7100. In California, contact the state Department of Health Services, telephone 1-510-231-7600.

b. Antibiotics are not recommended except for the treatment of secondary infections. Cathartics are not recommended.

C. **Decontamination** (p 50). Administer activated charcoal orally if conditions are appropriate (see Table I–38, p 54).

D. **Enhanced elimination.** There is no role for enhanced elimination; the toxin binds rapidly to nerve endings, and any free toxin can be readily detoxified with antitoxin.

► BROMATES

Thomas R. Sands, PharmD

Bromate poisoning was most common during the 1940s and 1950s, when bromate was a popular ingredient in home permanent neutralizers. Less toxic substances have been substituted for bromates in kits for home use, but poisonings still occur occasionally from professional products (bromate-containing permanent wave neutralizers have been ingested in suicide attempts by professional hairdressers). Commercial bakeries often use bromate salts to improve bread texture, and bromates are components of the fusing material for some explosives. Bromates previously were used in matchstick heads. Bromate-contaminated sugar was the cause of one reported epidemic of bromate poisoning.

I. **Mechanism of toxicity.** The mechanism is not known. The bromate ion is toxic to the cochlea, causing irreversible hearing loss, and nephrotoxic, causing acute tubular necrosis. Bromates may be converted to hydrobromic acid in the stomach, causing gastritis. Bromates are also strong oxidizing agents that are capable of oxidizing hemoglobin to methemoglobin.

II. **Toxic dose.** The acute ingestion of 200–500 mg of potassium bromate per kilogram is likely to cause serious poisoning. Ingestion of 2–4 oz of 2% potassium bromate solution caused serious toxicity in children. The sodium salt is believed to be less toxic.

III. **Clinical presentation**

A. Within 2 hours of ingestion, victims develop GI symptoms, including vomiting (occasionally hematemesis), diarrhea, and epigastric pain. This may be accompanied by restlessness, lethargy, coma, and convulsions.

B. An asymptomatic phase of a few hours may follow before overt renal failure develops. Anuria is usually apparent within 1–2 days of ingestion; renal failure may be irreversible.

C. Tinnitus and irreversible sensorineural deafness occur between 4 and 16 hours after ingestion in adults, but deafness may be delayed for several days in children.

D. Hemolysis and thrombocytopenia have been reported in some pediatric cases.

E. Methemoglobinemia (p 317) has been reported but is rare.

IV. **Diagnosis** is based on a history of ingestion, especially if accompanied by gastroenteritis, hearing loss, or renal failure.

A. **Specific levels.** Bromates may be reduced to bromide in the serum, but bromide levels do not correlate with the severity of poisoning. There are qualitative tests for bromates, but serum concentrations are not available.

B. **Other useful laboratory** studies include CBC, electrolytes, glucose, BUN, creatinine, urinalysis, audiometry, and methemoglobin (via co-oximetry analysis).

V. **Treatment**

A. **Emergency and supportive measures**

1. Maintain an open airway and assist ventilation if necessary (pp 1–7).
2. Treat coma (p 18) and seizures (p 23) if they occur.
3. Replace fluid losses, treat electrolyte disturbances caused by vomiting and diarrhea, and monitor renal function. Perform hemodialysis as needed for support of renal failure.

B. **Specific drugs and antidotes**

1. Sodium thiosulfate (p 629) theoretically may reduce bromate to the less toxic bromide ion. There are few data to support the use of thiosulfate, but in the recommended dose, it is benign. Administer 10% thiosulfate solution, 10–50 mL (0.2–1 mL/kg) IV.
2. Treat methemoglobinemia with methylene blue (p 579).

C. **Decontamination** (p 50). Sodium bicarbonate (baking soda), 1 tsp in 8 oz of water orally, may prevent formation of hydrobromic acid in the stomach. For large recent ingestions, consider gastric lavage with a 2% sodium bicarbonate solution to prevent formation of hydrobromic acid in the stomach. Activated charcoal may also be administered.

D. **Enhanced elimination.** The bromate ion may be removed by hemodialysis, but this treatment has not been evaluated carefully. Because bromates are primarily excreted renally, initiating hemodialysis early in the course of a documented large ingestion may be prudent therapy to prevent irreversible hearing loss and renal failure.

▶ BROMIDES

Hallam Gugelmann, MD, MPH

Compounds containing bromide ions—including potassium-, sodium-, and ammonium bromide—were once used as sedatives and anticonvulsants, and were a major ingredient in over-the-counter products (eg, Bromo-Seltzer, Dr. Miles' Nervine) until 1975. Bromides are still used to treat epilepsy in dogs. Bromism (chronic bromide intoxication) was once common; 10% of patients admitted to psychiatric hospitals once had measurable bromide levels. Bromism is now rare, but cases continue to be reported worldwide owing to bromide-based medications. Recent examples include: Cordial de Monell, a teething/colic medication recalled because of infant bromism (United States); pipobroman/Vercyte/Amedel, an alkylating agent used for polycythemia vera (UK); and bromovalerylurea/bromisoval, used as an analgesic (Taiwan); several of the aforementioned preparations are still available for purchase online or in certain countries. In 2007, table salt contamination led to the greatest recorded outbreak of bromide poisoning, with 467 officially recognized cases (Angola). Bromide is still found in photographic chemicals, in some well water, in bromide-containing hydrocarbons (eg, methyl bromide, ethylene dibromide, halothane), and in some soft drinks containing brominated vegetable oil. Foods fumigated with methyl bromide (p 321) may contain some residual bromide, but the amounts are too small to cause bromide toxicity.

I. Mechanism of toxicity

A. Bromide ions substitute for chloride in various membrane transport systems, particularly within the nervous system. Bromide ions diffuse more readily through $GABA_A$ receptor–mediated chloride channels, enhancing inhibitory neuronal effects. Bromide is preferentially reabsorbed over chloride by the kidney, and chloride excretion further increases when bromide ion intake exceeds elimination. Up to 45% of chloride may be replaced in the body. With high bromide levels, the membrane-depressant effect progressively impairs neuronal transmission.

B. Pharmacokinetics. The volume of distribution of bromide is 0.35–0.48 L/kg; bioavailability of bromide salts is nearly 100%. The half-life is 9–12 days, and bioaccumulation occurs with chronic exposure. Clearance is about 26 mL/kg/d; elimination is renal. Bromide is excreted in breast milk. It crosses the placenta, and neonatal bromism has been described.

II. Toxic dose. The adult therapeutic dose of bromide is 3–5 g. One death has been reported after ingestion of 100 g of sodium bromide. Chronic consumption of 0.5–1 g per day may cause bromism.

III. Clinical presentation. Death is rare. Acute oral overdose usually causes nausea and vomiting from gastric irritation. Chronic intoxication can result in a variety of neurologic, psychiatric, GI, and dermatologic effects.

A. Neurologic and **psychiatric** manifestations are protean and include restlessness, irritability, ataxia, confusion, memory impairment, hallucinations, schizophreniform psychosis, weakness, stupor, and coma.

B. Gastrointestinal effects include nausea and vomiting (acute ingestion) and anorexia and constipation (chronic use).

C. Dermatologic effects include acneiform, pustular, granulomatous, bullous, and erythematous rashes. Up to 25–30% of patients are affected.

IV. Diagnosis. Consider bromism in any confused or psychotic patient with a high serum chloride level and a low or negative anion gap. The **serum chloride level is often falsely elevated** (up to >200 mEq/L in some reports) due to interference by bromide in the analytic test. The degree of elevation varies with the method of chloride measurement.

A. Specific levels. Assays are not readily available from most clinical laboratories, although veterinary facilities may have measurement capabilities. Endogenous serum bromide does not usually exceed 5 mg/L (0.06 mEq/L). The threshold for detection by usual methods is 50 mg/L. Therapeutic levels are 50–100 mg/L (0.6–1.2 mEq/L); levels above 3,000 mg/L (40 mEq/L) may be fatal.

B. Other useful laboratory studies include electrolytes, glucose, BUN, creatinine, and abdominal radiography (bromide is radiopaque).

V. Treatment

A. Emergency and supportive measures

1. Protect the airway and assist ventilation if needed (pp 1–7).

2. Treat coma if it occurs (p 18).

B. **Specific drugs and antidotes.** There is no specific antidote. However, administering chloride will promote bromide excretion (see below).

C. **Decontamination** (p 50). After a recent large ingestion, gastric lavage may decrease further absorption. Activated charcoal does not adsorb inorganic bromide ions, but it may adsorb organic bromides.

D. **Enhanced elimination.** Bromide is eliminated entirely by the kidney. The serum half-life can be reduced dramatically with fluids and chloride loading. The goal of treatment is resolution of symptoms. Aggressive elimination can result in rebound due to redistribution from intracellular compartments.

1. Administer **sodium chloride** IV as normal saline (0.9% sodium chloride) at a rate sufficient to obtain a urine output of 2–4 mL/kg/h. **Furosemide**, 1 mg/kg, may assist urinary excretion.
2. **Hemodialysis** is effective and may be indicated in patients with renal insufficiency or severe toxicity; case reports indicate that hemodialysis may speed resolution of symptoms. Hemoperfusion is not effective.

▶ CADMIUM

Leslie M. Israel, DO, MPH

Cadmium (Cd) is found in sulfide ores, along with zinc and lead. Exposure is common during the mining and smelting of zinc, copper, and lead. The metallic form of Cd is used in electroplating because of its anticorrosive properties, the metallic salts are used as pigments and stabilizers in plastics, and Cd alloys are used in soldering, welding, nickel-cadmium batteries, and photovoltaic cells. Cd solder in water pipes and Cd pigments in pottery can be sources of contamination of water and acidic foods.

I. **Mechanism of toxicity.** Inhaled Cd is at least 60 times more toxic than the ingested form. Fumes and dust may cause delayed chemical pneumonitis and resultant pulmonary edema and hemorrhage. Ingested Cd, at very high levels, is a GI tract irritant. Once absorbed, Cd is bound to metallothionein and filtered by the kidney, where renal tubule damage may occur. Cd is a known human carcinogen (IARC Group 1).

II. **Toxic dose**

A. **Inhalation.** The ACGIH-recommended threshold limit value (TLV) for air exposure to Cd dusts and fumes is 0.01 (total dusts) to 0.002 (respirable dusts) mg/m^3 as an 8-hour time-weighted average. Exposure to 5 mg/m^3 inhaled for 8 hours may be lethal. The level considered immediately dangerous to life or health (IDLH) for Cd dusts or fumes is 9 mg/m^3.

B. **Ingestion.** Cd salts in solutions at concentrations greater than 15 mg/L may induce vomiting. The lethal oral dose ranges upward from 150 mg.

C. **Water.** The US Environmental Protection Agency has established a safe limit of 0.005 mg/L in drinking water.

III. **Clinical presentation**

A. **Direct contact** may cause local skin or eye irritation. There are no data on dermal absorption of Cd in humans.

B. **Acute inhalation** may cause cough, dyspnea, headache, fever, and, if severe, chemical pneumonitis and noncardiogenic pulmonary edema within 12–36 hours after exposure.

C. **Chronic inhalation** may result in bronchitis, emphysema, and fibrosis. Chronic inhalation at high levels is associated with lung cancer (IARC 2000).

D. **Acute ingestion** of Cd salts causes nausea, vomiting, abdominal cramps, and diarrhea, sometimes bloody, within minutes after exposure. Deaths after oral ingestion result from shock or acute renal failure.

E. **Chronic ingestion** has been associated with kidney damage and skeletal system effects. Environmental contamination of food and water in Japan's Jinzu River basin in the 1950s resulted in an endemic painful disease called *itai-itai* ("ouch-ouch").

IV. **Diagnosis** is based on a history of exposure and the presence of respiratory complaints (after inhalation) or gastroenteritis (after acute ingestion).

A. **Specific levels.** Whole-blood Cd levels may confirm recent exposure; normal levels, in unexposed nonsmokers, are less than 1 mcg/L. Very little Cd is excreted in the urine until binding of Cd in the kidney is exceeded or renal damage occurs. Urine Cd values are normally less than 1 mcg/g of creatinine. Measures of tubular microproteinuria (beta2-microglobulin, retinol-binding protein, albumin, and metallothionein) are used to monitor the early and toxic effects of Cd on the kidney.

B. **Other useful laboratory studies** include CBC, electrolytes, glucose, BUN, creatinine, arterial blood gases or oximetry, and chest radiography.

V. **Treatment**

A. **Emergency and supportive measures**

1. **Inhalation**. Monitor arterial blood gases and obtain chest radiograph. Observe for at least 6–8 hours and treat wheezing and pulmonary edema (pp 7–8) if they occur. After significant exposure, it may be necessary to observe for 1–2 days for delayed-onset noncardiogenic pulmonary edema.
2. **Ingestion**. Treat fluid loss caused by gastroenteritis with IV crystalloid fluids (p 15).

B. **Specific drugs and antidotes.** There is no evidence that chelation therapy is effective, although various chelating agents have been used following acute overexposure. BAL, penicillamine, and EDTA are contraindicated owing to the increased risk for renal damage.

C. **Decontamination**

1. **Inhalation.** Remove the victim from exposure and give supplemental oxygen if available.
2. **Ingestion** (p 50). Perform gastric lavage after significant ingestion. The effectiveness of activated charcoal is unknown.
3. **Skin and eyes.** Remove contaminated clothing and wash exposed skin with water. Irrigate exposed eyes with copious amounts of tepid water or saline (p 47).

D. **Enhanced elimination.** There is no role for dialysis, hemoperfusion, or repeat-dose charcoal.

▶ CAFFEINE

Ann Arens, MD and Neal L. Benowitz, MD

Caffeine is the most widely used psychoactive substance. Besides its well-known presence in coffee, tea, colas, and chocolate, it is available in many over-the-counter and prescription oral medications and as injectable caffeine sodium benzoate (occasionally used for neonatal apnea). Caffeine is widely used as an anorectant, a co-analgesic, a diuretic, and a sleep suppressant. Botanical forms of caffeine, including yerba mate, guarana (*Paullinia cupana*), kola nut (*Cola nitida*), and green tea extract, are common constituents of "thermogenic" dietary supplements that are widely touted for weight loss and athletic enhancement (see also p 261). Caffeine is occasionally combined in tablets with other stimulants, such as MDMA (methylenedioxymethamphetamine). Although caffeine has a wide therapeutic index and rarely causes serious toxicity, there are many documented cases of accidental, suicidal, and iatrogenic intoxication, some resulting in death.

In November of 2010, the FDA issued warnings to manufacturers of caffeinated alcoholic beverages to stop production due to public health safety concerns, and these have since been removed from sale in the United States.

I. Mechanism of toxicity

A. Caffeine is a trimethylxanthine that is closely related to theophylline. It acts primarily through nonselective inhibition of adenosine receptors. In addition, with overdose there is considerable beta$_1$- and beta$_2$-adrenergic stimulation secondary to release of endogenous catecholamines.

B. Addition of caffeine to alcoholic beverages can decrease subjective perception of alcohol intoxication without affecting objective markers of intoxication such as motor control, and may increase risky sexual behavior and injury.

C. Pharmacokinetics. Caffeine is rapidly and completely absorbed orally, with a volume of distribution of 0.7–0.8 L/kg. Its elimination half-life is approximately 4–6 hours but can range from 3 hours in healthy smokers to 10 hours in nonsmokers; after overdose, the half-life may be as long as 15 hours. In infants younger than 2–3 months old, metabolism is extremely slow, and the half-life may exceed 24 hours (see also Table II–66, p 462). Caffeine is metabolized in the liver by cytochrome P450 (CYP), primarily the CYP1A2 isoenzyme, and is subject to several potential drug interactions, including inhibition by oral contraceptives, cimetidine, norfloxacin, and alcohol. Tobacco (and marijuana) smoking accelerates caffeine metabolism.

II. Toxic dose. The reported lethal oral dose is 10 g (150–200 mg/kg), although one case report documents survival after a 24-g ingestion. In children, ingestion of 35 mg/kg may lead to moderate toxicity. Coffee contains 50–200 mg (tea, 40–100 mg) of caffeine per cup depending on how it is brewed. No-Doz and other sleep suppressants usually contain about 200 mg per tablet. "Thermogenic" dietary supplements, which are sold as energy beverages (eg, Red Bull), bars, capsules, tablets, or liquid drops, contain the equivalent of 40–200 mg of caffeine per serving as either concentrated plant extracts or synthetic caffeine (see Table II–17).

III. Clinical presentation

A. The earliest symptoms of **acute** caffeine poisoning are usually anorexia, tremor, and restlessness, followed by nausea, vomiting, tachycardia, and agitation. With serious intoxication, delirium, seizures, supraventricular and ventricular tachyarrhythmias, hypokalemia, and hyperglycemia may occur. Hypotension is caused by excessive beta$_2$-mediated vasodilation and is characterized by a low diastolic pressure and a wide pulse pressure. Ingestion of caffeine-containing diet aids has been associated with sudden death in people with bulimia or laxative abuse, most likely owing to aggravation of hypokalemia. Caffeine poisoning occasionally causes rhabdomyolysis and acute renal failure. Coronary vasospasm has also been described. Concomitant administration of caffeine with MDMA aggravated tachycardia and hyperthermia in animal.

B. Chronic high-dose caffeine intake can lead to "caffeinism" (nervousness, irritability, anxiety, tremulousness, muscle twitching, insomnia, palpitations, and hyperreflexia).

IV. Diagnosis is suggested by the history of caffeine exposure or the constellation of nausea, vomiting, tremor, tachycardia, seizures, and hypokalemia (also consider theophylline [p 435]).

A. Specific levels. Serum caffeine levels are not routinely available in hospital laboratories but can be determined at reference toxicology laboratories. Some pediatric hospitals may offer caffeine testing for monitoring therapeutic use in neonates. Toxic concentrations may be detected by cross-reaction with theophylline assays (see Table I–33, p 46). Coffee drinkers have caffeine levels of 1–10 mg/L, and levels exceeding 80 mg/L have been associated with death. The level associated with a high likelihood of seizures is unknown.

TABLE II–17. Caffeine Content of Some Common Beverages and Tablets

	Volume per Container (oz)	Volume (mL)	Caffeine Concentration (mg/mL)	Total Caffeine (mg)
Energy Drinks				
Red Bull	16	473	0.32	151
Monster	16	473	0.34	160
Rockstar	16	473	0.34	160
Full Throttle	16	473	0.34	160
Amp	16	473	0.33	142
NOS	16	473	0.34	160
Energy "Shots"				
5-hour ENERGY	1.93	57	3.5	200
NoDoz Energy Shots	1.89	56	2.05	115
Starbucks Coffee[a]				
Espresso (single shot)	1	30	2.5	75
Brewed ("Short")	8	236	0.75	175
Brewed ("Tall")	12	354	0.73	260
Brewed ("Grande")	16	473	0.70	330
Brewed ("Venti")	20	591	0.69	410
Starbucks Hot Chocolate[a]	8	236	0.04	10
Twinings Teas[b]				
Earl Grey	6	177	0.16	29
English Breakfast Tea	6	177	0.14	25
Irish Breakfast Tea	6	177	0.17	30
Soft Drinks[c]				
Coca-Cola Classic	12	355	0.10	34.5
Pepsi Cola	12	355	0.10	38
Mountain Dew	12	355	0.15	54
Caffeine Tablets				
MET-Rx	1 tablet			200
NoDoz	1 tablet			200
Xenadrine	1 tablet			100

[a]Based on nutritional facts provided by Starbucks®. Available at http://news.starbucks.com/uploads/documents/nutrition.pdf, accessed on 1/3/2015.

[b]Adapted from Chin JM, Merves ML, Goldberger BA, Sampson-Cone A, Cone EJ. Caffeine content of brewed teas. *J Anal Toxicol.* 2008;32(8):702–704. Based on 5-minute steep time.

[c]Adapted from Reissig CJ, Strain EC, Griffiths RR. Caffeinated energy drinks–a growing problem. *Drug Alcohol Depend.* 2009;99(1–3):1–10.

B. Other useful laboratory studies include electrolytes, glucose, ECG, and telemetry monitoring.

V. Treatment

A. Emergency and supportive measures

1. Maintain an open airway and assist ventilation if necessary (pp 1–7).
2. Treat seizures (p 23) and hypotension (p 15) if they occur. Extreme anxiety or agitation may respond to benzodiazepines such as IV lorazepam (p 516).
3. Hypokalemia usually resolves without treatment but in severe cases it may be necessary (see p 611) as it can contribute to life-threatening arrhythmias.
4. Monitor ECG and vital signs for at least 6 hours after ingestion.

B. Specific drugs and antidotes

1. Beta blockers effectively reverse cardiotoxic and hypotensive effects mediated by excessive beta-adrenergic stimulation. Treat tachyarrhythmias and hypotension with IV **propranolol**, 0.01–0.02 mg/kg (p 617), or **esmolol**, 0.025–0.1 mg/kg/min (p 552), beginning with low doses and titrating to effect. Because of its short half-life and cardioselectivity, esmolol is preferred for tachyarrhythmias in normotensive patients. Adenosine may not be effective in reversal of supraventricular tachycardias, because of adenosine receptor antagonism.
2. If vasopressor drugs are required, **vasopressin** (p 632) or **phenylephrine** (p 606) is recommended to avoid the potassium-lowering effects of catecholamines.

C. Decontamination (p 50). Administer activated charcoal orally if conditions are appropriate (see Table I–38, p 54). Gastric lavage is not necessary after small-to-moderate ingestions if activated charcoal can be given promptly.

D. Enhanced elimination. Repeat-dose activated charcoal (p 59) may enhance caffeine elimination. Seriously intoxicated patients (with multiple seizures, significant tachyarrhythmias, or intractable hypotension) may require hemodialysis (p 59).

▶ CALCIUM CHANNEL ANTAGONISTS

Neal L. Benowitz, MD

Calcium channel antagonists (also known as calcium channel blockers or calcium antagonists) are widely used to treat hypertension, angina pectoris, coronary spasm, hypertrophic cardiomyopathy, supraventricular cardiac arrhythmias, Raynaud phenomenon, and migraine headache. Toxicity from calcium antagonists may occur with therapeutic use (often owing to underlying cardiac conduction disease or drug interactions) or as a result of accidental or intentional overdose. Overdoses of calcium antagonists are frequently life-threatening and one of the most important sources of drug-induced mortality. As little as one tablet can be potentially life-threatening in a small child.

I. Mechanism of toxicity. Calcium antagonists decrease calcium entry through L-type cellular calcium channels, acting on vascular smooth muscle, the heart and pancreas. They can cause coronary and peripheral vasodilation, reduced cardiac contractility, slowed atrioventricular nodal conduction, and depressed sinus node activity. Lowering of blood pressure through a fall in peripheral vascular resistance may be moderated by reflex tachycardia, although this reflex response is often blunted by depressant effects on AV and sinus node activity. In addition, these agents are metabolic poisons causing increased dependence of the heart on carbohydrate metabolism rather than the usual free fatty acids. This toxic effect is compounded by the inhibition of pancreatic insulin release, making it difficult for the heart to use carbohydrates during shock.

A. In therapeutic doses, the dihydropyridines (amlodipine, felodipine, isradipine, nicardipine, nifedipine, and nisoldipine) act primarily on blood vessels (causing vasodilation), whereas the phenylalkylamines (verapamil) and benzothiazepines (diltiazem) also act on the heart, reducing cardiac contractility and heart rate. Overdoses of verapamil and diltiazem are generally most severe due to cardiogenic shock, while overdoses of dihydropyridines are usually less severe, manifesting as vasodilatory shock, although in massive overdose this selectivity may be lost.

B. Nimodipine has a greater action on cerebral arteries and is used to reduce vasospasm after recent subarachnoid hemorrhage.

C. Important **drug interactions** may result in toxicity. Hypotension is more likely to occur in patients taking beta blockers, nitrates, or both, especially if they are hypovolemic after diuretic therapy. Patients taking disopyramide or other cardiodepressant drugs and those with severe underlying myocardial disease are also at risk for hypotension. Macrolide antibiotics, grapefruit juice, and other inhibitors of the cytochrome P450 enzyme CYP3A4 can increase the blood levels of many calcium antagonists. Life-threatening bradyarrhythmias may occur when beta blockers and verapamil are given together, and asystole has occurred after parenteral administration. Fatal rhabdomyolysis has occurred with concurrent administration of diltiazem and statins.

D. Pharmacokinetics. Absorption is slowed with sustained-release preparations, and the onset of toxicity may be delayed several hours. Most of these agents are highly protein bound and have large volumes of distribution. They are eliminated mainly via extensive hepatic metabolism, and most undergo substantial first-pass removal. In a report on two patients with verapamil overdoses (serum levels, 2,200 and 2,700 ng/mL), the elimination half-lives were 7.8 and 15.2 hours (see also Table II–66, p 462).

II. Toxic dose. Usual therapeutic daily doses for each agent are listed in Table II–18. The toxic-therapeutic ratio is relatively small, and serious toxicity may occur with therapeutic doses. Any dose greater than the usual therapeutic range should be considered potentially life-threatening. Note that many of the common agents are

TABLE II–18. CALCIUM ANTAGONISTS

Drug	Usual Adult Daily Dose (mg)	Elimination Half-Life (h)	Primary Site(s) of Activity[a]
Amlodipine	2.5–10	30–50	V
Bepridil[b]	200–400	24	M, V
Diltiazem	90–360 (PO) 0.25 mg/kg (IV)	4–6	M, V
Felodipine	5–30	11–16	V
Isradipine	5–25	8	V
Nicardipine	60–120 (PO) 5–15 mg/h (IV)	8	V
Nifedipine	30–120	2–5	V
Nisoldipine	20–40	4	V
Nitrendipine	40–80	2–20	V
Verapamil	120–480 (PO) 0.075–0.15 mg/kg (IV)	2–8	M, V

[a]Major toxicity: M, myocardial (decreased contractility, AV block); V, vascular (vasodilation).
[b]Removed from US market.

available in sustained-release formulations, which can result in delayed onset or sustained toxicity.

III. Clinical presentation

A. The primary features of calcium antagonist intoxication are **hypotension** and **bradycardia.**

1. Hypotension may be caused by peripheral vasodilation (vasodilatory shock), reduced cardiac contractility and slowed heart rate (cardiogenic shock), or a combination. Dihydropyridines are most likely to cause vasodilatory shock, while verapamil and diltiazem cause combined vasodilatory and cardiogenic shock. Shock from calcium blocker overdoses may be refractory to usual supportive measures.
2. Bradycardia may result from sinus bradycardia, second- or third-degree AV block, or sinus arrest with junctional rhythm. These are seen most commonly with verapamil and diltiazem overdose.
3. Most calcium antagonists do not affect intraventricular conduction, so the QRS duration is usually not affected. The PR interval may be prolonged even with therapeutic doses of verapamil.
4. Noncardiogenic pulmonary edema and ischemic injury to bowel, brain, or kidney may complicate overdose and its management.

B. Noncardiac manifestations of intoxication include nausea and vomiting, metabolic acidosis (resulting from hypotension and/or cardiac metabolic derangements), and hyperglycemia (owing to blockade of insulin release). Hypoinsulinemia impairs myocardial glucose uptake, thereby reducing contractility and contributing to hypotension. In one study, the degree of hyperglycemia was correlated with the severity of the overdose. Mental status is usually normal, but in severe overdoses stupor, confusion and seizures may occur, probably related to cerebral hypoperfusion.

IV. Diagnosis. The findings of hypotension and bradycardia, particularly with sinus arrest or AV block, in the absence of QRS interval prolongation should suggest calcium antagonist intoxication. The differential diagnosis should include beta blockers, clonidine, and other sympatholytic drugs. The presence of hyperglycemia in a nondiabetic patient in combination with cardiac toxicity should suggest calcium antagonist toxicity.

A. Specific levels. Serum or blood drug levels are not widely available. Diltiazem and verapamil may be detectable in comprehensive urine toxicology screening.

B. Other useful laboratory studies include electrolytes, glucose, BUN, creatinine, arterial blood gases or oximetry, and ECG and cardiac monitoring. A bedside echocardiogram may help characterize the hemodynamic physiology and assist with planning therapy.

V. Treatment

A. Emergency and supportive measures

1. Maintain an open airway and assist ventilation if necessary (pp 1–7).
2. Treat coma (p 18), hypotension (p 15), and bradyarrhythmias (p 10) if they occur. The use of cardiopulmonary bypass or other cardiovascular assist devices to allow time for liver metabolism have been reported in patients with massive calcium blocker poisoning. Atropine (p 512) and cardiac pacing, although having variable success, can be considered for bradyarrhythmias that are contributing to hypotension.
3. Monitor the vital signs and ECG for at least 6 hours after alleged ingestion of immediate-release compounds. Sustained-release products, especially verapamil, require a longer observation period (24 hours for verapamil, 18 hours for others). Admit symptomatic patients for at least 24 hours.

B. Specific drugs and antidotes

1. **Calcium** (p 526) reverses the depression of cardiac contractility in some patients, but it does not affect sinus node depression or peripheral vasodilation

and has variable effects on AV nodal conduction. Administer **calcium chloride** 10%, 10 mL (0.1–0.2 mL/kg) IV, or **calcium gluconate** 10%, 20–30 mL (0.3–0.4 mL/kg) IV. Repeat every 5–10 minutes as needed. In case reports, doses as high as 10–15 g over 1–2 hours and 30 g over 12 hours have been administered without apparent calcium toxicity. Calcium chloride should be given only via a central line or secure peripheral IV line owing to the potential for skin necrosis.

2. **Hyperinsulinemia/euglycemia** (HIE) therapy is effective in animal models of severe verapamil intoxication and has been successful in multiple human case reports. The putative mechanism is enhanced transport of glucose, lactate, and oxygen into myocardial cells, and correction of calcium antagonist–induced hypoinsulinemia, leading to improved cell carbohydrate metabolism, which in turn increases myocardial contractility. Like calcium, HIE treatment is not likely to reverse calcium antagonist–induced vasodilation, conduction block, or bradycardia.
   a. A bolus of **insulin**, 1 U/kg (p 564), is followed by an infusion of 1–10 U/kg/h. To avoid hypoglycemia, the patient is given an initial bolus of **glucose** (25 g or 50 mL of $D_{50}W$; children: 0.5 g/kg as $D_{25}W$) followed by additional boluses and infusions to maintain the serum glucose between 100 and 200 mg/dL.
   b. Blood sugar levels should be checked every 10 minutes initially, then every 30–60 minutes. Hypokalemia may need correction.
3. **Intravenous lipid emulsion** (ILE) therapy (p 574) has shown promise in animal studies and a few case reports of severe verapamil and diltiazem poisoning. The usual dose is an IV bolus of 100 mL (1.5 mL/kg of lean body weight) of lipid emulsion 20% (preparation normally used for hyperalimentation), which can be repeated twice at 5-minute intervals for a total of three doses. The bolus can be followed by a continuous infusion of the drug at 0.25–0.5 mL/kg/min for an hour; a maximum of 10–12 mL/kg total over the first 30–60 minutes has been recommended.
4. **Vasopressors** are often needed to manage shock from calcium blockers. Sometimes extraordinarily high doses are required for refractory shock. While vasopressors are helpful in maintaining circulatory function, they carry a risk of causing ischemic events, which are not uncommon. It is recommended that calcium and HIE therapy be provided before high-dose pressors. The choice of pressor depends on the pathophysiology. For cardiogenic shock with bradycardia, epinephrine, glucagon, dobutamine, isoproterenol, and phosphodiesterase inhibitors (milrinone) should be considered. For vasodilatory shock, norepinephrine, phenylephrine, and vasopressin should be considered.
5. **Glucagon** (p 559) is reported to increase blood pressure in patients with refractory hypotension and may also help with bradyarrhythmias. It can be started as a bolus in adults at 5 mg (0.05 mg/kg), repeated in 10 minutes if no response, with caution for vomiting that may ensue.
6. **Emerging therapies** with evidence of benefit in animal studies but limited human experience: **levosimendan** (sensitizes myocardium to effects of calcium and increases contractility, but is also a vasodilator); **methylene blue** (inhibits nitric oxide release and may be useful for vasodilatory shock, particularly from amlodipine [see p 579]); **cyclodextrins**, such as sugammadex (may encapsulate and sequester verapamil from site of action).

C. **Decontamination** (p 50). Administer activated charcoal orally if conditions are appropriate (see Table I–38, p 54). For large ingestions of a sustained-release preparation, consider whole-bowel irrigation (p 55) in addition to repeated doses of charcoal (p 59).

D. **Enhanced elimination.** Owing to extensive protein binding and large volumes of distribution, dialysis and hemoperfusion are not effective.

▶ CAMPHOR AND OTHER ESSENTIAL OILS

Ilene B. Anderson, PharmD

Camphor is one of several essential oils (volatile oils) derived from natural plant products that have been used for centuries as topical rubefacients for analgesic and antipruritic purposes (Table II–19). Camphor and other essential oils are found in over-the-counter remedies such as BenGay, Vicks VapoRub, and Campho-Phenique. In addition, camphor is used for religious, spiritual, aromatic, folk medicinal, and insecticidal purposes, often in powder or cube form. Toxic effects have occurred primarily when essential oils have been intentionally administered orally for purported therapeutic effects and in accidental pediatric ingestions.

I. Mechanism of toxicity.

A. After topical application, essential oils produce dermal hyperemia followed by a feeling of comfort, but if ingested, they can cause systemic toxicity. Most essential oils cause CNS stimulation or depression. **Camphor** is a CNS stimulant that causes seizures soon after ingestion. The underlying mechanism is unknown; however, a transient decrease in hyperpolarization-activated conductance has been noted in human poisoning. Camphor is absorbed rapidly from the GI tract and metabolized by the liver. It is not known whether metabolites contribute to toxicity.

B. Overdose during pregnancy. Camphor crosses the placenta. There are case reports of overdose during pregnancy. One infant died 30 minutes after delivery but labor was complicated by pre-eclampsia, premature placental separation and breech presentation. Laboratory confirmation of camphor in the infant was documented. Two other cases involved maternal seizures but later delivery of health babies.

C. Pharmacokinetics. Well absorbed after inhalation, ingestion, or dermal application. Following ingestion, seizures may occur within 20–30 minutes. The volume of distribution is 2–4 L/kg. The half-life is 1.5–2.7 hours. Camphor is primarily metabolized by the liver and eliminated in the urine as the glucuronide form.

II. Toxic dose. Serious poisonings and death have occurred in children after ingestion of as little as 1 g of camphor. This is equivalent to just 10 mL of Campho-Phenique or 5 mL of camphorated oil (20%). Recovery after ingestion of 42 g in an adult has been reported. The concentrations of other essential oils range from 1% to 20%; doses of 5–15 mL are considered potentially toxic. Doses <30 mg/kg are unlikely to result in serious toxicity.

III. Clinical presentation (see also Table II–19)

A. Acute manifestations of oral overdose usually occur within 5–30 minutes. Burning in the mouth and throat occurs immediately, followed by nausea, vomiting, and abdominal discomfort. Camphor typically causes abrupt onset of seizures within 20–30 minutes after ingestion. Ataxia, drowsiness, dizziness, confusion, hallucinations, restlessness, delirium, muscle twitching, and coma may occur. Aspiration may result in pneumonitis. Death is rare and may result from respiratory arrest or complications of status epilepticus.

B. Chronic camphor exposure has resulted in myocarditis, granulomatous hepatitis, and death.

C. Dermal exposure may result in flushing and allergic reactions. Extensive pediatric dermal exposure has resulted in ataxia and seizures.

D. Smoking (eg, clove cigarettes) or inhaling essential oils may cause tracheobronchitis.

E. IV injection (eg, peppermint oil) can cause pulmonary edema and acute respiratory distress syndrome (ARDS).

IV. Diagnosis usually is based on a history of exposure. The pungent odor of camphor and other volatile oils is usually apparent.

A. Specific levels are not available.

TABLE II–19. ESSENTIAL OILS[a]

Name	Comments
Arnica Oil	Contains sesquiterpene lactones. Vomiting, diarrhea, CNS depression, hypertension, bradycardia or tachycardia, and bleeding reported after acute ingestion. May cause allergic contact dermatitis.
Birch oil	Contains 98% methyl salicylate (equivalent to 1.4 g of aspirin per milliliter; see "Salicylates," p 410).
Camphor	Pediatric toxic dose 1 g (see text).
Cinnamon oil	A potent sensitizing agent causing erythema, dermatitis, and stomatitis. A 7.5-year-old boy ingested 2 oz, which resulted in oral irritation, diplopia, dizziness, vomiting, and CNS depression that resolved within 5 hours. "Cinnamon challenge" (ingesting a spoonful of cinnamon powder without water) may result in coughing, choking, nasal and throat irritation, nausea, vomiting, and pneumonitis if aspirated.
Clove oil	Contains 80–90% eugenol. Metabolic acidosis, CNS depression, seizures, coagulopathy, and hepatotoxicity after acute ingestion. Fulminant hepatic failure in a 15-month-old boy after a 10-mL ingestion. *N*-Acetylcysteine may be beneficial in preventing or treating the hepatotoxicity. Smoking clove cigarettes may cause irritant tracheobronchitis, hemoptysis.
Eucalyptus oil	Contains 70% eucalyptol. Toxic dose is 5–10 mL. Ingestion causes epigastric burning, vomiting, hypoventilation, ataxia, seizures, or rapid CNS depression.
Guaiacol	Nontoxic.
Lavender oil	Mild headache, constipation, and reversible gynecomastia (in prepubertal boys) reported with chronic dermal application. CNS depression and confusion within 3 hours of ingestion in an 18-month-old male. Anticholinergic syndrome, supraventricular tachycardia after lavender stoechas tea ingestion.
Melaleuca oil	Tea tree oil. Toxic dose in children is 10 mL. Sedation, confusion, ataxia, and coma are reported after ingestion. Onset in 30–60 minutes. Contact dermatitis with dermal contact.
Menthol	An alcohol derived from various mint oils. Ingestion may cause oral mucosal irritation, vomiting, tremor, ataxia, and CNS depression.
Nutmeg	Myristica oil. Used as a hallucinogen and purported to have amphetamine-like effects; 2–4 tablespoons of ground nutmeg can cause psychogenic effects. Symptoms: abdominal pain, vomiting, lethargy, delirium, dizziness, agitation, hallucinations, seizures, miosis or mydriasis, tachycardia, and hypertension. Fatality reported with co-ingestion of flunitrazepam.
Pennyroyal oil	Moderate-to-severe toxicity with ingestion of more than 10 mL. Vomiting, abdominal cramping, syncope, coma, centrilobular hepatic necrosis, renal tubular degeneration, disseminated intravascular coagulation, multiple-organ failure, and death. *N*-Acetylcysteine may be effective in preventing hepatic necrosis.
Peppermint oil	Contains 50% menthol. Oral mucosal irritation, burning, and rarely mouth ulcers reported. Intravenous injection resulted in coma, cyanosis, pulmonary edema, and ARDS. Allergic contact dermatitis with dermal exposure. Nasal instillation in 2-month-old resulted in dyspnea, stridor, hyperextension, coma, and metabolic acidosis.
Thymol	Used as an antiseptic (see "Phenol," p 368). May cause allergic contact dermatitis.
Wintergreen oil	Contains methyl salicylate 98% (equivalent to 1.4 g of aspirin per milliliter; see "Salicylates," p 410).
Wormwood oil	Absinthe. Euphoria, vomiting, lethargy, confusion, agitation, hallucinations, seizures, rhabdomyolysis, renal failure, bradycardia, arrhythmias.

[a]Information primarily derived from case reports often lacking detailed or documented laboratory confirmation.

B. **Other useful laboratory studies** include electrolytes, glucose, liver aminotransferases, and arterial blood gases (if the patient is comatose or in status epilepticus).

V. **Treatment**

A. **Emergency and supportive measures**

1. Maintain an open airway and assist ventilation if necessary (pp 1–7).
2. Treat seizures (p 23) and coma (p 18) if they occur.

B. **Specific drugs and antidotes**. There are no specific antidotes for camphor. ***N*-acetylcysteine** (p 499) may be effective for preventing hepatic injury after pennyroyal and clove oil ingestion. Naloxone (p 584) may be effective for reversing the central nervous system and respiratory depression from eucalyptus oil ingestion.

C. **Decontamination** (p 50). Administer activated charcoal orally if conditions are appropriate (see Table I–38, p 54).

D. **Enhanced elimination.** The volumes of distribution of camphor and other essential oils are extremely large, and it is unlikely that any enhanced removal procedure will remove significant amounts of camphor. Poorly substantiated case reports have recommended hemoperfusion.

▶ CARBAMAZEPINE AND OXCARBAZEPINE

Thomas E. Kearney, PharmD

Carbamazepine (Tegretol), an iminostilbene compound, was introduced in the United States in 1974 for the treatment of trigeminal neuralgia. It has become a first-line drug for the treatment of generalized and partial complex seizure disorders and has found expanded use for pain syndromes, psychiatric illnesses, and drug withdrawal reactions. **Oxcarbazepine** (Trileptal) was approved by the US FDA in 2000 and is the 10-keto analog of carbamazepine. It is considered a prodrug with a principal metabolite, 10,11-dihydro-10-hydroxycarbazepine (monohydroxy derivative [MHD]) that is responsible for its principal therapeutic and toxic effects, which are similar to those of carbamazepine.

I. **Mechanism of toxicity**

A. **Carbamazepine.** Most toxic manifestations appear to be related to its CNS-depressant and anticholinergic effects. It also alters cerebellar-vestibular brainstem function. In addition, presumably because its chemical structure is similar to that of the tricyclic antidepressant imipramine, acute carbamazepine overdose can cause seizures and cardiac conduction disturbances.

B. **Oxcarbazepine** is a CNS depressant and seems to lack the toxicity profile of carbamazepine. This may be attributed to the limited rate of production of the active metabolite and lack of a toxic epoxide metabolite. The exception may be a dose-related nephrogenic dilutional hyponatremia.

C. **Pharmacokinetics** (see also Table II–66, p 462)

1. **Carbamazepine** is slowly and erratically absorbed from the GI tract, and peak levels may be delayed for 6–24 hours, particularly after an overdose (continued absorption for over 100 hours has been reported with extended-release preparations). The exception may be with oral suspension dosage forms, whose absorption may be rapid, with symptoms occurring within 30 minutes of ingestion. It is 75–78% protein bound with a volume of distribution of approximately 1.4 L/kg (up to 3 L/kg after overdose). Up to 28% of a dose is eliminated in the feces, and there is enterohepatic recycling. The parent drug is metabolized by cytochrome P450, and 40% is converted to its 10,11-epoxide, which is as active as the parent compound. The elimination half-life is variable and subject to autoinduction of cytochrome P450 enzymes; the half-life of carbamazepine is approximately 18–55 hours

(initially) to 5–26 hours (with long-term use). The half-life of the epoxide metabolite is approximately 5–10 hours.

2. **Oxcarbazepine** is well absorbed from the GI tract (bioavailability >95%) and metabolized rapidly (half-life of 1–5 hours) to its active metabolite, MHD, with peak levels achieved at 1–3 hours and 4–12 hours for the parent and the active metabolite, respectively. The active metabolite has 30–40% protein binding, a volume of distribution of 0.8 L/kg, and a half-life of 7–20 hours (average, 9 hours). The active metabolite is not subject to autoinduction.

II. Toxic dose

A. Carbamazepine. Acute ingestion of more than 10 mg/kg can result in a blood level above the therapeutic range of 4–12 mg/L. The recommended maximum daily dose is 1.6–2.4 g in adults (35 mg/kg/d in children). Death has occurred after adult ingestion of 3.2–60 g, but survival has been reported after an 80-g ingestion. Life-threatening toxicity occurred after ingestion of 5.8–10 g in adults and 2 g (148 mg/kg) in a 23-month-old child.

B. Oxcarbazepine. The recommended daily therapeutic dose is 0.6–1.2 g in adults (8–10 mg/kg/d in children, up to 600 mg/d) to a maximum of 2.4 g/d (which is poorly tolerated). Ingestion of 30.6 g by an adult and 15 g by a 13-year-old child resulted in only mild CNS depression. A 42-g ingestion by an adult required endotracheal intubation. However, an adult who ingested 3.3 g while on oxcarbazepine therapy developed CNS and cardiovascular symptoms.

III. Clinical presentation

A. Carbamazepine

1. Ataxia, nystagmus, ophthalmoplegia, movement disorders (dyskinesia, dystonia), mydriasis, and sinus tachycardia are common with mild-to-moderate overdose. With more serious intoxication, myoclonus, seizures (including status epilepticus), hyperthermia, coma, and respiratory arrest may occur. Atrioventricular block and bradycardia have been reported, particularly in the elderly. Based on its structural similarity to tricyclic antidepressants, carbamazepine may cause QRS- and QT-interval prolongation and myocardial depression; however, in case reports of overdose, QRS widening rarely exceeds 100–120 msec and is usually transient.
2. After an acute overdose, manifestations of intoxication may be delayed for several hours because of erratic absorption. Cyclic coma and rebound relapse of symptoms may be caused by continued absorption from a tablet mass as well as enterohepatic circulation of the drug.
3. Chronic use has been associated with bone marrow depression, hepatitis, renal disease, cardiomyopathy, hyponatremia, and exfoliative dermatitis. Individuals who have the HLA-B*1502 genotype are at much greater risk for developing Stevens–Johnson syndrome and toxic epidermal necrolysis. The prevalence rate of this mutation is highest among Asians, particularly Han Chinese and Thai. Carbamazepine also has been implicated in rigidity-hyperthermia syndromes (eg, neuroleptic malignant syndrome and serotonin syndrome) in combination with other drugs.

B. Oxcarbazepine. The primary side effects and overdose symptoms are CNS-related (drowsiness, ataxia, diplopia, tinnitus, dizziness, tremor, headache, and fatigue). Toxicity from acute overdose may be minimized owing to the rate-limiting production of the toxic metabolite, MHD. Status epilepticus was reported in patients with severe mental retardation. There is also a report of a dose-related dystonia (oculogyric crisis). Cardiovascular system–related effects (bradycardia and hypotension) were observed after an ingestion of 3.3 g. Significant hyponatremia (most commonly associated with high doses, elderly patients, concomitant use of other medications associated with hyponatremia, and polydipsia) may be a contributory cause of seizures and coma associated with oxcarbazepine. Hypersensitivity reactions—rash, eosinophilia, and leukopenia—have been reported and have 25–35% cross-reactivity with carbamazepine.

IV. Diagnosis is based on a history of exposure and clinical signs such as ataxia and stupor and, in the case of carbamazepine, tachycardia.

A. Specific levels. Obtain a stat serum carbamazepine level and repeat levels every 4–6 hours to rule out delayed or prolonged absorption.

1. Serum levels of carbamazepine greater than 10 mg/L are associated with ataxia and nystagmus. Serious intoxication (coma, respiratory depression, seizures) is likely with serum levels greater than 40 mg/L, although there is poor correlation between levels and severity of clinical effects.
2. The epoxide metabolite of carbamazepine may be produced in high concentrations after overdose. It is nearly equipotent and may cross-react with some carbamazepine immunoassays to a variable extent.
3. Carbamazepine can produce a false-positive test result for tricyclic antidepressants on drug screening.
4. Ingestion of oxcarbazepine doses of 15, 30.6, and 42 g have resulted in peak levels of 7.9, 31.6, and 12.45 mg/L for the parent drug and 46.6, 59, and 65.45 mg/L of the active metabolite, MHD, respectively. These ingestions did not exceed a level twofold greater than the therapeutic range (10–35 mg/L) for the active metabolite, MHD, and were delayed 6–8 hours.

B. Other useful laboratory studies include CBC, electrolytes (in particular sodium), glucose, arterial blood gases or oximetry, and ECG monitoring.

C. Genetic polymorphisms. Testing for the HLA-B*1502 genotype is available from reference laboratories

V. Treatment

A. Emergency and supportive measures

1. Maintain an open airway and assist ventilation if necessary (pp 1–7). Administer supplemental oxygen.
2. Treat seizures (p 23), coma (p 18), hyperthermia (p 21), arrhythmias (p 13), hyponatremia (p 37), and dystonias (p 26) if they occur.
3. Asymptomatic patients should be observed for a minimum of 6 hours after ingestion and for at least 12 hours if an extended-release preparation was ingested. Note that CNS depression after oxcarbazepine poisoning may progress over 24 hours owing to prolonged production of the active metabolite.

B. Specific drugs and antidotes. There is no specific antidote. Sodium bicarbonate (p 520) is of unknown value for QRS prolongation. Physostigmine is ***not*** recommended for anticholinergic toxicity.

C. Decontamination (p 50). Administer activated charcoal orally if conditions are appropriate (see Table I–38, p 54). Gastric lavage is not necessary after small-to-moderate ingestions if activated charcoal can be given promptly. For massive ingestions of carbamazepine, consider additional doses of activated charcoal and possibly whole-bowel irrigation (p 55).

D. Enhanced elimination

1. **Carbamazepine.** In contrast to tricyclic antidepressants, the volume of distribution of carbamazepine is small, making it accessible to enhanced removal procedures. These procedures should be considered in carbamazepine poisoned patients with high serum levels (eg, >40 mg/L) associated with severe intoxication (eg, status epilepticus, cardiotoxicity) unresponsive to standard treatment.
   a. Intermittent **hemodialysis** using newer, high flux and high efficiency dialyzer membranes is the preferred method of drug removal. Conventional dialysis machines are not as efficient.
   b. **Charcoal hemoperfusion** is highly effective for carbamazepine, but the availability of hemoperfusion columns may be limited.
   c. Continuous venovenous hemodiafiltration (CVVHDF), with or without albumin enhancement, has also been used but does not remove drug as quickly as hemodialysis or hemoperfusion.
   d. **Repeat-dose activated charcoal** may increase clearance of carbamazepine by up to 50% as well as prevent systemic absorption of pill

masses (pharmacobezoars) in the GI tract. However, it may be difficult to administer safely or effectively in a patient with obtundation and ileus.

e. Peritoneal dialysis does not remove carbamazepine effectively.

f. Plasma exchange has been used in children with carbamazepine poisoning.

2. **Oxcarbazepine.** The pharmacokinetics of its active metabolite, MHD, make it theoretically amenable to dialysis owing to low protein binding and small volume of distribution. However, current reported overdose experience suggests that supportive care is sufficient in most cases.

▶ CARBON DISULFIDE

Paul D. Blanc, MD, MSPH

Carbon disulfide is a volatile organic solvent that is used industrially as a starting material in rayon and cellophane manufacture in the viscose process. It was important historically as a pesticide fumigant and in the cold vulcanization of rubber. Although no longer used as a vulcanizing agent, carbon disulfide remains an industrial precursor in rubber industry chemical synthesis and has a number of other industrial applications. Carbon disulfide also is widely used as a solvent in a variety of laboratory settings. It is a metabolite of the drug disulfiram (p 226) and a spontaneous breakdown by-product of the pesticides metam sodium and sodium tetrathiocarbamate.

I. **Mechanism of toxicity.** Carbon disulfide toxicity appears to involve disruption of a number of metabolic pathways in various organ systems, including but not limited to the CNS. Although key toxic effects have been attributed to the functional disruption of enzymes, especially in dopamine-dependent systems, carbon disulfide is widely reactive with a variety of biologic substrates.

II. **Toxic dose**

A. Carbon disulfide is highly volatile (vapor pressure, 297 mm Hg), and inhalation is a major route of exposure. The OSHA workplace limit (permissible exposure limit—ceiling [PEL-C]) for carbon disulfide is 30 ppm (the PEL is 20 ppm with an allowable 15-minute peak to 100 ppm). The ACGIH recommended workplace exposure limit (threshold limit value—8-hour time-weighted average [TLV-TWA]) is considerably lower at 1 ppm. The NIOSH recommended exposure limit (REL) is also 1 ppm, and the short-term exposure limit (STEL) is 10 ppm. Various international standards are also in this range. Carbon disulfide is also well absorbed through the skin.

B. Acute carbon disulfide overexposure via ingestion is unusual, but if ingested, it is well absorbed. Chronic ingestion of therapeutic doses of disulfiram (200 mg/d) has been suspected to cause carbon disulfide–mediated toxicity, but this has not been firmly established.

III. **Clinical presentation**

A. Acute carbon disulfide exposure can cause eye and skin irritation and CNS depression.

B. Short-term (days to weeks) high-level exposure to carbon disulfide is associated with psychiatric manifestations ranging from mood change to frank delirium and psychosis.

C. Chronic exposure can cause parkinsonism and other poorly reversible CNS impairments, optic neuritis, peripheral neuropathy, and CNS and cardiac atherosclerosis. Epidemiologic studies indicate that carbon disulfide exposure also is associated with adverse reproductive function and outcomes.

IV. **Diagnosis** of carbon disulfide toxicity is based on a history of exposure along with consistent signs and symptoms of one of its toxic manifestations. Industrial hygiene data documenting airborne exposure, if available, are useful diagnostically and in initiating protective measures.

A. Specific levels. Biological monitoring for carbon disulfide can be performed using urinary 2-thiothiazolidine-4-carboxylic acid (TTCA) but this is not performed routinely in the United States.

B. Other useful laboratory studies can include nerve conduction studies if neuropathy is suspected and brain magnetic resonance imaging/magnetic resonance angiography (MRI/MRA) to assess the CNS. Chronic carbon disulfide exposure is associated with altered lipid profiles.

V. Treatment

A. Emergency and supportive measures. Severe acute exposure would present as nonspecific CNS depression.

1. Maintain an open airway and assist ventilation if necessary (pp 1–7). Administer supplemental oxygen.
2. Start an IV line and monitor the patient's vital signs and ECG closely.

B. Specific drugs and antidotes. There are no specific antidotes for carbon disulfide.

C. Decontamination after high-level exposure (p 50)

1. **Inhalation.** Remove the victim from exposure and give supplemental oxygen if available.
2. **Skin and eyes.** Remove contaminated clothing and wash exposed skin. Irrigate exposed eyes with copious amounts of tepid water or saline (p 51).
3. **Ingestion.** Administer activated charcoal if it is available and the patient is alert. Consider gastric lavage if the ingestion occurred within 60 minutes of presentation.

D. Enhanced elimination. There is no role for these procedures.

► CARBON MONOXIDE

Kent R. Olson, MD

Carbon monoxide (CO) is a colorless, odorless, tasteless, and nonirritating gas produced by the incomplete combustion of any carbon-containing material. Common sources of human exposure include smoke inhalation in fires; automobile exhaust fumes; faulty or poorly ventilated charcoal, kerosene, or gas stoves; and, to a lesser extent, cigarette smoke and methylene chloride (p 323). CO poisoning accounts for approximately 50,000 emergency department visits every year in the United States.

I. Mechanism of toxicity. Toxicity is a consequence of cellular hypoxia and ischemia.

A. CO binds to hemoglobin with an affinity 250 times that of oxygen, resulting in reduced oxyhemoglobin saturation and decreased blood oxygen-carrying capacity. In addition, the oxyhemoglobin dissociation curve is displaced to the left, impairing oxygen delivery at the tissues.

B. CO may also directly inhibit cytochrome oxidase, further disrupting cellular function, and it is known to bind to myoglobin, possibly contributing to impaired myocardial contractility.

C. In animal models of intoxication, damage is most severe in areas of the brain that are highly sensitive to ischemia and often correlates with the severity of systemic hypotension. Postanoxic injury appears to be complicated by lipid peroxidation, excessive release of reactive oxygen species and excitatory neurotransmitters, and inflammatory changes.

D. Fetal hemoglobin is more sensitive to binding by CO, and fetal or neonatal levels may be higher than maternal levels.

E. Pharmacokinetics. The carboxyhemoglobin (CO-Hgb) complex gradually dissociates after removal from exposure. The approximate half-life of elimination of CO-Hgb during treatment with high-flow oxygen by tight-fitting mask or endotracheal tube is 74 minutes (range, 24–148 minutes). In room air the approximate half-life is as much as 200 minutes, and during hyperbaric oxygen therapy it is as short as 12–20 minutes.

II. Toxic dose. The recommended workplace limit (ACGIH TLV-TWA) for carbon monoxide is 25 ppm as an 8-hour time-weighted average. The level considered immediately dangerous to life or health (IDLH) is 1,200 ppm (0.12%). However, the *duration* of exposure is very important. Whereas exposure to 1,000 ppm (0.1%) eventually will result in 50% saturation of CO-Hgb, it may take several hours to reach that level. In 1895, Haldane experimented on himself by breathing CO at 2,100 ppm for over an hour, and it was only after 34 minutes, when his level would have been approximately 25%, that he described a throbbing headache. Brief exposure to much higher levels may produce a more rapid rise in CO-Hgb.

III. Clinical presentation. Symptoms of intoxication are predominantly in organs with high oxygen consumption, such as the brain and heart.

- **A.** The majority of patients describe headache, dizziness, and nausea. Patients with coronary disease may experience angina or myocardial infarction. With more severe exposures, impaired thinking, syncope, coma, convulsions, cardiac arrhythmias, hypotension, and death may occur. Although blood CO-Hgb levels may not correlate reliably with the severity of intoxication, levels greater than 25% are considered significant, and levels greater than 40–50% usually are associated with obvious intoxication.
- **B.** Survivors of serious poisoning may experience numerous overt neurologic sequelae consistent with a hypoxic-ischemic insult, ranging from gross deficits such as parkinsonism and a persistent vegetative state to subtler personality and memory disorders. Some may have a delayed onset of several hours to days after exposure. Various studies suggest that the incidence of subtle neuropsychiatric sequelae, such as impaired memory and concentration and mood disorders, may be as high as 47%.
- **C.** Exposure during pregnancy may result in fetal demise.

IV. Diagnosis is not difficult if there is a history of exposure (eg, the patient was found in a car in a locked garage) but may be elusive if it is not suspected in less obvious cases. There are no specific reliable clinical findings; cherry-red skin coloration or bright red venous blood is highly suggestive but not frequently noted. The routine arterial blood gas instruments measure the partial pressure of oxygen dissolved in plasma (PO_2), but oxygen saturation is calculated from the PO_2 and is therefore unreliable in patients with CO poisoning. Conventional pulse oximetry also gives falsely normal readings because it is unable to distinguish between oxyhemoglobin and CO-Hgb. (A newer pulse CO-oximeter can detect CO-Hgb and methemoglobin; its accuracy and its role in diagnostic screening are being investigated.)

- **A. Specific levels.** Obtain a specific CO-Hgb concentration by co-oximetry with arterial or venous blood. ***Note:***
  1. The presence of the cyanide antidote hydroxocobalamin can falsely elevate CO-Hgb.
  2. Persistence of fetal hemoglobin may produce falsely elevated CO-Hgb levels in young infants.
- **B. Other useful laboratory studies** include electrolytes, glucose, BUN, creatinine, ECG, and pregnancy tests. Metabolic acidosis suggests more serious poisoning. With smoke inhalation, measure the blood methemoglobin level (use a co-oximeter) and cyanide level (not routinely available in clinical laboratories).

V. Treatment

- **A. Emergency and supportive measures**
  1. Maintain an open airway and assist ventilation if necessary (pp 1–7). If smoke inhalation has also occurred, consider early intubation for airway protection.
  2. Treat coma (p 18) and seizures (p 23) if they occur.
  3. Continuously monitor the ECG for several hours after exposure.
  4. Because smoke often contains other toxic gases, consider the possibility of cyanide poisoning (p 208), methemoglobinemia (p 317), and irritant gas injury (p 255).

TABLE II–20. CARBON MONOXIDE POISONING: PROPOSED INDICATIONS FOR HYPERBARIC OXYGEN[a]

Loss of consciousness
Carboxyhemoglobin >25%
Age older than 36 years
Severe metabolic acidosis
Abnormal neurologic examination (cerebellar dysfunction)[b]
Cardiovascular dysfunction
Exposure to carbon monoxide for more than 24 hours
Pregnancy

[a]From Weaver LK: Carbon monoxide poisoning. *N Eng J Med.* 2009;360:1217–1225.
[b]From Weaver LK et al: Hyperbaric oxygen for acute carbon monoxide poisoning. *N Engl J Med.* 2002;347:1057–1067.

B. Specific drugs and antidotes. Administer **oxygen** in the highest possible concentration (100%). Breathing 100% oxygen speeds the elimination of CO from hemoglobin to approximately 1 hour, compared with about 6 hours in room air. Use a tight-fitting mask and high-flow oxygen with a reservoir (nonrebreather) or administer the oxygen by endotracheal tube. Treat until the CO-Hgb level is less than 5%. Consider **hyperbaric oxygen** in severe cases (see below).

C. Decontamination. Remove the patient immediately from exposure and give supplemental oxygen. Rescuers exposed to potentially high concentrations of CO should wear self-contained breathing apparatus.

D. Enhanced elimination. Hyperbaric oxygen provides 100% oxygen under 2–3 atm of pressure and can enhance elimination of CO (half-life reduced to 20–30 minutes). In animal models, it reduces lipid peroxidation and neutrophil activation, and in one randomized controlled trial in humans, it reduced the incidence of subtle cognitive sequelae compared with normobaric 100% oxygen, although other similar studies found no benefit. Hyperbaric oxygen may be useful in patients with severe intoxication, especially when there is ready access to a chamber. It remains unclear whether its benefits over normobaric oxygen apply to victims who present many hours after exposure or have milder degrees of intoxication. Consult a regional poison control center (1-800-222-1222) for advice and for the location of nearby hyperbaric chambers. See Table II–20 for a list of proposed indications for hyperbaric oxygen.

► CARBON TETRACHLORIDE AND CHLOROFORM

Frederick Fung, MD, MS

Carbon tetrachloride (CCl4, tetrachloromethane) was once used widely as a dry cleaning solvent, degreaser, spot remover, fire extinguisher agent, and antihelminthic. Because of its liver toxicity and known carcinogenicity in animals, its role has become limited; it is now used mainly as an intermediate in chemical manufacturing.

Chloroform (trichloromethane) is a chlorinated hydrocarbon solvent used as a raw material in the production of freon and as an extractant and solvent in the chemical and pharmaceutical industries. Because of its hepatic toxicity, it is no longer used as a general anesthetic or antihelminthic agent. Chronic low-level exposure may occur in some municipal water supplies owing to chlorination of biologic methanes (trihalomethanes).

I. Mechanism of toxicity. Carbon tetrachloride and chloroform are CNS depressants and potent hepatic and renal toxins. They may also increase the sensitivity of the myocardium to arrhythmogenic effects of catecholamines. The mechanism of hepatic and renal toxicity is thought to be a result of a toxic free radical intermediate (trichloromethyl radical) of cytochrome P450 metabolism. This radical can bind to cellular molecules (nucleic acid, protein, lipid) and form DNA adducts. Bioactivation of CCl4 has become a model for chemical toxicity induced by free radicals. The toxic reactions are important to elucidate the mechanisms of apoptosis, fibrosis, and carcinogenicity. Chronic use of metabolic enzyme inducers such as phenobarbital and ethanol increases the toxicity of carbon tetrachloride. Carbon tetrachloride is a known animal and a suspected human carcinogen. Chloroform is embryotoxic and is an animal carcinogen.

II. Toxic dose

A. Toxicity from **inhalation** is dependent on the concentration in air and the duration of exposure.

1. **Carbon tetrachloride.** Symptoms have occurred after exposure to 160 ppm for 30 minutes. The recommended workplace limit (ACGIH TLV-TWA) is 5 ppm as an 8-hour time-weighted average, and the air level considered immediately dangerous to life or health (IDLH) is 200 ppm.
2. **Chloroform.** The air level considered immediately dangerous to life or health (IDLH) is 500 ppm. The recommended workplace limit (ACGIH TLV-TWA) is 10 ppm as an 8-hour time-weighted average.

B. Ingestion

1. **Carbon tetrachloride.** Ingestion of as little as 5 mL has been reported to be fatal.
2. **Chloroform.** The fatal **oral** dose may be as little as 10 mL, although survival after ingestion of more than 100 mL has been reported. The oral LD50 in rats is 2,000 mg/kg.

III. Clinical presentation

A. Persons exposed to carbon tetrachloride or chloroform from **acute inhalation, skin absorption, or ingestion** may present with nausea, vomiting, headache, dizziness, and confusion. Mucous membrane irritation is also seen with ingestion or inhalation. With serious intoxication, respiratory arrest, cardiac arrhythmias, and coma may occur.

B. Severe and sometimes fatal **renal and hepatic damage** may become apparent after 1–3 days.

C. Skin or eye contact results in irritation and a defatting type of dermatitis.

IV. Diagnosis is based on a history of exposure and the clinical presentation of mucous membrane irritation, CNS depression, arrhythmias, and hepatic necrosis. Carbon tetrachloride is radiopaque and may be visible on abdominal radiograph after acute ingestion.

A. Specific levels. Blood, urine, or breath concentrations may document exposure but are rarely available and are not useful for acute management. Qualitative urine screening for chlorinated hydrocarbons (Fujiwara test) may be positive after massive overdose.

B. Other useful laboratory studies include electrolytes, glucose, BUN, creatinine, liver aminotransferases, prothrombin time, and ECG monitoring.

V. Treatment

A. Emergency and supportive measures

1. Maintain an open airway and assist ventilation if necessary (pp 1–7).
2. Treat coma (p 18) and arrhythmias (pp 12–15) if they occur. ***Caution:*** Avoid the use of epinephrine or other sympathomimetic amines because they may induce or aggravate arrhythmias. Tachyarrhythmias caused by increased myocardial sensitivity may be treated with **propranolol**, 1–2 mg IV in adults (p 617), or **esmolol**, 0.025–0.1 mg/kg/min IV (p 552). Monitor patients for at least 4–6 hours after exposure and longer if they are symptomatic.

B. Specific treatment. *N*-acetylcysteine (p 499) may minimize hepatic and renal toxicity by acting as a scavenger for the toxic intermediate. Acetylcysteine has been used without serious side effects for carbon tetrachloride or chloroform poisoning based on limited human reports. If possible, it should be given within the first 12 hours after exposure. Animal studies also suggest possible roles for cimetidine, calcium channel blockers, and hyperbaric oxygen in reducing hepatic injury, but there is insufficient human experience with these treatments.

C. **Decontamination** (p 50)
   1. **Inhalation.** Remove from exposure and give supplemental oxygen, if available.
   2. **Skin and eyes.** Remove contaminated clothing and wash affected skin with copious soap and water. Irrigate exposed eyes with copious saline or water.
   3. **Ingestion.** Administer activated charcoal orally if conditions are appropriate (see Table I–38, p 54). Consider gastric lavage if the ingestion occurred within 60 minutes of presentation.

D. **Enhanced elimination.** There is no role for dialysis, hemoperfusion, or other enhanced removal procedures.

▶ CAUSTIC AND CORROSIVE AGENTS

Derrick Lung, MD, MPH

A wide variety of chemical and physical agents may cause corrosive injury. They include mineral and organic acids, alkalis, oxidizing agents, denaturants, some hydrocarbons, and agents that cause exothermic reactions. Although the mechanism and the severity of injury may vary, the consequences of mucosal damage and permanent scarring are shared by all these agents.

Button batteries are small, disk-shaped batteries used in watches, calculators, and cameras. They can generate an electrolytic current across a mucosal surface and contain caustic metal salts such as mercuric chloride that may cause corrosive injury.

I. **Mechanism of toxicity**
   A. **Acids** cause an immediate coagulation-type necrosis that creates an eschar, which tends to self-limit further damage.
   B. In contrast, **alkalis** (eg, Drano) cause a liquefactive necrosis with saponification and continued penetration into deeper tissues, resulting in extensive damage.
   C. **Other agents** may act by alkylating, oxidizing, reducing, or denaturing cellular proteins or by defatting surface tissues.
   D. **Button batteries** cause injury by corrosive effects resulting from leakage of the corrosive metal salts, and burns from local discharge of electric current at the site of impaction.

II. **Toxic dose.** There is no specific toxic dose or level because the concentration of corrosive solutions and the potency of caustic effects vary widely. For example, whereas the acetic acid concentration in most household vinegar is 5–10%, that of "Russian vinegar" may be as high as 70%. The pH or concentration of the solution may indicate the potential for serious injury. A pH lower than 2 or higher than 12 increases the risk for injury. For alkalis, the titratable alkalinity (concentration of the base) is a better predictor of corrosive effect than is the pH. Injury is also related to the volume ingested and duration of exposure.

III. **Clinical presentation**
   A. **Inhalation** of corrosive gases (eg, chlorine and ammonia) may cause upper respiratory tract injury, with stridor, hoarseness, wheezing, and noncardiogenic pulmonary edema. Pulmonary symptoms may be delayed after exposure to gases with low water solubility (eg, nitrogen dioxide and phosgene [p 255]).
   B. **Eye or skin** exposure to corrosive agents usually results in immediate pain and redness, followed by blistering. Conjunctivitis and lacrimation are common. Serious full-thickness burns and blindness can occur.
   C. **Ingestion** of corrosives can cause oral pain, dysphagia, drooling, and pain in the throat, chest, or abdomen. Esophageal or gastric perforation may occur, accompanied by severe chest or abdominal pain, signs of peritoneal irritation, or pancreatitis. Free air may be visible in the mediastinum or abdomen on radiograph. Hematemesis and shock may occur. Systemic acidosis has been reported after acid ingestion and may be caused partly by absorption of

TABLE II–21. CORROSIVE AGENTS WITH SYSTEMIC EFFECTS (SELECTED CAUSES)[a]

Corrosive Agent	Systemic Symptoms
Formaldehyde	Metabolic acidosis, formate poisoning (p 249)
Hydrofluoric acid	Hypocalcemia, hyperkalemia (p 269)
Methylene chloride	CNS depression, cardiac arrhythmias, converted to carbon monoxide (p 323)
Oxalic acid	Hypocalcemia, renal failure (p 360)
Paraquat	Pulmonary fibrosis (p 361)
Permanganate	Methemoglobinemia (p 317)
Phenol	Seizures, coma, hepatic and renal damage (p 368)
Phosphorus	Hepatic and renal injury (p 373)
Picric acid	Renal injury
Silver nitrate	Methemoglobinemia (p 317)
Tannic acid	Hepatic injury

[a]Edelman PA. Chemical and electrical burns. In: Achauer BM, ed. *Management of the Burned Patient,* pp 183–202. Appleton & Lange; 1987.

hydrogen ions. Scarring of the esophagus or stomach may result in permanent stricture formation and chronic dysphagia.

D. **Systemic toxicity** can occur after inhalation, skin exposure, or ingestion of a variety of agents (Table II–21).

E. **Button batteries** can cause serious injury if they become impacted in the esophagus, leading to perforation into the aorta or mediastinum. Most such cases involve larger (25-mm-diameter) batteries. If button batteries reach the stomach without impaction in the esophagus, they nearly always pass uneventfully via the stools within several days.

IV. **Diagnosis** is based on a history of exposure to a corrosive agent and characteristic findings of skin, eye, or mucosal irritation or redness and the presence of injury to the GI tract. Victims with oral or esophageal injury nearly always have drooling or pain on swallowing.

A. **Endoscopy.** Esophageal or gastric injury is unlikely after ingestion if the patient is completely asymptomatic, but studies have shown repeatedly that a small number of patients will have injury in the absence of oral burns or obvious dysphagia. For this reason, some authorities recommend endoscopy for all patients regardless of symptoms.

B. **Radiographs** of the chest and abdomen usually reveal impacted button batteries. Plain radiographs and CT scans may also demonstrate air in the mediastinum from esophageal perforation or free abdominal air from GI perforation.

C. **Specific levels.** See the specific chemical. Urine mercury levels have been reported to be elevated after button battery ingestion.

D. **Other useful laboratory studies** include CBC, electrolytes, glucose, arterial blood gases, and radiographic imaging.

V. **Treatment**

A. **Emergency and supportive measures**

1. **Inhalation.** Give supplemental oxygen and observe closely for signs of progressive airway obstruction or noncardiogenic pulmonary edema (pp 6–7).

2. **Ingestion**

a. Assessment of the **airway** is paramount. Early intubation should be considered to avoid progressive airway obstruction from oropharyngeal edema.

b. Otherwise, if tolerated, immediately give water or milk to drink. Provide **antiemetics** (eg, ondansetron, 8 mg IV in adults or 0.15 mg/kg in children [p 597]) to prevent additional esophageal injury from emesis.

c. If esophageal or gastric perforation is suspected, obtain immediate surgical or endoscopic consultation.

d. Patients with mediastinitis or peritonitis need broad-spectrum antibiotics and aggressive management of hemorrhage and septic shock.

B. **Specific drugs and antidotes.** For most agents, there is no specific antidote (see p 269 for hydrofluoric acid burns and p 368 for phenol burns). In the past, corticosteroids were used by many clinicians in the hope of reducing scarring, but this treatment has been proven ineffective. Moreover, steroids may be harmful in a patient with perforation because they mask early signs of inflammation and inhibit resistance to infection.

C. **Decontamination** (p 50). ***Caution:*** Rescuers should use appropriate respiratory and skin-protective equipment.

1. **Inhalation.** Remove from exposure; give supplemental oxygen if available.
2. **Skin and eyes.** Remove all clothing; wash skin and irrigate eyes with copious water or saline.
3. **Ingestion**

a. **Prehospital.** If tolerated, immediately give water or milk to drink. Do ***not*** induce vomiting or give pH-neutralizing solutions (eg, dilute vinegar or bicarbonate).

b. **Hospital. Gastric lavage** to remove the corrosive material is controversial but probably beneficial in acute liquid corrosive ingestion, and it will be required before endoscopy anyway. Use a soft, flexible tube and lavage with repeated aliquots of water or saline, frequently checking the pH of the washings.

c. In general, do ***not*** give activated charcoal, as it may interfere with visibility at endoscopy. Charcoal may be appropriate if the ingested agent can cause significant systemic toxicity.

d. **Button batteries** lodged in the esophagus must be removed immediately by endoscopy to prevent rapid perforation. Batteries in the stomach or intestine should not be removed unless signs of perforation or obstruction develop. Repeat radiographs are advised to ensure continued progression through the GI tract.

D. **Enhanced elimination.** In general, there is no role for any of these procedures (see specific chemical).

▶ CHLORATES

Thomas R. Sands, PharmD

Potassium chlorate is a component of some match heads, barium chlorate (see also p 152) is used in the manufacture of fireworks and explosives, sodium chlorate is still a major ingredient in some weed killers used in commercial agriculture, and other chlorate salts are used in dye production. Safer and more effective compounds have replaced chlorate in toothpaste and antiseptic mouthwashes. Chlorate poisoning is similar to bromate intoxication (p 165), but chlorates are more likely to cause intravascular hemolysis and methemoglobinemia.

I. **Mechanism of toxicity.** Chlorates are potent oxidizing agents and also attack sulfhydryl groups, particularly in red blood cells and the kidneys. Chlorates cause methemoglobin formation as well as increased fragility of red blood cell membranes, which may result in intravascular hemolysis. Renal failure probably is caused by a combination of direct cellular toxicity and hemolysis.

II. **Toxic dose.** The minimum toxic dose in children is not established but is estimated to range from 1 g in infants to 5 g in older children. Children may ingest up to

1–2 matchbooks without toxic effect (each match head may contain 10–12 mg of chlorate). The adult lethal dose was estimated to be 7.5 g in one case but is probably closer to 20–35 g. A 26-year-old woman survived a 150- to 200-g ingestion.

III. Clinical presentation. Within a few minutes to hours after ingestion, abdominal pain, vomiting, and diarrhea may occur. Methemoglobinemia is common (p 317). Massive hemolysis, hemoglobinuria, and acute tubular necrosis may occur over 1–2 days after ingestion. Coagulopathy and hepatic injury have been described.

IV. Diagnosis usually is based on a history of exposure and the presence of methemoglobinemia (via co-oximetry) and hemolysis.

- **A. Specific levels.** Blood levels are not available.
- **B. Other useful laboratory studies** include CBC, haptoglobin, plasma free hemoglobin, electrolytes, glucose, BUN, creatinine, bilirubin, methemoglobin level, prothrombin time, liver aminotransferases, and urinalysis.

V. Treatment

- **A. Emergency and supportive measures**
  1. Maintain an open airway and assist ventilation if necessary (pp 1–7).
  2. Treat coma (p 18), hemolysis, hyperkalemia (p 39), and renal (p 41) or hepatic failure (p 42) if they occur.
  3. Massive hemolysis may require blood transfusions. To prevent renal failure resulting from deposition of free hemoglobin in the kidney tubules, administer IV fluids and sodium bicarbonate.
- **B. Specific drugs and antidotes**
  1. Treat methemoglobinemia with 1% solution of **methylene blue** (p 579), 1–2 mg/kg (0.1–0.2 mL/kg). Methylene blue is reportedly most effective when used early in mild cases but has poor effectiveness in severe cases in which hemolysis has already occurred.
  2. IV **sodium thiosulfate** (p 629) may inactivate the chlorate ion and has been reported to be successful in anecdotal reports. However, this treatment has not been clinically tested. Administration as a lavage fluid may potentially produce some hydrogen sulfide, so it is contraindicated.
- **C. Decontamination** (p 50). Administer activated charcoal orally if conditions are appropriate (see Table I–38, p 54). Gastric lavage is not necessary after small-to-moderate ingestions if activated charcoal can be given promptly. ***Note:*** Spontaneous vomiting is common after significant ingestion.
- **D. Enhanced elimination.** Chlorates are eliminated mainly through the kidney; elimination may be hastened by hemodialysis, especially in patients with renal insufficiency. Exchange transfusion and peritoneal dialysis have been used in a few cases.

► CHLORINATED HYDROCARBON PESTICIDES

Darren H. Lew, PharmD

Chlorinated hydrocarbon pesticides are used widely in agriculture, structural pest control, and malaria control programs around the world. Lindane is used medicinally for the treatment of lice and scabies. Chlorinated hydrocarbons are of major toxicologic concern, and many (eg, DDT [dichloro-diphenyl-trichloroethane] and chlordane) have been banned from commercial use because they persist in the environment and accumulate in biological systems. Despite being banned decades ago, these substances are still being measured in the environment and food chain in ongoing studies. In 2002, sale of lindane was banned in California.

I. Mechanism of toxicity

- **A.** Chlorinated hydrocarbons are neurotoxins that interfere with transmission of nerve impulses, especially in the brain, resulting in behavioral changes, involuntary muscle activity, and depression of the respiratory center. They may

TABLE II–22. CHLORINATED HYDROCARBONS

Low Toxicity (Animal Oral LD_{50} >1 g/kg)	Moderately Toxic (Animal Oral LD_{50} >50 mg/kg)	Highly Toxic (Animal Oral LD_{50} <50 mg/kg)
Ethylan (Perthane)	Chlordane	Aldrin
Hexachlorobenzene	DDT	Dieldrin
Methoxychlor	Heptachlor	Endrin
	Kepone	Endosulfan
	Lindane	
	Mirex	
	Toxaphene	

also sensitize the myocardium to arrhythmogenic effects of catecholamines, and many can cause liver or renal injury, possibly owing to generation of toxic metabolites. In addition, some chlorinated hydrocarbons may be carcinogenic.

B. Pharmacokinetics. Chlorinated hydrocarbons are well absorbed from the GI tract, across the skin, and by inhalation. They are highly lipid soluble and accumulate with repeated exposure. Elimination does not follow first-order kinetics; compounds are released slowly from body stores over days to several months or years.

II. Toxic dose. The acute toxic doses of these compounds are highly variable, and reports of acute human poisonings are limited. Table II–22 ranks the relative toxicity of several common compounds.

A. Ingestion of as little as 1 g of lindane can produce seizures in a child, and 10–30 g is considered lethal in an adult. The estimated adult lethal oral doses of aldrin and chlordane are 3–7 g each; that of dieldrin, 2–5 g. A 49-year-old man died after ingesting 12 g of endrin. A 20-year-old man survived a 60-g endosulfan ingestion but was left with a chronic seizure disorder.

B. Skin absorption is a significant route of exposure, especially with aldrin, dieldrin, and endrin. Extensive or repeated (as little as two applications on two successive days) whole-body application of lindane to infants has resulted in seizures and death.

III. Clinical presentation. Shortly after acute ingestion, nausea and vomiting occur, followed by paresthesias of the tongue, lips, and face; confusion; tremor; obtundation; coma; seizures; and respiratory depression. Because chlorinated hydrocarbons are highly lipid soluble, the duration of toxicity may be prolonged.

A. Recurrent or delayed-onset seizures have been reported.

B. Arrhythmias may occur owing to myocardial sensitivity to catecholamines.

C. Metabolic acidosis may occur.

D. Signs of hepatitis or renal injury may develop.

E. Hematopoietic dyscrasias can develop late.

IV. Diagnosis is based on the history of exposure and clinical presentation.

A. Specific levels. Chlorinated hydrocarbons can be measured in the serum, but levels are not routinely available.

B. Other useful laboratory studies include electrolytes, glucose, BUN, creatinine, hepatic aminotransferases, prothrombin time, and ECG monitoring.

V. Treatment

A. Emergency and supportive measures

1. Maintain an open airway and assist ventilation if necessary (pp 1–7). Administer supplemental oxygen. As most liquid products are formulated in organic solvents, observe for evidence of pulmonary aspiration (see "Hydrocarbons," p 266).
2. Treat seizures (p 23), coma (p 18), and respiratory depression (p 5) if they occur. Ventricular arrhythmias may respond to beta-adrenergic blockers such as propranolol (p 617) and esmolol (p 552).

3. Attach an electrocardiographic monitor and observe the patient for at least 6–8 hours.

B. **Specific drugs and antidotes.** There is no specific antidote.

C. **Decontamination** (p 50)

1. **Skin and eyes**. Remove contaminated clothing and wash affected skin with copious soap and water, including hair and nails. Irrigate exposed eyes with copious tepid water or saline. Rescuers must take precautions to avoid personal exposure.
2. **Ingestion.** Administer activated charcoal orally if conditions are appropriate (see Table I–38, p 54). Gastric lavage is not necessary after small-to-moderate ingestions if activated charcoal can be given promptly.

D. **Enhanced elimination** (p 56)

1. Repeat-dose activated charcoal or cholestyramine resin may be administered to enhance elimination by interrupting enterohepatic circulation.
2. Exchange transfusion, peritoneal dialysis, hemodialysis, and hemoperfusion are not likely to be beneficial because of the large volume of distribution of these chemicals.

▶ CHLORINE

R. Steven Tharratt, MD, MPVM

Chlorine is a heavier-than-air yellowish-green gas with an irritating odor. It is used widely in chemical manufacturing, in bleaching, and (as hypochlorite) in swimming pool disinfectants and cleaning agents. **Hypochlorite** is an aqueous solution produced by the reaction of chlorine gas with water; most household bleach solutions contain 3–5% hypochlorite, and swimming pool disinfectants and industrial-strength cleaners may contain up to 20% hypochlorite. The addition of acid to hypochlorite solution may release chlorine gas. The addition of ammonia to hypochlorite solution may release chloramine, a gas with toxic properties similar to those of chlorine.

I. **Mechanism of toxicity.** Chlorine gas produces a corrosive effect on contact with moist tissues, such as those of the eyes and upper respiratory tract. Exposure to aqueous solutions causes corrosive injury to the eyes, skin, or GI tract (p 186). Chloramine is less water soluble and may produce more indolent or delayed irritation.

II. **Toxic dose**

A. **Chlorine gas.** The recommended workplace limit (ACGIH TLV-TWA) for chlorine gas is 0.5 ppm (1.5 mg/m^3) as an 8-hour time-weighted average. The short-term exposure limit (STEL) is 1 ppm. The level considered immediately dangerous to life or health (IDLH) is 10 ppm.

B. **Aqueous solutions.** Dilute aqueous hypochlorite solutions (3–5%) commonly found in homes rarely cause serious burns but are moderately irritating. However, more concentrated industrial cleaners (20% hypochlorite) are much more likely to cause serious corrosive injury.

III. **Clinical presentation**

A. **Inhalation of chlorine gas.** Symptoms are rapid in onset owing to the relatively high water solubility of chlorine. Immediate burning of the eyes, nose, and throat occurs, accompanied by coughing. Wheezing also may occur, especially in patients with pre-existing bronchospastic disease. With serious exposure, upper airway swelling may rapidly cause airway obstruction, preceded by croupy cough, hoarseness, and stridor. With massive exposure, noncardiogenic pulmonary edema (chemical pneumonitis) and adult respiratory distress syndrome (ARDS) may also occur.

B. **Skin or eye contact with gas or concentrated solution.** Serious corrosive burns may occur. Manifestations are similar to those of other acidic corrosive exposures (p 186).

C. **Ingestion of aqueous solutions.** Immediate burning in the mouth and throat is common, but no further injury is expected after ingestion of 3–5% hypochlorite. With more concentrated solutions, serious esophageal and gastric burns may occur, and victims often have dysphagia, drooling, and severe throat, chest, and abdominal pain. Hematemesis and perforation of the esophagus or stomach may occur.

IV. **Diagnosis** is based on a history of exposure and description of the typical irritating odor, accompanied by irritative or corrosive effects on the eyes, skin, or upper respiratory or GI tract.

A. **Specific levels** are not available.

B. **Other useful laboratory studies** include, with **ingestion,** CBC, electrolytes, and chest and abdominal radiographs; with **inhalation,** arterial blood gases or oximetry and chest radiography.

V. **Treatment**

A. **Emergency and supportive measures**

1. **Inhalation of chlorine gas**

a. Immediately give humidified supplemental oxygen. Observe carefully for signs of progressive upper airway obstruction and intubate the trachea if necessary (pp 1–7).

b. Use bronchodilators for wheezing and treat noncardiogenic pulmonary edema (pp 6–7) if it occurs.

2. **Ingestion of hypochlorite solution**. If a solution of 10% or greater has been ingested or if there are any symptoms of corrosive injury (dysphagia, drooling, or pain), flexible endoscopy is recommended to evaluate for serious esophageal or gastric injury. Obtain chest and abdominal radiographs to look for mediastinal or intra-abdominal air, which suggests perforation.

B. **Specific drugs and antidotes**. There is no proven specific treatment. Inhalation of sodium bicarbonate solutions continues to be advocated, although the few studies available show only modest objective benefits. Likewise, inhaled and systemic corticosteroids have not been shown to be helpful after inhalation or oral exposures, and may be harmful in patients with perforation or serious infection.

C. **Decontamination** (p 50)

1. **Inhalation.** Remove immediately from exposure and give supplemental oxygen if available. Administer inhaled bronchodilators if wheezing is present.

2. **Skin and eyes.** Remove contaminated clothing and flush exposed skin immediately with copious water. Irrigate exposed eyes with water or saline.

3. **Ingestion of hypochlorite solution.** Immediately give water by mouth. Do *not* induce vomiting. Gastric lavage may be useful after concentrated liquid ingestion in order to remove any corrosive material in the stomach and to prepare for endoscopy; use a small, flexible tube to avoid injury to damaged mucosa.

4. Do ***not*** use activated charcoal; it may obscure the endoscopist's view.

D. **Enhanced elimination**. There is no role for enhanced elimination.

▶ CHLOROPHENOXY HERBICIDES (2,4-D)

Michael A. O'Malley, MD, MPH

2,4-Dichlorophenoxyacetic acid (2,4-D) and its chemical derivatives are widely used herbicides. A large number of formulations are available containing different 2,4-D salts (sodium, amine, alkylamine, and alkanolamine) and esters (propanoic acid, butanoic acid, and other alkoxy compounds). The most frequently used agricultural product, based upon 2013 California pesticide use data, is the dimethylamine salt of 2,4-D. Current California registration data (November 2015) show 205 formulations for the dimethylamine salt, with concentrations ranging from 0.12% (for the most dilute home use product) to 46.8–96.9% (for agricultural formulations). Although some concentrated formulations of 2,4-D esters are wettable powders, others contain petroleum solvents (identified on the "first aid" statement on the pesticide label); even though these solvents are considered "inert" ingredients because they are not pesticides, they may have their own innate toxicity (see "Toluene and Xylene," p 437, and "Hydrocarbons," p 266).

Agent Orange was a mixture of the chlorophenoxy herbicides 2,4-D (dichlorophenoxyacetic acid) and 2,4,5-T (trichlorophenoxyacetic acid) that also contained small amounts of the highly toxic contaminant TCDD (2,3,7,8-tetrachlorodibenzo-*p*-dioxin [p 197]), derived from the process of manufacturing 2,4,5-T. Manufacture of 2,4-D by chlorination of phenol does not produce TCDD. Populations involved in the manufacture or handling of 2,4,5-T may show elevated levels of TCDD on serum testing and overall increased rates of cancer compared with the general population.

I. **Mechanism of toxicity.** In plants, the compounds act as growth hormone stimulators. The mechanism of toxicity is unclear but may involve mitochondrial injury. In animals, cell membrane damage, uncoupling of oxidative phosphorylation, and disruption of acetyl coenzyme A metabolism are found, widespread muscle damage occurs, and the cause of death is usually ventricular fibrillation. Toxicity is markedly increased at doses that exceed the capacity of the renal anion transport mechanism (approximately 50 mg/kg). Massive rhabdomyolysis has been described in human patients, most often in cases involving ingestion of formulations containing more than 10% active ingredient.

II. **Toxic dose.** 2,4-D doses of 5 mg/kg are reported to have no effect in human volunteer studies. The minimum toxic dose of 2,4-D in humans is 3–4 g or 40–50 mg/kg, and death has occurred after adult ingestion of 6.5 g. Less than 6% of 2,4-D applied to the skin is absorbed systemically, although dermal exposure may produce skin irritation. The degree of dermal absorption may be less with salt formulations than with 2,4-D esters.

III. **Clinical presentation**

A. **Acute ingestion.** Vomiting, abdominal pain, and diarrhea are common. Tachycardia, muscle weakness, and muscle spasms occur shortly after ingestion and may progress to profound muscle weakness and coma. Massive rhabdomyolysis, metabolic acidosis, and severe and intractable hypotension have been reported, resulting in death within 24 hours. (A review of 66 published cases reported 33% were fatal.) Neurotoxic effects include ataxia, hypertonia, seizures, and coma. Hepatitis and renal failure may occur.

B. **Dermal exposure** to 2,4-D may produce skin irritation. Exposures to formulations containing 2,4,5-T may also produce chloracne. Substantial dermal exposure has been reported to cause a mixed sensory-peripheral neuropathy after a latent period.

IV. **Diagnosis** depends on a history of exposure and the presence of muscle weakness and elevated serum creatine kinase (CK).

A. **Specific levels** of 2,4-D can be measured by specialty or agricultural laboratories but may not be available in a timely enough fashion to be of help in establishing the diagnosis. The elimination half-life of 2,4-D is 11.5 hours, and more than 75% is excreted by 96 hours after ingestion. More than 80% is excreted in the urine unchanged.

B. **Other useful laboratory studies** include electrolytes, glucose, BUN, creatinine, CK, urinalysis (occult heme test result positive in the presence of myoglobin), liver enzymes, 12-lead ECG, and ECG monitoring.

V. **Treatment**

A. **Emergency and supportive measures**

1. Maintain an open airway and assist ventilation if necessary (pp 1–7).
2. Treat coma (p 18), hypotension (p 15), and rhabdomyolysis (p 27) if they occur.
3. Monitor the patient closely for at least 6–12 hours after ingestion because of the potential for delayed onset of symptoms.

B. **Specific drugs and antidotes.** There is no specific antidote.

C. **Decontamination** (p 50)

1. **Skin or eye exposure.** Remove contaminated clothing and wash affected areas.
2. **Ingestion.** Administer activated charcoal orally if conditions are appropriate (see Table 1–38, p 54). If a delay of more than 60 minutes is expected before charcoal can be given, consider using ipecac or other emetic if it can be administered within a few minutes of exposure and there are no contraindications. Consider gastric lavage after a large recent ingestion.

D. **Enhanced elimination.** There is no proven role for these procedures, although alkalinization of the urine may promote excretion of 2,4-D. (As with other weak acids, alkalinization would be expected to promote ionization of the phenoxy acid and decrease reabsorption from the renal tubules.) Hemodialysis has been recommended on the basis of limited clinical data showing clearances similar to those of alkaline diuresis. Plasmapheresis was reported effective in a pediatric case of polyneuropathy associated with 2,4-D ingestion.

▶ CHLOROQUINE AND OTHER AMINOQUINOLINES

Timothy E. Albertson, MD, MPH, PhD

Chloroquine and other aminoquinolines are used in the prophylaxis of or therapy for malaria and other parasitic diseases. Chloroquine and hydroxychloroquine also are used in the treatment of autoimmune diseases including rheumatoid arthritis. Antimalarial and related drugs include chloroquine phosphate (Aralen), amodiaquine hydrochloride (Camoquin), hydroxychloroquine sulfate (Plaquenil), mefloquine (Lariam), primaquine phosphate, and quinacrine hydrochloride (Atabrine). Chloroquine overdose is common, especially in countries where malaria is prevalent, and the mortality rate is 10–30%. Quinine toxicity is described on p 400.

I. **Mechanism of toxicity**

A. **Chloroquine** blocks the synthesis of DNA and RNA and also has some quinidine-like cardiotoxicity. Hydroxychloroquine has similar actions but is considerably less potent.

B. **Primaquine** and **quinacrine** are oxidizing agents and can cause methemoglobinemia or hemolytic anemia (especially in patients with glucose-6-phosphate dehydrogenase [G6PD] deficiency).

C. **Pharmacokinetics.** Chloroquine and related drugs are highly tissue-bound (volume of distribution [Vd] = 150–250 L/kg) and are eliminated very slowly from the body. The half-life of chloroquine and hydroxychloroquine are variable and long at 75–278 hours and 15.5–31 hours, respectively. But the terminal half-life of chloroquine maybe as long as 2 months, and that of hydroxychloroquine maybe as long as 40 days. Primaquine, with a half-life of 3–8 hours, is extensively metabolized to an active metabolite that is eliminated much more slowly (half-life of 22–30 hours) and can accumulate with chronic dosing (see also Table II–66, p 462).

II. **Toxic dose.** The therapeutic dose of chloroquine phosphate is 500 mg once a week for malaria prophylaxis or 2.5 g over 2 days for the treatment of malaria. Deaths have been reported in children after ingesting one or two tablets—doses as low as 300 mg; the lethal dose of chloroquine for an adult is estimated at 30–50 mg/kg.

III. **Clinical presentation**

A. **Mild-to-moderate chloroquine overdose** results in dizziness, nausea and vomiting, abdominal pain, headache and visual/retinal disturbances (sometimes including irreversible blindness), auditory disturbances (sometimes leading to deafness), agitation, and neuromuscular excitability. The use of chloroquine and proguanil in combination is common and is associated with GI and neuropsychiatric side effects, including acute psychosis.

B. **Severe chloroquine overdose** may cause convulsions, coma, shock, and respiratory or cardiac arrest. Quinidine-like severe cardiotoxicity may be seen, including sinoatrial arrest, depressed myocardial contractility, QRS- and/or QT-interval prolongation, heart block, and ventricular arrhythmias. Severe hypokalemia can occur with either chloroquine or hydroxychloroquine and may contribute to arrhythmias.

C. **Primaquine** and **quinacrine** intoxication commonly causes GI upset and may also cause severe methemoglobinemia (p 317) or hemolysis; chronic treatment can cause ototoxicity and retinopathy. Cardiovascular toxicity is not associated with primaquine.

D. **Amodiaquine** in therapeutic doses has caused severe and even fatal neutropenia.

E. **Mefloquine** in therapeutic use or overdose may cause headache, dizziness, vertigo, insomnia, visual and auditory hallucinations, panic attacks, severe depression, psychosis, confusion, and seizures. Neuropsychiatric side effects generally resolve within a few days after withdrawal of mefloquine and with supportive pharmacotherapy, but occasionally symptoms persist for several weeks.

IV. **Diagnosis.** The findings of gastritis, visual disturbances, and neuromuscular excitability, especially if accompanied by hypokalemia, hypotension, QRS- or QT-interval widening, or ventricular arrhythmias, should suggest chloroquine overdose. Hemolysis or methemoglobinemia suggests primaquine or quinacrine overdose.

A. **Specific levels.** Chloroquine is usually not detected on comprehensive toxicology screening. Quantitative levels can be measured in blood but are not generally available. Because chloroquine is concentrated intracellularly, whole-blood measurements are fivefold higher than serum or plasma levels.

1. Plasma (trough) concentrations of 10–20 ng/mL (0.01–0.02 mg/L) are effective in the treatment of various types of malaria.
2. Cardiotoxicity may be seen with serum levels of 1 mg/L (1,000 ng/mL); serum levels reported in fatal cases have ranged from 1 to 210 mg/L (average, 60 mg/L).

B. **Other useful laboratory studies** include electrolytes (particularly potassium levels), glucose, BUN, creatinine, ECG, and ECG monitoring. With primaquine or quinacrine, also include CBC, free plasma hemoglobin, and methemoglobin.

V. **Treatment**

A. **Emergency and supportive measures**

1. Maintain an open airway and assist ventilation if necessary (pp 1–7).
2. Treat seizures (p 23), coma (p 18), hypotension (p 15), hypokalemia (p 39), and methemoglobinemia (p 317) if they occur.
3. Treat massive hemolysis with blood transfusions if needed and prevent hemoglobin deposition in the kidney tubules by alkaline diuresis (as for rhabdomyolysis [p 27]).
4. Continuously monitor the ECG for at least 6–8 hours or until ECG normalizes.

B. **Specific drugs and antidotes**

1. Treat cardiotoxicity as for quinidine poisoning (p 398) with **sodium bicarbonate** (p 520), 1–2 mEq/kg IV.
2. Potassium should be administered for severe hypokalemia but should be dosed with caution and with frequent serum potassium measurements, as hyperkalemia may exacerbate quinidine-like cardiotoxicity.
3. If dopamine and norepinephrine are not effective, **epinephrine** infusion (p 551) may be useful in treating hypotension via combined vasoconstrictor and inotropic actions. Dosing recommendations in one study were 0.25 mcg/kg/min, increased by increments of 0.25 mcg/kg/min until adequate blood pressure was obtained, along with administration of high-dose diazepam (see below) and mechanical ventilation.
4. High-dose benzodiazepines such as **diazepam** (2 mg/kg) IV given over 30 minutes after endotracheal intubation and mechanical ventilation has been reported to reduce mortality in animals and to relieve cardiotoxicity in human chloroquine poisonings. The mechanism of protection is unknown.

C. **Decontamination** (p 50). Administer activated charcoal orally if conditions are appropriate (see Table I–38, p 54). Perform gastric lavage for significant ingestions (eg, >30–50 mg/kg).

D. **Enhanced elimination.** Because of extensive tissue distribution, enhanced removal procedures are ineffective.

▶ CHROMIUM

Thomas J. Ferguson, MD, PhD

Chromium is a durable metal used in electroplating, paint pigments (chrome yellow), primers and corrosion inhibitors, wood preservatives, textile preservatives, and leather tanning agents. Chromium exposure may occur by inhalation, ingestion, or skin exposure. Although chromium can exist in a variety of oxidation states, most human exposures involve one of two types: trivalent (eg, chromic oxide, chromic sulfate) or hexavalent (eg, chromium trioxide, chromic anhydride, chromic acid, dichromate salts). Toxicity is associated most commonly with hexavalent compounds; however, fatalities have occurred after ingestion of compounds of either type, and chronic skin sensitivity probably is related to the trivalent form. Chromium picolinate is a trivalent chromium compound often promoted as a body-building agent.

I. **Mechanism of toxicity**

A. **Trivalent chromium** compounds are relatively insoluble and noncorrosive and are less likely to be absorbed through intact skin. Biological toxicity is estimated to be 10- to 100-fold lower than that of the hexavalent compounds.

B. **Hexavalent compounds** are powerful oxidizing agents and corrosive to the airway, skin, mucous membranes, and GI tract. Acute hemolysis and renal tubular necrosis may also occur. Chronic occupational exposure to less soluble hexavalent forms is associated with chronic bronchitis, dermatitis, and lung cancer.

C. **Chromic acid** is a strong acid, whereas some chromate salts are strong bases.

II. **Toxic dose**

A. **Inhalation.** The OSHA workplace permissible exposure limit (PEL, 8-hour time-weighted average) for chromic acid and hexavalent compounds is 0.05 mg/m^3 (carcinogen). For bivalent and trivalent chromium, the PEL is 0.5 mg/m^3.

B. **Skin.** Chromium salts can cause skin burns, which may enhance systemic absorption, and death has occurred after a 10% surface area burn.

C. **Ingestion.** Life-threatening toxicity has occurred from ingestion of as little as 500 mg of hexavalent chromium. The estimated lethal dose of chromic acid is 1–2 g, and of potassium dichromate 6–8 g. Drinking water standards for total chromium are set at 0.1 mg/L (100 ppb).

III. **Clinical presentation**

A. **Inhalation.** Acute inhalation can cause upper respiratory tract irritation, wheezing, and noncardiogenic pulmonary edema (which may be delayed for several hours to days after exposure). Chronic exposure to hexavalent compounds may lead to pulmonary sensitization, asthma, and cancer.

B. **Skin and eyes.** Acute contact may cause severe corneal injury, deep skin burns, and oral or esophageal burns. Hypersensitivity dermatitis may result. It has been estimated that chronic chromium exposure is responsible for about 8% of all cases of contact dermatitis. Nasal ulcers may also occur after chronic exposure.

C. **Ingestion.** Ingestion may cause acute hemorrhagic gastroenteritis; the resulting massive fluid and blood loss may cause shock and oliguric renal failure. Hemolysis, hepatitis, and cerebral edema have been reported. Chromates are capable of oxidizing hemoglobin, but clinically significant methemoglobinemia is relatively uncommon after acute overdose.

IV. **Diagnosis** is based on a history of exposure and clinical manifestations such as skin and mucous membrane burns, gastroenteritis, renal failure, and shock.

A. **Specific levels.** Blood levels are not useful in emergency management and are not widely available. Detection in the urine may confirm exposure; normal urine levels are less than 1 mcg/L.

B. **Other useful laboratory studies** include CBC, plasma free hemoglobin and haptoglobin (if hemolysis is suspected), electrolytes, glucose, BUN, creatinine, liver aminotransferases, urinalysis (for hemoglobin), arterial blood gases, cooximetry or pulse oximetry, methemoglobin, and chest radiography.

V. **Treatment**

A. **Emergency and supportive measures**

1. **Inhalation.** Give supplemental oxygen. Treat wheezing (p 8) and monitor the victim closely for delayed-onset noncardiogenic pulmonary edema (p 7). Delays in the onset of pulmonary edema of up to 72 hours have been reported after inhalation of concentrated solutions of chromic acid.
2. **Ingestion**
   a. Dilute immediately with water. Treat hemorrhagic gastroenteritis with aggressive fluid and blood replacement (p 16). Consider early endoscopy to assess the extent of esophageal or gastric injury.
   b. Treat hemoglobinuria resulting from hemolysis with alkaline diuresis as for rhabdomyolysis (p 27). Treat methemoglobinemia (p 317) if it occurs.

B. **Specific drugs and antidotes**

1. Chelation therapy (eg, with BAL [British anti-lewisite]) is not effective.
2. After oral ingestion of hexavalent compounds, **ascorbic acid** has been suggested to assist in the conversion of hexavalent to less toxic trivalent compounds. Although no definitive studies exist, the treatment is benign and may be helpful. In animal studies, the effective dose was 2–4 g of ascorbic acid orally per gram of hexavalent chromium compound ingested.
3. **Acetylcysteine** (p 499) has been used in several animal studies and one human case of dichromate poisoning.

C. **Decontamination** (p 50)

1. **Inhalation.** Remove the victim from exposure and give supplemental oxygen if available.
2. **Skin.** Remove contaminated clothing and wash exposed areas immediately with copious soap and water. EDTA (p 548) 10% ointment may facilitate removal of chromate scabs. A 10% topical solution of ascorbic acid has been advocated to enhance the conversion of hexavalent chromium to the less toxic trivalent state.
3. **Eyes.** Irrigate copiously with tepid water or saline and perform fluorescein examination to rule out corneal injury if pain or irritation persists.
4. **Ingestion.** Give milk or water to dilute corrosive effects. Do *not* induce vomiting because of the potential for corrosive injury. For large recent ingestions, perform gastric lavage. Activated charcoal is of uncertain benefit in adsorbing chromium and may obscure the view if endoscopy is performed.

D. **Enhanced elimination.** There is no evidence for the efficacy of enhanced removal procedures such as dialysis and hemoperfusion.

► CLONIDINE AND RELATED DRUGS

Cyrus Rangan, MD

Clonidine and the related centrally acting adrenergic inhibitors **guanabenz, guanfacine,** and **methyldopa** are commonly used for the treatment of hypertension. Clonidine also has been used to alleviate opioid and nicotine withdrawal symptoms. Clonidine overdose may occur after ingestion of pills or ingestion of the long-acting skin patches. **Oxymetazoline, naphazoline,** and **tetrahydrozoline** are nasal and conjunctival decongestants that may cause toxicity identical to that of clonidine.

Tizanidine is a chemically related agent used for the treatment of muscle spasticity. **Apraclonidine** and **brimonidine,** ophthalmic preparations for the treatment of glaucoma and ocular hypertension, may cause poisoning from ingestion and from systemic absorption after topical administration.

I. **Mechanism of toxicity.** All these agents decrease central sympathetic outflow by stimulating alpha$_2$-adrenergic presynaptic (inhibitory) receptors in the brain.

   A. **Clonidine, oxymetazoline,** and **tetrahydrozoline** may also stimulate peripheral alpha$_1$ receptors, resulting in vasoconstriction and transient hypertension.

   B. **Guanabenz** is structurally similar to guanethidine, a ganglionic blocker. **Guanfacine** is related closely to guanabenz and has more selective alpha$_2$ agonist activity than does clonidine.

   C. **Methyldopa** may further decrease sympathetic outflow by metabolism to a false neurotransmitter (alpha-methylnorepinephrine) or by decreasing plasma renin activity.

   D. **Tizanidine** is structurally related to clonidine but has low affinity for alpha$_1$ receptors.

   E. **Pharmacokinetics.** The onset of effects is rapid (30 minutes) after oral administration of clonidine. Other than methyldopa, these drugs are widely distributed with large volumes of distribution (see also Table II–66, p 462).

II. **Toxic dose**

   A. **Clonidine.** As little as one 0.1-mg tablet of clonidine has produced toxic effects in children; however, 10 mg shared by twin 34-month-old girls was not lethal. Adults have survived acute ingestions with as much as 100 mg. No fatalities from acute overdoses have been reported, but a child had permanent neurologic damage after a respiratory arrest.

   B. **Guanabenz.** Mild toxicity developed in adults who ingested 160–320 mg and in a 3-year-old child who ingested 12 mg. Severe toxicity developed in a 19-month-old child who ingested 28 mg. A 3-year-old child had moderate symptoms after ingesting 480 mg. All these children recovered by 24 hours.

   C. **Guanfacine.** Severe toxicity developed in a 25-year-old woman who ingested 60 mg. A 2-year-old boy ingested 4 mg and became lethargic within 20 minutes, but the peak hypotensive effect occurred 20 hours later.

   D. **Methyldopa.** More than 2 g in adults is considered a toxic dose, and death was reported in an adult after an ingestion of 25 g. However, survival was reported after ingestion of 45 g. The therapeutic dose of methyldopa for children is 10–65 mg/kg/d, and the higher dose is expected to cause mild symptoms.

   E. **Brimonidine and apraclonidine.** Recurrent episodes of unresponsiveness, hypotension, hypotonia, hypothermia, and bradycardia occurred in a 1-month-old infant receiving therapeutic dosing of brimonidine. A 2-week-old infant had severe respiratory depression after one drop was instilled into each eye. Both children recovered with supportive care in less than 24 hours. Apraclonidine ingestion in a 6-year-old girl led to respiratory depression requiring short-term intubation with uneventful recovery.

III. **Clinical presentation.** Manifestations of intoxication result from generalized sympathetic depression and include pupillary constriction, lethargy, coma, apnea, bradycardia, hypotension, and hypothermia. Paradoxical hypertension caused by stimulation of peripheral alpha1 receptors may occur with clonidine, oxymetazoline, and tetrahydrozoline (and possibly guanabenz) and is usually transient. The onset of symptoms is usually within 30–60 minutes, although peak effects may occur more than 6–12 hours after ingestion. Full recovery is usual within 24 hours. In an unusual massive overdose, a 28-year-old man who accidentally ingested 100 mg of clonidine powder had a three-phase intoxication over 4 days: initial hypertension, followed by hypotension, and then a withdrawal reaction with hypertension.

IV. **Diagnosis.** Poisoning should be suspected in patients with pinpoint pupils, respiratory depression, hypotension, and bradycardia. Although clonidine overdose may mimic an opioid overdose, it usually does not respond to administration of naloxone.

A. Specific levels. Serum drug levels are not routinely available or clinically useful. These drugs are not usually detectable on comprehensive urine toxicology screening.

B. Other useful laboratory studies include electrolytes, glucose, and arterial blood gases or oximetry.

V. Treatment. Patients usually recover within 24 hours with supportive care.

A. Emergency and supportive measures

1. Protect the airway and assist ventilation if necessary (pp 1–7).
2. Treat coma (p 18), hypotension (p 15), and bradycardia (p 9) if they occur. They usually resolve with supportive measures such as fluids, atropine, and dopamine. Hypertension is usually transient and does not require treatment. Treat lethargy and respiratory depression initially with intermittent tactile stimulation. Mechanical ventilation may be necessary in some patients.

B. Specific drugs and antidotes

1. Naloxone (p 584) has been reported to reverse signs and symptoms of clonidine overdose, but this has not been confirmed. Apparent arousal after naloxone administration may arise from competitive inhibition with endorphins and enkephalins. However, because the overdose mimics opioid intoxication, naloxone is indicated because of the possibility that narcotics may also have been ingested.
2. Tolazoline, a central $alpha_2$ receptor antagonist, was previously recommended, but the response has been highly variable, and it should ***not*** be used.

C. Decontamination (p 50). Administer activated charcoal orally if conditions are appropriate (see Table I–38, p 54). Gastric lavage is not necessary after small-to-moderate ingestions if activated charcoal can be given promptly. Consider whole-bowel irrigation after ingestion of clonidine skin patches.

D. Enhanced elimination. There is no evidence that enhanced removal procedures are effective.

▶ COBALT

Timur S. Durrani, MD, MPH, MBA

Cobalt is an essential trace metal element in the human diet, being an integral component of Vitamin B_{12} (cobalamin). It can be found in certain ores with other metals such as nickel, copper or arsenic. It has high melting and boiling points, approximately 1,500°C and 3,000°C, respectively. Cobalt has elemental, organic, and inorganic forms. When combined with tungsten carbide, the material is termed "hard metal" and is used for industrial cutting, drilling, and polishing. Cobalt is also found in jewelry alloys and has ferromagnetic properties making it a useful component in magnets.

Rubratope-57 (Cyanocobalamin Co 57 Capsules) is intended for the diagnosis of pernicious anemia and as a diagnostic adjunct in other defects of intestinal vitamin B12 absorption. Cobalt-60, a radionuclide of cobalt, is used as a source for radiation therapy, in industrial radiography, and in the sterilization of foods and spices, as well as in linear accelerators and leveling devices. Historically, inorganic cobalt salts were used for the treatment of anemia including during pregnancy and were also the cause of "beer drinkers cardiomyopathy" resulting from cobalt additives to beer to stabilize foam. More recently, an excess body burden of cobalt has been linked to failing cobalt alloy metal-on-metal hip joint replacements.

I. Mechanism of toxicity

A. Cobalt can exert toxic effects by interacting with a complex array of biological receptors and proteins to stimulate erythropoiesis, foster generation of reactive oxygen species, interfere with mitochondrial function, inhibit thyroidal iodine uptake, and alter calcium homeostasis.

B. Cobalt is considered a possible **carcinogen** (Class 2B by the International Agency for Research on Cancer).

C. Overdose during **pregnancy**. There are no reports of overdose in pregnancy. Cobalt had previously been used therapeutically to treat anemia in pregnancy. No fetal anomalies have been reported. A pregnant woman with bilateral metal on metal hips had blood cobalt concentrations of 138 and 143 mcg/L at 7 and 38 weeks gestation, and delivered a healthy male who showed normal development through age 14 weeks.

D. Pharmacokinetics. Cobalt is well absorbed via inhalation and variably absorbed by ingestion. It is distributed in serum, whole blood, liver, kidney, heart and spleen. The major route of elimination is renal, with half-lives on the order of several hours to a week. Lung retention of relatively insoluble cobalt compounds such as cobalt oxide may be prolonged, with pulmonary clearance half-lives of 1–2 years.

II. Toxic dose

A. Ingestion

1. Acute ingestion of 2.5 g of cobalt chloride by a 6-year-old child caused only abdominal pain. Hemoglobin and electrolytes remained normal.
2. Chronic doses of 45–90 mg per day were used to induce erythropoiesis in pregnancy, with no reported side effects. Fatal cases of dilated cardiomyopathy were reported among alcoholics who drank an average of 17 glasses of beer per day containing 0.5 ppm of cobalt (range of 0.0–5 ppm).

B. Inhalation of cobalt-containing dust may cause respiratory irritation at air concentrations between 0.002 and 0.01 mg/m^3. Concentrations greater than 0.01 mg/m^3 may cause "cobalt asthma," a reactive airway disease and occupational cause of adult onset asthma.

C. Dermal. Doses of 0.7–1.1 mcg/cm^2 can be released from handling 6% cobalt and 15% cobalt chloride metallic discs.

III. Clinical presentation

A. Ingestion

1. **Acute ingestion** may cause vomiting and abdominal pain.
2. **Chronic** ingestion of cobalt-adulterated beer caused "beer-drinkers' cardiomyopathy." Chronic use may also cause polycythemia.

B. Inhalation

1. Acute exposure can cause nasal irritation, cough and wheezing.
2. Chronic inhalation can cause a specific form of interstitial pulmonary fibrosis manifesting as giant cell pneumonitis ("hard metal/diamond polisher's disease"). It can also cause bronchiolitis obliterans and hypersensitivity pneumonitis. Onset of cough and exertional dyspnea may be insidious.

C. Dermal exposure may cause redness, scaling, blistering, formation of papules or pustules, exudation, and excoriation. Chronic exposure leads to fissures, lichenification, and hyperkeratosis. Cobalt is often alloyed in combination with other metals such as nickel and chromium in jewelry, and such alloys are a common cause of allergic contact dermatitis.

D. Metal-on-metal hip prostheses containing cobalt alloys have been associated with hypothyroidism, heart failure, and hearing and visual deficits. Symptoms occurred after an average of 19 months, with whole blood or serum concentrations ranging from 23 to 625 mcg/L.

IV. Diagnosis is based on a history of exposure and clinical findings consistent with cobalt toxicity.

A. Specific levels. Cobalt can be measured in serum, whole blood or urine.

1. Serum levels in nonexposed persons are about 0.9 ng/mL (roughly equivalent to ppb).
2. Urine cobalt levels averaged 0.375 mcg/L in the US population according to the National Health and Nutrition Examination Survey conducted in 2011–2012. Urinary measurements mainly reflect recent exposure, although substantial occupational exposures have produced elevated urinary levels for many weeks. Persons with occupational exposure to cobalt often have urinary cobalt levels that are many times higher than those of the general population.

3. **Metal-on-metal hip prostheses.** Patients with nonfailing hip prostheses will have higher cobalt concentrations than nonimplant patients, with whole blood levels of 4–10 mcg/L. Patients with **failing cobalt alloy hip replacements** generally will have levels greater than 10 mcg/L.

B. **Other useful laboratory studies** include a complete blood count to evaluate for polycythemia, thyroid studies to evaluate for hypothyroidism, creatinine to evaluate renal clearance ability, transthoracic echocardiogram to evaluate for dilated cardiomyopathy, and patch testing to evaluate allergic contact dermatitis.

C. **Occupational inhalation.** Pathognomonic multinucleated giant cells may be recovered from bronchoalveolar biopsy or lavage. Pulmonary function tests with and without methacholine and during and when away from work may be helpful in confirming workplace exposure sensitivity. Inhalational challenge with cobalt is the gold standard for diagnosis; however, this requires specialized facilities and is available at only a few centers.

V. Treatment

A. Emergency and supportive measures

1. After inhalational exposure, maintain an open airway, give bronchodilators as needed for wheezing, and assist ventilation if necessary. Once airway hyper-reactivity has been documented, further inhalation exposure to cobalt is contraindicated.
2. Prevention from further exposure may reverse acute disease, including asthma or allergic contact dermatitis, and prevent the development of chronic disease. Involve public health authorities to determine whether other workers are at increased risk through improper workplace controls.
3. Treat vomiting with antiemetics and replace volume losses with IV fluids.
4. Patients with mechanical symptoms (including pain, clicking or effusion) of a failing implanted hip prosthesis should be referred to their orthopedic surgeon for possible replacement. Patients who have no symptoms but have concern for cobalt toxicity can have their cobalt levels evaluated. However, the United Kingdom's Medicines and Healthcare Products Regulatory Agency recommends routine cobalt testing only for patients who are symptomatic or have stemmed metal-on-metal total hip replacements with a femoral head diameter ≥36 mm or Depuy ASR brand prostheses.

B. **Specific drugs and antidotes.** See chelation under item D, below.

C. **Decontamination.** Treatment of acute ingestion may include gastric decontamination (such as whole-bowel irrigation or endoscopic removal of cobalt containing magnets) and fluid repletion.

D. Enhanced elimination.

1. There are no reports of benefit via hemodialysis following cobalt exposure.
2. Chelation with EDTA (p 548), DTPA (p 547), and DMSA (p 624) has been suggested but indications are uncertain. Increased urine levels and apparent clinical improvement were reported with IV EDTA in an 11-year-old following a cobalt-containing magnet ingestion.

► COCAINE

Hallam M. Gugelmann, MD and Neal L. Benowitz, MD

Cocaine is one of the most popular drugs of abuse. It may be sniffed into the nose (snorted), smoked, or injected IV. Occasionally, it is combined with heroin and injected ("speedball"). Cocaine purchased on the street may contain adulterant drugs such as lidocaine or benzocaine (p 84) or stimulants such as caffeine (p 169), methamphetamine (p 81), ephedrine (p 394), and phencyclidine (p 365). Most illicit cocaine in the United States is adulterated with **levamisole,** an antiparasitic drug that can cause agranulocytosis and leukocytoclastic vasculitis.

The "**free base**" form of cocaine is preferred for smoking because it volatilizes at a lower temperature and is not as easily destroyed by heat as the crystalline hydrochloride salt. Free base is made by dissolving cocaine salt in an aqueous alkaline solution and then extracting the free base form with a solvent such as ether. Heat sometimes is applied to hasten solvent evaporation, creating a fire hazard. "**Crack**" is a free base form of cocaine produced by using sodium bicarbonate to create the alkaline aqueous solution, which is then dried.

I. Mechanism of toxicity. The primary actions of cocaine are local anesthetic effects (p 84), CNS stimulation, and inhibition of neuronal uptake of catecholamines.

A. Central nervous system stimulation and inhibition of catecholamine uptake result in a state of generalized sympathetic stimulation very similar to that of amphetamine intoxication (p 81).

B. Cardiovascular effects of high doses of cocaine, presumably related to blockade of cardiac cell sodium channels, include depression of conduction (QRS prolongation) and contractility. Cocaine-induced QT prolongation also has been described.

C. Pharmacokinetics. Cocaine is well absorbed from all routes, and toxicity has been described after mucosal application as a local anesthetic. Smoking and IV injection produce maximum effects within 1–2 minutes, whereas oral or mucosal absorption may take up to 20–30 minutes. Once absorbed, cocaine is eliminated by metabolism and hydrolysis, with a half-life of about 60 minutes. In the presence of ethanol, cocaine is transesterified to **cocaethylene,** which has similar pharmacologic effects and a longer half-life than cocaine (see also Table II–66, p 462).

II. Toxic dose. The toxic dose is highly variable and depends on individual tolerance, the route of administration, and the presence of other drugs, as well as other factors. Rapid IV injection or smoking may produce transiently high brain and heart levels, resulting in convulsions or cardiac arrhythmias, whereas the same dose swallowed or snorted may produce only euphoria.

A. The usual maximum recommended dose for intranasal local anesthesia is 100–200 mg (1–2 mL of 10% solution).

B. A typical "line" of cocaine to be snorted contains 20–30 mg or more. Crack usually is sold in pellets or "rocks" containing 100–150 mg.

C. Ingestion of 1 g or more of cocaine is likely to be fatal.

III. Clinical presentation

A. Central nervous system manifestations of toxicity may occur within minutes after smoking or IV injection or may be delayed for 30–60 minutes after snorting, mucosal application, or oral ingestion.

1. Initial euphoria may be followed by anxiety, agitation, delirium, psychosis, tremulousness, muscle rigidity or hyperactivity, and seizures. High doses may cause respiratory arrest.
2. Seizures are usually brief and self-limited; status epilepticus should suggest continued drug absorption (as from ruptured cocaine-filled condoms in the GI tract) or hyperthermia.
3. Coma may be caused by a postictal state, hyperthermia, or intracranial hemorrhage resulting from cocaine-induced hypertension.
4. Cocaine is the most common cause of drug-induced stroke. Stroke can be hemorrhagic (related to severe hypertension), embolic (resulting from atrial fibrillation or endocarditis), or ischemic (resulting from cerebral artery constriction and thrombosis). Stroke should be suspected if there is altered mental status and/or focal neurologic deficits.
5. With chronic cocaine use, insomnia, weight loss, and paranoid psychosis may occur. A "washed-out" syndrome has been observed in cocaine abusers after a prolonged binge, consisting of profound lethargy and deep sleep that may last for several hours to days, followed by spontaneous recovery.

B. **Cardiovascular toxicity** may also occur rapidly after smoking or IV injection and is mediated by sympathetic overactivity.
   1. Fatal ventricular tachycardia or fibrillation may occur. QRS-interval prolongation similar to that seen with tricyclic antidepressants may occur.
   2. Severe hypertension may cause hemorrhagic stroke or aortic dissection.
   3. Coronary artery spasm and/or thrombosis may result in myocardial infarction, even in patients with no coronary disease. Diffuse myocardial necrosis similar to catecholamine myocarditis and chronic cardiomyopathy have been described.
   4. Shock may be caused by myocardial, intestinal, or brain infarction; hyperthermia; tachyarrhythmias; or hypovolemia produced by extravascular fluid sequestration caused by vasoconstriction. Intestinal infarction may be complicated by severe, diffuse GI hemorrhage and hemoperitoneum.
   5. Renal failure may result from shock, renal arterial spasm and/or infarction, or rhabdomyolysis with myoglobinuria.

C. **Death** is usually caused by a sudden fatal arrhythmia, status epilepticus, intracranial hemorrhage, or hyperthermia. Hyperthermia is usually caused by seizures, muscular hyperactivity, or rigidity and typically is associated with rhabdomyolysis, myoglobinuric renal failure, coagulopathy, and multiple-organ failure. Severe hyperthermia is more common when the environmental temperature is high, particularly when a high ambient temperature is combined with physical hyperactivity.

D. A variety of **other effects** have occurred after smoking or snorting cocaine.
   1. Chest pain without ECG evidence of myocardial ischemia is common. The presumed basis is musculoskeletal, and it may be associated with ischemic necrosis of chest wall muscle.
   2. Pneumothorax and pneumomediastinum cause pleuritic chest pain, and the latter is often recognized by a "crunching" sound ("Hamman sign") heard over the anterior chest.
   3. Nasal septal perforation may occur after chronic snorting.
   4. Accidental subcutaneous injection of cocaine may cause localized necrotic ulcers ("coke burns"), and wound botulism (p 163) has been reported.
   5. Methemoglobinemia has been observed after the use of cocaine adulterated with benzocaine.

E. **Body "packers"** or **"stuffers."** Persons attempting to smuggle cocaine may swallow large numbers of tightly packed cocaine-filled condoms ("body packers"). Street vendors suddenly surprised by a police raid may quickly swallow their wares, often without carefully wrapping or closing the packets or vials ("body stuffers"). The swallowed condoms, packets, or vials may break open, releasing massive quantities of cocaine, causing severe intoxication. Intestinal obstruction may also occur. The packages are sometimes, but not always, visible on plain abdominal radiograph. Likewise, CT imaging of body stuffers or packers does not consistently confirm the presence or absence of ingested packets.

IV. **Diagnosis** is based on a history of cocaine use or typical features of sympathomimetic intoxication. Skin marks of chronic IV drug abuse, especially with scarring from coke burns, and nasal septal perforation after chronic snorting suggest cocaine use. Chest pain with electrocardiographic evidence of ischemia or infarction in a young, otherwise healthy person also suggests cocaine use. ***Note:*** Young adults, particularly young African-American men, have a high prevalence of normal J-point elevation on ECG, which can be mistaken for acute myocardial infarction. Otherwise unexplained seizures, coma, hyperthermia, stroke, or cardiac arrest should raise suspicion of cocaine poisoning.

A. **Specific levels.** Blood cocaine levels are not routinely available and do not assist in emergency management. Cocaine and its metabolite benzoylecgonine are easily detected in the urine for up to 72 hours after ingestion and provide qualitative confirmation of cocaine use.

B. Other useful laboratory studies include electrolytes, glucose, BUN, creatinine, creatine kinase (CK), urinalysis, urine myoglobin, cardiac troponin, ECG and ECG monitoring, CT head scan (if hemorrhage is suspected). Abdominal radiography (plain films or CT scanning) is not reliably sensitive enough to confirm or rule out ingested drug-filled packets.

V. Treatment

A. Emergency and supportive measures

1. Maintain an open airway and assist ventilation if necessary (pp 1–7).
2. Treat coma (p 18), agitation (p 24), seizures (p 23), hyperthermia (p 21), arrhythmias (pp 10–15), and hypotension (p 15) if they occur. Benzodiazepines (p 516) are a good choice for initial management of hypertension and tachycardia associated with agitation.
3. Angina pectoris may be treated with benzodiazepines, aspirin, nitrates, or calcium channel blockers. For acute myocardial infarction, thrombolysis has been recommended but is controversial. Supporting its use is the high prevalence of acute thrombosis, often superimposed on coronary spasm. Against its use is the excellent prognosis for patients with cocaine-induced infarction, even without thrombolysis, and concerns about increased risks for bleeding caused by intracranial hemorrhage or aortic dissection.
4. Monitor vital signs and ECG for several hours. Patients with suspected coronary artery spasm should be admitted to a coronary care unit, and because of reports of persistent or recurrent coronary spasm up to several days after initial exposure, consider the use of an oral calcium antagonist and/or cardiac nitrates for 2–4 weeks after discharge.

B. Specific drugs and antidotes. There is no specific antidote.

1. It is widely recommended that beta blockers be avoided in treating acute cocaine toxicity because propranolol, a nonselective beta blocker, may produce *paradoxical worsening* of hypertension because of blockade of $beta_2$-mediated vasodilation. However, if a beta blocker is needed (eg, for tachycardia not responsive to benzodiazepines and IV fluids, especially if associated with myocardial ischemia), it is reasonable to administer a cardioselective beta blocker such as **esmolol** (a very short-acting beta blocker [p 552]) or metoprolol. Beta blockers may also be used **in combination** with a vasodilator such as **phentolamine** (p 605) for management of hypertension.
2. **QRS prolongation** caused by sodium channel blockade can be treated with **sodium bicarbonate** (p 520). Wide-complex tachyarrhythmias may also respond to **lidocaine** (p 573).

C. Decontamination (p 50). Decontamination is not necessary after smoking, snorting, or IV injection. After **ingestion**, perform the following steps:

1. Administer activated charcoal orally if conditions are appropriate (see Table I–38, p 54).
2. Gastric lavage is not necessary after small-to-moderate ingestions if activated charcoal can be given promptly.
3. For ingestion of cocaine-filled condoms or packets, give repeated doses of activated charcoal and consider whole-bowel irrigation (p 55) unless there is evidence of bowel obstruction, bowel perforation, or severe GI hemorrhage. If large ingested packets (ie, Ziploc bags) are not removed by these procedures, laparotomy and surgical removal may be necessary. Surgical intervention to remove ingested packets may also be required for patients with persistent severe symptoms of cocaine intoxication or bowel obstruction.

D. Enhanced elimination. Because cocaine is extensively distributed to tissues and rapidly metabolized, dialysis and hemoperfusion procedures are not effective. Acidification of the urine does not significantly enhance cocaine elimination and may aggravate myoglobinuric renal failure.

▶ COLCHICINE

Mark Sutter, MD

Colchicine is FDA approved for the treatment and prophylaxis of gout and familial Mediterranean fever. It is also used for acute and recurrent pericarditis and a variety of inflammatory conditions such as Behçet disease. It is available in tablet form, and it is also found in certain plants, such as *Colchicum autumnale* (autumn crocus or meadow saffron) and *Gloriosa superba* (glory lily). The injectable form of colchicine was banned in 2009 by the FDA due to serious toxicity. Its antimitotic mechanism of action is similar to that of some chemotherapeutic agents, and colchicine overdoses are extremely serious, with considerable mortality.

I. Mechanism of toxicity. Colchicine inhibits microtubular formation and function, arresting dividing cells during mitosis. **Pharmacokinetics:** Colchicine is rapidly absorbed after oral administration and extensively distributed to body tissues. It is eliminated in the liver by CYP3A4 with a half-life of 4.4–31 hours (see also Table II–66, p 462).

II. Toxic dose. The maximum FDA-approved therapeutic dose of oral colchicine for acute gout is 1.2 mg followed by 0.6 mg after 1 hour, for a total dose of 1.8 mg. This is a significant reduction from the previously recommended maximum dose of 8 mg. In a series of 150 cases, doses of 0.5 mg/kg or less were associated with diarrhea and vomiting but not death, doses of 0.5–0.8 mg/kg were associated with bone marrow aplasia and 10% mortality, and ingestions greater than 0.8 mg/kg uniformly resulted in death. Fatalities, however, have been reported with single ingestions of as little as 7 mg, although other case reports describe survival after ingestions of more than 60 mg. Ingestions of parts of colchicine-containing plants have resulted in severe toxicity and death. The dose used for familial Mediterranean fever in adults is slightly higher at 1.2–2.4 mg per day. Dosing should be reduced for renal dysfunction for all uses of colchicine.

Prior to the ban on injectable colchicine, healthy individuals receiving a cumulative dose of greater than 4 mg of IV colchicine per treatment course were at risk for significant toxicity and death.

III. Clinical presentation. Colchicine poisoning affects many organ systems, with toxic effects occurring from hours to several days after exposure.

A. After an **acute overdose,** symptoms typically are delayed for 2–12 hours and include nausea, vomiting, abdominal pain, and severe bloody diarrhea. Shock results from depressed cardiac contractility and fluid loss into the GI tract and other tissues. Delirium, seizures, or coma may occur. Lactic acidosis related to shock and inhibition of cellular metabolism is common. Other manifestations of colchicine poisoning include acute myocardial injury, rhabdomyolysis with myoglobinuria, disseminated intravascular coagulation, and acute renal failure.

Chronic colchicine poisoning presents with a more insidious onset. Factors precipitating toxicity from chronic use include renal insufficiency, liver disease, and drug interactions (erythromycin, cimetidine, cyclosporine) that can inhibit colchicine clearance.

B. Death usually occurs after 8–36 hours and is caused by respiratory failure, intractable shock, and cardiac arrhythmias or sudden cardiac arrest.

C. Late complications include bone marrow suppression, particularly leukopenia and thrombocytopenia (4–5 days) and alopecia (2–3 weeks). Chronic colchicine therapy may produce myopathy (proximal muscle weakness and elevated creatine kinase [CK] levels) and polyneuropathy. This also has occurred after acute poisoning.

IV. Diagnosis. A syndrome beginning with severe gastroenteritis, leukocytosis, shock, rhabdomyolysis, and acute renal failure, followed by leukopenia and thrombocytopenia, should suggest colchicine poisoning. A history of gout or familial Mediterranean fever in the patient or a family member is also suggestive.

A. **Specific levels.** Colchicine levels in blood and urine are not readily available. However, levels may be useful for forensic purposes, especially in cases of unexplained pancytopenia and multiple-organ failure. Bone marrow biopsy may reveal metaphase arrest and "pseudo-Pelger–Huët" cells.

B. **Other useful laboratory studies** include CBC, electrolytes, hepatic enzymes, glucose, BUN, creatinine, CK, cardiac troponin (T or I), urinalysis, and ECG monitoring. Elevated serum levels of troponin suggest greater severity of myocardial necrosis and higher mortality.

V. **Treatment**

A. **Emergency and supportive measures.** Provide aggressive supportive care, with careful monitoring and treatment of fluid and electrolyte disturbances.

1. Anticipate sudden respiratory or cardiac arrest and maintain an open airway and assist ventilation if necessary (pp 1–7).
2. Treatment of shock (p 15) may require large amounts of crystalloid fluids and possibly blood (to replace losses from hemorrhagic gastroenteritis).
3. Infusion of sodium bicarbonate may be considered if there is evidence of rhabdomyolysis (p 27).
4. Bone marrow depression requires specialized intensive care. Severe neutropenia requires patient isolation and management of febrile episodes, as for other neutropenic conditions. Platelet transfusions may be required to control bleeding.

B. **Specific drugs and antidotes.** Colchicine-specific antibodies (Fab fragments) were used experimentally in France to treat a 25-year-old woman with severe colchicine overdose. Unfortunately, they were never commercially produced and are no longer available. Granulocyte colony–stimulating factor (G-CSF) has been used for the treatment of severe leukopenia.

C. **Decontamination** (p 50). Administer activated charcoal orally if conditions are appropriate (see Table I–38, p 54). If a delay of more than 60 minutes is expected before charcoal can be given, consider using ipecac to induce vomiting if it can be administered within a few minutes of the exposure. Gastric lavage is not necessary after small-to-moderate ingestions if activated charcoal can be given promptly.

D. **Enhanced elimination.** Because colchicine is highly bound to tissues, with a large volume of distribution, hemodialysis and hemoperfusion are ineffective. Colchicine undergoes enterohepatic recirculation, so **repeat-dose charcoal** might be expected to accelerate elimination, although this has not been documented. The use of rifampin to induce hepatic CYP3A4 elimination of colchicine has been suggested but not tested.

► COPPER

Timur S. Durrani, MD, MPH, MBA

Copper is widely used in its elemental metallic form, in metal alloys, and in the form of copper salts. Each of the copper forms has different physical properties, resulting in different toxicities. Elemental metallic copper is used in electrical wiring and plumbing materials and was formerly the main constituent of pennies (now mostly zinc). Copper salts such as copper sulfate, copper oxide, copper chloride, copper nitrate, copper cyanide, and copper acetate are used as pesticides and algaecides and in a variety of industrial processes. Because of its toxicity, copper sulfate is no longer used as an emetic. Copper levels may be elevated in persons who drink from copper containers or use copper plumbing. The increased acidity of beverages stored in copper alloy (eg, brass or bronze) containers enhances leaching of copper into the liquid.

I. **Mechanism of toxicity**

A. **Elemental metallic copper** is poorly absorbed orally and is essentially nontoxic. However, inhalation of copper dust or metallic fumes created when copper alloys are welded or brazed may cause chemical pneumonitis or a syndrome similar to metal fume fever (p 311). Metallic copper dust in the eye (chalcosis) may lead to corneal opacification, uveitis, ocular necrosis, and blindness unless the dust is removed quickly.

B. **Copper sulfate** salt is highly irritating, depending on the concentration, and may produce mucous membrane irritation and severe gastroenteritis.

C. **Systemic absorption** can produce hepatic and renal tubular injury. Hemolysis has been associated with copper exposure from hemodialysis equipment or absorption through burned skin.

II. **Toxic dose.** Copper is an essential trace metal. The daily adult requirement of 2 mg is supplied in a normal diet.

A. **Inhalation.** The recommended workplace limit (ACGIH TLV-TWA) for copper fumes is 0.2 mg/m^3; for dusts and mists, it is 1 mg/m^3. The air level considered immediately dangerous to life or health (IDLH) for dusts or fumes is 100 mg/m^3.

B. **Ingestion** of more than 250 mg of copper sulfate can produce vomiting, and larger ingestions potentially can cause hepatic and renal injury.

C. **Water.** The US Environmental Protection Agency (EPA) has established a safe limit of 1.3 mg/L in drinking water under the Lead and Copper Rule. According to the EPA, this has led to the reduction in risk of copper exposure that can cause stomach and intestinal distress, liver or kidney damage, and complications of Wilson disease in genetically predisposed people. The WHO (World Health Organization, 2004) guideline value for drinking water is 2 mg/L.

III. **Clinical presentation**

A. **Inhalation of copper fumes or dusts** initially produces a metallic taste and upper respiratory irritation (dry cough, sore throat, and eye irritation). Large exposures may cause severe cough, dyspnea, fever, leukocytosis, and pulmonary infiltrates (see also “Metal Fume Fever,” p 311).

B. **Ingestion of copper sulfate or other salts** causes the rapid onset of nausea and vomiting with characteristic blue-green vomit. Gastrointestinal bleeding may occur. Fluid and blood loss from gastroenteritis may lead to hypotension and oliguria. Intravascular hemolysis can result in acute tubular necrosis. Hepatitis has been reported, caused by centrilobular necrosis. Multisystem failure, shock, and death may occur. Chronic interstitial nephritis has been reported after parenteral copper sulfate poisoning. Methemoglobinemia is uncommon. Reduced serum cortisol level with adrenal insufficiency has been reported, but its relation to copper toxicity is uncertain.

C. **Chronic** exposure to Bordeaux mixture (copper sulfate with hydrated lime) may occur in vineyard workers. Pulmonary fibrosis, lung cancer, cirrhosis, angiosarcoma, and portal hypertension have been associated with this occupational exposure.

D. Ingestion of **organocopper** compounds is rare. Suicidal ingestion of an organocopper fungicide containing primarily copper-8-hydroxyquinolate caused lethargy, dyspnea, and cyanosis, with 34% methemoglobinemia.

E. Swimming in water contaminated with copper-based algaecides can cause green discoloration of the hair.

IV. **Diagnosis** is based on a history of acute ingestion or occupational exposure. Occupations at risk include those associated with handling algaecides, herbicides, wood preservatives, pyrotechnics, ceramic glazes, and electrical wiring, as well as welding or brazing copper alloys.

A. **Specific levels.** If copper salt ingestion is suspected, a serum copper level should be obtained. Normal serum copper concentrations average 1 mg/L, and this doubles during pregnancy. Serum copper levels above 5 mg/L are considered very toxic. Whole-blood copper levels may correlate better with acute intoxication because acute excess copper is carried in the red blood cells; however, whole-blood copper levels are not as widely available. Normal serum copper levels have been reported even in the face of severe acute toxicity.

B. **Other useful laboratory studies** include CBC, electrolytes, BUN, creatinine, hepatic aminotransferases (ALT and AST), arterial blood gases or oximetry, and chest radiograph. If hemolysis is suspected, send blood for type and cross-match, plasma-free hemoglobin, and haptoglobin and check urinalysis for occult blood (hemoglobinuria).

V. **Treatment**

A. **Emergency and supportive measures**

1. **Inhalation of copper fumes or dusts.** Give supplemental oxygen if indicated by arterial blood gases or oximetry and treat bronchospasm (p 7) and chemical pneumonitis (p 7) if they occur. Symptoms are usually short lived and resolve without specific treatment.
2. **Ingestion of copper salts**
   a. Treat shock caused by gastroenteritis with aggressive IV fluid replacement and, if necessary, pressor drugs (p 16).
   b. Consider endoscopy to rule out corrosive esophageal or stomach injury, depending on the concentration of the solution and the patient's symptoms.
   c. Blood transfusion may be needed if significant hemolysis or GI bleeding occurs.

B. **Specific drugs and antidotes**

1. **BAL** (dimercaprol [p 514]) and **penicillamine** (p 601) are effective chelating agents and should be used in seriously ill patients with large ingestions.
2. **Trientine hydrochloride** (Syprine) is a specific copper chelator approved for use in Wilson disease; although it is better tolerated than penicillamine, its role in acute ingestion or chronic environmental exposure has not been established.
3. **Unithiol** (DMPS, dimercaptopropanesulfonic acid [p 630]) has been used, but its efficacy is unclear. Because DMPS and its heavy metal complexes are excreted predominantly by the kidney, caution should be exercised in patients with renal failure.

C. **Decontamination** (p 50)

1. **Inhalation.** Remove the victim from exposure and give supplemental oxygen if available.
2. **Eyes.** Irrigate copiously and attempt to remove all copper from the surface; perform a careful slit-lamp examination and refer the case to an ophthalmologist urgently if any residual material remains.
3. **Ingestion.** Perform gastric lavage if there has been a recent ingestion of a large quantity of copper salts. There is no proven benefit for activated charcoal, and its use may obscure the view if endoscopy is performed.

D. **Enhanced elimination.** There is no role for hemodialysis, hemoperfusion, repeat-dose charcoal, or hemodiafiltration. Hemodialysis may be required for supportive care of patients with acute renal failure, and it can marginally increase the elimination of the copper–chelator complex.

▶ CYANIDE

Paul D. Blanc, MD, MSPH

Cyanide is a highly toxic chemical with a variety of uses, including chemical synthesis, laboratory analysis, and metal plating and polishing. Aliphatic nitriles (acrylonitrile and propionitrile) used in plastic manufacturing are metabolized to cyanide. The vasodilator drug nitroprusside releases cyanide upon exposure to light or through metabolism. Natural sources of cyanide (amygdalin and many other cyanogenic glycosides) are found in apricot pits, cassava, and many other plants and seeds, some of which may be important exposures, depending on ethnobotanical practices. Acetonitrile, a solvent that was a component of some artificial nail glue removers, has caused several pediatric deaths due to conversion to cyanide in the body.

Hydrogen cyanide gas is generated easily by mixing acid with cyanide salts and also is a common combustion by-product of burning plastics, wool, and many other natural and synthetic products. Hydrogen cyanide poisoning is an important cause of death from structural fires and deliberate cyanide exposure (through cyanide salts) remains an important instrument of homicide and suicide. Hydrogen cyanamide, an agricultural chemical used as a plant regulator, is a potent toxin that inhibits aldehyde dehydrogenase but does not act as a cyanide analog.

I. Mechanism of toxicity

- **A.** Cyanide is a chemical asphyxiant, blocking the aerobic utilization of oxygen by binding to cellular cytochrome oxidase.
- **B.** The bulk of unbound cyanide (80%) is detoxified by metabolism to thiocyanate, a much less toxic compound that is excreted in the urine.
- **C.** Pharmacokinetic data in humans are limited. Inhalation absorption of gas is almost immediate and oral absorption of salts is rapid (minutes). It has been estimated that in poisoning, 50% of cyanide is found in blood (98% in erythrocytes) and the remainder evenly divided between muscles and all other sites. Based on animal studies, the volume of distribution is approximately 0.8 L/kg and the elimination half-life is 23 minutes (predominantly first-order kinetics prior to sulfur-based detoxification saturation).

II. Toxic dose

- **A.** Exposure to **hydrogen cyanide gas** (HCN), even at low levels (150–200 ppm), can be fatal. The air level considered immediately dangerous to life or health (IDLH, NIOSH) is 25 mg/m^3. The Occupational Safety and Health Administration (OSHA) legal permissible exposure limit (PEL) for HCN is 5 mg/m^3. The recommended workplace ceiling limit (ACGIH TLV-C) is 4.7 ppm (5 mg/m^3 for cyanide salts). Cyanide salts in solution are well absorbed across the skin.
- **B.** Adult **ingestion** of as little as 200 mg of the sodium or potassium salt can be fatal. Solutions of cyanide salts are readily absorbed through intact skin.
- **C.** During nitroprusside infusions at normal rates and durations, cyanide poisoning is relatively rare.
- **D.** Dietary acute toxicity after ingestion of amygdalin-containing seeds (unless they have been pulverized) is uncommon, but unusual plant sources should be kept in mind. Chronic cyanide toxicity can characterize exposure through dietary sources.

III. Clinical presentation. Abrupt onset of profound toxic effects shortly after exposure is the hallmark of acute cyanide poisoning. Symptoms include headache, nausea, dyspnea, and confusion. Syncope, seizures, coma, agonal respirations, and cardiovascular collapse ensue rapidly after heavy exposure.

- **A.** A very brief delay may occur if the cyanide is ingested as a salt, especially if it is in a capsule or if there is food in the stomach.
- **B.** Delayed onset (minutes to hours) may occur after ingestion of nitriles and plant-derived cyanogenic glycosides because metabolism to cyanide is required.
- **C.** Chronic neurologic sequelae may follow severe acute cyanide poisoning, consistent with anoxic injury.
- **D.** Neurologic disease associated with chronic dietary exposure to cyanogenic glycosides (prototypically *Konzo* in cassava-dependent regions of Africa) is etiologically complex, differing in mechanism from acute cyanide poisoning.

IV. Diagnosis is based on a history of exposure or the presence of rapidly progressive symptoms and signs. Severe **lactic acidosis** is usually present with substantive exposure. The **measured venous oxygen saturation** may be elevated owing to blocked cellular oxygen consumption. The classic "bitter almond" odor of hydrogen cyanide may or may not be noted, in part because of genetic variability in the ability to detect the smell.

- **A. Specific levels.** Cyanide determinations are rarely of use in emergency management because they cannot be performed rapidly enough to influence initial treatment. In addition, they must be interpreted with caution because of a variety of complicating technical factors.

1. Whole-blood levels higher than 0.5–1 mg/L are considered toxic.
2. Cigarette smokers may have levels of up to 0.1 mg/L.
3. Rapid nitroprusside infusion may produce levels as high as 1 mg/L, accompanied by metabolic acidosis.
4. Measurement of exhaled cyanide can theoretically detect over-exposure but this is not a clinically relevant test.

B. **Other useful laboratory studies** include electrolytes, glucose, lactate, arterial blood gases, mixed venous oxygen saturation, and carboxyhemoglobin (via cooximetry, if the patient experienced smoke inhalation exposure).

V. **Treatment**

A. **Emergency and supportive measures.** Treat all cyanide exposures as potentially lethal.

1. Maintain an open airway and assist ventilation if necessary (pp 1–7). Administer supplemental oxygen.
2. Treat coma (p 18), hypotension (p 15), and seizures (p 23) if they occur.
3. **Gain** IV access and monitor the patient's vital signs and ECG closely.

B. **Specific drugs and antidotes.** There are only two FDA-approved cyanide antidotes in the United States:

1. **Hydroxocobalamin** (Cyanokit, p 563) binds and detoxifies free cyanide. It can interfere with multiple serum assays. Red chromaturia and skin erythema are nearly universal with treatment; rash is also common.
   a. In acute poisoning, give 5 g of hydroxocobalamin (children: 70 mg/kg) by IV infusion over 15 minutes.
   b. In severe cases, a second dose may be considered.
   c. For prophylaxis of cyanide toxicity from nitroprusside, recommended hydroxocabalamin dosing is 25 mg/h by IV infusion.
2. **Nithiodote** (p 592 and p 629) is an older cyanide treatment based on two modalities, one of which produces cyanide-scavenging methemoglobinemia while the second serves as a sulfur donor for cyanide metabolism.
   a. **Sodium nitrite i**njection, 300 mg/10 mL is administered IV at 2.5–5 mL/min (children 0.2 mL/kg of a 3% solution [6 mg/kg or 6–8 mL/m^2] not to exceed 300 mg). ***Caution:*** Nitrite-induced methemoglobinemia can be extremely dangerous and even lethal. Nitrite should not be given if the symptoms are mild or if the diagnosis is uncertain, especially if concomitant carbon monoxide poisoning is suspected.
   b. Following the sodium nitrite, **sodium thiosulfate,** 50 mL of a 25% solution (12.5 g) is administered IV (children 1 mL/kg 25% solution [250 mg/kg or 30–40 mL/m^2] not to exceed 12.5 g). Thiosulfate is relatively benign. Its use as an adjunct concomitant with hydroxocobalamin is not supported by experimental data.
3. Amyl nitrate is no longer approved by the FDA for the treatment of cyanide intoxication due to uncertain effectiveness and risk of diversion for abuse.
4. **Dicobalt edetate** is used outside the United States to treat cyanide but is associated with multiple adverse side effects.
5. **Hyperbaric oxygen** has no proven role in cyanide-poisoning treatment.

C. **Decontamination** (p 50). ***Caution:*** Avoid contact with cyanide-containing salts or solutions and avoid inhaling vapors from vomitus (which may give off hydrogen cyanide gas).

1. **Inhalation.** Remove victims from hydrogen cyanide exposure and give supplemental oxygen if available. Each rescuer should wear a positive-pressure, self-contained breathing apparatus and, if possible, chemical-protective clothing.
2. **Skin.** Remove and isolate all contaminated clothing and wash affected areas with copious soap and water.
3. **Ingestion** (p 53). Even though charcoal has a relatively low affinity for cyanide, it will effectively bind the doses typically ingested (eg, 100–500 mg).

a. **Prehospital.** Immediately administer activated charcoal if it is available and the patient is alert. Do *not* induce vomiting unless the victim is more than 30 minutes from a medical facility and charcoal is not available.

b. **Hospital.** Immediately place a gastric tube and administer activated charcoal, then perform gastric lavage. Give additional activated charcoal and a cathartic after the lavage.

D. **Enhanced elimination.** There is no role for hemodialysis or hemoperfusion in cyanide-poisoning treatment. Hemodialysis may be indicated in patients with renal insufficiency who develop high thiocyanate levels while on extended treatment with thiosulfate.

▶ DAPSONE

Kathryn H. Meier, PharmD

Dapsone is an antibiotic used for treatment of and prophylaxis against various infections, including leprosy, malaria, and *Pneumocystis carinii* pneumonia. The anti-inflammatory and immune-suppressant effects of dapsone make it valuable for the treatment of some rheumatologic and rare dermatologic disorders. A 5% topical formulation is used for treatment of acne vulgaris.

I. **Mechanism of toxicity.** The toxic effects are caused by oxidized cytochrome P450 (CYP) dapsone metabolites, which can lead to methemoglobinemia, sulfhemoglobinemia, and Heinz body hemolytic anemia, decreasing the oxygen-carrying capacity of the blood.

A. Methemoglobinemia occurs when dapsone metabolites oxidize the ferrous iron–hemoglobin complex to the ferric state.

B. **Sulfhemoglobinemia** occurs when dapsone metabolites irreversibly sulfate the pyrrole hemoglobin ring.

C. **Delayed hemolysis** secondary to erythrocyte oxidative stress may be preceded by the appearance of Heinz body precipitates on the blood smear.

D. **Pharmacokinetics.** Absorption of dapsone after overdose is delayed; peak plasma levels occur between 4 and 8 hours after ingestion. Bioavailability ranges from 84% to 100%. The volume of distribution is 1.5 L/kg, and protein binding is 70–90%. Dapsone is metabolized by two primary routes: acetylation and CYP oxidation. Both dapsone and its acetylated metabolite undergo enterohepatic recirculation and oxidation. Currently, the isoenzymes thought to be primarily responsible for oxidation are CYP2C19 >> CYP2B6 > CYP2D6 > CYP3A4. The average elimination half-life is dose dependent and variable: 10–50 hours with therapeutic doses and potentially more than 77 hours after an overdose (see also Table II–66, p 462). Dapsone concentrations persist in the liver and kidneys for up to 3 weeks after discontinuation of treatment.

II. **Toxic dose.** Although the adult therapeutic dose ranges from 50 to 300 mg/d, dosing and patient tolerance are limited by toxic effects. Chronic daily dosing of 100 mg can cause methemoglobin levels of 5–12%. Hemolysis has not been reported in adults with doses of less than 300 mg/d. Persons with glucose-6-phosphate dehydrogenase (G6PD) deficiency, congenital hemoglobin abnormalities, or underlying hypoxemia may experience greater toxicity at lower doses. Death has occurred after overdoses of 1.4 g and greater, although recovery from severe toxicity has been reported after ingestion of 7.5 g.

III. **Clinical presentation.** Manifestations of acute dapsone intoxication include vomiting, cyanosis, tachypnea, tachycardia, altered or depressed mental status, and seizures. Methemoglobinemia and sulfhemoglobinemia usually are observed within a few hours of the overdose, but intravascular hemolysis may be delayed. The illness lasts several days. Clinical manifestations are more severe in patients with underlying medical conditions that may contribute to hypoxemia.

A. **Methemoglobinemia** (p 317) causes cyanosis and dyspnea. Drawn blood may appear "chocolate" brown when the methemoglobin level is greater than 15–20%. Because of the long half-life of dapsone and its metabolites, methemoglobinemia may persist for several days, requiring repeated antidotal treatment.

B. **Sulfhemoglobinemia** also decreases oxyhemoglobin saturation and is unresponsive to methylene blue. Sulfhemoglobinemia can produce a cyanotic appearance at a lower percentage of total hemoglobin compared with methemoglobin, but the amount of sulfhemoglobin generated is rarely more than 5%.

C. **Hemolysis** may be delayed in onset, usually 2–3 days after acute overdose.

D. **Chronic toxicity.** Therapeutic doses may affect vision, peripheral motor neuronal, renal and hepatic functions. **Dapsone hypersensitivity syndrome** (fever, rash, and hepatitis) occurs in about 2% patients within 6 weeks of starting treatment, and has a reported mortality rate of 11%.

IV. **Diagnosis.** Overdose should be suspected in cyanotic patients with elevated methemoglobin levels, especially if there is a history of dapsone use or a diagnosis that is likely to be treated with dapsone. Although there are many agents that can cause methemoglobinemia, there are very few that produce both detectable sulfhemoglobin and a prolonged, recurrent methemoglobinemia. Dapsone was the leading cause of methemoglobinemia in one retrospective review of patients in an American hospital.

A. **Specific levels.** Dapsone levels are not routinely available. When plasma samples are analyzed by HPLC or LC-MS/MS (liquid chromatography—tandem mass spectrometry), both dapsone and monoacetyl dapsone can be measured.

1. **Methemoglobinemia** (p 317) is suspected when a cyanotic patient fails to respond to high-flow oxygen or cyanosis persists despite a normal arterial Po_2. Conventional two-wavelength pulse oximetry is not a reliable indicator of oxygen saturation in patients with methemoglobinemia. Specific methemoglobin concentrations can be measured by using a multiwave cooximeter. Qualitatively, a drop of blood on white filter paper will appear brown (when directly compared with normal blood) if the methemoglobin level is greater than 15–20%.
2. ***Note:*** Administration of the antidote **methylene blue** (see Item V.B.1 below) can cause transient false elevation of the measured methemoglobin level (up to 15%).
3. **Sulfhemoglobin** is difficult to detect, in part because its spectrophotometric absorbance is similar to that of methemoglobin on the cooximeter. A blood sample will turn red if a crystal of potassium cyanide is added but will not if significant sulfhemoglobin is present.
4. The oxygen-carrying capacity of the blood is dependent not only on oxygen saturation but also on total hemoglobin concentration. Interpret methemoglobin and sulfhemoglobin levels with reference to the degree of anemia.

B. **Other useful laboratory studies** include CBC (with differential smear to look for reticulocytes and Heinz bodies), glucose, electrolytes, liver aminotransferases, bilirubin, renal function (BUN, creatinine), and arterial blood gases. Consider testing for G6PD deficiency.

V. **Treatment**

A. **Emergency and supportive measures**

1. Maintain an open airway and assist ventilation if needed (pp 1–7). Administer supplemental oxygen.
2. If hemolysis occurs, administer IV fluids and consider alkalinizing the urine, as for rhabdomyolysis (p 27), to mitigate risk for acute renal tubular necrosis. For severe hemolysis, blood transfusions may be required.
3. Mild symptoms may resolve without intervention, but this may take 2–3 days.

B. Specific drugs and antidotes

1. **Methylene blue** (p 579) is indicated in a symptomatic patient with a methemoglobin level greater than 20% or with lower levels if even minimal compromise of oxygen-carrying capacity is potentially harmful (eg, severe pneumonia, anemia, or myocardial ischemia). Conventionally, methylene blue has been given intermittently every 6–8 hours as needed during prolonged dapsone intoxications. However, intermittent administration can produce wide swings in methemoglobin levels over the course of treatment, which can aggravate erythrocyte oxidative stress and worsen hemolysis. Maintenance infusions have been reported to provide better and more even methemoglobin control.
   a. **Loading dose:** Give methylene blue, 1–2 mg/kg (0.1–0.2 mL/kg of 1% solution) IV over 5 minutes. Conditions allowing, administer in 1-mg/kg increments, allowing 30 minutes for response. The goal is improved cyanosis and a methemoglobin level preferably under 10%. Then start the maintenance infusion.
   b. **Maintenance infusion** (dapsone intoxications only): 0.1–0.25 mg/kg/h, depending on the effective loading dose. After 48 hours, pause treatment to determine if significant methemoglobinemia returns over a 15-hour period. If it does, give another partial loading dose, titrating to effect, and restart another maintenance infusion. Treatment is usually required for at least 2–3 days.
   c. Methylene blue is ineffective for sulfhemoglobin and is contraindicated in patients with G6PD deficiency due to the risk of hemolysis. Methylene blue doses over 7 mg/kg may worsen methemoglobinemia.
2. **Cimetidine** (p 532), an inhibitor of several CYP isoenzymes, can decrease the production of toxic metabolites.
   a. During chronic dapsone therapy, cimetidine improved patient tolerance and decreased methemoglobin levels at oral doses of 400 mg three times daily.
   b. To date, no evaluation of cimetidine in acute dapsone overdose has been performed. If considered after acute overdose, administration of activated charcoal would necessitate IV dosing.
3. Supplemental therapies, such as alpha-lipoic acid, ascorbic acid, and vitamin E, have been proposed as antioxidants for dapsone toxicity, but their efficacy is unproven.

C. Decontamination (p 50). Administer activated charcoal orally if conditions are appropriate (see Table I–38, p 54). Gastric lavage may be considered for a patient with a very large overdose (>75 mg/kg) presenting within 2–3 hours of ingestion, but is not necessary after small-to-moderate ingestions if activated charcoal can be given promptly.

D. Enhanced elimination (p 56)

1. **Repeat-dose activated charcoal** interrupts enterohepatic recirculation and can effectively reduce the dapsone half-life (from 77 to 13.5 hours in one report), but it should be used with caution in persons with severely altered mental status and discontinued if intestinal ileus occurs. Continue repeat-dose charcoal for 48–72 hours. Do ***not*** use preformulated charcoal and sorbitol combinations.
2. **Extracorporeal interventions** may be considered in a severe intoxication unresponsive to conventional treatment. **Hemodialysis** clears very little dapsone and metabolites because of high protein binding, but in one recent case report symptomatic improvement was observed. **Charcoal hemoperfusion** efficiently clears dapsone and reduces the plasma dapsone half-life to 1.5 hours in overdose. **Continuous venovenous hemofiltration (CVVH)** with regional citrate anticoagulation for 72 hours effectively reduced dapsone and metabolite half-life to 12.6 hours after overdose.

▶ DETERGENTS

Michael J. Walsh, PharmD

Detergents, familiar and indispensable products in the home, are synthetic surface active agents that are chemically classified as **anionic, nonionic,** or **cationic** (Table II–23). Most of these products also contain bleaching (chlorine-releasing), bacteriostatic (having a low concentration of a quaternary ammonium compound), or enzymatic agents. Accidental ingestion of detergents by children is very common, but severe toxicity rarely occurs. However, the introduction of concentrated, single-use laundry detergent packets ("pacs" or "pods") in 2012 has resulted in an increase in reported serious ingestions, including some deaths. Overall, laundry detergent packet exposures are more severe than exposures to laundry nonpacket products. In addition, laundry packet exposures are more severe than both dishwasher packet and nonpacket exposures.

I. **Mechanism of toxicity.** Detergents may precipitate and denature protein, are irritating to tissues, and have keratolytic and corrosive actions.
   A. **Anionic** and **nonionic** detergents are only mildly irritating, but **cationic** detergents are more hazardous because quaternary ammonium compounds may be caustic (benzalkonium chloride solutions of 10% have been reported to cause corrosive burns).
   B. **Low-phosphate** detergents and **electric dishwasher** soaps often contain alkaline corrosive agents such as sodium metasilicate, sodium carbonate, and sodium tripolyphosphate.
   C. The **enzyme-containing** detergents may cause skin irritation and have sensitizing properties; they may release bradykinin and histamine, causing bronchospasm.

II. **Toxic dose.** Mortality and serious morbidity are rare, but the nature of the toxic effect varies with the ingredients and concentration of the specific product. Cationic and dishwasher detergents are more dangerous than anionic and nonionic products. For benzalkonium chloride solutions, ingestion of 100–400 mg/kg has been fatal.

III. **Clinical presentation.** Immediate spontaneous vomiting often occurs after oral ingestion. Large ingestions may produce intractable vomiting, diarrhea, and hematemesis. Corrosive injury to the lips, mouth, pharynx, and upper GI tract can occur. Exposure to the eye may cause mild to serious corrosive injury, depending on the specific product. Dermal contact generally causes a mild erythema or rash. Ingestions of laundry packets are more likely to cause respiratory symptoms and CNS depression requiring endotracheal intubation.
   A. Phosphate-containing products may produce hypocalcemia, hypomagnesemia, tetany, and respiratory failure.
   B. Methemoglobinemia was reported in a 45-year-old woman after copious irrigation of a hydatid cyst with a 0.1% solution of cetrimide, a cationic detergent.

IV. **Diagnosis** is based on a history of exposure and prompt onset of vomiting. A sudsy or foaming mouth may also suggest exposure. In laundry packet ingestion, drooling and stridor have been reported.
   A. **Specific levels.** There are no specific blood or urine levels.
   B. **Other useful laboratory studies** include electrolytes, glucose, calcium, magnesium and phosphate (after ingestion of phosphate-containing products),

TABLE II–23. CATIONIC DETERGENTS

Pyridinium Compounds	Quaternary Ammonium Compounds	Quinolinium Compounds
Cetalkonium chloride	Benzalkonium chloride	Dequalinium chloride
Cetrimide	Benzethonium chloride	
Cetrimonium bromide		
Cetylpyridinium chloride		
Stearalkonium chloride		

and methemoglobin (cationic detergents). Consider chest x-ray if pulmonary symptoms.

V. Treatment

A. Emergency and supportive measures

1. In patients with protracted vomiting or diarrhea, administer IV fluids to correct dehydration and electrolyte imbalance (p 16).
2. If corrosive injury is suspected, consult a gastroenterologist for possible endoscopy. Ingestion of products containing greater than 5–10% cationic detergents is more likely to cause corrosive injury.

B. Specific drugs and antidotes. If symptomatic hypocalcemia occurs after ingestion of a phosphate-containing product, administer IV **calcium** (p 526). If methemoglobinemia occurs, administer **methylene blue** (p 579).

C. Decontamination (p 50)

1. **Ingestion.** Dilute orally with small amounts of water or milk. A significant ingestion is unlikely if spontaneous vomiting has not already occurred.
   a. Do ***not*** induce vomiting because of the risk for corrosive injury.
   b. Consider gentle gastric lavage with a small, flexible tube after very large ingestions of cationic, corrosive, or phosphate-containing detergents.
   c. Activated charcoal is not effective. Oral aluminum hydroxide can potentially bind phosphate in the GI tract.
2. **Eyes and skin.** Irrigate with copious amounts of tepid water or saline. Consult an ophthalmologist if eye pain persists or if there is significant corneal injury on fluorescein examination.

D. Enhanced elimination. There is no role for these procedures.

▶ DEXTROMETHORPHAN

Ilene B. Anderson, PharmD

Dextromethorphan is a common antitussive agent found in many over-the-counter (OTC) cough and cold preparations. Dextromethorphan is often found in combination products containing antihistamines (p 110), decongestants (p 394), ethanol (p 231), or acetaminophen (p 73). *Common combination products containing dextromethorphan* include Coricidin HBP Cough & Cold Tablets, Robitussin DM, and NyQuil Nighttime Cold Medicine. Dextromethorphan is well tolerated at therapeutic doses, and serious toxicity rarely occurs, even with moderate-to-high doses. However, major toxicity and death have been reported, caused either by dextromethorphan as a sole agent or more commonly by coingestants, drug–drug interactions, or genetic polymorphism. Intentional abuse, especially among adolescents and young adults, has been a continuing problem owing to the hallucinogenic potential at high doses. *Common slang terms* include "triple C," "CCC," "skittles," "robo," "DXM," and "dex." "Crystal Dex" and "DXemon Juice" refer to dextromethorphan extracted from the other ingredients in OTC cold medications using simple home acid–base extraction techniques.

I. Mechanism of toxicity. Although dextromethorphan is structurally related to opioids (its active metabolite is the *d*-isomer of levorphanol) and it has antitussive activity approximately equal to that of codeine, it has no apparent activity at mu or kappa receptors and does not produce a typical opioid syndrome in overdose.

A. Dextromethorphan is metabolized in the liver by the cytochrome P450 isoenzyme CYP2D6 to dextrorphan. Both dextromethorphan and dextrorphan antagonize *N*-methyl-D-aspartate (NMDA) glutamate receptors, although dextrorphan is more potent and primarily responsible for the psychoactive effects of high-dose dextromethorphan. Genetic polymorphism of CYP2D6 may explain the variable clinical responses reported; extensive metabolizers are more likely to experience the "desirable" psychoactive effects with recreational use.

B. Dextromethorphan and dextrorphan inhibit reuptake of serotonin and may lead to **serotonin syndrome** (p 21), especially in patients taking agents that increase serotonin levels, such as selective serotonin reuptake inhibitors (p 104) and monoamine oxidase inhibitors (p 326). Serotoninergic effects, as well as NMDA glutamate receptor inhibition, may explain the acute and chronic abuse potential of dextromethorphan.

C. Dextromethorphan hydrobromide can cause **bromide** poisoning (p 166).

D. Many of the combination preparations contain **acetaminophen,** and overdose or abuse may result in hepatotoxicity (p 73).

E. **Pharmacokinetics.** Dextromethorphan is well absorbed orally, and effects are often apparent within 15–30 minutes (peak, 2–2.5 hours). The volume of distribution is approximately 5–6 L/kg. The rate of metabolism is dependent on CYP2D6 polymorphism. Dextromethorphan has a plasma half-life of about 3–4 hours in extensive metabolizers versus a half-life exceeding 24 hours in slow metabolizers (about 10% of the population). In addition, dextromethorphan competitively inhibits CYP2D6-mediated metabolism of other drugs, leading to many potential drug interactions (see also Table II–66, p 462).

II. **Toxic dose.** Establishing a clear correlation between dose and clinical effects is problematic, given wide patient variability, genetic polymorphism, and the fact that most of the scientific literature is comprised of self-reported poisonings involving combination products lacking laboratory confirmation. Moderate symptoms usually occur when the amount of dextromethorphan exceeds 10 mg/kg. Severe poisoning is associated with ingestions of more than 20–30 mg/kg. The usual recommended adult daily dose of dextromethorphan is 60–120 mg/d; children age 2–5 years can be given up to 30 mg/d.

III. **Clinical presentation**

A. **Mild-to-moderate intoxication.** Nausea, vomiting, nystagmus, mydriasis or miosis, tachycardia, hypertension, dizziness, lethargy, agitation, ataxia, euphoria, dysphoria, and auditory and visual hallucinations ("CEVs," or closed-eye visualizations, often described as color changes) have been reported.

B. **Severe poisoning.** Disorientation, stupor, psychosis, dissociative hallucinations, seizures, coma, hyperthermia, QT prolongation, respiratory depression, pulmonary and cerebral edema, and death can occur.

C. **Serotonin syndrome** (p 21). Severe hyperthermia, muscle rigidity, altered mental status, and hypertension may occur, especially with concomitant use of agents that increase serotonin or catecholamine levels as well as CYP2D6 inhibitors that may increase dextromethorphan levels.

D. **Withdrawal syndrome.** Abdominal pain, vomiting, diarrhea, tachycardia, hypertension, depression, dysphoria, diaphoresis, insomnia, tremor, myalgias, restlessness, and drug craving have been reported.

E. **Chronic poisoning.** Psychosis, mania, and cognitive deterioration have been reported following chronic DXM abuse. Chronic ingestion of the hydrobromide salt has resulted in bromism (see p 166).

IV. **Diagnosis** should be considered with ingestion of any over-the-counter cough suppressant, especially when the clinical presentation is consistent and toxicology screening is positive for phencyclidine (PCP; dextromethorphan cross-reacts with many PCP immunoassays). Because dextromethorphan often is combined with other ingredients (eg, antihistamines, phenylpropanolamine, or acetaminophen), suspect mixed ingestion.

A. **Specific levels.** Assays exist for serum and urinalysis but are not generally available. In five teenage fatalities (ages 17–19 years) secondary to recreational dextromethorphan use, postmortem blood concentrations ranged from 950–3,230 ng/mL (median, 1,890 ng/mL). Despite its structural similarity to opioids, dextromethorphan is not likely to produce a false-positive urine opioid immunoassay screen. However, it may produce a false-positive result on methadone and PCP immunoassays. Dextromethorphan is readily detected by comprehensive urine toxicology screening.

B. Other useful laboratory studies include electrolytes, glucose, and arterial blood gases (if respiratory depression is suspected). Blood ethanol and acetaminophen levels should be obtained if those drugs are contained in the ingested product.

V. Treatment

A. Emergency and supportive measures. Most patients with mild symptoms (ie, restlessness, ataxia, or mild drowsiness) can be observed for 4–6 hours and discharged if their condition is improving.

1. Maintain an open airway and assist ventilation if needed (pp 1–7).

2. Treat seizures (p 23) and coma (p 18) if they occur.

B. Specific drugs and antidotes. Although **naloxone** (p 584) has been reported to be effective in doses of 0.06–0.4 mg, other cases have failed to respond to doses up to 2.4 mg.

C. Decontamination (p 50). Administer activated charcoal orally if conditions are appropriate (see Table I–38, p 54). Gastric lavage is not necessary after small-to-moderate ingestions if activated charcoal can be given promptly.

D. Enhanced elimination. The volume of distribution of dextromethorphan is very large, and there is no role for enhanced removal procedures.

▶ DIABETIC DRUGS

Susan Kim-Katz, PharmD

Recent advances have resulted in a dramatic increase in the number and types of drugs used to manage diabetes. These agents can be divided broadly into parenteral and oral drugs. Table II–24 lists the various available antidiabetic agents. Metformin is also discussed in a separate chapter (see p 313). Other drugs and poisons can also cause hypoglycemia (see Table I–25, p 36).

TABLE II–24. DIABETIC DRUGS[a]

Agent	Onset (h)	Peak (h)	Duration[b] (h)	Hypoglycemia[c]
Insulins				
Regular insulin	0.5–1	2–3	8–12	Y
Regular insulin Inhaled (Afrezza)		0.9	3	Y
Rapid insulin zinc (semilente)	0.5	4–7	12–16	Y
Insulin lispro (Humalog)	0.25	0.5–1.5	6–8	Y
Insulin aspart (Novolog)	0.25	1–3	3–5	Y
Insulin glulisine (Apidra)	0.3	0.6–1	5	Y
Isophane insulin (NPH)	1–2	8–12	18–24	Y
Insulin zinc (lente)	1–2	8–12	18–24	Y
Insulin glargine (Lantus)	1.5	Sustained effect	22–24	Y
Insulin detemir (Levemir)	1	6–8	20	Y
Extended zinc insulin (ultralente)	4–8	16–18	36	Y
Protamine zinc insulin (PZI)	4–8	14–20	36	Y
Amylin analog				
Pramlintide acetate (Symlin)		0.3–0.5	3	N

(*continued*)

TABLE II–24. DIABETIC DRUGS[a] (CONTINUED)

Agent	Onset (h)	Peak (h)	Duration[b] (h)	Hypoglycemia[c]
GLP-1 agonists				
Albiglutide (Tanzeum)		3–5 days	[Half-life 5 days]	+/–
Exenatide (Byetta)		2	6–8	+/–
Exenatide (Bydureon, extended-release formulation)		Biphasic: 2 weeks then 6–7 weeks	10 weeks	+/–
Liraglutide (Victoza)		8–12	[Half-life 13 h]	+/–
Sulfonylureas				
Acetohexamide	2	4	12–24	Y
Chlorpropamide	1	3–6	24–72[b]	Y
Glimepiride	2–3		24	Y
Glipizide [extended-release form]	0.5 [2–3]	1–2 [6–12]	<24 [45]	Y
Glyburide [micronized form]	0.5	4 [2–3]	24[b]	Y
Tolazamide	1	4–6	14–20	Y
Tolbutamide	1	5–8	6–12	Y
Meglitinides				
Nateglinide (Starlix)	0.25	1–2	[Half-life 1.5–3 h]	Y
Repaglinide (Prandin)	0.5	1–1.5	[Half-life 1–1.5 h]	Y
Biguanide				
Metformin (see p 313)		2	[Half-life 2.5–6 h]	+/–
Alpha-glucosidase inhibitors				
Acarbose (Precose)		N/A (<2% of an oral dose absorbed systemically)		N
Miglitol (Glyset)		2–3	[Half-life 2 h]	N
Glitazones (thiazolidinediones)				
Pioglitazone (Actos)		2–4	[Half-life 3–7 h]	N
Rosiglitazone (Avandia)		1–3.5	[Half-life 3–4 h]	N
Dipeptidyl peptidase-4 inhibitors				
Alogliptin (Nesina)		1–2	[Half-life 21 h]	N
Linagliptin (Tradjenta)		1.5	[Half-life >100 h]	N
Sitagliptin (Januvia)		1–4	[Half-life 12.4 h]	+/–
Saxagliptin (Onglyza)			[Half-life 2.5 h]	N
Sodium-glucose cotransporter 2 inhibitors				
Canagliflozen (Invokana)		1–2	[Half-life 10.6-13.1 h]	N
Dapagliflozen (Farxiga)		2	[Half-life 12.9 h]	N

[a]See also Table II–66, p 462.
[b]Duration of hypoglycemic effects after overdose may be much longer, especially with glyburide, chlorpropamide, and extended-release products (case report of 45-hour duration in a 6-year-old child after ingestion of extended-release glipizide).
[c]Hypoglycemia likely after an acute overdose as a single agent.

I. **Mechanism of toxicity**

A. **Parenteral agents**

1. **Insulin.** Blood glucose is lowered directly by the stimulation of cellular uptake and metabolism of glucose. Cellular glucose uptake is accompanied by an intracellular shift of potassium and magnesium. Insulin also promotes glycogen formation and lipogenesis. **Insulin** products are mostly given by the parenteral route. An orally inhaled delivery system for regular insulin was recently approved in the United States. All insulin produce effects similar to those of endogenous insulin; they differ in antigenicity and in onset and duration of effect.

2. **Amylin analogs. Pramlintide** is a synthetic analog of amylin, a peptide hormone synthesized by and excreted from pancreatic beta cells along with insulin during the postprandial period. Amylin slows gastric emptying and suppresses glucagon secretion.

3. **Glucagon-like Peptide 1 (GLP-1) Receptor Agonists.** GLP-1 is released from the intestines in response to oral glucose intake. Stimulation of the GLP-1 receptors in pancreatic beta cells leads to increased insulin release in the presence of elevated glucose concentrations, while glucagon secretion is blocked.

   a. **Exenatide** is a GLP-1 mimetic that improves glycemic control through a combination of mechanisms.

   b. **Liraglutide,** an analog of human GLP-1, is a GLP-1 receptor agonist.

   c. **Albiglutide** is comprised of two copies of modified human GLP-1 fused to human albumin, allowing for once-weekly injections.

B. **Oral agents**

1. **Sulfonylureas** lower blood glucose primarily by stimulating endogenous pancreatic insulin secretion and secondarily by enhancing peripheral insulin receptor sensitivity and reducing glycogenolysis.

2. **Meglitinides** also increase pancreatic insulin release and can cause hypoglycemia in overdose.

3. **Biguanides.** Metformin (see p 313) decreases hepatic glucose production (gluconeogenesis) and intestinal absorption of glucose while increasing peripheral glucose uptake and utilization. It does not stimulate insulin release.

4. **Alpha-glucosidase inhibitors** delay the digestion of ingested carbohydrates, reducing postprandial blood glucose concentrations.

5. **Glitazones** decrease hepatic glucose output and improve target cell response to insulin. Hepatotoxicity has been reported with chronic therapy for all the drugs in this class and led to removal of troglitazone from the US market.

6. **Dipeptidyl peptidase-4 (DDP-4) inhibitors.** Incretin hormones are rapidly inactivated by the enzyme DDP-4. Inhibition of these enzymes produces increased and prolonged active incretin levels, leading to increased insulin release and decreased glucagon levels in the circulation in a glucose-dependent manner.

7. **Sodium-glucose co-transporter 2 inhibitors (SGLT2).** Expressed in the proximal renal tubules, SGLT2 is responsible for the majority of the reabsorption of filtered glucose from the tubular lumen. Inhibition of SGLT2 reduces reabsorption of filtered glucose and lowers the renal threshold for glucose, increasing urinary glucose excretion.

8. ***Note:*** Although alpha-glucosidase inhibitors, glitazones, GLP-1 agonists, DDP-4 inhibitors and SGLT2 inhibitors are not likely to cause hypoglycemia after an acute overdose, they may contribute to the hypoglycemic effects of sulfonylureas, meglitinides, or insulin. Metformin (p 313) inhibits gluconeogenesis, and there are a few reports of hypoglycemia after overdose with this agent even when taken alone.

C. **Pharmacokinetics** (see Tables II–24 and II–66)

II. Toxic dose

A. Insulin.

1. Severe hypoglycemic coma and permanent neurologic sequelae have occurred after injections of 800–3,200 units of insulin. Deliberate subcutaneous injection of 800 units of insulin lispro and 3,800 units of insulin glargine by a diabetic adult resulted in prolonged hypoglycemia. Plasma insulin levels returned to normal at 108 hours. A 26-year-old type 1 diabetic male who injected 4,800 units of insulin glargine and was treated with approximately 800 g per day of glucose supplementation developed acute hepatic injury. On day 4, a depot of insulin was excised from the patient's abdominal wall, with subsequent reduction in glucose requirements and improvement in liver function.
2. Orally administered insulin is poorly absorbed and is generally not toxic. However, intentional ingestion of 3,000 units of insulin aspart, lispro, and glargine produced symptomatic hypoglycemia within 1 hour in a nondiabetic 51-year-old male.
3. Drug interactions: Albuterol increased the absorption of orally inhaled insulin by 25% in patients with asthma.

B. Pramlintide. Hypoglycemia is not expected from the drug alone but is possible when coadministered with other hypoglycemic agents. A 10-mg dose in healthy volunteers caused nausea, vomiting, vasodilation, and dizziness.

C. Deliberate injection of 1,800 mcg (90 times the maximum daily dose) of **exenatide** resulted in sustained nausea for 24 hours, during which the patient required insulin for the management of hyperglycemia. Overdose of 17.4 mg of **liraglutide** (10 times the maximum recommended dose) caused severe nausea and vomiting. Hypoglycemia was not reported.

D. Sulfonylureas. Toxicity depends on the agent and the total amount ingested. Toxicity may also occur owing to drug interactions, resulting in impaired elimination of the oral agent.

1. **Ingestion of a single tablet** of chlorpropamide (250 mg), glipizide (5 mg), or glyburide (2.5 mg) in each case produced hypoglycemia in children 1–4 years old. Two 500-mg tablets of acetohexamide caused hypoglycemic coma in an adult. In a 79-year-old nondiabetic person, 5 mg of glyburide caused hypoglycemic coma.
2. **Interactions** with the following drugs may increase the risk for hypoglycemia: other hypoglycemic agents, fluoroquinolones (gatifloxacin and levofloxacin), sulfonamides, propranolol, salicylates, clofibrate, probenecid, pentamidine, valproic acid, dicumarol, cimetidine, monoamine oxidase (MAO) inhibitors, and alcohol. In addition, co-ingestion of alcohol may occasionally produce a disulfiram-like interaction (p 226).
3. **Hepatic** or **renal insufficiency** may impair drug elimination and result in hypoglycemia.

E. Meglitinides. A 4-mg dose of **repaglinide** produced hypoglycemia in a nondiabetic 18-year-old. Ingestion of 3,420 mg of **nateglinide** in a nondiabetic adult resulted in hypoglycemia lasting 6 hours.

F. DDP-4 Inhibitors. In a review of 650 cases of DDP-4 inhibitor ingestions, 3 patients, including 2 nondiabetics, developed hypoglycemia. A 27-year-old female who ingested 700 mg of sitagliptin complained of abdominal discomfort but did not become hypoglycemic. A 70-year-old female remained asymptomatic after ingestion of 1,800 mg of sitagliptin.

G. Metformin. See p 313.

III. Clinical presentation

A. Hypoglycemia may be delayed in onset, depending on the agent used and the route of administration (ie, subcutaneous vs. intravenous). Manifestations of hypoglycemia include agitation, confusion, coma, seizures, tachycardia, and diaphoresis. Serum potassium and magnesium levels may also be depressed.

Note: In patients receiving beta-adrenergic–blocking agents (p 158), many of the manifestations of hypoglycemia (tachycardia, diaphoresis) may be blunted or absent.

B. **SGLT2 inhibitors** may cause hypotension due to intravascular volume depletion, and elevations in serum potassium, magnesium, and phosphate may occur.

C. **Metformin** can cause severe lactic acidosis (see p 313), and occasionally hypoglycemia.

IV. **Diagnosis.** Overdose involving a sulfonylurea, meglitinide, or insulin should be suspected in any patient with hypoglycemia. Other causes of hypoglycemia that should be considered include alcohol ingestion (especially in children) and fulminant hepatic failure.

A. **Specific levels**

1. Serum concentrations of many agents can be determined in commercial toxicology laboratories but have little utility in acute clinical management.
2. Exogenously administered animal insulin can be distinguished from endogenous insulin (ie, in a patient with hypoglycemia caused by insulinoma) by determination of C-peptide (present with endogenous insulin secretion).

B. **Other useful laboratory studies** include glucose, electrolytes, magnesium, and ethanol. If metformin is suspected, obtain a venous blood lactate level (gray-top tube).

V. **Treatment.** Observe asymptomatic patients for a minimum of 8 hours after ingestion of a sulfonylurea. Because of the potential for a delay in onset of hypoglycemia if the patient has received food or IV glucose, it is prudent to observe children overnight or otherwise ensure that finger stick blood glucose checks can be obtained frequently at home for up to 24 hours.

A. **Emergency and supportive measures**

1. Maintain an open airway and assist ventilation if necessary (pp 1–7).
2. Treat coma (p 18) and seizures (p 23) if they occur.
3. Obtain finger stick blood glucose levels every 1–2 hours until stabilized.
4. Monitor serum potassium, magnesium, and phosphate in patients with SGLT-2 inhibitor overdose.

B. **Specific drugs and antidotes**

1. If the patient is hypoglycemic, administer concentrated **glucose** (p 562) orally or IV. In adults, give 50% dextrose ($D_{50}W$), 1–2 mL/kg; in children, use 25% dextrose ($D_{25}W$), 2–4 mL/kg. Give repeated glucose boluses and administer 5–10% dextrose (D_5–D_{10}) as needed to maintain normal serum glucose concentrations (60–110 mg/dL).
2. For patients with a sulfonylurea or meglitinide overdose, consider use of **octreotide** (p 596) if 5% dextrose infusions do not maintain satisfactory glucose concentrations.
3. Maintaining serum glucose concentrations above 90–100 mg/dL for the first 12 hours of therapy or longer is often necessary to prevent recurrent hypoglycemia. However, once hypoglycemia resolves (usually 12–24 hours after the ingestion) and the patient no longer requires dextrose infusions, serum glucose concentrations should be allowed to normalize. Follow serum glucose levels closely for several hours after the last dose of dextrose.

C. **Decontamination** (p 50)

1. **Oral agents.** Administer activated charcoal orally if conditions are appropriate (see Table I–38, p 54). Gastric lavage is not necessary after small-to-moderate ingestions if activated charcoal can be given promptly.
2. **Insulin.** Orally ingested insulin is very poorly absorbed (<1% bioavailability), thus gut decontamination is not usually necessary.

D. **Enhanced elimination**

1. **Sulfonylureas.** Alkalinization of the urine increases the renal elimination of chlorpropamide. Forced diuresis and dialysis procedures are of no known value for other hypoglycemic agents. The high degree of protein binding of

the sulfonylureas suggests that dialysis procedures would not generally be effective. However, charcoal hemoperfusion reduced the serum half-life of chlorpropamide in a patient with renal failure.

2. **Metformin** (see p 313) can be removed by hemodialysis.

▶ DIGOXIN AND OTHER CARDIAC GLYCOSIDES

Neal L. Benowitz, MD

Cardiac glycosides and related cardenolides are found in several plants, including digitalis, oleander, foxglove, *Cerbera spp* (pong pong), lily of the valley, red squill, dogbane, and rhododendron, and in toad venom (bufadienolides, *Bufo* species), which may be found in some Chinese herbal medications and herbal aphrodisiacs. Cardiac glycosides are used therapeutically in tablet form as digoxin and digitoxin. Digoxin is also available in liquid-filled capsules with greater bioavailability.

I. **Mechanism of toxicity**

A. Cardiac glycosides inhibit the function of the sodium-potassium-ATPase pump. After acute overdose, this results in hyperkalemia (with chronic intoxication, the serum potassium level is usually normal or low owing to concurrent diuretic therapy).

B. Direct effects and potentiation of vagal tone result in slowing of the sinus rate and decreased sinus and atrioventricular (AV) node conduction velocity.

C. Increased atrial and ventricular automaticity occurs because of accumulation of intracellular calcium, enhanced diastolic depolarization, and development of afterdepolarizations. These effects are augmented by hypokalemia and hypomagnesemia.

D. **Pharmacokinetics.** The bioavailability of digoxin ranges from 60% to 80%; for digitoxin, more than 90% is absorbed. The volume of distribution (Vd) of digoxin is very large (5–10 L/kg), whereas for digitoxin the Vd is small (~0.5 L/kg). Peak effects occur after a delay of 6–12 hours. The elimination half-life of digoxin is 30–50 hours, and is dependent on renal function. The elimination of digitoxin is via the liver; its half-life is 5–8 days (owing to enterohepatic recirculation; see also Table II–66, p 462).

E. **Drug interactions.** A number of drugs that are often co-administered with digitalis inhibit its metabolism and/or its cellular transport (via P-glycoprotein), increasing serum levels, and may induce toxicity. These include amiodarone, verapamil, diltiazem, quinidine, macrolide antibiotics, and others.

II. **Toxic dose.** Acute ingestion of as little as 1 mg of digoxin in a child or 3 mg of digoxin in an adult can result in serum concentrations well above the therapeutic range. More than these amounts of digoxin and other cardiac glycosides may be found in just a few leaves of oleander or foxglove. Generally, children appear to be more resistant than adults to the cardiotoxic effects of cardiac glycosides.

III. **Clinical presentation.** Intoxication may occur after acute accidental or suicidal ingestion or with chronic therapy. Signs and symptoms depend on the chronicity of the intoxication.

A. With **acute overdose**, nausea, vomiting, hyperkalemia, and cardiac arrhythmias are often seen. Bradyarrhythmias include sinus bradycardia, sinoatrial arrest, second- or third-degree AV block, and asystole. Tachyarrhythmias include paroxysmal atrial tachycardia with AV block, accelerated junctional tachycardia, ventricular bigeminy, ventricular tachycardia, bidirectional ventricular tachycardia, and ventricular fibrillation.

B. With **chronic intoxication**, nausea, anorexia, abdominal pain, visual disturbances (flashing lights, halos, green-yellow perceptual impairment), weakness, fatigue, sinus bradycardia, atrial fibrillation with slowed ventricular response rate or junctional escape rhythm, and ventricular arrhythmias (ventricular bigeminy or trigeminy, ventricular tachycardia, bidirectional tachycardia, and ventricular fibrillation) are common. Accelerated junctional tachycardia and paroxysmal atrial tachycardia with block are seen frequently. Hypokalemia and hypomagnesemia from chronic diuretic use may be evident and appear to worsen the tachyarrhythmias. Mental status changes are common in the elderly and include confusion, depression, and hallucinations.

IV. Diagnosis is based on a history of recent overdose or characteristic arrhythmias (eg, bidirectional tachycardia and accelerated junctional rhythm) in a patient receiving chronic therapy. Hyperkalemia suggests acute ingestion but also may be seen with very severe chronic poisoning. Serum potassium levels higher than 5.5 mEq/L are associated with severe poisoning, with the extent of hyperkalemia a predictor of mortality.

A. Specific levels. Therapeutic levels of digoxin are 0.5–1 ng/mL, and those of digitoxin are 10–30 ng/mL.

1. Stat serum digoxin and/or digitoxin levels are recommended, although they may not correlate accurately with the severity of intoxication. This is especially true after acute ingestion, when the serum level is high for 6–12 hours before tissue distribution is complete. Serum levels taken more than 6 hours after ingestion are better correlated with digoxin effects.
2. After use of digitalis-specific antibodies, the immunoassay digoxin level is falsely markedly elevated.
3. The presence of human anti-mouse antibodies may falsely elevate digoxin levels in some patients if older immunoassays are used. Levels as high as 45.9 ng/mL have been reported.
4. Even in the absence of digoxin use, false-positive digoxin can also occur for some immunoassays for selected patient populations (uremia, hypertension, liver disease, and preeclampsia) owing to the presence of digoxin-like immunoreactive factor (DLIF).

B. Other useful laboratory studies include electrolytes, BUN, creatinine, serum magnesium, and ECG and ECG monitoring.

V. Treatment

A. Emergency and supportive measures

1. Maintain an open airway and assist ventilation if necessary (pp 1–7).
2. Monitor the patient closely for at least 12–24 hours after significant ingestion because of delayed tissue distribution.
3. Treat **hyperkalemia** (p 39) with digoxin-specific antibodies (see below); calcium (calcium gluconate 10%, 10–20 mL or 0.2–0.3 mL/kg, or calcium chloride 10%, 5–10 mL or 0.1–0.2 mL/kg, slowly IV); sodium bicarbonate, 1 mEq/kg; glucose, 0.5 g/kg IV, with insulin, 0.1 U/kg IV; and/or sodium polystyrene sulfonate (Kayexalate), 0.5 g/kg orally.
   a. ***Note:*** Although it is widely recommended that calcium be avoided in patients with cardiac glycoside toxicity because of concern that it will worsen ventricular arrhythmias, this warning is based on old and very weak case reports and is not substantiated by animal studies. Calcium is the drug of first choice for life-threatening cardiac toxicity due to hyperkalemia.
   b. Mild hyperkalemia may actually protect against tachyarrhythmias.
4. Hypokalemia and hypomagnesemia should be corrected, as these may contribute to cardiac toxicity.
5. Treat **bradycardia** or **heart block** with atropine, 0.5–2 mg IV (p 512). Temporary transvenous cardiac pacemaker may be needed for persistent symptomatic bradycardia, but because a pacemaker may trigger serious arrhythmias in patients with digitalis toxicity, pacing is recommended only after failure or unavailability of digoxin-specific antibodies.
6. **Ventricular tachyarrhythmias** may respond to correction of low potassium or magnesium. Lidocaine (p 573) and phenytoin (p 608) have been used,

but digoxin-specific antibody is the preferred treatment for life-threatening arrhythmias. Avoid quinidine, procainamide, and other type Ia or type Ic antiarrhythmic drugs.

B. **Specific drugs and antidotes.** Fab fragments of **digoxin-specific antibodies** (eg, DigiFab, p 542) are highly effective in reversing digoxin toxicity and are indicated for significant poisoning. This includes hyperkalemia (>5 mEq/L), symptomatic arrhythmias, high-degree AV block, ventricular arrhythmias, and hemodynamic instability. Digoxin antibodies should also be considered in digoxin-toxic patients with renal failure and for prophylactic treatment in a patient with massive oral overdose and high serum levels. Digoxin antibodies rapidly bind to digoxin and, to a lesser extent, digitoxin and other cardiac glycosides. The inactive complex that is formed is excreted rapidly in the urine. Details of dose calculation and infusion rate are given on p 542.

C. **Decontamination** (p 50). Administer activated charcoal orally if conditions are appropriate (see Table I–38, p 54). Gastric lavage is not necessary after small-to-moderate ingestions if activated charcoal can be given promptly.

D. **Enhanced elimination**

1. Because of its large volume of distribution, **digoxin** is not effectively removed by dialysis or hemoperfusion. Repeat-dose activated charcoal or cholestyramine may be useful in patients with severe renal insufficiency, in whom clearance of digoxin is markedly diminished.
2. **Digitoxin** has a small volume of distribution and also undergoes extensive enterohepatic recirculation, and its elimination can be markedly enhanced by repeat-dose charcoal or cholestyramine.

▶ DIOXINS

Stephen C. Born, MD, MPH

Polychlorinated dibenzodioxins (PCDDs) and dibenzofurans (PCDFs) are a group of highly toxic substances commonly known as dioxins. Dioxins are not produced commercially. They are formed during the production of certain organochlorines (eg, trichlorophenoxyacetic acid [2,4,5-T], hexachlorophene, pentachlorophenol); and by the combustion of these and other compounds, such as polychlorinated biphenyls (PCBs [p 393]), as well as the incineration of medical and municipal waste. Agent Orange, an herbicide used by the United States during the Vietnam War, contained dioxins (most importantly, 2,3,7,8-tetrachlorodibenzo-*p*-dioxin [TCDD], the most toxic and extensively researched dioxin) as contaminants. There are 75 PCDD and 135 PCDF congeners. Some PCBs have biological activity similar to that of dioxins and are identified as "dioxin-like." The most common route of exposure to dioxins in the United States is through dietary consumption.

I. **Mechanism of toxicity.** Dioxins are highly lipid soluble and are concentrated in fat, and they bioaccumulate in the food chain. Dioxins are known to bind to the aryl hydrocarbon receptor protein (AhR) in cytoplasm, form a heterodimer with nuclear proteins, and induce transcription of multiple genes. AhR activation by dioxins causes disruption of biochemical pathways involved in development and homeostasis. As a result, the timing of exposure as well as dose determines toxicity. Dioxins also have endocrine disruptor effects, and exposure may result in reproductive and developmental defects, immunotoxicity, and liver damage. Some dioxins are known animal carcinogens and are classified as human carcinogens by the EPA, the National Toxicology Program, and the IARC. TCDD is classified by IARC as a Group 1 human carcinogen. Human exposure leads to an overall increase in the rates of all cancers in exposed individuals.

II. **Toxic dose.** Dioxins are extremely potent animal toxins. With the discovery of significant noncancer developmental abnormalities in environmentally exposed animals, the "no effect" level for exposure to dioxins is under reevaluation and is likely to be within an order of magnitude of current human dietary exposure. The oral 50% lethal dose (LD_{50}) in animals varies from 0.0006 to 0.045 mg/kg. Daily dermal exposure to 10–30 ppm in oil or 100–3,000 ppm in soil produces toxicity in animals. Chloracne is likely with daily dermal exposure exceeding 100 ppm. The greatest source of exposure for the general population is food, which is contaminated in minute quantities, usually measured in picograms (trillionths of a gram). Higher exposures have occurred through industrial accidents or intentional poisoning.

III. Clinical presentation

A. Acute symptoms after exposure include irritation of the skin, eyes, and mucous membranes and nausea, vomiting, and myalgias.

B. After a latency period that may be prolonged (up to several weeks or more), chloracne, porphyria cutanea tarda, hirsutism, or hyperpigmentation may occur. Elevated levels of hepatic transaminases and blood lipids may be found. Polyneuropathies with sensory impairment and lower extremity motor weakness have been reported. The Ukrainian president, Viktor Yushchenko, was poisoned with TCDD in 2004 and exhibited many of the classic signs and symptoms, including chloracne.

C. Death in laboratory animals occurs a few weeks after a lethal dose and is caused by a "wasting syndrome" characterized by reduced food intake and loss of body weight. Death from acute toxicity in humans is rare, even in cases of intentional poisoning.

IV. Diagnosis is difficult and rests mainly on a history of exposure; the presence of chloracne (which is considered pathognomonic for exposure to dioxins and related compounds) provides strong supporting evidence. Although many products previously contaminated with dioxins are no longer produced in the United States, exposures to PCDDs and PCDFs occur during many types of chemical fires, and the possibility of exposure can cause considerable public and individual anxiety. Dioxins are classified by the WHO as among the most environmentally persistent of all organic pollutants.

A. Specific levels. It is difficult and expensive to detect dioxins in human blood or tissue, and there is no established correlation with symptoms. There are many congeners of PCDDs, PCDFs, and PCBs; the individual contribution of each one to toxicity is assessed by using toxic equivalence factors (TEFs) established by the World Health Organization, based on relative potency estimates for each congener (TCDD by definition has a TEF of 1). Testing is not clinically indicated unless there has been a massive exposure. The WHO is a source of information regarding certified laboratories outside the United States; testing in the United States is performed by the CDC/NCEH (National Center for Environmental Health). As a result of more stringent controls over environmental exposures, the human body burden of dioxins has decreased over the last 30 years. Unexposed persons have a mean of 5.38 pg of 2,3,7,8-TCDD per gram of serum lipid, compared with workers producing trichlorophenols, who had a mean of 220 pg/g. The highest recorded level is 144,000 pg/g of blood fat in a patient with few adverse health effects other than chloracne.

B. Other useful laboratory studies include glucose, electrolytes, BUN, creatinine, liver transaminases, CBC, and uroporphyrins (if porphyria is suspected).

V. Treatment

A. Emergency and supportive measures. Treat skin, eye, and respiratory irritation symptomatically.

B. Specific drugs and antidotes. There is no specific antidote.

C. Decontamination (p 50)

1. **Inhalation.** Remove victims from exposure and give supplemental oxygen if available.
2. **Eyes and skin.** Remove contaminated clothing and wash affected skin with copious soap and water; irrigate exposed eyes with copious tepid water or

saline. Personnel involved in decontamination should wear protective gear appropriate to the suspected level of contamination.

3. **Ingestion.** Administer activated charcoal if conditions are appropriate (see Table I–38, p 54). Gastric emptying is not necessary if activated charcoal can be given promptly.

D. **Enhanced elimination.** Since dioxins are lipid soluble, lactation significantly enhances elimination. Elimination of dioxins may be enhanced through administration of **olestra,** a nonabsorbable fat substitute that increases fecal excretion. Low-density lipoprotein (LPL)-apheresis has also been used to lower body burden of dioxins, but entails risk. Unfortunately, clinical studies of methods to enhance elimination have been extremely limited and are not conclusive; however, olestra administration has lowered the half-life of TCDD from 5–10 years to 1–2 years.

▶ DISULFIRAM

Richard J. Geller, MD, MPH, MS

Disulfiram (tetraethylthiuram disulfide [CASRN 97-77-8], or Antabuse) is an antioxidant industrial chemical produced since 1881 for the vulcanization of rubber. Introduced in the 1930s into clinical medicine as a vermicide and scabicide, it has been used in the United States since 1951 as a drug in the treatment of alcoholism. Ingestion of ethanol while taking disulfiram causes a well-defined unpleasant reaction, the fear of which provides a negative incentive to drink alcohol. Clinical toxicity is caused by overdose or occurs as a result of a disulfiram–ethanol drug interaction. Disulfiram is being investigated for the treatment of cocaine addiction, drug-resistant fungal infections, and malignancies. The toxicities resulting from disulfiram overdose differ from those of disulfiram–ethanol interaction.

I. **Mechanism of toxicity**

A. Disulfiram causes inhibition of two critical enzymes. It binds irreversibly to aldehyde dehydrogenase, leading to accumulation of toxic acetaldehyde after ethanol ingestion. Inhibition of dopamine beta-hydroxylase (necessary for norepinephrine synthesis from dopamine) results in norepinephrine depletion at presynaptic sympathetic nerve endings, leading to vasodilation and orthostatic hypotension. The resulting surplus of dopamine may potentiate psychosis and provides a theoretic basis for the use of disulfiram in treating cocaine dependence.

B. Disulfiram is metabolized via cytochrome P450-mediated phase I oxidation, and by phase II methylation and glucuronidation. A metabolite is carbon disulfide (see also p 181), which may play a role in central and peripheral nervous system toxicity.

C. Disulfiram and its metabolites contain either sulfhydryl (S–H) or thiocarbonyl (C=S) moieties common to chelating agents. Chronic use may cause depletion of certain essential metals (copper, zinc). This may in part be the cause of the enzyme-inhibiting effects of disulfiram, as both of these enzymes require copper as a cofactor. Idiosyncratic fulminant hepatic failure or distal sensory-motor and optic neuropathy may also occur with chronic use.

D. **Pharmacokinetics.** Disulfiram is absorbed rapidly and completely, but because enzyme inhibition is the mechanism of action, peak effects may be delayed for 8–12 hours. Although the elimination half-life is 7–8 hours, clinical effects may persist for days because of high lipid solubility and slow enzyme resynthesis. Disulfiram is metabolized in the liver. It inhibits multiple cytochrome P450 enzymes, thus inhibiting the metabolism of many other drugs, including isoniazid, phenytoin, theophylline, warfarin, and many benzodiazepines.

II. Toxic dose

A. Disulfiram overdose. A typical therapeutic dose of disulfiram is 250 mg/day. Ingestion of 2.5 g or more has caused toxicity in children after a delay of 3–12 hours.

B. Disulfiram–ethanol interaction. Ingestion of as little as 7 mL of ethanol can cause a severe reaction in patients taking as little as 200 mg of disulfiram per day. Mild reactions have been reported after use of cough syrup, aftershave lotions, and other alcohol-containing products.

III. Clinical presentation

A. Acute disulfiram overdose (without ethanol) is uncommon and exhibits primarily neurologic symptoms, with headache, ataxia, confusion, lethargy, seizures, and prolonged coma. Multiple authors report neuropathy and basal ganglia lesions. Neuropsychological impairment may be chronic. A garlic-like breath odor, vomiting, and hypotension have been reported with acute disulfiram overdose.

B. Disulfiram–ethanol interaction. The severity of the reaction usually depends on the doses of disulfiram and ethanol. Mild reactions (mild headache, facial flushing) may occur almost immediately after ethanol ingestion or at a plasma ethanol level of 10 mg/dL. Moderate reactions occur with ethanol levels of about 50 mg/dL and manifest with anxiety, nausea, tachycardia, hypotension, throbbing headache, and dyspnea. Severe reactions have resulted in coma and seizures as well as respiratory and cardiovascular failure and death. Reactions do not usually occur unless the patient has been on oral disulfiram therapy for at least 1 day; the reaction may occur up to 14 days after the last dose of disulfiram, as aldehyde dehydrogenase is resynthesized very slowly.

IV. Diagnosis of disulfiram overdose is based on a history of acute ingestion and the presence of CNS symptoms with vomiting. The **disulfiram–ethanol interaction** is diagnosed in a patient with a history of disulfiram use and possible exposure to ethanol who exhibits a characteristic hypotensive flushing reaction.

A. Specific levels. A plasma ethanol level may help predict the degree of a disulfiram–ethanol reaction. Plasma disulfiram levels are not of value in diagnosis or treatment. Plasma acetaldehyde levels may be elevated during the disulfiram–ethanol reaction, but this information is of little value in acute management.

B. Other useful laboratory studies include electrolytes, glucose, BUN, creatinine and liver aminotransferases.

V. Treatment

A. Emergency and supportive measures

1. Acute disulfiram overdose

a. Maintain an open airway and assist ventilation if necessary (pp 1–7).

b. Treat coma (p 18) and seizures (p 23) if they occur.

2. Disulfiram–ethanol interaction

a. Maintain an open airway and assist ventilation if necessary (pp 1–7).

b. Treat hypotension with supine position and IV fluids (eg, saline). If a pressor agent is needed, a direct-acting agent such as norepinephrine (p 595) is preferred over indirect-acting drugs such as dopamine because neuronal norepinephrine stores are reduced.

c. Administer benzodiazepine anxiolytics (lorazepam is preferred [p 516]) and reassurance as needed.

d. Treat vomiting with a 5-HT_3 receptor antagonist or metoclopramide (p 581) and headache with IV analgesics if needed. Avoid phenothiazine antiemetics (which have an alpha receptor–blocking effect) such as prochlorperazine.

e. Histamine receptor antagonists may alleviate flushing.

B. Specific drugs and antidotes. There is no specific antidote. Fomepizole would be expected to block formation of the acetaldehyde and was shown in one small study to relieve the symptoms of the disulfiram–ethanol reaction.

C. **Decontamination** (p 50)
1. **Acute disulfiram overdose.** Administer activated charcoal orally if conditions are appropriate (see Table I–38, p 54). Rapid drug absorption argues against gastric lavage except for ingestions both large and very recent.
2. **Disulfiram–ethanol interaction.** Decontamination procedures are not likely to be of benefit once symptoms occur.

D. **Enhanced elimination.** Hemodialysis is not indicated for disulfiram overdose, but it may remove ethanol and acetaldehyde and has been reported to be effective in treating the acute disulfiram–ethanol interaction. This is not likely to be necessary in patients receiving adequate fluid and pressor support.

▶ DIURETICS

Joyce Go, PharmD

Diuretics are prescribed commonly for the management of essential hypertension, congestive heart failure, ascites, and chronic renal insufficiency. Adverse effects from chronic use or misuse (in sports, dieting, and anorexia) are more frequently encountered than those from acute overdose. Overdoses are generally benign, and no serious outcomes have resulted from acute ingestion. Common currently available diuretics are listed in Table II–25.

I. **Mechanism of toxicity**

A. The toxicity of these drugs is associated with their pharmacologic effects, which decrease fluid volume and promote electrolyte loss; these include dehydration, hypokalemia (or hyperkalemia with spironolactone and triamterene), hypomagnesemia, hyponatremia, and hypochloremic alkalosis. Electrolyte imbalance may lead to cardiac arrhythmias and may enhance digitalis toxicity (p 222). Diuretics are classified on the basis of the pharmacologic mechanisms by which they affect solute and water loss (see Table II–25).

B. **Pharmacokinetics** (see Table II–66, p 462)

II. **Toxic dose.** Minimum toxic doses have not been established. Significant dehydration or electrolyte imbalance is unlikely if the amount ingested is less than

TABLE II–25. DIURETICS

Drug	Maximum Adult Daily Dose (mg)	Drug	Maximum Adult Daily Dose (mg)
Carbonic anhydrase inhibitors		**Thiazides**	
Acetazolamide	1,000	Bendroflumethiazide	5
Methazolamide	300	Chlorothiazide	2,000
Loop diuretics		Chlorthalidone	200
Bumetanide	10	Hydrochlorothiazide	200
Ethacrynic acid	400	Indapamide	5
Furosemide	600	Metolazone	20
Torsemide	200		
Osmotic diuretics			
Mannitol[a]	200 g		
Potassium-sparing diuretics			
Amiloride	20		
Spironolactone	400		
Triamterene	300		
Eplerenone	100		

[a]Note: Mannitol doses >200 g/day or doses resulting in serum osmolality >320 mOsm/L can cause acute kidney injury.

the usual recommended daily dose (see Table II–25). High doses of intravenous ethacrynic acid and furosemide can cause ototoxicity, especially when administered rapidly and to patients with renal failure.

III. Clinical presentation. Gastrointestinal symptoms including nausea, vomiting, and diarrhea are common after acute oral overdose. Lethargy, weakness, hyporeflexia, and dehydration (and occasionally hypotension) may be present if volume loss and electrolyte disturbances are present, although the onset of symptoms may be delayed for 2–4 hours or more until diuretic action is obtained. Spironolactone is very slow, with maximal effects after the third day.

A. Hypokalemia may cause muscle weakness, cramps, and tetany. Severe hypokalemia may result in flaccid paralysis and rhabdomyolysis. Cardiac rhythm disturbances may also occur.

B. Spironolactone and other potassium-sparing agents may cause hyperkalemia and hyperchloremic metabolic acidosis, especially in patients with renal insufficiency.

C. Hypocalcemia and hypomagnesemia may also cause tetany.

D. Hyponatremia, hyperglycemia, hypercalcemia, and hyperuricemia may occur, especially with thiazide diuretics.

E. Carbonic anhydrase inhibitors may induce metabolic acidosis. Drowsiness and paresthesias are commonly seen in renal insufficiency or the elderly.

F. Rapid administration of mannitol (an osmotic diuretic) may cause excessive intravascular volume expansion and circulatory overload resulting in CHF or pulmonary edema. Rapid diuresis may result in fluid and electrolyte imbalances, dehydration and hypovolemia. Mannitol can also transiently increase the osmol gap (see p 33).

IV. Diagnosis is based on a history of exposure and evidence of dehydration and acid–base or electrolyte imbalance. Note that patients on diuretics may also be taking other cardiac and antihypertensive medications.

A. Specific levels are not routinely available or clinically useful.

B. Other useful laboratory studies include electrolytes (including calcium and magnesium), glucose, BUN, creatinine, and ECG.

V. Treatment

A. Emergency and supportive measures

1. Replace fluid loss with IV crystalloid solutions and correct electrolyte abnormalities (pp 36–39). Correction of sodium in patients with diuretic-induced hyponatremia should be limited to 1–2 mEq/h to avoid central pontine myelinolysis unless seizures or coma is present. In this case, 3% hypertonic saline should be used for a more rapid correction.

2. Monitor the ECG until the potassium level is normalized.

B. Specific drugs and antidotes. There are no specific antidotes.

C. Decontamination (p 50). Administer activated charcoal orally if conditions are appropriate (see Table I–38, p 54). Gastric lavage is not necessary after small-to-moderate ingestions if activated charcoal can be given promptly. Cathartics have not been shown to be beneficial in preventing absorption and may worsen dehydration.

D. Enhanced elimination. No experience with extracorporeal removal of diuretics has been reported.

► ERGOT DERIVATIVES

Neal L. Benowitz, MD, Charles W. O'Connell, MD

Ergot derivatives are used to treat migraine headache and enhance uterine contraction postpartum. Ergots are produced by the fungus *Claviceps purpurea,* which may grow on rye and other grains. Natural or synthetic ergot drugs include ergotamine (Cafergot, Ergomar, Gynergen, and Ergostat), dihydroergotamine (DHE45), methysergide

(Sansert), methylergonovine (Methergine), and ergonovine (Ergotrate). Some ergoloid derivatives (dihydroergocornine, dihydroergocristine, and dihydroergocryptine) have been used in combination (Hydergine and Deapril-ST) for the treatment of dementia. Bromocriptine (Parlodel [p 524]) and pergolide (Permax) are ergot derivatives with dopamine agonist activity that are used to treat Parkinson disease. Bromocriptine is also used to treat hyperprolactinemic states.

I. Mechanism of toxicity

A. Ergot derivatives have very complex pharmacologic properties, including varying degrees of central and peripheral agonist, antagonist or mixed activity at serotonergic, dopaminergic and alpha-adrenergic receptors. Ergots directly stimulate vasoconstriction and uterine contraction and may indirectly dilate some vessels via CNS sympatholytic action. The relative contribution of each of these mechanisms to toxicity depends on the particular ergot alkaloid and its dose. **Sustained vasoconstriction** causes most of the serious toxicity; reduced blood flow causes local tissue hypoxia and ischemic injury, resulting in tissue edema and local thrombosis, worsening ischemia, and leading to further injury. At a certain point, reversible vasospasm progresses to irreversible vascular insufficiency and limb gangrene.

B. Pharmacokinetics (see Table II–66, p 462). Ergot alkaloids are extensively metabolized and highly tissue-bound, the latter characteristic accounting for protracted clinical ergot poisoning after the drug is stopped. Most of the ergots undergo hepatic metabolism. Ergotism has occurred in people taking **HIV protease inhibitors** in combination with ergots for migraine, presumably owing to inhibition of ergot metabolism via CYP3A4.

II. Toxic dose. Death has been reported in a 14-month-old child after acute ingestion of 12 mg of ergotamine. However, most cases of severe poisoning occur with chronic overmedication for migraine headaches rather than acute single overdoses. Daily doses of 10 mg or more of ergotamine are usually associated with toxicity. There are many case reports of vasospastic complications with normal therapeutic dosing.

III. Clinical presentation

A. Ergotamine and related agents. Mild intoxication causes nausea and vomiting. Serious poisoning results in vasoconstriction that may involve many parts of the body. Owing to persistence of ergots in tissues, vasospasm may continue for up to 10–14 days.

1. Involvement of the extremities causes paresthesias, pain, pallor, coolness, and loss of peripheral pulses in the hands and feet; gangrene may ensue.
2. Other complications of vasospasm include coronary ischemia and myocardial infarction, abdominal angina and bowel infarction, renal infarction and failure, visual disturbances and blindness, and stroke. Psychosis, seizures, and coma occur rarely.
3. Iatrogenic neonatal ergot poisoning has occurred when methylergonovine meant for the mother after delivery was administered mistakenly to the baby. Manifestations include respiratory failure, apnea, cyanosis, hypotension, peripheral ischemia, oliguria, and seizures.

B. Bromocriptine intoxication may present with hallucinations, paranoid behavior, hypertension, and tachycardia. Involuntary movements, hallucinations, and hypotension are reported with **pergolide**.

C. Chronic use of **methysergide** occasionally causes retroperitoneal fibrosis.

IV. Diagnosis is based on a history of ergot use and clinical findings.

1. **Specific levels**. Ergotamine levels are not widely available, and blood concentrations do not correlate well with toxicity.
2. **Other useful laboratory studies** include CBC, electrolytes, BUN, creatinine, and ECG. Arteriography of the affected vascular bed is indicated occasionally.

V. **Treatment**

A. **Emergency and supportive measures**

1. Maintain an open airway and assist ventilation if necessary (pp 1–7).
2. Treat coma (p 18) and convulsions (p 23) if they occur.
3. Immediately discontinue ergot treatment. Hydration and analgesia should be provided. Hospitalize patients with vasospastic symptoms and treat promptly to prevent complications.

B. **Specific drugs and antidotes**

1. **Peripheral ischemia** requires prompt vasodilator therapy and anticoagulation to prevent local thrombosis.
   a. There is no standard first-line choice for management of critical limb ischemia with ergotism. Options include IV **nitroprusside** (p 593), starting with 1–2 mcg/kg/min, or IV **phentolamine** (p 605), starting with 0.5 mg/min; increase the infusion rate until ischemia is relieved or systemic hypotension occurs. Intra-arterial infusion is occasionally required. Nifedipine or other vasodilating calcium antagonists may also enhance peripheral blood flow. Case reports have also noted successful use of intravenous iloprost, a synthetic prostaglandin I_2 analog, intra-arterial infusion of prostaglandin E1, and oral sildenafil.
   b. Administer **heparin**, 5,000 units IV followed by 1,000 units/h (in adults), with adjustments in the infusion rate to maintain the activated coagulation time (ACT) or the activated partial thromboplastin time (aPTT) at approximately 2 times the baseline.
2. **Coronary spasm.** Administer **nitroglycerin**, 0.15–0.6 mg sublingually or 5–20 mcg/min IV. Intracoronary artery nitroglycerin may be required if there is no response to IV infusion. Also consider using a calcium antagonist.

C. **Decontamination** after acute ingestion (p 50). Administer activated charcoal orally if conditions are appropriate (see Table I–38, p 54). Gastric lavage is not necessary after small-to-moderate ingestions if activated charcoal can be given promptly.

D. **Enhanced elimination.** Dialysis and hemoperfusion are not effective. Repeat-dose charcoal has not been studied, but because of extensive tissue distribution of ergots, it is not likely to be useful.

▶ ETHANOL

Allyson Kreshak, MD

Commercial beer, wine, and liquors contain various amounts of ethanol. Ethanol is also found in a variety of colognes, perfumes, aftershaves, and mouthwashes; some rubbing alcohols; many food flavorings (eg, vanilla, almond, and lemon extracts); pharmaceutical preparations (eg, elixirs); hand sanitizers; and many other products. Ethanol is frequently ingested recreationally and is the most common coingestant with other drugs in suicide attempts. Ethanol may also serve as a competitive substrate in the emergency treatment of methanol and ethylene glycol poisonings (p 314 and 234).

I. **Mechanism of toxicity**

A. **Central nervous system (CNS) depression** is the principal effect of acute ethanol intoxication. Ethanol has additive effects with other CNS depressants, such as barbiturates, benzodiazepines, opioids, antidepressants, and antipsychotics.

B. **Hypoglycemia** may be caused by impaired gluconeogenesis in patients with depleted or low glycogen stores (particularly small children and poorly nourished persons).

C. Ethanol intoxication and chronic alcoholism also predispose patients to trauma, exposure-induced hypothermia, injurious effects of alcohol on the GI tract and nervous system, and a number of nutritional disorders and metabolic derangements.

D. In **pregnancy**, ethanol is absorbed by the mother and crosses the placenta. Fetal concentrations of ethanol rapidly approach those of the mother. Fetal excretion of ethanol into the amniotic fluid can lead to fetal reabsorption. Ethanol is a category C drug and ingestion during pregnancy can lead to fetal alcohol syndrome.

E. **Pharmacokinetics.** Ethanol is readily absorbed (peak, 30–120 minutes) and distributed into the body water (volume of distribution, 0.5–0.7 L/kg or ~50 L in the average adult). Elimination is mainly by oxidation in the liver and follows zero-order kinetics. The average adult can metabolize about 7–10 g of alcohol per hour, or about 12–25 mg/dL/h. This rate varies among individuals and is influenced by polymorphisms of the alcohol dehydrogenase enzyme and the activity of the microsomal ethanol-oxidizing systems.

II. **Toxic dose.** Generally, 0.7 g/kg of pure ethanol (approximately 3–4 drinks) will produce a blood ethanol concentration of 100 mg/dL (0.1 g/dL). The legal limit for adult drivers of noncommercial vehicles in the United States is 80 mg/dL (0.08 g/dL).

A. A level of 100 mg/dL decreases reaction time and judgment and may be enough to inhibit gluconeogenesis and cause hypoglycemia in children and patients with liver disease, but by itself it is not enough to cause coma.

B. The level sufficient to cause deep coma or respiratory depression is highly variable, depending on the individual's degree of tolerance to ethanol. Although levels above 300 mg/dL usually cause coma in novice drinkers, persons with chronic alcoholism may be awake with levels of 500–600 mg/dL or higher.

III. **Clinical presentation**

A. **Acute intoxication**

1. With **mild**-to-moderate intoxication, patients exhibit euphoria, mild incoordination, ataxia, nystagmus, and impaired judgment and reflexes. Social inhibitions are loosened, and boisterous or aggressive behavior is common. Hypoglycemia may occur, especially in children and persons with reduced hepatic glycogen stores.
2. With **deep intoxication**, coma, respiratory depression, and pulmonary aspiration may occur. In these patients, the pupils are usually small, and the temperature, blood pressure, and pulse rate are often decreased. Rhabdomyolysis may result from prolonged immobility.

B. **Chronic ethanol abuse** is associated with numerous complications:

1. **Hepatic toxicity** includes fatty infiltration of the liver, alcoholic hepatitis, and eventually cirrhosis. Liver injury can lead to portal hypertension, ascites, bleeding from esophageal varices and hemorrhoids; hyponatremia from fluid retention; and bacterial peritonitis. Production of clotting factors is impaired, leading to prolonged prothrombin time. Hepatic metabolism of drugs and endogenous toxins is impaired and may contribute to hepatic encephalopathy.
2. **Gastrointestinal** bleeding may result from alcohol-induced gastritis, esophagitis, and duodenitis. Other causes of massive bleeding include Mallory–Weiss tears of the esophagus and esophageal varices. Acute pancreatitis is a common cause of abdominal pain and vomiting.
3. **Cardiac** disorders include various dysrhythmias, such as atrial fibrillation, that may be associated with potassium and magnesium depletion and poor caloric intake ("holiday heart"). Cardiomyopathy has been associated with long-term alcohol use. (Cardiomyopathy was also historically associated with ingestion of cobalt used to stabilize beer.)
4. **Neurologic** toxicity includes cerebral atrophy, cerebellar degeneration, and peripheral stocking-glove sensory neuropathy. Nutritional disorders such as thiamine (vitamin B_1) deficiency can cause Wernicke encephalopathy or Korsakoff psychosis.

5. **Hematologic** toxicity may manifest as leukopenia, thrombocytopenia and macrocytosis with or without anemia. These hematologic effects result from ethanol's direct toxicity as well as its interference with folate metabolism.
6. **Alcoholic ketoacidosis** is characterized by anion gap metabolic acidosis and elevated levels of beta-hydroxybutyrate and, to a lesser extent, acetoacetate. The osmolar gap may also be elevated, causing this condition to be mistaken for methanol or ethylene glycol poisoning.

C. **Alcohol withdrawal.** Sudden discontinuation after chronic high-level alcohol use often causes headache, tremulousness, anxiety, palpitations, and insomnia. Brief, generalized seizures may occur, usually within 6–12 hours of decreased ethanol consumption. Sympathetic nervous system overactivity may progress to **delirium tremens**, a life-threatening syndrome characterized by tachycardia, diaphoresis, hyperthermia, and delirium, which usually manifests 48–72 hours after cessation of heavy alcohol use. The "DTs" may cause significant morbidity and mortality if untreated.

D. **Other problems.** Ethanol abusers sometimes intentionally or accidentally ingest ethanol substitutes, such as isopropyl alcohol (p 282), methanol (p 314), and ethylene glycol (p 234). In addition, ethanol may serve as the vehicle for swallowing large numbers of pills in a suicide attempt. Disulfiram (p 226) use can cause a serious acute reaction with ethanol ingestion.

IV. **Diagnosis** of ethanol intoxication is usually simple, based on the history of ingestion, the characteristic smell of fresh alcohol or the fetid odor of acetaldehyde and other metabolic products, and the presence of nystagmus, ataxia, and altered mental status. However, other disorders may accompany or mimic intoxication, such as hypoglycemia, head trauma, hypothermia, meningitis, Wernicke encephalopathy, and intoxication with other drugs or poisons.

A. **Specific levels**. Serum ethanol levels are usually available at most hospital laboratories and, depending on the method used, are accurate and specific. Note that serum levels are approximately 12–18% higher than corresponding whole-blood values.

1. In general, there is only rough correlation between blood levels and clinical presentation; however, an ethanol level below 300 mg/dL in a comatose patient should initiate a search for alternative causes.
2. If ethanol levels are not readily available, the ethanol concentration may be estimated by calculating the osmol gap (p 33).
3. The metabolite ethyl glucuronide is present in urine for up to 24 hours after ethanol ingestion.

B. **Suggested laboratory studies** in the acutely intoxicated patient may include glucose, electrolytes, BUN, creatinine, liver aminotransferases, prothrombin time (PT/INR), magnesium, arterial blood gases or oximetry, and chest radiography (if pulmonary aspiration is suspected). Consider CT scan of the head if the patient has focal neurologic deficits or altered mental status inconsistent with the degree of blood alcohol elevation.

V. **Treatment**

A. **Emergency and supportive measures**

1. **Acute intoxication.** Treatment is mainly supportive.
   a. Protect the airway to prevent aspiration and intubate and assist ventilation if needed (pp 1–7).
   b. Give glucose and thiamine (pp 562 and 628), and treat coma (p 18) and seizures (p 23) if they occur. Glucagon is not effective for alcohol-induced hypoglycemia.
   c. Correct hypothermia with gradual rewarming (p 20).
   d. Most patients will recover within 4–6 hours. Observe children until their blood alcohol level is below 50 mg/dL and there is no evidence of hypoglycemia.

2. **Alcoholic ketoacidosis.** Treat with volume replacement, thiamine (p 628), and supplemental glucose. Most patients recover rapidly.
3. **Alcohol withdrawal.** Treat with benzodiazepines (eg, diazepam, 5–10 mg IV initially and repeat as needed [p 516]) and/or phenobarbital (p 604).

B. **Specific drugs and antidotes.** There is no available specific ethanol receptor antagonist.

C. **Decontamination** (p 50). Because ethanol is rapidly absorbed, gastric decontamination is usually not indicated unless other drug ingestion is suspected. Consider aspirating gastric contents with a small, flexible tube if the alcohol ingestion was massive and recent (within 30–45 minutes). Activated charcoal does not effectively adsorb ethanol but may be given if other drugs or toxins were ingested.

D. **Enhanced elimination.** Metabolism of ethanol normally occurs at a fixed rate of approximately 12–25 mg/dL/h. Elimination rates are faster in persons with chronic alcoholism and at serum levels above 300 mg/dL. Hemodialysis efficiently removes ethanol, but enhanced removal is rarely needed because supportive care is usually sufficient. Hemoperfusion and forced diuresis are not effective.

▶ ETHYLENE GLYCOL AND OTHER GLYCOLS

Ilene B. Anderson, PharmD

Ethylene glycol is the primary ingredient (up to 95%) in antifreeze. It sometimes is consumed intentionally as an alcohol substitute by alcoholics and is tempting to children and pets because of its sweet taste. Intoxication by ethylene glycol itself causes inebriation and mild gastritis; more importantly, its metabolic products cause metabolic acidosis, renal failure, and death. Other glycols may also produce toxicity (Table II–26).

I. **Mechanism of toxicity**

A. **Ethylene glycol** is metabolized by alcohol dehydrogenase to glycoaldehyde, which is then metabolized to glycolic, glyoxylic, and oxalic acids. These acids, along with excess lactic acid, are responsible for the anion gap metabolic acidosis. Oxalate readily precipitates with calcium to form insoluble calcium monohydrate oxalate crystals. Tissue injury is caused by widespread deposition of oxalate crystals and the toxic effects of glycolic and glyoxylic acids. Calcium oxalate monohydrate crystal accumulation in the kidney is responsible for the renal tubular necrosis.

B. **Overdose in pregnancy.** Ethylene glycol crosses the placenta. Fetal toxicity is expected to mimic maternal toxicity in overdose.

C. **Pharmacokinetics**. Ethylene glycol is well absorbed orally. The volume of distribution is about 0.6–0.8 L/kg. It is not protein bound. Metabolism is by alcohol dehydrogenase, with a half-life of about 3–5 hours. In the presence of fomepizole or ethanol (see below), both of which block ethylene glycol metabolism, elimination is entirely renal with a reported half-life of 14.2–17 hours.

D. **Other glycols** (see Table II–26). Propylene and dipropylene glycols are of relatively lower toxicity, although metabolism of propylene glycol creates lactic acid. Polypropylene glycol and other high–molecular-weight polyethylene glycols are poorly absorbed and virtually nontoxic. However, diethylene glycol and glycol ethers produce toxic metabolites with toxicity similar to that of ethylene glycol.

II. **Toxic dose.** The approximate lethal oral dose of 95% ethylene glycol (eg, antifreeze) is 1.0–1.5 mL/kg; however, survival has been reported after an ingestion of 2 L in a patient who received treatment within 1 hour of ingestion.

TABLE II–26. OTHER GLYCOLS

Compounds	Toxicity and Comments	Treatment
Diethylene glycol (DEG)	Highly nephrotoxic and neurotoxic. Epidemic poisonings have occurred when DEG has been inappropriately used in consumer products or as a diluent for water insoluble pharmaceuticals. Toxicity has also occurred after large acute ingestion and repeated dermal application in burn patients with extensive injuries. Clinical presentation includes initial ethanol-like inebriation and gastritis, metabolic acidosis, acute renal injury, dysphonia, cranial nerve VII paresis or paralysis, facial and peripheral extremity weakness, coma and death. Metabolic acidosis may be delayed for 12 hours or longer after ingestion. DEG is primarily metabolized to 2-hydroxyethoxyacetic acid and diglycolic acid. Diglycolic acid is likely responsible for the nephrotoxicity; however, DEG itself may also be toxic. Molecular weight is 106. Vd 1 L/kg (animal).	Ethanol and fomepizole may limit toxicity due to DEG metabolites. Hemodialysis is indicated for patients with large ingestions, anuric renal failure or severe metabolic acidosis nonresponsive to medical treatments.
Dioxane (dimer of ethylene glycol)	May cause coma, liver and kidney damage. The vapor (>300 ppm) may cause mucous membrane irritation. Dermal exposure to the liquid may have a defatting action. Metabolites unknown. Molecular weight is 88.	Role of ethanol and fomepizole is unknown, but they may be effective.
Dipropylene glycol	Relatively low toxicity. Central nervous system depression, hepatic injury, and renal damage have occurred in animal studies after massive exposures. There is a human report of acute renal failure, polyneuropathy, and myopathy after an ingestion of dipropylene glycol fog solution but no reports of acidosis or lactate elevation. Molecular weight is 134.	Supportive care. There is no role for ethanol or fomepizole therapy.
Ethylene glycol monobutyl ether (EGBE, 2-butoxyethanol, butyl cellosolve)	Clinical toxic effects include lethargy, coma, anion gap metabolic acidosis, hyperchloremia, elevated lactate, hypotension, respiratory depression, hemolysis, renal and hepatic dysfunction; rare disseminated intravascular coagulation (DIC), noncardiogenic pulmonary edema, and acute respiratory distress syndrome (ARDS). Oxalate crystal formation and osmolar gap elevation have been reported, but not in all cases. Serum levels in poisoning cases have ranged from 0.005 to 432 mg/L. Butoxyethanol is metabolized by alcohol dehydrogenase to butoxyaldehyde and butoxyacetic acid (BAA); however, the affinity of alcohol dehydrogenase for butoxyethanol is unknown. Molecular weight is 118.	Ethanol, fomepizole, and hemodialysis may be effective.
Ethylene glycol monoethyl ether (EGEE, 2-ethoxyethanol, ethyl cellosolve)	Calcium oxalate crystals have been reported in animals. Animal studies indicate that EGEE is metabolized in part to ethylene glycol; however, the affinity of alcohol dehydrogenase is higher for EGEE than for ethanol. One patient developed vertigo, unconsciousness, metabolic acidosis, renal insufficiency, hepatic damage, and neurasthesia after ingesting 40 mL. Teratogenic effect has been reported in humans and animals. Molecular weight is 90.	Ethanol and fomepizole may be effective.

(continued)

TABLE II–26. OTHER GLYCOLS (CONTINUED)

Compounds	Toxicity and Comments	Treatment
Ethylene glycol monomethyl ether (EGME, 2-methoxyethanol, methyl cellosolve)	Delayed toxic effects (8 and 18 hours after ingestion) similar to those of ethylene glycol have been reported. Calcium oxalate crystals may or may not occur. Cerebral edema, hemorrhagic gastritis, and degeneration of the liver and kidneys were reported in one autopsy. Animal studies indicate that EGME is metabolized in part to ethylene glycol; however, the affinity of alcohol dehydrogenase is about the same for EGME as for ethanol. Oligospermia has been reported with chronic exposure in humans. Teratogenic effects have been reported in animals. Molecular weight is 76.	Effectiveness of ethanol and fomepizole uncertain; in one report, fomepizole did not prevent acidosis.
Polyethylene glycols	Very low toxicity. A group of compounds with molecular weights ranging from 200 to more than 4,000. High–molecular-weight compounds (>500) are poorly absorbed and rapidly excreted by the kidneys. Low–molecular-weight compounds (200–400) may result in metabolic acidosis, renal failure, and hypercalcemia after massive oral ingestions or repeated dermal applications in patients with extensive burn injuries. Acute respiratory failure occurred after accidental nasogastric infusion into the lung of a pediatric patient. Alcohol dehydrogenase metabolizes polyethylene glycols.	Supportive care.
Propylene glycol (PG)	Relatively low toxicity. Lactic acidosis, central nervous system depression, coma, hypoglycemia, seizures, and hemolysis have been reported rarely after massive exposures or chronic exposures in high-risk patients. Risk factors include renal insufficiency, small infants, epilepsy, burn patients with extensive dermal application of propylene glycol, and patients in alcohol withdrawal receiving ultra-high doses of IV lorazepam or diazepam. Osmolar gap, anion gap, and lactate are commonly elevated. PG levels of 6–42 mg/dL did not result in toxicity after acute infusion. A PG level of 1,059 mg/dL was reported in an 8-month-old with extensive burn injuries after repeated dermal application (the child experienced cardiopulmonary arrest). A level of 400 mg/dL was measured in an epileptic patient who experienced status epilepticus, respiratory depression, elevated osmolar gap, and metabolic acidosis. Metabolites are lactate and pyruvate. Molecular weight is 76.	Supportive care, sodium bicarbonate. There is no role for ethanol or fomepizole therapy. Hemodialysis is effective but rarely indicated unless renal failure or severe metabolic acidosis unresponsive to medical treatment. Discontinue any drugs containing PG.
Triethylene glycol	Uncommon intoxication in humans. Coma, metabolic acidosis with elevated anion gap, osmolar gap of 7 mOsm/L reported 1–1.5 hours after ingestion of one “gulp.” Treated with ethanol and recovered by 36 hours.	Ethanol and fomepizole may be effective.

III. Clinical presentation

A. Ethylene glycol

1. **During the first few hours** after acute ingestion, the victim may appear intoxicated as if by ethanol. The osmol gap (p 33) is increased, but there is no initial acidosis. Gastritis with vomiting may also occur.
2. **After a delay of 4–12 hours**, evidence of intoxication by metabolic products occurs, with anion gap acidosis, hyperventilation, convulsions, coma, cardiac conduction disturbances, and arrhythmias. Renal failure is common but usually reversible. Pulmonary edema and cerebral edema may also occur. Hypocalcemia with tetany has been reported.
3. **After a delay of days to weeks**, delayed neurologic sequelae have been reported albeit rare. Examples include cranial nerve VII and VIII neuropathies, cerebral edema, Parkinson's disease, diaphragmatic paralysis, gastroparesis, and postural hypotension.

B. Other glycols (see Table II–26). Diethylene glycol and glycol ethers are extremely toxic and may produce central nervous system depression, acute renal failure, metabolic acidosis and neurotoxicity. Calcium oxalate crystals may or may not be present.

IV. Diagnosis of ethylene glycol poisoning usually is based on the history of antifreeze ingestion, typical symptoms, and elevation of the osmol and anion gaps. Oxalate or hippurate crystals may be present in the urine (calcium oxalate crystals may be monohydrate [cigar-shaped] or dihydrate [cuboidal]). Glycol ethers increase plasma osmolality but the increase may be too small to reflect clinical risk. Because many antifreeze products contain fluorescein, the urine may exhibit fluorescence under a Wood lamp. However, false-positive and false-negative Wood lamp results have been reported.

A. Specific levels. Tests for ethylene glycol levels are usually available from regional commercial toxicology laboratories but are difficult to obtain quickly.

1. Serum levels higher than 50 mg/dL usually are associated with serious intoxication, although lower levels do not rule out poisoning if the parent compound has already been metabolized (in such a case, the anion gap should be markedly elevated). Calculation of the osmol gap (p 33) may be used to estimate the ethylene glycol level.
2. **False-positive ethylene glycol levels** can be caused by elevated triglycerides (see Table I–33, p 46) and by 2,3-butanediol, lactate, glycerol, and other substances when glycerol dehydrogenase is used in some enzymatic assays. An elevated ethylene glycol level should be confirmed by gas chromatography (GC). Falsely negative EG levels may occur in the presence of glycerol or propylene glycol, using some enzymatic assays.
3. Elevated concentrations of the toxic metabolite **glycolic acid** are a better measure of toxicity but are not widely available. Levels less than 10 mmol/L are not toxic. ***Note:*** Glycolic and glyoxylic acid can produce a false-positive result for lactic acid in some point-of-care assays.
4. In the absence of a serum ethylene glycol level, if the osmol and anion gaps are both normal and the patient is asymptomatic, serious ingestion is not likely to have occurred.

B. Other useful laboratory studies include electrolytes, lactate, ethanol, glucose, BUN, creatinine, calcium, hepatic aminotransferases (ALT, AST), urinalysis (for crystals), measured osmolality, arterial blood gases, and ECG monitoring. Serum **beta-hydroxybutyrate** levels may help distinguish ethylene glycol poisoning from **alcoholic ketoacidosis**, which also may cause increased anion and osmol gaps. (Patients with alcoholic ketoacidosis may not have markedly positive tests for ketones, but the beta-hydroxybutyrate level will usually be elevated.)

V. Treatment

A. Emergency and supportive measures

1. Maintain an open airway and assist ventilation if necessary (pp 1–7). Administer supplemental oxygen.

2. Treat coma (p 18), convulsions (p 23), cardiac arrhythmias (pp 10–15), and metabolic acidosis (p 35) if they occur. Observe the patient for several hours to monitor for development of metabolic acidosis, especially if the patient is symptomatic or there is known co-ingestion of ethanol.
3. Treat hypocalcemia with IV calcium gluconate or calcium chloride (p 526).

B. **Specific drugs and antidotes**

1. Administer **fomepizole** (p 558) or **ethanol** (p 553) to saturate the enzyme alcohol dehydrogenase and prevent metabolism of ethylene glycol to its toxic metabolites. Indications for therapy include the following:
   a. Ethylene glycol level is higher than 20 mg/dL.
   b. History of ethylene glycol ingestion is accompanied by an osmol gap greater than 10 mOsm/L not accounted for by ethanol or other alcohols.
2. Administer **pyridoxine** (p 621), **folate** (p 557), and **thiamine** (p 628), cofactors required for the metabolism of ethylene glycol that may alleviate toxicity by enhancing metabolism of glyoxylic acid to nontoxic metabolites.

C. **Decontamination** (p 50). Perform lavage (or simply aspirate gastric contents with a small, flexible tube) if the ingestion was recent (within 30–60 minutes). Activated charcoal is not likely to be of benefit because the required effective dose is large and ethylene glycol is rapidly absorbed, but it may be given if other drugs or toxins were ingested.

D. **Enhanced elimination.** The volume of distribution of ethylene glycol is 0.6–0.8 L/kg, making it accessible to enhanced elimination procedures. **Hemodialysis** efficiently removes ethylene glycol and its toxic metabolites and rapidly corrects acidosis and electrolyte and fluid abnormalities. Continuous venovenous hemodiafiltration (CVVHDF) was reported effective in one case report, although the rate of elimination is slower.

1. **Indications for hemodialysis** include the following:
   a. Suspected ethylene glycol poisoning with an osmol gap greater than 10 mOsm/L not accounted for by ethanol or other alcohols and accompanied by metabolic acidosis (pH <7.25–7.30) unresponsive to therapy.
   b. Ethylene glycol intoxication accompanied by renal failure.
   c. Ethylene glycol serum concentration greater than 50 mg/dL unless the patient is asymptomatic and is receiving fomepizole or ethanol therapy.
   d. Severe metabolic acidosis in a patient with a history of ethylene glycol ingestion, even if the osmol gap is not elevated (late presenter).
2. **End point of treatment.** The minimum serum concentration of ethylene glycol associated with serious toxicity is not known. In addition, ethylene glycol levels are reported to rebound after dialysis ceases. Therefore, treatment with fomepizole or ethanol should be continued until the osmol and anion gaps are normalized or (if available) serum ethylene glycol and glycolic acid levels are no longer detectable.

► ETHYLENE OXIDE

Stephen C. Born, MD, MPH

Ethylene oxide is a highly penetrating, chemically reactive flammable gas or liquid that is used widely as a sterilizer of medical equipment and supplies. It is also an important industrial chemical that is used as an intermediate in the production of ethylene glycol, solvents, surfactants, and multiple other industrial chemicals. Ethylene oxide liquid has a boiling point of 10.7°C (760 mm Hg) and is readily miscible with water and organic solvents. Ethylene oxide in air poses a risk for fire/explosion at concentrations greater than 2.6%.

I. **Mechanism of toxicity.** Ethylene oxide is an alkylating agent and reacts directly with proteins and DNA to cause cell death. Direct contact with the gas causes irritation of the eyes, mucous membranes, and lungs. Ethylene oxide is mutagenic, teratogenic, and carcinogenic (regulated as a carcinogen by OSHA and categorized by IARC as a known human carcinogen). It may be absorbed through intact skin.

II. Toxic dose. Occupational exposure to ethylene oxide is regulated by OSHA, whose standard and excellent supporting documentation can be found at www.osha.gov. The workplace permissible exposure limit (PEL) in air is 1 ppm (1.8 mg/m^3) as an 8-hour time-weighted average (TWA). The air level immediately dangerous to life or health (IDLH) is 800 ppm. Occupational exposure above OSHA-determined trigger levels (0.5 ppm as an 8-hour TWA) requires medical surveillance (29 CFR 1910.1047). The odor threshold is approximately 500 ppm, giving the gas poor warning properties. High levels of ethylene oxide can occur when sterilizers malfunction or during opening or replacing ethylene oxide tanks. Exposure may also occur when fumigated or sterilized materials are inadequately aerated. A minute amount of ethylene oxide is produced endogenously in humans from the metabolism of ethylene. Levels are also increased by cigarette smoking.

III. Clinical presentation

- **A.** Ethylene oxide is a potent mucous membrane irritant and can cause eye and oropharyngeal irritation, bronchospasm, and pulmonary edema. Cataract formation has been described after significant eye exposure. Exposure to ethylene oxide in solution can cause vesicant injury to the skin. Ethylene oxide can cause CNS depression, seizures, or coma.
- **B.** Neurotoxicity, including convulsions and delayed peripheral neuropathy, may occur after exposure.
- **C.** Other systemic effects include cardiac arrhythmias when ethylene oxide is used in combination with freon (p 251) as a carrier gas.
- **D.** Leukemia has been described in workers chronically exposed to ethylene oxide.
- **E.** Hypersensitivity may occur in those who are chronically exposed to small amounts of ethylene oxide, and often has a similar presentation to latex hypersensitivity.

IV. Diagnosis is based on a history of exposure and typical upper airway irritant effects. Detection of ethylene oxide odor indicates significant exposure. Industrial hygiene sampling is necessary to document air levels of exposure.

- **A. Specific levels.** Blood levels are transient and not commercially available. Ethylene oxide DNA or hemoglobin adducts indicate exposure but few laboratories are set up to measure these (hydroxyethylvaline can be measured at RTI International: www.rti.org). IgE testing is commercially available from multiple laboratories.
- **B. Other useful laboratory studies** include CBC, glucose, electrolytes, arterial blood gases or pulse oximetry, and chest radiography.

V. Treatment

- **A. Emergency and supportive measures.** Monitor closely for several hours after exposure.
  1. Maintain an open airway and assist ventilation if necessary (pp 1–7). Treat bronchospasm (p 7), anaphylaxis (p 28), and pulmonary edema (p 7) if they occur.
  2. Treat coma (p 18), convulsions (p 23), and arrhythmias (pp 10–15) if they occur.
- **B. Specific drugs and antidotes.** There is no specific antidote. Treatment is supportive.
- **C. Decontamination** (p 50)
  1. Remove the victim from the contaminated environment immediately and administer oxygen. Rescuers should wear self-contained breathing apparatus and chemical-protective clothing.

2. Remove all contaminated clothing and wash exposed skin. For eye exposures, irrigate copiously with tepid water or saline.

D. **Enhanced elimination.** There is no role for these procedures.

▶ FLUORIDE

Kathryn H. Meier, PharmD

Fluoride-liberating chemicals are found in some automobile wheel cleaners, rust removers, glass-etching solutions, pesticides, agents used in aluminum production, dietary supplements, drugs used to prevent dental caries, and the antifungal voriconazole. It is also found in hydrogen fluoride and hydrofluoric acid, which have additional dermal and inhalational hazards and are discussed separately (p 269). By ingestion, soluble fluoride salts are rapidly absorbed and are more acutely toxic than poorly soluble compounds (Table II–27). Most toothpaste contains up to 5 mg of fluoride per teaspoon, and tea can contain 0.3–5.1 mg of fluoride per liter. Although low fluoride concentrations added to public drinking water decreases tooth decay, in some parts of the world high concentrations of fluoride contaminating drinking water causes a number of chronic health problems including skeletal fluorosis.

I. **Mechanism of toxicity**

A. In addition to its direct cytotoxic and metabolic effects, fluoride binds avidly to calcium and magnesium, causing hypocalcemia and hypomagnesemia and generates reactive oxygen species. Fluoride toxicity disrupts many intracellular mechanisms, including glycolysis, G-protein–mediated signaling, oxidative phosphorylation, adenosine triphosphate (ATP) production, function of Na^+/K^+-ATPase, and potassium channels.

B. **Pharmacokinetics.** Fluoride is a weak acid (pKa = 3.4) that is passively absorbed from the stomach and small intestine. In an acidic environment, more fluoride is present as hydrogen fluoride (HF), which is absorbed more rapidly than ionized fluoride. Fasting peak absorption occurs in 30–60 minutes. The volume of distribution is 0.5–0.7 L/kg. Fluoride is not protein bound but binds readily to magnesium and calcium in blood and tissues and is deposited in bone. The elimination half-life is 2.4–4.3 hours and is prolonged in patients with renal failure.

II. **Toxic dose.** Vomiting and abdominal pain are common with acute ingestions of elemental fluoride of 3–5 mg/kg (see Table II–27); hypocalcemia and muscular symptoms appear with ingestions of 5–10 mg/kg. Death has been reported in a 3-year-old child after ingestion of 16 mg/kg and in adults with doses in excess of 32 mg/kg. Although chronic total fluoride intake above 14 mg per day is

TABLE II–27. FLUORIDE-CONTAINING COMPOUNDS

Compound	Elemental Fluoride (%)
Soluble salts	
Ammonium bifluoride	67
Hydrogen fluoride	95
Sodium fluoride	45
Sodium fluosilicate	61
Less soluble salts	
Cryolite	54
Sodium monofluorophosphate	13
Stannous fluoride	24

associated with a clear excess risk of skeletal adverse effects, a threshold closer to 6 mg per day has been suggested by the World Health Organization, International Programme on Chemical Safety.

III. Clinical presentation

A. Acute poisoning. Nausea and vomiting frequently occur within 1 hour of ingestion. Symptoms of serious fluoride intoxication include skeletal muscle weakness, tetanic contractions, respiratory muscle weakness, and respiratory arrest. Hypocalcemia, hypomagnesemia, hyperkalemia, and increased QT interval can occur. Death is due to intractable cardiac dysrhythmias and usually occurs within 6–12 hours.

B. Chronic effects. The recommended daily limit for children is 2 mg and for adults is 4 mg. Minor overexposure in children younger than age 10 can cause tooth discoloration. Chronic overexposure can cause crippling skeletal fluorosis (osteosclerosis), increased bone density and ligament calcification. Recent studies are evaluating chronic effects on cardiovascular and neurologic systems.

IV. Diagnosis usually is based on a history of ingestion. Symptoms of GI distress, muscle weakness, hypocalcemia, and hyperkalemia suggest acute fluoride intoxication.

A. Specific levels. The normal serum fluoride concentration is less than 20 mcg/L (ng/mL) but varies considerably with diet and water source. Serum fluoride concentrations are generally difficult to obtain and thus are of limited utility for acute overdose management.

B. Other useful laboratory studies include electrolytes, glucose, BUN, creatinine, calcium (and ionized calcium), magnesium, and ECG. For evaluation of chronic exposure, parathyroid hormone levels and bone imaging may be considered.

V. Treatment

A. Emergency and supportive measures

1. Maintain an open airway and assist ventilation if necessary (pp 1–7).
2. Monitor ECG and serum calcium, magnesium, and potassium for at least 4–6 hours. Admit patients who have electrolyte abnormalities, ECG abnormalities, or muscular symptoms to an intensive care setting with cardiac monitoring.

B. Specific drugs and antidotes. For hypocalcemia, administer **IV calcium gluconate** (p 526), 10–20 mL (children: 0.2–0.3 mL/kg), monitor ionized calcium levels, and titrate further doses as needed. To date, early IV calcium administration is the only treatment that has increased survival in an animal model. Treat hypomagnesemia with IV **magnesium sulfate**, 1–2 g given over 10–15 minutes (children: 25–50 mg/kg diluted to <10 mg/mL). Treat hyperkalemia with IV calcium and other standard measures (p 39). Antioxidants have not been evaluated in the treatment of acute poisoning.

C. Decontamination (p 50)

1. **Prehospital.** Do ***not*** induce vomiting because of the risk for abrupt onset of seizures and arrhythmias. Administer an antacid containing **calcium** (eg, calcium carbonate [Tums, Rolaids]) orally to raise gastric pH and complex free fluoride, impeding absorption. Milk, rich in calcium, has been shown to bind small fluoride doses and may be useful in the field if calcium carbonate is not available. There are little data documenting the effectiveness of magnesium-containing antacids.
2. **Hospital.** Administer antacids containing **calcium** as described above. Consider gastric lavage for large recent ingestions. Activated charcoal does not adsorb fluoride.

D. Enhanced elimination. Because fluoride rapidly binds to free calcium and bone and has a short elimination half-life, the effectiveness of prompt hemodialysis for acute poisoning remains unclear.

▶ FLUOROACETATE

Steven R. Offerman, MD

Fluoroacetate, also known as compound 1080, sodium monofluoroacetate (SMFA), and sodium fluoroacetate, is one of the most toxic substances known. In the past, it was used primarily as a rodenticide by licensed pest control companies, but it largely has been removed from the US market because of its hazardous nature. Compound 1080 use is currently restricted to livestock protection collars designed to protect sheep and cattle from coyotes. Occasionally, unlicensed product may be encountered. It is also still used commonly in Australia and New Zealand for vertebrate pest control. It is a tasteless, odorless water-soluble white crystalline powder. Fluoroacetamide (compound 1081) is a similar compound with similar toxicity.

I. Mechanism of toxicity

- **A.** Fluoroacetate is metabolized to the toxic compound fluorocitrate, which blocks cellular metabolism by binding and inhibiting the aconitase enzyme within the Krebs cycle. This impairs ATP production leading to lactic acid production and metabolic acidosis. Krebs inhibition also causes citrate accumulation, which chelates calcium cations resulting in hypocalcemia.
- **B. Pharmacokinetics.** The onset of effect is reported to be 30 minutes to several hours after ingestion. Fluoroacetate is rapidly and well absorbed orally. There is little to no absorption through intact skin. The time to peak effect, volume of distribution, duration of action, and elimination half-life in humans are unknown, but there are reports of late-onset coma (36 hours in one report). In sheep the serum half-life is 6.6–13.3 hours, and up to 33% may be excreted unchanged in urine over 48 hours.

II. Toxic dose. Inhalation or ingestion of as little as 1 mg of fluoroacetate is sufficient to cause serious toxicity. Death is likely after ingestion of more than 2–10 mg/kg.

III. Clinical presentation. After a delay of minutes to several hours (most patients develop symptoms in 3–6 hours, although onset of coma was 36 hours in one report), manifestations of diffuse cellular poisoning become apparent; nausea, vomiting, diarrhea, metabolic acidosis (lactic acidosis), shock, renal failure, agitation, confusion, seizures, coma, respiratory arrest, pulmonary edema, and ventricular dysrhythmias may occur. One case series reported a high incidence of hypocalcemia and hypokalemia. Hypotension, acidemia, and elevated serum creatinine are the most sensitive predictors of mortality. Death is usually the result of respiratory failure or ventricular dysrhythmia.

IV. Diagnosis is based on a history of ingestion and clinical findings. Fluoroacetate poisoning may mimic other cellular toxins, such as hydrogen cyanide and hydrogen sulfide, although with these poisons the onset of symptoms is usually more rapid.

- **A.** Specific levels. There is no assay available.
- **B.** Other useful laboratory studies include electrolytes, glucose, BUN, creatinine, calcium, arterial blood gases, ECG, and chest radiography. Perform continuous ECG monitoring.

V. Treatment

- **A. Emergency and supportive measures**
  1. Maintain an open airway and assist ventilation if necessary (pp 1–7). Administer supplemental oxygen.
  2. Replace fluid losses from gastroenteritis with IV saline or other crystalloids.
  3. Treat shock (p 15), seizures (p 23), and coma (p 18) if they occur. Because of the reported potential delay in the onset of serious symptoms, it is prudent to monitor the patient for at least 36–48 hours.
- **B. Specific drugs and antidotes.** Although several antidotes have been investigated, none has been proven effective in humans. Ethanol and monoacetin (glyceryl monoacetate) are thought to act as antidotes by increasing blood acetate levels, which may inhibit fluorocitrate conversion.

1. In animal studies, **ethanol** is effective only if given within minutes of exposure. Ethanol has been used in humans. Although conclusive evidence of benefit is lacking, it is reasonable to attempt ethanol infusion (p 553) with a target level of 100 mg/dL.
2. **Monoacetin** has been used experimentally in monkeys but is not available or recommended for human use. Animal evidence suggests that **hypocalcemia** may worsen fluoroacetate toxicity. Although its importance in human poisoning is uncertain, meticulous monitoring and correction of low serum calcium is recommended.

C. **Decontamination** (p 50)

1. **Prehospital.** If it is available and the patient is alert, immediately administer activated charcoal.
2. **Hospital.** Immediately administer activated charcoal. Consider gastric lavage if it can be performed within 60 minutes of ingestion.
3. **Skin exposure.** Fluoroacetate is poorly absorbed through intact skin, but a significant exposure could occur through broken skin. Remove contaminated clothing and wash exposed skin thoroughly.

D. **Enhanced elimination.** There is no role for any enhanced removal procedure.

▶ FOOD POISONING: BACTERIAL

Susan Kim-Katz, PharmD

Food-borne bacteria and bacterial toxins are a common cause of epidemic gastroenteritis. In general, the illness is relatively mild and self-limited, with recovery within 24 hours. However, severe and even fatal poisoning may occur with listeriosis, salmonellosis, or **botulism** (p 163) and with certain strains of *Escherichia coli.* Poisoning after the consumption of **fish and shellfish** is discussed on p 246. **Mushroom** poisoning is discussed on p 330. **Viruses** such as the Norwalk virus and Norwalk-like caliciviruses, enteroviruses, and rotaviruses are the causative agent in as many as 80% of food-related illness. Other microbes that can cause food-borne illness include *Cryptosporidium* and *Cyclospora,* which can cause serious illness in immunocompromised patients. However, in over half of reported food-borne outbreaks, no microbiological pathogens are identified.

I. **Mechanism of toxicity.** Gastroenteritis may be caused by invasive bacterial infection of the intestinal mucosa or by a toxin elaborated by bacteria. Bacterial toxins may be preformed in food that is improperly prepared and improperly stored before use or may be produced in the gut by the bacteria after they are ingested (Table II–28).

II. **Toxic dose.** The toxic dose depends on the type of bacteria or toxin and its concentration in the ingested food as well as individual susceptibility or resistance. Some of the preformed toxins (eg, staphylococcal toxin) are heat resistant and once in the food are not removed by cooking or boiling.

III. **Clinical presentation.** Commonly, a delay or "incubation period" of 2 hours to 3 days precedes the onset of symptoms (see Table II–28).

A. **Gastroenteritis** is the most common finding, with nausea, vomiting, abdominal cramps, and diarrhea. Vomiting is more common with preformed toxins. Significant fluid and electrolyte abnormalities may occur, especially in young children or elderly patients.

B. **Fever, bloody stools, and fecal leukocytosis** are common with invasive bacterial infections.

C. **Systemic infection** can result from *Bacillus cereus, Campylobacter, E. coli, Listeria, Salmonella, or Shigella.*

1. Rapid onset of fulminant hepatic failure and severe rhabdomyolysis has been reported with ingestion of ***B. cereus*** emetic toxin.

TABLE II–28. BACTERIAL FOOD POISONING

Organism	Incubation Period	Common Symptoms[a] and Mechanism	Common Foods
Bacillus cereus	1–6 h (emetic) 8–16 h (diarrheal)	V > D, S; toxins produced in food and gut	Reheated fried rice, improperly refrigerated meats.
Campylobacter jejuni	1–8 d	D+, F; invasive and possibly toxin produced in gut	Poultry, water, milk; direct contact (eg, food handlers).
Clostridium perfringens	6–16 h	D > V; toxin produced in food and gut	Meats, gravy, dairy products.
Escherichia coli "enterotoxigenic"	12–72 h	D > V; toxin produced in gut	"Traveler's diarrhea": water, various foods; direct contact (eg, food handlers).
E. coli "enteroinvasive"	24–72 h	D+; invasive infection	Water, various foods; direct contact (eg, food handlers).
E. coli "enterohemorrhagic" (STEC, eg, 0157:H7)	1–8 d	D+, S; toxin produced in gut	Water, ground beef, salami and other meats, unpasteurized milk and juice, contaminated lettuce and sprouts; direct contact (eg, food handlers).
Listeria monocytogenes	Varies	D+, S; invasive infection	Milk, soft cheeses, raw meat.
Salmonella spp	12–36 h	D+, F; invasive infection	Meat, dairy, eggs, water, sprouts; direct contact (eg, food handlers).
Shigella spp	1–7 d	D+, S; invasive infection	Water, fruits, vegetables; direct contact (eg, food handlers, contact with contaminated reptiles/frogs).
Staphylococcus aureus	1–6 h	V > D; toxin preformed in food; heat-resistant	Very common: meats, dairy, bakery foods; direct contact (eg, food handlers).
Vibrio parahemolyticus	8–30 h	V, D+; invasive and toxin produced in gut	Shellfish, water.
Yersinia enterocolitica	3–7 d	D+; invasive infection	Water, meats, dairy.

[a]D, diarrhea; D+, diarrhea with blood and/or fecal leukocytes; F, fever; S, systemic manifestations; V, vomiting.

2. ***Campylobacter*** infections sometimes are followed by Guillain–Barré syndrome or reactive arthritis.
3. **Listeriosis** can cause sepsis and meningitis, particularly in children, the elderly, and immunocompromised persons, with an estimated fatality rate of 20–30% among these high-risk individuals. Infection during pregnancy produces a mild flulike illness in the mother but serious intrauterine infection resulting in fetal death, neonatal sepsis, or meningitis.
4. ***Salmonella*** infection has led to rhabdomyolysis and acute renal failure, and it can also trigger acute reactive arthritis.
5. ***Shigella*** and Shiga toxin–producing ***E. coli*** (STEC) strains (eg, **O157:H7, O154:H4**) may cause acute hemorrhagic colitis complicated by hemolytic-uremic syndrome, renal failure, and death, especially in children and immunocompromised adults. Seizures have been reported in 10–45% of pediatric patients with shigellosis.

IV. Diagnosis. Bacterial food poisoning is often difficult to distinguish from common viral gastroenteritis unless the incubation period is short and there are multiple victims who ate similar foods at one large gathering. The presence of many white blood cells in a stool smear suggests invasive bacterial infection. With any epidemic gastroenteritis, consider other food-borne illnesses, such as those caused by viruses or parasites, illnesses associated with seafood (p 246), botulism (p 163), and ingestions of certain mushrooms (p 330).

A. Specific levels

1. In most laboratories, routine stool cultures may differentiate *E. coli*, *Salmonella, Shigella,* and *Campylobacter* infections. Recent advances provide more accurate and faster detection of enteric pathogens or their toxins, using enzyme immunoassay (EIA), polymerase chain reaction (PCR), and other methods. The FDA recently approved a qualitative PCR assay that simultaneously detects 15 different pathogens in human stool samples, including viruses and protozoa. PCR assays yield results in 3 hours or less, compared to 2 or more days required for conventional stool cultures.
2. **Blood and cerebrospinal fluid (CSF)** may grow invasive organisms, especially *Listeria* (and rarely *Salmonella* or *Shigella*).
3. **Food samples** should be saved for bacterial culture and toxin analysis, primarily for use by public health investigators.

B. Other useful laboratory studies include CBC, electrolytes, glucose, BUN, and creatinine.

V. Treatment

A. Emergency and supportive measures

1. Replace fluid and electrolyte losses with IV saline or other crystalloid solutions (patients with mild illness may tolerate oral rehydration). Patients with hypotension may require large-volume IV fluid resuscitation (p 15).
2. Antiemetic agents are acceptable for symptomatic treatment, but strong antidiarrheal agents such as Lomotil (diphenoxylate plus atropine) should not be used in patients with suspected invasive bacterial infection (fever and bloody stools).

B. Specific drugs and antidotes. There are no specific antidotes.

1. In patients with invasive bacterial infection, antibiotics may be used once the stool testing reveals the specific bacteria responsible, although antibiotics do not always shorten the course of illness. In fact, quinolones can prolong the carrier state in salmonellosis, and antibiotics may increase the risk for hemolytic-uremic syndrome from *E. coli* 0157:H7 infection. Empiric treatment with trimethoprim-sulfamethoxazole (TMP/SMX) or quinolones is often initiated while awaiting culture results. However, 88–100% of *Shigella* strains isolated during outbreaks in Kansas, Missouri, and Kentucky in 2005 were resistant to ampicillin and TMP/SMX.
2. Pregnant women who have eaten *Listeria*-contaminated foods should be treated empirically, even if they are only mildly symptomatic, to prevent serious intrauterine infection. The antibiotic of choice is IV ampicillin, with gentamicin added for severe infection.

C. Decontamination procedures are not indicated in most cases.

D. Enhanced elimination. There is no role for enhanced removal procedures.

SELECTED INTERNET WEBSITES WITH MORE INFORMATION ABOUT FOOD POISONING

Centers for Disease Control website on food-related illnesses: http://emergency. cdc. gov/agent/food

U.S. Food and Drug Administration foodborne illness website: http://www.fda.gov/ Food/ FoodSafety/FoodborneIllness/default.htm

▶ FOOD POISONING: FISH AND SHELLFISH

Susan Kim-Katz, PharmD

A variety of illnesses can occur after ingestion of, and less commonly from dermal or inhalational contact with, fish or shellfish toxins. The most common types of seafood-related toxins include **ciguatera, scombroid, neurotoxic shellfish poisoning, paralytic shellfish poisoning,** and **tetrodotoxin.** Less commonly encountered toxins will be discussed briefly. Shellfish-induced bacterial gastroenteritis is described on p 243 (Table II–28).

I. **Mechanism of toxicity.** The mechanism varies with each toxin. Marine toxins are generally tasteless, odorless, and heat-stable. Therefore, cooking the seafood does not prevent illness.
   A. **Ciguatera.** The toxins, ciguatoxin and related compounds such as maitotoxin, are produced by dinoflagellates, which are then consumed by reef fish. Ciguatoxin binds to voltage-sensitive sodium channels, causing increased sodium permeability and depolarization of excitable membranes. Stimulation of central or ganglionic cholinergic receptors may also be involved.
   B. **Diarrheic shellfish** poisoning is caused by several identified toxins, all of which appear to be produced by marine dinoflagellates. Suspected toxins include okadaic acid, dinophysistoxins, pectenotoxins, and azaspiracids. Yessotoxin is often classified as a diarrheic toxin, although animal testing suggests that its target organ is the heart.
   C. **Domoic acid,** the causative agent for amnesic shellfish poisoning, is produced by phytoplankton, which are concentrated by filter-feeding fish and shellfish. The toxin is thought to bind to glutamate receptors, causing neuroexcitatory responses.
   D. **Neurotoxic shellfish** poisoning is caused by ingestion of brevetoxins, which are produced by "red tide" dinoflagellates. The mechanism appears to involve stimulation of sodium channels, resulting in depolarization of nerve fibers.
   E. **Palytoxin** and its analogs are potent toxins first isolated from the coral genus *Palythoa* and produced by the dinoflagellate genus *Ostreopsis*. Through complicated mechanisms, one of which is disruption of the Na^+/K^+-ATPase pump, the toxin alters normal ion homeostasis, causing abnormal depolarization and contraction of smooth, skeletal, and cardiac muscles. It is also a potent vasoconstrictor.
   F. **Paralytic shellfish.** Dinoflagellates ("red tide"), and less commonly cyanobacteria from fresh water, produce saxitoxin and 21 other related toxins, which are concentrated by filter-feeding clams and mussels and rarely by nontraditional vectors such as puffer fish, crabs, and lobsters. Saxitoxin binds to voltage-gated, fast sodium channels in nerve cell membranes, blocking neuromuscular transmission.
   G. **Scombroid.** Scombrotoxin is a mixture of histamine and histamine-like compounds produced when histidine in fish tissue decomposes.
   H. **Tetrodotoxin,** produced primarily by marine bacteria, is found in puffer fish (fugu), California newts, some gastropod mollusks, horseshoe crab eggs, and some South American frogs. It blocks the voltage-dependent sodium channel in nerve cell membranes, interrupting neuromuscular transmission.

II. **Toxic dose.** The concentration of toxin varies widely, depending on geographic and seasonal factors. The amount of toxin necessary to produce symptoms is unknown in most cases. An oral dose of 0.1 mcg of ciguatoxin can produce symptoms in a human adult. Saxitoxin is extremely potent; the estimated lethal dose in humans is 0.3–1 mg, and contaminated mussels may contain 15–20 mg. For many marine toxins (eg, ciguatoxin, tetrodotoxin), ingestion of the organs or viscera is associated with greater symptom severity than eating only the fillet.

III. **Clinical presentation.** The onset of symptoms and clinical manifestations vary with each toxin (Table II–29). In the majority of cases, the seafood appears normal, with no adverse smell or taste (scombroid may have a peppery taste; palytoxin may be bitter).

TABLE II–29. FISH AND SHELLFISH INTOXICATIONS

Type	Onset	Common Sources	Syndrome
Amnesic shellfish poisoning (domoic acid)	Minutes to hours (mean 5.5 hours)	Mussels, clams, anchovies	Gastroenteritis, headache, myoclonus, seizures, coma, persistent neuropathy, and memory impairment
Ciguatera poisoning (ciguatoxin, maitotoxin)	1–6 hours; milder cases may be delayed	Barracuda, red snapper, grouper	Gastroenteritis, hot and cold sensation reversal, itching, paresthesias, myalgias, weakness, hypotension, bradycardia
Clupeotoxism (palytoxin, clupeotoxin)	Hours	Parrotfish, crabs, mackerel, sardines, seaweed	Gastroenteritis, paresthesias, severe muscle spasms, rhabdomyolysis, seizures, respiratory distress, myocardial damage
Diarrheic shellfish poisoning (various toxins)	30 minutes–2 hours	Bivalve mollusks, crabs	Nausea, vomiting, diarrhea
Neurotoxic shellfish poisoning (brevetoxin)	Minutes (inhalation) to 3 hours	Bivalve shellfish, whelks (conchs)	Gastroenteritis, ataxia, paresthesias, seizures, respiratory tract irritation from inhalation
Paralytic shellfish poisoning (saxitoxin and related)	Within 30 minutes	Bivalve shellfish, puffer fish, crab	Gastroenteritis, paresthesias, ataxia, respiratory paralysis
Scombroid poisoning (scombrotoxin)	Minutes to hours	Tuna, mahi-mahi, bonito, mackerel	Gastroenteritis, flushed skin, hypotension, urticaria, wheezing
Tetrodotoxin	Within 30–40 minutes	Puffer fish ("fugu"), sun fish, porcupine fish, California newt	Vomiting, paresthesias, muscle twitching, diaphoresis, weakness, respiratory paralysis

A. Ciguatera. Intoxication produces vomiting and watery diarrhea 1–6 hours after ingestion, followed by headache, malaise, myalgias, paresthesias of the mouth and extremities, ataxia, blurred vision, photophobia, temperature-related dysesthesia (hot and cold sensation reversal), extreme pruritus, hypotension, bradycardia, and rarely seizures and respiratory arrest. Although symptoms generally resolve after several days, some sensory and neuropsychiatric symptoms can last for weeks to months. Ciguatoxins in contaminated fish from the Pacific and Indian Oceans are generally more potent and cause more neurologic symptoms than those in fish from the Caribbean; the latter are associated with more prominent GI symptoms in the initial stages.

B. Diarrheic shellfish poisoning causes nausea, vomiting, stomach cramps, and severe diarrhea. The illness is usually self-limiting, lasting 3–4 days. Intoxication from azaspiracids is sometimes characterized as a distinct poisoning because in animal studies it causes neurologic symptoms and liver damage, but GI symptoms predominate in humans. In animal studies, pectenotoxins cause liver necrosis, and yessotoxins damage cardiac muscle.

C. Domoic acid. Symptoms begin from 15 minutes to 38 hours after ingestion and consist of gastroenteritis accompanied by unusual neurologic toxicity, including fasciculations, mutism, severe headache, hemiparesis, and myoclonus. Coma, seizures, hypotension, and profuse bronchial secretions have been reported with severe intoxication, with a human fatality rate estimated at 3%. Long-term sequelae include persistent severe anterograde memory loss, motor neuropathy, and axonopathy.

D. **Neurotoxic shellfish.** Onset is within a few minutes to 3 hours. Gastroenteritis is accompanied by paresthesias of the mouth, face, and extremities; muscular weakness and spasms; seizures; and rarely respiratory arrest. Hot and cold sensation reversal has been reported. Inhalation of aerosolized brevetoxins can cause throat irritation, sneezing, coughing, and irritated eyes, and it may worsen respiratory symptoms in persons with asthma. Dermal exposure to contaminated ocean waters or aerosols can cause skin irritation and pruritus.

E. Clinical presentation of **palytoxin** poisoning may initially mimic that of ciguatera poisoning. However, palytoxin produces greater morbidity and mortality as a result of severe muscle spasms, seizures, rhabdomyolysis, coronary vasospasm, hypertension, arrhythmias, and acute respiratory failure. Severe hyperkalemia and hyperphosphatemia were seen in a fatal case of palytoxin poisoning confirmed by laboratory analysis. Milder versions of human poisonings have occurred from dermal and inhalational exposure to the toxin; respiratory symptoms include hypoxia and persistent dyspnea. **Clupeotoxism,** a highly toxic marine poisoning associated with ingestion of sardines and herring, is thought to be caused by palytoxin. Symptoms include abrupt onset of generalized paralysis, convulsions and acute respiratory distress.

F. **Paralytic shellfish.** Vomiting, diarrhea, and facial paresthesias usually begin within 30 minutes of ingestion. Headache, myalgias, dysphagia, weakness, and ataxia have been reported. In serious cases, respiratory arrest may occur after 1–12 hours.

G. **Scombroid.** Symptoms begin rapidly (minutes to 3 hours) after ingestion. Gastroenteritis, headache, and skin flushing sometimes are accompanied by urticaria, bronchospasm, tachycardia, and hypotension.

H. **Tetrodotoxin.** Symptoms occur within 30–40 minutes after ingestion and include vomiting, paresthesia, salivation, twitching, diaphoresis, weakness, and dysphagia. Hypotension, bradycardia, flaccid paralysis, and respiratory arrest may occur up to 6–24 hours after ingestion.

I. Other unusual poisonings from marine toxins include **Haff disease,** unexplained rhabdomyolysis after ingestion of buffalo fish or salmon; **hallucinatory fish poisoning (ichthyoallyeinotoxism),** characterized by hallucinations and nightmares from ingestion of several families of fish (sometimes known locally as "dreamfish"); and **chelonitoxism,** a potentially fatal poisoning involving multiorgan-system failure resulting from ingestion of marine turtles. The causative toxins in these poisonings have not been definitively identified.

IV. **Diagnosis** depends on a history of ingestion and is more likely to be recognized when multiple victims present after consumption of a seafood meal. Scombroid may be confused with an allergic reaction because of the histamine-induced urticaria.

A. **Specific levels** are not generally available. However, when epidemic poisoning is suspected, state public health departments, the Food and Drug Administration, or the Centers for Disease Control may be able to analyze suspect food for toxins.

B. Cigua-Check®, a commercially available monoclonal antibody screening test for ciguatoxin-1, was determined to be poorly reliable in a recent study.

C. **Other useful laboratory studies** include electrolytes, glucose, BUN, creatinine, CPK, arterial blood gases, ECG monitoring, and stool for bacterial culture.

V. **Treatment**

A. **Emergency and supportive measures.** Most cases are mild and self-limited and require no specific treatment. However, because of the risk for respiratory arrest, all patients should be observed for several hours (except patients with diarrheic shellfish poisoning).

1. Maintain an open airway and assist ventilation if necessary (pp 1–7).
2. Replace fluid and electrolyte losses from gastroenteritis with IV crystalloid fluids.

B. Specific drugs and antidotes

1. **Ciguatera.** There are anecdotal reports of successful treatment with IV mannitol 20%, 0.5–1 g/kg infused over 30 minutes, particularly when instituted within 48–72 hours of symptom onset (p 578). Although a randomized study showed no difference in outcome between mannitol and saline therapy, inclusion of late-presenting patients may have clouded the data. Gabapentin, 400 mg 3 times daily, has also been reported anecdotally to relieve symptoms of neuropathy.
2. **Neurotoxic shellfish.** Atropine (p 512) may help reverse bronchospasm and bradycardia due to brevetoxin.
3. **Scombroid** intoxication can be treated symptomatically with both H_1 and H_2 histamine blockers, such as diphenhydramine (p 544) and cimetidine, 300 mg IV (p 532). Rarely, bronchodilators may also be required.
4. **Tetrodotoxin.** Some authors recommend IV neostigmine for the treatment of muscle weakness. However, its effectiveness is unproven, and its routine use cannot be recommended.

C. Decontamination (p 50) procedures are not indicated in most cases. However, consider using activated charcoal if immediately available after ingestion of a highly toxic seafood (eg, fugu fish).

D. Enhanced elimination. There is no role for these procedures.

▶ FORMALDEHYDE

John R. Balmes, MD

Formaldehyde is a gas with a pungent odor that is used commonly in the processing of paper, fabrics, and wood products and for the production of urea foam insulation. Low-level formaldehyde exposure has been found in stores selling clothing treated with formaldehyde-containing crease-resistant resins, in mobile homes, and in tightly enclosed rooms built with large quantities of formaldehyde-containing products used in construction materials. Formaldehyde aqueous solution (formalin) is used in varying concentrations (usually 37%) as a disinfectant and tissue fixative. Stabilized formalin may also contain 6–15% methanol (p 314).

I. Mechanism of toxicity

A. Formaldehyde causes precipitation of proteins and will cause coagulation necrosis of exposed tissue. The gas is highly water soluble. When inhaled, it produces immediate local irritation of the upper respiratory tract and has been reported to cause spasm and edema of the larynx.

B. Metabolism of formaldehyde produces formic acid, which may accumulate and produce metabolic acidosis if sufficient formaldehyde was ingested.

C. Formaldehyde has been listed by the International Agency for Research on Cancer (IARC) as a known human carcinogen associated with nasal sinus and nasopharyngeal cancer. NIOSH also considers formaldehyde a carcinogen.

II. Toxic dose

A. Inhalation. The OSHA workplace permissible exposure limit (PEL) is 0.75 ppm (8-hour TWA) and the short-term exposure limit (STEL) is 2 ppm. The NIOSH-recommended exposure limit (REL) is 0.016 ppm (8-hour TWA); the ceiling for a 15-minute exposure is 0.1 ppm. The air level considered immediately dangerous to life or health (IDLH) is 20 ppm.

B. Ingestion of as little as 30 mL of 37% formaldehyde solution has been reported to have caused death in an adult.

III. Clinical presentation

A. Formaldehyde gas exposure produces irritation of the eyes, and inhalation can produce cough, wheezing, and noncardiogenic pulmonary edema.

B. Ingestion of formaldehyde solutions may cause severe corrosive esophageal and gastric injury, depending on the concentration. Lethargy and coma have been reported. Metabolic (anion gap) acidosis may be caused by formic acid accumulation from metabolism of formaldehyde or methanol.

C. Hemolysis has occurred when formalin was accidentally introduced into the blood through contaminated hemodialysis equipment.

IV. Diagnosis is based on a history of exposure and evidence of mucous membrane, respiratory, or GI tract irritation.

A. Specific levels

1. Plasma formaldehyde levels are available in plasma, but formate levels may better indicate the severity of intoxication.

2. Methanol (p 314) and formate levels may be helpful in cases of intoxication by formalin solutions containing methanol.

B. Other useful laboratory studies include arterial blood gases, electrolytes, glucose, BUN, creatinine, osmolality, and calculation of the osmole gap (p 32).

V. Treatment

A. Emergency and supportive measures

1. Maintain an open airway and assist ventilation if necessary (pp 1–7).

2. Inhalation. Treat bronchospasm (p 8) and pulmonary edema (p 7) if they occur. Administer supplemental oxygen and observe for at least 4–6 hours.

3. Ingestion

a. Treat coma (p 18) and shock (p 15) if they occur.

b. Administer IV saline or other crystalloids to replace fluid losses caused by gastroenteritis. Avoid fluid overload in patients with inhalation exposure because of the risk for pulmonary edema.

c. Treat metabolic acidosis with sodium bicarbonate (p 35).

B. Specific drugs and antidotes

1. If a **methanol**-containing solution has been ingested, evaluate and treat with **ethanol** or **fomepizole** as for methanol poisoning (p 314).

2. Formate intoxication caused by formaldehyde alone should be treated with **folic acid** (p 557), but ethanol and **fomepizole** are not effective.

C. Decontamination (p 50). Rescuers should wear self-contained breathing apparatus and appropriate chemical-protective clothing when handling a heavily contaminated patient.

1. Inhalation. Remove victims from exposure and give supplemental oxygen if available.

2. Skin and eyes. Remove contaminated clothing and wash exposed skin with soap and water. Irrigate exposed eyes with copious tepid water or saline; perform fluorescein examination to rule out corneal injury if pain and lacrimation persist.

3. Ingestion. Give plain water to dilute concentrated solutions of formaldehyde. Perform aspiration of liquid formaldehyde from the stomach if large quantities were swallowed. Depending on the concentration of solution and patient symptoms, consider endoscopy to rule out esophageal or gastric injury. Activated charcoal is of uncertain benefit and may obscure the endoscopist's view.

D. Enhanced elimination

1. Hemodialysis is effective in removing methanol and formate and in correcting severe metabolic acidosis. Indications for hemodialysis include severe acidosis and an osmol gap (p 33) greater than 10 mOsm/L.

2. Alkalinization of the urine helps promote excretion of formate.

▶ FREONS AND HALONS

Tanya Mamantov, MD, MPH

Freons (fluorocarbons and chlorofluorocarbons [CFCs]) historically have been widely used as aerosol propellants, in refrigeration units, in the manufacture of plastics, in foam blowing, metal and electronics cleaning, mobile air conditioning, and sterilization. Although the use of CFCs is being phased out to avoid further depletion of stratospheric ozone, freons remain in older refrigeration and air conditioning systems, and illicit importation of freons occurs. Most freons are gases at room temperature, but some are liquids (freons 11, 21, 113, and 114) and may be ingested. Specialized fire extinguishers contain closely related compounds known as **halons,** which contain bromine, fluorine, and chlorine. HCFCs (Hydrochlorofluorocarbons) and HFCs (hydrofluorocarbons) are being used as transitional refrigerants because they break down more easily in the atmosphere than CFCs.

I. Mechanism of toxicity

A. Freons are mild CNS depressants and asphyxiants that displace oxygen from the ambient environment. Freons are well absorbed by inhalation or ingestion and are usually rapidly excreted in the breath within 15–60 minutes.

B. Like chlorinated hydrocarbons, freons may potentiate cardiac arrhythmias by sensitizing the myocardium to the effects of catecholamines.

C. Direct freezing of the skin, with frostbite, may occur if the skin is exposed to rapidly expanding gas as it escapes from a pressurized tank.

D. Freons and halons are mild irritants and may produce more potent irritant gases and vapors (eg, phosgene, hydrochloric acid, hydrofluoric acid, and carbonyl fluoride) when heated to high temperatures, as may happen in a fire or if a refrigeration line is cut by a welding torch or electric arc.

E. Some agents are hepatotoxic after large acute or chronic exposure.

II. Toxic dose

A. Inhalation. The toxic air level is quite variable, depending on the specific agent (see Table IV–4, p 659). Freon 21 (dichlorofluoromethane; TLV, 10 ppm [42 mg/m^3]) is much more toxic than freon 12 (TLV, 2,000 ppm). In general, anesthetic or CNS-depressant doses require fairly large air concentrations, which can also displace oxygen, leading to asphyxia. The air level of dichloromonofluoromethane considered immediately dangerous to life or health (IDLH) is 5,000 ppm. Other TLV and IDLH values can be found in Table IV–4 (p 659).

B. Ingestion. The toxic dose by ingestion is not known.

III. Clinical presentation

A. Skin or mucous membrane exposure can cause pharyngeal, ocular, and nasal irritation. Dysesthesia of the tongue is commonly reported. Frostbite may occur after contact with rapidly expanding compressed gas. Chronic exposure may result in skin defatting and erythema.

B. Respiratory effects can include cough, dyspnea, bronchospasm, hypoxemia, and pneumonitis.

C. Systemic effects of moderate exposure include dizziness, headache, nausea and vomiting, confusion, impaired speech, tinnitus, ataxia, and incoordination. More severe intoxication may result in coma or respiratory arrest. Ventricular arrhythmias may occur even with moderate exposures. A number of deaths, presumably caused by ventricular fibrillation, have been reported after freon abuse by "sniffing" or "huffing" freon products from plastic bags or air conditioning fluid. Hepatic injury may occur.

IV. Diagnosis is based on a history of exposure and clinical presentation. Many chlorinated and aromatic hydrocarbon solvents may cause identical symptoms.

A. Specific levels. Expired-breath monitoring is possible, and blood levels may be obtained to document exposure, but these procedures are not useful in emergency clinical management.

B. Other useful laboratory studies include arterial blood gases or oximetry, ECG monitoring, and liver enzymes.

V. **Treatment**

A. **Emergency and supportive measures**

1. Remove the individual from the contaminated environment.
2. Maintain an open airway and assist ventilation if necessary (pp 1–7).
3. Treat coma (p 18) and arrhythmias (pp 10–15) if they occur. Avoid epinephrine or other sympathomimetic amines that may precipitate ventricular arrhythmias. Tachyarrhythmias caused by increased myocardial sensitivity may be treated with **propranolol** (p 617), 1–2 mg IV, or **esmolol** (p 552), 0.025–0.1 mg/kg/min IV.
4. Monitor the ECG for 4–6 hours.

B. **Specific drugs and antidotes.** There is no specific antidote. Steroids have been used in inhalational exposure but have no proven benefit.

C. **Decontamination** (p 50)

1. **Inhalation.** Remove victim from exposure and give supplemental oxygen if available.
2. **Ingestion.** Do *not* give charcoal or induce vomiting because freons are rapidly absorbed and there is a risk for abrupt onset of CNS depression. Consider gastric lavage (or simply aspirate liquid from stomach) if the ingestion was very large and recent (<30–45 minutes). The efficacy of activated charcoal is unknown.

D. **Enhanced elimination.** There is no documented efficacy for diuresis, hemodialysis, hemoperfusion, or repeat-dose charcoal.

▶ GAMMA-HYDROXYBUTYRATE (GHB)

Jo Ellen Dyer, PharmD

Gamma-hydroxybutyrate (GHB) originally was investigated as an anesthetic agent during the 1960s but was abandoned because of side effects including myoclonus and emergence delirium. In 2002, it was approved by the FDA as a treatment for cataplexy and in 2005 for excessive daytime sleepiness in patients with narcolepsy. For abuse purposes, GHB is readily available through the illicit drug market and can be made in home laboratories by using recipes posted on the Internet. As a result of increasing abuse, GHB without a legitimate prescription is regulated as a Schedule I substance. Chemical precursors that are converted to GHB in the body, including **gamma-butyrolactone (GBL)** and **1,4-butanediol (1,4-BD),** are also regulated as Schedule I analogs (when intended for human consumption). These chemicals often are sold under constantly changing product names with intentionally obscure chemical synonyms (Table II–30), and to avoid the legal consequences of selling an analog intended for human consumption, they may be sold as a cleaner, paint stripper, nail polish remover, or solvent, labeled "not for ingestion."

GHB has been promoted as a growth hormone releaser, muscle builder, diet aid, soporific, euphoriant, hallucinogen, antidepressant, alcohol substitute, and enhancer of sexual potency. GHB use in dance clubs and at "rave" parties commonly involves ingestion along with ethanol and other drugs. GHB has also become known as a "date rape" drug because it can produce a rapid incapacitation or loss of consciousness, facilitating sexual assault.

I. **Mechanism of toxicity**

A. **GHB** is a structural analog of the neurotransmitter gamma-aminobutyric acid (GABA) with agonist activity at both GABA(B) and GHB receptors. It readily crosses the blood–brain barrier, leading to general anesthesia and respiratory depression. Death results from injury secondary to abrupt loss of consciousness, apnea, pulmonary edema, or pulmonary aspiration of gastric contents.

TABLE II–30. GHB AND RELATED CHEMICALS

Chemical	Chemical or Legitimate Names
Gamma-hydroxybutyric acid CASRN 591-81-1 $C_4H_8O_3$ MW 104.11	Gamma-hydroxybutyric acid; 4-hydroxybutanoic acid
Gamma-hydroxybutyrate, sodium salt CASRN 502-85-2 $C_4H_7NaO_3$ MW 126.09	Gamma-hydroxybutyrate, sodium; 4-hydroxybutyrate, sodium *Prescription drug formulations:* sodium oxybate (generic name); Gamma OH (France); Somsanit (Germany); Alcover (Italy); and Xyrem (United States)
Gamma-butyrolactone CASRN 96-48-0 $C_4H_6O_2$ MW 86.09	1,2-butanolide; 1,4-butanolide; 3-hydroxybutyric acid lactone; alpha-butyrolactone; blon; butyric acid lactone; butyric acid; 4-hydroxygamma-lactone; butyrolactone; butyryl lactone; dihydro-2(3H) furanone; gamma-bl; gamma butanolide; gammabutyrolactone; gammadeoxytetronic acid; gamma hydroxybutanoic acid lactone; gamma-hydroxybutyric acid cyclic ester; gamma-hydroxybutyric acid lactone; gamma-hydroxybutyric acid; gamma-lactone; gamma-hydroxy butyrolactone; gamma-lactone 4-hydroxybutanoic acid; gamma 6480; nci-c55875; tetrahydro-2-furanone
1,4-Butanediol CASRN 110-63-4 $C_4H_{10}O_2$ MW 90.1	1,4-butylene glycol; 1,4-dihydroxybutane; 1,4-tetramethylene glycol; butane-1,4-diol; butanediol; BD; BDO; butylene glycol; diol 1–4 B; sucol B; tetramethylene 1,4-diol; tetramethylene glycol

Fatal potentiation of the depressant effects of GHB has occurred with ethanol and other depressant drugs.

B. Gamma-butyrolactone (GBL), a solvent now regulated by the Drug Enforcement Administration (DEA) as a List I chemical, can be chemically converted by sodium hydroxide to GHB. In addition, GBL is rapidly converted in the body by peripheral lactonases to GHB within minutes.

C. 1,4-Butanediol (1,4-BD), an intermediate for chemical synthesis, is readily available through chemical suppliers. 1,4-BD is converted in vivo by alcohol dehydrogenase to gamma-hydroxybutyraldehyde, then by aldehyde dehydrogenase to GHB.

D. Pharmacokinetics. Onset of CNS-depressant effects begins within 10–15 minutes after oral ingestion of GHB and 2–8 minutes after IV injection. Peak levels occur within 25–45 minutes, depending on the dose. A recent meal may reduce systemic bioavailability by 37% compared with the fasting state. The duration of effect is 1–2.5 hours after anesthetic doses of 50–60 mg/kg and about 2.5 hours in nonintubated accidental overdoses seen in the emergency department (range, 15 minutes–5 hours). The rate of elimination of GHB is saturable. Plasma blood levels of GHB are undetectable within 4–6 hours after therapeutic doses. The volume of distribution is variable owing to saturable absorption and elimination. GHB is not protein bound (see also Table II–66, p 462).

II. Toxic dose

A. GHB. Response to low oral doses of GHB is unpredictable, with variability between patients and in the same patient. Narcolepsy studies with 30 mg/kg have reported effects including abrupt onset of sleep, enuresis, hallucinations, and myoclonic movements. Anesthetic studies reported unconsciousness with 50 mg/kg and deep coma with 60 mg/kg. Fasting, ethanol, and other depressants enhance the effects of GHB.

B. GBL, a nonionized molecule, has greater bioavailability than GHB when given orally in the same doses. A dose of 1.5 g produced sleep lasting 1 hour.

C. **1,4-BD** is equipotent to GHB, although in the presence of ethanol, competition for the metabolic enzyme alcohol dehydrogenase may delay or decrease the peak effect.

III. **Clinical presentation.** Patients with acute GHB overdose commonly present with coma, bradycardia, and myoclonic movements.

A. **Soporific effects and euphoria** usually occur within 15 minutes of an oral dose; unconsciousness and deep coma may follow within 30–40 minutes. When GHB is ingested alone, the duration of coma is usually short, with recovery within 2–4 hours and complete resolution of symptoms within 8 hours.

B. **Delirium and agitation** are common. **Seizures** occur rarely. Bradypnea with increased tidal volume is seen frequently. Cheyne–Stokes respiration and loss of airway-protective reflexes occur. Vomiting is seen in 30–50% of cases, and incontinence may occur. Stimulation may cause tachycardia and mild hypertension, but bradycardia is more common.

C. **Alkaline corrosive burns** result from misuse of the home manufacture kits; a dangerously basic solution is produced when excess base is added, the reaction is incomplete, or there is inadequate back titration with acid. (The solution can also be acidic from excessive back titration.)

D. Frequent use of GHB in high doses may produce tolerance and dependence. A **withdrawal syndrome** has been reported when chronic use is discontinued. Symptoms include tremor, paranoia, agitation, confusion, delirium, visual and auditory hallucinations, tachycardia, and hypertension. Rhabdomyolysis, myoclonus, seizure, and death have occurred.

E. See also the discussion of **drug-facilitated assault** (p 70).

IV. **Diagnosis** is usually suspected clinically in a patient who presents with abrupt onset of coma and recovers rapidly within a few hours.

A. **Specific levels.** Laboratory tests for GHB levels are not readily available but can be obtained from a few national reference laboratories. Serum levels greater than 50 mg/L are associated with loss of consciousness, and levels over 260 mg/L usually produce unresponsive coma. In a small series of accidental overdoses, awakening occurred as levels fell into the range of 75–150 mg/L. GBL and 1,4BD are rapidly converted in vivo to GHB. The duration of detection of GHB in blood and urine is short (6 and 12 hours, respectively, after therapeutic doses).

B. **Other useful laboratory studies** include glucose, electrolytes, and arterial blood gases or co-oximetry. Consider urine toxicology screening and blood ethanol to rule out other common drugs of abuse that may enhance or prolong the course of poisoning.

V. **Treatment**

A. **Emergency and supportive measures**

1. Protect the airway and assist ventilation if needed. Note that patients who require intubation are often awake and are extubated within a few hours.
2. Treat coma (p 18), seizures (p 23), bradycardia (p 9), and corrosive burns (p 186) if they occur.
3. Evaluate for and treat drug-facilitated assault (p 70).

B. **Specific drugs and antidotes.** There are no specific antidotes available. Flumazenil and naloxone are not clinically effective. GHB withdrawal syndrome is managed with benzodiazepine (p 516) sedation as in other depressant withdrawal syndromes. Large doses may be needed. Withdrawal refractory to benzodiazepines is not uncommon and may benefit from the addition of barbiturates (pp 602–604), baclofen (a GABA(B) agonist) or propofol (p 613).

C. **Decontamination**

1. **Prehospital.** Do ***not*** give charcoal or induce vomiting because of the risk for rapid loss of consciousness and loss of airway-protective reflexes, which may lead to pulmonary aspiration.
2. **Hospital.** The small doses of GHB usually ingested are rapidly absorbed, and gastric lavage and activated charcoal are of doubtful benefit and may

increase the risk for pulmonary aspiration. Consider activated charcoal administration only for recent, large ingestions or when significant co-ingestion is suspected.

D. Enhanced elimination. There is no role for enhanced removal procedures such as dialysis and hemoperfusion.

▶ GASES, IRRITANT

John R. Balmes, MD

A vast number of compounds produce irritant effects when inhaled in the gaseous form. The most common source of exposure to irritant gases is industry, but significant exposures may occur in a variety of circumstances, such as after mixing cleaning agents at home, with smoke inhalation in structural fires, or after highway tanker spills.

I. Mechanism of toxicity. Irritant gases often are divided into two major groups on the basis of their water solubility (Table II–31).

A. Highly soluble gases (eg, ammonia and chlorine) are readily adsorbed by the upper respiratory tract and rapidly produce their primary effects on moist mucous membranes in the eyes, nose, and throat.

TABLE II–31. IRRITANT TOXIC GASES

Gas	TLV[a] (ppm)	IDLH[b] (ppm)
High water solubility		
Ammonia	25	300
Chloramine[c]	N/A	N/A
Formaldehyde	0.3(C)	20
Hydrogen chloride	2(C)	50
Hydrogen fluoride	2(C)	30
Nitric acid	2	25
Sulfur dioxide	0.25(S)	100
Moderate water solubility		
Acrolein	0.1(C)	2
Chlorine	0.5	10
Fluorine	1	25
Low water solubility		
Nitric oxide	25	100
Nitrogen dioxide	3	20
Ozone	0.2[d]	5
Phosgene	0.1	2

[a]Threshold limit value, ACGIH-recommended exposure limit as an 8-hour time-weighted average for a 40-hour workweek (TLV-TWA). "(C)" indicates ceiling limit, which should not be exceeded at any time (TLV-C). "(S)" indicates short-term exposure limit.

[b]Air level considered immediately dangerous to life or health (IDLH), defined as the maximum air concentration from which one could reasonably escape within 30 minutes without any escape-impairing symptoms or any irreversible health effects.

[c]Chloramine is formed when chlorine or hypochlorite is added to water containing ammonia. It is usually a mixture of mono-, di-, and trichloramines. (N/A: TLV and IDLH are not established.)

[d]For exposure of no more than 2 hours (all workloads).

B. **Less soluble gases** (eg, phosgene and nitrogen dioxide) are not rapidly adsorbed by the upper respiratory tract and can be inhaled deeply into the lower respiratory tract to produce delayed-onset pulmonary toxicity.

II. **Toxic dose.** The toxic dose varies with the properties of the gas. Table II–31 illustrates the workplace exposure limits (TLV-TWA) and the levels immediately dangerous to life or health (IDLH) for several common irritant gases.

III. **Clinical presentation.** All these gases may produce irritant effects in the upper and/or lower respiratory tract, but warning properties and the onset and location of primary symptoms depend largely on the water solubility of the gas and the concentration of exposure.

A. **Highly soluble gases.** Because of the good warning properties (upper respiratory tract irritation) of highly soluble gases, voluntary prolonged exposure to even low concentrations is unlikely.

1. Low-level exposure causes rapid onset of mucous membrane and upper respiratory tract irritation; conjunctivitis, rhinitis, skin erythema and burns, sore throat, cough, wheezing, and hoarseness are common.
2. With high-level exposure, laryngeal edema, tracheobronchitis, and abrupt airway obstruction may occur. Irritation of the lower respiratory tract and lung parenchyma causes tracheobronchial mucosal sloughing, chemical pneumonitis, and noncardiogenic pulmonary edema.

B. **Less soluble gases.** Because of poor warning properties owing to minimal upper respiratory tract effects, prolonged exposure to moderate levels of these gases often occurs; therefore, chemical pneumonitis and pulmonary edema are more common. The onset of pulmonary edema may be delayed up to 12–24 hours or even longer.

C. **Sequelae.** Although most patients who suffer toxic inhalation injury recover without any permanent impairment, bronchiectasis, bronchiolitis obliterans, persistent asthma, and pulmonary fibrosis can occur.

IV. **Diagnosis** is based on a history of exposure and the presence of typical irritant upper or lower respiratory effect. Arterial blood gases and chest radiograph may reveal early evidence of chemical pneumonitis or pulmonary edema. Whereas highly soluble gases have good warning properties and the diagnosis is not difficult, less soluble gases may produce minimal symptoms shortly after exposure; therefore, a high index of suspicion and repeated examinations are required.

A. **Specific levels.** There are no specific blood or serum levels available.

B. **Other useful laboratory studies** include arterial blood gases or oximetry, chest radiography, spirometry, and peak expiratory flow measurement.

V. **Treatment**

A. **Emergency and supportive measures**

1. Immediately assess the airway; hoarseness or stridor suggests laryngeal edema, which necessitates direct laryngoscopy and endotracheal intubation if swelling is present (p 4). Assist ventilation if necessary (p 6).
2. Give supplemental oxygen, and treat bronchospasm with aerosolized bronchodilators (p 8).
3. Monitor arterial blood gases or oximetry, chest radiographs, and pulmonary function. Treat pulmonary edema if it occurs (p 7).
4. For victims of smoke inhalation, consider the possibility of concurrent intoxication by carbon monoxide (p 182) or cyanide (p 208).

B. **Specific drugs and antidotes**. There is no specific antidote for any of these gases.

C. **Decontamination** (p 50). Remove the victim from exposure and give supplemental oxygen if available. Rescuers should take care to avoid personal exposure; in most cases, self-contained breathing apparatus should be worn.

D. **Enhanced elimination**. There is no role for enhanced elimination.

► GLYPHOSATE

Craig Smollin, MD

Glyphosate (*N*-[phosphonomethyl]glycine) is an herbicide that is used widely in agriculture, forestry, and commercial weed control. It is one of the first herbicides against which crops have been genetically modified to increase their tolerance. U.S. poison control center data from 2014 report glyphosate to be the most common herbicide exposure. There are over 750 commercial glyphosate-based products (Roundup, Vantage, and many others) marketed for sale in the United States. Concentrations of glyphosate range from 0.5% to 41% or higher and most products consist of an aqueous mixture of the isopropylamino salt of glyphosate, a surfactant, and various minor components. Concentrated Roundup, the most commonly used glyphosate preparation in the United States, contains 41% glyphosate and 15% polyoxyethyleneamine (POEA).

I. Mechanism of toxicity. The precise mechanisms of toxicity of glyphosate formulations are complicated. There are five different glyphosate salts, and commercial formulations contain surfactants that vary in chemical structure and concentration.

- **A.** It has been hypothesized that toxicity is related to the presence of the surfactant rather than to the glyphosate itself. Surfactants may impair cardiac contractility and increase pulmonary vascular resistance.
- **B.** Some have postulated that glyphosate or the surfactants may uncouple mitochondrial oxidative phosphorylation.
- **C.** Glyphosate is a phosphorus-containing compound, but it does not inhibit acetylcholinesterase.

II. Toxic dose. Glyphosate itself has very low toxicity by the oral and dermal routes, with 50% lethal dose (LD_{50}) values in animals of more than 5,000 and more than 2,000 mg/kg, respectively. However, the surfactant (POEA) is more toxic, with an oral LD_{50} of 1,200 mg/kg. Ingestion of >85 mL of a concentrated formulation is likely to cause significant toxicity in adults.

III. Clinical presentation. Most patients with acute unintentional glyphosate exposures are asymptomatic or have only mild toxicity, and basic supportive care is generally effective. However, large intentional ingestions may cause serious toxicity and death. The case fatality rate in acute intentional poisoning has been documented in various studies to be between 3% and 8%. In one large prospective observational study involving 601 patients, there were 19 deaths. Death was associated with older age (>40 years), larger ingestions (>190 mL) and high plasma glyphosate concentrations on admission. Gastrointestinal symptoms, respiratory distress, hypotension, altered level of consciousness, and oliguria were observed in fatal cases.

- **A. Dermal exposure.** Prolonged exposure to the skin can cause dermal irritation. Severe skin burns are rare. Glyphosate is poorly absorbed across the skin, with only 3% of patients with dermal exposure developing systemic symptoms.
- **B. Ocular exposure** can cause a mild conjunctivitis and superficial corneal injury. No serious eye injury occurred among 1,513 consecutive ocular exposures reported to a poison control center.
- **C. Inhalation** is a minor route of exposure. Aerosolized mist can cause oral or nasal discomfort and throat irritation.
- **D. Ingestion.** After acute ingestion of a large amount of a glyphosate/surfactant-containing product, serious GI, cardiopulmonary, and other organ system toxicity may occur.
  1. **Gastrointestinal corrosive effects** include mouth, throat, and epigastric pain and dysphagia. Vomiting and diarrhea are common. Esophageal and gastric mucosal injury may occur.
  2. **Cardiovascular.** Glyphosate/surfactant-induced myocardial depression can result in cardiogenic shock.

3. **Ventilatory insufficiency** can occur secondary to pulmonary aspiration of the product or noncardiogenic pulmonary edema.
4. **Other.** Renal and hepatic impairment and a diminished level of consciousness may occur secondary to reduced organ perfusion, although a direct toxic effect of glyphosate or surfactant may contribute. Dilated pupils, convulsions, confusion, a neutrophil leukocytosis, fever, and increased serum amylase have also been reported. In a series of 131 cases of glyphosate ingestion, metabolic acidosis was present in 48% of cases and ECG abnormalities (sinus tachycardia and/or nonspecific ST-T–wave changes most commonly) occurred in up to 20% of cases.

IV. Diagnosis is based on the history of contact with or ingestion of glyphosate-containing products.

A. Specific levels. Although unlikely to affect clinical management, serum and urine glyphosate levels may be obtained from a reference laboratory or the manufacturer of Roundup (Monsanto, St. Louis, MO). Initial serum concentrations greater than 731 mcg/mL were associated with fatal outcome in one case series.

B. Other useful laboratory studies include chest radiography, electrolytes, renal function studies, and arterial blood gases or pulse oximetry to assess oxygenation.

V. Treatment

A. Emergency and supportive measures

1. Maintain an open airway and assist ventilation if necessary (pp 1–7).
2. Treat hypotension (p 15) and coma (p 18) if they occur. Intravenous lipid emulsion (p 574) was effective in reversing hypotension in one reported case.
3. If corrosive injury to the GI tract is suspected, consult a gastroenterologist for possible endoscopy.

B. Specific drugs and antidotes. No specific antidote is available.

C. Decontamination (p 50)

1. **Skin and eyes.** Remove contaminated clothing and wash exposed skin with water. Flush exposed eyes with copious tepid water or saline.
2. **Ingestion.** For small ingestions of a diluted or low-concentration product, no decontamination is necessary. For larger ingestions, place a flexible nasogastric tube and aspirate gastric contents, then lavage with tepid water or saline. The efficacy of activated charcoal is unknown.

D. Enhanced elimination. Extracorporeal techniques are not expected to augment the clearance of the surfactant due to its large molecular weight. Several case reports describe the use of hemodialysis primarily to support renal function, to treat significant acidosis, and to correct electrolyte abnormalities. There is insufficient evidence to routinely recommend its use.

▶ HEPARINS

Janna H. Villano, MD

Heparins (Table II–32) have been used for many years as injectable anticoagulants for prophylaxis of thromboembolic disease and management of multiple conditions including hypercoagulable disorders, venous thromboembolic disease, acute coronary syndrome, and to maintain patency in intravascular access and hemodialysis machines. Conventional or **unfractionated heparin** (UFH) is primarily administered in health care settings and thus intentional overdoses are rare; most cases involve inadvertent iatrogenic administration errors. **Low–molecular-weight-heparins** (LMWHs) are obtained from UFH and have greater bioavailability, longer half-life, predictable anticoagulation with a fixed-dose schedule, and are more easily self-administered by patients in outpatient settings.

TABLE II–32. HEPARINS

Heparin	Half-Life[a] (hours)	Duration of Anticoagulant Effect[a] (hours)	Anti Xa/IIa Ratio
Unfractionated heparin (UFH)	1–2.5	1–3	1.2
Low–molecular-weight heparins (LMWH)[b]			
Enoxaparin	3–6	3–5	3.9
Dalteparin	3–5	3.5–4.5	2.5
Tinzaparin	3–4	4–5	1.6

[a]Half-life and duration of effect as measured when administered intravenously (UFH) or subcutaneously (LMWHs).
[b]Other LMWHs not currently available in the United States include parnaparin, reviparin, nadroparin, certoparin, and bemiparin.

I. Mechanism of toxicity

A. UFH causes anticoagulation by binding to and activating antithrombin III, which then inactivates thrombin (factor II) and other proteases involved in coagulation, including factors IX, Xa, XI, XII, kallikrein, and thrombin.

B. LMWHs act similar to UFH, but exhibit greater factor Xa inhibition and less inhibition of thrombin.

C. Heparins do not cross the placenta and have been used during pregnancy to treat hypercoagulable states, thromboembolic disease, and to prevent miscarriage in patients with recurrent fetal loss.

D. Pharmacokinetics

1. UFH remains largely in the intravascular compartment (Vd 0.06 L/kg) bound to proteins and fibrinogen. Elimination half-life is dose-dependent and ranges from 1 to 2.5 hours. Elimination is largely hepatic via a heparinase enzyme.
2. LMWHs have high bioavailability (90%) when administered via the subcutaneous route. Elimination half-life ranges from 3 to 6 hours depending on the specific preparation. Peak anticoagulant effect occurs between 3 and 5 hours after administration. LMWHs are hepatically metabolized and renally eliminated. (See also Table II–66, p 462).

II. Toxic dose

A. The toxic dose is highly variable and depends on several patient-dependent and administration factors. Any patient receiving anticoagulation therapy is at risk for bleeding, even at therapeutic doses.

B. Patients at increased risk for bleeding include those receiving warfarins or other newer anticoagulants, antiplatelet agents, nonsteroidal anti-inflammatory drugs, and (with LMWHs) patients taking selective serotonin reuptake inhibitors. Patients with renal insufficiency are at increased risk of LMWH toxicity.

III. Clinical presentation.

A. After **acute exposure**, anticoagulant effects may be subclinical in nature. However, significant bleeding may occur. Reported complications have included abdominal wall and other subcutaneous hematomas, intrahepatic hemorrhage, gastrointestinal hemorrhage, spinal hematoma, post-traumatic compartment syndrome, and intracranial hemorrhage. Fatalities are rare but have been reported.

B. In addition to bleeding complications, **chronic exposure** to heparin infrequently predisposes patients to necrotic skin lesions, aldosterone suppression leading to hyperkalemia, and osteoporosis.

C. Heparin-induced thrombocytopenia (HIT) is an uncommon but potentially serious complication of therapeutic use of heparins. It is more common with UFH but can occur with LMWH.

1. **Type 1 HIT** occurs in the first few days after heparin is started and usually normalizes with continued heparin administration.

2. **Type 2 HIT** is less common but more serious. It occurs 4–10 days after starting heparin, is immune-mediated and may include thrombosis as well as bleeding (HIT with thrombosis, or HITT). It is more common in females, nonwhites, and the elderly.
3. Treatment includes discontinuation of heparin products and use of alternative anticoagulants.

IV. Diagnosis.

A. Specific levels.

1. **UFH.** Serial measurement of activated PTT (aPTT) is most useful in evaluating the anticoagulant activity.
2. **LMWH.** Specific anti-factor Xa activity is the preferred test if available, although aPTT can also be monitored.

B. Other useful laboratory studies include electrolytes (evaluate for hyperkalemia), BUN, creatinine, and complete blood count. Thrombin time, fibrinogen, and prothrombin time (PT/INR) may be useful in consideration of other causes of bleeding.

V. Treatment

A. Emergency and supportive measures

1. If clinically significant bleeding occurs, be prepared to treat shock with blood transfusion and fresh-frozen plasma.
2. Obtain immediate neurosurgical consultation if intracranial bleeding is suspected.

B. Specific drugs and antidotes

1. Studies and case reports are conflicting as to the use of reversal agents when clinically significant bleeding has not occurred.
2. **Protamine**
   a. **UFH.** Given heparin's short duration of action, clinically insignificant bleeding may be managed by discontinuation of heparin infusion and monitoring alone. When severe bleeding occurs, UFH is effectively reversed by **protamine sulfate** (see p 619).
      i. Protamine has a rapid onset of action and effects last up to 2 hours. Redosing may be necessary.
      ii. Dosage calculation is based on time of last dose of heparin and volume of heparin administered.
      iii. Protamine should be used with caution in pregnant patients as an anaphylactoid reaction or hypotension could result in fetal harm.
   b. **LMWH. Protamine** can effectively neutralize the antithrombin activity of LMWH, but only partially neutralizes anti-Xa activity (20–60%). Animal studies demonstrate conflicting results of the ability of protamine to reverse LMWH-associated hemorrhage, and human cases of only partial hemorrhage control have been described. Still, protamine is recommended for patients with LMWH anticoagulation and significant hemorrhage.
      i. Dosing is based on the type of LMWH administered and the number of equivalent anti-factor Xa international units (see p 619). Protamine administration should ideally be within 8 hours of LMWH administration.
      ii. Anti-Xa activity should be measured prior to and 5–15 minutes after protamine is given.
3. **Other drugs**
   a. **Activated factor VII** has been reported to partially reverse the anticoagulant effects of LMWHs in patients with clinically significant bleeding.
   b. **Tranexamic acid** has been used anecdotally in cases of LMWH overdose associated with hemorrhagic complications.
   c. Animal studies have also demonstrated success with use of adenosine triphosphate, synthetic protamine variants, heparinase, and other compounds that are not yet widely available.

C. Decontamination (p 50). Not required. Oral bioavailability of UFH and LMWH is low, and gastrointestinal decontamination is not indicated.

D. Enhanced elimination. Heparin has a small volume of distribution and exchange transfusion has been used in neonates. However, due to its short duration of action and the availability of a rapidly effective reversal agent (protamine) in cases of significant bleeding, neither exchange transfusion nor hemodialysis is generally used in heparin toxicity.

► HERBAL AND ALTERNATIVE PRODUCTS

Richard Ko, PharmD, PhD

The use of herbal medicines, dietary supplements, and other alternative products has risen sharply since passage of the Dietary Supplement Health and Education Act (DSHEA) in 1994. In contrast to prescription or nonprescription drugs, these products do not require FDA approval before marketing. Premarketing evaluation of safety and efficacy is not mandated, and adherence to good manufacturing practices and quality control standards is not enforced. Consumers often mistakenly believe that these "natural" products are free of harm and may unknowingly be at risk for illness from the products and herb–drug and herb–disease interactions, particularly with "polysupplement" use. Table II–33 lists common selected products that are available as herbal remedies or dietary supplements or that have alternative uses, along with their potential toxicities.

I. Mechanism of toxicity

A. Adulterants. A number of poisonings related to herbal preparations have been caused by **heavy metals** such as cadmium, lead, arsenic, and mercury or pharmaceutical adulterants such as diazepam, acetaminophen, phenylbutazone, and prednisone. An epidemic of "eosinophilia-myalgia syndrome" in the late 1980s apparently was caused by contaminants associated with mass production of the amino acid L-tryptophan, and similar contaminants have been identified in some melatonin products. Currently, a number of male sexual enhancement supplements are adulterated with sildenafil analogs (eg, acetildenafil), which are difficult to identify in the laboratory. As a general rule, if the product results in an immediate effect, it may mean that the product contains pharmaceutical rather than natural herbal ingredients.

B. Misidentification. Some herbs are intrinsically toxic, and poisoning may occur as a result of misidentification or mislabeling of plant materials, as occurred with a Belgian slimming formulation contaminated with the herb *Stephania fangchi* containing the nephrotoxin aristolochic acid.

C. Improper or nontraditional processing. Many herbs must be processed to remove the toxins before they are consumed. Aconite roots (p 77) contain cardiotoxic and neurotoxic alkaloids, and they must be processed to reduce the amounts of the toxic substances. Green tea extract (concentrated through processing, different from regular green tea) has been linked to a number of hepatitis cases and should not be taken on an empty stomach.

D. Herb–drug interactions. Herbal products may potentiate or diminish the effects of drugs with narrow therapeutic margins. **Ginseng (*Panax ginseng*), *Salvia miltiorrhiza*** (Danshen), nattokinase, and *Ginkgo biloba* appear to have anticoagulant effects and should not be used concomitantly with warfarin, aspirin, or other anticoagulant or antiplatelet therapies. St. John wort has been shown to have several clinically significant pharmacokinetic interactions with substrates for *p*-glycoprotein and the cytochrome P450 system, resulting in decreased plasma levels of drugs such as indinavir, cyclosporine, digoxin, and oral contraceptives.

E. Allergic reactions. Raw botanical herbs may cause allergic reactions. Many herbs are treated with sulfur as a preservative and should be used with caution in consumers who have known sulfur allergy.

F. Pesticides are commonly used on botanical products, and consumers may be unknowingly exposed to these chemicals resulting in acute or chronic poisoning.

TABLE II–33. DIETARY SUPPLEMENTS AND ALTERNATIVE REMEDIES[a]

Product	Source or Active Ingredient	Common or Purported Use(s)	Clinical Effects and Potential Toxicity
Aconite (monkshood)	Aconitine, mesaconitine, and hypaconitine	Rheumatism, pain	Nausea, vomiting, paresthesia, numbness; hypotension, palpitations, ventricular tachycardia, ventricular arrhythmias.
Androstenedione	Sex steroid precursor	Increase muscle size and strength	Virilization in women, increased estrogen in men.
Anabolic steroids	Methandrostenolone, oxandrolone, testolactone, many other steroid derivatives	Body building	Virilization; feminization; cholestatic hepatitis; aggressiveness, mania, or psychosis; hypertension; acne; hyperlipidemia; immune suppression.
Azarcon (Greta)	Lead salts	Hispanic folk remedy for abdominal pain, colic	Lead poisoning (p 286).
Bitter orange	*Citrus aurantium* (source of synephrine)	Weight loss, athletic enhancement	Synephrine: alpha-adrenergic agonist (p 394); may cause vasoconstriction, hypertension.
Bufotoxin	Bufotenine (toad venom); "love stone"; Chan su	Purported aphrodisiac, hallucinogen	Cardiac glycosides (p 222).
Cascara sagrada	*Rhamnus purshiana*	Cathartic in some diet aids	Abdominal cramps, diarrhea; fluid and electrolyte loss.
Chitosan	Derived from marine exoskeletons	Weight loss	Dyspepsia, oily stools, shellfish hypersensitivity reaction.
Chondroitin sulfate	Shark or bovine cartilage or synthetic	Osteoarthritis	Possible anticoagulant activity.
Chromium	Chromium picolinate	Glucose and cholesterol lowering, athletic performance enhancement	Renal insufficiency, possibly mutagenic in high doses, niacin-like flushing reaction with picolinate salt (p 445).
Comfrey	*Symphytum officinale*	Anti-inflammatory, gastritis, diarrhea	Hepatic veno-occlusive disease, possible teratogen/carcinogen. (***Note:*** Many other plants also contain hepatotoxic pyrrolizidine alkaloids; see Table II–52, p 377.)
Creatine	Creatine monohydrate, creatine monophosphate	Athletic performance enhancement	Nausea, diarrhea, muscle cramping, rhabdomyolysis, renal dysfunction.
Danshen	*Salvia miltiorrhiza*	Cardiovascular diseases, menstrual problem, wound healing	Anticoagulant effect; may potentiate cardiac glycoside toxicity

(*continued*)

TABLE II–33. DIETARY SUPPLEMENTS AND ALTERNATIVE REMEDIES[a] (CONTINUED)

Product	Source or Active Ingredient	Common or Purported Use(s)	Clinical Effects and Potential Toxicity
DHEA	Dehydroepiandrosterone (an adrenal steroid)	Anticancer, antiaging	Possible androgenic effects.
Echinacea	*Echinacea angustifolia* *Echinacea pallida* *Echinacea purpurea*	Immune stimulation, prevention of colds	Allergic reactions, possible exacerbation of autoimmune diseases.
Fenugreek	*Trigonella foenum-graecum*	Increase appetite, promote lactation	Hypoglycemia in large doses, anticoagulant effects possible.
Feverfew	*Tanacetum parthenium*	Migraine prophylaxis	Allergic reactions, antiplatelet effects.
Garlic	*Allium sativum*	Hyperlipidemia, hypertension	Anticoagulant effect, gastrointestinal irritation, body odor.
Ginkgo	Extract of *Ginkgo biloba*	Memory impairment, tinnitus, peripheral vascular disease	Gastrointestinal irritation, antiplatelet effects.
Ginseng	*Panex ginseng, Panex quinquefolium*	Fatigue/stress, immune stimulation	Decreases glucose, increases cortisol; *ginseng abuse syndrome*: nervousness, insomnia, gastrointestinal distress.
Glucosamine	Marine exoskeletons or synthetic	Osteoarthritis	Possibly decreased insulin production.
Goldenseal	*Hydrastis canadensis*	Dyspepsia, postpartum bleeding, drug test adulterant	Nausea, vomiting, diarrhea, paresthesia, seizures; use during pregnancy/lactation can cause kernicterus in infants.
Grape seed extract	Procyanidins	Circulatory disorders, antioxidant	None described.
Green tea extract (concentrated)	*Camellia sinensis*	Mental alertness, stomach disorder, weight loss, cancer	Standardized extract has been associated with hepatitis. May interact with drugs and supplements, including iron.
Guarana	Caffeine	Athletic performance enhancement, appetite suppressant	Tachycardia, tremor, vomiting (see "Caffeine," p 169).
Jin bu huan	L-Tetrahydropalmatine	Chinese traditional medicine	Acute CNS depression and bradycardia, chronic hepatitis.
Kava	*Piper methysticum*	Anxiety, insomnia	Drowsiness; hepatitis, cirrhosis, acute liver failure; habituation; reversible skin rash.
Kratom	*Mitragyna speciosa*	Mood enhancer, opioid substitute	Low doses: euphoria, mild stimulant; high doses: dizziness, dysphoria, somnolence; may cause seizures and coma.

(*continued*)

TABLE II–33. DIETARY SUPPLEMENTS AND ALTERNATIVE REMEDIES[a] (CONTINUED)

Product	Source or Active Ingredient	Common or Purported Use(s)	Clinical Effects and Potential Toxicity
Ma huang	Ephedrine (various *Ephedra* spp)	Stimulant, athletic Performance enhancement, appetite suppressant	Insomnia; hypertension, tachycardia, cardiac dysrhythmias, stroke; psychosis, seizures (p 394).
Melatonin	Pineal gland	Circadian rhythm sleep disorders	Drowsiness, headache, transient depressive symptoms.
Milk thistle	*Silybum marianum*	Toxic hepatitis and other liver diseases	Mild GI distress, possible allergic reaction.
Nattokinase	Enzyme extracted from natto, a Japanese fermented soybean product	Anticoagulant, fibrinolytic; also promoted for Alzheimer disease	Bleeding; additive anticoagulant effect with other drugs.
Phenibut	Beta-phenyl-GABA	Anxiety, insomnia	GABA-B agonist: lethargy, stupor, respiratory depression, mydriasis, hypothermia; withdrawal syndrome after prolonged use.
SAMe	S-Adenosyl-L methionine	Depression	Mild gastrointestinal distress, mania (rare).
Saw palmetto	*Serenoa repens*	Benign prostatic hypertrophy	Antiandrogenic, headache.
Senna	*Cassia angustifolia, Cassia acutifolia*	Weight loss, laxative	Watery diarrhea, abdominal cramps, fluid and electrolyte loss.
Shark cartilage	Pacific Ocean shark *Squalus acanthias*	Cancer, arthritis	Bad taste, hepatitis, hypercalcemia, hyperglycemia.
Spirulina	Some blue-green algae	Body building	Niacin-like flushing reaction.
St. John wort	*Hypericum perforatum*	Depression	Possible mild MAO inhibition (p 326), photosensitivity, P-glycoprotein and P450 enzyme induction.
Tea tree oil	*Melaleuca alternifolia*	Lice, scabies, ringworm, vaginitis, acne	Sedation and ataxia when taken orally; contact dermatitis, local skin irritation.
L-Tryptophan	Essential amino acid	Insomnia, depression	Eosinophilia-myalgia syndrome due to contaminants in tryptophan reported in 1989; similar contaminants found in 5-hydroxytryptophan and melatonin.
Valerian root	*Valeriana officinalis, Valeriana edulis*	Insomnia	Sedation, vomiting.
Vanadium	Vanadyl sulfate	Body building	Greenish discoloration of tongue, intestinal cramps, diarrhea, renal dysfunction.

(*continued*)

TABLE II–33. DIETARY SUPPLEMENTS AND ALTERNATIVE REMEDIES[a] (CONTINUED)

Product	Source or Active Ingredient	Common or Purported Use(s)	Clinical Effects and Potential Toxicity
Xanthium	*Xanthium sibiricum*	Hyperglycemia, hypertension, pain, anticoagulant, rhinitis	Headache, dizziness, nausea, vomiting, bradycardia, tachycardia; hepatic toxins leading to hepatic failure.
Yohimbine	*Corynanthe yohimbe*	Sexual dysfunction	Hallucinations, tachycardia, tremor, hypertension, irritability, gastrointestinal irritation.
Zinc	Zinc gluconate lozenges	Flu/cold symptoms	Nausea, mouth/throat irritation, anosmia.

[a]Most of these products are legally considered food supplements and therefore are not as tightly regulated by the FDA as pharmaceuticals (Dietary Supplement Health and Education Act [DSHEA] of 1994). Toxicity may be related to the active ingredient(s) or to impurities, contaminants, or adulterants in the product. See also "Caffeine," (p 169) "Camphor and Other Essential Oils," (p 176) "Salicylates," (p 410) and "Vitamins" (p 445).

II. Clinical presentation depends on the toxic constituent of the herbal product and may be acute in onset (eg, with the cardiac-stimulant effects of ephedra or guarana) or delayed (as with Chinese herbal nephropathy caused by *Aristolochia*). Allergic reactions to botanical products may manifest with skin rash (including urticaria), bronchospasm, and even anaphylaxis.

III. Diagnosis is based on a history of use of alternative products and exclusion of other medical/toxicologic causes. Identification of an unknown herb may be facilitated by consulting with a local Chinese herbalist, acupuncturist, or naturopathic practitioner. In some cases, chemical analysis of the product may confirm the presence of the suspected causative constituent or contaminant.

- **A. Specific levels.** Quantitative levels are not available for most alternative medicine toxins. Ephedrine can be measured in the blood and urine of people taking *Ma huang*. Some immunoassays for amphetamines are sensitive to ephedrine.
- **B. Laboratory studies.** Serum electrolytes including glucose, BUN, creatinine, liver aminotransferases, and prothrombin time are useful in cases of suspected organ toxicity resulting from alternative therapies. Heavy metals screening is recommended if consistent with poisoning.

IV. Treatment

- **A. Emergency and supportive measures.** Toxic effects of herbal medicines should be managed with the same approach taken with other ingestions.
  1. Replace fluid losses caused by diarrhea or vomiting with IV crystalloid fluids (p 16).
  2. Treat hypertension (p 17), tachycardia (p 12), and arrhythmias (pp 10–15) if they occur.
  3. Treat anxiety, agitation, or seizures (p 23) caused by stimulant herbs with IV benzodiazepines (p 516).
  4. Maintain an open airway and assist ventilation if necessary in cases of CNS depression or coma related to sedative herb use.
- **B. Specific drugs and antidotes.** There are no specific antidotes for toxicity related to herbal and alternative products.
- **C. Decontamination** (p 50). Administer activated charcoal orally if conditions are appropriate (see Table I–38, p 54). Gastric lavage is not necessary after small-to-moderate ingestions if activated charcoal can be given promptly.
- **D. Enhanced elimination.** The effectiveness of these procedures in removing herbal and alternative medicine toxins has not been studied.

ONLINE SOURCES OF INFORMATION ABOUT HERBAL AND ALTERNATIVE PRODUCTS

Alternative Medicine Foundation: HerbMed, an evidence-based scientific database on herbal medicines supported by the nonprofit Alternative Medicine Foundation. http://www.herbmed.org/

FDA Office of Food Safety and Nutrition: Consumer alerts and health professional advisories about safety concerns related to botanical products and other dietary supplements. http://www.cfsan.fda.gov

▶ HYDROCARBONS

Derrick Lung, MD, MPH

Hydrocarbons are used widely as solvents, degreasers, fuels, and lubricants. Besides inadvertent exposure, poisoning also commonly occurs from inhalation of volatile hydrocarbon gases used as drugs of abuse. Hydrocarbons include organic compounds derived from petroleum distillation as well as many other sources, including plant oils, animal fats, and coal. Subcategories of hydrocarbons include aliphatic (saturated carbon structure), aromatic (containing one or more benzene rings), halogenated (containing chlorine, bromine, or fluorine atoms), alcohols and glycols, ethers, ketones, carboxylic acids, and many others. This chapter emphasizes toxicity caused by common household hydrocarbons. See specific chemicals elsewhere in Section II and in Table IV–4 (p 659).

I. **Mechanism of toxicity.** Hydrocarbons may cause direct injury to the lung after pulmonary aspiration or systemic intoxication after ingestion, inhalation, or skin absorption (Table II–34). Many hydrocarbons are also irritating to the eyes and skin.
   A. **Pulmonary aspiration.** Chemical pneumonitis is caused by direct tissue damage and disruption of surfactant. Aspiration risk is greatest for hydrocarbons with low viscosity and low surface tension (eg, petroleum naphtha, gasoline, turpentine).

TABLE II–34. HYDROCARBON INGESTION

Common Compounds	Risk for Systemic Toxicity After Ingestion	Risk for Chemical Aspiration Pneumonia	Treatment
No systemic toxicity, high viscosity Petrolatum jelly, motor oil	Low	Low	Supportive.
No systemic toxicity, low viscosity Gasoline, kerosene, petroleum naphtha, mineral seal oil, petroleum ether	Low	High	Observe for pneumonia; do ***not*** empty stomach.
Unknown or uncertain systemic toxicity Turpentine, pine oil	Uncertain	High	Observe for pneumonia; consider removal by nasogastric suction and/or administration of activated charcoal if ingestion is more than 2 mL/kg.
Systemic toxins Camphor, phenol, halogenated or aromatic compounds	High	High	Observe for pneumonia; consider removal by nasogastric suction and/or administration of activated charcoal.

B. Ingestion

1. **Aliphatic hydrocarbons** and **simple petroleum distillates** such as lighter fluid, kerosene, furniture polish, and gasoline are poorly absorbed from the GI tract and do not pose a significant risk for systemic toxicity after ingestion as long as they are not aspirated.
2. In contrast, many **aromatic** and **halogenated hydrocarbons, alcohols, ethers, ketones,** and other **substituted or complex hydrocarbons** are capable of causing serious systemic toxicity, such as coma, seizures, and cardiac dysrhythmias.

C. Inhalation of hydrocarbon vapors in an enclosed space may cause intoxication as a result of systemic absorption or displacement of oxygen from the atmosphere; in addition, sensitization of the myocardium to catecholamines can cause cardiac dysrhythmias.

D. Injection of hydrocarbons into skin, subcutaneous tissue, or muscle may cause a severe local inflammatory reaction and liquefaction necrosis.

E. Skin and eye contact can cause local irritation. Dermal absorption can be significant for some agents but is insignificant for most of the simple aliphatic compounds.

II. Toxic dose. The toxic dose is variable, depending on the agent involved and whether it is aspirated, ingested, injected, or inhaled.

A. Pulmonary aspiration of as little as a few milliliters may produce chemical pneumonitis.

B. Ingestion of as little as 10–20 mL of some systemic toxins, such as camphor and carbon tetrachloride, may cause serious or fatal poisoning.

C. For recommended **inhalation exposure limits** for common hydrocarbons, see Table IV–4 (p 659).

D. Injection of less than 1 mL can cause significant local tissue inflammation.

E. Dermal absorption is insignificant for most simple aliphatic compounds but may occur with other agents.

III. Clinical presentation

A. Pulmonary aspiration usually causes immediate onset of coughing or choking. This may progress within minutes or hours to a chemical pneumonitis characterized by respiratory distress, including tachypnea, retractions, grunting, wheezing, rales, hypoxia, and hypercarbia. Death may ensue from respiratory failure, secondary bacterial infection, and other respiratory complications.

B. Ingestion often causes abrupt nausea and vomiting, occasionally with hemorrhagic gastroenteritis. Some compounds may be absorbed and produce systemic toxicity.

C. Systemic toxicity caused by hydrocarbon ingestion, inhalation, intravenous injection, or dermal absorption is highly variable, depending on the compound, but often includes confusion, ataxia, lethargy, and headache. With significant exposure, syncope, coma, and respiratory arrest may occur. Cardiac dysrhythmias may occur as a result of myocardial sensitization, especially with halogenated and aromatic compounds. Atrial fibrillation, ventricular fibrillation, and sudden cardiac death are reported. Many agents also may cause hepatic and renal injury.

D. Injection of hydrocarbons can cause local tissue inflammation, pain, and necrosis. Severe scarring and loss of function have occurred after injection into a finger with a paint gun or another high-pressure spray device containing a hydrocarbon solvent. Often, the puncture wound and local swelling appear minor, but tracking of hydrocarbon solvent down fascial planes into the palm and forearm may cause widespread inflammation and injury.

E. Skin or eye contact may cause local irritation, burns, or corneal injury. Chronic skin exposure often causes a defatting dermatitis (resulting from removal of oils from the skin). Some agents are absorbed through the skin and can produce systemic effects.

IV. Diagnosis

A. Aspiration pneumonitis. Diagnosis is based on a history of exposure and the presence of respiratory symptoms such as coughing, tachypnea, and wheezing. Chest radiograph and arterial blood gases or oximetry may assist in the diagnosis of chemical pneumonitis, although chest radiographic findings may be delayed for more than 24 hours.

B. Systemic intoxication. Diagnosis is based on a history of ingestion or inhalation, accompanied by the appropriate systemic clinical manifestations.

C. Specific levels. Specific levels are generally not available or useful.

D. Other useful laboratory studies. For suspected aspiration pneumonitis, obtain arterial blood gases or oximetry and a chest radiograph; for suspected systemic toxicity, obtain electrolytes, glucose, BUN, creatinine, and liver transaminases and perform ECG monitoring.

V. Treatment

A. Emergency and supportive measures

1. **General.** Provide basic supportive care for all symptomatic patients.
   - **a.** Maintain an open airway and assist ventilation if necessary (pp 1–7). Administer supplemental oxygen.
   - **b.** Monitor arterial blood gases or oximetry, chest radiographs, and ECG and admit symptomatic patients to an intensive care setting.
   - **c.** Use epinephrine and other beta-adrenergic medications with caution in patients with significant hydrocarbon intoxication because dysrhythmias may be induced.
2. **Pulmonary aspiration.** Patients who remain completely asymptomatic after 4 hours of observation may be discharged. In contrast, if the patient is coughing on arrival, aspiration probably has occurred.
   - **a.** Administer supplemental oxygen and treat bronchospasm (p 8) and hypoxia (p 7) if they occur.
   - **b.** Do ***not*** use steroids or prophylactic antibiotics. A randomized, controlled trial of antibiotics for aspiration pneumonitis in children demonstrated ***no*** benefit.
3. **Ingestion.** In the vast majority of accidental childhood ingestions, less than 5–10 mL is actually swallowed and systemic toxicity is rare. Treatment is primarily supportive.
4. **Injection.** For injections into the fingertip or hand, especially those involving a high-pressure paint gun, consult with a plastic or hand surgeon immediately, as prompt wide exposure, irrigation, and debridement are often required.

B. Specific drugs and antidotes

1. There is no specific antidote for aspiration pneumonitis; antibiotics and corticosteroids are of no proven value.
2. Specific drugs or antidotes may be available for systemic toxicity of some hydrocarbons (eg, acetylcysteine for carbon tetrachloride and methylene blue for methemoglobin formers) or their solutes (eg, chelation therapy for leaded gasoline and antidotes for pesticides).

C. Decontamination (p 50)

1. **Inhalation.** Move the victim to fresh air and administer oxygen if available.
2. **Skin and eyes.** Remove contaminated clothing and wash exposed skin with water and soap. Irrigate exposed eyes with copious water or saline and perform fluorescein examination for corneal injury.
3. **Ingestion**. For agents with no known systemic toxicity, gut decontamination is neither necessary nor desirable because it increases the risk for aspiration. For systemic toxins, consider aspiration of the liquid via nasogastric tube and administration of activated charcoal. Take precautions to prevent pulmonary aspiration if the patient is obtunded.
4. **Injection.** See Item A.4 above.

D. Enhanced elimination. There is no known role for any of these procedures.

▶ HYDROGEN FLUORIDE AND HYDROFLUORIC ACID

Janna H. Villano, MD and Binh T. Ly, MD

Hydrogen fluoride (HF) is an irritant gas that liquefies at 19.5°C; in an aqueous solution, it produces hydrofluoric acid. HF gas is used in chemical manufacturing. In addition, it may be released from fluorosilicates, fluorocarbons, or Teflon when heated to over 350°C. Hydrofluoric acid (aqueous HF solution) is widely used as a rust remover, in glass etching, and in the manufacture of silicon semiconductor chips. Hydrofluoric acid events at the workplace were shown to be two times more likely to involve injuries compared with other acids. Poisoning usually occurs after dermal exposure, usually on the hands, although ingestions and inhalations occasionally occur. There has been one case report of chemical colitis due to a hydrofluoric acid enema. Similar toxicity can result from exposure to ammonium bifluoride and sodium fluoride.

I. Mechanism of toxicity. HF is a dermal and respiratory irritant. Hydrofluoric acid is a relatively weak acid (the dissociation constant is about 1,000 times less than that of hydrochloric acid), and toxic effects result primarily from the highly reactive fluoride ion.

- **A.** HF is able to penetrate tissues deeply before dissociating into hydrogen and fluoride ions. The highly cytotoxic fluoride ion is released and cellular destruction occurs.
- **B.** Fluoride ion binds strongly to calcium and magnesium, resulting in their systemic depletion; this may cause systemic hypocalcemia, hypomagnesemia, and local bone demineralization.

II. Toxic dose. Toxicity depends on the air levels and duration of exposure to HF gas or the concentration and extent of exposure to aqueous HF solutions.

- **A. HF gas.** The recommended workplace ceiling limit (ACGIH TLV-C) for HF gas is 3 ppm (2.5 mg/m^3); 30 ppm is considered immediately dangerous to life or health (IDLH). A 5-minute exposure to air concentrations of 50–250 ppm is likely to be lethal.
- **B. Aqueous solutions.** Solutions of 50–70% are highly toxic and produce immediate pain. Concomitant inhalation exposure may occur with exposure to higher concentrations caused by the release of HF gas. Intermediate concentrations (20–40%) may cause little pain initially but result in deep injury after a delay of 1–8 hours. Weak solutions (5–15%) cause almost no pain on contact but may cause serious delayed injury after 12–24 hours. Most household products containing aqueous HF contain 5–8% or less.

III. Clinical presentation. Symptoms and signs depend on the type of exposure (gas or liquid), concentration, duration, and extent of exposure.

- **A. Inhalation** of HF gas produces ocular and nasopharyngeal irritation, coughing, and bronchospasm. After a delay of up to several hours, chemical pneumonitis and noncardiogenic pulmonary edema may occur. Corneal injury may result from ocular exposure.
- **B. Skin exposure.** After acute exposure to weak (5–15%) or intermediate (20–40%) solutions, there may be no symptoms because the pH effect is not pronounced. Concentrated (50–70%) solutions have better warning properties because of immediate pain. After a delay of 1–12 hours, progressive redness, swelling, skin blanching, and pain occur owing to penetration to deeper tissues by the fluoride ion. The exposure is typically through a pinhole-size defect in a rubber glove, and the fingertip is the most common site of injury. The pain is progressive and unrelenting. Severe deep-tissue destruction may occur, including full-thickness skin loss and destruction of underlying bone.
- **C. Ingestion** of HF may cause corrosive injury to the mouth, esophagus, and stomach.
- **D. Systemic, life-threatening hypocalcemia and hypomagnesemia** may occur after ingestion or skin burns involving a large body surface area or highly concentrated solution (can occur with exposure to >2.5% body surface

area and a highly concentrated solution). **Hyperkalemia** may occur as a result of fluoride-mediated inactivation of the Na-K ATPase, activation of the Na-Ca ion exchanger and/or tissue injury. These electrolyte imbalances, either alone or in combination, can lead to cardiac dysrhythmias, the primary cause of death in HF exposures. Prolonged QT interval may be the initial manifestation of hypocalcemia or hypomagnesemia.

IV. Diagnosis is based on a history of exposure and typical findings. Immediately after exposure to weak or intermediate solutions, there may be few or no symptoms, even though potentially severe injury may develop later.

A. Specific levels. Serum fluoride concentrations are not useful after acute exposure but may be used in evaluating chronic occupational exposure. Normal serum fluoride is less than 20 mcg/L but varies considerably with dietary and environmental intake. In workers, pre-shift urine excretion of fluoride should not exceed 3 mg/g of creatinine.

B. Other useful laboratory studies include electrolytes, BUN, creatinine, calcium, magnesium, and continuous ECG monitoring.

V. Treatment

A. Emergency and supportive measures

1. **All HF ingestions should be considered potentially life-threatening**. Maintain an open airway and assist ventilation if necessary (pp 1–7). Administer supplemental oxygen. Treat pulmonary edema (p 7) if it occurs.
2. Patients with HF ingestion should be evaluated for corrosive injury, with consultation by a gastroenterologist for consideration of endoscopic evaluation (p 186).
3. Monitor the ECG and serum calcium, magnesium, and potassium concentrations; give IV calcium (p 526; also see below) if there is evidence of hypocalcemia or severe hyperkalemia; replace magnesium as indicated.

B. Specific drugs and antidotes. Calcium (p 526) rapidly precipitates fluoride ions and is an effective antidote for dermal exposures and systemic hypocalcemia resulting from absorbed fluoride. In addition, serum magnesium should be monitored and replaced aggressively as appropriate.

1. **Skin burns.** For exposures involving the hands or fingers, immediately consult an experienced hand surgeon, a medical toxicologist or a poison control center (1-800-222-1222). Historically, fingernail removal was used, but this can result in disfiguring morbidity. Occasionally, **calcium gluconate** will have to be given by the intra-arterial route or by intravenous Bier block technique. This can result in significant pain relief. ***Caution:*** Do ***not*** use calcium ***chloride*** salt for subcutaneous, Bier block, or intra-arterial injections; this form contains a larger proportion of calcium ion compared with the gluconate salt and may cause vasospasm and tissue necrosis.
   a. **Topical.** Apply a gel containing calcium gluconate or carbonate (p 526), using an occlusive dressing or a rubber glove to enhance skin penetration. Some experts add dimethyl sulfoxide (DMSO) to enhance skin penetration of the calcium, although evidence is anecdotal. Alternately, soak in a quaternary benzalkonium chloride solution such as Zephiran (1.3 g/L of water) or a magnesium sulfate solution such as Epsom salt solution. If pain is not significantly relieved within 30–60 minutes, consider subcutaneous or intra-arterial injection.
   b. **Subcutaneous.** Inject calcium gluconate 5–10% subcutaneously in affected areas, using a 27- or 30-gauge needle and no more than 0.5 mL per digit or 1 mL/cm^2 in other regions.
   c. **Intra-arterial.** Injection of calcium by the intra-arterial route (p 526) may be necessary for burns involving several digits or subungual areas, or if topical therapy fails.
   d. **Bier block.** This intravenous regional perfusion technique has been reported to be useful (see "Calcium," p 526).

e. **Surgical excision.** Early burn excision has been used in cases of non-hand exposures in which pain is uncontrollable despite topical or subcutaneous calcium therapy.

2. **Systemic hypocalcemia or hyperkalemia.** Administer calcium gluconate 10%, 0.2–0.4 mL/kg IV, or calcium chloride 10%, 0.1–0.2 mL/kg IV.

C. **Decontamination** (p 50). Rescuers entering a contaminated area should wear self-contained breathing apparatus and appropriate personal protective equipment to avoid exposure.

1. **Inhalation.** Immediately remove victims from exposure and give supplemental oxygen if available. The use of 2.5% calcium gluconate by nebulization is recommended by some authorities.
2. **Skin.** Immediately remove contaminated clothing and flood exposed areas with copious amounts of water. Then soak in a solution of Epsom salts (magnesium sulfate) or calcium; immediate topical use of calcium or magnesium may help prevent deep burns. Some facilities that frequently manage HF cases purchase or prepare a 2.5% calcium gluconate gel (in water-based jelly). This intervention can be highly effective if applied immediately.
3. **Eyes.** Flush with copious amounts of water or saline. The effectiveness of a weak (1–2%) calcium gluconate solution is not established. Consult with an ophthalmologist if there is evidence or suspicion of ocular exposure.
4. **Ingestion**
   a. **Prehospital.** Immediately give any available calcium-containing (calcium carbonate or milk) or magnesium-containing (Epsom salts, magnesium hydroxide) substance by mouth. Do ***not*** induce vomiting because of the risk for corrosive injury. Activated charcoal is not effective.
   b. **Hospital.** Consider gastric suctioning with a nasogastric tube. Administer magnesium- or calcium-containing substance as in Item 4.a above.

D. **Enhanced elimination.** There is no role for enhanced elimination procedures.

▶ HYDROGEN SULFIDE

Stephen W. Munday, MD, MPH, MS

Hydrogen sulfide is a highly toxic, flammable, colorless gas that is heavier than air. It is produced naturally by decaying organic matter and is also a by-product of many industrial processes. Hazardous levels may be found in petroleum refineries, tanneries, mines, pulp-making factories, sulfur hot springs, carbon disulfide production, commercial fishing holds, hot asphalt fumes, and pools of sewage sludge or liquid manure. It sometimes is referred to as "pit gas." There have been reports of suicide by mixing acid-containing household cleaners with calcium sulfide–containing bath salts to generate hydrogen sulfide gas.

I. **Mechanism of toxicity.** Hydrogen sulfide causes cellular asphyxia by inhibition of the cytochrome oxidase system, similar to the action of cyanide. Because it is absorbed rapidly by inhalation, symptoms occur nearly immediately after exposure, leading to rapid unconsciousness, or "knockdown." Hydrogen sulfide is also a mucous membrane irritant.

II. **Toxic dose.** The characteristic rotten egg odor of hydrogen sulfide is detectable at concentrations as low as 0.025 ppm. The recommended workplace limit (ACGIH TLV-TWA) is 10 ppm (14 mg/m^3) as an 8-hour time-weighted average, with a short-term exposure limit (STEL) of 15 ppm (21 mg/m^3). The federal OSHA permissible exposure limit (PEL) is 20 ppm as a 15-minute ceiling during an 8-hour workday. Marked respiratory tract irritation occurs with levels of 50–100 ppm. Olfactory nerve paralysis occurs with levels of 100–150 ppm. The level considered immediately dangerous to life or health (IDLH) is 100 ppm. Pulmonary edema occurs at levels of 300–500 ppm. Levels of 600–800 ppm are rapidly fatal.

III. Clinical presentation

A. Irritant effects. Upper airway irritation, burning eyes, and blepharospasm may occur at relatively low levels. Skin exposure can cause painful dermatitis. Chemical pneumonitis and noncardiogenic pulmonary edema may occur after a delay of several hours.

B. Acute systemic effects include headache, nausea and vomiting, dizziness, confusion, seizures, and coma. Massive exposure may cause immediate cardiovascular collapse, respiratory arrest, and death. Survivors may be left with serious neurologic impairment.

IV. Diagnosis is based on a history of exposure and rapidly progressive manifestations of airway irritation and cellular asphyxia, with sudden collapse. The victim or coworkers may describe the smell of rotten eggs, but because of olfactory nerve paralysis, the absence of this odor does not rule out exposure. Silver coins in the pockets of victims have been blackened (by conversion to silver sulfide). Greenish discoloration of the brain has been reported at autopsy.

A. Specific levels are not generally available (sulfide is unstable in vitro), although elevated whole-blood sulfide and thiosulfate have been measured postmortem. Sulfhemoglobin is not thought to be produced after hydrogen sulfide exposure.

B. Other useful laboratory studies include electrolytes, glucose, arterial blood gases, and chest radiography.

V. Treatment

A. Emergency and supportive measures. *Note:* Rescuers should use self-contained breathing apparatus to prevent personal exposure.

1. Maintain an open airway and assist ventilation if necessary (pp 1–7). Administer high-flow humidified supplemental oxygen. Observe for several hours for delayed-onset chemical pneumonia or pulmonary edema (p 7).
2. Treat coma (p 18), seizures (p 23), and hypotension (p 15) if they occur.

B. Specific drugs and antidotes

1. Theoretically, administration of **nitrites** (p 592) to produce methemoglobinemia may promote conversion of sulfide ions to sulfmethemoglobin, which is far less toxic. However, there is limited evidence for the effectiveness of nitrites, and they can cause hypotension and impaired oxygen delivery.
2. Animal data and limited human case reports have suggested that **hyperbaric oxygen** (p 599) may be helpful if it is provided early after exposure, but this therapy remains unproven.
3. **Hydroxocobalamin** (p 563) has been approved for the treatment of cyanide poisoning and theoretically could be expected to be of benefit in hydrogen sulfide poisoning, but human data are lacking. A study in mice showed improved survival. In this same study, nitrite use was not found to enhance survival.

C. Decontamination (p 50). Remove the victim from exposure and give supplemental oxygen if available.

D. Enhanced elimination. There is no role for enhanced elimination procedures. Although hyperbaric oxygen therapy has been promoted for the treatment of hydrogen sulfide poisoning, this is based on anecdotal cases, and there is no convincing rationale or scientific evidence for its effectiveness.

► HYMENOPTERA

Richard F. Clark, MD

Venomous insects are grouped into four families of the order Hymenoptera: Apidae (honeybees), Bombidae (bumblebees), Vespidae (wasps, hornets, and yellow jackets), and Formicidae (ants). With the exception of Vespidae, most Hymenoptera sting only when disturbed or when the hive is threatened. Yellow jackets and other vespids may attack without provocation and are the most common cause of insect-induced anaphylactic reactions.

I. **Mechanism of toxicity.** The venoms of Hymenoptera are complex mixtures of enzymes and are delivered by various methods. The venom apparatus is located in the posterior abdomen of the female.

A. The terminal end of the stinger of the **Apidae** (honeybees) is barbed, so the stinger remains in the victim and some or all of the venom apparatus is torn from the body of the bee, resulting in its death as it flies away. The musculature surrounding the venom sac continues to contract for several minutes after evisceration, causing venom to be ejected persistently. The **Bombidae** and **Vespidae** have stingers that are barbed but remain functionally intact after a sting, resulting in their ability to inflict multiple stings.

B. The envenomating **Formicidae** have secretory venom glands in the posterior abdomen and envenomate either by injecting venom through a stinger or by spraying venom from the posterior abdomen into a bite wound produced by their mandibles.

II. **Toxic dose.** The dose of venom delivered per sting may vary from none to the entire contents of the venom gland. The toxic response is highly variable, depending on individual sensitivity. Some Hymenoptera, such as wasps, have the ability to sting several times, increasing the venom load. Africanized bee attacks may result in over 1,000 stings. Disturbing a fire ant nest may result in as many as 3,000–5,000 stings within seconds.

III. **Clinical presentation.** The patient may present with local or systemic signs of envenomation or an allergic reaction.

A. **Envenomation.** Once venom is injected, there is usually an immediate onset of severe pain, followed by a local inflammatory reaction that may include erythema, wheal formation, ecchymosis, edema, vesiculation and blisters, itching, and a sensation of warmth. Multiple stings, and very rarely severe single stings, may also produce vomiting, diarrhea, hypotension, syncope, cyanosis, dyspnea, rhabdomyolysis, coagulopathy, and death.

B. **Allergic reactions.** Numerous deaths occur annually in the United States from immediate hypersensitivity (anaphylactic) reactions characterized by urticaria, angioedema, bronchospasm, and shock. Most anaphylactic reactions occur within 15 minutes of envenomation. Rarely, delayed-onset reactions may occur, including Arthus reactions (arthralgias and fever), nephritis, transverse myelitis, and Guillain–Barré syndrome. Cross-sensitivity to fire ant venom can exist in some patients with Apidae or Vespidae allergies.

IV. **Diagnosis** is usually obvious from the history of exposure and typical findings.

A. **Specific levels.** Not relevant.

B. **Other useful laboratory studies.** Creatine kinase (CK), the CK-MB isoenzyme, cardiac troponin T or I, and renal function should be checked in severe cases of multiple stings.

V. **Treatment**

A. **Emergency and supportive measures**

1. Monitor the victim closely for at least 30–60 minutes.
2. Treat anaphylaxis (p 28), if it occurs, with epinephrine (p 551) and diphenhydramine (p 544) or hydroxyzine. Persistent urticaria may respond to the addition of ranitidine, 50 mg IV or 150 mg orally, or another histamine$_2$ (H_2) receptor antagonist (p 532). Standard doses of prednisone (1 mg/kg/day for 5 days) may also be considered for persistent allergic signs or symptoms. Persons known to be sensitive to Hymenoptera venom should wear medical alert jewelry and carry an epinephrine emergency kit at all times.
3. In most cases, the painful localized tissue response will resolve in a few hours without therapy. Some symptomatic relief may be obtained by topical application of ice, papain (meat tenderizer), or creams containing corticosteroids or antihistamines.
4. Provide tetanus prophylaxis if appropriate.

B. **Specific drugs and antidotes.** There is no available antidote.

C. **Decontamination.** Examine the sting site carefully for any retained stingers; stingers can be removed by gentle scraping with a sharp edge (eg, a knife blade) or with tweezers (venom gland contents have almost always been quickly and completely expelled). Wash the area with soap and water.

D. **Enhanced elimination.** These procedures are not applicable.

▶ IODINE

Mariam Qozi, PharmD

The chief use of iodine is for its antiseptic property. It is bactericidal, sporicidal, protozoacidal, cysticidal, and virucidal. Liquid formulations of iodine are usually prepared in ethanol (tincture of iodine) to increase solubility and concentration. Lugol solution is 5% iodine and 10% iodide in water. Iodoform is triiodomethane (CHI_3). Iodophors such as povidone-iodine (Betadine) consist of iodine linked to a large–molecular-weight molecule. These are usually less toxic owing to the slow release of iodine from the carrier molecule. Radioactive iodine is used in the treatment of thyroid cancer. The antiarrhythmic drug amiodarone releases iodine and may cause either thyrotoxicosis or hypothyroidism after prolonged use. Iodine is also used in the manufacture of dyes and photographic reagents. Table salt is fortified with iodine.

I. **Mechanism of toxicity.** Toxicity can occur through skin or mucosal absorption, ingestion, or inhalation. When ingested, iodine can cause severe corrosive injury to the GI tract owing to its oxidative properties. In the body, iodine is converted rapidly to iodide and stored in the thyroid gland.

II. **The toxic dose** depends on the product and the route of exposure. Iodophors and iodoform are generally less toxic, as iodine is released more slowly. However, significant systemic absorption can occur in patients receiving povidone-iodine treatment on areas of skin breakdown or when used for internal irrigation of an infected area or as a dye.

   A. **Iodine vapor.** The ACGIH-recommended workplace ceiling limit (TLV-C) for iodine vapor is 0.1 ppm (1 mg/m^3). The air level considered immediately dangerous to life or health (IDLH) is 2 ppm.

   B. **Skin and mucous membranes.** Strong iodine tincture (7% iodine and 5% potassium iodide in 83% ethanol) may cause burns, but USP iodine tincture (2% iodine and 2% sodium iodide in 50% ethanol) is not likely to produce corrosive damage. Povidone-iodine 10% can also cause burns especially with prolonged exposure (1–8 hours). Systemic absorption of iodine is more likely to occur after an acute application of strong iodine tincture or after chronic applications of less concentrated products; however, it can also occur from internal applications of the 2% povidone-iodine.

   C. **Ingestion.** Reported fatal doses vary from 200 mg to more than 20 g of iodine; an estimated mean lethal dose is approximately 2–4 g of free iodine. USP iodine tincture contains 100 mg of iodine per 5 mL, and strong iodine tincture contains 350 mg of iodine per 5 mL. Iodine ointment contains 4% iodine. Povidone-iodine 10% contains 1% free iodine. Consider ethanol toxicity with large exposures (p 231).

III. **Clinical presentation.** The manifestations of acute iodine ingestion are related largely to the corrosive effect on mucous membranes and the GI tract.

   A. **Inhalation** of iodine vapor can cause severe pulmonary irritation, which can lead to pulmonary edema.

   B. **Skin** and eye exposures may result in severe corrosive burns.

   C. **Ingestion** can cause corrosive gastroenteritis with vomiting, hematemesis, and diarrhea, which can result in significant volume loss and circulatory collapse. Pharyngeal swelling and glottic edema have been reported. Mucous membranes are usually stained brown, and the vomitus may be blue if starchy foods are already present in the stomach.

D. **Chronic** ingestions or absorption may result in hypothyroidism and goiter, or hyperthyroidism. Systemic absorption has also caused hypernatremia, metabolic acidosis, increased osmolality and hyperchloremia (due to iodine's interference with the chloride assay). Iodides cross the placenta, and neonatal hypothyroidism and death from respiratory distress secondary to goiter have been reported.

E. Chronic iodine deficiency can lead to hypothyroidism and goiter.

IV. **Diagnosis** is based on a history of exposure and evidence of corrosive injury. Mucous membranes are usually stained brown, and vomitus may be blue.

A. **Specific levels.** Blood levels are not clinically useful but may confirm exposure

B. **Other useful laboratory studies** for serious corrosive injury include CBC, electrolytes, BUN, and creatinine. For inhalational exposure, arterial blood gases or oximetry and chest radiography are useful.

V. **Treatment**

A. **Emergency and supportive measures**

1. Maintain an open airway and perform endotracheal intubation if airway edema is progressive (pp 1–7). Treat bronchospasm (p 8) and pulmonary edema (p 7) if they occur.
2. Treat fluid loss from gastroenteritis aggressively with IV crystalloid solutions.
3. If corrosive injury to the esophagus or stomach is suspected, consult a gastroenterologist to perform endoscopy.

B. **Specific drugs and antidotes.** Sodium thiosulfate may convert iodine to iodide and tetrathionate but is not recommended for intravenous use because iodine is converted rapidly to iodide in the body.

C. **Decontamination** (p 50)

1. **Inhalation.** Remove the victim from exposure.
2. **Skin and eyes.** Remove contaminated clothing and flush exposed skin with water. Irrigate exposed eyes copiously with tepid water or saline for at least 15 minutes.
3. **Ingestion.** Do ***not*** induce vomiting because of the corrosive effects of iodine. Administer a starchy food (potato, flour, or cornstarch) or milk to lessen GI irritation. Activated charcoal does bind iodine in vitro but is of unknown efficacy.

D. **Enhanced elimination.** Since iodine is converted rapidly to iodide once absorbed into the circulation, enhanced drug removal is usually unnecessary. However, hemodialysis was performed (calculated dialysis clearance 120 mL/min) in a patient with hepatic and renal dysfunction and high blood levels (>1,000 mcg/dL) after mediastinal irrigation with povidone-iodine.

▶ IPECAC SYRUP

Nasim Ghafouri, PharmD

Ipecac syrup is an alkaloid derivative of the ipecacuanha plant (*Cephaline ipecacuanha*). The principal alkaloids, emetine and cephaline, both have emetogenic properties. The emetine extract has been used for the treatment of amebiasis. Syrup of ipecac is no longer widely available over the counter, nor is it recommended for home use by pediatricians.

I. **Mechanism of toxicity**

A. **Mechanism of action.** Ipecac causes vomiting in two ways: by direct irritation of the gastric mucosa, and by systemic absorption and stimulation of the central chemoreceptor trigger zone.

B. **Acute ingestion** can cause profuse vomiting and diarrhea, especially ingestion of the more concentrated fluid extract (no longer available in the United States).

C. The effects of **overdose during pregnancy** are not well studied.

D. With **chronic repeated dosing**, the emetine component of ipecac causes inhibition of protein synthesis, which is particularly demonstrated in cardiac and skeletal muscle cells. Another proposed mechanism for cellular toxicity is blockade of sodium and calcium channels.

E. **Pharmacokinetics.** Ipecac syrup causes emesis within 15–30 minutes of ingestion, and symptoms may last up to 1 hour in some cases. Ipecac is absorbed systemically; however, the rate and extent of absorption varies considerably among individuals. Emetine may be detectable in the urine for up to several weeks after chronic use.

II. **Toxic dose.** Toxicity depends on the formulation and whether the exposure is acute or chronic.

A. **Acute ingestion** of 60–120 mL of **syrup of ipecac** is not likely to cause serious poisoning. However, the **fluid extract,** which is approximately 14 times more potent than syrup of ipecac, has caused death after ingestion of as little as 10 mL.

B. **Chronic dosing** results in cumulative toxicity because of the slow elimination of emetine. Repeated ingestion over time, as in cases of Munchausen by proxy or eating disorders, has been reported to cause myotoxicity with total accumulated doses of 600–1,250 mg. Daily ingestion of 90–120 mL of syrup of ipecac for 3 months caused death from cardiomyopathy.

III. **Clinical presentation**

A. **Acute ingestion** of ipecac causes nausea and vomiting. In patients with depressed airway-protective reflexes, pulmonary aspiration of gastric contents may occur. Prolonged or forceful vomiting may cause gastritis, gastric rupture, pneumomediastinum, retropneumoperitoneum, or Mallory–Weiss tears of the cardioesophageal junction. One fatal case of intracerebral hemorrhage was reported in an elderly patient after a single therapeutic dose of ipecac syrup.

B. **Chronic intoxication.** In patients with chronic misuse, dehydration and electrolyte abnormalities (eg, hypokalemia) occur as a result of frequent vomiting and diarrhea, and myopathy or cardiomyopathy may develop. Symptoms of myopathy include muscle weakness and tenderness, hyporeflexia, and elevated serum CPK. Cardiomyopathy, with congestive heart failure and arrhythmias, may be fatal.

1. **"Munchausen by proxy."** Children intentionally poisoned with ipecac typically have a history of recurrent hospitalizations for vomiting that seems refractory to outpatient medical treatment. The symptoms usually decrease in the hospital but worsen when the child returns home. Progressive weight loss and loss of developmental milestones are common. Physical examination reveals muscle weakness and other signs of chronic myopathy. Some children have been reported to develop a secondary eating disorder, such as rumination, as a result of their recurrent vomiting.

2. **Adults with an eating disorder** and frequent use of ipecac often present with a history of recent weight loss. Malnutrition and chronic vomiting may cause electrolyte disturbances, dental changes, and skin changes associated with various vitamin deficiencies.

IV. **Diagnosis** is based on a careful history of ingestion. Chronic ipecac poisoning should be suspected in any patient with an eating disorder and evidence of dehydration, electrolyte imbalance, or myopathy or in a young child with repeated unexplained episodes of vomiting, diarrhea, and failure to thrive. The electrocardiogram may show prolonged QRS and QT intervals, flat or inverted T waves, and supraventricular and ventricular arrhythmias.

A. **Specific levels.** Emetine may be detected in the urine for up to several weeks after ingestion, and its presence may provide qualitative confirmation of ipecac exposure but does not correlate with the degree of effect. It is not part of a routine comprehensive toxicology screen and must be requested specifically. Levels as low as 95 ng/mL in urine and 21 ng/mL in blood have been found in cases of confirmed Munchausen by proxy. A urinary level of 1,700 ng/mL was found in a 4-year-old child who died after chronic vomiting, diarrhea, and failure to thrive. Pathologic findings of the heart muscle included marked autolytic changes with swollen mitochondria and fragmented, irregular alignment of Z bands.

B. **Other useful laboratory studies** include electrolytes, BUN, creatinine, creatine kinase (CK), lactate dehydrogenase (LDH), and ECG.

V. **Treatment**

A. **Emergency and supportive measures**

1. Correct fluid and electrolyte abnormalities with IV fluids and potassium as needed.
2. Diuretics and pressor support may be required in patients with congestive cardiomyopathy.
3. Monitor the ECG for 6–8 hours and admit patients with evidence of myopathy or cardiomyopathy. Treat arrhythmias with standard drugs (pp 10–15).

B. **Specific drugs and antidotes.** There is no specific antidote.

C. **Decontamination** (acute ingestions only [p 51]). Consider using activated charcoal orally, but only if it can be given within a few minutes after a large ipecac ingestion.

D. **Enhanced elimination.** There is no known role for enhanced elimination. The alkaloids are highly bound to tissue.

▶ IRON

Michael Young, DO

Iron is used for the treatment of anemia and as a prenatal or daily mineral supplement. Owing to its wide availability as an over-the-counter nutritional supplement, it remains a common (and potentially fatal) ingestion. Introduction of blister packages and smaller dosages have led to an overall decline in iron poisonings. Currently, there are many iron preparations that contain various amounts of iron salts. Most children's preparations contain 10–18 mg of elemental iron per dose, and most adult preparations contain 60–90 mg of elemental iron per dose. The following description of the toxicity of iron relates to the ingestion of ferrous iron salts (eg, sulfate, gluconate, fumarate). Two elemental iron products, carbonyl iron and iron polysaccharide complex, have not been reported to produce the same toxicity as iron salts.

I. **Mechanism of toxicity.** Toxicity results from direct corrosive effects and cellular toxicity.

A. Iron has a direct corrosive effect on mucosal tissue and may cause hemorrhagic necrosis and perforation. Fluid loss from the GI tract results in severe hypovolemia.

B. Absorbed iron, in excess of protein-binding capacity, causes cellular dysfunction and death, resulting in lactic acidosis and organ failure. Iron-induced reactive oxygen species cause oxidative and free radical injury and disrupt cellular process such as mitochondrial oxidative phosphorylation.

II. **Toxic dose.** The acute lethal dose in animal studies is 150–200 mg/kg of elemental iron. The lowest reported lethal dose was in a 21-month-old child who was said to have ingested between 325 and 650 mg of elemental iron in the form of ferrous sulfate. Symptoms are unlikely if less than 20 mg/kg of elemental iron has been ingested. Doses of 20–30 mg/kg may produce self-limited vomiting, abdominal pain, and diarrhea. Ingestion of more than 40 mg/kg is considered potentially serious, and more than 60 mg/kg is potentially lethal. Even though they contain iron salts, there are no reported cases of serious or fatal poisoning from the ingestion of children's chewable vitamins with iron. The reason for this is likely from its lower iron per tablet dosage than typical iron supplements.

III. **Clinical presentation.** Iron poisoning is usually described in five stages. However, clinical manifestations may overlap and patients do not necessarily pass through the same temporal stages.

A. **First stage.** Shortly after ingestion, the corrosive effects of iron cause abdominal pain, vomiting, and diarrhea, often bloody. Massive fluid or blood loss into the GI tract may cause serious hemodynamic instability. Absence of GI symptoms within the first 6 hours of ingestion essentially excludes serious iron toxicity.

B. **Second stage.** Patients who pass the first stage may experience a latent period of apparent GI improvement over 6–24 hours. However, ongoing cellular toxicities still occur and patients continue to demonstrate tachycardia and lethargy along with evidence of metabolic acidosis.

C. **Third stage.** This may occur within the first few hours of massive ingestion or 12–24 hours after a moderate ingestion. Systemic toxicities such as coma, shock, seizures, metabolic acidosis, and coagulopathy are among the common findings. *Yersinia enterocolitica* sepsis may also occur (see below).

D. **Fourth stage.** This stage is characterized by hepatic failure that occurs 1–3 days postingestion. Coagulopathy worsens and it may complicate bleeding and hypovolemia.

E. **Fifth stage.** If the victim survives, scarring from the initial corrosive injury may result in pyloric stricture or other intestinal obstruction within 2–8 weeks postingestion.

F. Patients with iron poisoning treated with deferoxamine are at risk of *Yersinia enterocolitica* infection. Iron is a required growth factor for this bacteria and deferoxamine is a siderophore that fosters its growth. Patients with fever, abdominal pain, and bloody diarrhea after resolution of iron toxicity should be evaluated for Yersinia infection.

IV. **Diagnosis** is based on a history of exposure and the presence of vomiting, diarrhea, hypotension, and other clinical signs. Radiopaque pills may be visible on abdominal radiographs.

A. **Specific levels.**

1. **Serum iron** levels greater than 300–500 mcg/dL are common in patients with GI symptoms. Serum levels between 500 and 1,000 mcg/dL are associated with systemic toxicities. Iron levels greater than 1,000 mcg/dL represent significant poisoning and are associated with high morbidity and mortality. Obtain serum iron level 4–6 hours after ingestion and repeat iron levels every 4–6 hours maybe necessary to rule out delayed absorption (eg, from a sustained-release tablet or a tablet bezoar).
2. The conventional method of measuring total iron-binding capacity (TIBC) is unreliable in iron overdose and should not be used to estimate free iron levels.
3. Serum or plasma ferritin level is a more reliable marker for chronic iron toxicity and should not be used in acute settings.

B. **Other useful laboratory studies** include CBC, venous or arterial blood gases (to assess pH), electrolytes, glucose, BUN, creatinine, hepatic aminotransferases (AST and ALT), lactic acid, coagulation studies, and abdominal radiography.

V. **Treatment.** Patients who have self-limited mild GI symptoms or who remain asymptomatic for 6 hours after ingestion are unlikely to develop serious intoxication. In contrast, those with serious ingestion must be managed promptly and aggressively.

A. **Emergency and supportive measures**

1. Maintain an open airway and assist ventilation if necessary (pp 1–7).
2. Treat shock caused by hemorrhagic gastroenteritis aggressively with IV crystalloid fluids (p 16) and replace blood if needed. Patients are often markedly hypovolemic owing to GI losses and third spacing of fluids into

the intestinal wall and interstitial space. Vasopressors may be needed if patients are unresponsive to crystalloid fluids and/or blood transfusions.

3. Treat coma (p 18), seizures (p 23), and metabolic acidosis (p 35) if they occur.

B. **Specific treatment.** For seriously intoxicated victims (eg, shock, severe acidosis, and/or serum iron >500 mcg/dL), administer IV **deferoxamine** (p 539). Monitor the urine for the characteristic orange or pink-red ("*vin rosé*") color of the chelated deferoxamine–iron complex, although this may not always be seen. Therapy may be stopped when the urine color returns to normal or when the serum iron level decreases below 500 mcg/dL. Prolonged deferoxamine therapy (>32–72 hours) has been associated with adult respiratory distress syndrome (ARDS) and *Yersinia* sepsis.

1. The IV route is preferred. Give 15 mg/kg/h by constant infusion; faster rates (up to 45 mg/kg/h) reportedly have been well tolerated in single cases, but rapid boluses usually cause hypotension. The manufacturer's recommended maximum daily dose is 6 g, but larger amounts have been given safely in massive iron overdoses.
2. Deferoxamine has also been given intramuscularly. However, in acute poisonings, absorption of the drug by this route is unreliable and is not recommended.

C. **Decontamination** (p 50). Activated charcoal is not effective. Ipecac is not recommended because it can aggravate iron-induced GI irritation and interfere with whole-bowel irrigation (see below).

1. Gastric lavage has limited value and is usually not effective. Intact tablets may not pass through a lavage tube. Do ***not*** use phosphate-containing solutions for lavage; they may result in life-threatening hypernatremia, hyperphosphatemia, and hypocalcemia. Sodium bicarbonate lavage has resulted in severe hypernatremia, alkalosis, and death. Deferoxamine lavage is not effective and may enhance iron absorption.
2. **Whole-bowel irrigation** (p 55) is potentially effective for ingested tablets and may be considered if large numbers of pills are visible on plain abdominal radiograph.
3. **Activated charcoal does not adsorb iron** and is not recommended unless other drugs have been co-ingested.
4. Large ingestions may result in tablet concretions or bezoars. Repeated or prolonged whole-bowel irrigation may be considered. Endoscopy or surgical gastrotomy is rarely required but has been used.

D. **Enhanced elimination**

1. **Hemodialysis** and **hemoperfusion** are not effective at removing iron but may be necessary to remove deferoxamine–iron complex in patients with renal failure.
2. **Exchange transfusion** is used occasionally for massive pediatric ingestion, but it may not be tolerated in patients with hemodynamic instability.

E. **Other chelators**

1. **Deferiprone** and **deferasirox** are two oral chelators used in patients with chronic iron overload. Although there are no studies addressing their use in acute iron poisoning, they might be considered in patients where deferoxamine therapy is contraindicated or inadequate.
   a. **Deferiprone:** Combining deferiprone (75 mg/kg/day divided every 8 hours) with deferoxamine appeared to improve outcome in studies with chronic iron overload. Adverse effects include neutropenia (5%) and agranulocytosis (<1%).
   b. **Deferasirox:** Studies on chronic iron overloaded thalassemic patients showed deferasirox (30 mg/kg/day once daily) was effective. Gastrointestinal symptoms are the most common adverse effects but acute renal insufficiency has been reported.

▶ ISOCYANATES

Paul D. Blanc, MD, MSPH

Toluene diisocyanate (TDI), methylene diisocyanate (MDI), hexamethylene diisocyanate (HDI), isophorone diisocyanate (IPDI), and related chemicals are industrial components in the polymerization of urethane coatings and insulation materials. Urethanes have widespread uses in sealants, coatings, finishes, glues, and even medical applications (eg, casts). Most two-part urethane products contain some amount of one of these chemicals, and lesser amounts contaminate one-part systems. **Methyl isocyanate** (the toxin released in the disaster in Bhopal, India) is a carbamate insecticide precursor; it is not used in urethanes, has actions different from those of the TDI group of chemicals, and is not discussed here (see Table IV–4, p 659).

I. **Mechanism of toxicity.** TDI and related isocyanates act as irritants and sensitizers at very low concentrations. The mechanism is poorly understood. They may act as haptens or through cell-mediated immune pathways. Inhalation is the typical route of sensitization but skin contact may also play a role. Once a person is sensitized to one isocyanate, cross-reactivity to others often occurs.

II. **Toxic dose.** The ACGIH-recommended 8-hour TLV–time-weighted averages (TWA) and the California OSHA permissible exposure limits (PELs) for TDI, MDI, HDI, and IPDI are all 0.005 ppm (Federal OSHA limits are less stringent for TDI and MDI and not established for HDI and IPDI). These exposure limits are intended to prevent acute irritant effects. In individuals with prior sensitivity, however, even this level may induce asthma responses. The level considered immediately dangerous to life or health (IDLH) for TDI is 2.5 ppm. Other isocyanates (eg, MDI, HDI) are less volatile, but exposure can occur from inhalation of spray aerosols and skin contact.

III. **Clinical presentation**

   A. **Acute exposure** to irritant levels causes skin and upper respiratory tract toxicity. Burning eyes and skin, cough, and wheezing are common. Noncardiogenic pulmonary edema may occur with severe exposure. Symptoms may occur immediately with exposure or may be delayed several hours.

   B. **Low-level chronic exposure** may produce dyspnea, wheezing, and other signs and symptoms consistent with asthma. A late-phase symptom onset in a sensitized individual may occur hours following exposure (eg, overnight after a work day). Interstitial lung responses, with radiographic infiltrates and hypoxemia, may occur less commonly as a hypersensitivity pneumonitis syndrome.

IV. **Diagnosis** requires a careful occupational history. Pulmonary function testing may document an obstructive deficit or less commonly restriction (if pneumonitis is present), or the results may be normal. Variable airflow or changing measures of airway reactivity (methacholine or histamine challenge) temporally linked to exposure strongly support the diagnosis of isocyanate-induced asthma.

   A. **Specific levels.** There are no routine clinical blood or urine tests for isocyanates.

      1. Test inhalation challenge to isocyanate is not advised except in experienced laboratories owing to the danger of severe asthma attack.

      2. Isocyanate antibody testing, although used in research, is difficult to interpret in an individual patient and may not correlate with illness.

   B. **Other useful laboratory studies** may include co-oximetry or arterial blood gases or chest radiography in selected clinical scenarios.

V. **Treatment**

   A. **Emergency and supportive measures**

      1. After acute high-intensity inhalational exposure, maintain an open airway (pp 1–4), give bronchodilators as needed for wheezing (p 8), and observe for 8–12 hours for pulmonary edema (p 7).

      2. Once airway hyperreactivity has been documented, further exposure to isocyanate is contraindicated. Involve public health or OSHA agencies

to determine whether other workers also are at increased risk through improper workplace controls.

B. Specific drugs and antidotes. There is no specific antidote.

C. Decontamination after high-level exposure (p 50)

1. **Inhalation.** Remove the victim from exposure and give supplemental oxygen if available.
2. **Skin and eyes.** Remove contaminated clothing (liquid or heavy vapor exposure) and wash exposed skin with copious soap and water. Irrigate exposed eyes with saline or tepid water.

D. Enhanced elimination. There is no role for these procedures.

▶ ISONIAZID (INH)

Alicia B. Minns, MD

Isoniazid (INH), a hydrazide derivative of isonicotinic acid, is an inexpensive and effective treatment for tuberculosis. INH is well known for its propensity to cause hepatitis with chronic use. Acute INH overdose is a well-known cause of drug-induced seizures and metabolic acidosis.

I. Mechanism of toxicity

A. Acute overdose. In the central nervous system, GABA is the predominant inhibitory neurotransmitter. Pyridoxal 5'-phosphate (the active form of vitamin B_6) is a necessary coenzyme in the synthesis of GABA. Isoniazid depletes vitamin B_6 by inhibiting pyridoxine phosphokinase, the enzyme that converts pyridoxine to its active form, pyridoxal 5'-phosphate. Isoniazid also reacts with pyridoxal 5'-phosphate to form an inactive complex that is renally excreted. This functional deficiency of pyridoxine in turn impairs the synthesis of GABA and increases susceptibility to seizures. INH may also inhibit the hepatic conversion of lactate to pyruvate, exacerbating the lactic acidosis resulting from seizures.

B. Chronic toxicity. The overall incidence of adverse effects from chronic INH use is approximately 5%. Peripheral neuropathy and optic neuritis are thought to be caused by pyridoxine deficiency. Peripheral neuropathy is the most common complication of chronic INH therapy and is more commonly seen in patients with comorbidities such as malnutrition, alcoholism, diabetes, and uremia. It presents in a stocking-glove distribution that progresses proximally. INH has also been associated with other CNS findings such as hallucinations, ataxia, psychosis, and coma.

The most serious adverse effect of INH is hepatocellular necrosis. The mechanism of INH-induced hepatitis involves two pathways: an autoimmune mechanism that is thought to be idiopathic, and more commonly, direct hepatic injury by INH and its metabolites. Asymptomatic elevation of aminotransferases is common in the first few months of treatment.

C. Pharmacokinetics. Peak absorption occurs in 1–2 hours. The volume of distribution is 0.6–0.7 L/kg, with insignificant protein binding. INH is metabolized via the cytochrome P450 system, with 75–95% of metabolites renally eliminated. The half-life is 0.5–1.6 hours in fast acetylators and 2–5 hours in slow acetylators (see also Table II–66, p 462).

II. Toxic dose

A. Acute ingestion of as little as 15–40 mg/kg can produce toxicity. Doses larger than this often cause seizures. Ingestion of 80–150 mg/kg is associated with increased mortality.

B. With **chronic use,** 10–20% of patients will develop hepatic toxicity when the dose is 10 mg/kg/d, but fewer than 2% will develop this toxicity if the dose is 3–5 mg/kg/d. Older persons are more susceptible to chronic toxicity.

III. Clinical presentation

A. After **acute overdose,** nausea, vomiting, slurred speech, ataxia, depressed sensorium, coma, respiratory depression, and seizures may occur rapidly (usually within 30–120 minutes). Profound anion gap metabolic acidosis (pH, 6.8–6.9) often occurs after only one or two seizures and is likely the result of lactic acidosis due to seizure activity. The lactate usually clears slowly, even after the seizure activity is controlled. Liver injury may occur after an acute overdose and may be delayed up to several days. Hemolysis may occur in patients with glucose-6-phosphate dehydrogenase (G6PD) deficiency. Rhabdomyolysis can be a complication of recurrent seizures. Coma may occur, which can last for 24–36 hours even after the resolution of seizures and acidemia.

B. **Chronic therapeutic** INH use may cause peripheral neuritis, hepatitis, hypersensitivity reactions including drug-induced lupus erythematosus, and pyridoxine deficiency.

IV. **Diagnosis** usually is made by history and clinical presentation. INH toxicity should be considered in any patient with acute-onset seizures, especially if they are unresponsive to routine anticonvulsant medications and accompanied by profound metabolic acidosis.

A. **Specific levels.** INH usually is not detected in routine toxicology screening. Specific levels may be obtained but are rarely available or helpful for the management of acute overdoses.

B. **Other useful laboratory studies** include electrolytes, glucose, BUN, creatinine, creatine kinase (CK), and arterial blood gases. In chronic INH use, hepatic aminotransferases should be regularly monitored.

V. **Treatment**

A. **Emergency and supportive measures**

1. Maintain an open airway and assist ventilation if necessary (pp 1–7).
2. Treat coma (p 18), seizures (p 23), and metabolic acidosis (p 35) if they occur. Administer diazepam, 0.1–0.2 mg/kg IV, for treatment of seizures.

B. **Specific drugs and antidotes. Pyridoxine** (vitamin B6) is a specific antidote and usually terminates seizures. Administer 5 g IV (p 621) if the amount of INH ingested is not known; if the amount is known, give an equivalent amount in grams of pyridoxine to grams of ingested INH. This may be repeated if seizures persist. Benzodiazepines should also be given with pyridoxine, as they may have a synergistic effect in terminating seizures. If no pyridoxine is available, high-dose diazepam (0.3–0.4 mg/kg) may be effective for status epilepticus. Pyridoxine treatment may also hasten the resolution of metabolic acidosis. Pyridoxine tablets may be crushed and administered with fluids via a nasogastric tube if the IV formulation is not available in sufficient quantities. Pyridoxine does not reverse hepatic injury in chronic INH use. However, it is effective in both prevention and treatment of neurologic toxicity.

C. **Decontamination** (p 50). Administer activated charcoal orally if conditions are appropriate (see Table I–38, p 54). Consider gastric lavage for massive ingestions.

D. **Enhanced elimination.** Forced diuresis and hemodialysis have been reported to be successful but are unnecessary for most cases because the half-life of INH is relatively short and toxicity usually can be easily managed with pyridoxine and benzodiazepines. Symptoms generally resolve over a course of 8–24 hours.

► ISOPROPYL ALCOHOL

James Chenoweth, MD

Isopropyl alcohol is a clear, colorless liquid with a bitter taste used widely in a solvent, an antiseptic, and a disinfectant and is commonly available in the home as a 70% solution (rubbing alcohol). It is often ingested by alcoholics as a cheap substitute for liquor. Unlike the other common alcohol substitutes methanol and ethylene glycol, isopropyl alcohol is not metabolized to highly toxic organic acids and therefore does not produce a profound anion gap acidosis.

I. Mechanism of toxicity

A. Isopropyl alcohol is a potent depressant of the CNS, and intoxication by ingestion or inhalation may result in coma and respiratory arrest. It is metabolized to acetone (dimethyl ketone), which may contribute to and prolong CNS depression.

B. Very large doses of isopropyl alcohol may cause hypotension secondary to vasodilation and possibly myocardial depression.

C. Isopropyl alcohol is irritating to the GI tract and commonly causes gastritis.

D. Chronic inhalation of isopropyl alcohol can cause respiratory tract irritation. Chronic exposure has also been associated with elevated hepatic transaminases, dementia, cerebellar dysfunction, and myopathy.

E. Pregnancy. Isopropyl alcohol crosses the placenta and is associated with decreased birth weight in animals.

F. Pharmacokinetics. Isopropyl alcohol is rapidly absorbed with peak levels 30 minutes after ingestion. It can also be absorbed dermally and by inhalation. It distributes into body water (volume of distribution, 0.6 L/kg). It is metabolized (half-life, 2.5–8 hours) by alcohol dehydrogenase to acetone. Up to 20% is excreted unchanged in the urine.

II. Toxic dose. Isopropyl alcohol is approximately two- to threefold more potent than ethanol.

A. Ingestion. The toxic oral dose is about 0.5–1 mL/kg of rubbing alcohol (70% isopropyl alcohol) but varies depending on individual tolerance and whether any other depressants were ingested. Fatalities have occurred after adult ingestion of 240 mL, but patients with ingestions of up to 1 L have recovered with supportive care.

B. Inhalation. The odor of isopropyl alcohol can be detected at an air level of 40–200 ppm. The OSHA Permissible Exposure Limit (PEL) is 400 ppm (983 mg/m^3) as an 8-hour time-weighted average. The air level considered immediately dangerous to life or health (IDLH) is 2,000 ppm. Toxicity has been reported in children after isopropyl alcohol sponge baths, probably as a result of inhalation rather than skin absorption.

III. Clinical presentation. Intoxication mimics drunkenness from ethanol, with slurred speech, ataxia, and stupor followed in large ingestions by coma, hypotension, and respiratory arrest.

A. Because of the gastric-irritant properties of isopropyl alcohol, abdominal pain and vomiting are common, and hematemesis occasionally occurs.

B. Metabolic acidosis may occur but is usually mild. The osmol gap is usually elevated (p 33). The serum creatinine may be falsely elevated (eg, 2–3 mg/dL) owing to interference with the laboratory method.

C. Isopropyl alcohol is metabolized to **acetone,** which contributes to CNS depression and gives a distinct odor to the breath (in contrast, methanol and ethylene glycol and their toxic metabolites are odorless). Acetone is also found in nail polish remover and is used widely as a solvent in industry and chemical laboratories. Acetone is metabolized through several organic acid intermediates, which may explain the occasional report of anion gap metabolic acidosis after acute isopropyl alcohol poisoning.

IV. Diagnosis usually is based on a history of ingestion and the presence of an elevated osmol gap, the absence of severe acidosis, and the characteristic smell of isopropyl alcohol or its metabolite, acetone. Ketonemia and ketonuria may be present within 1–3 hours of ingestion.

A. Specific levels. Serum isopropyl alcohol and acetone levels are usually available from commercial toxicology laboratories. The serum level may also be estimated by calculating the osmol gap (see Table I–22, p 33). Isopropyl alcohol levels higher than 150 mg/dL usually cause coma, but patients with levels up to 560 mg/dL have survived with supportive care and dialysis. Serum acetone concentrations may be elevated.

B. **Other useful laboratory studies** include electrolytes, glucose, BUN, creatinine (may be falsely elevated), serum osmolality and osmol gap, and arterial blood gases or oximetry.

V. **Treatment**

A. **Emergency and supportive measures**

1. Maintain an open airway and assist ventilation if necessary (pp 1–4). Administer supplemental oxygen if needed.
2. Treat coma (p 18), hypotension (p 15), and hypoglycemia (p 36) if they occur.
3. Admit and observe symptomatic patients for at least 6–12 hours.

B. **Specific drugs and antidotes.** There is no specific antidote. Fomepizole or ethanol therapy is ***not*** indicated because isopropyl alcohol does not produce a toxic organic acid metabolite.

C. **Decontamination** (p 50). Because isopropyl alcohol is absorbed rapidly after ingestion, gastric-emptying procedures are not likely to be useful if the ingestion is small (a swallow or two) or if more than 30 minutes has passed. For a large, recent ingestion, consider performing aspiration of gastric contents with a small, flexible tube.

D. **Enhanced elimination**

1. **Hemodialysis** effectively removes isopropyl alcohol and acetone but is rarely indicated because the majority of patients can be managed with supportive care alone. Dialysis should be considered when levels are extremely high (eg, >400–500 mg/dL), if hypotension does not respond to fluids and vasopressors, and in acute renal failure.
2. Hemoperfusion, repeat-dose charcoal, and forced diuresis are not effective.

▶ JELLYFISH AND OTHER CNIDARIA

Michael A. Darracq, MD, MPH

The phylum Cnidaria (coelenterates), numbering over 10,000 species, includes fire coral, jellyfish (including Portuguese man-o-war, box jellyfish, sea nettle), and anemones. Despite considerable morphologic variation, all these organisms deliver venom through specialized microscopic organelles called nematocysts. Of the 10,000 different species of cnidaria, 100 are known to injure humans with nematocysts capable of penetrating the human dermis

I. **Mechanism of toxicity.** Each nematocyst contains a small, ejectable thread soaking in venom. The thread has a barb on the tip and is fired from the nematocyst with enough velocity to pierce human skin. The nematocysts are contained in outer sacs (cnidoblasts) arranged along the tentacles of jellyfish or along the surface of fire coral and the finger-like projections of sea anemones. When the cnidoblasts are opened by hydrostatic pressure, physical contact, changes in osmolarity, or chemical stimulants that have not been identified, they release their nematocysts, which eject the thread and spread venom into the skin of the victim. The venom contains numerous chemical components, including neuromuscular toxins, cardiotoxins, hemolysins, dermonecrotoxins, and histamine-like compounds.

II. **Toxic dose.** Each time a nematocyst is opened, all the contained venom is released. The extent of toxicity is dependent on the number of nematocysts that successfully discharge venom, the envenomation site, the contact time, the particular species involved, and individual patient sensitivity. Hundreds of thousands of nematocysts may be discharged with a single exposure.

A. Deaths from jellyfish stings in the Northern Hemisphere are rare and almost always are due to the **Portuguese man-o-war** (*Physalia physalis*), although *Chiropsalmus quadrumanus* (a type of box jellyfish) was implicated in the death of a child off the coast of Texas.

B. The **Australian box jellyfish** (*Chironex fleckeri,* "Assassin's Hand") is the most venomous marine animal and responsible for numerous fatalities. It should not be confused with the Hawaiian box jellyfish (*Carybdea alata*), a related but significantly less toxic species.

III. Clinical presentation

A. Acute effects

1. Stinging produces immediate burning pain, pruritus, papular lesions, and local tissue inflammation, which may progress to pustules and desquamation.
2. Nausea, vertigo, dizziness, muscle cramping, myalgia, arthralgia, anaphylactic and anaphylactoid reactions, and transient elevation in liver transaminases may follow.
3. Severe envenomation may result in respiratory distress, severe muscle cramping with hypotension, arrhythmias, shock, and pulmonary edema. Lethal outcomes are associated with rapid onset of cardiovascular collapse. Fulminant hepatic failure and renal failure have been reported after sea anemone stings.
4. **"Irukandji syndrome"** is associated with stings from *Carukia barnesi,* found mostly in the oceans off Australia's Northern Territory and less commonly near Hawaii and Florida. These stings can induce a severe catecholamine rush that often leads to severe hypertension, cardiac dysrhythmias, pulmonary edema, cardiac myopathy, and death. Skin findings are often absent. Muscle spasms, frequently involving the back preferentially and coming in waves, are described as unbearable and parenteral analgesia is often necessary.
5. Envenomation by ***C. fleckeri*** results in severe pain with systemic symptoms including nausea, vomiting, muscle spasms, headache, malaise, fever, and chills. Death is often rapid, preventing victims from reaching shore. Cardiac arrest and pulmonary edema are reported in young healthy victims without any known cardiopulmonary disease.
6. Exposure to the larvae of ***Linuche Unguiculata*** can cause pruritic papular rash affecting seabathers along the Eastern United States coast. This **"seabather's eruption"** often occurs in areas covered by bathing suits as a result of larvae being trapped close to the skin. An immediate stinging sensation is followed by prolonged itching after leaving the water. Itching is often severe and may interfere with sleep. New lesions may erupt in the first 72 hours following exposure. Systemic symptoms such as malaise, fatigue, nausea, vomiting, headache, and chills may occur. Symptoms may last up to 2 weeks.

B. Potential long-term sequelae of cnidaria envenomation include skin necrosis, infections, cosmetic tissue damage (fat atrophy and hyperpigmentation), contractures, paresthesias, neuritis, recurrent cutaneous eruptions, paralysis, and regional vasospasm with vascular insufficiency.

C. Corneal stings from the sea nettle are usually painful but resolve within 1–2 days. However, there are reports of prolonged iritis, elevated intraocular pressure, mydriasis, and decreased visual acuity lasting months to years.

IV. Diagnosis is based on the history and observation of characteristic lines of inflammation along the sites of exposure ("tentacle tracks").

A. Specific levels. Specific toxin levels are not available.

B. Other useful laboratory studies include CBC, electrolytes, glucose, BUN, creatinine, creatine kinase (CK), liver aminotransferases, and urinalysis for hemoglobin. Serial cardiac enzymes are recommended in patients with Irukandji stings or in patients with significant cardiovascular manifestations of toxicity.

V. Treatment. Treatment should be directed at the alleviation of symptoms as well as prevention of further nematocyst discharge which may intensify pain or enhance toxicity. Symptomatic care is generally sufficient for most envenomations, even that of the box jellyfish.

A. Emergency and supportive measures

1. Maintain an open airway and assist ventilation if necessary (pp 1–7). Administer supplemental oxygen.

2. Treat hypertension (p 17) or hypotension (p 15), arrhythmias (pp 10–15), coma (p 18), and seizures (p 23) if they occur.
3. Hot water immersion (40–42°C), topical lidocaine (4%), and cold/ice packs have all been recommended for the treatment of pain resulting from cnidaria envenomation. The "optimal" therapy remains unclear and is controversial.

B. **Specific drugs and antidotes.** Box jellyfish *(Chironex fleckeri)* antivenom from Australia can terminate acute pain and cardiovascular symptoms, prevent tissue effects, and may be located by a regional poison control center (in the United States, 1-800-222-1222) for use in severe cases. Local marine biologists can help identify indigenous species for the planning of specific therapy.

C. **Decontamination.** Avoid thrashing about, scratching, scraping, or other mechanical maneuvers that may break open the nematocysts. Without touching the affected areas, wash them with cold sea or salt water. ***Do not use fresh water*** because it may cause nematocysts to discharge.

1. The most commonly recommended topical treatment for jellyfish envenomation is **vinegar**. It has been demonstrated to rapidly inhibit nematocyst discharge from *C. fleckeri* and *C. barnesi*. However, vinegar has no effect on nematocyst discharge from *Physalia* utriculus ("Blue bottle"), and it may *increase* nematocyst discharge from *Cyanea capillata* ("Lion's Mane"), *Chrysaora quinquecirrha* ("American sea nettle"), *Pelaiga noctiluca* ("Mauve Stinger") and *Physalia physalis* ("Portuguese man-o-war"), although some studies have suggested that vinegar provided better pain control than other topical therapies after *P. physalia* envenomation.
2. In the absence of clear identification of the offending "jellyfish," the optimal decontamination method can be guided by geographic location:
   a. In **Indo-Pacific region** (where *C. fleckeri* and *C. barnesi* are of greatest concern), apply **vinegar** liberally by spraying or soaking the affected area, then carefully remove adherent tentacles with a gloved hand, forceps, towel, or gentle scraping with a credit card, knife or other similar straight-edged tool.
   b. In the **United States** (where *P. physalia* and *C. quinquecirrha* are of greatest concern), **do not use vinegar**; instead, wash with **sea water** and gently remove adherent tentacles as described earlier.
3. Application of **urine** or **ethanol** is **not advised**; it has been shown to increase nematocyst discharge from *C. Fleckeri* and *C. barnesi.*

D. **Enhanced Elimination.** These procedures are not applicable.

▶ LEAD

Michael J. Kosnett, MD, MPH

Lead is a soft, malleable metal that is obtained chiefly by the primary smelting and refining of natural ores or by the widespread practice of recycling and secondary smelting of scrap lead products. Recycling accounts for nearly 85% of domestic lead consumption, approximately 85% of which is used in the manufacture of lead-acid batteries. Lead is used for weights and radiation shielding, and lead alloys are used in the manufacture of pipes; cable sheathing; brass, bronze, and steel; ammunition; and solder (predominantly electric devices and older automotive radiators). Lead compounds are added as pigments, stabilizers, or binders in paints, ceramics, glass, and plastic.

Although the use of lead in house paint has been curtailed since the 1970s, industrial use of corrosion-resistant lead-based paint continues, and high-level exposure may result from renovation, sandblasting, torching, or demolition. Corrosion of lead plumbing in older homes may increase the lead concentration of tap water. Young children are particularly at risk from repeated ingestion of lead-contaminated house dust, yard soil, or paint chips or from mouthing toy jewelry or other decorative items containing lead. Children may also be exposed to lead carried into the home on contaminated work clothes worn by adults. Regular consumption of game meat harvested with lead ammunition and contaminated with lead residues may increase blood lead above background levels, particularly in children.

Lead exposure may occur from the use of lead-glazed ceramics or containers for food or beverage preparation or storage. Certain folk medicines (eg, the Mexican remedies *azarcon* and *greta,* the Dominican remedy *litargirio,* and some Indian Ayurvedic preparations) may contain high amounts of lead salts.

Consumer protection legislation enacted in 2008 lowered the permissible concentration of lead in paint and other surface coatings for consumer use to 0.009% (90 ppm). Since 2011, the lead content of children's products must not exceed 100 ppm.

I. Mechanism of toxicity

A. The multisystem toxicity of lead is mediated by several mechanisms, including inactivation or alteration of enzymes and other macromolecules by binding to sulfhydryl, phosphate, or carboxyl ligands and interaction with essential cations, most notably calcium, zinc, and iron. Pathologic alterations in cellular and mitochondrial membranes, neurotransmitter synthesis and function, heme synthesis, cellular redox status, and nucleotide metabolism may occur. Adverse impacts on the nervous, renal, GI, hematopoietic, reproductive, and cardiovascular systems can result.

B. Pharmacokinetics. Inhalation of lead fume or other fine, soluble particulate results in rapid and extensive pulmonary absorption, the major although not exclusive route of exposure in industry. Nonindustrial exposure occurs predominantly by ingestion, particularly in children, who absorb 45–50% of soluble lead, compared with approximately 10–15% in adults. After absorption, lead is distributed via the blood (where 99% is bound to the erythrocytes) to multiple tissues, including transplacental transport to the fetus, and CNS transport across the blood–brain barrier. Clearance of lead from the body follows a multicompartment kinetic model, consisting of "fast" compartments in the blood and soft tissues (half-life, 1–2 months) and slow compartments in the bone (half-life, years to decades). Approximately 70% of lead excretion occurs via the urine, with smaller amounts eliminated via the feces and scant amounts via the hair, nails, and sweat. Greater than 90% of the lead burden in adults and more than two-thirds of the burden in young children occur in the skeleton. Slow redistribution of lead from bone to soft tissues may elevate blood lead concentrations for months to years after a patient with chronic high-dose exposure has been removed from external sources. In patients with a high bone lead burden, pathologic states associated with rapid bone turnover or demineralization, such as hyperthyroidism and immobilization osteoporosis, have resulted in symptomatic lead intoxication.

II. Toxic dose

A. Dermal absorption is minimal with inorganic lead but may be substantial with organic lead compounds, which may also cause skin irritation.

B. Ingestion. In general, absorption of lead compounds is directly proportional to solubility and inversely proportional to particle size. Gastrointestinal lead absorption is increased by iron deficiency and low dietary calcium. Absorption can increase substantially in a fasted state.

1. Acute symptomatic intoxication is rare after a single exposure but may occur within hours after ingestion of gram quantities of soluble lead compounds or days after GI retention of swallowed lead objects, such as fishing weights and curtain weights.
2. Studies have not established a low-dose threshold for adverse subclinical effects of lead. Recent epidemiologic studies in children have observed effects of lead on cognitive function at blood lead concentrations of less than 5 mcg/dL, and other studies suggest that background levels of lead exposure in recent decades may have been associated with hypertension

and increased cardiovascular mortality in some adults. The geometric mean blood lead concentration in the United States during 2011–2012 was estimated to be 0.973 mcg/dL; background dietary lead intake may be in the range of 1–4 mcg/d.

3. The US Environmental Protection Agency (EPA) action level for lead in drinking water is 15 ppb (parts per billion). However, the maximum contaminant level (MCL) goal for drinking water is 0 ppb, and EPA has set no "reference dose" for lead because of the lack of a recognized low-dose threshold for adverse effects.

C. **Inhalation.** Unprotected exposure to the massive airborne lead levels (>2,500 mcg/m^3) encountered during abrasive blasting, welding, or torch cutting metal surfaces coated with lead-based paint poses an acute hazard and has resulted in symptomatic lead intoxication from within a day to a few weeks. The OSHA workplace permissible exposure limit (PEL) for inorganic lead dusts and fumes is 50 mcg/m^3 as an 8-hour time-weighted average. The level considered immediately dangerous to life or health (IDLH) is 100 mg/m^3.

III. **Clinical presentation.** The multisystem toxicity of lead presents a spectrum of clinical findings ranging from overt, life-threatening intoxication to subtle, subclinical effects.

A. **Acute ingestion** of very large amounts of lead (gram quantities) may cause abdominal pain, anemia (usually hemolytic), toxic hepatitis, and encephalopathy.

B. **Subacute or chronic exposure** is more common than acute poisoning.

1. **Constitutional** effects include fatigue, malaise, irritability, anorexia, insomnia, weight loss, decreased libido, arthralgias, and myalgias.
2. **Gastrointestinal** effects include cramping abdominal pain (lead colic), nausea, constipation, or (less commonly) diarrhea.
3. **Central nervous system** manifestations range from impaired concentration, headache, diminished visual-motor coordination, and tremor to overt encephalopathy (a life-threatening emergency characterized by agitated delirium or lethargy, ataxia, convulsions, and coma). Chronic low-level exposure in infants and children may lead to decreased intelligence and impaired neurobehavioral development, stunted growth, and diminished auditory acuity. Recent studies in adults suggest that lead may accentuate age-related decline in cognitive function.
4. **Cardiovascular effects** of chronic lead exposure include blood pressure elevation and an increased risk for hypertension. Recent studies have detected elevated cardiovascular mortality in populations whose long-term blood lead concentrations were likely in the range of 10–25 mcg/dL.
5. **Peripheral motor neuropathy,** affecting mainly the upper extremities, can cause severe extensor muscle weakness ("wrist drop").
6. **Hematologic** effects include normochromic or microcytic anemia, which may be accompanied by basophilic stippling. Hemolysis may occur after acute or subacute high-dose exposure.
7. **Nephrotoxic** effects include reversible acute tubular dysfunction (including Fanconi-like aminoaciduria in children) and chronic interstitial fibrosis. Hyperuricemia and gout may occur.
8. **Adverse reproductive outcomes** may include diminished or aberrant sperm production, increased rate of miscarriage, preterm delivery, decreased gestational age, low birth weight, and impaired neurologic development.

C. **Repeated, intentional inhalation of leaded gasoline** has resulted in ataxia, myoclonic jerking, hyperreflexia, delirium, and convulsions.

IV. **Diagnosis.** Although overt encephalopathy or abdominal colic associated with a suspect activity may readily suggest the diagnosis of severe lead poisoning, the nonspecific symptoms and multisystem signs associated with mild or moderate intoxication may be mistaken for a viral illness or another disorder. Consider lead poisoning in any patient with multisystem findings that include abdominal pain, headache, anemia, and, less commonly, motor neuropathy, gout, and renal insufficiency. Consider lead encephalopathy in any child or adult with delirium or convulsions (especially with coexistent anemia), and chronic lead poisoning in any child with neurobehavioral deficits or developmental delays.

A. Specific levels. The **whole-blood lead** level is the most useful indicator of lead exposure. Relationships between blood lead levels and clinical findings generally have been based on subacute or chronic exposure, not on transiently high values that may result immediately after acute exposure. In addition, there may be considerable interindividual variability. ***Note:*** *Blood lead samples must be drawn and stored in* ***lead-free*** *syringes and tubes* ("trace metals" tube or royal blue stopper tube containing heparin or EDTA).

1. Blood lead levels are less than 5 mcg/dL in populations without occupational or specific environmental exposure. Levels between 1 and 25 mcg/dL have been associated with subclinical decreases in intelligence and impaired neurobehavioral development in children exposed in utero or in early childhood. The dose-response for IQ decrement is log-linear, such that IQ loss per mcg/dL is steepest at low dose. Studies in adults indicate that long-term blood lead concentrations in the range of 10–25 mcg/dL (and possibly lower) pose a risk for hypertension and cardiovascular mortality and may possibly contribute to age-related decline in cognitive function.
2. Blood lead levels of 25–60 mcg/dL may be associated with headache, irritability, difficulty concentrating, slowed reaction time, and other neuropsychiatric effects. Anemia may occur, and subclinical slowing of motor nerve conduction may be detectable.
3. Blood levels of 60–80 mcg/dL may be associated with GI symptoms and subclinical renal effects.
4. With blood levels in excess of 80 mcg/dL, serious overt intoxication may occur, including abdominal pain (lead colic) and nephropathy. Encephalopathy and neuropathy usually are associated with levels over 100 mcg/dL.

B. Elevations in **free erythrocyte protoporphyrin (FEP) or zinc protoporphyrin (ZPP)** (>35 mcg/dL) reflect lead-induced inhibition of heme synthesis. Because only actively forming and not mature erythrocytes are affected, elevations typically lag lead exposure by a few weeks. High blood levels of lead in the presence of a normal FEP or ZPP level therefore suggests very recent exposure. Protoporphyrin elevation is not specific for lead and may also occur with iron deficiency. Protoporphyrin levels are not sensitive for low-level exposure (blood lead <30 mcg/dL).

C. Urinary lead excretion increases and decreases more rapidly than blood lead. In the CDC's "Fourth National Report on Human Exposure to Environmental Chemicals" (http://www.cdc.gov/exposurereport), the geometric mean urinary lead concentration of subjects age 6 and older was 0.360 mcg/L. Normal, baseline urinary lead excretion for the general population is less than 3 mcg/d. Several empiric protocols that measure 6- or 24-hour urinary lead excretion after calcium EDTA challenge have been developed to identify persons with elevated body lead burdens. However, because chelatable lead predominantly reflects lead in soft tissues, which in most cases already correlates satisfactorily with blood lead, chelation challenges are seldom indicated in clinical practice.

D. Noninvasive in vivo **x-ray fluorescence measurement of lead in bone,** a test predominantly available in research settings, may provide the best index of long-term cumulative lead exposure and total-body lead burden.

E. Other tests. Nonspecific laboratory findings that support the diagnosis of lead poisoning include anemia (normocytic or microcytic) and basophilic stippling of erythrocytes, a useful but insensitive clue. Acute high-dose exposure sometimes may be associated with transient azotemia (elevated BUN and serum creatinine) and mild-to-moderate elevation in serum aminotransferases.

Recently ingested lead paint, glazes, chips, or solid lead objects may be visible on abdominal radiographs. CT or MRI of the brain often reveals cerebral edema in patients with lead encephalopathy. Because iron deficiency increases lead absorption, iron status should be evaluated.

V. Treatment

A. Emergency and supportive measures

1. Treat seizures (p 23) and coma (p 18) if they occur. Provide adequate fluids to maintain urine flow (optimally 1–2 mL/kg/h) but avoid overhydration, which may aggravate cerebral edema. Avoid phenothiazines for delirium, as they may lower the seizure threshold.
2. Patients with increased intracranial pressure may benefit from corticosteroids (eg, dexamethasone, 10 mg IV) and mannitol (0.25–1.0 g/kg IV as a 20–25% solution) or hypertonic saline. Intubation and short-term hyperventilation initially targeted to a $PaCO_2$ of 30–35 mm Hg may also be beneficial.

B. Specific drugs and antidotes. Treatment with chelating agents decreases blood lead concentrations and increases urinary lead excretion. Although chelation has been associated with relief of symptoms and decreased mortality, controlled clinical trials demonstrating efficacy are lacking, and *treatment recommendations have been largely empiric.*

1. **Encephalopathy.** Administer IV **calcium EDTA** (p 548). Some clinicians initiate treatment with a single dose of **BAL** (p 514), followed 4 hours later by concomitant administration of calcium EDTA and BAL.
2. **Symptomatic without encephalopathy.** Administer oral **succimer** (DMSA, p 624) or parenteral **calcium EDTA** (p 548). Calcium EDTA is preferred as initial treatment if the patient has severe GI toxicity (eg, lead colic) or if the blood lead concentration is extremely elevated (eg, >150 mcg/dL). **Unithiol** (p 630) may be considered as an alternative to DMSA.
3. **Asymptomatic children with elevated blood lead levels.** The CDC recommends treatment of children with levels of 45 mcg/dL or higher. Use oral **succimer** (DMSA, p 624). A large randomized, double-blind, placebo-controlled trial of DMSA in children with blood lead concentrations between 25 and 44 mcg/dL found no evidence of clinical benefit.
4. **Asymptomatic adults.** The usual treatment is removal from exposure and observation. Consider oral **succimer** (DMSA, p 624) for patients with markedly elevated levels (eg, >80–100 mcg/dL).
5. Although **D-penicillamine** (p 601) is an alternative oral treatment, it may be associated with more side effects and less efficient lead diuresis.
6. **Blood lead monitoring during chelation.** Obtain a blood lead measurement immediately before chelation and recheck the measurement within 24–48 hours after starting chelation to confirm that levels are declining. Recheck measurements 1 day and from 7 to 21 days after chelation to assess the extent of rebound in blood lead level associated with redistribution of lead from high bone stores and/or the possibility of re-exposure. Additional courses of treatment and further investigation of exposure sources may be warranted.

C. Decontamination (p 50)

1. **Acute ingestion.** Because even small items (eg, a paint chip or a sip of lead-containing glaze) may contain tens to hundreds of milligrams of lead, gut decontamination is indicated after acute ingestion of virtually any lead-containing substance.
   a. Administer activated charcoal (although efficacy is unknown).
   b. If lead-containing material is still visible on abdominal radiograph after initial treatment, consider whole-bowel irrigation (p 55).
   c. Consider endoscopic or surgical removal of lead foreign bodies that exhibit prolonged GI retention.

2. **Lead-containing buckshot, shrapnel, or bullets** in or adjacent to a synovial space or a fluid-filled space, such as a paravertebral pseudocyst or a subscapular bursa, should be surgically removed if possible, particularly if associated with evidence of systemic lead absorption.

D. **Enhanced elimination.** There is no role for dialysis, hemoperfusion, or repeat-dose charcoal. However, in anuric patients with chronic renal failure, limited study suggests that calcium EDTA (1 g in 250 cc normal saline infused over 1 hour) followed immediately by hemofiltration or high-flux hemodialysis (eg, using an F160 membrane) may increase lead clearance.

E. **Other required measures.** Remove the patient from the source of exposure and institute control measures to prevent repeated intoxication. Other possibly exposed persons (eg, coworkers or siblings or playmates of young children) should be evaluated promptly.

1. **Infants and children.** The CDC no longer recommends universal blood lead screening for low-income or Medicaid-eligible children, but instead urges state and local officials to target screening toward specific groups of children in their area at higher risk for elevated blood lead levels. In 2012, CDC agreed with an advisory committee recommendation that a reference value based on the 97.5th percentile of the NHANES-generated blood lead level distribution in children 1–5 years old (currently 5 mcg/dL) be used to identify children with elevated blood lead levels. Exposure assessment and follow-up monitoring of children with a blood lead level at or above the reference value is recommended.

2. **Adults with occupational exposure**

   a. Federal OSHA standards for workers exposed to lead provide specific guidelines for periodic blood lead monitoring and medical surveillance (www.osha-slc.gov/OshStd toc/OSHA Std toc 1910.html). Under the general industry standard, workers must be removed from exposure if a single blood lead level exceeds 60 mcg/dL or if the average of three successive levels exceeds 50 mcg/dL. In construction workers, removal is required if a single blood lead level exceeds 50 mcg/dL. Workers may not return to work until the blood lead level is below 40 mcg/dL and any clinical manifestations of toxicity have resolved. Prophylactic chelation is prohibited. OSHA standards mandate that workers removed from work because of elevated blood lead levels retain full pay and benefits.

   b. Medical removal parameters in the OSHA standards summarized earlier were established in the late 1970s and are outdated based on current background blood levels and recent concern about the hazards of lower-level exposure. The standards explicitly empower physicians to order medical removal at lower blood lead levels. It is prudent and feasible for employers to maintain workers' blood lead levels below 20 mcg/dL and possibly below 10 mcg/dL. California and some other state OSHA programs are proceeding with plans to develop and implement occupational lead standards that are more protective than those promulgated by federal OSHA. Under EPA regulations effective in 2010, contractors performing renovation, repair, and painting projects that disturb lead-based paint in homes, child care facilities, and schools built before 1978 must be certified and must follow specific work practices to prevent lead contamination.

   c. The CDC recommends that pregnant women with blood lead concentrations of 5 mcg/dL or higher undergo exposure reduction, nutritional counseling, and follow-up testing, and that pregnant women with blood lead concentrations of 10 mcg/dL or higher be removed from occupational lead exposure. A guidance document is available at http://www.cdc.gov/nceh/lead/publications/leadandpregnancy2010.pdf

► LIONFISH AND OTHER SCORPAENIDAE

Richard F. Clark, MD

The family Scorpaenidae are saltwater fish that are mostly bottom dwellers noted for their ability to camouflage themselves and disappear into the environment. There are 30 genera and about 300 species, some 30 of which can envenomate humans. Although they once were considered an occupational hazard only to commercial fishing, increasing contact with these fish by scuba divers and home aquarists has increased the frequency of envenomations. In addition, due to changing water temperatures and introduction of exotic species, some of these fish can now be found in aquatic environments where they previously weren't present, such as the recent proliferation of lionfish in the Gulf of Mexico.

I. **Mechanism of toxicity.** Envenomation usually occurs when the fish is being handled or stepped on or when the aquarist has hands in the tank. The dorsal, anal, and pectoral fins are supported by spines that are connected to venom glands. The fish will erect its spines and jab the victim, causing release of venom (and often sloughing of the integumentary sheath of the spine into the wound). The venom of all these organisms is a heat-labile mixture that is not completely characterized.

II. **Toxic dose.** The dose of venom involved in any sting is variable. Interspecies difference in the severity of envenomation is generally the result of the relation between the venom gland and the spines.

 A. ***Synanceja*** (Australian stonefish) have short, strong spines with the venom gland located near the tip; therefore, large doses of venom can be delivered, and severe envenomation can result.

 B. ***Pterois*** (lionfish, turkeyfish) have long delicate spines with poorly developed venom glands near the base of the spine and therefore are usually capable of delivering only small doses of venom.

III. **Clinical presentation.** Envenomation typically produces immediate onset of sharp, throbbing, intense, excruciating pain. In untreated cases, the intensity of pain peaks at 60–90 minutes, and the pain may persist for 1–2 days.

 A. **Systemic intoxication** associated mainly with stonefish envenomation can include the rapid onset of hypotension, tachycardia, cardiac arrhythmias, myocardial ischemia, syncope, diaphoresis, nausea, vomiting, abdominal cramping, dyspnea, pulmonary edema, cyanosis, headache, muscular weakness, and spasticity.

 B. **Local tissue effects** include erythema, ecchymosis, and swelling. Infection may occur owing to retained portions of the integumentary sheath. Hyperalgesia, anesthesia, or paresthesias of the affected extremity may occur, and persistent neuropathy has been reported.

IV. **Diagnosis** usually is based on a history of exposure, and the severity of envenomation is usually readily apparent.

 A. **Specific levels.** There are no specific toxin levels available.

 B. **Other useful laboratory studies** for severe intoxication include electrolytes, glucose, BUN, creatinine, creatine kinase (CK), urinalysis, ECG monitoring, and chest radiography. Soft-tissue radiographs of the sting site may occasionally demonstrate a retained integumentary sheath or other foreign material but should not be substituted for direct exploration of the wound when indicated.

V. **Treatment**

 A. **Emergency and supportive measures**

  1. After severe stonefish envenomation:

   a. Maintain an open airway and assist ventilation if needed (pp 1–7). Administer supplemental oxygen.

   b. Treat hypotension (p 15) and arrhythmias (pp 10–15) if they occur.

  2. General wound care:

a. Clean the wound carefully and remove any visible integumentary sheath. Monitor wounds for development of infection.
b. Give tetanus prophylaxis if needed.

B. **Specific drugs and antidotes.** Immediately immerse the extremity in **hot water** (45°C [113°F]) for 30–60 minutes. This should result in prompt relief of pain within several minutes. For stonefish envenomations, a specific antivenin can be located by a regional poison control center (in the United States, 1-800-222-1222), but most of these cases can be managed successfully with hot water immersion and supportive symptomatic care.

C. **Decontamination** procedures are not applicable.

D. **Enhanced elimination.** There is no role for these procedures.

▶ LITHIUM

Jonathan B. Ford, MD

Lithium is used for the treatment of bipolar depression and other psychiatric disorders and occasionally to raise the white blood cell count in patients with leukopenia. Serious toxicity is caused most commonly by chronic overmedication in patients with renal impairment. Acute overdose, in contrast, is generally less severe.

I. **Mechanism of toxicity**

A. Lithium is a naturally occurring alkali metal and a monovalent cation that enters cells and substitutes for sodium or potassium. The mechanisms by which lithium produces its therapeutic and toxic effects are not completely understood. Lithium has a similar size to magnesium and competes with magnesium as a cofactor for several key enzymes. Specific enzymes involved in intracellular signaling pathways are inhibited. Newer research suggests that the serotonergic system is strongly involved and the dopaminergic system may be as well. Lithium is also thought to stabilize cell membranes. With excessive levels, it depresses neural excitation and synaptic transmission.

B. **Pharmacokinetics.** Lithium is completely absorbed within 6–8 hours of ingestion. The initial volume of distribution (Vd) is about 0.5 L/kg, with slow entry into tissues and a final Vd of 0.7–1.4 L/kg. Entry into the brain is slow; this explains the delay between peak blood levels and CNS effects after an acute overdose. Elimination is virtually entirely by the kidney, with a half-life of 14–30 hours. Thyroxine enhances tubular reabsorption, which may increase lithium levels in patients with hyperthyroidism.

II. **Toxic dose.** The usual daily dose of lithium ranges from 300 to 2,400 mg (8- 64 mEq/d), and the therapeutic serum lithium level is 0.6–1.2 mEq/L. The toxicity of lithium depends on whether the overdose is acute, acute-on-chronic, or chronic.

A. **Acute ingestion** of 1 mEq/kg (40 mg/kg) will produce a blood level after tissue equilibration of approximately 1.2 mEq/L. Acute ingestion of more than 20–30 tablets by an adult potentially can cause serious toxicity.

B. **Acute-on-chronic** ingestions occur when patients regularly taking lithium ingest an acute overdose. Because the patient's tissues are already saturated with lithium, toxicity is potentially more serious than an acute overdose in a patient not regularly using lithium.

C. **Chronic intoxication** may occur in patients on therapeutic doses. Lithium is excreted by the kidneys, where it is handled like sodium; any state that causes dehydration, sodium depletion, or excessive sodium reabsorption may lead to increased lithium reabsorption, accumulation, and possibly intoxication. Common states causing lithium retention include acute gastroenteritis, diuretic use (particularly thiazides), use of nonsteroidal anti-inflammatory drugs or angiotensin-converting enzyme (ACE) inhibitors, and lithium-induced nephrogenic diabetes insipidus.

III. Clinical presentation. Severity of toxicity is proportional to the duration of lithium exposure and the amount ingested. Mild-to-moderate intoxication results in lethargy, muscular weakness, slurred speech, ataxia, tremor, and myoclonic jerks. Rigidity and extrapyramidal effects may be seen. Severe intoxication may result in agitated delirium, coma, convulsions, and hyperthermia. Recovery is often very slow, and patients may remain confused or obtunded for several days to weeks. Rarely, cerebellar and cognitive dysfunction is persistent and is referred to as syndrome of irreversible lithium-effectuated neurotoxicity (SILENT). Cases of rapidly progressive dementia, similar to Jakob–Creutzfeldt disease, have occurred and are usually reversible. Serotonin syndrome may occur in patients concurrently taking another serotonergic medication. The ECG commonly shows T-wave flattening or inversions and depressed ST segments in the lateral leads; less commonly, bradycardia, sinus node arrest, complete heart block, and unmasking of Brugada pattern may occur. The white cell count often is elevated (15–20,000/mm^3).

- **A. Acute ingestion** may cause initial mild nausea and vomiting, but systemic signs of intoxication are minimal and usually are delayed for several hours while lithium distributes into tissues, particularly the nervous system. Initially high serum levels fall by 50–70% or more with tissue equilibration. In general, this ingestion is less severe and is well tolerated.
- **B. Acute-on-chronic ingestions** are potentially more serious because of additive effects with lithium in tissues.
- **C.** Patients with **chronic intoxication** usually already have systemic manifestations on admission, and toxicity may be severe with levels only slightly above therapeutic levels. Typically, patients with chronic intoxication have elevated BUN and creatinine levels and other evidence of dehydration or renal insufficiency.
- **D. Nephrogenic diabetes insipidus** (p 37) is a recognized complication of chronic lithium therapy and may lead to dehydration and hypernatremia.
- **E.** Other effects of lithium include hyperparathyroidism (with hypercalcemia), hypothyroidism, and rarely hyperthyroidism.

IV. Diagnosis. Lithium intoxication should be suspected in any patient with a known psychiatric history who is confused, ataxic, or tremulous.

- **A. Specific levels.** The diagnosis is supported by an elevated lithium level.
  - **1.** Most hospital clinical laboratories can perform a stat serum lithium concentration. However, the serum lithium level is not an accurate predictor of toxicity.
    - **a.** With acute-on-chronic and chronic poisoning, toxicity may be associated with levels only slightly above the therapeutic range.
    - **b.** In contrast, peak levels as high as 9.3 mEq/L have been reported early after acute ingestion without signs of intoxication owing to measurement before final tissue distribution.
    - **c.** ***Note:*** Specimens obtained in a green-top tube (lithium heparin) will give a markedly false elevation of the serum lithium level due to the lithium content found in the tube itself.
  - **2.** Cerebrospinal fluid lithium levels higher than 0.4 mEq/L were associated in one case report with CNS toxicity. However, CSF lithium levels generally do not correlate with toxicity and are not clinically useful.
- **B. Other useful laboratory studies** include electrolytes (the anion gap may be narrowed owing to elevated chloride or bicarbonate), calcium, glucose, BUN, creatinine, thyroid function tests, and ECG monitoring.

V. Treatment

- **A. Emergency and supportive measures**
  - **1.** In obtunded patients, maintain an open airway and assist ventilation if necessary (pp 1–7). Administer supplemental oxygen.
  - **2.** Treat coma (p 18), seizures (p 23), and hyperthermia (p 21) if they occur.
  - **3.** In dehydrated patients, replace fluid deficits with IV crystalloid solutions. Initial treatment should include repletion of sodium and water with 1–2 L of

normal saline (children: 10–20 mL/kg). Once fluid deficits are replaced, give hypotonic (eg, half-normal saline) solutions because continued administration of normal saline often leads to hypernatremia, especially in patients with lithium-induced nephrogenic diabetes insipidus.

B. **Specific drugs and antidotes.** There is no specific antidote. Thiazides and indomethacin have been used for the treatment of nephrogenic diabetes insipidus (p 37); amiloride may also be effective.

C. **Decontamination** (p 50) measures are appropriate after acute ingestions and acute-on-chronic ingestions but not chronic intoxication.

1. Activated charcoal does not adsorb lithium but may be useful if other drug ingestion is suspected.
2. Whole-bowel irrigation (p 55) may enhance gut decontamination, especially in cases involving sustained-release preparations.
3. Oral administration of sodium polystyrene sulfonate (SPS; Kayexalate) has been advocated to reduce lithium absorption, but there is insufficient evidence of safety or effectiveness. Serum potassium levels must be monitored closely in patients given this therapy.

D. **Enhanced elimination** (p 56). Lithium is excreted exclusively by the kidneys. The clearance is about 25% of the glomerular filtration rate and is reduced by sodium depletion or dehydration.

1. **Hemodialysis (HD)** removes lithium effectively and is indicated for intoxicated patients with seizures or severely abnormal mental status and for patients unable to excrete lithium renally (ie, anephric or anuric patients). Repeated and prolonged HD may be necessary because of slow movement of lithium out of the CNS. Serum levels may rebound as tissue redistribution does occur. Serum levels and symptoms should be monitored following HD. There is some disagreement on the serum level of lithium at which one must initiate HD for lithium toxicity. The decision to initiate HD should be made using patient's symptoms, duration of lithium exposure, and kidney function in addition to the serum lithium level.
2. **Continuous venovenous hemodiafiltration** (CVVHDF) has been shown to be effective in removing lithium in several human cases. The clearance of lithium via CVVHDF is 28–62 mL/min compared with a normal renal clearance of 20–25 mL/min. (The clearance of lithium during HD is 60–170 mL/min.) Advantages of CVVHDF over HD include its wide availability in many intensive care units, reduced risk in patients with hemodynamic instability, and no postdialysis rebound in lithium concentrations as equilibration between the tissue and vascular compartments occurs between runs of dialysis.
3. **Forced diuresis** only slightly increases lithium excretion compared with normal hydration and is not recommended. However, establishing normal urine output may bring the urinary lithium clearance to 25–30 mL/min.
4. **Oral sodium polystyrene sulfonate** (SPS, Kayexalate) enhances elimination of lithium in animal models, and in one human retrospective study of chronic intoxication the half-life was reduced by nearly 50%. Mild hypokalemia was observed in one-half of the patients receiving SPS.
5. Hemoperfusion and repeat-dose charcoal are not effective.

▶ LOMOTIL AND OTHER ANTIDIARRHEALS

Ilene B. Anderson, PharmD

Lomotil is a combination product containing diphenoxylate and atropine that is prescribed commonly for symptomatic treatment of diarrhea. Children are especially sensitive to small doses of Lomotil and may develop delayed toxicity after accidental ingestion. **Motofen** is a similar drug that contains difenoxin and atropine. **Loperamide** (Imodium) is a nonprescription drug with similar properties.

I. Mechanism of toxicity

A. Diphenoxylate is an opioid analog of meperidine. It is metabolized to difenoxin (diphenoxylic acid), which has fivefold the antidiarrheal activity of diphenoxylate. Both agents have opioid effects (p 350) in overdose.

B. Atropine is an anticholinergic agent (p 97) that may contribute to lethargy and coma. It also slows drug absorption and may delay the onset of symptoms.

C. Loperamide is a synthetic piperidine derivative that is structurally similar to diphenoxylate and haloperidol. It may produce opioid-like toxicity in overdose.

D. Pharmacokinetics. See Table II–66, p 462. Absorption and peak effects of Lomotil may be slowed in overdose, resulting in delayed apnea especially in children.

II. Toxic dose

A. Lomotil. The toxic dose is difficult to predict because of wide individual variability in response to drug effects and promptness of treatment. The lethal dose is unknown, but death in children has been reported after ingestion of **fewer than five tablets.**

B. Loperamide. A single acute ingestion of less than 0.4 mg/kg is not likely to cause serious toxicity in children older than 1 year of age. Fatalities, abdominal distention, and paralytic ileus have been reported in children younger than 1 year of age after ingestion of 0.6–3 mg/d.

III. Clinical presentation.

A. Acute ingestion. Depending on the individual and the time since ingestion, manifestations may be those of primarily anticholinergic or opioid intoxication.

1. **Atropine** intoxication may occur before, during, or after opioid effects. Anticholinergic effects include lethargy or agitation, flushed face, dry mucous membranes, mydriasis (dilated pupils), ileus, hyperpyrexia, and tachycardia.
2. **Opioid intoxication** produces small pupils, coma, and respiratory arrest, and the onset of these effects often is delayed for several hours after ingestion.
3. All the antidiarrheals may cause vomiting, abdominal distention, and paralytic ileus.

B. Chronic, high-dose abuse of loperamide has been associated with QT prolongation and life-threatening ventricular arrhythmias (torsade de pointes). Discontinuation of the loperamide resulted in resolution of the rhythm disturbances.

IV. Diagnosis is based on the history and signs of anticholinergic or opioid intoxication.

A. Specific levels. Specific serum levels are not available.

B. Other useful laboratory studies include electrolytes, glucose, and arterial blood gases (if respiratory insufficiency is suspected).

V. Treatment

A. Emergency and supportive measures

1. Maintain an open airway and assist ventilation if necessary (pp 1–7).
2. Treat coma (p 18) and hypotension (p 15) if they occur.
3. Because of the danger of abrupt respiratory arrest, observe all children with Lomotil or Motofen ingestion in an intensive care unit for 18–24 hours. Similar precautions should be taken for patients with very large ingestions of loperamide.

B. Specific drugs and antidotes

1. Administer **naloxone,** 1–2 mg IV (p 584), to patients with lethargy, apnea, or coma. Repeated doses of naloxone may be required because its duration of effect ($\leq$1–2 hours) is much shorter than that of the opioids in these products.
2. There is no evidence that **physostigmine** (p 609) is beneficial for this overdose, although it may reverse signs of anticholinergic poisoning.

C. Decontamination (p 50). Administer activated charcoal orally if conditions are appropriate (see Table I–38, p 54). Gastric lavage is not necessary after small-to-moderate ingestions if activated charcoal can be given promptly.

D. Enhanced elimination. There is no role for these procedures.

► LYSERGIC ACID DIETHYLAMIDE (LSD) AND OTHER HALLUCINOGENS

Patil Armenian, MD

Patients who seek medical care after self-administering mind-altering substances may have used any of a large variety of compounds. Several of these agents are discussed elsewhere in this manual (eg, amphetamines [p 81], cocaine [p 201], marijuana [p 304], phencyclidine and ketamine [p 365], and toluene [p 437]). Many of the drugs discussed in this chapter are *entactogens* ("to touch within"), enhancing sensations and promoting illusions (eg, LSD, MDMA). Others have primarily sympathomimetic characteristics, with hallucinations a smaller part of the overall experience (eg, cathinones, PMA). Several have been used widely for personal experimentation as well as clinically to facilitate psychotherapy. Although the use of traditional hallucinogens such as LSD has declined over the past decades, there is a current resurgence of hallucinogen use from novel compounds, such as the 2C-NBOMe series and synthetic cathinones. Table II–35 lists some common and uncommon hallucinogens.

I. **Mechanism of toxicity.** Despite many intriguing theories and much current research, the biochemical mechanism of hallucinations is not known. The hallucinogenic effects of LSD are thought to be mediated by 5-HT2 receptor activation, and many other agents are thought to alter the activity of serotonin and dopamine in the brain. Central and peripheral sympathetic stimulation may account for some of the side effects, such as anxiety, agitation, psychosis, dilated pupils, tachycardia, and hyperthermia. Some agents (eg, MDMA) are directly neurotoxic.

II. **Toxic dose.** The toxic dose is highly variable, depending on the agent and the circumstances (see Table II–35). LSD is a highly potent hallucinogen. In general, entactogenic effects do not appear to be dose related; therefore, increasing the dose does not intensify the desired effects. Likewise, paranoia or panic attacks may occur with any dose and depend on the surroundings and the patient's current emotional state. In contrast, hallucinations, visual illusions, and sympathomimetic side effects are dose related. The toxic dose may be only slightly greater than the recreational dose. In human volunteers receiving recreational doses of MDMA, elimination was nonlinear, implying that small increases in dosing may increase the risk for toxicity.

III. **Clinical presentation**

A. Mild-to-moderate intoxication

1. A person experiencing a panic reaction or "bad trip" is conscious, coherent, and oriented but is anxious and fearful and may display paranoid or bizarre reasoning. The patient may also be tearful, combative, or self-destructive. Delayed intermittent "flashbacks" may occur after the acute effects have worn off and are usually precipitated by use of another mind-altering drug.
2. A person with dose-related sympathomimetic side effects may also exhibit hyperthermia, tachycardia, hypertension, mydriasis (dilated pupils), diaphoresis, bruxism, short attention span, tremor, and hyperreflexia.

B. Life-threatening toxicity

1. Intense sympathomimetic stimulation can cause seizures, severe hyperthermia, hypertension, intracranial hemorrhage, and cardiac arrhythmias. Hyperthermic patients are usually obtunded, agitated or thrashing about, diaphoretic, and hyperreflexic. Untreated, hyperthermia may result in hypotension, coagulopathy, rhabdomyolysis, and hepatic and other organ failure (p 21). Hyperthermia has been associated with LSD, methylene dioxyamphetamine (MDA), MDMA, and paramethoxyamphetamine (PMA).
2. Severe hyponatremia has been reported after use of MDMA and may result from excess water intake, excessive sweating (eg, dancing) and inappropriate secretion of antidiuretic hormone.
3. The use of 2,5-dimethoxy-4-bromoamphetamine (DOB) has resulted in ergot-like vascular spasm, circulatory insufficiency, and gangrene (p 229).

TABLE II–35. HALLUCINOGENS

Common Name(s)	Chemical Name	Classification[a]	Comments
Bufotenine	5-Hydroxy-*N,N*-dimethyltryptamine	N, T	From skin and secretions of the toad *Bufo alvarius* (Colorado river toad), which may also contain cardiac glycosides.
DMT	*N,N*-Dimethyltryptamine	N, S, T	Smoked, insufflated, injected or ingested in combination with MAOIs (harmaline, harmine) in ayahuasca.
DOB	2,5-Dimethoxy-4-bromoamphetamine	S, A[b]	Long time to onset (up to 3 h), may last up to 24 h. Potent ergot-like vasoconstriction may result in ischemia, gangrene.
DOM, STP ("Serenity, Tranquility, Peace")	2,5-Dimethoxy-4-methylamphetamine	S, P	Potent sympathomimetic.
Harmaline	4,9-Dihydro-7-methoxy-1-methyl-3-pyrido-(3,4)-indole	N, M	South American religious and cultural drink called yage or ayahuasca (along with DMT). Prevents metabolism and enhances effects of DMT in ayahuasca. Sympathomimetic effects.
LSD, "Acid"	Lysergic acid diethylamide	S, E	Potent hallucinogen. Average dose of 50–150 mcg in tablets, blotter papers. Effects may last up to 12 h.
MBDB	*n*-Methyl-1-(1,3-benzodioxol-5-yl)-2-butanamine	S, A[b]	Nearly pure entactogen without hallucinosis or sympathomimetic stimulation.
MDA	3,4-Methylenedioxyamphetamine	S, A[b]	Potent sympathomimetic. Several hyperthermic deaths reported. MDMA analog and metabolite. Sometimes found in "Ecstasy" tablets.
MDE, MDEA, "Eve"	3,4-Methylenedioxy-*N*-ethylamphetamine	S, A[b]	MDMA analog but reportedly less pronounced empathogen. Sometimes found in "Ecstasy" tablets.
MDMA, "Ecstasy," "Molly," "Adam"	3,4-Methylenedioxy-methamphetamine	S, A[b]	Sympathomimetic: hyperthermia, seizures, cerebral hemorrhage, and arrhythmias reported; hyponatremia. Associated with interpersonal closeness, emotional awareness, euphoria.
MDPV, "Energy 1," "Ivory wave"	3,4-Methylenedioxypyrovalerone	S, C	Stimulant drug sold as "bath salts" or "research chemicals" but really intended for ingestion or inhalation.
Mephedrone, "Bubbles," "M-Cat, "Meow-Meow"	4-methylmethcathinone	S, C	Stimulant drug sold as "bath salts" or "research chemicals" but really intended for ingestion or inhalation.

Mescaline	3,4,5-Trimethoxyphenethylamine	N, S, P	Derived from peyote cactus. Used by some Native Americans in religious ceremonies. GI distress common.
Methylone	3,4-Methylenedioxymethcathinone	S, C	Stimulant drug sold as "bath salts" or "research chemicals" but really intended for ingestion or inhalation.
Morning glory, *Ipopmoea violacea*	D-Lysergic acid amide (LSA)	N, E	Seeds contain LSA, a close relative of LSD.
Myristicin, nutmeg	Methoxysafrole	N, Ac	Anticholinergic presentation with tachycardia, agitation. Toxic dose of nutmeg is 1–3 seeds. Must be ground or crushed to release potent oils.
NBOME Series (2C-I-NBOMe, 2C-C-NBOMe, 2C-B-NBOMe), "Smiles"	4-X-2,5-dimethoxy-N-(2-methoxybenzyl) phenethylamine X=Iodo, Chloro, Bromo, respectively	S, P	Extremely active at low doses and sold on blotter paper similar to, and thus frequently mistaken for, LSD.
PMA, "Dr Death"	p-Methoxyamphetamine	S, A	Contaminant or adulterant in some pills sold as MDMA; very potent sympathomimetic. High morbidity and mortality associated with overdose.
Psilocybin	4-Phosphoryloxy-*N*-*N*-dimethyltryptamine	N, T	From *Psilocybe* and other mushrooms. Stable compound, retained in dried mushrooms and boiled extract. Some stalks characteristically turn blue after handling.
Salvia, *Salvia divinorum*	Salvinorin A	N	Soft-leaved plant native to southern Mexico. Chewed or smoked. Short duration of 15–40 min.
2C-B	4-bromo-2,5-dimethoxyphenethylamine	S, P	Most popular in a series of compounds in the 2C group.
5-MeO-DIPT, "Foxy Methoxy"	N,N-Diisopropyl-5-methoxytryptamine	S, T	Some stimulant effects. GI distress occurs.

[a]N, naturally derived; T, tryptamine; S, synthetically produced; P, phenethylamine; M, monoamine oxidase inhibitor; E, ergot-like; C, cathinone; A, amphetamine; Ac, anticholinergic.
[b]Although classified as a phenethylamine in many sources, chemical structure is actually an amphetamine.

IV. Diagnosis is based on a history of use and the presence of signs of sympathetic stimulation or the appearance of responding to internal stimuli. Diagnosis of hyperthermia requires a high level of suspicion and use of a thermometer that accurately measures core temperature (eg, rectal probe).

A. Specific levels. Serum drug levels are neither widely available nor clinically useful in emergency management. The amphetamine derivatives (eg, DOB, STP, MDA, MDMA) cross-react with many of the available screening procedures for amphetamine-class drugs. However, LSD and the other nonamphetamine hallucinogens listed in Table II–35 are not identified on routine toxicology screening. Recently, several LSD screening immunoassays have become available, although they are of limited use because of false-positive and false-negative results and a short window of detection (4–12 hours).

B. Other useful laboratory studies include electrolytes, glucose, BUN, and creatinine. In hyperthermic patients, obtain prothrombin time, hepatic transaminases, creatine kinase (CK), and urinalysis for occult blood (myoglobinuria will be present).

V. Treatment

A. For a patient with a "bad trip" or panic reaction, provide gentle reassurance and relaxation techniques in a quiet environment.

1. Treat agitation (p 24) or severe anxiety states with benzodiazepines such as midazolam, lorazepam, or diazepam (p 516). Butyrophenones such as haloperidol (p 503) are useful despite a small theoretic risk of lowering the seizure threshold.
2. Treat seizures (p 23), hyperthermia (p 21), rhabdomyolysis (p 27), hypertension (p 17), and cardiac arrhythmias (pp 10–15) if they occur.

B. Specific drugs and antidotes. There is no specific antidote. Sedating doses of benzodiazepines such as diazepam (2–10 mg) may alleviate anxiety, and hypnotic doses (10–20 mg) can induce sleep for the duration of the "trip."

C. Decontamination (p 50). Most of these drugs are taken orally in small doses, and decontamination procedures are relatively ineffective and likely to aggravate psychological distress. Consider the use of activated charcoal or gastric lavage only after recent (within 30–60 minutes) large ingestions.

D. Enhanced elimination. These procedures are not useful. Although urinary acidification may increase the urine concentration of some agents, it does not significantly enhance total-body elimination and may aggravate myoglobinuric renal failure.

▶ MAGNESIUM

Kathryn H. Meier, PharmD

Magnesium (Mg) is a divalent cation that is required for a variety of intracellular processes and is an essential ion for proper neuromuscular functioning. Oral magnesium salts are widely available in over-the-counter antacids (eg, Maalox and Mylanta) and cathartics (milk of magnesia and magnesium citrate and sulfate). IV magnesium sulfate is used to treat toxemia of pregnancy, polymorphous ventricular tachycardia, refractory ventricular arrhythmias, and severe bronchospasm.

I. Mechanism of toxicity

A. The toxic effects of magnesium involve mainly the cardiovascular, skeletal muscle, and central nervous systems.

1. **Cardiovascular** effects include altered automaticity and conduction due to effects on both potassium and calcium ion channels; decreased myocardial contractility by alteration of intracellular calcium mobility; vascular smooth muscle relaxation by reduction in available intracellular calcium; and impaired catecholamine release by inhibition of calcium-mediated exocytosis.

2. **Skeletal muscle** effects are probably mediated by antagonizing calcium permeable channels, calcium binding proteins, and calcium-mediated release of acetylcholine.
3. Toxic effects in the **central nervous system** are less well defined but probably involve stimulation of NDMA and $GABA_{-A}$ receptors, increased calcitonin gene-related peptide, and possibly inhibited production of nitrous oxide and substance P.

B. Pharmacokinetics. The average adult body content of magnesium is approximately 24 g. Because magnesium is found primarily in bone, muscle, and intracellular fluids, serum levels may not accurately represent body stores. Magnesium transport channels are located in the ileum and colon and account for most dietary absorption. The oral bioavailability ranges from 20% to 40% depending on the salt form. Although best modeled with two-compartment pharmacokinetics, the average volume of distribution is about 0.5 L/Kg, and the elimination half-life averages 4–5 hours in healthy adults. Magnesium is primarily excreted by the kidney, and impaired elimination can occur when the creatinine clearance is less than 30 mL/min.

II. Toxic dose. The adult recommended daily allowance for magnesium is 320–420 mg per day. Although most acute or chronic overexposures do not result in hypermagnesemia, poisoning has been reported after IV overdose, enemas, or massive oral overdose. Toxicity after standard doses has been observed in patients with renal insufficiency and in patients with impaired neuromuscular functioning (myasthenia gravis or treatment with neuromuscular blocking drugs).

A. Commonly available antacids (Maalox, Mylanta, and others) contain 12.5–37.5 mEq of magnesium per 15 mL (1 tablespoon), milk of magnesia contains about 40 mEq/15 mL, and magnesium sulfate (in Epsom salts and IV preparations) contains 8 mEq/g.

B. Ingestion of 200 g of magnesium sulfate caused coma in a young woman with normal renal function. Pediatric deaths have been reported after the use of Epsom salt enemas.

III. Clinical presentation. Orally administered magnesium causes diarrhea, usually within 3 hours. Repeated or excessive doses of magnesium-containing cathartics can cause serious fluid and electrolyte abnormalities. Moderate toxicity may cause nausea, vomiting, muscle weakness, and cutaneous flushing. Higher levels can cause cardiac conduction abnormalities (bradycardia, QT prolongation, and intraventricular conduction delay leading to heart block), hypotension, severe muscle weakness, and lethargy. Very high levels can cause coma, respiratory arrest, and asystole (Table II–36).

IV. Diagnosis should be suspected in a patient who presents with hypotonia, hypotension, and CNS depression, especially if there is a history of using magnesium-containing antacids or cathartics or renal insufficiency.

TABLE II–36. MAGNESIUM POISONING

Magnesium (mg/dL)	Magnesium (mEq/L)	Magnesium (mmol/L)	Possible Clinical Effects
1.7–2.4	1.5–2	0.7–1.0	Range of normal serum magnesium
>3.5	>3	>1.5	Nausea, vomiting, weakness, cutaneous flushing
>6	>5	>2.5	ECG changes: prolonged PR, QRS, QT intervals
8–12	7–10	3.5–5	Hypotension, loss of deep tendon reflexes, sedation
>12	>10	>5	Muscle paralysis, respiratory arrest, hypotension, arrhythmias
>17	>14	>7	Death from respiratory arrest or asystole

A. **Specific levels.** Determination of total serum magnesium concentration is rapidly available. The normal range of total magnesium is 1.7–2.4 mg/dL (0.7–1.0 mmol/L, or 1.5–2.0 mEq/L). Therapeutic levels of total magnesium for the treatment of toxemia of pregnancy (eclampsia) are 5–7.4 mg/dL (2–3 mmol/L, or 4–6 mEq/L). Ionized levels correlate with total magnesium levels and are not needed to assess overdose, nor are they widely available.

B. **Other useful laboratory studies** include electrolytes, calcium, BUN, creatinine, serum osmolality and osmolar gap (magnesium may elevate the osmolar gap), calcium, arterial blood gases (if respiratory depression is suspected), and ECG.

V. **Treatment**

A. **Emergency and supportive measures**

1. Maintain an open airway and assist ventilation if necessary (pp 1–7).
2. Replace fluid losses and correct electrolyte abnormalities caused by excessive catharsis.
3. Treat hypotension with IV fluids and vasopressors (p 15).

B. **Specific drugs and antidotes.** There is no specific antidote. However, administration of IV **calcium** (p 526) may temporarily alleviate respiratory depression, hypotension, and arrhythmias.

C. **Decontamination** (p 50). Activated charcoal is not effective. Consider gastric emptying with a nasogastric tube for large recent ingestions. Do ***not*** administer a cathartic.

D. **Enhanced elimination**

1. **Hemodialysis** rapidly removes magnesium and is the only route of elimination in anuric patients. Continuous renal replacement therapy (CRRT) has not been evaluated in the setting of magnesium overdose.
2. Hemoperfusion and repeat-dose charcoal are not effective.
3. Forced diuresis with IV furosemide and normal saline may enhance magnesium elimination, but there are insufficient human data to recommend it.

► MANGANESE

Paul D. Blanc, MD, MSPH

Although manganese (Mn) is an essential trace nutrient, intoxication is caused by chronic overexposure. Sources of inorganic manganese exposure include mining, metal working, smelting, foundries, and welding. There is a potential link between organic manganese fungicides (Maneb and Mancozeb) and chronic neurologic toxicity. An organic manganese gasoline additive, methylcyclopentadienyl manganese tricarbonyl (MMT) is in limited use in the United States and in wider use elsewhere. Parenteral exposure to inorganic manganese can occur through injection drug abuse of potassium permanganate–adulterated substances, through manganese-containing total parenteral nutrition, and administration of the manganese-releasing pharmaceutical mangafodipir.

I. **Mechanism of toxicity.**

A. The precise mechanism of chronic toxicity is not known. The CNS is the target organ, specifically regions within the basal ganglia.

B. Pharmacokinetic data in humans are limited. Manganese is well absorbed by inhalation. Metallic inorganic Mn is poorly absorbed from the GI tract of adults, although relative bioavailability is increased in infants and in iron deficiency. The volume of distribution is approximately 1 L/kg, with extensive peripheral distribution including in the liver and kidneys. Excretion is primarily via the bile. Bone can be a major site of long-term storage (estimated 8.5-year half-life in humans).

II. **Toxic dose.**

A. The primary route of exposure is inhalation, but there is evidence that absorption to the CNS through the olfactory system may play a role in CNS toxicity.

Potassium permanganate ingestion can cause systemic toxicity. MMT can be absorbed across the skin.

B. Workplace exposure limits. The Federal OSHA workplace limit (permissible exposure limit—ceiling [PEL-C]) for inorganic manganese is 5 mg/m^3; the California OSHA PEL is 0.2 mg/m^3 (respirable fraction) and the ACGIH-recommended workplace exposure limit (threshold limit value–8-hour time-weighted average [TLV-TWA]) is considerably lower at 0.02 mg/m^3 (respirable fraction). For MMT, the Federal OSHA PEL-C is 5 mg/m^3 and the ACGIH TLV-TWA is 0.2 mg/m^3 (skin). The NIOSH air level of manganese considered immediately dangerous to life or health (IDLH) is 500 mg/m^3.

III. Clinical presentation. Acute high-level manganese inhalation can produce an irritant-type pneumonitis, but this is rare (p 255). More typically, toxicity occurs after chronic exposure to low levels over months or years. The time course following injection of manganese (eg, in contaminated parenteral drug abuse substances) is considerably shorter. The patient may present with a psychiatric disorder that can be misdiagnosed as schizophrenia or atypical psychosis. Signs of neurologic toxicity, such as parkinsonism and other extrapyramidal movement disorders, usually appear later, up to years after any primarily psychiatric presentation. Ingestion of potassium permanganate can cause severe acute hepatic and renal toxicity and methemoglobinemia. Ingestion of Maneb or Mancozeb is associated with acute toxicity attributed to its carbamate structure, although a subacute picture linked to manganese has been reported.

IV. Diagnosis depends on a thorough occupational, drug abuse, and psychiatric history.

A. Specific levels. Testing of whole blood, serum, or urine may be performed, but the results should be interpreted with caution, as they may not correlate with clinical effects. Whole-blood levels are 20 times higher than levels in serum or plasma, and red blood cell contamination can falsely elevate serum or plasma levels.

1. Normal serum manganese concentrations are usually less than 1.2 mcg/L.
2. Elevated urine manganese concentrations (>2 mcg/L) may confirm recent acute exposure. Exposures at the OSHA PEL usually do not raise urinary levels above 8 mcg/L. Chelation challenge does not have a role in diagnosis.
3. Hair and nail levels are not useful as clinical tests.

B. Other useful laboratory studies include arterial blood gases or oximetry and chest radiography (after acute, heavy, symptomatic inhalation exposure if acute lung injury is suspected). Magnetic resonance imaging (MRI) of the brain may show findings suggestive of manganese deposition.

V. Treatment

A. Emergency and supportive measures

1. **Acute inhalation.** Administer supplemental oxygen. Treat bronchospasm (p 8) and noncardiogenic pulmonary edema (p 7) if they occur.
2. **Chronic intoxication.** Psychiatric and neurologic effects are treated with the usual psychiatric and antiparkinsonian drugs but often respond poorly.

B. Specific drugs and antidotes. Calcium EDTA and other chelators have ***not*** been proven effective after chronic neurologic damage has occurred. The efficacy of chelators early after acute exposure has not been studied.

C. Decontamination (p 50)

1. **Acute inhalation.** Remove the victim from exposure and give supplemental oxygen if available.
2. **Ingestion.** Because inorganic metallic manganese is so poorly absorbed from the GI tract, gut decontamination is probably not necessary. For massive ingestions, particularly of organic compounds (eg, Maneb, Mancozeb, or MMT) or of potassium permanganate, gut decontamination may be appropriate but has not been studied.

D. Enhanced elimination. There is no known role for dialysis or hemoperfusion.

► MARIJUANA

Neal L. Benowitz, MD

Marijuana consists of the leaves and flowering parts of the plant *Cannabis sativa*. It usually is smoked in cigarettes ("joints" or "reefers") or pipes or added to food (usually cookies, brownies, or tea). Resin from the plant may be dried and compressed into blocks called hashish. Marijuana contains a number of cannabinoids; the primary psychoactive one is delta-9-tetrahydrocannabinol (THC). THC is available by prescription in capsule form (dronabinol [Marinol]) and is available in liquid form for inhalation using electronic cigarette devices. Marijuana can also be inhaled using a vaporizer (such as Volcano), which vaporizes THC without combusting marijuana. THC is used medically as an appetite stimulant for patients with such conditions as AIDS-related anorexia; it also is used as treatment for vomiting associated with cancer chemotherapy, for chronic pain, and for multiple sclerosis, glaucoma, and other disorders. In some US states cannabis products are legal for medical use, and in others for recreational use.

Synthetic cannabinoid analogs such as JWH-018 and many similar compounds, sold as "K2" or "Spice" and in some so-called "herbal" preparations, are banned in some states but available via the Internet. These may produce acute toxicity similar to that seen with THC; some have been associated with seizures.

Cannabinoid **antagonists** include rimonabant (a CB_1 selective antagonist) which was developed as medication to reduce appetite and weight, and also for smoking cessation. It was marketed briefly in Europe and then withdrawn due to psychiatric side effects, particularly depression and suicidal ideation.

I. Mechanism of toxicity

A. THC, which binds to cannabinoid (anandamide) CB_1 and CB_2 receptors in the brain, may have stimulant, sedative, or hallucinogenic actions, depending on the dose and time after consumption. Both catecholamine release (resulting in tachycardia) and inhibition of sympathetic reflexes (resulting in orthostatic hypotension) may be observed.

B. Pharmacokinetics. Only about 10–20% of ingested THC is absorbed into the bloodstream, with onset of effects within 30–60 minutes and peak absorption at 2–4 hours. It is metabolized by hydroxylation to active and inactive metabolites. Blood THC levels decline rapidly after inhalation due to tissue redistribution, followed by an elimination half-life of 20–30 hours, which may be longer in chronic users.

II. Toxic dose. Typical marijuana cigarettes contain 1–4% THC, but more potent varieties may contain up to 25% THC. Hashish contains 3–6% and hashish oil 30–50% THC. Dronabinol is available in 2.5-, 5-, and 10-mg capsules. Toxicity is dose related, but there is much individual variability, influenced in part by prior experience and degree of tolerance.

III. Clinical presentation

A. Subjective effects after smoking a marijuana cigarette include euphoria, palpitations, heightened sensory awareness, and altered time perception, followed after about 30 minutes by sedation. More severe intoxication may result in anxiety, impaired short-term memory, depersonalization, visual hallucinations, and acute paranoid psychosis. Cannabis use may precipitate or exacerbate psychosis in individuals with schizophrenia or bipolar disorder. Occasionally, even with low doses of THC, subjective effects may precipitate a panic reaction. Acute cannabis intoxication may result in impaired driving and motor vehicle accidents. Cannabis dependence, both behavioral and physical, occurs in 5–10% of users. A cannabis withdrawal syndrome is seen after stopping use in heavy chronic users, consisting of irritability, anxiety, fatigue, sleep disturbance often with abnormal dreams, and depression.

B. Physical findings may include tachycardia, orthostatic hypotension, conjunctival injection, incoordination, slurred speech, and ataxia. Stupor with pallor, conjunctival injection, fine tremor, and ataxia have been observed in children after they have eaten marijuana cookies. Seizures have been reported in children but are rare.

C. **Other health problems.** Marijuana use has been associated with precipitation of acute myocardial infarction, usually in people with underlying coronary disease, but sometimes in those without, as well as arrhythmias including marked sinus tachycardia, atrial fibrillation, and ventricular tachycardia and fibrillation. Salmonellosis and pulmonary aspergillosis are reported from use of contaminated marijuana. Marijuana may be contaminated by paraquat, but paraquat is destroyed by pyrolysis, and there have been no reports of paraquat toxicity from smoking marijuana. Chronic heavy marijuana use has been associated with various psychiatric disorders, chronic bronchitis, increased risk for coronary heart disease, and several types of cancer. Chronic heavy marijuana use can also cause recurrent nausea, abdominal pain and vomiting, termed cannabinoid hyperemesis syndrome, which resolves after cessation of cannabis use.

D. **Intravenous use** of marijuana extract or hashish oil may cause dyspnea, abdominal pain, fever, shock, disseminated intravascular coagulation, acute renal failure, and death.

IV. **Diagnosis** usually is based on the history and typical findings, such as tachycardia and conjunctival injection, combined with evidence of altered mood or cognitive function.

A. **Specific levels.** Blood THC levels are available but are not commonly measured. Cannabinoid metabolites may be detected in the urine by enzyme immunoassay up to several days after a single acute exposure or several weeks after chronic THC exposure. Urine levels do not correlate with the degree of intoxication or functional impairment, but blood THC levels of 2.5–5 ng/mL or higher are very suggestive of intoxication. Hemp and hemp seed products (eg, hemp seed nutrition bars) may provide alternative explanations for positive urine testing; however, they have no pharmacologic effect.

B. **Other useful laboratory studies** include electrolytes and glucose.

V. **Treatment**

A. **Emergency and supportive measures**

1. Most psychological disturbances can be managed by simple reassurance, possibly with adjunctive use of lorazepam, diazepam, or midazolam (p 516).
2. Sinus tachycardia usually does not require treatment but, if necessary, may be controlled with beta blockers.
3. Orthostatic hypotension responds to head-down position and IV fluids.

B. **Specific drugs and antidotes.** There is no currently available specific antidotes.

C. **Decontamination** after ingestion (p 50). Administer activated charcoal orally if conditions are appropriate (see Table I–38, p 54). Gastric lavage is not necessary if activated charcoal can be given promptly.

D. **Enhanced elimination.** These procedures are not effective owing to the large volume of distribution of cannabinoids.

► MERCURY

Michael J. Kosnett, MD, MPH

Mercury (Hg) is a naturally occurring metal that is mined chiefly as HgS in cinnabar ore. It is converted to three primary forms, each with a distinct toxicology: elemental (metallic) mercury (Hg^0), inorganic mercury salts (eg, mercuric chloride [$HgCl_2$]), and organic (alkyl and aryl) mercury (eg, methylmercury). Approximately one-half to one-third of commercial mercury use is in the manufacture of chlorine and caustic soda, one-half to one-third in electric equipment, and the remainder in various applications, such as dental amalgam, fluorescent lamps, switches, thermostats, and artisanal gold production. In the United States, mercury use in batteries and paints has been discontinued. Previous use in pharmaceuticals and biocides has declined sharply, although mercuric chloride is still used as a stool fixative, and some organomercury compounds (such as mercurochrome, phenylmercuric acetate, and thimerosal) are still used as topical antiseptics or preservatives. Some folk medicines contain inorganic mercury compounds, and some Latin American and Caribbean communities have used elemental mercury in religious or cultural rituals. Hazardous exposure has resulted from dermal use of imported skin lightening creams formulated with inorganic mercury salts. Aquatic organisms can convert inorganic mercury into methylmercury, with resulting bioaccumulation in large carnivorous fish such as swordfish. Mercury is released to the environment from the burning of coal and from fugitive emissions during the large-scale mining of gold. In an effort to curtail the use of elemental mercury in artisanal gold mining and other pathways of environmental mercury pollution, the European Union has enacted a ban on the export of most inorganic mercury effective 2011; a US ban on export of elemental mercury took effect in 2013.

I. **Mechanism of toxicity.** Mercury reacts with sulfhydryl (SH) groups, resulting in enzyme inhibition and pathologic alteration of cellular membranes.
   A. Elemental mercury and methylmercury are particularly toxic to the CNS. Metallic mercury vapor is also a pulmonary irritant. Methylmercury is associated with neurodevelopmental disorders.
   B. Inorganic mercuric salts are corrosive to the skin, eyes, and GI tract and are nephrotoxic.
   C. Inorganic and organic mercury compounds may cause contact dermatitis.

II. **Toxic dose.** The pattern and severity of toxicity are highly dependent on the form of mercury and the route of exposure, mostly because of different pharmacokinetic profiles. Chronic exposure to any form may result in toxicity (see Table II–37 for a summary of absorption and toxicity).
   A. **Elemental (metallic) mercury** is a volatile liquid at room temperature.
      1. **Hg^0 vapor** is absorbed rapidly by the lungs and distributed to the CNS. Airborne exposure to 10 mg/m^3 is considered immediately dangerous to life or health (IDLH), and chemical pneumonitis may occur at levels in excess of 1 mg/m^3. In occupational settings, overt signs and symptoms of elemental mercury intoxication generally have required months to years of sustained daily exposure to airborne mercury levels of 0.05–0.2 mg/m^3. The recommended workplace limit (ACGIH TLV-TWA) is 0.025 mg/m^3 as an 8-hour time-weighted average; however, some studies suggest that subclinical effects on the CNS and kidneys may occur below this level. The US Agency for Toxic Substances and Disease Registry (ATSDR) recommends

TABLE II–37. MERCURY COMPOUNDS

Form	Absorption		Toxicity	
	Oral	Inhalation	Neurologic	Renal
Elemental (metallic) mercury				
Hg^0 liquid	Poor	N/A[a]	Rare	Rare
Hg^0 vapor	N/A[a]	Good	Likely	Possible
Inorganic mercuric salts				
Hg^{2+}	Good	Rare but possible	Rare	Likely
Organic (alkyl) mercury				
RHg^+	Good	Rare but possible	Likely	Possible

[a]N/A, not applicable.

evacuation from residences at 0.01 mg/m^3 and avoidance of long-term occupancy if levels exceed 0.001 mg/m^3.

2. **Liquid metallic mercury** is poorly absorbed from the GI tract, and acute ingestion has been associated with poisoning only in the presence of abnormal gut motility that markedly delays normal fecal elimination or after peritoneal contamination.

B. **Inorganic mercuric salts.** The acute lethal oral dose of mercuric chloride is approximately 1–4 g. Severe toxicity and death have been reported after use of peritoneal lavage solutions containing mercuric chloride in concentrations of 0.2–0.8%. Weeks to years of dermal application of skin lightening creams and other topical preparations containing 0.1% to >10% inorganic mercury (often as mercurous chloride or mercuric ammonium chloride) has resulted in neurotoxicity or nephrotoxicity.

C. **Organic mercury**

1. **Mercury-containing antiseptics** such as mercurochrome have limited skin penetration; however, in rare cases, such as topical application to an infected omphalocele, intoxication has resulted. Oral absorption is significant and may also pose a hazard.
2. **Methylmercury** is well absorbed after inhalation, ingestion, and probably dermal exposure. Ingestion of 10–60 mg/kg may be lethal, and chronic daily ingestion of 10 mcg/kg may be associated with adverse neurologic and reproductive effects. The US Environmental Protection Agency reference dose (RfD), the daily lifetime dose believed to be without potential hazard, is 0.1 mcg/kg/d. The RfD was derived from studies of neuropsychological deficits arising from in utero exposure in humans. To minimize neurodevelopmental risk while optimizing nutrition, the US EPA and FDA in 2014 issued revised draft guidance advising pregnant women, women who may become pregnant, nursing mothers, and young children to avoid consumption of fish with high levels of mercury (eg, swordfish) and to limit consumption of albacore tuna to 6 oz a week, but to otherwise consume 8–12 oz of fish per week.
3. **Dimethylmercury,** a highly toxic synthetic liquid used in analytic chemistry, is well absorbed through the skin, and cutaneous exposure to only a few drops has resulted in a delayed but fatal encephalopathy.

III. **Clinical presentation**

A. **Acute inhalation of high concentrations of metallic mercury vapor** may cause severe chemical pneumonitis and noncardiogenic pulmonary edema. Acute gingivostomatitis may also occur.

B. **Chronic intoxication from inhalation of mercury vapor** produces a classic triad of tremor, neuropsychiatric disturbances, and gingivostomatitis.

1. Early stages feature a fine intention tremor of the fingers, but involvement of the face and progression to choreiform movements of the limbs may occur.
2. **Neuropsychiatric manifestations** include fatigue, insomnia, anorexia, and memory loss. There may be an insidious change in mood to shyness, withdrawal, and depression, combined with explosive irritability and frequent blushing ("erethism").
3. Subclinical changes in peripheral nerve function and renal function have been reported, but frank neuropathy and nephropathy are rare.
4. **Acrodynia,** a rare idiosyncratic reaction to chronic mercury exposure, occurs mainly in children and has the following features: pain in the extremities, often accompanied by pinkish discoloration and desquamation ("pink disease"); hypertension; profuse sweating; anorexia, insomnia, irritability, and/or apathy; and a miliary rash.

C. **Acute ingestion of inorganic mercuric salts,** particularly mercuric chloride, causes an abrupt onset of hemorrhagic gastroenteritis and abdominal pain. Intestinal necrosis, shock, and death may ensue. Acute oliguric renal failure from acute tubular necrosis may occur within days. Chronic exposure may result in CNS toxicity.

D. **Organic mercury compounds,** particularly short-chain alkyl compounds such as methylmercury, primarily affect the CNS, causing paresthesias, ataxia, dysarthria, hearing impairment, and progressive constriction of the visual fields. Symptoms first become apparent after a latent interval of several weeks or months.

1. **Ethylmercury** undergoes less CNS penetration than does methylmercury and has faster total-body clearance. In addition to neurotoxicity, symptoms of acute poisoning may include gastroenteritis and nephrotoxicity. Thimerosal (ethylmercury thiosalicylate), a preservative that undergoes metabolism to ethylmercury, was removed from most childhood vaccines in the United States on a precautionary basis. No causal link between thimerosal-containing vaccines and neurodevelopmental disorders has been established. A 2004 Institute of Medicine report concluded that evidence favors *rejection* of a causal relationship between thimerosal-containing vaccines and autism.
2. **Phenylmercury** compounds, which undergo deacylation in vivo, produce a pattern of toxicity intermediate between those of alkyl mercury and inorganic mercury.
3. **Methylmercury** is a potent reproductive toxin, and perinatal exposure has caused mental retardation and a cerebral palsy–type syndrome in offspring.

IV. **Diagnosis** depends on integration of characteristic findings with a history of known or potential exposure and the presence of elevated mercury blood levels or urinary excretion.

A. **Specific levels.** Elemental mercury and inorganic mercury follow a biphasic elimination rate (initially rapid, then slow), and both urinary and fecal excretion occur. The urinary elimination half-life is approximately 40 days. ***Note:*** Urine mercury may be reported as the mass of the metal per volume of urine (ie, micrograms per liter) or as the mass of the metal per gram of creatinine (ie, micrograms per gram of creatinine). Adjustment for creatinine, which reduces the impact of variation in urine flow rate, can be of value in comparing serial measurements obtained in the same individual (eg, workplace biomonitoring) or in evaluating dose–response trends in small population studies. However, when one is assessing a "creatinine-corrected" result, the urine concentration of the metal (grams of mercury per liter) and of creatinine (grams of creatinine per liter) should also be reviewed individually. Specimens in which the creatinine concentration is very low (eg, <0.5 g/L) or very high (>3 g/L) may be unreliable and should be interpreted cautiously. The urine creatinine concentration of adults is on average close to 1 g/L, and therefore urine mercury values expressed as micrograms per gram of creatinine will often be similar to values expressed as micrograms per liter. In infants, creatinine-corrected values may appear anomalously elevated owing to infants' relatively low rate of creatinine excretion.

1. **Metallic and inorganic mercury.** Whole-blood and urine mercury levels are useful in confirming exposure. Shortly after acute exposures, whole-blood mercury values may rise faster than urine mercury levels. Decline in blood mercury then follows a biphasic pattern, with respective half-times of approximately 4 and 45 days. Urine mercury levels, reflecting the mercury content of the kidneys, are in general a better biomarker of chronic exposure. In most people without occupational exposure, whole-blood mercury is less than 5 mcg/L and urine mercury is less than 3 mcg/L. The median urine mercury concentration for the US general population in the 2009–2010 National Health and Nutrition Examination Survey (NHANES) was 0.400 mcg/L. Based on the ACGIH biological exposure index for workers exposed to elemental or inorganic mercury, it has been recommended that end-of-workweek blood mercury levels remain less than 15 mcg/L

and that the urine mercury level remain less than 35 mcg/g of creatinine. Studies have noted a small, reversible increase in urinary *N*-acetyl-glucosaminidase, a biomarker of perturbation in renal tubular function, in workers with urinary mercury levels of 25–35 mcg/L. Overt neurologic effects have occurred in persons with chronic urine mercury levels greater than 100–200 mcg/L, although lower levels have been reported in some pediatric cases of acrodynia. In patients with acute inorganic mercury poisoning resulting in gastroenteritis and acute tubular necrosis, blood mercury levels are often greater than 500 mcg/L. Two randomized trials of dental amalgam in children detected no overall adverse effect of low-level elemental mercury exposure (urine mercury <5 mcg/L) on neurocognitive development, although further analysis of one trial suggested effects may be influenced by genetic polymorphisms.

2. **Organic mercury.** Methylmercury undergoes biliary excretion and enterohepatic recirculation, with 90% eventually excreted in the feces; as a result, urine levels are not useful. The half-life of methylmercury in blood is variable but averages 50 days. Whole-blood mercury levels greater than 200 mcg/L have been associated with symptoms. In a 2001 analysis, the US EPA considered umbilical cord blood mercury levels of 46–79 mcg/L to represent lower-boundary estimates of levels associated with a significant increase in adverse neurodevelopmental effects in children. The geometric mean total blood mercury concentration in the US population assessed in the 2011–2012 NHANES was 0.703 mcg/L; the 95th percentile was 4.40 mcg/L (≈90% present as methylmercury). Among a subset of women ages 16–49 years studied in NHANES 1999–2000 who consumed fish and/or shellfish two times or more per week, the 95th percentile whole-blood organomercury level (almost entirely methylmercury) was 12.1 mcg/L. Because methylmercury undergoes bioconcentration across the placenta, umbilical cord blood mercury levels are on average 1.7 times higher than maternal whole-blood mercury levels.

   Hair levels have been used to document remote or chronic exposure to methylmercury. In US females age 16–49 years (NHANES 1999–2000), the geometric mean hair mercury concentration was 0.20 mcg/g and the 95th percentile was 1.73 mcg/g.

B. **Other useful laboratory studies** include electrolytes, glucose, BUN, creatinine, liver aminotransferases, urinalysis, chest radiography, and arterial blood gases (if pneumonitis is suspected). Urinary markers of early nephrotoxicity (microalbuminuria, retinol-binding protein, beta$_2$-microglobulin, alpha-1-microglobulin, and *N*-acetylglucosaminidase) may aid in the detection of early adverse effects. Formal visual field examination may be useful for organic mercury exposure. ***Note:*** Empiric protocols that measure urine mercury concentration after administration of a single dose of a chelating agent such as unithiol (DMPS) have been described, but their diagnostic or prognostic utility has not been established. After administration of a dose of unithiol, urine mercury concentration may transiently increase on the order of 10-fold regardless of whether basal (prechallenge) levels are low or high.

V. Treatment

A. Emergency and supportive measures

1. **Inhalation.** Observe closely for several hours for the development of acute pneumonitis and pulmonary edema (p 7) and give supplemental oxygen if indicated.
2. **Mercuric salt ingestion.** Anticipate severe gastroenteritis and treat shock aggressively with IV fluid replacement (p 15). Vigorous hydration may also help maintain urine output. Acute renal failure is usually reversible, but hemodialysis may be required for 1–2 weeks.
3. **Organic mercury ingestion.** Provide symptomatic supportive care.

B. Specific drugs and antidotes

1. **Metallic (elemental) mercury.** In acute or chronic poisoning, oral **succimer** (DMSA, p 624) or oral **unithiol** (DMPS, p 630) may enhance urinary mercury excretion (although its effect on clinical outcome has not been fully studied). Although **penicillamine** (p 601) is an alternative oral treatment, it may be associated with more side effects and less efficient mercury excretion.
2. **Inorganic mercury salts.** Treatment with IV **unithiol** (DMPS [p 630]) or IM **BAL** (p 514), if begun within minutes to a few hours after ingestion, may reduce or avert severe renal injury. Because prompt intervention is necessary, do not delay treatment while waiting for specific laboratory confirmation. Oral **succimer** (DMSA [p 624]) is also effective, but its absorption may be limited by gastroenteritis and shock, and it is more appropriately used as a follow-up to DMPS or BAL treatment.
3. **Organic mercury.** In methylmercury intoxication, limited data suggest that oral **succimer** (DMSA [p 624]) and oral ***N*-acetylcysteine** (NAC [p 499]) may be effective in decreasing mercury levels in tissues, including the brain.
4. Because BAL may redistribute mercury to the brain from other tissue sites, it should not be used in poisoning by metallic or organic mercury because the brain is a key target organ.

C. Decontamination (p 50)

1. **Inhalation**
   a. Immediately remove the victim from exposure and give supplemental oxygen if needed.
   b. Even minute indoor spills (eg, 1 mL) of metallic mercury can result in hazardous chronic airborne levels. Cover the spill with powdered sulfur and carefully clean up and discard all residue and contaminated carpeting, porous furniture, and permeable floor covering. Do ***not*** use a home vacuum cleaner, as this may disperse the liquid mercury, increasing its airborne concentration. Professional guidance and cleanup with self-contained vacuum systems is recommended for spills of more mercury than the amount present in a thermometer or compact fluorescent light. Instruments that provide instantaneous (real-time) measurement of mercury vapor concentration are available for monitoring contamination and cleanup. Guidance on the management of mercury spills and contaminated buildings and residences is available from ATSDR (http://www.atsdr.cdc.gov/emergency_response/action_levels_for_elemental_mercury_spills_2012.pdf). The EPA provides instructions for the clean-up of small spills (https://www.epa.gov/mercury/what-do-if-mercury-thermometer-breaks#instructions). Spills of more than 1 lb (2 tablespoons) of elemental mercury should be reported to the US government's National Response Center, available 24 hours a day, 7 days a week at 1-800-424-8802 (telephone) or http://www.nrc. uscg.mil/nrchp.html (online reporting tool).
2. **Ingestion of metallic mercury.** In healthy persons, metallic mercury passes through the intestinal tract with minimal absorption, and there is no need for gut decontamination after minor ingestions. With large ingestions or in patients with abnormally diminished bowel motility or intestinal perforation, there is a risk for chronic intoxication. Whole-bowel irrigation (p 55) or even surgical removal may be necessary, depending on radiographic evidence of mercury retention or elevated blood or urine mercury levels.
3. **Ingestion of inorganic mercuric salts**
   a. **Prehospital.** Administer activated charcoal if available. Do ***not*** induce vomiting because of the risk for serious corrosive injury.
   b. **Hospital.** Consider gastric lavage. Administer activated charcoal, which has a very high adsorbent capacity for mercuric chloride.
   c. Arrange for endoscopic examination if corrosive injury is suspected.

4. **Ingestion of organic mercury.** After acute ingestion, perform gastric lavage and administer activated charcoal. Immediately stop breastfeeding but continue to express and discard milk, as some data suggest this may accelerate reduction of blood mercury levels.

D. **Enhanced elimination**

1. There is no role for dialysis, hemoperfusion, or repeat-dose charcoal in removing metallic or inorganic mercury. However, dialysis may be required for supportive treatment of renal failure, and it may slightly enhance removal of the mercury–chelator complex in patients with renal failure (hemodialysis clearance of the mercury–BAL complex is about 5 mL/min). A somewhat higher rate of mercury clearance (10 mL/min) was described when high-flux continuous venovenous hemodiafiltration was combined with unithiol in the treatment of mercuric sulfate–induced acute renal failure.
2. In patients with chronic methylmercury intoxication, repeated oral administration of an experimental polythiol resin was effective in enhancing mercury elimination by interrupting enterohepatic recirculation.

▶ METAL FUME FEVER

Paul D. Blanc, MD, MSPH

Metal fume fever is an acute febrile illness caused by the inhalation of respirable particles (fume) of zinc oxide. Although metal fume fever is invoked as a generic effect of exposure to numerous other metal oxides (copper, cadmium, iron, magnesium, and manganese), there is little evidence to support this (although some of those metals can cause acute lung injury). Metal fume fever usually occurs in workplace settings involving welding, melting, or flame-cutting galvanized metal (zinc-coated steel), or in brass foundry operations. Zinc chloride from smoke bombs can cause severe lung injury, but does not cause metal fume fever.

I. **Mechanism of toxicity.** Metal fume fever results from inhalation of zinc oxide (neither ingestion nor parenteral administration induces this syndrome, although other toxicity may result from those routes of exposure). The mechanism is uncertain but may be cytokine mediated. It does not involve sensitization (it is not an allergy) and can occur with first exposure (in persons previously naïve to inhaled zinc oxide).

II. **Toxic dose.** The toxic dose is variable. Resistance to the condition develops after repeated days of exposure (tachyphylaxis) but wears off rapidly when exposure ceases. The ACGIH-recommended workplace exposure limit (TLV-TWA) for zinc oxide fumes is 2 mg/m^3 as an 8-hour time-weighted average with a short-term exposure limit (STEL) of 10 mg/m^3, which is intended to prevent metal fume fever in most exposed workers. Welding on galvanized metal without appropriate ventilation easily can exceed these limits. The air level considered immediately dangerous to life or health (IDLH) is 500 mg/m^3.

III. **Clinical presentation**

A. Symptoms typically begin 4–8 hours after exposure with fever, malaise, myalgia, and headache. The white blood cell count may be elevated (12,000–16,000/mm^3). The chest radiograph is usually normal. Typically, all symptoms resolve on their own within 24–36 hours.

B. Rare asthmatic or allergic responses to zinc oxide fume have been reported. These responses are not part of the metal fume fever syndrome.

C. Pulmonary infiltrates and hypoxemia are not consistent with pure metal fume fever. If present, this suggests possible heavy metal pneumonitis resulting from cadmium or other toxic inhalations (eg, phosgene and nitrogen oxides) associated with metal working, foundry operations, or welding.

IV. **Diagnosis.** A history of welding, especially on galvanized metal, and typical symptoms and signs are sufficient to make the diagnosis.

A. **Specific levels.** There are no specific tests to diagnose or exclude metal fume fever. Blood or urine zinc determinations do not have a role in clinical diagnosis of the syndrome.

B. **Other useful laboratory studies** include CBC. Oximetry or arterial blood gases and chest radiography are used to exclude other disorders manifested as acute lung injury, if this is suspected.

V. **Treatment**

A. **Emergency and supportive measures**

1. Administer supplemental oxygen and give bronchodilators if there is wheezing and consider other diagnoses, such as an allergic response (p 8). If hypoxemia or wheezing is present, consider other toxic inhalations (p 255).
2. Provide symptomatic care (eg, acetaminophen or another antipyretic) as needed; symptoms are self-limited.

B. **Specific drugs and antidotes.** There is no specific antidote.

C. **Decontamination** is not necessary; by the time symptoms develop, the exposure has usually been over for several hours.

D. **Enhanced elimination.** There is no role for these procedures.

▶ METALDEHYDE

Kathryn H. Meier, PharmD

Metaldehyde is a cyclic tetramer of acetaldehyde primarily used as a molluscicide for snails and slugs. It may be formulated in combination with other pesticides. Metaldehyde might rarely be found in solid fuel or fire starter pellets (up to 100% metaldehyde) or novelty products used to colorize flames (up to 90% metaldehyde) marketed outside of the United States. Because of its menthol-like odor and taste, poisonings have occurred when pellets were mistaken for edibles. The United States limits metaldehyde content in molluscicides to 4% and since 2001 has required the addition of the bittering agent denatonium benzoate, but other countries permit higher concentrations. Some products sold in the United States include Cory's Slug and Snail Death, Deadline for Slugs and Snails, and Bug Geta Snail and Slug Pellets.

I. **Mechanism of toxicity**

A. The mechanism of toxicity is not well understood. Metaldehyde, like paraldehyde, is a polymer of acetaldehyde, but depolymerization into acetaldehyde does not account for most of its toxic effects. Although metaldehyde's CNS actions have not been fully elucidated, animal models have shown decreased GABA concentrations and increased MAO activity.

B. **Pharmacokinetics.** Metaldehyde is readily absorbed, and onset of symptoms usually begins within a few hours. However, case reports of large ingestions have suggested a prolonged absorption phase, and high levels did not begin to drop for 35 hours in one case. Volume of distribution and protein binding are not known. The elimination half-life is approximately 27 hours.

II. **Toxic dose.** Small 5–10 mg/kg doses cause mild GI upset, but doses of 50 mg/kg or above are associated with CNS toxicity. Ingestion of 100–150 mg/kg may cause myoclonus and convulsions, and ingestion of more than 400 mg/kg is potentially lethal. Death occurred in a child after ingestion of 3 g.

III. **Clinical presentation.** Symptoms usually begin within 1–3 hours after ingestion, but might be delayed after lower doses. Symptoms continue to progress over several hours.

A. Small ingestions (5–10 mg/kg) cause salivation, facial flushing, vomiting, abdominal cramps, diarrhea, and fever.

B. Larger doses may produce irritability, ataxia, drowsiness, myoclonus, opisthotonus, convulsions, and coma. Seizure activity may be delayed as long as 10–14 hours based on current reports. Rhabdomyolysis and hyperthermia may result from seizures or excessive muscle activity. Liver and kidney damage has been reported.

C. Metabolic acidosis and an elevated osmol gap have been reported.

IV. **Diagnosis** is based on a history of ingestion and clinical presentation. The vomitus or breath may have an aldehyde odor because some of the metaldehyde can decompose into acetaldehyde in the stomach.

A. **Specific levels.** Serum levels are not generally available.

B. **Other useful laboratory studies** include electrolytes, glucose, BUN, creatinine, osmolality (osmol gap may be elevated), and liver enzymes. If rhabdomyolysis is suspected, also perform a urine dipstick for occult blood (myoglobin is positive) and obtain a serum creatine kinase (CK).

V. **Treatment**

A. **Emergency and supportive measures**

1. Maintain an open airway and assist ventilation if necessary (pp 1–7).
2. Treat coma (p 18) and seizures (p 23) if they occur.
3. Treat fluid loss from vomiting or diarrhea with IV crystalloid fluids (p 15).
4. Monitor asymptomatic patients for at least 4–6 hours after ingestion. If any symptoms are noted during this time, observation should be extended to monitor for progression.

B. **Specific drugs and antidotes.** There is no specific antidote.

C. **Decontamination** (p 50). Do ***not*** induce vomiting because of the risk for abrupt onset of seizures. Gastric lavage is not necessary after small-to-moderate ingestions if activated charcoal can be given promptly. Administer activated charcoal orally if conditions are appropriate (see Table I–38, p 54). Activated charcoal has been shown to bind metaldehyde and reduce absorption in animal studies. Adequate charcoal to toxin ratio (10:1) may be difficult to achieve after large toxic doses.

D. **Enhanced elimination.** The clinical benefit from dialysis or hemoperfusion is unknown. A recent in vitro study showed enhanced plasma clearance with both hemodialysis and hemoperfusion. Forced diuresis and repeat-dose charcoal has not been studied.

▶ METFORMIN

Suad A. Al-Abri, MD

Metformin is a biguanide antihyperglycemic agent that is recommended as the initial drug treatment in patients with type II diabetes. Metformin toxicity can occur after acute overdose or in the setting of chronic use in patients with renal impairment.

I. **Mechanism of toxicity**

A. Metformin acts by inhibiting gluconeogenesis and glycogen breakdown, decreasing glucose absorption and improving peripheral insulin sensitivity.

B. Other pharmacologic actions include inhibition of fatty acid oxidation and oxidative phosphorylation, and increased intestinal lactate production.

C. **Pharmacokinetics.** Peak absorption occurs 2–6 hours after ingestion but may be delayed after ingestion of sustained-release formulations. The volume of distribution (Vd) has been reported as high as several hundred liters but is probably closer to 80 L in an adult. Elimination is entirely renal, with a half-life of 2.5–6 hours.

II. **Toxic dose**

A. **Adults.** Lactic acidosis occurred 9 hours after ingestion of 25 g of metformin by an 83-year-old, and fatal lactic acidosis and cardiovascular collapse occurred 4 hours after ingestion of 35 g by a 33-year-old.

B. **Children.** Based on a multicenter pediatric case series, unintentional ingestion of less than 1,700 mg is unlikely to cause significant toxicity.

III. Clinical presentation

A. The most common effects after acute metformin overdose are nausea, vomiting, lethargy, and abdominal pain. More serious poisoning is associated with coma, seizures, and cardiovascular collapse.

B. Lactic acidosis is common with serious intoxication and may be fatal. The risk increases in the presence of renal dysfunction.

C. Pancreatitis has been reported in both therapeutic use and overdose of metformin.

D. Hypoglycemia is not common (metformin does not increase insulin release) but has been reported, even in the absence of other hypoglycemic drugs such as sulfonylureas or insulin.

IV. Diagnosis. Metformin toxicity should be suspected in any patient with severe lactic acidosis.

A. Specific levels. Serum metformin levels can be measured in specialty laboratories but are not readily available in most hospitals. The therapeutic plasma concentration is 0.5–2.5 mg/L. Levels greater than 50 mg/L were associated with serious toxicity and high mortality.

B. Other useful laboratory studies. Arterial blood gases, renal function tests, electrolytes, glucose, and lactate level.

V. Treatment

A. Emergency and supportive measures

1. Maintain an open airway and assist ventilation if necessary (p 1–7).

2. Treat hypotension (p 15), coma (p 18), seizures (p 23), or hypoglycemia (p 36) if they occur.

3. Closely monitor lactate levels, renal function, and glucose.

B. Specific drugs and antidotes. No specific antidotes are available. Lactic acidosis can be treated with sodium bicarbonate; however, bicarbonate infusions alone are often ineffective and patients with severe acidosis may require hemodialysis.

C Decontamination. Administer activated charcoal orally if conditions are appropriate (see Table I–38, p 54).

D. Enhanced elimination.

1. Hemodialysis is recommended for correction of severe acidosis and also enhances the clearance of metformin (170 mL/min).

2. Continuous venovenous hemofiltration (CVVH) has been used successfully in hemodynamically unstable patients, with a reported clearance of 50.4 mL/min.

3. Rebound lactic acidosis may occur and may require prolonged dialysis or CVVH, especially in patients with renal dysfunction.

▶ METHANOL

Ilene B. Anderson, PharmD

Methanol (wood alcohol) is a common ingredient in many solvents, windshield-washing solutions, duplicating fluids, and paint removers. It sometimes is used as an ethanol substitute by alcoholics. Although methanol produces mainly inebriation, its metabolic products may cause metabolic acidosis, blindness, and death after a characteristic latent period of 6–30 hours.

I. Mechanism of toxicity

A. Methanol is slowly metabolized by alcohol dehydrogenase to formaldehyde and subsequently by aldehyde dehydrogenase to formic acid (formate). Systemic acidosis is caused by both formate and lactate, whereas blindness is caused primarily by formate. Both ethanol and methanol compete for the enzyme alcohol dehydrogenase, and saturation with ethanol (or the antidote fomepizole) blocks the metabolism of methanol to its toxic metabolites.

B. Overdose during Pregnancy. Methanol crosses the placenta, and severe fetal methanol toxicity and death associated with maternal methanol poisoning has been reported.

C. Pharmacokinetics. Methanol is readily absorbed and quickly distributed to the body water (Vd = 0.6–0.77 L/kg). It is not protein bound. It is metabolized slowly by alcohol dehydrogenase via zero-order kinetics at a rate about one-tenth that of ethanol. The reported "half-life" ranges from 2.5 to 87 hours, depending on methanol serum concentration (the higher the serum level, the longer the half-life) and whether metabolism is blocked (eg, by ethanol or fomepizole). Only about 3% is excreted unchanged by the kidneys, and less than 10–20% through the breath. Endogenous formate half-life ranges from 1.9 to 9.3 hours; during dialysis, the half-life decreases to 1.5–3.1 hours.

II. Toxic dose.

A. Acute ingestion. The fatal oral dose of methanol is estimated to be 30–240 mL (20–150 g). The minimum toxic dose is approximately 100 mg/kg. Elevated serum methanol levels have been reported after extensive dermal exposure and concentrated inhalation.

B. Inhalation. The ACGIH-recommended workplace exposure limit (TLV-TWA) for inhalation is 200 ppm as an 8-hour time-weighted average, and the level considered immediately dangerous to life or health (IDLH) is 6,000 ppm.

III. Clinical presentation

A. In the first few hours after acute ingestion, methanol-intoxicated patients present with inebriation and gastritis. Acidosis is not usually present because metabolism to toxic products has not yet occurred. There may be a noticeable elevation in the osmol gap (p 33); an osmol gap as low as 10 mOsm/L is consistent with toxic concentrations of methanol.

B. After a latent period of up to 30 hours, severe anion gap metabolic acidosis, visual disturbances, blindness, seizures, coma, acute renal failure with myoglobinuria, and death may occur. Patients describe the visual disturbance as blurred vision, haziness, or "like standing in a snowfield." Funduscopic examination may reveal optic disc hyperemia or pallor, venous engorgement, peripapilledema, and retinal or optic disc edema. The latent period is longer when ethanol has been ingested concurrently with methanol. Visual disturbances may occur within 6 hours in patients with a clear sensorium. Findings on magnetic resonance imaging (MRI) and computed tomography (CT), such as putaminal necrosis and hemorrhage, may be present; however, these changes are nonspecific and can change over time and therefore are not diagnostic of methanol poisoning.

IV. Diagnosis usually is based on the history, symptoms, and laboratory findings because stat methanol levels are rarely available. Calculation of the osmol and anion gaps (p 33) can be used to estimate the methanol level and predict the severity of the ingestion. A large anion gap not accounted for by elevated lactate suggests possible methanol (or ethylene glycol) poisoning because the anion gap in these cases is mostly nonlactate.

A. Specific levels

1. **Serum methanol** levels higher than 20 mg/dL should be considered toxic, and levels higher than 40 mg/dL should be considered very serious. After the latent period, a low or nondetectable methanol level does not rule out serious intoxication in a symptomatic patient because all of the methanol may already have been metabolized to formate. If serum methanol levels are not available, an estimation can be calculated from the osmol gap (see Table I–23, p 33); an osmol gap greater than 10 mOsm/L is consistent with a toxic methanol level.
2. Elevated **serum formate** concentrations may confirm the diagnosis and are a better measure of toxicity, but formate levels are rarely available. ***Note:***

if co-ingested ethanol is transiently preventing methanol metabolism, the formate level may be low initially.

B. Other useful laboratory studies include electrolytes (and anion gap), glucose, BUN, creatinine, serum osmolality and osmol gap, arterial blood gases, ethanol level, and lactate level.

V. Treatment

A. Emergency and supportive measures

1. Maintain an open airway and assist ventilation if necessary (pp 1–7).
2. Treat coma (p 18) and seizures (p 23) if they occur.
3. Treat metabolic acidosis with IV sodium bicarbonate (p 520). Correction of acidosis should be guided by arterial blood gases.

B. Specific drugs and antidotes

1. Administer **fomepizole** (p 558) or **ethanol** (p 553) to saturate the enzyme alcohol dehydrogenase and prevent formation of the toxic metabolites of methanol. Therapy is indicated in patients with the following:
   a. A history of significant methanol ingestion when methanol serum levels are not immediately available and the osmol gap is greater than 10 mOsm/L.
   b. Metabolic acidosis (arterial pH <7.3, serum bicarbonate <20 mEq/L) and an osmol gap greater than 10 mOsm/L not accounted for by ethanol or isopropanol.
   c. A methanol blood concentration greater than 20 mg/dL.
2. **Leucovorin** (p 572) or **folic acid** (p 557) may enhance the conversion of formate to carbon dioxide and water. A suggested dose of either leucovorin or folic acid is 1 mg/kg (up to 50 mg) IV every 4 hours.

C. Decontamination (p 50). Aspirate gastric contents if this can be performed within 30–60 minutes of ingestion. Activated charcoal is not likely to be useful because the effective dose is very large and methanol is absorbed rapidly from the GI tract.

D. Enhanced elimination. Hemodialysis rapidly removes both methanol (half-life reduced to 3–6 hours) and formate.

1. The indications for dialysis when methanol is suspected include elevated serum methanol level, elevated osmol gap, severe acidosis, coma ,or seizures (see Table II–38).
2. Dialysis, fomepizole, or ethanol should be continued until the methanol concentration is less than 20 mg/dL and the osmol and anion gaps are normalized.

TABLE II–38. GUIDELINES FOR HEMODIALYSIS IN METHANOL POISONING

The Extracorporeal Treatments in Poisoning (EXTRIP) Workgroup[a] recommends hemodialysis for methanol if ANY of the following conditions are present:

- Coma or seizures
- New vision deficits
- Blood pH ≤7.15
- Persistent metabolic acidosis despite adequate supportive measures and antidotes
- Serum anion gap higher than 24 mmol/L
- Serum methanol >700 mg/L or 21.8 mmol/L in the context of fomepizole therapy
- Serum methanol >600 mg/L or 18.7 mmol/L in the context of ethanol treatment
- Serum methanol >500 mg/L or 15.6 mmol/L in the absence of fomepizole or ethanol
- Elevated osmole gap
- Impaired kidney function

[a]Adapted, with permission from Roberts DM, Yates C, Megarbane B, et al. Recommendations for the role of extracorporeal treatments in the management of acute methanol poisoning: a systematic review and consensus statement. *Crit Care Med.* 2015;43(2):461–472.

▶ METHEMOGLOBINEMIA

Paul D. Blanc, MD, MSPH

Methemoglobin is an oxidized form of hemoglobin. Many oxidant chemicals and drugs are capable of inducing methemoglobinemia. Selected agents include nitrites and nitrates, bromates and chlorates, aniline derivatives, some pesticides (indoxacarb, metaflumizone, propanil), antimalarial agents, rasburicase, sulfonamides, dapsone, and local anesthetics (exposure to these can occur topically) (Table II–39). High-risk occupations include chemical and munitions work. An important environmental source for methemoglobinemia in infants is nitrate-contaminated well water. Amyl nitrite and butyl nitrite are abused for their alleged sexual enhancement properties. Oxides of nitrogen and other oxidant combustion products make smoke inhalation an important potential cause of methemoglobinemia.

I. Mechanism of toxicity

A. Methemoglobin inducers act by oxidizing ferrous (Fe^{2+}) to ferric (Fe^{3+}) hemoglobin. This abnormal hemoglobin is incapable of carrying oxygen, inducing a functional anemia. In addition, the shape of the oxygen–hemoglobin dissociation curve is altered, aggravating cellular hypoxia.

B. Methemoglobinemia does not cause hemolysis directly; however, many oxidizing agents that induce methemoglobinemia may also cause hemolysis through either hemoglobin (Heinz body) or cell membrane effects, particularly in patients with low tolerance for oxidative stress (eg, those with glucose-6-phosphate dehydrogenase [G6PD] deficiency).

II. Toxic dose. The dose required to induce methemoglobinemia is highly variable and depends on the substance and the route of exposure. Neonates and persons with congenital methemoglobin reductase deficiency or G6PD deficiency have an impaired ability to regenerate normal hemoglobin and are therefore more likely to accumulate methemoglobin after oxidant exposure. Concomitant hemolysis suggests either heavy oxidant exposure or increased cell vulnerability.

III. Clinical presentation. The severity of symptoms usually correlates with measured methemoglobin levels (Table II–40).

A. Symptoms and signs are caused by decreased blood oxygen content and cellular hypoxia and include headache, dizziness, and nausea; with greater compromise, these progress to dyspnea, confusion, seizures, and coma. Even at low levels, skin discoloration ("chocolate cyanosis"), especially of the nails, lips, and ears, can be striking.

B. Typically, mild methemoglobinemia (<15–20%) is well tolerated and will resolve spontaneously. This presumes that pre-existing anemia has not already

TABLE II–39. METHEMOGLOBINEMIA (SELECTED CAUSES)

Local Anesthetics	Other Pharmaceuticals	Industrial Chemicals and Pesticides
Benzocaine	4-Dimethyl-amino-phenol(4-DMAP)	Aminophenol
Lidocaine	Metoclopramide	Aniline, *p*-chloroaniline
Prilocaine	Nitric oxide	Bromates
Antimicrobials	Rasburicase	Chlorates
Chloroquine	Pegloticase	Indoxacarb
Dapsone	Phenazopyridine	Metaflumizone
Primaquine	**Nitrites and nitrates**	Naphthalene
Sulfonamides	Ammonium nitrate	Nitrobenzene
Trimethoprim	Amyl nitrite	Nitroethane
Analgesics	Butyl nitrite	Nitrogen dioxide
Phenazopyridine	Isobutyl nitrite	Nitroglycerin
Phenacetin	Potassium nitrate	Potassium permanganate
	Sodium nitrate	Propanil

TABLE II–40. METHEMOGLOBIN LEVELS

Methemoglobin Level (%)[a]	Typical Symptoms
<15	Often asymptomatic
15–20	Cyanosis, mild symptoms
20–45	Marked cyanosis, moderate symptoms
45–70	Severe cyanosis, severe symptoms
>70	Usually lethal

[a]These percentages assume normal-range total hemoglobin concentrations without other abnormalities. Concomitant anemia may lead to greater severity at lower proportional methemoglobinemia.

compromised the patient, thus making a smaller proportional impairment more clinically relevant. Continued metabolism yielding oxidant compounds from a long-acting parent compound (eg, dapsone) may lead to prolonged effects (2–3 days).

IV. Diagnosis. A patient with mild-to-moderate methemoglobinemia appears markedly cyanotic yet may be relatively asymptomatic. The arterial oxygen partial pressure (PO_2) is normal. The diagnosis is suggested by the finding of "chocolate brown" blood (dry a drop of blood on filter paper and compare with normal blood), which is usually apparent when the methemoglobin level exceeds 15%. Differential diagnosis includes other causes of cellular hypoxia (eg, carbon monoxide, cyanide, and hydrogen sulfide) and sulfhemoglobinemia.

A. Specific levels. The co-oximeter type of arterial blood gas analyzer directly measures oxygen saturation and methemoglobin percentages (measure as soon as possible because levels fall rapidly in vitro).

1. ***Note:*** Sulfhemoglobin and the antidote methylene blue both can lead to erroneous co-oximeter measurements; a dose of 2 mL/kg methylene blue can lead to a false-positive methemoglobin reading of approximately 15%.
2. The routine arterial blood gas machine measures the serum PO_2 (which is normal) and calculates a falsely normal oxygen saturation in the face of methemoglobinemia.
3. Routine 2-wavelength pulse oximetry is ***not*** reliable; it does not accurately reflect the degree of hypoxemia in a patient with severe methemoglobinemia (or sulfhemoglobinemia) and may appear falsely abnormal in a patient who has been given methylene blue. Newer multi-wavelength pulse oximetry devices may be able to better assess methemoglobin, but their reliability compared to co-oximetry remains uncertain.

B. Other useful laboratory studies include electrolytes and glucose. Consider testing for G6PD deficiency. If hemolysis is suspected, add CBC, haptoglobin, peripheral smear, and urinalysis dipstick for occult blood (free hemoglobin is positive). With substantial hemolysis, carboxyhemoglobin levels may be elevated in the 5–10% range.

V. Treatment

A. Emergency and supportive measures

1. Maintain an open airway and assist ventilation if necessary (pp 1–7). Administer supplemental oxygen.
2. Usually, mild methemoglobinemia (<15–20%) will resolve spontaneously and requires no intervention.

B. Specific drugs and antidotes

1. **Methylene blue** (p 579) is indicated in a symptomatic patient with methemoglobin levels higher than 20% or for whom even minimal compromise of oxygen-carrying capacity is potentially harmful (eg, pre-existing anemia, congestive heart failure, *Pneumocystis* pneumonia, angina pectoris). Give

methylene blue, 1–2 mg/kg (0.1–0.2 mL/kg of 1% solution), over several minutes. ***Caution:*** Methylene blue can slightly worsen methemoglobinemia when given in excessive amounts; in patients with G6PD deficiency, it may substantially aggravate methemoglobinemia and cause hemolysis.

2. **Ascorbic acid,** which can reverse methemoglobin by an alternate metabolic pathway, is of minimal use acutely because of its slow action.

C. **Decontamination** (p 50) depends on the specific agent involved.

D. **Enhanced elimination** (p 55)

1. If methylene blue is contraindicated (eg, G6PD deficiency) or has not been effective, **exchange transfusion** may rarely be necessary in patients with severe methemoglobinemia.
2. **Hyperbaric oxygen** is theoretically capable of supplying sufficient oxygen independently of hemoglobin and may be useful in extremely serious cases that do not respond rapidly to antidotal treatment.

▶ METHOTREXATE

Hallam Gugelmann, MD, MPH

Methotrexate, or *N*-(4-{[(2,4-diamino-6-pteridinyl)methyl]-methylamino}benzoyl)-L-glutamic acid, is an antimetabolite chemotherapeutic agent that is also used for psoriasis, rheumatoid arthritis, systemic sclerosis, placenta accreta, and ectopic pregnancy. Most toxicity is caused by chronic oral overmedication. Inadvertent high-dose intrathecal, intravenous, and intramuscular methotrexate administration and acute intentional overdose have been reported.

I. **Mechanism of toxicity**

A. Methotrexate is a folic acid antagonist that inhibits dihydrofolic acid reductase in the synthesis of purine nucleotide and thymidylate. It interferes with DNA synthesis and repair and with cellular replication. Tissues with active proliferation are more sensitive to this effect. It may affect immune function, but this mechanism remains unknown.

B. **Pharmacokinetics.** Peak serum level occurs within 1–2 hours after ingestion. Bioavailability is 60% at a dose of 30 mg/m^2 but significantly decreases at doses greater than 80 mg/m^2. Peak serum concentration occurs 30–60 minutes after IM injection. The steady-state volume of distribution is 0.4–0.8 L/kg, with approximately 50% protein bound. Drugs such as trimethoprim-sulfamethoxazole (TMP/SMX), probenecid, and salicylates can compete with methotrexate for protein-binding sites, raising free levels. Methotrexate does not penetrate the blood–cerebrospinal fluid (CSF) barrier in therapeutic doses given orally or parenterally. The terminal half-life is approximately 3–10 hours with low doses ($<$15 mg/m^2) and 8–15 hours after higher doses. Methotrexate accumulates in third-space fluid, so a prolonged half-life and clinical effects can be observed in patients with ascites, pleural effusion, and pericardial effusion. Ninety percent of the absorbed dose is excreted unchanged in the urine within 48 hours.

II. **Toxic dose**

A. **Therapeutic doses** vary widely, depending on the indication. Adults with rheumatoid arthritis often take 5–20 mg once a week. Ectopic pregnancy is treated with doses of 15–30 mg/d for 5 days. Neoplastic disease is treated with much higher doses (eg, 8–12 g/m^2 IV for some sarcomas). Intrathecal doses of 0.2–0.5 mg/kg are given for some CNS neoplasms.

B. **Toxic doses are variable, depending on the route and chronicity.** Bone marrow suppression can occur in 25% of patients receiving therapeutic doses used for the treatment of cancers. **Intrathecal injection** of more than 500 mg is associated with severe morbidity or death. Toxicity often occurs after prolonged use ($>$2 years) or after a total oral dose of 1.5 g. Alcoholism, obesity, diabetes, advanced age, and decreased renal function are risk factors associated with chronic hepatic toxicity.

III. Clinical presentation. Acute unintentional ingestion is generally benign. Chronic oral overmedication may occur in patients who misunderstand and take their weekly doses daily for several days. Severe toxicity usually results from an inadvertent high dose of intrathecal or IV methotrexate. Causes of death in severe toxicity are sepsis and multiple-organ failure.

A. Gastrointestinal effects including nausea, vomiting, diarrhea, and ulcerative stomatitis are the most common reported adverse effects from oral methotrexate toxicity.

B. Hematologic effects such as leukopenia, anemia, thrombocytopenia, and pancytopenia occur within a week after exposure and resolve in 2 weeks. Bone marrow suppression can lead to fatal systemic infections.

C. Hepatic manifestations include acute elevated aminotransaminases and chronic fibrosis or cirrhosis after prolonged use.

D. Neurologic toxicity is usually seen only in patients with intrathecal or IV methotrexate overdose. Serious neurotoxicity includes generalized or local seizures and coma. Acute chemical arachnoiditis following intrathecal dosing presents as headache, back pain, nuchal rigidity, and fever; paraparesis and paraplegia can occur. Chronic leukoencephalopathy may cause confusion, irritability, somnolence, ataxia, dementia, seizure, and coma, and may be mistaken for acute ischemic stroke with restricted diffusion seen on magnetic resonance imaging (MRI).

E. Interstitial pneumonitis manifests with a dry or nonproductive cough.

F. Renal damage from high-dose IV methotrexate results from deposition of methotrexate and its metabolite in the renal tubules.

G. Dermatologic reactions include toxic epidermal necrosis, Stevens–Johnson syndrome, exfoliative dermatitis, skin necrosis, and erythema multiforme.

H. Teratogenic effects and fetal death are well documented. Methotrexate is categorized as Pregnancy Category X by the FDA.

IV. Diagnosis. Methotrexate intoxication should be suspected in any patient with nausea, vomiting, abdominal discomfort, elevated aminotransaminases, and/or bone marrow suppression.

A. Specific levels. A serum methotrexate level greater than 1 mcmol/L is potentially toxic. The level should be monitored every 24 hours after overdose.

B. Other useful laboratory studies include CBC with differential and platelet count, BUN, creatinine, electrolytes, liver function test, and chest radiography if indicated.

V. Treatment

A. Emergency and supportive measures

1. Maintain an open airway and assist ventilation if necessary (pp 1–7). Administer supplemental oxygen.
2. Treat coma (p 18), seizures (p 23), and infection if they occur.
3. Treat nausea and vomiting with ondansetron (p 597) or metoclopramide (p 581) and fluid loss with IV crystalloid solutions.
4. Bone marrow suppression should be treated with the assistance of an experienced hematologist or oncologist. Granulocyte colony–stimulating factor and transfusion of red cells or platelets may be considered if appropriate.
5. Remove third-space fluid (eg, ascites, pleural effusion) in severe methotrexate overdose to prevent prolonged toxic effects.
6. **Intrathecal overdose**. Intrathecal leucovorin administration may be fatal. Treatment strategies in reported cases include CSF drainage to remove methotrexate via lumbar puncture, CSF exchange, or ventriculolumbar perfusion. IV (not intrathecal) leucovorin (100 mg every 6 hours for 4 doses), IV dexamethasone (4 mg every 6 hours for 4 doses), and intrathecal glucarpidase (2,000 units over 5 minutes) have been used. ***Note:*** Patients who

have received less than 100 mg of methotrexate intrathecally are unlikely to develop severe toxicity and probably do not require intervention.

B. Specific drugs and antidotes

1. **Leucovorin** (folinic acid [p 572]) should be administered as soon as possible to patients with significant risk for toxicity. ***Note:*** Do not wait for methotrexate levels to initiate therapy after acute poisoning. Leucovorin "rescue" is routinely used for patients receiving high-dose methotrexate (>500 mg/m^2).
2. **Glucarpidase** (p 561) is a recombinant enzyme that rapidly hydrolyzes methotrexate to the inactive metabolite 2,4-diamino-N10-methylpteroic acid (DAMPA) and glutamic acid. It rapidly lowers serum methotrexate levels by IV and intrathecal administration. Glucarpidase does not counteract the intracellular effects of methotrexate; leucovorin rescue is still necessary.
3. Administration of corticosteroids (dexamethasone 4 mg IV every 6 hours for 4 doses) may be of utility.

C. Decontamination (p 50) measures are appropriate after acute ingestion but not chronic intoxication. Administer activated charcoal orally if conditions are appropriate (see Table I–38, p 54). Gastric lavage is not necessary after small-to-moderate ingestions if activated charcoal can be given promptly.

D. Enhanced elimination from the systemic circulation (p 56)

1. Effective clearance of methotrexate by means of acute intermittent hemodialysis (with a high-flux dialyzer) and by use of continuous venovenous hemodialysis have been reported. It is recommended for patients who have renal failure and are anticipated to have prolonged high serum methotrexate levels.
2. Urine alkalinization is recommended to increase elimination and decrease precipitation of methotrexate and its metabolite in the renal tubules.
3. Multiple-dose activated charcoal is reported to decrease the elimination half-life of methotrexate but has not been shown to affect outcomes.

▶ METHYL BROMIDE

Timur S. Durrani, MD, MPH, MBA

Methyl bromide, a potent alkylating agent, is an odorless, colorless, extremely toxic gas used as a fumigant in soil, perishable foods, cargo containers, and nonresidential buildings. Commercially known as Halon 1001, methyl bromide was used (until the 1960s) as a refrigerant and fire extinguisher. Fields or buildings to be fumigated are evacuated and covered with a tarp, and the gas is introduced. After 12–24 hours, the tarp is removed, and the area is ventilated and then tested for residual methyl bromide before reoccupation. Methyl bromide is a major source of ozone-destroying bromine in the stratosphere, and most production and use were scheduled to be phased out by 2005 in developed countries and by 2015 in developing countries; however, it is still being used in the United States owing to EPA critical use exemptions.

I. Mechanism of toxicity

A. Methyl bromide is a potent, nonspecific alkylating agent with a special affinity for sulfhydryl and amino groups. Limited data indicate that toxicity is the result of direct alkylation of cellular components (eg, glutathione, proteins, or DNA) or formation of toxic metabolites from methylated glutathione. Animal data clearly indicate that its toxicity does not result from the bromide ion.

B. Pharmacokinetics. Inhaled methyl bromide is distributed rapidly to all tissues and metabolized. In sublethal animal studies, approximately 50% is eliminated as exhaled carbon dioxide, 25% is excreted in urine and feces, and 25% is bound to tissues as a methyl group. The elimination half-life of the bromide ion is 9–15 days.

II. Toxic dose. Methyl bromide is threefold heavier than air, may accumulate in low-lying areas, and may seep via piping or conduits from fumigated buildings into adjacent structures. It may condense to a liquid at cold temperatures (3.6°C [38.5°F]), then vaporize when temperatures rise. Methyl bromide gas lacks warning properties, so the lacrimator chloropicrin (2%) usually is added. However, chloropicrin has a different vapor pressure and may dissipate at a different rate, limiting its warning properties.

A. **Inhalation** is the most important route of exposure. The ACGIH-recommended workplace exposure limit (TLV-TWA) in air is 1 ppm (3.9 mg/m^3) as an 8-hour time-weighted average. Toxic effects generally are seen at levels of 200 ppm, and the air level considered immediately dangerous to life or health (IDLH) is 250 ppm. NIOSH considers methyl bromide a potential occupational carcinogen.

B. **Skin** irritation and absorption may occur, causing burns and systemic toxicity. Methyl bromide may penetrate clothing and some protective gear. Retained gas in clothing and rubber boots can be a source of prolonged dermal exposure.

III. **Clinical presentation**

A. **Acute irritant effects** on the eyes, mucous membranes, and upper respiratory tract are attributed to the added lacrimator chloropicrin. (Lethal exposures can occur without warning if chloropicrin has not been added.) Moderate skin exposure can result in dermatitis and, in severe cases, chemical burns.

B. **Acute systemic effects** usually are delayed by 2–24 hours. Initial toxicity may include malaise, visual disturbances, headache, nausea, vomiting, and tremor, which may advance to intractable seizures and coma. Death may be caused by fulminant respiratory failure with noncardiogenic pulmonary edema or complications of status epilepticus. Sublethal exposure may result in flulike symptoms, respiratory complaints, or chronic effects.

C. **Chronic neurologic sequelae** can result from chronic exposure or a sublethal acute exposure. A wide spectrum of neurologic and psychiatric problems may occur that may be reversible (months to years) or irreversible. They include agitation, delirium, dementia, psychoneurotic symptoms, psychosis, visual disturbances, vertigo, aphasia, ataxia, peripheral neuropathies, myoclonic jerking, tremors, and seizures.

IV. **Diagnosis** is based on a history of exposure to the compound and on clinical presentation.

A. **Specific levels.** Bromide levels in patients with acute methyl bromide exposure are usually well below the toxic range for bromism and may be only mildly elevated compared with levels in unexposed persons (see "Bromides," p 166). Nontoxic serum bromide levels do not rule out methyl bromide poisoning. Levels of methylated proteins or DNA have been investigated as possible biomarkers for methyl bromide exposure.

B. **Other useful laboratory studies** include electrolytes, glucose, BUN, and creatinine. If there is respiratory distress, also perform arterial blood gases or oximetry and chest radiography.

V. **Treatment**

A. **Emergency and supportive measures**

1. Administer supplemental oxygen and treat bronchospasm (p 8), pulmonary edema (p 7), seizures (p 23), and coma (p 18) if they occur. Intractable seizures usually predict a fatal outcome. Consider induction of barbiturate coma with a short-acting agent such as pentobarbital (p 602) and consult a neurologist as soon as possible.
2. Monitor patients for a minimum of 6–12 hours to detect development of delayed symptoms, including seizures and noncardiogenic pulmonary edema.

B. **Specific drugs and antidotes.** Theoretically, *N*-acetylcysteine (NAC [p 499]) or dimercaprol (BAL [p 514]) can offer a reactive sulfhydryl group to bind free methyl bromide, although neither agent has been critically tested. There were strikingly different outcomes for two patients with the same exposure but different glutathione transferase activity, suggesting that NAC can possibly exacerbate toxicity. Neither agent can be recommended at this time.

C. Decontamination (p 50). Properly trained personnel should use self-contained breathing apparatus and chemical-protective clothing before entering contaminated areas. The absence of irritant effects from chloropicrin does not guarantee that it is safe to enter without protection.

1. Remove victims from exposure and administer supplemental oxygen if available.
2. If exposure is to liquid methyl bromide, remove contaminated clothing and wash affected skin with soap and water. Irrigate exposed eyes with copious water or saline.

D. Enhanced elimination. There is no role for these procedures.

▶ METHYLENE CHLORIDE

Binh T. Ly, MD and Charles W. O'Connell MD

Methylene chloride (dichloromethane, DCM) is a volatile, colorless liquid with a chloroform-like odor. Even though DCM is thought to be one of the least toxic chlorinated hydrocarbons, it can cause substantial toxic effects and mortality when used improperly. It has a wide variety of industrial uses, many of which are based on its solvent properties, including paint stripping, bathtub refinishing, pharmaceutical manufacturing, metal cleaning and degreasing, adhesives, film base production, agricultural fumigation, and plastics manufacturing. Methylene chloride is metabolized to carbon monoxide in vivo and may produce phosgene, chlorine, or hydrogen chloride upon combustion.

I. Mechanism of toxicity

A. Solvent effects. Like other hydrocarbons, DCM is an irritant to mucous membranes, defats the skin epithelium, and may sensitize the myocardium to the dysrhythmogenic effects of catecholamines.

B. Anesthetic effects. Like other halogenated hydrocarbons, DCM can cause CNS depression ranging from mild sedation to coma.

C. Carbon monoxide (CO) is generated in vivo during metabolism by mixed-function oxidases (CYP2E1) in the liver. Elevated carboxyhemoglobin (CO-Hgb) levels may be delayed and prolonged. CO-Hgb levels associated with DCM are usually lower than severe exogenous exposures to CO, but a level as high as 50% has been reported (see also "Carbon Monoxide," p 182).

D. Methylene chloride is a **suspected human carcinogen** (IARC Group 2B).

II. Toxic dose. Toxicity may occur after inhalation or ingestion.

A. Inhalation. Inhalation toxicity typically occurs when DCM is used in poorly ventilated, enclosed areas. The permissible exposure limit (PEL) is 25 ppm as an 8-hour time-weighted average. The ACGIH workplace threshold limit value (TLV-TWA) is 50 ppm (174 mg/m^3) for an 8-hour shift, which may result in a CO-Hgb level of 3–4%. The short-term exposure limit (STEL) is 125 ppm. The air level considered immediately dangerous to life or health (IDLH) is 2,300 ppm. The odor threshold is about 100–200 ppm.

B. Ingestion. The acute oral toxic dose is approximately 0.5–5 mL/kg.

III. Clinical presentation

A. Inhalation is the most common route of exposure and may cause irritation of mucous membranes, upper airway and skin, nausea, vomiting, tachypnea, sweating, and headache. Ocular exposure can cause conjunctival irritation. Severe exposure may lead to pulmonary edema or hemorrhage, cardiac dysrhythmias, and CNS and respiratory depression.

B. Ingestion can cause corrosive injury to the GI tract and systemic intoxication. Renal and hepatic injury and pancreatitis have been reported.

C. Dermal exposure can cause dermatitis or chemical burns, and systemic symptoms can result from skin absorption.

D. **Chronic exposure** can cause bone marrow, hepatic, and renal toxicity. Methylene chloride is a known animal and a suspected human carcinogen (IARC Group 2B).

IV. **Diagnosis** is based on a history of exposure and clinical presentation.

A. **Specific levels**

1. **Carboxyhemoglobin** levels should be obtained serially as CO-Hgb levels may have a delayed peak and prolonged elimination.
2. Expired air and blood or urine levels of **methylene chloride** may be obtained to assess workplace exposure but are not useful in clinical management.

B. **Other useful laboratory studies** include CBC, electrolytes, glucose, BUN, creatinine, liver aminotransferases, and ECG monitoring.

V. **Treatment**

A. **Emergency and supportive measures**

1. Maintain an open airway and assist ventilation if necessary (pp 1–7).
2. Administer supplemental oxygen and treat coma (p 18) and pulmonary edema (p 7) if they occur.
3. Monitor the ECG for at least 4–6 hours and treat dysrhythmias (pp 10–15) if they occur. Avoid the use of catecholamines (eg, epinephrine, dopamine), which may precipitate cardiac dysrhythmias. Tachydysrhythmias caused by myocardial sensitization may be treated with **esmolol** (p 552), 0.025–0.1 mg/kg/min IV, or **propranolol** (p 617), 1–2 mg IV.
4. If corrosive injury is suspected after ingestion, consult a gastroenterologist regarding possible endoscopic evaluation.

B. **Specific drugs and antidotes.** Administer 100% **oxygen** by tight-fitting mask or endotracheal tube if the CO-Hgb level is elevated. Consider hyperbaric oxygen (p 599) if the CO-Hgb level is elevated and the patient has findings of CNS toxicity.

C. **Decontamination** (p 50)

1. **Inhalation.** Remove the victim from exposure and give supplemental oxygen, if available.
2. **Skin and eyes.** Remove contaminated clothing and wash exposed skin with soap and water. Irrigate exposed eyes with copious saline or water.
3. **Ingestion.** Activated charcoal is of limited value and may make endoscopic evaluation difficult if corrosive injury is suspected. Perform nasogastric suction (if there has been a large, recent ingestion).

D. **Enhanced elimination.** There is no documented efficacy for repeat-dose activated charcoal, hemodialysis, or hemoperfusion. Although treatment with hyperbaric oxygen may enhance elimination of carbon monoxide, its efficacy for patients with acute methylene chloride poisoning remains unproven.

▶ MOLDS

John R. Balmes, MD

Fungi are ubiquitous in all environments and play a critical ecologic role by decomposing organic matter. "Mold" is the common term for multicellular fungi that grow as a mat of intertwined microscopic filaments (hyphae). Molds are pervasive in the outdoor environment but may also be present indoors under certain conditions, primarily in the presence of excessive moisture from leaks in roofs or walls, plant pots, or pet urine. The most common indoor molds are *Cladosporium, Penicillium, Aspergillus,* and *Alternaria.* Other molds that can grow indoors include *Fusarium, Trichoderma,* and *Stachybotrys;* the presence of these molds often indicates a long-standing problem with water leakage or damage.

I. **Mechanism of toxicity.** Molds and other fungi may affect human health adversely through three processes: allergy, infection, and toxicity.

A. **Allergy.** Outdoor molds are generally more abundant and important in allergic disease than indoor molds. The most important indoor allergenic molds are *Penicillium* and *Aspergillus* species. Outdoor molds, such as *Cladosporium* and *Alternaria,* often can be found at high levels indoors if there is abundant access for outdoor air (eg, open windows). Excessive moisture or water damage in homes and buildings can lead to enhanced growth of allergenic fungi.

B. **Infection.** Several fungi cause superficial infections involving the skin or nails. A very limited number of pathogenic fungi (eg, *Blastomyces, Coccidioides, Cryptococcus,* and *Histoplasma*) can infect nonimmunocompromised individuals. Persons with severe immune dysfunction (eg, cancer patients on chemotherapy, organ transplant patients on immunosuppressive drugs, patients with HIV infection) are at increased risk for both the pathogenic fungal infections listed earlier and more severe opportunistic fungal infections (eg, with *Candida* and *Aspergillus*).

C. **Mycotoxins and glucans.** Some species of fungi are capable of producing mycotoxins, whereas most molds have one of a group of substances known as glucans in their cell walls. Serious veterinary and human mycotoxicoses have been documented after ingestion of foods heavily overgrown with toxigenic mold species. Inhalational exposure to high concentrations of mixed organic dusts (often in occupational settings) is associated with **organic dust toxic syndrome** (ODTS), an acute febrile illness. This self-limited condition generally is attributed to bacterial endotoxins and potentially to mold glucans rather than to mycotoxins. Exposure to mycotoxins has been documented in indoor environments, but currently there is insufficient evidence to confirm that inhalational exposures result in human disease. Cases of acute idiopathic pulmonary hemorrhage (AIPH) in infants have been attributed to home contamination by *Stachybotrys chartarum*, but this apparent association has not been definitively confirmed. Ingestion of certain mycotoxins (eg, aflatoxins) has been associated with hepatocarcinogenesis.

D. **Volatile organic compounds** (VOCs), including low–molecular-weight alcohols, aldehydes, and ketones, are generated by molds and are often responsible for the musty, disagreeable odor associated with indoor molds. A role for these VOCs in some building-related symptoms is possible.

II. **Toxic dose.** Because mycotoxins are not volatile, exposure would require inhalation of aerosolized spores, mycelial fragments, or contaminated substrates. The toxic inhaled dose of mycotoxin for humans is not known. Based on experimental data from single-dose in vivo studies, *Stachybotrys chartarum* spores (intranasally in mice or intratracheally in rats) in high doses (>30 million spores per kilogram) can produce pulmonary inflammation and hemorrhage. The no-effect dose in rats (3 million spores per kilogram) corresponds to a continuous 24-hour exposure to 2.1 million spores per cubic meter for infants, 6.6 million spores per cubic meter for a school-age child, or 15.3 million spores per cubic meter for an adult. These spore concentrations are much higher than those measured in building surveys.

III. **Clinical presentation**

A. **Mold allergy** occurs in atopic individuals who develop IgE antibodies to a wide range of indoor and outdoor allergens, including animal dander, dust mites, and weed, tree, and grass pollens. Allergic responses are most commonly experienced as asthma or allergic rhinitis ("hay fever"). A much less common but more serious immunologic condition, **hypersensitivity pneumonitis** (HP), may follow exposure (often occupational) to relatively high concentrations of fungal (and other microbial) proteins.

B. **Infection** caused by pathogenic fungi is generally unrelated to exposure to molds from identifiable point sources and is beyond the scope of this chapter.

C. **Organic dust toxic syndrome** presents as a flulike illness with an onset 4–8 hours after a heavy exposure (eg, shoveling compost). Symptoms resolve without treatment over 24 hours.

D. **"Sick building syndrome,"** or "nonspecific building-related illness," comprises a poorly defined set of symptoms that are attributed to a building's indoor environment and can include neurologic, GI, dermatologic, and respiratory complaints. The potential role of building-associated exposure to molds in some of these cases is suspected, but the mechanism is not clear. Existing data do not support a specific role for mycotoxins in this syndrome.

IV. **Diagnosis.** A history of recurrent respiratory symptoms associated with a specific building environment is consistent with either asthma or HP. Inquire about home, school, or work building conditions. If the conditions suggest the likelihood of mold contamination, consult with a specialist trained in the evaluation of building environments (eg, an industrial hygienist or a structural engineer). Mold risk is increased with a history of prior water damage or leak even when it is not ongoing, especially in the context of damaged drywall or carpeting on concrete.

A. **Specific tests.** Allergen skin prick testing or radioallergosorbent testing (RAST) can confirm the presence of specific IgE-mediated allergy to common fungi. Testing for the presence of IgG precipitating antibodies can confirm exposure to HP-inducing fungi, but a positive test does not confirm the diagnosis of HP. There are no specific blood or urine tests for mycotoxin exposure.

B. **Other useful laboratory studies.** Pulmonary function testing is helpful in distinguishing asthma (obstructive pattern with a normal diffusing capacity) from HP (restrictive pattern with a low diffusing capacity). Chest imaging may suggest the presence of interstitial lung disease consistent with HP or active or past fungal infection. Histologic examination of lung tissue obtained from transbronchial or open-lung biopsy may be necessary to confirm the diagnosis of HP.

C. **Environmental evaluation.** Indoor air samples with contemporaneous outdoor air samples can assist in evaluating whether there is mold growth indoors; air samples may also assist in evaluating the extent of potential indoor exposure. Bulk, wipe, and wall cavity samples may indicate the presence of mold but do not adequately characterize inhalational exposures of building occupants.

V. **Treatment**

A. **Emergency and supportive measures.** Treat bronchospasm (p 8) and hypoxemia (p 7) if they are present.

B. **Specific drugs and antidotes.** None.

C. **Decontamination of the environment (remediation).** Mold overgrowth in indoor environments should be remediated not only because it may produce offensive odors and adverse health effects but also because mold physically destroys the building materials on which it grows. A patient with HP caused by sensitization to a specific fungus present in a building environment is not likely to get better until excess exposure is eliminated. Once the source of moisture that supports mold growth has been eliminated, active mold growth can be halted. Colonized porous materials such as clothing and upholstery can be cleaned by washing or dry cleaning as appropriate and need not be discarded unless cleaning fails to restore an acceptable appearance and odor. Carpeting, drywall, and other structural materials, once contaminated, may present a greater remediation challenge.

D. **Enhanced elimination.** Not relevant.

► MONOAMINE OXIDASE INHIBITORS

Neal L. Benowitz, MD

Most monoamine oxidase (MAO) inhibitors are used primarily for severe depression resistant to other antidepressant drugs, but are also used to treat phobias and anxiety disorders. First-generation MAO inhibitors include **isocarboxazid** (Marplan), **phenelzine** (Nardil), and **tranylcypromine** (Parnate). Newer-generation MAO inhibitors with

TABLE II–41. MONOAMINE OXIDASE INHIBITOR INTERACTIONS[a]

Drugs		Foods
Amphetamines	Metaraminol	Beer
Buspirone	Methyldopa	Broad bean pods and fava beans
Clomipramine	Methylphenidate	Cheese (natural or aged)
Cocaine	Paroxetine	Chicken liver
Dextromethorphan	Phenylephrine	Pickled herring
Ephedrine	Phenylpropanolamine	Smoked, pickled, or aged meats
Fluvoxamine	Reserpine	Snails
Fluoxetine	Sertraline	Spoiled or bacterially contaminated foods
Guanethidine	Tramadol	Summer sausage
L-Dopa	Trazodone	Wine (red)
LSD (lysergic acid diethylamide)	Tryptophan	Yeast (dietary supplement and Marmite)
MDMA	Venlafaxine	
Meperidine (Demerol)		

[a]Possible interactions based on case reports or pharmacologic considerations.

lower toxicity include **selegiline** (Eldepryl, Emsam, Zelapar) and rasagiline (Azilect), also used in the treatment of Parkinson's disease, and **moclobemide** (Aurorix, Manerix), a much less toxic antidepressant that is available in many countries, but not in the United States. Multiple other MAO inhibitors are marketed outside the United States to treat depression, anxiety disorders, Parkinson's disease, and bacterial infections. Serious toxicity from MAO inhibitors occurs with overdose or owing to interactions with certain other drugs or foods (Table II–41).

Drugs of other classes may have MAO-inhibiting activity, including **procarbazine** (Matulane), **linezolid** (Zyvox), the recreational drugs paramethoxyamphetamine (PMA) and methylenedioxymethamphetamine (MDMA, "ecstasy" [p 81]), and **methylene blue** (p 579). The popular herbal product used for depression, **St. John's wort** (*Hypericum perforatum*), appears to act in part as an MAO inhibitor and has been implicated in interactions with medications such as selective serotonin reuptake inhibitors (SSRIs). A number of other plant products containing tryptamines, harmines, and hydroxyindole have also been shown to have MAO-inhibiting activity, including such popular herbals as resveratrol piperine (found in pepper), ginkgo biloba, ginseng, and berberine.

I. Mechanism of toxicity. MAO inhibitors inactivate MAO, an enzyme responsible for degradation of catecholamines within CNS neurons. MAO is an enzyme with two major subtypes, MAO-A and MAO-B. MAO-A is also found in the liver and intestinal wall, where it metabolizes tyramine and therefore limits its entry into the systemic circulation.

A. Toxicity results from the release of excessive neuronal stores of vasoactive amines, inhibition of metabolism of catecholamines, or absorption of large amounts of dietary tyramine (which in turn releases catecholamines from neurons).

1. Selegiline was developed as a *selective* MAO-B inhibitor that does not require a restrictive diet. (MAO-B selectivity is lost at doses above 20 g/d; thus, overdose with selegiline resembles that of the older MAO inhibitors.) Antidepressant treatment with transdermal selegiline (Emsam) is feasible because higher doses of selegiline reach the CNS owing to bypass of hepatic first-pass metabolism. A recent study showed that at low transdermal doses (6 mg/24 h), no dietary restrictions were required, although the potential for drug interactions (see below) remains.

2. Older MAO inhibitors and selegiline are *irreversible* inhibitors of the enzyme. Because effects can last up to 2 weeks, concomitant or delayed drug and food interactions are common and potentially fatal with the first-generation drugs. However, **moclobemide** is a *reversible* competitive MAO-A inhibitor. As a result, it does not require food restrictions, has much less potential for drug interactions, and is much safer in overdose than are the older MAO inhibitors.

B. Toxic reactions to MAO inhibitors can be classified into four distinct types: food interactions, interactions with certain drugs, serotonin syndrome, and acute overdose.

1. **Food interactions.** Tyramine is a dietary monoamine that normally is degraded by gastrointestinal MAO-A. MAO inhibition allows excessive absorption of tyramine, which acts indirectly to release norepinephrine, causing a hyperadrenergic syndrome. Patients taking therapeutic oral doses of the MAO-B–specific selegiline or the reversible inhibitor moclobemide (up to 900 mg/d) are not susceptible to this interaction and can eat a nonrestrictive diet.
2. **Interactions with indirectly acting monoamine drugs.** MAO inhibits degradation of presynaptic norepinephrine, so that increased amounts are stored in the nerve endings. Drugs that act indirectly to release norepinephrine, such as pseudoephedrine and phenylephrine, can cause marked hypertension and tachycardia in people taking MAO inhibitors. Selegiline is not likely to cause this reaction because MAO-B has a much greater effect on brain dopamine than on norepinephrine levels.
3. **Serotonin syndrome.** Severe muscle hyperactivity, clonus, and hyperthermia may occur when patients receiving MAO inhibitors use even therapeutic doses of drugs such as meperidine, tramadol, dextromethorphan, tricyclic antidepressants, SSRIs, venlafaxine, lithium, buspirone, methylene blue, tryptophan, or MDMA ("ecstasy"). It appears to involve elevation of CNS serotonin levels via multiple mechanisms.
4. **Acute overdose** involving any MAO inhibitor is very serious and can be fatal. Selectivity for MAO-B is lost in selegiline overdose. In addition, selegiline is metabolized to L-amphetamine, which can contribute to hyperadrenergic symptoms in overdose.

C. ***Note:*** Because of irreversible MAO inhibition, adverse drug interactions may occur for up to 2 weeks after discontinuation of older MAO inhibitors. Interactions may also occur when MAO inhibitors are started within 2–3 weeks after stopping fluoxetine, owing to the long half-life of fluoxetine.

II. Toxic dose. First-generation MAO inhibitors have a low therapeutic index; acute ingestion of 2–3 mg or more of tranylcypromine, isocarboxazid, or phenelzine per kilogram should be considered potentially life-threatening. In contrast, overdoses of up to 13 times the daily starting dose of moclobemide alone (~28 mg/kg) typically result in mild or no symptoms. (However, overdose of moclobemide at lower doses, if taken along with SSRIs, can result in life-threatening toxicity.)

III. Clinical presentation. Symptoms may be delayed by 6–24 hours after acute overdose but occur rapidly after ingestion of interacting drugs or foods in a patient on chronic MAO inhibitor therapy. Because of irreversible inactivation of MAO, toxic effects (and the potential for drug or food interactions) may persist for several days when first-generation drugs are involved.

A. Drug or food interactions typically cause tachycardia, hypertension, anxiety, flushing, diaphoresis, and headache. Hypertensive crisis can lead to ischemia and end-organ damage such as intracranial hemorrhage, myocardial infarction, or renal failure.

B. With the **serotonin syndrome,** an altered mental status with both neuromuscular and autonomic instability, such as hyperthermia, tremor, myoclonic jerking, hyperreflexia, and shivering, may develop. Lower extremity clonus and sometimes ocular clonus is often reported, and patients are usually agitated, diaphoretic, and/or delirious. Severe hyperthermia can lead to acute cardiovascular collapse and multiple-organ failure (p 21).

C. **Acute overdose** can cause a clinical syndrome characterized by elements of both adrenergic hyperactivity and excessive serotonin activity, including severe hypertension, delirium, hyperthermia, dysrhythmias, seizures, obtundation, and eventually hypotension and cardiovascular collapse with multisystem failure. One case documented drug-induced myocarditis with shock and severely depressed ventricular function. Other findings may include mydriasis, nystagmus, hallucinations, and tachypnea.

D. **Hypotension,** particularly when the patient is in an upright position (orthostatic hypotension), is seen with therapeutic dosing and also may occur with overdose.

IV. **Diagnosis** is based on clinical features of sympathomimetic drug intoxication with a history of MAO inhibitor use, particularly in combination with drugs or foods known to interact. Serotonin syndrome (p 21) is suspected when the patient has an altered mental status with signs of autonomic and neuromuscular instability, especially clonus.

A. **Specific levels.** Drug levels are not generally available. Most agents are not detectable on comprehensive urine toxicology screening. Selegiline is metabolized to L-amphetamine, which may be detected on some urine toxicology screening tests. In one reported case, elevated urinary serotonin levels correlated temporally with symptoms.

B. Other useful laboratory studies include electrolytes, glucose, BUN, creatinine, creatine kinase (CK), troponin, 12-lead ECG, and ECG monitoring. If intracranial hemorrhage is suspected, perform a CT head scan.

V. **Treatment**

A. **Emergency and supportive measures**

1. Maintain an open airway and assist ventilation if necessary (pp 1–7). Administer supplemental oxygen.
2. Treat hypertension (p 17), coma (p 18), seizures (p 23), and hyperthermia (p 21) if they occur.
   a. Use titratable intravenous antihypertensives such as nitroprusside (p 593) and phentolamine (p 605) because of the potential for rapid changes in hemodynamics.
   b. If hypotension occurs, it may reflect depletion of neuronal catecholamine stores, and in this case the directly acting agent norepinephrine is preferred over the indirectly acting drug dopamine.
3. Continuously monitor temperature, other vital signs, and ECG for a minimum of 6 hours in asymptomatic patients and admit all symptomatic patients for continuous monitoring for 24 hours.

B. **Specific drugs and antidotes**

1. Because the hypertension is catecholamine-mediated, alpha-adrenergic blockers (eg, phentolamine [p 605]) or combined alpha- and beta-adrenergic blockers (eg, labetalol [p 571]) are particularly useful. ***Note:*** Use of nonselective beta blockers without a vasodilator may cause paradoxical worsening of hypertension owing to unopposed alpha-adrenergic effects.
2. **Serotonin syndrome** should be treated with supportive care, sedation, and cooling. Anecdotal case reports suggest benefit with cyproheptadine (Periactin), 12 mg orally (PO) initially followed by 4 mg every hour for 3–4 doses (p 537). Chlorpromazine 25–50 mg IV has also been used.

C. **Decontamination.** Administer activated charcoal orally if conditions are appropriate (see Table I–38, p 54). Consider gastric lavage if the patient presents early after a very large ingestion of a first-generation drug or selegiline.

D. **Enhanced elimination.** Dialysis and hemoperfusion are not effective. Repeat-dose activated charcoal has not been studied.

▶ MUSHROOMS

Annamariam Pajouhi, PharmD

There are more than 5,000 varieties of mushrooms, of which about 50–100 are known to be toxic and only 200–300 are known to be safely edible. The majority of toxic mushrooms cause mild-to-moderate self-limited gastroenteritis. A few species may cause severe or even fatal reactions. The major categories of poisonous mushrooms are described in Table II–42. *Amanita phalloides* and other amatoxin-containing mushrooms are discussed on p 333.

I. Mechanism of toxicity. The various mechanisms thought to be responsible for poisoning are listed in Table II–42. The majority of toxic incidents are caused by GI irritants that produce vomiting and diarrhea shortly after ingestion.

II. Toxic dose. This is not known. The amount of toxin varies considerably among members of the same species, depending on local geography and weather conditions. In most cases, the exact amount of toxic mushroom ingested is unknown because the victim has unwittingly added a toxic species to a meal of edible fungi.

III. Clinical presentation. The various clinical presentations are described in Table II–42. These presentations often can be recognized by onset of action. If symptom onset is within 6 hours, the likely categories will be GI irritants, cholinergic syndrome, hallucinogenic, isoxazole syndrome, immunohemolytic, allergic pneumonitis, or allenic norleucine class.

Mushrooms that cause symptoms from 6 to 24 hours after ingestion include those containing amatoxins or monomethylhydrazine and those causing erythromelalgia.

Onset of symptoms more than 24 hours after ingestion suggests poisoning by the orellanines that cause kidney damage, mushrooms causing rhabdomyolysis, or mushrooms causing delayed CNS toxicity. Mushrooms in the coprine category do not cause symptoms unless the patient ingests alcohol. This disulfiram-like effect can occur from 30 minutes to as long as 5 days after ingestion.

IV. Diagnosis may be difficult because the victim may not realize that the illness was caused by mushrooms, especially if symptoms are delayed by 12 or more hours after ingestion. If leftover mushrooms are available, obtain assistance from a mycologist through a local university or mycologic society. However, note that the mushrooms brought for identification may not be the same ones that were eaten.

History is key to determining the category of toxic mushroom. It is important to get a description of the mushroom and the environment from which it was obtained. Was the mushroom dish cooked or eaten raw? Were several types of mushrooms ingested? What was the time of ingestion in relation to the onset of symptoms? Was alcohol ingested after the mushrooms were eaten? Is everyone who ate the mushroom ill? Are those who did not eat the mushroom also ill? Were the mushrooms eaten several times? Were they stored properly? The suspected mushroom should be kept in a paper bag in the refrigerator labeled "do not eat" in case more identification is required.

A. Specific levels. Qualitative detection of the toxins of several mushroom species has been reported, but these tests are not routinely available.

B. Other useful laboratory studies include CBC, electrolytes, glucose, BUN, creatinine, liver aminotransferases, and prothrombin time (PT/INR). Obtain a methemoglobin level if gyromitrin-containing mushrooms are suspected or the patient is cyanotic. Obtain a chest radiograph if allergic pneumonitis syndrome is suspected, and serial creatine kinase (CK) levels for suspected rhabdomyolysis.

V. Treatment

A. Emergency and supportive measures

1. Treat hypotension from gastroenteritis with intravenous crystalloid solutions (p 15) and supine positioning. Treat agitation (p 24), hyperthermia (p 21), rhabdomyolysis (p 27), and seizures (p 27) if they occur. Antiemetics should be given to patients with nausea and/or vomiting.

TABLE II–42. MUSHROOM TOXICITY

Syndrome	Toxin(s)	Causative Mushrooms	Symptoms and Signs
Delayed gastroenteritis and liver failure	Amatoxins (p 333)	*Amanita phalloides, Amanita ocreata, Amanita verna, Amanita virosa, Amanita bisporigera, Galerina autumnalis, Galerina marginata,* and some *Lepiota* and *Conocybe* spp	Delayed onset 6–24 hours: vomiting, severe diarrhea, abdominal cramps, hypovolemic shock, followed by fulminant hepatic failure after 2–3 days.
Delayed gastroenteritis, CNS abnormalities, hemolysis, hepatitis	Monomethylhydrazine	*Gyromitra (Helvella) esculenta,* others	Delayed onset 5–10 hours: nausea, vomiting, diarrhea, abdominal cramps, followed by dizziness, weakness, headache, ataxia, delirium, seizures, coma; hemolysis, methemoglobinemia, hepatic and renal injury may also occur.
Cholinergic syndrome	Muscarine	*Clitocybe dealbata, Clitocybe cerrusata, Inocybe cincinnata*	Onset 15 minutes–2 hours: diaphoresis, bradycardia, bronchospasm, lacrimation, salivation, sweating, vomiting, diarrhea, miosis. Treat with atropine (p 512).
Disulfiram-like reaction with alcohol	Coprine	*Coprinus atramentarius, Clitocybe claviceps*	Within 30 minutes to a few hours after ingestion of alcohol: nausea, vomiting, flushing, tachycardia; risk for reaction up to 5 days after ingestion. (see "Disulfiram," p 226).
Isoxazole syndrome	Ibotenic acid, muscimol	*Amanita muscaria, Amanita pantherina,* others	Onset 30 minutes–2 hours: nausea, vomiting, lethargy or hyperactivity, muscular jerking, hallucinations, delirium, rarely seizures. May last up to 12 hours.
Gastritis and renal failure	Allenic norleucine	*Amanita smithiana, Amanita proxima, others*	Abdominal pain, vomiting within 30 minutes–12 hours, followed by progressive acute renal failure within 2–3 days. Some elevation in hepatic enzymes may occur.
Delayed-onset gastritis and renal failure	Orellanine	*Cortinarius orellanus,* other *Cortinarius* spp	Abdominal pain, anorexia, vomiting starting after 24–36 hours, followed by progressive acute renal failure (tubulointerstitial nephritis) 3–14 days later.
Hallucinogenic	Psilocybin, psilocyn	*Psilocybe cubensis, panaeolina foenisecii,* others	Onset 30 minutes–2 hours: visual hallucinations, sensory distortion, tachycardia, mydriasis, occasionally seizures.

(continued)

TABLE II–42. MUSHROOM TOXICITY (CONTINUED)

Syndrome	Toxin(s)	Causative Mushrooms	Symptoms and Signs
Gastrointestinal irritants	Unidentified	*Chlorophyllum molybdites, Boletus satanas,* many others	Vomiting, diarrhea within 30 minutes–2 hours of ingestion; symptoms resolve within 6–24 hours.
Immunohemolytic anemia	Unidentified	*Paxillus involutus, Clitocybe claviceps, Boletus luridus*	GI irritant for most, but a few people develop immune-mediated hemolysis within 2 hours of ingestion.
Allergic pneumonitis (inhaled spores)	Lycoperdon spores	*Lycoperdon* spp	Inhalation of dry spores can cause acute nausea, vomiting, and nasopharyngitis, followed within days by fever, malaise, dyspnea, and inflammatory pneumonitis.
Erythromelalgia	Acromelic acids	*Clitocybe acromelalga, Clitocybe amoenolens*	Onset hours to several days after ingestion: severe burning pain, paresthesias, redness and edema in the hands and feet; may persist for several weeks.
Rhabdomyolysis	Unidentified	*Tricholoma equestre, Russula subnigricans*	Onset 24–72 hours: fatigue, muscle weakness, myalgias, rhabdomyolysis, renal insufficiency, and myocarditis.
Delayed CNS toxicity	Polyporic acid	*Hapalopilus rutilans*	Onset after 12–24 hours: nausea, vomiting, headache, malaise, blurred or double vision, nystagmus, ataxia, weakness, somnolence.

2. Monitor patients for 12–24 hours for delayed-onset gastroenteritis associated with amatoxin or monomethylhydrazine poisoning.
3. Monitor renal function for 1–2 weeks after suspected *Cortinarius* species ingestion, or 2–4 days after *Amanita smithiana* ingestion. Provide supportive care, including hemodialysis if needed, for renal dysfunction.

B. Specific drugs and antidotes

1. For seizures following **monomethylhydrazine** poisoning, treat with IV benzodiazepines (lorazepam or diazepam), and give pyridoxine, 25 mg/kg IV (p 621); treat methemoglobinemia with methylene blue, 1–2 mg/kg IV (p 579).
2. For **muscarine** intoxication with cholinergic symptoms, give atropine, 1–2 mg IV for adults and 0.02 mg/kg IV for children (p 512).
3. **Allergic pneumonitis** may benefit from corticosteroid administration.
4. Treat **amatoxin-type** poisoning as described on p 333.
5. For coprine-associated disulfiram-like reaction, treat with fluids (see Disulfiram, p 226).

C. Decontamination (p 50). If the mushroom is potentially toxic or unidentified, administer activated charcoal orally if conditions are appropriate (see Table I–38, p 54).

1. Charcoal is probably not warranted after a trivial ingestion (eg, a lick or a nibble) of an unknown mushroom by a toddler.
2. Repeat-dose activated charcoal (p 59) may be helpful after amatoxin ingestion (p 333).

D. Enhanced elimination. There is no accepted role for these procedures.

▶ MUSHROOMS, AMATOXIN-TYPE

Kent R. Olson, MD

Amatoxins are a group of highly toxic peptides found in several species of mushrooms, including Amanita phalloides, Amanita virosa, Amanita bisporigera, Amanita ocreata, Amanita verna, Galerina autumnalis, Galerina marginata, and some species of Lepiota and Conocybe. This category of mushrooms is responsible for more than 90% of mushroom deaths worldwide.

This group is also referred to as cyclopeptide-containing mushrooms. The three cyclopeptides are amatoxin, phallotoxin, and virotoxin. Amatoxins, principally alpha-amanitin, are the most toxic and responsible for hepatic and renal toxicity. Phallotoxins are not well absorbed and cause GI symptoms. Virotoxins are not implicated in human poisoning.

I. Mechanism of toxicity. Amatoxins are highly stable and resistant to heat and are not removed by any form of cooking. They bind to DNA-dependent RNA polymerase II and inhibit the elongation essential to transcription. The result is a decrease in mRNA that causes an arrest of protein synthesis and cell death. Metabolically active tissue dependent on high rates of protein synthesis, such as cells of the GI tract, hepatocytes, and the proximal convoluted tubules of the kidney, are disproportionately affected. Cellular damage has also been found in the pancreas, adrenal glands, and testes.

A. Pharmacokinetics. Amatoxins are readily absorbed from the intestine and transported across the hepatocytes by bile transport carriers. About 60% undergo enterohepatic recirculation. They have limited protein binding and are eliminated in urine, vomitus, and feces. Toxins are detectable in urine within 90–120 minutes after ingestion. No metabolites of amatoxin have been detected. The half-life in humans is unknown, but there is a rapid decrease in serum, bile and urine levels in animals, with most of the toxin eliminated within the first 24 hours.

II. Toxic dose. Amatoxins are among the most potent toxins known; the minimum lethal dose is about 0.1 mg/kg. One *Amanita phalloides* cap may contain 10–15 mg. In contrast, *Galerina* species contain far less toxin; 15–20 caps would be a fatal dose for an adult.

III. Clinical presentation. Amatoxin poisoning can be divided into three phases, although not all patients experience phases 2 and 3. There is an initial phase of delayed GI toxicity, followed by a false "recovery" period and then late-onset hepatic failure.

A. Phase 1. Onset of symptoms is 6–24 hours after ingestion. Symptoms include vomiting, severe abdominal cramps, and explosive watery diarrhea, which may become grossly bloody. This GI phase may cause severe volume depletion and hypotension, leading to acute renal failure. Death may occur within the first 24 hours from massive fluid loss.

B. Phase 2 occurs 18–36 hours after ingestion. There is a period of transient clinical improvement in the gastroenteritis but liver enzymes (transaminases) are often rising.

C. Phase 3 begins 2–4 days after ingestion and is characterized by markedly elevated transaminases, hyperbilirubinemia, coagulopathy, hypoglycemia, acidosis, hepatic encephalopathy, hepatorenal syndrome, multiple-organ failure, disseminated intravascular coagulation, and convulsions. Death usually occurs 6–16 days after ingestion. Encephalopathy, metabolic acidosis, severe coagulopathy, and hypoglycemia are grave prognostic signs and usually predict a fatal outcome.

IV. Diagnosis is usually based on a history of wild mushroom ingestion and a delay of 6–24 hours before the onset of severe gastroenteritis (see also monomethylhydrazine toxin, Table II–42, p 331). However, if a variety of mushrooms have been eaten, stomach upset may occur much earlier owing to ingestion of a different toxic species, making diagnosis of amatoxin poisoning more difficult.

Any available mushroom specimens that may have been ingested should be examined by a mycologist. Pieces of mushroom retrieved from the vomit or even mushroom spores found on microscopic examination may provide clues to the ingested species.

A. Specific levels

1. Amatoxin can be detected in serum, urine, and gastric fluids by radioimmunoassay or high-performance liquid chromatography (HPLC) with mass spectrometry (LC-MS), but these methods are not readily available to assist in treatment decisions.
2. A qualitative test (Meixner test) may determine the presence of amatoxins in mushroom specimens. Juice from the mushroom is dripped onto newspaper or other high–lignin-content paper and allowed to dry. A single drop of concentrated hydrochloric acid is then added; a blue color suggests the presence of amatoxins. ***Caution:*** This test has unknown reliability and can be misinterpreted or poorly performed; it should not be used to determine the edibility of mushroom specimens. In addition, false-positive reactions can be caused by drying at a temperature higher than 63°C, exposure of the test paper to sunlight, or the presence of psilocybin, bufotenin, or certain terpenes.

B. Other useful laboratory studies include electrolytes, glucose, BUN, creatinine, liver aminotransferases (AST and ALT), bilirubin, and prothrombin time (PT/INR). Aminotransferases usually peak 60–72 hours after ingestion. Measures of liver function such as the INR are more useful in evaluating the severity of hepatic failure.

V. Treatment. The mortality rate is approximately 6–10% with intensive supportive care.

A. Emergency and supportive measures

1. Maintain an open airway and assist ventilation if necessary (pp 1–7). Administer supplemental oxygen.
2. Treat fluid and electrolyte losses aggressively because massive fluid losses may cause circulatory collapse. Administer normal saline or another crystalloid solution, 10- to 20-mL/kg boluses, with monitoring of central venous pressure to guide fluid therapy.

3. Provide vigorous supportive care for hepatic failure (p 42); orthotopic **liver transplant** may be lifesaving in patients who develop fulminant hepatic failure. Contact a liver transplant service for assistance.
4. Use of an extracorporeal bioartificial liver has shown some promise in stabilizing a patient until spontaneous liver regeneration occurs or in serving as a bridge to liver transplant.

B. **Specific drugs and antidotes.** No antidote has been proven effective for amatoxin poisoning, although over the years many therapies have been promoted. Consult a medical toxicologist or a regional poison control center (1-800-222-1222 in the United States) for further information.
   1. Animal studies and retrospective case series in humans suggest that early treatment with IV **silibinin** (an extract of milk thistle that is used in Europe [p 623]) may be effective in reducing hepatocyte uptake of amatoxin. The product (brand name, Legalon SIL) can be obtained as an emergency Investigational New Drug by calling 1-866-520-4412.
   2. **Other unproven therapies.** High doses of penicillin given before the poisoning showed some hepatoprotective effects in dog and rat studies, but controlled human studies are lacking. A retrospective analysis of 20 years of amatoxin treatment found that high-dose penicillin was the most frequently used chemotherapy but showed little efficacy. The therapies that the authors of this review thought were probably most effective were silibinin, *N*-acetylcysteine, and detoxification procedures. There are no data to support the use of cimetidine or steroids, and thioctic acid can cause severe hypoglycemia. Amatoxin-specific Fab fragments actually increased of amatoxins in mice.

C. **Decontamination** (p 50). Administer activated charcoal orally. Gastric lavage may not remove mushroom pieces.

D. **Enhanced elimination.** There is no proven role for forced diuresis, hemoperfusion, hemofiltration, or hemodialysis in the removal of amatoxins.
   1. Repeat-dose activated charcoal may trap small quantities of amatoxin undergoing enterohepatic recirculation and may be considered in the first 48 hours.
   2. Cannulation of the bile duct or gall bladder to remove bile has been reported effective in dog studies and a few human case reports, but is not without risk, especially in patients with coagulopathy. There has been no direct comparison of the effectiveness of biliary drainage versus repeated-dose activated charcoal.

▶ NAPHTHALENE AND PARADICHLOROBENZENE

Kai Li, MD

Naphthalene and paradichlorobenzene are common ingredients in diaper pail and toilet bowl deodorizers, insecticides, and mothballs. Both compounds have a similar pungent odor and are clear-to-white crystalline substances; therefore, they are difficult to distinguish visually. Naphthalene, 10% in oil, was used as a scabicide in the past. Naphthalene is no longer commonly used because it largely has been replaced by the less toxic paradichlorobenzene. While formulations and sizes vary, most moth repellent products contain nearly 100% naphthalene or paradichlorobenzene.

I. **Mechanism of toxicity.** Both compounds sublimate into vapor and enter the atmosphere upon being opened, and are well absorbed through the GI and respiratory tracts. Both compounds cause GI upset, and both may cause CNS stimulation. In addition, naphthalene may produce hemolysis, especially in patients with glucose-6-phosphate dehydrogenase (G6PD) deficiency.

II. **Toxic dose**

A. **Naphthalene.** As little as 250–500 mg may produce hemolysis in a patient with G6PD deficiency. The amount necessary to produce lethargy or seizures is not known but may be as little as 1–2 g. Several infants developed serious poisoning from clothes and bedding that had been stored in naphthalene mothballs. The LD_{50} is 1.8 g/kg in adult rats.

B. Paradichlorobenzene is much less toxic than naphthalene; up to 20-g ingestions have been well tolerated in adults. The oral LD_{50} for adult rats is 3.8 g/kg.

C. Pharmacokinetics. Both compounds are rapidly absorbed orally or by inhalation. Dermal absorption is believed to be very low.

III. Clinical presentation. Acute ingestion usually causes prompt nausea and vomiting. Both compounds are volatile, and inhalation of vapors may cause eye, nose, and throat irritation.

A. Naphthalene.

1. Agitation, headaches, confusion, lethargy, and seizures may occur with naphthalene ingestion.
2. Hemolytic anemia, particularly in children following ingestion and in patients with G6PD deficiency, has been well documented.
3. Nausea, vomiting, diarrhea (occasionally bloody), hematuria, and jaundice (as a consequence of hemolysis) have also been noted.

B. Paradichlorobenzene

1. Acute ingestions of small amounts in children are virtually always innocuous.
2. Exposure to the vapor can cause ocular irritation and GI upset.
3. Prolonged direct contact can cause a burning sensation to the skin. Paradichlorobenzene decomposes to hydrochloric acid; this may explain some of its irritant effects.
4. Unlike naphthalene, there is no clear evidence of hematologic effects even in chronic exposures.
5. A single case report from the 1950s reports hepatic necrosis and death in two people living in a home saturated with paradichlorobenzene for several months; other symptoms included headaches, clumsiness, slurred speech, diarrhea, and weight loss. No air measurements were taken and no other possible causes of their symptoms were discussed.

IV. Diagnosis usually is based on a history of ingestion and the characteristic "mothball" smell around the mouth and in the vomitus. Differentiation between naphthalene and paradichlorobenzene by odor or color is difficult. In an in vitro x-ray study, paradichlorobenzene was radiopaque but naphthalene was not visible. In a saturated salt solution (about 1 tablespoon of salt in 4 oz of water), naphthalene will float and paradichlorobenzene will sink.

A. Specific levels. Serum and urine testing is not widely available. Paradichlorobenzene breakdown products (2,5-dichlorophenol) can be found in the urine and blood. Similarly, naphthalene, 1-methylnaphthalene, 2-methylnaphthalene, or their breakdown products can be found in samples of urine, stool, blood, milk, or body fat. Elevated levels indicate that a patient was exposed but are not correlated with clinical outcome.

B. Other useful laboratory studies include CBC, hepatic transaminases and, if hemolysis is suspected, haptoglobin, free hemoglobin, and urine dipstick for occult blood (positive with hemoglobinuria).

V. Treatment

A. Emergency and supportive measures

1. Maintain an open airway and assist ventilation if necessary (pp 1–7).
2. Treat coma (p 18) and seizures (p 23) if they occur.
3. Treat hemolysis and resulting hemoglobinuria, if they occur, by intravenous hydration and urinary alkalinization (see "Rhabdomyolysis," p 27).

B. Specific drugs and antidotes. There is no specific antidote.

C. Decontamination (p 50)

1. **Naphthalene.** Administer activated charcoal orally if conditions are appropriate (see Table I–38, p 54). Gastric lavage is not necessary after small-to-moderate ingestions if activated charcoal can be given. Do not induce

vomiting because of risk for lethargy and seizures. Do not administer milk, fats, or oil, which may enhance absorption.

2. **Paradichlorobenzene.** Gut emptying and charcoal are not necessary unless a massive dose has been ingested. Do not administer milk, fats, or oils, which may enhance absorption.
3. **Inhalation.** With either agent, remove the victim from exposure; fresh air is all that is required.

D. Enhanced elimination. There is no role for these procedures.

▶ NICOTINE

Neal L. Benowitz, MD

Nicotine poisoning may occur in children after they ingest tobacco or drink saliva expectorated by a tobacco chewer (which is often collected in a can or other containers), in children or adults after accidental or suicidal ingestion of nicotine-containing pesticides (eg, Black Leaf 40, which contains 40% nicotine sulfate), occasionally after cutaneous exposure to nicotine, such as occurs among tobacco harvesters ("green tobacco sickness"), and most recently after ingestions of nicotine-containing liquids used in electronic cigarettes. Nicotine chewing gum (Nicorette and generics), transdermal delivery formulations (Habitrol, Nicoderm, Nicotrol, and generics), and nicotine nasal spray, inhalers, and lozenges are widely available as adjunctive therapy for smoking cessation. Nicotine is found in various smokeless tobacco products (snuff and chewing tobacco), including compressed dissolvable tobacco tablets that look like candy. Alkaloids similar to nicotine (anabasine, cytisine, coniine, and lobeline) are found in several plant species (see "Plants," p 375). **Neonicotinoid insecticides** (imidacloprid and others) are widely used both in agriculture and for flea control in dogs and cats.

I. Mechanism of toxicity

A. Nicotine binds to nicotinic cholinergic receptors, resulting initially, via actions on autonomic ganglia, in predominantly sympathetic nervous stimulation. With higher doses, parasympathetic stimulation and then ganglionic and neuromuscular blockade may occur. Direct effects on the brain may also result in vomiting and seizures.

B. Pharmacokinetics. Nicotine is absorbed rapidly by all routes and enters the brain quickly. The apparent volume of distribution is 3 L/kg. It is rapidly metabolized and to a lesser extent excreted in the urine, with a half-life of 120 minutes. Neonicotinoids penetrate the CNS less well than nicotine and therefore are less toxic than nicotine at low levels of exposure.

II. Toxic dose. Owing to presystemic metabolism and spontaneous vomiting, which limit absorption, the bioavailability of nicotine that is swallowed is about 30–40%. The LD_{50} for nicotine is estimated to be between 6.5 and 13 mg/kg. Rapid absorption of 2–5 mg can cause nausea and vomiting, particularly in a person who does not use tobacco habitually.

A. Tobacco. Cigarette tobacco contains about 1.5% nicotine, or 10–15 mg of nicotine per cigarette. Moist snuff is also about 1.5% nicotine; most containers hold 30 g of tobacco. Chewing tobacco contains 2.5–8% nicotine. Compressed tobacco tablets typically contain 1 mg of nicotine. In a child, ingestion of one cigarette or three cigarette butts should be considered potentially toxic, although serious poisoning from ingestion of cigarettes is very uncommon. Ingestions of smokeless tobacco products are a common cause of nicotine poisoning in infants and children.

B. Electronic cigarettes. E-cigarettes are devices that heat a solution, usually containing nicotine, propylene glycol and/or vegetable glycerin, to generate a vapor that is inhaled like a tobacco cigarette. Many devices are refillable, and the refills (e-liquids) can be purchased in small bottles. Most e-liquids are flavored and potentially attractive to children. E-liquids typically contain 10–20-mg nicotine per mL, such that a 5-mL bottle can contain 100 mg, which could be lethal to an infant or small child. The number of poison center calls regarding nicotine toxicity from e-cigarettes has risen exponentially in recent years, with 50% of calls involving children 5 years or younger. The most common routes of exposure are ingestion, inhalation, ocular exposure, and skin exposure. The most common toxicities are nausea, vomiting, and eye irritation. There have been a few deaths from ingestion or IV injection of e-liquids.

C. **Nicotine gum** contains 2 or 4 mg per piece, but owing to its slow absorption and high degree of presystemic metabolism, nicotine intoxication from these products is uncommon.

D. **Transdermal nicotine patches** deliver an average of 5–22 mg of nicotine over the 16–24 hours of intended application, depending on the brand and size. Transdermal patches may produce intoxication in light smokers or in nonsmokers, particularly children to whom a used patch inadvertently sticks. Ingestion of a discarded patch may also potentially produce poisoning.

E. **Nicotine nasal spray** delivers about 1 mg (a single dose is one spray in each nostril).

F. **Nicotine inhaler systems** consist of a plastic mouthpiece and replaceable cartridges containing 10 mg of nicotine. If accidentally ingested, the cartridge will release the nicotine slowly, and no serious intoxication has been reported.

G. **Nicotine lozenges** contain 2–4 mg of nicotine, and ingestion can cause serious toxicity in a child.

H. **Neonicotinoids** are relatively nontoxic in small doses, but intentional ingestions of 30 mL or more have been associated with serious and even fatal toxicity.

III. **Clinical presentation.** Nicotine intoxication commonly causes dizziness, nausea, vomiting, pallor, and diaphoresis. Abdominal pain, salivation, lacrimation, diarrhea, and muscle weakness may be noted. Pupils may be dilated or constricted. Confusion, agitation, lethargy, and convulsions are seen with severe poisonings. Initial tachycardia and hypertension may be followed by bradycardia and hypotension. Respiratory muscle weakness with respiratory arrest is the most likely cause of death. Symptoms usually begin within 15 minutes after acute liquid nicotine ingestion and resolve in 1 or 2 hours, although more prolonged symptoms may be seen with higher doses or cutaneous exposure, with the latter resulting in continued absorption from the skin. Delayed onset and prolonged symptoms may also be seen with nicotine gum or transdermal patches.

IV. **Diagnosis** is suggested by vomiting, pallor, and diaphoresis, although these symptoms are nonspecific. The diagnosis usually is made by a history of tobacco, insecticide, or therapeutic nicotine product exposure. Nicotine poisoning should be considered in a small child with unexplained vomiting whose parents consume tobacco or e-cigarettes.

A. **Specific levels.** Nicotine and its metabolite cotinine are detected in comprehensive urine toxicology screens, but because they are so commonly present, they will not usually be reported unless a specific request is made. Commercial screening assays for urinary cotinine are also available but are not widely implemented in hospital-based clinical laboratories. Serum levels of nicotine can be performed but are not useful in acute management. Anabasine levels (found in *Nicotiana glauca,* or tree tobacco) can be measured by some laboratories.

B. **Other useful laboratory studies** include electrolytes, glucose, and arterial blood gases or oximetry.

V. **Treatment**

A. **Emergency and supportive measures**

1. Maintain an open airway and assist ventilation if necessary (pp 1–7). Administer supplemental oxygen.

2. Treat seizures (p 23), coma (p 18), hypotension (p 15), hypertension (p 17), and arrhythmias (pp 10–15) if they occur.
3. Observe for at least 4–6 hours to rule out delayed toxicity, especially after skin exposure. For ingestion of intact gum, tablets, or transdermal patches, observe for a longer period (up to 12–24 hours).

B. Specific drugs and antidotes

1. **Mecamylamine** (Inversine) is a specific antagonist of nicotine actions; however, it is available only in tablets, a form not suitable for a patient who is vomiting, convulsing, or hypotensive.
2. Signs of muscarinic stimulation (eg, bradycardia, salivation, wheezing), if they occur, may respond to **atropine** (p 512).

C. Decontamination (p 50). ***Caution:*** Rescuers should wear appropriate skin-protective gear when treating patients with oral or skin exposure to liquid nicotine.

1. **Skin and eyes.** Remove all contaminated clothing and wash exposed skin with copious soap and water. Irrigate exposed eyes with copious saline or water.
2. **Ingestion.** Administer activated charcoal orally if conditions are appropriate (see Table I–38, p 54). Gastric lavage is not necessary after tobacco ingestions if activated charcoal can be given promptly. Consider gastric lavage for large recent ingestions of liquid nicotine.
   a. For asymptomatic small-quantity cigarette ingestions, no gut decontamination is necessary.
   b. For ingestion of transdermal patches or large amounts of gum, consider repeated doses of charcoal (p 59) and whole-bowel irrigation (p 55).

D. Enhanced elimination. These procedures are not likely to be useful because the endogenous clearance of nicotine is high, its half-life is relatively short (2 hours), and the volume of distribution is large.

▶ NITRATES AND NITRITES

Neal L. Benowitz, MD

Organic nitrates (eg, nitroglycerin, isosorbide dinitrate, and isosorbide mononitrate) are widely used as vasodilators for the treatment of ischemic heart disease and heart failure. Organic nitrates such as nitroglycerin also are used in explosives. Bismuth subnitrate, ammonium nitrate, and silver nitrate are used in antidiarrheal drugs, cold packs, and topical burn medications, respectively. Sodium and potassium nitrate and nitrite are used in preserving cured foods and may also occur in high concentrations in some well water and in antifreeze mixtures. Butyl, amyl, ethyl, and isobutyl nitrites often are sold as "room deodorizers" or "liquid incense" and sometimes are inhaled for abuse purposes.

I. Mechanism of toxicity. Nitrates and nitrites both cause vasodilation, which can result in hypotension.

A. Nitrates relax veins at lower doses and arteries at higher doses. Nitrates may be converted into nitrites in the GI tract, especially in infants.

B. Nitrites are potent oxidizing agents. Oxidation of hemoglobin by nitrites may result in methemoglobinemia (p 317), which hinders oxygen-carrying capacity and oxygen delivery. Many organic nitrites (eg, amyl nitrite and butyl nitrite) are volatile and may be inhaled.

II. Toxic dose. In the quantities found in food, nitrates and nitrites are generally not toxic; however, infants may develop methemoglobinemia after ingestion of sausages or well water because they readily convert nitrate to nitrite and because their hemoglobin is more susceptible to oxidation than is that of adults. Severe methemoglobinemia has occurred in adults when sodium nitrite marketed as a food additive or preservative is applied directly to foods and ingested. Methemoglobinemia induced by nitrite may be more severe and associated with hemolysis in the presence of G6PD deficiency.

A. **Nitrates.** The estimated adult lethal oral dose of nitroglycerin is 200–1,200 mg. Hypotension occurs at low doses, but massive doses of nitroglycerin are usually required to produce methemoglobinemia.

B. **Nitrites.** Ingestion of as little as 15 mL of butyl nitrite produced 40% methemoglobinemia in an adult. The estimated adult lethal oral dose of sodium nitrite is 1 g.

III. **Clinical presentation.** Headache, skin flushing, and orthostatic hypotension with reflex tachycardia are the most common adverse effects of nitrates and nitrites and occur commonly, even with therapeutic doses of organic nitrates.

A. **Hypotension** may aggravate or produce symptoms of cardiac ischemia or cerebrovascular disease and may even cause seizures. However, fatalities from hypotension are rare.

B. Workers or patients regularly exposed to nitrates may develop tolerance and may develop **angina** or **myocardial infarction** owing to rebound coronary vasoconstriction upon sudden withdrawal of the drug. Inhaled nitrites are flammable and their accidental ignition (such as after lighting a cigarette that had been dipped a nitrite solution) has resulted in serious burns.

C. **Methemoglobinemia** (p 317) is most common after nitrite exposure; the skin is cyanotic even at levels low enough for the individual to be otherwise asymptomatic (eg, 15%).

D. Use of **sildenafil** (Viagra) and other selective phosphodiesterase inhibitors (tadalafil [Cialis], vardenafil [Levitra]) used to treat erectile dysfunction can prolong and intensify the vasodilating effects of nitrates, causing severe hypotension.

IV. **Diagnosis** is suggested by hypotension with reflex tachycardia and headache. Methemoglobinemia of 15% or more may be diagnosed by noting cyanosis with a low oxygen saturation in the absence of respiratory disease. A chocolate brown coloration of the blood when it is dried on filter paper may be seen.

A. **Specific levels.** Blood levels are not commercially available. With a urine nitrite dipstick (normally used to detect bacteria in urine), nitrite can be detected in the serum of patients intoxicated by alkyl nitrites.

B. **Other useful laboratory studies** include electrolytes, glucose, arterial blood gases or oximetry, methemoglobin concentration, and ECG monitoring. Note that arterial blood gases and conventional pulse oximetry do not measure methemoglobin. (A newer pulse co-oximeter can detect carboxyhemoglobin and methemoglobin.)

V. **Treatment**

A. **Emergency and supportive measures**

1. Maintain an open airway and assist ventilation if necessary (pp 1–7). Administer supplemental oxygen.
2. Treat hypotension with supine positioning, IV crystalloid fluids, and low-dose pressors if needed (p 15).
3. Monitor vital signs and ECG for 4–6 hours.

B. **Specific drugs and antidotes.** Symptomatic methemoglobinemia may be treated with **methylene blue** (p 579).

C. **Decontamination** (p 50)

1. **Inhalation.** Remove victims from exposure and administer supplemental oxygen if available.
2. **Skin and eyes.** Remove contaminated clothing and wash with copious soap and water. Irrigate exposed eyes with water or saline.
3. **Ingestion.** Administer activated charcoal orally if conditions are appropriate (see Table I–38, p 54). Gastric lavage is not necessary after small-to-moderate ingestions if activated charcoal can be given promptly.

D. **Enhanced elimination.** Hemodialysis and hemoperfusion are not effective. Severe methemoglobinemia in infants not responsive to methylene blue therapy may require **exchange transfusion.**

▶ NITROGEN OXIDES

Paul D. Blanc, MD, MSPH

Nitrogen oxides (nitric oxide and nitrogen dioxide, ***not*** *nitrous* oxide [p 343]) are gases commonly released from nitrous or nitric acid, from reactions between nitric acid and organic materials, from burning of nitrocellulose and many other products, as a by-product of detonations, and as a breakdown reactant of the rocket fuel dinitrogen tetroxide. Exposure to nitrogen oxides occurs in electric arc welding (especially gas-shielded), electroplating, and engraving. Nitrogen oxides are found in engine exhaust, and they are produced when grain with a high nitrite content is filled into storage silos. Nitric oxide used as a therapeutic agent can react with oxygen (particularly in the presence of hyperoxia) to form nitrogen dioxide and other oxidants.

I. Mechanism of toxicity. Nitrogen oxides are irritant gases with relatively low water solubility. Nitrogen oxides cause delayed-onset chemical pneumonitis. In addition, they can oxidize hemoglobin to methemoglobin.

II. Toxic dose. The Federal OSHA legal permissible exposure limit—ceiling (PEL-C) for nitrogen dioxide is 5.0 ppm; California OSHA has a short-term exposure limit (STEL) of 1 ppm; and the ACGIH-recommended workplace exposure limit (threshold limit value–8-hour time-weighted average [TLV-TWA]) for nitrogen dioxide is 0.2 ppm. The OSHA PEL and the ACGIH TLV-TWA for nitric oxide is 25 ppm. The air levels considered immediately dangerous to life or health (IDLH) for nitrogen dioxide and nitric oxide are 20 and 100 ppm, respectively.

III. Clinical presentation. Because of the poor water solubility of nitrogen oxides, there is very little mucous membrane or upper respiratory irritation at low levels (<10 ppm for nitrogen dioxide). This allows prolonged exposure with few warning symptoms other than mild cough or nausea. With more concentrated exposures, upper respiratory symptoms such as burning eyes, sore throat, and cough may occur.

- **A.** After a delay of up to 24 hours, chemical pneumonitis may develop, with progressive hypoxemia and pulmonary edema. The onset may be more rapid after exposure to higher concentrations. Some cases may evolve to bronchiolitis obliterans in the days after an initial improvement.
- **B.** After recovery from acute chemical pneumonitis and after chronic low-level exposure to nitrogen oxides, permanent lung disease from tissue damage may become evident.
- **C.** Methemoglobinemia (p 317) has been described in victims exposed to nitrogen oxides in smoke during major structural fires.
- **D.** Inhaled nitric oxide (eg, used for therapeutic purposes as a pulmonary vasodilator) can have extrapulmonary effects, including reduced platelet aggregation, methemoglobinemia, and systemic vasodilation.

IV. Diagnosis is based on a history of exposure, if known. Because of the potential for delayed effects, all patients with significant smoke inhalation should be observed for several hours.

- **A. Specific levels.** There are no specific blood levels.
- **B. Other useful laboratory studies** include arterial blood gases with co-oximetry to assess concomitant methemoglobinemia, chest radiography, and pulmonary function tests.

V. Treatment

A. Emergency and supportive measures

1. Observe closely for signs of upper airway obstruction, and intubate the trachea and assist ventilation if necessary (pp 1–7). Administer humidified supplemental oxygen.
2. Observe symptomatic victims for a minimum of 24 hours after exposure and treat pneumonitis and noncardiogenic pulmonary edema (p 7) if they occur.

B. Specific drugs and antidotes

1. The role of corticosteroids is most clearly indicated for later onset of bronchiolitis obliterans. In acute lung injury from chemical inhalation, including inhalation of nitrogen oxide, a beneficial role of steroids has not been established.
2. Treat methemoglobinemia with **methylene blue** (p 579).

C. Decontamination (p 50). Rescuers should wear self-contained breathing apparatus and, if there is the potential for high-level gas exposure or exposure to liquid nitric acid (as a source of nitrogen dioxide), chemical-protective clothing.

1. **Inhalation.** Remove victims from exposure immediately and give supplemental oxygen, if available.
2. **Skin and eyes.** Remove any wet clothing and flush exposed skin with water. Irrigate exposed eyes with copious water or saline.

D. Enhanced elimination. There is no role for enhanced elimination procedures.

▶ NITROPRUSSIDE

Neal L. Benowitz, MD

Sodium nitroprusside is a short-acting, parenterally administered vasodilator that is used to treat severe hypertension and cardiac failure. It also is used to treat hypertension in postoperative cardiac surgery patients and to induce hypotension for certain surgical procedures. Toxicity may occur with acute high-dose nitroprusside treatment or with prolonged infusions.

I. Mechanism of toxicity. Nitroprusside is rapidly hydrolyzed (half-life, 11 minutes) and releases free cyanide, which normally is converted quickly to thiocyanate by rhodanese enzymes in the liver and blood vessels. Cardiopulmonary bypass–associated free hemoglobin release accelerates the release of free cyanide and may increase the risk for cyanide toxicity.

A. Acute cyanide poisoning (p 208) may occur with short-term high-dose nitroprusside infusions (eg, >10–15 mcg/kg/min for ≥1 hour).

B. Thiocyanate is eliminated by the kidneys and may accumulate in patients with renal insufficiency, especially after prolonged infusions.

II. Toxic dose. The toxic dose depends on renal function and the rate of infusion.

A. Clinical cyanide poisoning is uncommon at nitroprusside infusion rates of less than 8–10 mcg/kg/min, but a dose of 2 mcg/kg/min has been used as a threshold for possible cyanide toxicity. One study in children receiving nitroprusside after cardiac surgery found that a dose of 1.8 mcg/kg/min or greater predicted elevated blood cyanide levels, although not necessarily clinical toxicity.

B. Thiocyanate toxicity does not occur with acute brief use in persons with normal renal function but may result from prolonged infusions (eg, >3 mcg/kg/min for ≥48 hours), especially in persons with renal insufficiency (with rates as low as 1 mcg/kg/min).

III. Clinical presentation. The most common adverse effect of nitroprusside is hypotension, which often is accompanied by reflex tachycardia. Peripheral and cerebral hypoperfusion can lead to lactic acidosis and altered mental status.

A. Cyanide poisoning may be accompanied by headache, dizziness, nausea, vomiting, anxiety, agitation, delirium, psychosis, tachypnea, tachycardia, hypotension, loss of consciousness, seizures, and metabolic acidosis. ECG may reveal ischemic patterns.

B. Thiocyanate accumulation causes somnolence, confusion, delirium, tremor, and hyperreflexia. Seizures and coma may rarely occur with severe toxicity.

C. Methemoglobinemia occurs rarely and is usually mild.

IV. Diagnosis. Lactic acidosis, altered mental status, or seizures during short-term high-dose nitroprusside infusion should suggest cyanide poisoning, whereas confusion or delirium developing gradually after several days of continuous use should suggest thiocyanate poisoning.

A. **Specific levels.** Cyanide levels may be obtained but are not usually available rapidly enough to guide treatment when cyanide poisoning is suspected. Cyanide levels may not reflect toxicity accurately because of simultaneous production of methemoglobin, which binds some of the cyanide. Whole-blood cyanide levels higher than 0.5 mg/L are considered elevated, and levels higher than 1 mg/L usually produce lactic acidosis. **Thiocyanate** levels higher than 50–100 mg/L may cause delirium and somnolence.

B. **Other useful laboratory studies** include electrolytes, glucose, BUN, creatinine, serum lactate, ECG, arterial blood gases and measured arterial and venous oxygen saturation (see "Cyanide," p 208), and methemoglobin level (with use of a co-oximeter).

V. **Treatment**

A. **Emergency and supportive measures**

1. Maintain an open airway and assist ventilation if necessary (pp 1–7). Administer supplemental oxygen.
2. For hypotension, stop the infusion immediately and administer IV fluids and pressors if necessary (p 15).

B. **Specific drugs and antidotes.** If cyanide poisoning is suspected, administer **sodium thiosulfate** (p 629). Sodium nitrite treatment may aggravate hypotension and should not be used. **Hydroxocobalamin** (p 563), 25-mg/h IV infusion, sometimes is co-administered with high-dose nitroprusside as prophylaxis against cyanide toxicity.

C. **Decontamination.** These procedures are not relevant because the drug is administered only parenterally.

D. **Enhanced elimination.** Nitroprusside and cyanide are both metabolized rapidly, so there is no need to consider enhanced elimination for them. Hemodialysis may accelerate **thiocyanate** elimination and is especially useful in patients with renal failure.

► NITROUS OXIDE

Aaron Schneir, MD

Nitrous oxide, or laughing gas, is used as an adjuvant for general anesthesia, an anesthetic and analgesic agent for minor procedures, and a propellant in many commercial products, such as whipped cream and cooking oil spray. ("Whippets" are small cartridges of nitrous oxide that can be purchased at restaurant supply stores, grocery convenience stores, and "head shops.") Nitrous oxide is used by many US dentists, in some cases without adequate scavenging equipment. Abuse of nitrous oxide is not uncommon in the medical and dental professions.

I. **Mechanism of toxicity**

A. **Acute toxicity** after exposure to nitrous oxide is caused mainly by asphyxia if adequate oxygen is not supplied with the gas.

B. **Chronic toxicity** to the hematologic and nervous systems results from inactivation of vitamin B_{12} after irreversible oxidation of its cobalt atom. Vitamin B_{12} is required for the synthesis of methionine from homocysteine and for the production of tetrahydrofolate. Methionine is essential for myelin production, and tetrahydrofolate is essential for DNA synthesis. Use of nitrous oxide can precipitate neurologic symptoms in patients with subclinical B_{12} or folic acid deficiency.

C. **Adverse reproductive** outcomes have been reported in workers chronically exposed to nitrous oxide.

II. **Toxic dose.** The toxic dose is not established. Chronic occupational exposure to 2,000 ppm nitrous oxide produced asymptomatic but measurable depression of vitamin B_{12} in dentists. The ACGIH-recommended workplace exposure limit (TLV-TWA) is 50 ppm (90 mg/m^3) as an 8-hour time-weighted average.

III. Clinical presentation

A. Signs of **acute toxicity** are related to **asphyxia,** and include headache, dizziness, confusion, syncope, seizures, and cardiac arrhythmias. Interstitial emphysema and pneumomediastinum have been reported after forceful inhalation from a pressurized whipped cream dispenser.

B. Chronic nitrous oxide abuse may produce megaloblastic anemia, thrombocytopenia, leukopenia, peripheral neuropathy, and myelopathy (especially posterior column findings), similar to the effects of vitamin B_{12} deficiency. Symptoms of neuropathy (eg, ataxia) are often the presenting complaints and physical examination may reveal abnormal vibratory sensation and proprioception.

IV. Diagnosis is based on a history of exposure and clinical presentation (eg, evidence of asphyxia and an empty can or tank). It also should be considered in a patient with manifestations suggesting chronic vitamin B_{12} deficiency but with normal vitamin B_{12} levels.

A. Specific levels. Specific levels are not generally available and are unreliable owing to off-gassing.

B. Other useful laboratory studies include CBC with manual differential, vitamin B_{12}, folic acid, nerve conduction studies, and MRI if the patient has neuropathy. Elevated homocysteine and methylmalonic acid levels have been documented in nitrous oxide abusers who had normal vitamin B_{12} levels.

V. Treatment

A. Emergency and supportive measures

1. Maintain an open airway and assist ventilation if necessary (see pp 1–7). Administer high-flow supplemental oxygen.
2. After significant asphyxia, anticipate and treat coma (see p 18), seizures (p 23), and cardiac arrhythmias (pp 10–15).

B. Specific drugs and antidotes. Chronic effects may resolve over 2–3 months after discontinuation of exposure. Vitamin B_{12} and folinic acid supplementation is indicated to correct underlying deficiencies. Successful treatment with methionine has been reported.

C. Decontamination. Remove victims from exposure and give supplemental oxygen if available.

D. Enhanced elimination. These procedures are not effective.

▶ NONSTEROIDAL ANTI-INFLAMMATORY DRUGS

Craig Smollin, MD

The nonsteroidal anti-inflammatory drugs (NSAIDs) are a chemically diverse group of agents that have similar pharmacologic properties and are widely used for their anti-inflammatory, antipyretic, and analgesic properties (Table II–43). Overdose by most of the agents in this group usually produces only mild GI upset. However, toxicity may be more severe after overdose with **oxyphenbutazone, phenylbutazone, mefenamic acid, piroxicam,** or **diflunisal.**

I. Mechanism of toxicity

A. NSAIDs produce their pharmacologic and most toxicologic effects by inhibiting the enzyme cyclooxygenase (isoforms COX-1 and COX-2); this results in decreased production of prostaglandins and decreased pain and inflammation. Central nervous system, hemodynamic, pulmonary, and hepatic dysfunction also occurs with some agents, but the relationship to prostaglandin production remains uncertain. Prostaglandins are also involved in maintaining the integrity of the gastric mucosa and regulating renal blood flow; thus, acute or chronic intoxication may affect these organs.

TABLE II–43. NSAIDs

Drug	Maximum Daily Adult Dose (mg)	Half-life (h)	Comments
Carboxylic acids			
Bromfenac sodium	150	1–2	Chronic use associated with severe liver injury.
Carprofen	4 mg/kg (PO or SC)	4–10 (PO) 12 (IV)	Approved for use in dogs only.
Diclofenac	200	2	
Diflunisal	1,500	8–12	Overdose produces toxicity resembling salicylate poisoning
Etodolac	1,000	7	
Fenoprofen	3,200	3	Acute renal failure.
Ibuprofen[a]	3,200	2–4	Massive overdose may cause coma, renal failure, metabolic acidosis, and cardiorespiratory depression.
Indomethacin	200	3–11	
Ketoprofen	300	2–4	Large overdoses may cause respiratory depression, coma, and seizures.
Ketorolac	40 (PO) 60–120 (IV)	4–6	High risk for renal failure.
Meclofenamate	400	1–3	
Mefenamic acid	1,000	2	Seizures, twitching.
Naproxen[a]	1,500	12–17	Seizures, acidosis.
Oxaprozin	1,800	42–50	
Sulindac	400	7–16	Extensive enterohepatic recirculation.
Tolmetin	1,800	1	
Enolic acids			
Nabumetone	2,000	24	
Oxyphenbutazone	600	27–64	Seizures, acidosis.
Phenylbutazone	600	50–100	Seizures, acidosis.
Piroxicam	20	45–50	Seizures, coma.
Meloxicam	15	15–20	
COX-2 inhibitors			
Celecoxib	400	11	
Rofecoxib	50	17	Removed from US market owing to concern for increased risk for cardiovascular events.
Valdecoxib	40	8–11	Removed from US market in 2005 owing to concern for increased risk for cardiovascular events and serious skin reactions.

[a]Currently available in the United States as nonprescription formulations.

B. The newest generation of NSAIDs, known as the COX-2 inhibitors, selectively inhibit the COX-2 isoform, with no COX-1 inhibition at therapeutic doses. Because COX-1 is involved in GI mucosal protection, the likelihood of GI bleeding is less with these drugs than with conventional NSAIDs. However, COX-2 selective inhibitors have been associated with an increased risk of cardiovascular disease (both rofecoxib and valdecoxib were voluntarily withdrawn from the US market in 2004 for this reason).

C. **Pharmacokinetics.** NSAIDs are generally well absorbed, and volumes of distribution are relatively small (eg, 0.15 L/kg for ibuprofen). COX-2 inhibitors have larger volumes of distribution (eg, 400 L for celecoxib). Most of these agents are highly protein bound, and most are eliminated through hepatic metabolism and renal excretion, with variable half-lives (eg, 1.5–2.5 hours for ibuprofen and 12–17 hours for naproxen; see also Table II–66, p 462).

II. **Toxic dose.** Human data are insufficient to establish a reliable correlation between amount ingested, plasma concentrations, and clinical toxic effects. Generally, significant symptoms occur after ingestion of more than 5–10 times the usual therapeutic dose.

III. **Clinical presentation.** In general, patients with NSAID overdose are asymptomatic or have mild GI upset (nausea, vomiting, abdominal pain, sometimes hematemesis). Occasionally, patients exhibit drowsiness, lethargy, ataxia, nystagmus, tinnitus, and disorientation.

A. With the more toxic agents **oxyphenbutazone, phenylbutazone, mefenamic acid,** and **piroxicam** and with massive **ibuprofen** or **fenoprofen** overdose, seizures, coma, renal failure, and cardiorespiratory arrest may occur. Hepatic dysfunction, hypoprothrombinemia, and metabolic acidosis are also reported.

B. **Diflunisal** overdose produces toxicity resembling salicylate poisoning (p 410).

C. Chronic use of **bromfenac** for more than 10 days has resulted in fatal hepatotoxicity.

D. **Phenylbutazone** and **antipyrine** use has been associated with agranulocytosis and other blood dyscrasias.

E. There is limited information regarding overdoses of COX-2 inhibitors. Rofecoxib and valdecoxib were removed from the US market because of concerns about increased risk for cardiovascular events (including myocardial infarctions and strokes). There was also an increased risk for serious skin reactions with valdecoxib.

IV. **Diagnosis** usually is based primarily on a history of ingestion of NSAIDs because symptoms are mild and nonspecific, and quantitative levels are not usually available.

A. **Specific levels** are not usually readily available and do not contribute to clinical management.

B. **Other useful laboratory studies** include CBC, electrolytes, glucose, BUN, creatinine, liver aminotransferases, prothrombin time (PT/INR), acetaminophen level, and urinalysis.

V. **Treatment**

A. **Emergency and supportive measures**

1. Maintain an open airway and assist ventilation if necessary (pp 1–7). Administer supplemental oxygen.
2. Treat seizures (p 23), coma (p 18), and hypotension (p 15) if they occur.
3. Antacids may be used for mild GI upset. Replace fluid losses with IV crystalloid solutions.

B. **Specific drugs and antidotes.** There is no antidote. Vitamin K (p 633) may be used for patients with elevated prothrombin time caused by hypoprothrombinemia.

C. **Decontamination** (p 50). Administer activated charcoal orally if conditions are appropriate (see Table I–38, p 54). Gastric lavage is not necessary after small-to-moderate ingestions if activated charcoal can be given promptly.

D. **Enhanced elimination.** NSAIDs are highly protein bound and extensively metabolized. Thus, hemodialysis, peritoneal dialysis, and forced diuresis are not likely to be effective.

1. **Charcoal hemoperfusion** may be effective for **phenylbutazone** overdose, although there are limited clinical data to support its use and the procedure is not widely available.

2. Repeat-dose activated charcoal therapy may enhance the elimination of meloxicam, oxyphenbutazone, phenylbutazone, and piroxicam.
3. Repeated oral doses of cholestyramine have been reported to increase the clearance of meloxicam and piroxicam.

▶ NONTOXIC OR MINIMALLY TOXIC HOUSEHOLD PRODUCTS

Eileen Morentz and Jay Schrader

A variety of products commonly found around the home are completely nontoxic or cause little or no toxicity after typical accidental exposures. Treatment is rarely required because the ingredients are not toxic, the concentrations of potentially toxic ingredients are minimal, or the construction or packaging of the product is such that a significant dose of a harmful ingredient is extremely unlikely.

Table II–44 lists a number of products considered nontoxic. However, the taste or texture of the product may be disagreeable or cause mild stomach upset. Also, some of the products listed can create a foreign-body effect or a choking hazard, depending on the formulation and the age of the child. Table II–45 provides examples of products that may cause mild GI upset but are generally not considered toxic after small ingestions. Stomach cramps, vomiting, or diarrhea may occur, but each of these is usually mild and self-limited. Table II–46 lists several other products that often are

TABLE II–44. NONTOXIC OR MINIMALLY TOXIC PRODUCTS[a]

Air fresheners	Diapers, disposable	Plastic
Aluminum foil	Erasers	Playdoh
Antiperspirants	Eye makeup	Putty
Ashes, wood/fireplace	Felt tip markers and pens	Rouge
Aspartame	Fingernail polish (dry)	Rust
Baby lotion (***Note:*** Baby oil can cause aspiration pneumonitis; see p 266.)	Glitter	Saccharin
Baby powder (without talc)	Glow stick/jewelry	Shellac (dry)
Baby wipes	Gum	Sheetrock
Ballpoint pen ink	Gypsum	Shoe polish
Calamine lotion	Incense	Silica gel
Candles	Indelible markers	Silly putty
Chalk[b]	Ink (without aniline dyes)	Soil
Charcoal	Kitty litter	Stamp pad ink
Charcoal briquettes	Lip balm	Starch
Cigarette ashes	Lipstick	Styrofoam
Cigarette filter tips (unsmoked)	Magic markers	Superglue
Clay	Makeup	Teething rings
Cold packs (for large ingestions, see "Nitrates," p 339)	Mascara	Thermometers (phthalates/alcohol, gallium)
Crayons	Matches (<3 paper books)	Wall board
Cyanoacrylate glues	Mylar balloons	Watercolor paints
Deodorants	Newspaper	Wax
Desiccants	Paraffin	Zinc oxide ointment
	Pencils (contain graphite, not lead)	
	Photographs	
	Plaster	

[a]These items are virtually nontoxic in small-to-moderate exposures. However, the taste or texture of the product may result in mild stomach upset. In addition, some of the products may cause a foreign-body effect or choking hazard, depending on the size of the product and the age of the child.
[b]Plain drawing chalk. (Old pool-cue chalk may contain lead. "Chinese chalk" contains pyrethrins.)

TABLE II–45. MILD GASTROINTESTINAL IRRITANTS[a]

A & D Ointment	Corticosteroids	Lanolin
Antacids	Dishwashing liquid soaps (not electric dishwasher type)	Latex paint
Antibiotic ointments	Fabric softeners	Liquid soaps
Baby bath	Fertilizers (nitrogen, phosphoric acid, and potash)	Miconazole
Baby shampoo	Glycerin	Petroleum jelly
Bar soap	Guaifenesin	Plant food
Bath oil beads	Hair shampoos	Prednisone
Bleach (household, <6% hypochlorite)	Hand soaps	Shaving cream
Body lotions and creams	Hydrocortisone cream	Simethicone
Bubble bath	Hydrogen peroxide 3%	Spermicides (nonoxynol-9 <10%)
Bubbles	Kaolin	Steroid creams
Carbamide peroxide 6.5%	Lactase	Sunscreen/suntan lotions (allergic reactions possible)
Chalk (calcium carbonate)		Toothpaste (without fluoride)
Clotrimazole cream		

[a]The items in this list usually have little or no effect in small ingestions. In moderate-to-large ingestions, gastrointestinal effects such as diarrhea, constipation, stomach cramps, and vomiting may occur. The effects are usually mild and rarely require medical intervention.

TABLE II–46. OTHER LOW-TOXICITY PRODUCTS[a]

Products	Comments
Holiday hazards	
Angel hair	Finely spun glass. Dermal or ocular irritation or corneal abrasion is possible.
Bubble lights	May contain a tiny amount of methylene chloride.
Christmas tree ornaments	Can cause foreign-body effect or choking hazard. Antique or foreign-made ornaments may be decorated with lead-based paint.
Christmas tree preservatives	Homemade solutions may contain aspirin, bleach, or sugar. Commercial products usually contain only concentrated sugar solution.
Easter egg dyes	Most of these contain nontoxic dyes and sodium bicarbonate. Older formulations may contain sodium chloride, which can cause hypernatremia if a large amount is ingested (p 37).
Fireplace crystals	May contain salts of copper, selenium, arsenic, and antimony. Small amounts can cause irritation to the mouth or stomach. (Larger ingestions could conceivably result in heavy metal poisoning; see specific heavy metal.)
Halloween candy	Tampering rarely occurs. Radiograph of candy provides a false sense of security; although it may reveal radiopaque glass or metallic objects, most poisons are radiolucent. Prudent approach is to discard candy or food items if they are not commercially packaged or if the package is damaged.
Snow scenes	The "snow" is composed of insoluble particles of calcium carbonate that are not toxic. The fluid may have bacterial growth.
Snow sprays	Sprays may contain hydrocarbon solvent or a methylene chloride (pp 266 and 323) vehicle. Inhalation may cause headache and nausea. Once dried, the snow is not toxic.

(continued)

TABLE II–46. OTHER LOW-TOXICITY PRODUCTS[a] (CONTINUED)

Products	Comments
Miscellaneous	
Capsaicin sprays	These products contain capsaicin, the main ingredient in chili peppers. Exposure causes intense mucous membrane irritation and a burning sensation. Treat with topical liquid antacids.
Cyanoacrylate glues	Ingestion is harmless. Cyanide is not released. Corneal abrasions may occur after ocular exposure. Adhesion of skin and eyelids is possible after dermal exposure. Treat adhesions with petrolatum-based ointment.
Fire extinguishers	The two common types contain sodium bicarbonate (white powder) or monoammonium phosphate (yellow powder). Small ingestions result in little to no effect. Mucous membrane irritation is common. Major risk is pneumonitis after extensive inhalation.
Fluorescent light bulbs	Contain inert gases and nontoxic powder that may be irritating to mucous membranes.
Oral contraceptives	Birth control pills contain varying amounts of estrogens and progesterones. In excessive amounts, these may cause stomach upset and in females transient vaginal spotting. Some formulations may contain iron.
Thermometers (mercury)	Household fever thermometers contain less than 0.5 mL of liquid mercury, which is harmless if swallowed. Clean up cautiously to avoid dispersing mercury as mist or vapor (ie, do not vacuum).
Household pesticides	Numerous formulations. Some contain hydrocarbon solvents; others are water-based. Pesticides used may include pyrethrins, organophosphates, or carbamates, but generally of low potency and in concentrations of less than 1.5%. The risk for pesticide poisoning is very low unless there is intentional massive exposure. Symptoms after exposure are due mainly to inhalation of the hydrocarbon solvent
Topical monthly flea control products	Formulations include fipronil and imidacloprid. Low oral toxicity after ingestion of less than 2–3 mL. Dermal and ocular irritation may occur.
Respiratory irritants	
Baby powders (talc containing), spray starch	These products have little or no toxicity when ingested. However, if aspirated into the lungs, they can cause an inflammatory pneumonitis.

[a]These products may contain small amounts of potentially toxic ingredients but rarely cause problems because of the small concentrations or conditions of exposure.

ingested by small children with minimal effect. Although they may contain potentially toxic ingredients, the concentration or packaging makes it very unlikely that symptoms will occur after a small exposure.

In all cases involving exposures to these substances, attempt to confirm the identity and/or ingredients of the product and ensure that no other, more toxic products were involved. Determine whether there are any unexpected symptoms or evidence of choking or foreign-body effect. Advise the parent that mild GI upset may occur. Water or another liquid may be given to reduce the taste or texture of the product. For symptomatic eye exposures, follow the instructions for ocular decontamination (p 51).

► OPIATES AND OPIOIDS

Timothy E. Albertson, MD, MPH, PhD

Opiates are a group of naturally occurring compounds derived from the juice of the poppy *Papaver somniferum.* Morphine and codeine are classic opiate derivatives used widely in medicine; heroin (diacetylmorphine) is a well-known semi-synthetic, highly addictive street narcotic. The term *opioid* refers to opiates and semi-synthetic derivatives of naturally occurring opium (eg, morphine, heroin, codeine, and hydrocodone) as well as new, totally synthetic opiate analogs (eg, fentanyl, butorphanol, meperidine, and methadone [Table II–47]). A wide variety of prescription medications contain opioids, often in combination with aspirin or acetaminophen. **Dextromethorphan** (p 215) is an opioid derivative with potent antitussive but no analgesic or addictive properties. **Tramadol** (Ultram) is an analgesic that is unrelated chemically to the opiates but acts on mu-opioid receptors and blocks serotonin reuptake. **Butorphanol** is available as a nasal spray with rapid absorption. **Buprenorphine** is a partial opioid agonist that is approved for the treatment of opioid addiction. **Suboxone** is a sublingual tablet containing buprenorphine plus naloxone to reduce intravenous abuse. **Tapentadol**

TABLE II–47. OPIATES AND OPIOIDS[a]

Drug	Type of Activity	Usual Adult Dose[a] (mg)	Elimination Half-life (h)	Duration of Analgesia (h)
Buprenorphine	Agonist[b]	2–8	20–70	24–48
Butorphanol	Mixed	2	5–6	3–4
Codeine	Agonist	60	2–4	4–6
Fentanyl	Agonist	0.2	1–5	0.5–2
Heroin[c]	Agonist	4	N/A[c]	3–4
Hydrocodone	Agonist	5	3–4	4–8
Hydromorphone	Agonist	1.5	1–4	4–5
Loperamide	Agonist	4–16	9–14	Unknown
Meperidine	Agonist[d]	100	2–5	2–4
Methadone	Agonist	10	20–30	4–8[e]
Morphine	Agonist	10	2–4	3–6[f]
Nalbuphine	Mixed	10	5	3–6
Oxycodone	Agonist	4.5	2–5	4–6[f]
Oxymorphone	Agonist	1–10	7–11	3–6[f]
Pentazocine	Mixed	50	2–3	2–3
Propoxyphene[g]	Agonist	100	6–12	4–6
Tapentadol	Agonist[h]	50–100	4	4–6
Tramadol	Agonist[d]	50–100	6–7.5	4–6

[a]Usual dose: dose equivalent to 10 mg of morphine.
[b]Partial agonist that slowly dissociates from mu-opioid receptor.
[c]Rapidly hydrolyzed to 6-acetylmorphine and morphine.
[d]Also inhibits serotonin reuptake.
[e]Sedation and coma may last 2–3 days.
[f]Longer durations of analgesia seen with slow-release products.
[g]Discontinued by the FDA.
[h]Also blocks norepinephrine reuptake.

(Nucynta) is a mu-opioid agonist that also inhibits the reuptake of norepinephrine. The alkaloid mitragynine is the active component of **kratom** found in the Southeast Asian tree *Mitragyna speciosa Kroth*; it has stimulant and opioid-like effects, and has been used for self-treatment of opioid withdrawal.

I. Mechanism of toxicity

A. In general, opioids share the ability to stimulate a number of specific opiate receptors in the CNS, causing sedation and respiratory depression. Death results from respiratory failure, usually as a result of apnea or pulmonary aspiration of gastric contents. In addition, acute noncardiogenic pulmonary edema may occur by unknown mechanisms. In addition to its opioid-like effects, kratom may also stimulate postsynaptic alpha-2 adrenergic and serotonergic ($5HT_{2A}$) receptors.

B. Pharmacokinetics. Usually, peak effects occur within 2–3 hours, but absorption may be slowed by the pharmacologic effects of opioids on GI motility. Slow-release preparations of morphine (eg, MS Contin), oxymorphone (eg, Opana ER) or oxycodone (eg, OxyContin) may have a delayed onset of action and prolonged effects. With fentanyl patches, dermal absorption can continue even after removal. Smoking or ingesting fentanyl patches can result in rapid and high levels. Most of these drugs have large volumes of distribution (3–5 L/kg). The rate of elimination is highly variable, from 1 to 2 hours for fentanyl derivatives to 15–30 hours for methadone (see also Tables II–47 and II–66). Some patients have been found to be rapid metabolizers of codeine (to morphine through the hepatic enzyme CYP2D6), which may increase the risk for acute intoxication.

II. Toxic dose. The toxic dose varies widely, depending on the specific compound, the route and rate of administration, and tolerance to the effects of the drug as a result of chronic use. Some newer fentanyl derivatives have potency up to 2,000 times that of morphine.

III. Clinical presentation

A. With mild or moderate overdose, lethargy is common. The pupils are usually small, often of "pinpoint" size. Blood pressure and pulse rate are decreased, bowel sounds are diminished, and the muscles are usually flaccid.

B. With higher doses, coma is accompanied by respiratory depression, and apnea often results in sudden death. Noncardiogenic pulmonary edema may occur, often after resuscitation and administration of the opiate antagonist naloxone.

C. Seizures are not common after opioid overdose but occur occasionally with certain compounds (eg, codeine, dextromethorphan, kratom, meperidine, methadone, propoxyphene, and tramadol). Seizures may occur in patients with renal compromise who receive repeated doses of meperidine owing to accumulation of the metabolite normeperidine.

D. A leukoencephalopathy with typical magnetic resonance imaging (MRI) changes has been reported in some heroin smokers ("chasing the dragon").

E. Cardiotoxicity similar to that seen with tricyclic antidepressants (p 107) and quinidine (p 398) can occur in patients with severe **propoxyphene** intoxication. Prolonged QTc intervals and torsade de pointes have been reported with **methadone** and may account for some of the sudden deaths associated with its use. The *R*-enantiomer of methadone is apparently more active at the mu receptor and less likely to affect the hERG channel (and thus the QTc interval) compared with the *S*-enantiomer.

F. Some newer synthetic opioids have mixed agonist and antagonist effects, with unpredictable results in overdose. **Buprenorphine** causes less maximal opioid effect than morphine does, and because of strong binding to opioid receptors it can cause acute withdrawal symptoms in persons on high doses of conventional opioids.

G. Opioid **withdrawal syndrome** can cause anxiety, piloerection (goose bumps), heightened sensation of pain, abdominal cramps and diarrhea, and insomnia.

IV. Diagnosis is simple when typical manifestations of opiate intoxication are present (pinpoint pupils and respiratory and CNS depression) and is confirmed when the patient quickly awakens after administration of naloxone. Signs of intravenous drug abuse (eg, needle track marks) may be present.

A. Specific levels are not usually performed because of poor correlation with clinical effects. Qualitative screening of the urine is an effective way to confirm recent use (codeine, morphine, hydrocodone, hydromorphone). Fentanyl derivatives, tramadol, and some other synthetic opioids are not detected by routine toxicologic screens (see Table I–31, p 45). Separate immunoassays are available for oxycodone/oxymorphone and 6-acetylmorphine (heroin-specific metabolite).

B. Other useful laboratory studies include electrolytes, glucose, arterial blood gases or oximetry, chest radiography, and stat serum acetaminophen or salicylate levels (if the ingested overdose was of a combination product.)

C. Genetic polymorphisms. Individuals who are ultra-rapid metabolizers for CYP2D6 (eg, *1 gene duplication) are at risk for morphine toxicity at therapeutic codeine doses. CYP 2D6 tests are available through reference laboratories.

V. Treatment

A. Emergency and supportive measures

1. Maintain an open airway and assist ventilation if necessary (pp 1–7). Administer supplemental oxygen.
2. Treat coma (p 18), seizures (p 23), hypotension (p 15), ventricular arrhythmias (p 13) and noncardiogenic pulmonary edema (p 7) if they occur.

B. Specific drugs and antidotes

1. **Naloxone** (p 584) is a specific opioid antagonist with no agonist properties of its own; large doses may be given safely.
   a. As little as 0.2–0.4 mg IV or IM is usually effective for heroin overdose. Repeat doses every 2–3 minutes if there is no response, up to a total dose of 10–20 mg if an opioid overdose is strongly suspected. Intranasal naloxone is effective but not as effective as IM naloxone in the prehospital setting
   b. ***Caution:*** The duration of effect of naloxone (1–2 hours) is shorter than that of many opioids. Therefore, do not release a patient who has awakened after naloxone treatment until at least 3–4 hours has passed since the last dose of naloxone. In general, if naloxone was required to reverse opioid-induced coma, it is safer to admit the patient for at least 6–12 hours of observation.
2. **Nalmefene** (p 584) is an opioid antagonist with a longer duration of effect (3–5 hours).
   a. Nalmefene may be given in doses of 0.1–2 mg IV, with repeated doses of up to 10–20 mg if an opioid overdose is strongly suspected.
   b. ***Caution:*** Although the duration of effect of nalmefene is longer than that of naloxone, it is still much shorter than that of methadone. If a methadone overdose is suspected, the patient should be observed for at least 8–12 hours after the last dose of nalmefene.
3. **Sodium bicarbonate** (p 520) may be effective for QRS-interval prolongation or hypotension associated with propoxyphene poisoning.

C. Decontamination (p 50). Administer activated charcoal orally if conditions are appropriate (see Table I–38, p 54). Gastric lavage is not necessary after small-to-moderate ingestions if activated charcoal can be given promptly. Consider whole-bowel irrigation after ingestion of sustained-release products (eg, MS Contin, OxyContin, Opana ER).

D. Enhanced elimination. Because of the very large volumes of distribution of the opioids and the availability of an effective antidotal treatment, there is no role for enhanced elimination procedures.

▶ ORGANOPHOSPHORUS AND CARBAMATE INSECTICIDES

Rais Vohra, MD

Organophosphorus (OP) compounds and carbamates, also known as *cholinesterase inhibitors,* are widely used pesticides. These agents, which comprise thousands of structurally related substances, are responsible for a large number of suicidal or accidental poisonings, with the greatest mortality (an estimated 200,000 deaths per year) in rural areas of developing countries.

During the 1930s, German military scientists synthesized numerous OP compounds, including parathion and several highly potent **chemical warfare agents** (eg, GA [tabun], GB [sarin], and GD [soman]; see p 452 and Table II–64). Because these chemical weapons affect the autonomic nervous system, they are sometimes referred to as "nerve agents." Terrorist attacks in Japan (1994 and 1995) affected thousands of urban civilians who were exposed to the OP compound sarin. Accidental poisoning with cholinesterase inhibitors can also occur from the contamination of food or beverages.

Carbamates, although less deadly than OP agents, are used frequently as pesticides, fungicides, herbicides, rodenticides, and medications (eg, pyridostigmine) to treat neurologic disorders such as myasthenia gravis.

I. Mechanism of toxicity

A. Organophosphorus compounds inhibit two enzymes: acetylcholinesterase (AChE), found in synaptic junctions and in red blood cells (RBCs), and butyrylcholinesterase, also known as pseudocholinesterase (PChE) or plasma cholinesterase, found in the blood. Each of these enzymes breaks down acetylcholine.

1. Blockade of AChE is the most clinically significant effect of OPs and carbamates because this leads to the accumulation of excessive amounts of acetylcholine at muscarinic receptors (found on various cholinergic secretory cells), at nicotinic receptors (located on skeletal neuromuscular junctions and autonomic ganglia), and in the CNS.
2. Permanent inhibition of AChE ("**aging**") may occur when there is covalent binding by the OP to the enzyme. The rate of aging is highly variable, from several minutes to days, depending on the route of exposure as well as the specific OP. Dimethyl OP compounds (eg, dimethoate) generally age more quickly than diethyl agents (eg, chlorpyrifos), and lipophilic OP compounds can be released into the systemic circulation from fat stores for many days to weeks following exposure, prolonging both the duration of clinical toxicity and the aging window. Antidotal treatment with an oxime (see "Pralidoxime," p 613) is considered beneficial only if administered before aging occurs.

B. Carbamates also inhibit the AChEs and lead to accumulation of acetylcholine, with similar acute clinical effects.

1. CNS effects from carbamates are often less pronounced because they have more difficulty crossing the blood–brain barrier.
2. Carbamates do not "age" the AChE enzyme, and toxicity is usually more brief and self-limited than with the OP compounds.
3. Patients with myasthenia gravis and related neurologic disorders may be at increased risk for carbamate-induced cholinergic toxicity because they are frequently prescribed the carbamate **pyridostigmine** or related "-stigmine" compounds.
4. **Aldicarb** is relatively more potent and is translocated systemically by certain plants (eg, melons) and concentrated in their fruit. An acute outbreak of poisoning occurred in California in 1985 after ingestion of watermelons that had been grown in a field previously sprayed with aldicarb. The use of an imported rodenticide (Tres Pasitos, "three little steps") led to an epidemic of aldicarb poisoning in New York in 1994–1997.

C. In addition, the effects of the **hydrocarbon solvents** in which these compounds are frequently formulated (eg, **xylene, cyclohexanone, naphtha**) must also be considered in evaluating the clinical toxicity from these compounds.

D. **Pharmacokinetics.** Signs and symptoms of acute OP poisoning may be immediate or delayed several hours, depending on the agent, route, co-ingested toxins, and degree of exposure. Most OPs and carbamates can be absorbed by any route: inhalation, ingestion, or absorption through the skin. **Highly lipophilic organophosphates** (disulfoton, fenthion, and others) are stored in fat tissue, with the potential to cause prolonged toxicity. The severity and tempo of intoxication are also affected by the rate of exposure (acute vs. chronic), the ongoing metabolic degradation and elimination of the agent, and, for some OP compounds (eg, malathion, parathion), the rate of metabolism to their clinically active "oxon" derivatives.

II. **Toxic dose.** There is a wide spectrum of relative potency of the OP and carbamate compounds (Tables II–48, II–49, and II–50).

TABLE II–48. ORGANOPHOSPHORUS AND CARBAMATE PESTICIDES

Agent	CAS Number	Chemical Structure[a]	WHO Classification[b]	GHS Classification[c]
Acephate	30560-19-1	OP (diM)	II	4
Alanycarb	83130-01-2	C	II	4
Aldicarb	116-06-3	C	Ia	1
Anilofos	64249-01-0	OP (diM)	II	4
Azamethiphos	35575-96-3	OP (diM)	II	4
Azinphos-methyl	86-50-0	OP (dM)	Ib	2
Azinphos-ethyl	2642-71-9	OP (diE)	Ib	2
Bendiocarb	22781-23-3	C	II	3
Benfuracarb	82560-54-1	C	II	3
Bensulide	741-58-2	OP	II	3
Butamifos	36335-67-8	OP	II	4
Butocarboxim	34681-10-2	C	Ib	3
Butoxycarboxim	34681-23-7	C	Ib	3
Cadusafos	95465-99-9	OP	Ib	2
Carbetamide	16118-49-3	C	U	5
Carbaryl	63-25-2	C	II	3
Carbofuran	1563-66-2	C	Ib	1
Carbosulfan	55285-14-8	C	II	3
Chlorethoxyfos	54593-83-8	OP (diE)	Ia	1
Chlorfenvinphos	470-90-6	OP (diE)	Ib	2
Chlormephos	24934-91-6	OP (diE)	Ia	2
Chlorpropham	101-21-3	C	U	5
Chlorpyrifos	2921-88-2	OP (diE)	II	3
Chlorpyrifos-methyl	5598-13-0	OP (diM)	III	5
Coumaphos	56-72-4	OP (diE)	Ib	2
Cyanophos	2636-26-2	OP (diM)	II	4

(continued)

TABLE II–48. ORGANOPHOSPHORUS AND CARBAMATE PESTICIDES (CONTINUED)

Agent	CAS Number	Chemical Structure[a]	WHO Classification[b]	GHS Classification[c]
Demeton-*S*-methyl	919-86-8	OP (diM)	Ib	2
Diazinon	333-41-5	OP (diE)	II	4
Dichlorvos (DDVP)	62-73-7	OP (diM)	Ib	3
Dicrotophos	141-66-2	OP (diM)	Ib	2
Dimethoate	60-51-5	OP (dM)	II	3
Disulfoton	298-04-4	OP (diE)	Ia	1
Edifenphos	17109-49-8	OP	Ib	3
EPN	2104-64-5	OP	Ia	2
Ethiofencarb	29973-13-5	C	Ib	3
Ethion	563-12-2	OP (diE)	II	3
Ethoprophos	13194-48-4	OP	Ia	2
Famphur	52-85-7	OP (diM)	Ib	2
Fenamiphos	22224-92-6	OP	Ib	2
Fenitrothion	122-14-5	OP (diM)	II	4
Fenobucarb	3766-81-2	C	II	4
Fenoxycarb	79127-80-3	C	U	5
Fenthiocarb	62850-32-2	C	II	4
Fenthion	55-38-9	OP (diM)	II	3
Formetanate	22259-30-9	C	Ib	2
Fosamine	25954-13-6	OP	III	5
Furathiocarb	65907-30-4	C	Ib	2
Heptenophos	23560-59-0	OP (diM)	Ib	3
Isoprocarb	2631-40-5	C	II	4
Isoxathion	18854-04-8	OP (diE)	Ib	3
Malathion	121-75-5	OP (diM)	III	5
Mecarbam	2595-54-2	C	Ib	2
Methacrifos	62610-77-9	OP (diM)	II	4
Methamidophos	10265-92-6	OP (diM)	Ib	2
Methidathion	950-37-8	OP (diM)	Ib	2
Methiocarb	2032-65-7	C	Ib	2
Methomyl	16752-77-5	C	Ib	2
Metolcarb	1129-41-5	C	II	3
Mevinphos	26718-65-0	OP (diM)	Ia	1
Monocrotophos	6923-22-4	OP (diM)	Ib	2
MPMC (xylylcarb)	2425-10-7	C	II	4
Naled	300-76-5	OP (diM)	II	4
Omethoate	1113-02-6	OP (diM)	Ib	2
Oxamyl	23135-22-0	C	Ib	2

(*continued*)

TABLE II–48. ORGANOPHOSPHORUS AND CARBAMATE PESTICIDES (CONTINUED)

Agent	CAS Number	Chemical Structure[a]	WHO Classification[b]	GHS Classification[c]
Oxydemeton-methyl	301-12-2	OP (diM)	Ib	3
Parathion	56-38-2	OP (diE)	Ia	1
Parathion-methyl	298-00-0	OP (diM)	Ia	1
Phenthoate	2597-03-7	OP (diM)	II	4
Phorate	298-02-2	OP (diE)	Ia	1
Phosalone	2310-17-0	OP (diE)	II	3
Phosmet	732-11-6	OP (diM)	II	3
Phosphamidon	13171-21-6	OP (diM)	Ia	2
Phoxim	14816-18-3	OP (diE)	II	4
Piperophos	24151-93-7	OP	II	4
Pirimicarb	23103-98-2	C	II	3
Primiphos-methyl	29232-93-7	OP	II	4
Profenofos	41198-08-7	OP	II	4
Propetamphos	31218-83-4	OP	Ib	3
Propoxur	114-26-1	C	II	3
Prothiofos	34643-46-4	OP	II	4
Pyraclofos	77458-01-6	OP	II	3
Pyrazophos	13457-18-6	OP (diE)	II	4
Pyridaphenthion	119-12-0	OP (diE)	II	4
Quinalphos	13593-03-8	OP (diE)	II	3
Sulfotep	3689-24-5	OP (diE)	Ia	1
Tebuprimifos	96182-53-5	OP (diE)	Ia	1
Temephos	3383-96-8	OP (diM)	III	5
Terbufos	13071-79-9	OP (diE)	Ia	1
Tetrachlorvinphos	22248-79-9	OP (diM)	III	5
Thiodicarb	59669-26-0	C	II	3
Thiofanox	39196-18-4	C	Ib	2
Thiometon	640-5-3	OP (diM)	Ib	3
Triazophos	24017-47-8	OP (diM)	Ib	3
Trichlorfon	52-68-6	OP (diM)	II	3
Vamidothion	2275-23-2	OP (diM)	Ib	3
XMC (cosban)	2655-14-3	C	II	4

[a]C, carbamate; OP (diM), dimethyl organophosphate; OP (diE), diethyl organophosphate. ***Note:*** Some organophosphates have a chemical structure other than dimethoxy or diethoxy. For example, ethoprophos is a dipropyl compound.
[b]World Health Organization (WHO) Pesticide Classification Scheme (based on oral LD_{50} values in the rat): Class I, extremely or highly hazardous; Class II, moderately hazardous; Class III, slightly hazardous (see Table II–49).
[c]Globally Harmonized System (GHS) for classification and labeling: range of toxicity 1–5, with 1 indicating the most hazardous and 5 indicating the least hazardous based on the best available toxicity (eg, LD_{50}) data (see Table II–50).
Note: The likelihood of serious toxicity depends not only on the dose and type of pesticide but also on the route of exposure, circumstances of the exposure, type of co-ingested solvents, and pre-existing cholinesterase activity. In addition, agents that are highly lipid soluble, such as fenthion and sulfoton, may cause prolonged intoxication.

TABLE II–49. DEFINITION OF WORLD HEALTH ORGANIZATION HAZARD CLASSIFICATION[a]

		LD_{50} for the Rat (mg/kg of body weight)	
WHO Class		Oral	Dermal
Ia	Extremely hazardous	<5	<50
Ib	Highly hazardous	5–50	50–200
II	Moderately hazardous	50–2,000	200–2,000
III	Slightly hazardous	>2,000	>2,000
U	Unlikely to present acute hazard	≥5,000	≥5,000

[a]Reproduced, with permission, from World Health Organization: The WHO Recommended Classification of Pesticides by Hazard and Guidelines to Classification: 2009, p 5. Geneva: World Health Organization; 2010.

III. Clinical presentation. Respiratory failure is a major cause of mortality in patients with acute cholinesterase inhibitor toxicity. Acute clinical manifestations may be classified into muscarinic, nicotinic, and CNS effects (see below), all of which can contribute to respiratory failure. In addition, acute lung injury, pulmonary edema, and chemical pneumonitis due to aspiration of hydrocarbon solvents (p 266) may compound the multiple respiratory derangements that characterize cholinesterase inhibitor poisoning.

A. Muscarinic manifestations include bronchospasm, bradycardia, abdominal pain, vomiting, diarrhea, miosis, and excessive sweating. Fluid losses can result in shock. ***Note:*** Cholinesterase inhibition can produce either bradycardia or tachycardia, and either miosis or mydriasis, as a result of the competing effects of ganglionic stimulation of both parasympathetic and sympathetic pathways.

B. Nicotinic effects are mainly due to acetylcholine excess in skeletal muscles and include muscle weakness and tremors/fasciculations. Respiratory muscle weakness, complicated by bronchorrhea and bronchospasm due to muscarinic effects, can be fatal unless aggressive and timely care is rendered. These effects resemble toxicity from nicotine and related alkaloids (p 337).

C. Central nervous system manifestations include agitation, seizures, and coma. Respiratory center dysfunction can also cause apneic episodes.

D. Late peripheral neuropathy. Some cholinesterase inhibitors may cause a delayed, often permanent peripheral neuropathy affecting the long motor axons of the legs (OP-induced delayed neuropathy, or OPIDN). The mechanism appears to be the result of inhibition of neuropathy target esterase (NTE), an

TABLE II–50. GLOBALLY HARMONIZED SYSTEM CLASSIFICATION[c]

	Oral Classification Criteria		Dermal Classification Criteria	
GHS Category	LD_{50} (mg/kg)[a]	Hazard Statement	LD_{50} (mg/kg)[b]	Hazard Statement
1	<5	Fatal if swallowed	<50	Fatal in contact with skin
2	5–50	Fatal if swallowed	50–200	Fatal in contact with skin
3	50–300	Toxic if swallowed	200–1,000	Toxic in contact with skin
4	300–2,000	Harmful if swallowed	1,000–2,000	Harmful in contact with skin
5	2,000–5,000	May be harmful if swallowed	2,000–5,000	May be harmful in contact with skin

[a]For oral data, the rat is the preferred species, although data from other species may be appropriate when their use is scientifically justified.
[b]For dermal data, the rat or the rabbit is the preferred species, although data from other species may be appropriate when their use is scientifically justified.
[c]Reproduced, with permission, from World Health Organization: The WHO Recommended Classification of Pesticides by Hazard and Guidelines to Classification: 2009, p 10. Geneva: World Health Organization; 2010.

enzyme in nervous tissues distinct from other AChEs. The epidemic outbreak of "ginger jake paralysis" in the 1930s was due to drinking rum contaminated with triorthocresyl phosphate (TOCP). More recent outbreaks have been reported from Asia in which contaminated cooking oils were implicated.

E. **Intermediate syndrome.** Patients can develop proximal motor weakness 2–4 days after exposure, termed "intermediate" because it coincides with resolution of the acute cholinergic crisis but occurs before the period during which delayed peripheral neuropathy typically manifests. Weakness in neck flexion ("broken neck" sign) can progress to bulbar and proximal limb weakness. This syndrome is important to recognize early because fatal respiratory muscle weakness may occur abruptly. Although the pathophysiology of this entity is unclear, the intermediate syndrome is theorized to be a sequela of toxin redistribution (eg, liberation of lipophilic pesticide from fat stores), inadequate oxime therapy, or a complication of cholinergic myopathy. Symptoms may last 1–3 weeks and do not usually respond to additional treatment with oximes or atropine.

F. **Miscellaneous toxic effects** of cholinesterase inhibitor pesticides have been reported in acute or chronic toxicity, with unclear pathophysiologic mechanisms. These relatively rare complications include the Guillain–Barré syndrome, mononeuritis, cognitive-behavioral or choreiform movement disorders, parkinsonian symptoms, glucose abnormalities, metabolic acidosis, acute coronary syndrome, hypotension, pancreatitis, and infertility.

IV. **Diagnosis** is based on the history of exposure and the presence of characteristic muscarinic, nicotinic, and CNS manifestations of acetylcholine excess. In the majority of cases, the most prominent symptoms are due to excessive muscarinic stimulation. (A useful mnemonic for muscarinic toxicity is DUMBBELSS: diarrhea, urinary incontinence, miosis, bronchospasm, bronchorrhea, emesis, lacrimation, salivation, and sweating.) There may be a solvent odor, and some agents have a strong "garlic" odor. A Glasgow Coma Scale (GCS) score of 13 or lower at presentation is considered a poor prognostic indicator. Several other scoring systems for critically ill patients (such as APACHE II Score and Simplified Acute Physiology Score) have also been advocated to help with prediction of clinical outcomes from cholinesterase inhibitor poisoning. Other drugs or toxins that increase cholinergic activity, such as nicotine alkaloids, should be considered in the differential diagnosis.

A. **Specific levels**

1. **Organophosphorus compounds** depress plasma pseudocholinesterase (PChE) and red blood cell acetylcholinesterase (AChE) activities. In emergency practice, these tests are not readily available, nor are they considered central to management. Moreover, because of wide interindividual variability, significant depression of enzyme activity may occur but still fall within the "normal" range. It is most helpful if the patient had a pre-exposure baseline measurement for comparison (eg, as part of a workplace health surveillance program). Proper storage and handling of specimens must be maintained after venipuncture because enzyme activity can continue to be affected by the toxin in vitro or artifactually depressed by fluoride preservatives in certain blood tubes. A point-of-care test for bedside measurement of cholinesterase activity is currently being investigated.

   a. The RBC AChE activity provides a more reliable measure of the toxic effect; a 50% or greater depression in activity from baseline generally indicates a true exposure effect. The level of RBC AChE activity can be altered in patients using oral contraceptive agents or antimalarial drugs, those with pernicious anemia, and infants younger than 4 months of age.

   b. PChE activity is a sensitive indicator of exposure but is not as specific as AChE activity. PChE may be depressed owing to genetic deficiency, pregnancy, medical illness, malnutrition, or chronic OP exposure. PChE activity usually falls before RBC AChE and recovers faster.

2. **Carbamate** poisoning produces reversible cholinesterase inhibition, and spontaneous recovery of enzyme activity may occur within several hours, making both of the above tests less useful.
3. Assay of blood, urine, gastric lavage fluid, and excrement for specific agents and their metabolites may also provide evidence of exposure, but these tests are not widely available.

B. **Other useful laboratory studies to consider:** arterial blood gases, pulse oximetry, ECG, electrolytes, glucose, BUN, creatinine, lactic acid, creatine kinase (CK), lipase and liver function tests, and chest radiography.
1. Respiratory function tests such as spirometry and negative inspiratory force (NIF) can help assess the severity of respiratory weakness.
2. Electromyographic and nerve stimulation studies can identify patients at high risk for respiratory failure due to intermediate syndrome or rebound toxicity due to continued absorption or redistribution.

V. **Treatment**

A. **Emergency and supportive measures.** ***Caution:*** Rescuers and health care providers should take measures to prevent direct contact with the skin or clothing of contaminated victims because secondary contamination and serious illness may result, especially with nerve agents or potent pesticides (Section IV, p 636). In addition, respiratory protective measures must be taken by persons working in areas contaminated by nerve agent vapors or aerosols.
1. Maintain an open airway and assist ventilation if necessary (pp 1–7). Administer supplemental oxygen. Pay careful attention to respiratory muscle weakness and the presence of bronchial secretions. Respiratory arrest is often preceded by increasing weakness of neck flexion muscles. If intubation is required, a nondepolarizing agent (p 586) should be used because the effect of succinylcholine will be markedly prolonged secondary to the inhibition of PChE.
2. Anticipate and treat hydrocarbon pneumonitis (p 266), bradycardia and other dysrhythmias (pp 9–15), hypotension (p 15), seizures (p 23), and coma (p 18) if they occur. Seizures should be treated with a benzodiazepine such as diazepam (p 516).
3. Observe asymptomatic patients for at least 8–12 hours to rule out delayed-onset symptoms, especially after extensive skin exposure or ingestion of a highly fat-soluble agent.

B. **Specific drugs and antidotes.** Specific treatment includes the antimuscarinic agent **atropine** and the enzyme reactivator **pralidoxime.** These agents are also packaged together as an auto-injector kit (Mark-1 or Nerve Agent Antidote Kit) for prehospital, disaster, or military settings.
1. Give **atropine in escalating doses** until clinical improvement is evident. Begin with 2–5 mg IV initially (p 512), and double the dose administered every 5 minutes until respiratory secretions have cleared. ***Note:*** Atropine will reverse muscarinic but not nicotinic effects.
   a. Reassess the patient's secretions, oxygen saturation, and respiratory rate every 5–10 minutes. The most important indication for redosing atropine is persistent wheezing or bronchorrhea. Tachycardia is not necessarily a contraindication to additional atropine in the context of severe respiratory secretions.
   b. Once the respiratory secretions have been initially controlled, continuous infusions of atropine may be useful in selected cases, but clinical vigilance is required to prevent over-atropinization. Large cumulative doses of atropine (up to 100 mg or more) may be required in severe cases.
   c. Other antimuscarinic agents (eg, glycopyrrolate) have been demonstrated to reverse the peripheral muscarinic toxicity of OP agents, but they do not penetrate the CNS and are thus less beneficial than atropine, which has good CNS penetration.

2. **Pralidoxime** (p 613) is an oxime that reactivates the cholinesterase enzymes when administered before enzyme aging. Evidence regarding the use of oximes is inconclusive. Oximes may be more effective against *diethyl* compounds than against *dimethyl* agents, which cause a faster aging of the AChE enzyme. Recent evidence from placebo-controlled clinical trials indicates that pralidoxime may not benefit some OP-poisoned patients; however, oximes are still recommended in the treatment of OP poisoning until more selective and evidence-based guidelines are formulated.
   a. Pralidoxime should be given as a loading dose (30–50 mg/kg, total of 1–2 g in adults) over 30 minutes, followed by a continuous infusion of 8–20 mg/kg/h (up to 650 mg/h). It is most effective if started early, before irreversible phosphorylation of the cholinesterase occurs (aging), but may still be effective if given later, particularly after exposure to highly lipid-soluble compounds released into the blood from fat stores over days to weeks. It is unclear how long oxime therapy should be continued, but it seems reasonable to continue pralidoxime for 24 hours after the patient becomes asymptomatic, or at least as long as atropine infusion is required.
   b. Pralidoxime generally is not recommended for carbamate intoxication because in such cases the cholinesterase inhibition is spontaneously reversible and short lived. However, if the exact agent is not identified and the patient has significant toxicity, pralidoxime should be given empirically.
3. Many **other treatments** (magnesium, clonidine, bicarbonate, glutamate antagonists, fresh-frozen plasma, exogenous hydrolases, hemoperfusion) have been proposed and/or are currently being investigated.

C. **Decontamination** (p 50). ***Note:*** Rescuers should wear chemical-protective clothing and gloves when handling a grossly contaminated victim. If there is heavy liquid contamination with a volatile solvent such as xylene or toluene, clothing removal and victim decontamination should be carried out outdoors or in a room with high-flow ventilation. However, decontamination procedures must not delay the administration of atropine and airway management in the severely poisoned patient.
1. **Skin and mucous membranes.** Remove all contaminated clothing and wash exposed areas with soap and water, including the hair and under the nails. Irrigate exposed eyes with copious tepid water or saline.
2. **Ingestion.** Gastric lavage or aspiration of liquid stomach contents by a small nasogastric tube may be appropriate soon after moderate-to-large ingestions, but because of the possibility of seizures or rapidly changing mental status, lavage should be done only after the airway has been secured. Administer activated charcoal orally if conditions are appropriate (see Table I–38, p 54).

D. **Enhanced elimination.** Dialysis and hemoperfusion generally are not indicated because of the large volume of distribution of organophosphates.

▶ OXALIC ACID

Kent R. Olson, MD

Oxalic acid and oxalates are used as bleaches, metal cleaners, and rust removers and in chemical synthesis and leather tanning. A laundry powder containing sachets of oxalic acid and potassium permanganate was reported to cause an epidemic of fatal self-poisonings in Sri Lanka. Soluble and insoluble oxalate salts are found in several species of plants.

I. **Mechanism of toxicity**

A. **Oxalic acid solutions** are highly irritating and corrosive. Ingestion and absorption of oxalate cause acute hypocalcemia resulting from precipitation of the insoluble calcium oxalate salt. Calcium oxalate crystals may then deposit in the brain, heart, kidneys, and other sites, causing serious systemic damage.

B. **Insoluble calcium oxalate** salt found in *Dieffenbachia* and similar plants is not absorbed, but it causes local mucous membrane irritation.

II. **Toxic dose.** Ingestion of 5–15 g of oxalic acid has caused death. The recommended workplace limit (ACGIH TLV-TWA) for oxalic acid vapor is 1 mg/m^3 as an 8-hour time-weighted average. The short-term exposure limit (STEL), a level that should not be exceeded for more than 15 minutes, is 2 mg/m^3. The level considered immediately dangerous to life or health (IDLH) is 500 mg/m^3.

III. **Clinical presentation.** Toxicity may occur as a result of skin or eye contact, inhalation, or ingestion.

A. **Acute skin or eye contact** causes irritation and burning, which may lead to serious corrosive injury if the exposure and concentration are high.

B. **Inhalation** may cause sore throat, cough, and wheezing. Large exposures may lead to chemical pneumonitis or pulmonary edema.

C. **Ingestion** of soluble oxalates may result in weakness, tetany, convulsions, and cardiac arrest due to profound hypocalcemia. The QT interval may be prolonged, and variable conduction defects may occur. Oxalate crystals may be found on urinalysis. Insoluble oxalate crystals are not absorbed but can cause irritation and swelling in the oropharynx and esophagus.

IV. **Diagnosis** is based on a history of exposure and evidence of local or systemic effects or oxalate crystalluria.

A. **Specific levels.** Serum oxalate levels are not available.

B. **Other useful laboratory studies** include electrolytes, glucose, BUN, creatinine, calcium, ECG monitoring, and urinalysis.

V. **Treatment**

A. **Emergency and supportive measures**

1. Protect the airway (p 1), which may become acutely swollen and obstructed after a significant ingestion or inhalation. Administer supplemental oxygen and assist ventilation if necessary (pp 1–7).
2. Treat coma (p 18), seizures (p 23), and arrhythmias (pp 10–15) if they occur.
3. Monitor the ECG and vital signs for at least 6 hours after significant exposure and admit symptomatic patients to an intensive care unit.

B. **Specific drugs and antidotes.** Administer 10% **calcium solution** (chloride or gluconate) to counteract symptomatic hypocalcemia (p 526).

C. **Decontamination** (p 50)

1. **Insoluble oxalates** in plants. Flush exposed areas. For ingestions, dilute with plain water; do not induce vomiting or give charcoal.
2. **Oxalic acid or strong commercial oxalate solutions.** Immediately flush with copious water. Do ***not*** induce vomiting because of the risk for aggravating corrosive injury; instead, give water to dilute, and on arrival in the hospital perform gastric lavage.
3. **Plants containing soluble oxalates.** Attempt to precipitate ingested oxalate in the stomach by administering calcium (calcium chloride or gluconate, 1–2 g, or calcium carbonate [Tums], several tablets) orally or via a gastric tube. The effectiveness of activated charcoal is unknown.

D. **Enhanced elimination.** Maintain high-volume urine flow (3–5 mL/kg/h) to help prevent calcium oxalate precipitation in the tubules. Oxalate is removed by hemodialysis, but the indications for this treatment are not established.

▶ PARAQUAT AND DIQUAT

Richard J. Geller, MD, MPH

Paraquat dichloride (CAS # 1910-42-5) and diquat dibromide (CAS # 85-00-7) are dipyridyl herbicides used for weed control and as preharvest (desiccant) defoliants. Product formulations differ by country. In the United States, Syngenta currently markets Gramoxone Inteon (30.1% paraquat dichloride) and Reward (37.3% diquat dibromide).

Other, less concentrated formulations of diquat are also marketed. Roundup QuikPro is a water-soluble granular formulation (73.3% glyphosate and 2.9% diquat). In the United States, paraquat poisonings greatly outnumber diquat poisonings.

I. **Mechanism of toxicity**

A. **Paraquat and diquat** are di-cations whose toxic effects are similar. Concentrated solutions (eg, >20%) may cause severe corrosive injury when ingested, injected, or applied to the skin, eyes, or mucous membranes. The dipyridyl herbicides are extremely potent systemic toxins and cause multiple-system organ damage. Engaging in a nicotinamide adenosine dinucleotide phosphate (NADPH)–powered reduction and oxidation cycle, dipyridyls spawn highly reactive free radicals, including superoxide and hydroxyl anions, leading to cell death and tissue destruction via lipid peroxidation. Renal failure is a common feature of both poisonings. Hepatic and cardiovascular failure may occur.

1. In addition, **paraquat** is selectively taken up and concentrated by pulmonary alveolar cells, leading to cell necrosis followed (within days) by connective tissue proliferation and pulmonary fibrosis.
2. **Diquat** is not taken up by pulmonary alveolar cells and does not cause pulmonary fibrosis, but it has been associated with CNS hemorrhagic infarctions.

B. **Pharmacokinetics**

1. **Absorption.** Paraquat and diquat are rapidly (but incompletely) absorbed from the GI tract, and peak serum levels are reached within 2 hours of ingestion. The presence of food may reduce or delay absorption significantly. Although absorption is poor through intact skin, the dipyridyl herbicides can be taken up through abraded skin or after prolonged contact with concentrated solutions. Fatalities usually result from ingestion but have been reported after intramuscular injection, after vaginal and percutaneous exposure, and rarely after inhalation. Dipyridyls are contact herbicides not systemically incorporated into plants. Once applied to plants or soil, they are rapidly bound and unlikely to be toxic.
2. **Distribution.** Paraquat has an apparent volume of distribution of 1.2–1.6 L/kg. It is taken up most avidly by lung, kidney, liver, and muscle tissue. In the lungs, paraquat is actively taken up against a concentration gradient.
3. **Elimination.** Paraquat is eliminated renally, with more than 90% excreted unchanged within 12–24 hours if renal function is normal. Diquat is eliminated renally and via the GI tract.

II. **Toxic dose.** Diquat is slightly less toxic than paraquat. However, this distinction may be of little comfort, as both compounds are extremely poisonous.

A. **Paraquat.** Ingestion of as little as 2–4 g, or 10–20 mL, of concentrated 20% paraquat solution has resulted in death. The estimated lethal dose of 20% paraquat is 10–20 mL for adults and 4–5 mL for children. The mean oral 50% lethal dose (LD_{50}) in monkeys is approximately 50 mg/kg.

B. **Diquat.** Diquat deaths have been reported after ingestions of 15, 20, and 50 mL of 20% diquat, and after 30 mL of 14% diquat. The oral LD_{50} in monkeys is approximately 100–300 mg/kg.

III. **Clinical presentation**

A. **Paraquat.** After ingestion of concentrated solutions, there is pain and swelling in the mouth and throat, and oral ulcerations may be visible. Nausea, vomiting, and abdominal pain are common. Severe gastroenteritis and GI fluid sequestration may cause massive fluid and electrolyte loss that contributes to renal failure. The severity and tempo of illness depend on the dose. Ingestion of more than 40 mg/kg (~14 mL of a 20% solution in an adult) leads to corrosive GI injury, rapid onset of renal failure, myonecrosis, shock, and death within hours to a few days. Ingestion of 20–40 mg/kg causes a more indolent course evolving over several days, with most patients dying of pulmonary fibrosis after days to weeks. Patients with ingestions of less than 20 mg/kg usually recover fully.

B. **Diquat** causes very similar initial symptoms but does not cause pulmonary fibrosis. Agitation, seizures, and coma have been described. Cerebral and brainstem hemorrhagic infarctions may occur.

IV. **Diagnosis** is based on a history of ingestion and the presence of oral burns, gastroenteritis, and multiple-organ system failure. Pulmonary fibrosis suggests paraquat poisoning and may be rapidly progressive or delayed.

A. **Specific levels.** The prognosis may be correlated with specific plasma levels, but these levels are not likely to be available in a time frame useful for emergency management. Plasma and urine paraquat and diquat levels can be performed by Syngenta (US: 1-800-888-8372; Canada: 1-800-327-8633), although turnaround times may be very long. Plasma paraquat levels may be interpreted via the Hart nomogram or with assistance from a poison control center. A rapid qualitative test to detect paraquat or diquat adds sodium bicarbonate (2 g) and sodium dithionite (1 g) to 10 mL of the patient's urine a blue or greenish grey color change is consistent with paraquat ingestion and a green color is seen with diquat ingestion.

B. **Other useful laboratory studies** include liver, renal and electrolyte studies, CBC, arterial blood gas, and upright chest radiography (for fibrosis, pneumomediastinum, or GI perforation). Rapid rise of creatinine (out of proportion to the BUN) has been seen.

V. **Treatment**

A. **Emergency and supportive measures.** The **Syngenta Agricultural Products Emergency Information Network (1-800-327-8633)** is a resource for managing dipyridyl exposures and is available 24 hours a day, 7 days a week.

1. Maintain an open airway and assist ventilation if needed (pp 1–7).
2. Treat fluid and electrolyte imbalance caused by GI losses and third spacing with IV crystalloid solutions.
3. Avoid excessive oxygen administration, as oxygen is the substrate from which dipyridyls create harmful free radical species. Treat significant hypoxemia with supplemental oxygen, but use only the lowest amount needed to achieve a PO_2 of about 60 mm Hg.
4. Treat pain due to corrosive injury with adequate doses of opioids.
5. Obtain consultation and support from social and pastoral care services for patients with life-threatening poisoning.

B. **Specific drugs and antidotes.** In recent years, a large number of studies have examined proposed treatments for dipyridyl poisoning, but at present, no specific antidote can be recommended. Treatment with cyclophosphamide and glucocorticoids has been effective for moderate-to-severe paraquat poisoning in a few small clinical trials but benefit has not been definitively proven.

C. **Decontamination** (p 50)

1. **Skin and eyes.** Remove all contaminated clothing and wash exposed skin with soap and water. Irrigate exposed eyes with copious saline or water.
2. **Ingestion.** Immediate and aggressive GI decontamination is probably the only treatment that may affect the outcome significantly after paraquat or diquat ingestion.
   a. **Prehospital.** Prompt ingestion of food may provide some protection if charcoal is not immediately available.
   b. **Hospital.** Immediately administer 100 g of activated charcoal and repeat the dose in 1–2 hours. Gastric lavage may be helpful if performed within several hours of the ingestion. If herbicide is observed on back aspiration from an orogastric or nasogastric tube, consider several consecutive cycles of activated charcoal followed by lavage, until the herbicide is no longer observed. Various clays, such as bentonite and fuller's earth, also adsorb paraquat and diquat but are probably no more effective than charcoal.

D. **Enhanced elimination** (p 56). Although charcoal hemoperfusion has been advocated and early animal studies and human case reports suggested benefits, no controlled study has demonstrated improved outcome, and the current consensus is that the procedure is not indicated. Hemodialysis and forced diuresis do not enhance elimination, although renal failure may necessitate hemodialysis.

▶ PENTACHLOROPHENOL AND DINITROPHENOL

Kathy Vo, MD

Pentachlorophenol (penchloro, penta, PCP, others) is a chlorinated aromatic hydrocarbon that has been used as a pesticide to preserve wood products from insect and fungal damage (eg, power line poles). Since 1984, its use in the United States has been restricted to industrial purposes by certified applicators. It is a ubiquitous environmental contaminant detectable in the general population. It appears to be an endocrine and immune disrupter. It is a probable carcinogen (EPA). It is formed as a by-product during water disinfection with chlorinated oxidants. Moreover, it was noted that children living in the areas of pentachlorobenzene and hexachlorobenzene emissions had elevated pentachlorophenol serum and urine concentrations.

Dinitrophenols (dinosam, DNOC, DNP, and analogs) have been used as insecticides, herbicides, fungicides, and chemical intermediaries and are used in some explosives, dyes, and photographic chemicals. Dinitrophenol has also been taken orally for weight reduction. The use of dinitrophenol as a pesticide or as a weight-reducing agent is banned in the United States, although the chemical appears to be available over the Internet.

I. **Mechanism of toxicity**
   A. Pentachlorophenol and dinitrophenols uncouple oxidative phosphorylation in the mitochondria. Substrates are metabolized, but the energy produced is dissipated as heat instead of producing adenosine triphosphate (ATP). The basal metabolic rate increases, placing increased demands on the cardiorespiratory system. Excess lactic acid results from anaerobic glycolysis.
   B. Dinitrophenols may oxidize hemoglobin to methemoglobin (p 317).
   C. In animal studies, pentachlorophenol is mutagenic, teratogenic, and carcinogenic. DNP is mutagenic, teratogenic, and may be weakly carcinogenic.

II. **Toxic dose.** These agents are readily absorbed through the skin, lungs, and GI tract.
   A. **Inhalation.** The air level of pentachlorophenol considered immediately dangerous to life or health (IDLH) is 2.5 mg/m^3. The ACGIH-recommended workplace air exposure limit (TLV-TWA) is 0.5 mg/m^3 as an 8-hour time-weighted average.
   B. **Skin.** This is the main route associated with accidental poisoning. An epidemic of intoxication occurred in a neonatal nursery after diapers were inadvertently washed in 23% sodium pentachlorophenate.
   C. **Ingestion.** The minimum lethal oral dose of pentachlorophenol for humans is not known, but death occurred after ingestion of 2 g. Ingestion of 1–3 g of dinitrophenol in an adult is considered lethal.

III. **Clinical presentation.** The toxic manifestations of pentachlorophenol and dinitrophenol are nearly identical. Profuse sweating, fever, tachypnea, and tachycardia are universally reported in serious poisonings and can manifest as early as 3.5 hours after intentional overdose.
   A. **Acute exposure** causes irritation of the skin, eyes, and upper respiratory tract. Systemic absorption may cause headache, vomiting, weakness, and lethargy. Profound sweating, hyperthermia, tachycardia, tachypnea, convulsions, and coma are associated with severe or fatal poisonings. Pulmonary edema,

intravascular hemolysis, pancreatitis, jaundice, and acute renal failure have been reported. Death usually is caused by cardiovascular collapse or hyperthermia. After death, an extremely rapid onset of rigor mortis is reported frequently. Dinitrophenol may also induce methemoglobinemia and yellow-stained skin.

B. Chronic exposure may present in a similar manner as acute systemic poisoning and may cause weight loss, GI disturbances, fevers and night sweats, weakness, flulike symptoms, contact dermatitis and chloracne, and aplastic anemia (rare). In addition, impaired fertility and hypothyroidism have been reported. Cataracts and glaucoma have been associated with dinitrophenol.

IV. Diagnosis is based on history of exposure and clinical findings and should be suspected in patients with fever, metabolic acidosis, diaphoresis, and tachypnea.

A. Specific levels. Blood levels are not readily available or useful for emergency management.

B. Other useful laboratory studies include CBC, electrolytes, glucose, BUN, creatinine, creatine kinase (CK), liver aminotransferases, amylase and/or lipase, urine dipstick for occult blood (positive with hemolysis or rhabdomyolysis), arterial blood gases, methemoglobin level, and chest radiography.

V. Treatment

A. Emergency and supportive measures

1. Maintain a patent airway and assist ventilation if necessary (pp 1–7).
2. Treat coma (p 18), seizures (p 23), hypotension (p 15), and hyperthermia (p 21) if they occur. Dehydration from tachypnea, fever, and sweating is common and may require large-volume fluid replacement.
3. Monitor asymptomatic patients for at least 6 hours after exposure.
4. Do ***not*** use salicylates or anticholinergic agents, as they may worsen hyperthermia. Paralysis with neuromuscular blockers may not be helpful because of the intracellular mechanism for hyperthermia. Barbiturates (pp 602–604) may be of some value.

B. Specific drugs and antidotes. There is no specific antidote. Treat methemoglobinemia with methylene blue (p 579).

C. Decontamination (p 50)

1. **Inhalation.** Remove the victim from exposure and administer supplemental oxygen if available.
2. **Skin and eyes.** Remove contaminated clothing and store in a plastic bag; wash exposed areas thoroughly with soap and copious water. Irrigate exposed eyes with copious saline or tepid water. Rescuers should wear appropriate protective clothing and respirators to avoid exposure.
3. **Ingestion.** Administer activated charcoal orally if conditions are appropriate (see Table I–38, p 54). Gastric lavage is not necessary after small-to-moderate ingestions if activated charcoal can be given promptly.

D. Enhanced elimination. There is no evidence that enhanced elimination procedures are effective.

▶ PHENCYCLIDINE (PCP) AND KETAMINE

Patil Armenian, MD

Phencyclidine, or PCP [1-(1-phenylcyclohexyl)-piperidine], is an arylcyclohexylamine dissociative anesthetic agent with stimulant properties. It was previously marketed for veterinary use and became popular as an inexpensive street drug in the late 1960s. PCP is most commonly smoked but may also be snorted, ingested, or injected. It is frequently substituted for or added to illicit psychoactive drugs such as THC (tetrahydrocannabinol, or marijuana) and rarely, mescaline or LSD. PCP is known by a variety of street names, including “peace pill,” “angel dust,” “hog,” “goon,” and “animal tranquilizer.” “Sherms” is slang for Sherman cigarettes laced with PCP, and a “KJ” is a marijuana cigarette laced with PCP. Various structural analogs of PCP have been synthesized, including PCC (1-piperidonocyclohexanecarbinol), PCE (eticyclidine; 1-phenyl-cyclohexylethylamine), PHP (rolicyclidine; phenylcyclohexylpyrrolidine), and TCP (tenocyclidine; 1-(1-cyclohexyl) piperidine).

Ketamine [2-(2-chlorophenyl)-2-(methylamino)cyclohexanone] shares many structural, pharmacologic, and clinical characteristics with PCP. Although currently used as an anesthetic agent and for procedural sedation, ketamine is a popular drug of abuse owing to its dissociative, analgesic, and hallucinogenic properties. It was first used as a street drug in the 1970s and gained popularity in the club scene of the 1990s. Street names for ketamine include "K," "special K," "vitamin K," "jet," "special LA coke," and "super C." A severe ketamine intoxication is referred to as "falling into the K-hole." **Methoxetamine** [MXE; 2-(3-methoxyphenyl)-2-(amino)cyclohexanone] is a structural analog of ketamine that may be associated with worse side effects of cerebellar ataxia and mood disturbances.

I. Mechanism of toxicity

A. PCP, ketamine, and their analogs are dissociative anesthetics that produce generalized loss of pain perception with little or no depression of airway reflexes or ventilation. Psychotropic effects are primarily mediated through *N*-methyl-D-aspartate (NMDA) receptor antagonism. They also inhibit reuptake of dopamine, norepinephrine, and serotonin and block potassium conductance in the brain. PCP stimulates the sigma-opioid receptor, and ketamine stimulates the mu-, delta-, sigma-, and kappa-opioid receptors. PCP also binds to a site within the L-type calcium channel, thus attenuating the influx of calcium when excitatory neurotransmitters bind to this receptor.

B. Pharmacokinetics

1. PCP is absorbed rapidly by inhalation or ingestion. It is highly lipophilic and has a large volume of distribution (Vd) of about 6 L/kg. The duration of clinical effects after an overdose is highly variable and ranges from 11 to 14 hours in one report to 1–4 days in another. PCP is eliminated mainly by hepatic metabolism, although renal and gastric excretion accounts for a small fraction and is pH-dependent (see also Table II–66).

2. Ketamine is well absorbed after snorting and injection and poorly with oral and rectal ingestion. Effect onset occurs 30 seconds to 30 minutes after use and lasts up to 3 hours, depending on the route of administration. It is metabolized by the liver. The kidney is an important route of elimination for norketamine, the active metabolite of ketamine. The volume of distribution of ketamine is approximately 2–4 L/kg.

3. Methoxetamine effects occur 30–90 minutes after use and last 5–7 hours.

II. Toxic dose

A. PCP. In tablet form, the usual street dose is 1–6 mg, which results in hallucinations, euphoria, and disinhibition. Ingestion of 6–10 mg causes toxic psychosis and signs of sympathomimetic stimulation. Acute ingestion of 150–200 mg has resulted in death. Smoking PCP produces a rapid onset of effects, and may be an easier route for users to titrate to the desired level of intoxication.

B. Ketamine. Usual therapeutic anesthetic doses are 1–2 mg/kg IV or 4–10 mg/kg IM (see p 569). Recreational doses range from 10 to 250 mg nasally, 40 to 450 mg orally or rectally, and 10 to 100 mg IM.

III. Clinical presentation. Clinical effects may be seen within minutes of smoking PCP and can last 24 hours or longer, depending on the dose. Because users of PCP and ketamine may have also been using many other drugs simultaneously (eg, cocaine, marijuana, alcohol, methamphetamine), the initial presentation may be difficult to discern from other toxidromes. Although the clinical effects of PCP and ketamine are similar, reports of ketamine causing similar degrees of agitation and violent behavior are lacking.

A. Mild intoxication causes lethargy, euphoria, hallucinations, and occasionally bizarre or violent behavior. Hypersalivation and lacrimation may occur. Patients may abruptly swing between quiet catatonia and loud or agitated behavior. Vertical and horizontal nystagmus may be prominent with PCP intoxication.

B. Severe intoxication produces signs of adrenergic hyperactivity, including hypertension, tachycardia, diaphoresis, hyperthermia, rigidity, localized dystonic reactions, pulmonary edema, convulsions, and coma. The pupils are sometimes paradoxically small. Death from PCP may occur as a result of self-destructive behavior or as a complication of hyperthermia and subsequent multiple-organ system dysfunction (eg, rhabdomyolysis, renal failure, coagulopathy, or brain damage). Sudden death, probably from ventricular arrhythmia, has occurred during restraint for agitated delirium (such as in police custody). Acute methoxetamine intoxication has resulted in cerebellar ataxia.

C. Chronic ketamine abuse may cause dependence and tolerance, memory impairment, impaired concentration, and depression. It has been linked to urinary problems from bladder wall fibrosis. Animal studies have shown similar chronic bladder effects from methoxetamine.

IV. Diagnosis is suggested by the presence of rapidly fluctuating behavior, vertical nystagmus, and sympathomimetic signs.

A. Specific levels

1. Specific serum PCP levels are not readily available and do not correlate reliably with the degree of intoxication. Levels of 30–100 ng/mL have been associated with toxic psychosis. Specific serum ketamine levels are not readily available.
2. Qualitative urine screening for PCP is widely available; however, most PCP immunoassays produce false-positive results to venlafaxine, dextromethorphan, diphenhydramine, and many other drugs. PCP analogs may not be detected on routine screening, although they can cross-react in some immunologic assays (see Table I–33, p 46). Ketamine and its analogs are not detected on routine urine drug screening.

B. Other useful laboratory studies include electrolytes, glucose, BUN, creatinine, creatine kinase (CK), and urinalysis dipstick for occult blood (positive with myoglobinuria).

V. Treatment

A. Emergency and supportive measures

1. Maintain an open airway and assist ventilation if necessary (pp 1–7).
2. Treat coma (p 18), seizures (p 23), hypertension (p 17), hyperthermia (p 21), and rhabdomyolysis (p 27) if they occur.
3. Agitated behavior (p 24) may respond to limiting sensory stimulation but may require sedation with high doses of benzodiazepines (midazolam, lorazepam, or diazepam [p 516]) and haloperidol or other antipsychotic drugs (p 503). In the initial management of an extremely agitated patient, midazolam or haloperidol may be given IM if IV access is absent.
4. Monitor temperature and other vital signs for a minimum of 6 hours and admit all patients with hyperthermia or other evidence of significant intoxication.

B. Specific drugs and antidotes. There is no specific antidote. Clonidine at a dose of 2.5–5 mcg/kg orally has been used to attenuate the sympathomimetic effects of ketamine seen during anesthesia.

C. Decontamination. No decontamination measures are necessary after snorting, smoking, or injecting PCP or ketamine. For ingestion, administer activated charcoal if conditions are appropriate (see Table I–38, p 54). Gastric lavage is not necessary after small-to-moderate ingestions if activated charcoal can be given promptly.

D. Enhanced elimination. Because of their large volume of distribution, PCP and ketamine are not effectively removed by dialysis, hemoperfusion, or other enhanced removal procedures.

1. Repeat-dose activated charcoal has not been studied but may marginally increase elimination by adsorbing PCP partitioned into the acidic stomach

fluid. Continuous nasogastric suction has also been proposed for removal of gastrically partitioned PCP.

2. Although urinary acidification increases the urinary concentration of PCP, there is no evidence that this significantly enhances systemic elimination, and it may be dangerous because urinary acidification can aggravate myoglobinuric renal failure.

▶ PHENOL AND RELATED COMPOUNDS

Gary W. Everson, PharmD

Phenol (carbolic acid) was introduced into household use as a potent germicidal agent but today is found in fewer products because less toxic compounds have replaced it. Phenol can be found in topical skin products (eg, Campho-phenique containing 4.7% phenol) and in surface deodorizers and disinfectants (eg, Creolin®). Phenol is used in the production of fertilizers, wood preservatives, paint removers, and other chemicals. **Hexachlorophene** is a chlorinated biphenol that was used widely as a topical antiseptic and preoperative scrub until its adverse neurologic effects were recognized. Other phenolic compounds include **creosote, creosol, cresol, cresylic acid, hydroquinone, eugenol,** and chloroxylenol, the active ingredient in Dettol®. **Pentachlorophenol** and **dinitrophenols** are discussed on p 364.

I. **Mechanism of toxicity.** Phenol denatures protein, disrupts the cell wall, and produces a coagulative tissue necrosis. It may cause corrosive injury to the eyes, skin, and respiratory tract. Systemic absorption may result in cardiac arrhythmias and CNS stimulation, but the mechanisms of these effects are not known. Some phenolic compounds (eg, dinitrophenol and hydroquinone) may induce hemolysis and **methemoglobinemia** (p 317).

II. **Toxic dose.** The minimum toxic and lethal doses are not well defined. Most phenolic compounds can be absorbed following inhalation, skin exposure, and ingestion.

   A. **Inhalation.** The OSHA recommended workplace permissible exposure limit for pure phenol is 5 ppm (19 mg/m^3) as an 8-hour time-weighted average. The level considered immediately dangerous to life or health (IDLH) is 250 ppm.

   B. **Skin application.** Death has occurred in infants from repeated dermal applications of small doses. A 9-year-old child developed brief runs of ventricular tachycardia, became obtunded and required intubation after application of Creolin® to her head and upper torso. Cardiac arrhythmias occurred after dermal application of 3 mL of an 88% phenol solution. Solutions of more than 5% can be corrosive.

   C. **Ingestion.** Deaths have occurred after adult ingestions of 1–32 g of phenol; however, survival after ingestion of 45–65 g has been reported. As little as 50– 500 mg has been reported as fatal in infants.

   D. **Pharmacokinetics.** Phenol is rapidly absorbed by all routes. Its elimination half-life is 0.5–4.5 hours.

III. **Clinical presentation.** Toxicity may result from inhalation, skin or eye exposure, or ingestion.

   A. **Inhalation.** Vapors from phenol may cause respiratory tract irritation and chemical pneumonia. Smoking of clove cigarettes (clove oil contains the phenol derivative eugenol) may cause severe tracheobronchitis.

   B. **Skin and eyes.** Dermal exposure may produce a deep white patch that turns red, after which the skin stains brown. This lesion is often initially painless. Irritation and severe corneal damage may occur if concentrated phenolic compounds come in contact with eyes.

   C. **Ingestion** usually causes vomiting and diarrhea, and diffuse corrosive GI tract injury may occur. Systemic absorption may cause a mild transaminitis, agitation, confusion, seizures, coma, hypotension, arrhythmias, and respiratory arrest.

D. **Injection.** Accidental injection of high concentrations of phenol has resulted in acute renal failure and acute respiratory distress syndrome.

IV. **Diagnosis** is based on a history of exposure, the presence of a characteristic odor, and painless skin burns with white discoloration. Dark colored urine has also been seen after skin exposure and ingestion.

A. **Specific levels.** Normal urine phenol levels are less than 20 mg/L. Urine phenol levels may be elevated in workers exposed to benzene and after the use of phenol-containing throat lozenges and mouthwashes. These tests are not routinely available in hospital laboratories.

B. **Other useful laboratory studies** include CBC, electrolytes, glucose, BUN, creatinine, chest x-ray, and ECG. Obtain a methemoglobin level after hydroquinone exposures.

V. **Treatment**

A. **Emergency and supportive measures**

1. Maintain an open airway and assist ventilation if necessary (pp 1–7).
2. Treat coma (p 18), seizures (p 23), hypotension (p 15), and arrhythmias (pp 10–15) if they occur.
3. If corrosive injury to the GI tract is suspected, consult a gastroenterologist for possible endoscopy.

B. **Specific drugs and antidotes.** No specific antidote is available. If **methemoglobinemia** occurs, administer methylene blue (p 579).

C. **Decontamination** (p 50)

1. **Inhalation.** Remove victims from exposure and administer supplemental oxygen if available.
2. **Skin and eyes.** Remove contaminated clothing and wash exposed skin with very soapy water or, if available, polyethylene glycol 300, mineral oil, or olive oil. Immediately flush exposed eyes with copious tepid water or normal saline for at least 15 minutes.
3. **Ingestion.** Administer activated charcoal orally if conditions are appropriate (see Table I–38, p 54). Use caution because phenol can cause convulsions, increasing the risk for pulmonary aspiration. Charcoal may also interfere with endoscopy. Gastric lavage is not necessary after small-to-moderate ingestions if activated charcoal can be given promptly.

D. **Enhanced elimination.** Enhanced removal methods are generally not effective because of the large volume of distribution of these lipid-soluble compounds. Hexachlorophene is excreted in the bile, and repeat-dose activated charcoal (p 59) may possibly be effective in increasing its clearance from the gut.

▶ PHENYTOIN

Craig Smollin, MD

Phenytoin is used orally for the prevention of generalized (grand mal) and partial complex seizures. Intravenous phenytoin is used to treat status epilepticus and occasionally as an antiarrhythmic agent. Oral formulations include suspensions, capsules, extended-release capsules, and tablet preparations. The brand Dilantin Kapseals exhibits delayed absorption characteristics not usually shared by generic products.

I. **Mechanism of toxicity.** Toxicity may be caused by the phenytoin itself or by the propylene glycol diluent used in parenteral preparations. (To make it soluble for IV use, phenytoin must be dissolved in 40% propylene glycol and 10% ethanol at pH 12.)

A. **Phenytoin** suppresses high-frequency neuronal firing, primarily by increasing the refractory period of voltage-dependent sodium channels. Toxic levels usually cause CNS depression.

B. The **propylene glycol** diluent in parenteral preparations may cause myocardial depression and cardiac arrest when infused rapidly (>40–50 mg/min [0.5–1 mg/kg/min]). The mechanism is not known. The injectable form of phenytoin also is highly alkaline and can cause tissue necrosis if it infiltrates ("purple glove syndrome").

C. **Fosphenytoin,** a water-soluble prodrug, does not contain the propylene glycol diluent and does not cause these toxic effects. As a result, it can be given at rates twice as fast as those for phenytoin. It does not appear to provide faster times to peak plasma phenytoin concentration or to result in fewer adverse effects compared with phenytoin.

D. **Pharmacokinetics.** Absorption may be slow and unpredictable. The time to peak plasma levels varies with the dosage. The volume of distribution is about 0.5–0.8 L/kg. Protein binding is about 90% at therapeutic levels. Since only free drug is pharmacologically active, the phenytoin level should be corrected for the serum albumin. Phenytoin is metabolized by hepatic microsomal enzymes (CYP2C9 and CYP2C19) to inactive metabolites. Hepatic elimination is saturable (zero-order kinetics) at levels near the therapeutic range, so the apparent "half-life" increases as levels rise: 26 hours at 10 mg/L, 40 hours at 20 mg/L, and 60 hours at 40 mg/L (see also Table II–66, p 462).

II. **Toxic dose.** The minimum acute toxic oral overdose is approximately 20 mg/kg. Because phenytoin exhibits dose-dependent elimination kinetics, accidental intoxication can easily occur in patients on chronic therapy owing to drug interactions or slight dosage adjustments.

III. **Clinical presentation.** Toxicity caused by phenytoin may be associated with acute oral overdose or chronic accidental overmedication. In acute oral overdose, absorption and peak effects may be delayed.

A. **Mild-to-moderate intoxication** commonly causes nystagmus, ataxia, and dysarthria. Nausea, vomiting, diplopia, hyperglycemia, agitation, and irritability have also been reported.

B. **Severe intoxication** can cause stupor, coma, and respiratory arrest. Although seizures have been reported, seizures in a phenytoin-intoxicated patient should prompt a search for other causes (eg, anoxia, hyperthermia, or an overdose of another drug). Death from isolated oral phenytoin overdose is extremely rare.

C. **Rapid intravenous injection,** usually at rates exceeding 50 mg/min, can cause profound hypotension, bradycardia, arrhythmias, and cardiac arrest. These effects have previously been attributed to the propylene glycol diluent. However, serious arrhythmias have also been reported with rapid administration of fosphenytoin, which does not contain propylene glycol. In contrast, oral overdose does not produce cardiovascular toxicity.

IV. **Diagnosis** is based on a history of ingestion or is suspected in any epileptic patient with altered mental status or ataxia.

A. **Specific levels.** Serum phenytoin concentrations are generally available in hospital clinical laboratories. Obtain repeated blood samples because slow absorption may result in delayed peak levels. The therapeutic concentration range is 10–20 mg/L.

1. At levels above 20 mg/L, nystagmus is common. At levels above 30 mg/L, ataxia, slurred speech, and tremor are common. With levels higher than 40 mg/L, lethargy, confusion, and stupor ensue. Survival has been reported in three patients with levels above 100 mg/L.
2. Because phenytoin is highly protein bound and most laboratories measure total (bound and free) drug levels, patients with hypoalbuminemia may experience toxicity at lower serum levels. A corrected phenytoin level can be obtained by using the following equation:

$$\text{Corrected phenytoin} = \frac{\text{Measured serun phenytoin}}{([\text{Adjustment} \times \text{Albumin}] + 0.1)}$$

where the adjustment = 0.2 (normal renal function) or the adjustment = 0.1 (for patients with creatinine clearance <20 mL/min). Free (unbound) serum phenytoin levels are available in some but not most clinical laboratories.

B. **Other useful laboratory studies** include electrolytes, glucose, BUN, creatinine, serum albumin, and ECG monitoring (during IV infusion).

C. **Genetic polymorphisms.** Individuals with the HLA-B*1502 genotype are at greater risk for developing Stevens–Johnson syndrome and toxic epidermal necrolysis. The prevalence rate of this mutation is highest among Asians, particularly Han Chinese and Thai. Testing available through reference laboratories.

V. **Treatment**

A. **Emergency and supportive measures**

1. Maintain an open airway and assist ventilation if necessary (pp 1–7). Administer supplemental oxygen.
2. Treat stupor and coma (p 15) if they occur. Protect the patient from self-injury caused by ataxia.
3. If seizures occur, consider an alternative diagnosis and treat with other usual anticonvulsants (p 23).
4. If hypotension occurs with intravenous phenytoin administration, immediately stop the infusion and administer IV fluids and vasopressors (p 15) if necessary.

B. **Specific drugs and antidotes.** There is no specific antidote.

C. **Decontamination** (p 50). Administer activated charcoal orally if conditions are appropriate (see Table I–38, p 54). Gastric lavage is not necessary after small-to-moderate ingestions if activated charcoal can be given promptly.

D. **Enhanced elimination.** Repeat-dose activated charcoal (p 59) may enhance phenytoin elimination, but does not result in improved clinical outcomes and may increase the risk for aspiration pneumonitis in drowsy patients. There is no role for diuresis, dialysis, or hemoperfusion.

▶ PHOSGENE

John R. Balmes, MD

Phosgene originally was manufactured as a war gas. It is now used in the manufacture of dyes, resins, and pesticides. It is also commonly produced when chlorinated compounds are burned, such as in a fire, or in the process of welding metal that has been cleaned with chlorinated solvents.

I. **Mechanism of toxicity.** Phosgene is an irritant. However, because it is poorly water soluble, in lower concentrations it does not cause immediate upper airway or skin irritation. Thus, an exposed individual may inhale phosgene for prolonged periods deeply into the lungs, where it is slowly hydrolyzed to hydrochloric acid. This results in necrosis and inflammation of the small airways and alveoli, which may lead to noncardiogenic pulmonary edema.

II. **Toxic dose.** The ACGIH-recommended workplace exposure limit (TLV-TWA) is 0.1 ppm (0.4 mg/m^3) as an 8-hour time-weighted average. The level considered immediately dangerous to life or health (IDLH) by NIOSH is 2 ppm. Exposure to 50 ppm may be rapidly fatal.

III. **Clinical presentation.** Exposure to moderate concentrations of phosgene causes mild cough and minimal mucous membrane irritation. After an asymptomatic interval of 30 minutes to 8 hours (depending on the duration and concentration of exposure), the victim develops dyspnea and hypoxemia. Pulmonary edema may be delayed up to 24 hours. Permanent pulmonary impairment may be a sequela of serious exposure.

IV. **Diagnosis** is based on a history of exposure and the clinical presentation. Many other toxic gases may cause delayed-onset pulmonary edema (p 7).

A. **Specific levels.** There are no specific blood or urine levels.
B. **Other useful laboratory studies** include chest radiography and arterial blood gases or oximetry.

V. **Treatment**
A. **Emergency and supportive measures**
1. Maintain an open airway and assist ventilation if necessary (pp 1–7). Administer supplemental oxygen, and treat noncardiogenic pulmonary edema (p 7) if it occurs.
2. Monitor the patient for at least 12–24 hours after exposure because of the potential for delayed-onset pulmonary edema.

B. **Specific drugs and antidotes.** There is no specific antidote.
C. **Decontamination.** Remove the victim from exposure and give supplemental oxygen if available. Rescuers should wear self-contained breathing apparatus.
D. **Enhanced elimination.** These procedures are not effective.

▶ PHOSPHINE AND PHOSPHIDES

Paul Khasigian, PharmD

Phosphine is a colorless gas that is heavier than air. It is odorless in its pure form, but impurities give it a characteristic fishy or garlic-like odor. It has been used for fumigation, and it is a serious potential hazard in operations producing metal phosphides, in which phosphine can be released in the chemical reaction of water and metal alloys. Workers at risk include metal refiners, acetylene workers, firefighters, pest control operators, and those in the semiconductor industry. **Magnesium phosphide** and **aluminum phosphide** are available in pellets or tablets and are used as fumigants and rodenticides. **Zinc phosphide** is a crystalline, dark gray powder mixed into food as rodent bait. Phosphides are a leading cause of fatal suicides and accidental ingestions in India and many developing countries.

I. **Mechanism of toxicity.** Phosphine is a highly toxic gas, especially to the lungs, brain, kidneys, heart, and liver. The pathophysiologic action of phosphine is not clearly understood but may be related to inhibition of electron transport in mitochondria. Phosphides liberate phosphine gas upon contact with moisture, and this reaction is enhanced in the acidity of the stomach. Phosphine is then absorbed through the GI and respiratory tracts.

II. **Toxic dose**
A. **Phosphine gas.** The ACGIH-recommended workplace exposure limit (TLVTWA) is 0.3 ppm (0.42 mg/m^3), which is much lower than the minimal detectable (fishy odor) concentration of 1–3 ppm. Hence, the odor threshold does not provide sufficient warning of dangerous concentrations. An air level of 50 ppm is considered immediately dangerous to life or health (IDLH). Chronic exposure to sublethal concentrations for extended periods may produce toxic symptoms.
B. **Phosphides.** Ingestion of as little as 500 mg of **aluminum phosphide** has caused death in an adult. In a reported case series, survivors had ingested about 1.5 g (range, 1.5–18 g), whereas fatal cases had ingested an average of 2.3 g (range, 1.5–36 g). The 50% lethal dose (LD_{50}) for **zinc phosphide** in rats is 40 mg/kg; the lowest reported lethal dose in humans is 4 g. A 36-year-old man who ingested 6 mg/kg of zinc phosphide and was treated with ipecac and activated charcoal remained asymptomatic.

III. **Clinical presentation.** Inhalation of phosphine gas is associated with cough, dyspnea, headache, dizziness, and vomiting. Phosphide ingestion may cause nausea, vomiting, diarrhea, hypotension unresponsive to pressors, and a rotten fish or garlicky odor sensed by caregivers. Adult respiratory distress syndrome (ARDS), acute renal failure, hepatitis, seizures, and coma may occur. Myocardial injury manifested by elevated cardiac enzymes, ST-T–wave changes, global hypokinesia, and various atrial and ventricular arrhythmias have been reported, as well as pericardial and pleural effusions, adrenal necrosis, and pancreatitis. Methemoglobinemia has also been reported. The onset of symptoms is usually rapid, although delayed onset of pulmonary edema has been described. Survivors of acute poisoning have been reported to develop esophageal complications including esophageal strictures and tracheoesophageal fistula.

IV. Diagnosis is based on a history of exposure to the agent. ***Caution:*** Pulmonary edema may have a delayed onset, and initial respiratory symptoms may be mild or absent.

  A. Specific levels. Body fluid phosphine levels are not clinically useful.

  B. Other useful laboratory studies include BUN, creatinine, electrolytes, liver aminotransferases, arterial blood gases or oximetry, and chest radiography.

V. Treatment

  A. Emergency and supportive measures

    1. Maintain an open airway and assist ventilation if necessary (pp 1–7). Administer supplemental oxygen and treat noncardiogenic pulmonary edema (p 7) if it occurs.
    2. Treat seizures (p 23) and hypotension (p 15) if they occur.
    3. Patients with a history of significant phosphine inhalation or phosphide ingestion should be admitted and observed for 48–72 hours for delayed onset of pulmonary edema.
    4. IV **magnesium** has been used to treat cardiac arrhythmias otherwise unresponsive to treatment.
    5. In severe poisoning, adrenal function may be compromised, and IV **hydrocortisone** should be considered, especially if hypotension does not respond to IV fluids and vasopressors.

  B. Specific drugs and antidotes. There is no specific antidote.

  C. Decontamination

    1. Caregivers are at a low risk for secondary contamination, but off-gassing of phosphine may occur if the patient vomits or if gastric lavage fluid is not isolated.
    2. Administer activated charcoal orally if conditions are appropriate (see Table I–38, p 54), although studies have not determined its binding affinity for phosphides. Consider gastric lavage for large recent ingestion. Use of 3–5% sodium bicarbonate in the lavage fluid has been proposed (to reduce stomach acid and resulting production of phosphine) but is not of proven benefit.

  D. Enhanced elimination. Dialysis and hemoperfusion have not been shown to be useful in hastening elimination of phosphine.

▶ PHOSPHORUS

Allyson Kreshak, MD

There are two naturally occurring types of elemental phosphorus: red and white. **Red phosphorus** is not well absorbed and has limited toxicity. In contrast, **white phosphorus** (also called **yellow phosphorus**) is a highly toxic cellular poison. White phosphorus is a colorless or yellow wax-like crystalline solid with a garlic-like odor and is almost insoluble in water but glows with exposure to air.

White phosphorous is used in the manufacture of fertilizers, food additives, cleaning compounds, and incendiaries in military ammunition. Historically, it has been used as a rodenticide and in the manufacture of fireworks. Red phosphorous is used in the manufacture of methamphetamine.

I. Mechanism of toxicity

  A. White phosphorous ignites spontaneously in air to form phosphorous pentoxide, which reacts with water to form phosphoric acid. White phosphorus is also a cellular poison.

B. Toxicity resulting from red phosphorous is largely associated with methamphetamine production. This process may involve the inadvertent conversion of red phosphorous to white phosphorous and the generation of phosphine gas.

II. **Toxic dose**

A. **Ingestion.** The fatal oral dose of yellow/white phosphorus is approximately 1 mg/kg.

B. **Inhalation.** The ACGIH-recommended workplace limit (TLV-TWA) for white phosphorus is 0.1 mg/m^3 (0.02 ppm) as an 8-hour time-weighted average. The air level considered immediately dangerous to life or health (IDLH) is 5 mg/m^3. Occupational exposure limits are not well established for red phosphorous.

III. **Clinical presentation** (white phosphorous)

A. **Acute inhalation** may cause mucous membrane irritation, cough, wheezing, chemical pneumonitis, and noncardiogenic pulmonary edema.

B. **Skin or eye contact** with phosphorous may cause conjunctivitis or severe dermal or ocular burns. Large burns can result in systemic absorption and toxicity.

C. **Acute ingestion** may cause GI burns, inflammation and hemorrhage, severe vomiting and abdominal pain, and diarrhea with "smoking" stools (due to spontaneous combustion on exposure to air).

D. Systemic effects include headache, delirium, shock, seizures, coma, and arrhythmias (atrial fibrillation, QRS and QT prolongation, ventricular tachycardia and fibrillation). Acute renal injury and electrolyte derangements including hypocalcemia, hyperkalemia, and hyperphosphatemia may occur. Phosphorous is a hepatotoxin, and fulminant hepatic failure may occur after 2–3 days after exposure.

E. Chronic exposure to phosphorous is associated with "phossy jaw" or mandibular osteonecrosis.

IV. **Diagnosis** is based on a history of exposure and the clinical presentation. Cutaneous burns, a garlic odor of the vomitus, and "smoking" or luminescent stools and vomitus caused by spontaneous combustion of elemental phosphorus suggest ingestion. Wood lamp examination of the skin will cause embedded phosphorus particles to fluoresce.

A. **Specific levels.** Serum phosphorous concentrations are not useful in diagnosing phosphorous poisoning.

B. **Other useful laboratory studies** include BUN, creatinine, potassium, calcium, liver aminotransferases, urinalysis, blood gases or oximetry, ECG, and chest radiography (after acute inhalation).

V. **Treatment**

A. **Emergency and supportive measures**

1. Observe a victim of inhalation closely for signs of upper airway injury and perform endotracheal intubation and assist ventilation if necessary (p 4). Administer supplemental oxygen. Treat bronchospasm (p 8) and pulmonary edema (p 7) if they occur.
2. Treat fluid losses from gastroenteritis with aggressive IV crystalloid fluid replacement.
3. Consider endoscopy if oral, esophageal, or gastric burns are suspected (p 186).

B. **Specific drugs and antidotes.** There is no specific antidote.

C. **Decontamination** (p 50). Rescuers should wear appropriate protective gear to prevent accidental skin, eye, or inhalation exposure. Solid phosphorus or phosphorous particles should be covered with water. Contaminated clothing should be put under water.

1. **Inhalation.** Remove the victim from exposure and give supplemental oxygen.
2. **Skin and eyes**
   a. Remove contaminated clothing and wash exposed areas thoroughly with soap and water.
   b. Covering exposed areas with moist dressings or submersion in water may help prevent spontaneous combustion of white phosphorus.

c. Manually debride remaining phosphorus particles. A Wood lamp may help visualize embedded phosphorus, which fluoresces under ultraviolet light. The use of dilute copper sulfate or silver nitrate solutions to bind to or coat the phosphorus and aid in removal has been proposed, but the safety and effectiveness of these treatments have not been established.

3. **Ingestion.** Consider gastric lavage (p 52) and whole bowel irrigation (p 55) after acute white phosphorus ingestion. Activated charcoal is of unknown benefit.

D. **Enhanced elimination.** There is no effective method of enhanced elimination.

► PLANTS

Joanne M. Goralka, PharmD and Timothy E. Albertson, MD, MPH, PhD

Ingestion of plants is one of the top 10 causes of poisoning nationwide. Decorative plants are found in many homes, and home landscaped yards provide access to a variety of attractive and potentially toxic plants. Fortunately, serious poisoning from plants is rare in children because the quantity of plant material required to cause serious poisoning is greater than what a small child ingests. Serious toxicity or death from plant ingestion is usually a result of intentional abuse (eg, jimson weed), misuse (eg, various teas steeped from plants), or suicide attempts (eg, oleander).

I. **Mechanism of toxicity.** Plants can be categorized by their potential toxicity. Table II–51 describes the effects of various plant toxins, and Table II–52 provides an alphabetical list of many potentially toxic plants and herbs.

A. **Group 1** plants contain systemically active poisons that may cause serious intoxication (see Table II–51).

B. **Group 2a** plants contain insoluble calcium oxalate crystals that may cause burning pain and swelling of the mucous membranes. Many houseplants are found in this category.

C. **Group 2b** plants contain soluble oxalate salts (sodium or potassium) that can produce acute hypocalcemia, renal injury, and other organ damage secondary to precipitation of calcium oxalate crystals in various organs. Mucous membrane irritation is rare, making it possible to ingest sufficient quantities to cause systemic toxicity. Gastroenteritis may also occur (see also p 360).

D. **Group 3** plants contain various toxins that generally produce mild-to-moderate GI irritation after ingestion or dermatitis after skin contact.

II. **Toxic dose.** The amount of toxin ingested is usually unknown. Concentrations of the toxic agent may vary depending on the plant part, the season, and soil conditions. In general, childhood ingestions of a single leaf or a few petals, even of Group 1 plants, results in little or no toxicity because of the small amount of toxin absorbed. Steeping the plant in hot water (eg, an "herbal" tea) may allow very large amounts of toxin to be absorbed.

III. **Clinical presentation** depends on the active toxic agent (see Table II–51), although even nontoxic plants can cause coughing, choking, or gagging if a large piece is swallowed.

A. **Group 1.** In most cases, vomiting, abdominal pain, and diarrhea occur within 60–90 minutes of a significant ingestion, but systemic symptoms may be delayed a few hours while toxins are activated in the gut (eg, cyanogenic glycosides) or distributed to tissues (eg, cardiac glycosides). With some toxins (eg, ricin), severe gastroenteritis may result in massive fluid and electrolyte loss and GI sloughing.

B. **Group 2a.** Insoluble calcium oxalate crystals cause immediate oral burning, pain, and stinging upon contact with mucous membranes. Swelling of the lips, tongue, and pharynx may occur. In rare cases, glottic edema may result in airway obstruction. Symptoms usually resolve within a few hours.

TABLE II–51. PLANTS: SOME TOXIC COMPONENTS

Toxin or Source	Clinical Effects
Aconite	Paresthesias, gastroenteritis, skeletal muscle paralysis, ventricular arrhythmias, respiratory paralysis, shock, death (see p 77).
Aesculin	Single seed can cause gastroenteritis. Larger amounts can cause ataxia, gastroenteritis, CNS depression, and paralysis.
Anthraquinone	Severe diarrhea with GI bleeding, renal damage, dyspnea, and seizures.
Chinaberry	Gastroenteritis, lethargy, coma, respiratory failure, seizures, paralysis.
Cicutoxin	Seizures, tremors, tachycardia, mydriasis, fever, vomiting, diarrhea, rhabdomyolysis, death.
Coniine	Similar to nicotine (p 337): vomiting, seizures, rhabdomyolysis, muscle paralysis, and respiratory arrest.
Cyanogenic glycosides	Dyspnea, cyanosis, weakness, seizures, coma, cardiovascular collapse. Symptoms may be delayed for 3–4 hours or more as glycoside is hydrolyzed to cyanide (see p 208).
Cytisine	Vomiting, hallucinations, hypotension, tachycardia, paralysis, seizures, respiratory depression.
Daphne	GI and skin irritant; vomiting bloody diarrhea; delirium, seizures, coma.
Euphorbiaceae	Oral irritation, gastroenteritis. Erythema, edema, followed by vesicle and blister formation. Eye exposure may result in corneal ulceration, iritis, conjunctivitis, and temporary blindness. Systemic symptoms: seizures, coma, and death.
Gelsemium indole alkaloids	Headache, sweating, muscular weakness or rigidity, seizures, dyspnea, bradycardia, respiratory arrest.
Grayanotoxin	Burning, tingling of mouth, vomiting; hypotension, bradycardia, coma, seizures.
Hydroquinone	Vomiting, jaundice, dizziness, headache, delirium, pallor, anoxia, seizures, respiratory failure, cyanosis, cardiovascular collapse. Allergic contact dermatitis.
Lobeline	Similar to nicotine (p 337).
Nicotine alkaloids	Vomiting and diarrhea; agitation, seizures followed by coma and respiratory arrest. Initial hypertension and tachycardia followed by hypotension and bradycardia. See p 337.
Nitrites	Hypotension, tachycardia, methemoglobinemia (see p 317).
Protoanemonin	Acrid burning taste, oral ulceration, gastroenteritis, hematemesis.
Psoralens	Ultraviolet light-induced erythema, burns, pigmentation.
Pyrrolizidine alkaloids	Gastroenteritis; hepatic injury due to veno-occlusive disease.
Quinolizidine	Some lupines can cause anticholinergic syndrome.
Sanguinaria	Gastroenteritis, CNS depression, dyspnea, edema, respiratory paralysis.
Saponin	GI and skin irritant, mydriasis, hyperthermia, muscle weakness, dyspnea, coma.
Solanine	Gastroenteritis; less commonly drowsiness, coma, hypotension, bradycardia.
Tannin	Abdominal pain, vomiting, bloody diarrhea, liver and kidney injury.
Toxalbumin	Severe gastroenteritis; shock; multiple-organ injury (see Ricin, p 447).
Veratrum alkaloids	Gastroenteritis, bradycardia, AV block, syncope, paresthesias.

TABLE II–52. PLANTS: ALPHABETICAL LIST

Common Name	Botanical Name	Toxic Group[a]	Remarks (see text and Table II–51)
Acacia, black	*Robinia pseudoacacia*	1	Toxalbumin
Ackee	*Blighia sapida*	1	Hypoglycemia, encephalopathy, seizures, vomiting, hypotonia
Aconite	*Aconitum* spp	1	Aconitum (p 77)
Acorn	*Quercus* spp	3	Tannin; dermatitis
Agapanthus	*Agapanthus* spp	3	Dermatitis; GI irritant
Agave	*Agave* spp	3	Saponin; dermatitis
Alder, American	*Alnus crispa*	3	Dermatitis
Alder buckthorn	*Rhamnus frangula*	1	Anthraquinone
Almond, bitter	*Prunus dulcis var amara*	1	Cyanogenic glycosides (p 208)
Aloe vera	*Aloe vera*	3	GI upset, skin irritant
Amaryllis[b]	*Amaryllidaceae*	3	GI upset
Amaryllis[b]	*Hippeastrum equestre*	3	GI upset
American bittersweet	*Celastrus scandens*	1,3	GI upset; convulsions, coma
American ivy	*Parthenocissus* spp	2b	Soluble oxalates
Anemone	*Anemone* spp	1,3	Protoanemonin; dermatitis
Angelica	*Angelica archangelica*	3	Dermatitis, photosensitive (psoralens)
Angel's trumpet	*Brugmansia arborea, Datura* spp	1,3	Anticholinergic alkaloids (p 97)
Anthurium	*Anthurium* spp	2a	Calcium oxalate crystals
Apple (chewed seeds)	*Malus* spp	1	Cyanogenic glycosides (p 208)
Apricot (chewed pits)	*Prunus* spp	1	Cyanogenic glycosides (p 208)
Arrowhead vine	*Syngonium podophyllum*	2a	Calcium oxalate crystals
Artemisia	*Artemisia*	1,3	Some species are toxic: vomiting, diarrhea, vertigo, visual color distortion, sweating, seizures, respiratory failure
Arum	*Arum* spp	1,2a	Calcium oxalate crystals. *Arium maculatum* can cause flushing, mydriasis, drowsiness, tachycardia
Ash, white	*Fraxinus Americana*	3	Dermatitis
Aspen tree	*Populus tremuloides*	3	Dermatitis
Autumn crocus	*Colchicum autumnale*	1	Colchicine (p 205)
Avocado (leaves and seeds)	*Persea americana*	1	Ripe fruit is edible, but leaves and seeds have caused illness in animals (unknown toxin): hyperexcitability, anorexia, cerebral and pulmonary hemorrhage
Azalea	*Rhododendron* genus	1	Grayanotoxin
Azalea honey ("mad honey")	*Rhododendron* genus	1	Grayanotoxin

(continued)

TABLE II–52. PLANTS: ALPHABETICAL LIST (CONTINUED)

Common Name	Botanical Name	Toxic Group[a]	Remarks (see text and Table II–51)
Bahia	*Bahia oppositifolia*	1	Cyanogenic glycosides (p 208)
Balsam apple[b]	*Clusia rosea*	3	GI upset
Balsam apple[b]	*Momordica balsamina*	3	GI upset
Baneberry	*Actaea* spp	1,3	Irritant oil protoanemonin; dermatitis and severe gastroenteritis
Barbados nut, purge nut	*Jatropha curcas*	1	Toxalbumin, Euphorbiaceae
Barberry	*Berberis* spp	1,3	GI upset, hypotension, paresthesias, seizures
Bear's grape, bearberry	*Arctostaphylos uvo-ursi*	1,3	Hydroquinone; berries edible
Beech, European	*Fagus sylvatica*	3	Saponin-like
Beech, Japanese	*Fagus crenta*	3	Saponin-like
Begonia	*Begonia rex*	2a	Calcium oxalate crystals
Belladonna	*Atropa belladonna*	1	Atropine (p 97)
Bellyache bush	*Jatropha gossypifolia*	1	Euphorbiaceae
Be-still tree	*Thevetia peruviana*	1	Cardiac glycosides (p 222)
Big root	*Marah oreganus*	1,3	GI upset, muscle cramping, shock, coagulopathy
Birch (bark, leaves)	*Betula* spp	1,3	Methyl salicylate (p 410), irritant oils causing GI upset
Bird of paradise[b]	*Poinciana gillesi*	1,3	GI upset; vertigo and drowsiness
Bird of paradise flower[b]	*Streelizia reginae*	3	GI upset
Black cohosh	*Cimicifuga* spp	3	GI upset
Black-eyed Susan[b]	*Abrus precatorius*	1	Toxalbumin
Black-eyed Susan[b]	*Rudbeckia hirta*	3	Dermatitis
Black henbane	*Hyoscyamus niger*	1	Anticholinergic alkaloids (p 97)
Black lily	*Dracunculus vulgaris*	2a	Calcium oxalate crystals
Black locust	*Robinia pseudoacacia*	1	Toxalbumin
Black nightshade	*Solanum nigrum*	1	Solanine
Black snakeroot[b]	*Cimicifuga racemosa*	3	GI upset; bradycardia
Black snakeroot	*Zigadenus venenosus*	1	Veratrum alkaloids
Bleeding heart	*Dicentra Formosa*	1,3	Dermatitis; in animals may cause tremor, ataxia, salivation, convulsions with large ingestions
Bloodroot	*Sanguinaria canadensis*	3	Sanguinaria
Blue bonnet	*Lupinus* spp	1	Quinolizidine
Blue cohosh	*Caulophyllum thalictroides*	1,3	Cytisine; dermatitis. Saponin with weak nicotinelike activity
Boston ivy	*Parthenocissus* spp	2b	Soluble oxalates

(continued)

TABLE II–52. PLANTS: ALPHABETICAL LIST (CONTINUED)

Common Name	Botanical Name	Toxic Group[a]	Remarks (see text and Table II–51)
Bougainvillea	*Bougainvillea glabra*	3	Dermatitis
Box elder	*Acer negundo*	3	Dermatitis
Boxwood	*Buxus sempervirens*	3	GI upset, dermatitis
Bracken fern	*Pteridium aquilinum*	1	Potential carcinogen
Bradford pear	*Pyrus calleryana*	3	Dermatitis
Buckeye, California	*Aesculus* spp	1,3	Aesculin
Buckthorn	*Karwinski humboltiana*	1	Chronic ingestion may cause ascending paralysis; latent onset several weeks
Buckthorn	*Rhamnus frangula*	3	Anthraquinone
Bunchberry	*Cornus canadensis*	3	Dermatitis
Burdock	*Arctium lappa*	1,3	Rarely causes anticholinergic syndrome (p 97)
Burning bush[b]	*Dictamnus albus*	3	Dermatitis, photosensitive
Burning bush[b]	*Euonymus atropurpurea*	3	GI upset
Burning bush[b]	*Kochia scoparia*	1,2a,2b,3	Soluble and insoluble oxalates; dermatitis; in animals may cause elevated bilirubin, polyuria
Buttercup	*Ranunculus* spp	3	Protoanemonin
Cactus (thorn)	*Cactus*	3	Dermatitis, cellulitis (abscess may result)
Cactus, pencil	*Euphorbia tirucalli*	3	Euphorbiaceae
Cactus, peyote	*Lophophora williamsii*	1	Vomiting, tachycardia, hallucinations
Caladium	*Caladium* spp	2a	Calcium oxalate crystals
California geranium	*Senecio petasitis*	1,3	Hepatotoxic pyrrolizidine alkaloids; dermatitis
California poppy	*Eschscholzia californica*	3	Potentially mildly sedating, no recorded toxicity (does not contain opium)
California privet	*Ligustrum ovalifolium*	3	Saponin
Calla lily	*Zantedeschia* spp	2a	Calcium oxalate crystals
Candlenut	*Aleurites moluccana*	1,3	Euphorbiaceae
Cannabis	*Cannabis sativa*	1	Mild hallucinogen (see "Marijuana," p 304)
Cardinal flower	*Lobelia cardinalis*	1	Lobeline
Carnation	*Dianthus caryophyllus*	3	Dermatitis; possible GI upset
Carolina allspice	*Calycanthus* spp	1	Strychnine-like alkaloid (p 429)
Cascara	*Rhamnus* spp	3	Anthraquinone cathartic
Cassava	*Manihot esculenta*	1,3	Cyanogenic glycosides (p 208); euphorbiaceae; dermatitis
Castor bean	*Ricinus communis*	1	Toxalbumin (ricin, p 447)

(*continued*)

TABLE II–52. PLANTS: ALPHABETICAL LIST (CONTINUED)

Common Name	Botanical Name	Toxic Group[a]	Remarks (see text and Table II–51)
Catnip	*Nepeta cataria*	1,3	Mild hallucinogen; GI upset
Cedar, giant	*Thuja plicata*	3	Dermatitis
Celery	*Apium graveolens var dulce*	3	Dermatitis, photosensitive; leaves contain nitrites and fatalities reported in cattle ingesting large quantities
Century plant	*Agave americana*	3	Thorns can cause cellulitis, sap causes dermatitis
Chamomile	*Anthemis cotula*	3	Dermatitis (severe bullous dermatitis reported); GI upset
Cherry (chewed pits)	*Prunus* spp	1	Cyanogenic glycosides (p 208)
Chili pepper	*Capsicum* spp	3	Irritant to skin, eyes, mucous membranes
Chinaberry	*Melia azedarach*	1,3	Chinaberry; severe GI upset, seizures
Chokecherry (chewed pits)	*Prunus virginiana*	1	Cyanogenic glycosides (p 208)
Christmas rose	*Helleborus niger*	1,3	Protoanemonin; saponin; possibly cardiac glycosides (see p 222); dermatitis
Chrysanthemum; mum	*Chrysanthemum* spp	3	Dermatitis, GI upset
Clematis	*Clematis* spp	3	Protoanemonin
Clover, white[b]	*Trifolium repens*	1	Cyanogenic glycosides (p 208)
Clover, sweet[b]	*Melilotus alba and M officinalis*	1	Coumarins (p 459)
Coffeeberry	*Rhamnus californica*	3	Anthraquinone
Coffee tree	*Polyscias guilfoyei*	3	Saponin
Cola nut	*Cola nitida*	1	Caffeine (p 169)
Comfrey	*Symphytum officinale*	1,3	Hepatotoxic pyrrolidine alkaloids
Conquerer root	*Exogonium purga*	3	GI upset
Coral bean	*Erythrina herbacea*	1	Cyanogenic glycosides (p 208)
Coralberry[b]	*Rivina humulis*	3	GI upset
Coralberry[b]	*Symphoricarpos orbiculatus*	3	GI upset
Coriaria	*Coriaria japonica* spp	1	Contains convulsant similar to picrotoxin
Cotoneaster	*Cotoneaster*	1,3	Cyanogenic glycosides (p 208)
Cottonwood	*Populus deltoides*	3	Dermatitis
Coyotillo	*Karwinskia humboldtiana*	1	Chronic ingestion may cause ascending paralysis; latent onset several weeks
Crab apples (chewed pits)	*Malus* spp	1	Cyanogenic glycosides

(*continued*)

TABLE II–52. PLANTS: ALPHABETICAL LIST (CONTINUED)

Common Name	Botanical Name	Toxic Group[a]	Remarks (see text and Table II–51)
Creeping Charlie	*Glechoma hederacea*	1,3	GI upset; rarely toxic but horses poisoned after large ingestion: dilated pupils, sweating, slobbering
Crocus, wild or prairie	*Anemone* spp	3	Protoanemonin
Croton[b] (houseplant)	*Codiaeum* spp	3	GI upset, dermatitis
Croton[b]	*Croton tiglium*	1	Euphorbiaceae
Crowfoot	*Ranunculus repens*	1	Protoanemonin
Crown of thorns	*Euphorbia* spp	1,3	Euphorbiaceae
Cyclamen	*Cyclamen*	3	GI upset
Daffodil (bulb)	*Narcissus* spp	2a,3	Calcium oxalate crystals; GI upset
Dagga	*Cannabis sativa*	1	Mild hallucinogen
Daisy[b]	*Chrysanthemum* spp	3	GI upset, dermatitis (see "Pyrethrins," p 397)
Daisy, butter[b]	*Ranunculus repens*	1	Protoanemonin
Daisy, seaside[b]	*Erigeron karvinskianus*	3	Dermatitis
Daphne	*Daphne* spp	3	Daphne
Datura	*Datura* spp	1	Anticholinergic alkaloids (p 97)
Deadly nightshade[b]	*Atropa belladonna*	1	Atropine (p 97)
Deadly nightshade[b]	*Solanum* spp	1	Solanine
Death camas	*Zigadenus venenosus*	1	Veratrum alkaloids
Devil's apple[b]	*Several spp*	1	Common name for several toxic species, including *Datura, Solanum, Podophyllum*
Devil's apple[b], devil's trumpet	*Datura stramonium*	1	Anticholinergic alkaloids (p 97)
Devils ivy	*Scindapsus aureus, Epipremnum aureum*	2a	Calcium oxalate crystals
Dieffenbachia	*Dieffenbachia* spp	2a	Calcium oxalate crystals
Dill	*Anethum graveolens*	3	Dermatitis
Dogbane	*Apocynum* spp	1	Possibly cardiac glycosides (p 222)
Dogwood, bloodtwig	*Cornus sanguinea*	3	Dermatitis
Doll's-eyes	*Actaea* spp	3	Irritant oil protoanemonin; severe gastroenteritis, dermatitis
Dragon root	*Arisaema dracontium*	2a,3	Calcium oxalate crystals; dermatitis
Dumbcane	*Dieffenbachia* spp	2a	Calcium oxalate crystals
Dusty miller	*Senecio leucostachys*	1	Hepatotoxic pyrrolizidine alkaloids
Echium	*Echium vulgare*	1	Hepatotoxic pyrrolizidine alkaloids
Eggplant (green parts)	*Solanum melongena*	1	Solanine
Elderberry	*Sambucus* spp	1,3	Unripe berries, leaves, stems, bark cause diarrhea; cyanogenic glycosides (p 208)

(*continued*)

TABLE II–52. PLANTS: ALPHABETICAL LIST (CONTINUED)

Common Name	Botanical Name	Toxic Group[a]	Remarks (see text and Table II–51)
Elephant's ear, taro	*Alacasia* spp, *Colocasia* spp, *Philodendron* spp	2a	Calcium oxalate crystals
Elm, Chinese	*Ulmus parvifolia*	3	Dermatitis
English ivy	*Hedera helix*	3	Saponin; dermatitis
English laurel	*Prunus laurocerasus*	1	Cyanogenic glycosides (p 208)
Eucalyptus	*Eucalyptus*	3	GI upset
False hellebore	*Veratrum* spp	1,3	Veratrum alkaloids
False parsley[b] (water hemlock)	*Cicuta maculata*	1	Cicutoxin: seizures
False parsley[b] (lesser hemlock)	*Aethusa cynapium*	1	Coniine
Fava bean	*Vicia faba*	1	Hemolytic anemia in G6PD-deficient persons
Ficus (sap)	*Ficus* spp	3	Dermatitis
Fiddle-leaf fig	*Ficus* spp	3	Dermatitis
Fig	*Ficus carica*	3	Dermatitis
Fig, creeping or climbing	*Ficus pumila*	3	Dermatitis
Firethorn	*Pyracantha*	3	GI upset, thorn injury
Flag	*Iris* spp	3	GI upset, dermatitis
Flax	*Linum usitatisimum*	1	Cyanogenic glycosides (p 208)
Fleabane	*Erigeron* spp	3	Dermatitis
Fool's parsley	*Aethus cyanapium*	1	Coniine, nicotine-like alkaloid (p 337)
Four o'clock	*Mirabilis jalapa*	1,3	Seeds may have hallucinogenic effects; dermatitis, GI upset
Foxglove	*Digitalis purpurea*	1	Cardiac glycosides (p 222)
Garden sorrel	*Rumex acetosa*	2b,3	Soluble oxalates; dermatitis
Geranium[b]	*Pelargonium* spp	3	Dermatitis
Geranium, California[b]	*Senecio petasitis*	1,3	Hepatotoxic pyrrolizidine alkaloids; dermatitis
Ginkgo	*Ginkgo biloba*	1,3	Dermatitis, mucous membrane irritation; GI upset; chronic use can increase bleeding time
Goldenrod, rayless	*Haplopappus heterophyl-lus*	1	CNS depression reported in range animals
Golden chain	*Laburnum anagyroides*	1	Cytisine
Goldenseal	*Hydrastis spp*	1,3	GI upset; possible systemic toxicity based on animal studies (hypertension, seizures, respiratory failure)
Gordoloba	*Achillea millefolium*	3	GI upset, dermatitis
Gotu kola	*Hydrocotyle asiatica*	1,3	CNS depression, dermatitis
Grape ivy	*Cissus rhombifolia*	3	Dermatitis

(*continued*)

TABLE II–52. PLANTS: ALPHABETICAL LIST (CONTINUED)

Common Name	Botanical Name	Toxic Group[a]	Remarks (see text and Table II–51)
Groundsel	*Senecio* spp	1,3	Hepatotoxic pyrrolizidine alkaloids; dermatitis
Guaiac	*Guaiacum officinale*	3	Saponin
Harmaline	*Banisteriopsis* spp	1	Harmaline (hallucinogen)
Harmel	*Peganum harmala*	1	Harmaline (hallucinogen)
Hawaiian woodrose	*Merremia tuberosa*	1	Hallucinogen (may contain LSD [see p 297])
Hawaiian baby woodrose	*Argyreia nervosa*	1	Hallucinogen (may contain LSD [see p 297])
Heart leaf philodendron	*Philodendron* spp	2a	Calcium oxalate crystals
Heath	*Calluna vulggaris*	1	Grayanotoxin
Heliotrope	*Heliotropium* spp	1	Pyrrolizidine alkaloids; hepatotoxicity
Hell's bells	*Datura stramonium*	1	Anticholinergic
Hemlock[b] (poison hemlock)	*Conium maculatum*	1	Coniine
Hemlock[b] (water hemlock)	*Cicuta maculata*	1	Cicutoxin: seizures
Henbane, black henbane	*Hyoscyamus niger*	1	Anticholinergic alkaloids (p 97)
Holly (berry)	*Ilex* spp	3	GI upset. Many contain saponins
Hop, European	*Humulus lupulus*	3	Dermatitis
Hop, wild	*Bryonia* spp	3	GI upset, dermatitis
Horse chestnut	*Aesculus* spp	1,3	Aesculin
Horsetail	*Equisetum* spp	1	Chronic use: hyponatremia, hypokalemia and muscle weakness, possible symptoms nicotine-like
Hyacinth	*Hyacinthus* spp	3	GI upset, dermatitis
Hydrangea	*Hydrangea* spp	1,3	Cyanogenic glycosides (p 208); GI upset; allergic contact dermatitis
Indian currant	*Symphoricarpos albus*	3	GI upset
Indian tobacco	*Lobelia inflata*	1,3	Lobeline, nicotine-like alkaloid (p 337); dermatitis
Indigo weed, wild indigo	*Baptisia tinctora*	1	Cytisine
Inkberry	*Ilex glabra*	3	Saponin
Inkberry (pokeweed)	*Phytolacca americana*	3	Saponin
Iris	*Iris*	3	GI upset, dermatitis
Ithang	*Mitragyna* spp	1	Kratom: sedative and stimulant effects, depending on dose
I-thien-hung	*Emilia sonchifolia*	1	Pyrrolizidine alkaloids
Ivy[b]	*Hedera helix*	3	GI upset, dermatitis

(continued)

TABLE II–52. PLANTS: ALPHABETICAL LIST (CONTINUED)

Common Name	Botanical Name	Toxic Group[a]	Remarks (see text and Table II–51)
Ivy bush[b]	*Kalmia* spp	1	Grayanotoxin
Jack-in-the-pulpit	*Arisaema triphyllum*	2a,3	Calcium oxalate crystals; dermatitis
Jaggery palm	*Caryota urens*	2a	Calcium oxalate crystals
Jalap root	*Exogonium purga*	3	GI upset
Jasmine, Carolina	*Gelsemium spp*	1	Gelsemium
Jequirity bean	*Abrus precatorius*	1	Toxalbumin (abrin)
Jerusalem cherry	*Solanum pseudocapsicum*	1	Solanine and possibly anticholinergic alkaloids (p 97)
Jessamine, Carolina or yellow[b]	*Gelsemium spp*	1	Gelsemium
Jessamine, day blooming[b]	*Cestrum diurnum*	1	Solanine and anticholinergic alkaloids (p 97)
Jessamine, night blooming[b]	*Cestrum nocturnum*	1	Solanine and anticholinergic alkaloids (p 97)
Jessamine, poet's[b]	*Jasminum officianale*	3	Dermatitis
Jimmy weed	*Haplopappus heterophyl-lus*	1	CNS depression reported in range animals
Jimsonweed	*Brugmansia arborea, Datura*	1	Anticholinergic alkaloids (p 97)
Juniper	*Juniperus Virginia and sabina*	1,3	GI upset, dermatitis; chronic ingestion of *J sabina* may cause renal toxicity
Kaffir lily	*Clivia miniata*	3	GI upset
Kanna	*Sceletium tortuosum*	1	Mild hallucinogen
Kava-kava	*Piper methysticum*	1	Acute: sedation, ataxia; chronic: dermatitis (scaling skin) and hepatotoxicity
Kentucky coffee tree	*Gymnocladus dioica*	1	Cytisine, similar to nicotine (p 337)
Khat	*Catha edulis*	1	Mild stimulant: euphoria, mydriasis, tachycardia, anorexia
Kratom	*Mitragyna* spp	1	Sedative and stimulant effects, depending on dose
Lady's slipper[b]	*Cypripedium* spp	3	Dermatitis
Lady's slipper[b]	*Pedilanthus tithymaloides*	1,3	Euphorbiaceae; GI, skin and eye irritant
Lantana	*Lantana camara*	1	Mild GI upset; rarely CNS and respiratory depression
Larkspur	*Delphinium*	1	Aconitum-like
Laurel[b]	*Kalmia spp*	1	Grayanotoxin
Laurel[b]	*Laurus nobilis*	3	Dermatitis, GI upset
Licorice[b]	*Glycyrrhiza lepidata*	1,3	Hypokalemia, water retention usually after chronic use but has occurred after single large ingestion; GI upset

(*continued*)

TABLE II–52. PLANTS: ALPHABETICAL LIST (CONTINUED)

Common Name	Botanical Name	Toxic Group[a]	Remarks (see text and Table II–51)
Licorice, wild[b]	*Abrus precatorius*	1	Toxalbumin
Lily of the Nile	*Agapanthus*	3	GI upset, dermatitis
Lily-of-the-valley[b]	*Convallaria spp*	1	Cardiac glycosides (p 222)
Lily-of-the-valley bush[b]	*Pieris japonica*	1	Grayanotoxin
Lion's ear	*Leonotis leonurus*	1	Mild hallucinogen
Lobelia	*Lobelia berlandieri*	1	Lobeline
Locoweed[b]	*Astragalus* spp	1	Pyrrolizidine alkaloids
Locoweed[b]	*Datura stramonium*	1	Anticholinergic alkaloids (p 97)
Locoweed[b]	*Cannabis sativa*	1	Mild hallucinogen (p 304)
Lupine	*Lupines* spp	1	Quinolizidine
Mad honey	*Rhododendron* genus	1	Grayanotoxin
Mandrake[b]	*Mandragora officinarum*	1	Anticholinergic alkaloids (see p 97)
Mandrake[b]	*Podophyllum peltatum*	1,3	Oil is keratolytic, irritant; podophyllotoxin is similar to colchicine (p 184)
Marble queen pothos	*Scindapsus aureus; Epipremnum aurem*	2a	Calcium oxalate crystals
Marijuana	*Cannabis sativa*	1	Mild hallucinogen
Marsh marigold	*Caltha palustris*	3	Protoanemonin
Mate	*Ilex paraguariensis*	1	Caffeine
Mayapple	*Podophyllum peltatum*	1,3	Oil is keratolytic, irritant; podophyllotoxin is similar to colchicine (p 205)
Meadow crocus	*Colchicum autumnale*	1	Colchicine (p 205)
Mescal bean[b]	*Sophora secundiflora*	1	Cytisine, similar to nicotine (p 337)
Mescal button[b]	*Lophophora williamsii*	1	Hallucinogen (p 297)
Mexican breadfruit	*Monstera deliciosa*	2a	Calcium oxalate crystals
Milkweed	*Asclepias* spp	1,3	Cardiac glycosides (p 222); GI upset, CNS depressant, seizures
Mistletoe, American[b]	*Phoradendron flavescens*	3	GI upset. Systemic toxicity rarely reported
Mistletoe, European[b]	*Viscum album*	1,3	Seizures (rare), GI upset
Mock azalea[b]	*Menziesia ferruginea*	1	Grayanotoxin
Mock azalea[b]	*Adenium obesum*	1	Cardiac glycosides (p 222)
Monkshood	*Aconitum napellus*	1	Aconite (p 77)
Moonflower[b]	*Ipomoea alba*	3	Dermatitis
Moonflower[b]	*Datura inoxia*	1,3	Anticholinergic alkaloids; dermatitis
Moonseed[b]	*Menispermaceae*	1	Picrotoxin-like seizures
Moonseed, Carolina[b]	*Cocculus carolinus*	1	Seizures possible
Mormon tea	*Ephedra viridis*	1	Ephedra; tachycardia, hypertension (p 394)

(continued)

TABLE II–52. PLANTS: ALPHABETICAL LIST (CONTINUED)

Common Name	Botanical Name	Toxic Group[a]	Remarks (see text and Table II–51)
Morning glory	*Ipomoea violacea*	1	Seeds hallucinogenic (LSD, see p 297)
Morning, noon, and night	*Brunfelsia australis*	1	Seizures
Mountain laurel	*Kalmia* spp	1	Grayanotoxin
Naked lady	*Amaryllis belladonna, Lycoris* spp	3	GI upset, dermatitis
Narcissus	*Narcissus* spp	2a,3	GI upset, possibly calcium oxalates
Nectarine (chewed pits)	*Prunus* spp	1	Cyanogenic glycosides (p 208)
Needlepoint ivy	*Hedera helix*	3	GI upset, dermatitis
Nephthytis	*Syngonium podophyllum*	2a	Calcium oxalate crystals
Nettles, stinging	*Urtica* spp	3	Dermatitis
Nicotiana, ornamental	*Nicotiana longiflora*	1	Nicotine (p 337)
Nightshade	*Solanum* spp	1	Solanine and anticholinergic alkaloids (p 97)
Nightshade, black	*Solanum nigrum*	1	Solanine, anticholinergic alkaloids (p 97)
Nightshade, deadly[b]	*Atropa belladonna*	1	Atropine (p 97)
Nightshade, deadly[b]	*Solanum nigrum*	1	Solanine, anticholinergic alkaloids (p 97)
Nutmeg	*Myristica fragrans*	1	Hallucinogen (p 297); tachycardia, dry mouth, miosis, abdominal pain
Oak	*Quercus* spp	1	Tannin
Oakleaf ivy[b]	*Hedera helix*	1,3	GI upset, dermatitis; saponins
Oakleaf ivy[b], grape ivy	*Cissus rhombifolia*	3	Dermatitis
Oleander	*Nerium oleander*	1	Cardiac glycosides (p 222)
Oleander, yellow	*Thevetia peruviana*	1	Cardiac glycosides (p 222), more toxic than *Nerium*
Olive	*Olea europaea*	3	Dermatitis
Ornamental cherry (chewed seeds)	*Prunus* spp	1	Cyanogenic glycosides (p 208)
Ornamental crab apple (chewed seeds)	*Malus* spp	1	Cyanogenic glycosides (p 208)
Ornamental pear, Bradford pear	*Pyrus calleryana*	3	Dermatitis
Ornamental pepper[b]	*Capsicum annuum*	3	Skin, eye and GI irritant
Ornamental pepper[b]	*Solanum pseudocapsicum*	1	Solanine
Ornamental plum (chewed seeds)	*Prunus* spp	1	Cyanogenic glycosides (p 208)
Oxalis	*Oxalis* spp	2b	Soluble oxalates
Palm (thorns or spines)	Various	3	Cellulitis, synovitis

(continued)

TABLE II–52. PLANTS: ALPHABETICAL LIST (CONTINUED)

Common Name	Botanical Name	Toxic Group[a]	Remarks (see text and Table II–51)
Paper white narcissus	*Narcissus* spp	2a,3	GI upset; may contain calcium oxalates; no reports of systemic toxicity in humans
Paradise tree	*Melia azedarach*	1,3	Chinaberry; severe GI upset, seizures
Paraguay tea	*Ilex paraguaiensis*	1	Caffeine (p 169)
Parsnip	*Pastinaca sativa*	3	Dermatitis, photosensitive
Passion flower	*Passiflora caerulea*	1	Extract caused CNS depression, prolonged QT and ventricular tachycardia
Pasque flower	*Anemone* spp	1	Protoanemonin
Peace lily	*Spathiphyllum*	2a	Calcium oxalate crystals
Peach (chewed pits)	*Prunus* spp	1	Cyanogenic glycosides (p 208)
Pear (chewed seeds)	*Pyrus* spp	1	Cyanogenic glycosides (p 208)
Pecan	*Carya illinonensis*	3	Dermatitis
Pelargonium	*Pelargonium* spp	3	Possible dermatitis
Pennyroyal (oil)	*Mentha pulegium*	1	Hepatic injury, coagulopathy, multiple-system failure (p 176)
Periwinkle	*Vinca rosea*	1	Contains vincristine, vinblastine (p 114)
Periwinkle, rose	*Catharanthus roseus*	1	Contains vincristine, vinblastine (p 114)
Peruvian lily	*Alstroemeria aurantiaca*	3	GI upset, dermatitis
Peyote, mescal	*Lophophora williamsii*	1	Mescaline, hallucinogen (p 297); vomiting, tachycardia, mydriasis, agitation
Pheasant's-eye	*Adonis vernalis*	1	Possibly cardiac glycosides (p 222)
Philodendron	*Philodendron* spp	2a	Calcium oxalate crystals
Photinia	*Photinia arbutifolia*	1	Cyanogenic glycosides
Pigeonberry[b]	*Duranta repens*	3	Saponin
Pigeonberry[b]	*Cornus canadensis*	3	Dermatitis
Pigeonberry[b]	*Rivina humilis*	3	Saponin
Pigeonberry[b]	*Phytolacca americana*	3	Saponin
Pinks	*Dianthus caryophyllus*	3	Dermatitis, possible GI upset
Plum (chewed pits)	*Prunus* spp	1	Cyanogenic glycosides (p 208)
Poinsettia	*Euphorbia pulcherrima*	3	Possible GI upset
Poison hemlock	*Conium maculatum*	1	Coniine
Poison ivy, poison oak, poison sumac, poison vine	*Toxicodendron* spp	3	Urushiol oleoresin; contact dermatitis (*Rhus* dermatitis)
Pokeweed (unripe berries)	*Phytolacca americana*	3	Saponin

(*continued*)

TABLE II–52. PLANTS: ALPHABETICAL LIST (CONTINUED)

Common Name	Botanical Name	Toxic Group[a]	Remarks (see text and Table II–51)
Poplar	*Populus* spp	3	Dermatitis
Poppy, California[b]	*Eschscholzia californica*	1	No recorded human toxicity (does not contain opium); sedating and anxiolytic in mice
Poppy, common[b]	*Papaver somniferum*	1	Opiates (p 350)
Poppy, Oriental[b]	*Papaver orientale*	1	Opiates (p 350)
Potato (green parts, sprouts)	*Solanum tuberosum*	1	Solanine and anticholinergic alkaloids (p 97)
Pothos, Pothos vine	*Epipremnum aureum*	2a	Calcium oxalate crystals
Prayer bean	*Abrus prectorius*	1	Toxalbumin
Pregnant onion	*Ornithogalum caudatum*	1,3	Contains digoxin-like substances (p 222); dermatitis
Prickly pear (thorn)	*Opuntia* spp	3	Dermatitis, cellulitis, thorn injury
Prickly poppy	*Argemone mexicana*	1	Sanguinaria
Pride of China, pride of India	*Melia azedarach*	1	Chinaberry; severe GI upset, seizures
Pride of Madeira	*Echium* spp	1	Pyrrolizidine alkaloids; hepatotoxicity
Primrose	*Primula vulgaris*	3	Dermatitis
Privet, common privet, California privet	*Ligustrum* spp	3	Saponin
Purge nut	*Jatropha curcas*	1	Toxalbumin, Euphorbiaceae
Purslane, milk	*Euphorbia* spp	3	Euphorbiaceae
Pussy willow	*Salix caprea*	3	Dermatitis
Pyracantha	*Pyracantha*	3	GI upset; thorn stab wounds can cause cellulitis
Queen Anne's lace	*Daucus carota*	3	Dermatitis (psoralens)
Queen's delight, queen's root	*Stillingia sylvatica*	3	Euphorbiaceae
Ragweed	*Ambrosia artemisiifolia*	3	Dermatitis
Ragwort, tansy	*Senecio* spp	1	Hepatotoxic pyrrolizidine alkaloids
Ranunculus	*Ranunculus* spp	1	Protoanemonin
Rattlebox	*Crotalaria spectabilis*	1	Hepatotoxic pyrrolizidine alkaloids
Rattlebush	*Baptista tinctoria*	1	Cytisine
Redwood tree	*Sequoia sempervirens*	3	Dermatitis
Rhododendron, including honey made from rhododendron ("mad honey")	*Rhododendron* genus	1	Grayanotoxin
Rhubarb (leaves)	*Rheum rhaponticum*	2b	Soluble oxalates
Rosary pea, rosary bean	*Abrus precatorius*	1	Toxalbumin (abrin)
Rose (thorn)	*Rosa* spp	3	Cellulitis, dermatitis, thorn injury

(continued)

TABLE II–52. PLANTS: ALPHABETICAL LIST (CONTINUED)

Common Name	Botanical Name	Toxic Group[a]	Remarks (see text and Table II–51)
Rubber plant	*Ficus elastica*	3	Dermatitis
Rue	*Ruta graveolens*	3	Dermatitis; possible abortifacient
Rush	*Equisetum* spp	1	Chronic use: hyponatremia, hypokalemia, and muscle weakness; possible nicotine-like symptoms
Rustyleaf	*Menziesia ferruginea*	1	Grayanotoxins
Sagebrush	*Artemisia* spp	1,3	GI upset; CNS stimulant
Salvia	*Salvia divinorum*	1	Hallucinogen
Sassafras	*Sassafras* spp	1	Abortifacient, narcotic
Scotch broom	*Cytisus scoparius*	1,3	Cytisine
Shamrock	*Oxalis* spp	2b	Soluble oxalates
Silvercup	*Solandra grandiflora*	1	Solanine and anticholinergic alkaloids
Skullcap	*Scutellaria lateriflora*	1	Hepatotoxicity, possible seizures
Skunk cabbage[b]	*Symplocarpus foetidus*	2a	Calcium oxalate crystals
Skunk cabbage[b]	*Veratrum* spp	1,3	Veratrum alkaloids
Sky flower	*Duranta repens*	3	Saponin
Smoke tree, smoke bush	*Cotinus coggygria*	1,3	Tannins, hydroquinone; dermatitis
Snakeroot[b]	*Eupatorium rugosum*	1	Hepatotoxic pyrrolizidine alkaloids
Snakeroot[b] (water hemlock)	*Cicuta maculata*	1	Cicutoxin; seizures
Snakeroot[b]	*Aristolochia serpentina*	1,3	GI upset; delayed onset kidney injury
Snowberry	*Symphoricarpos* spp	3	GI upset
Sorrel	*Oxalis* spp, *Rhumex* spp	2b	Soluble oxalates
Soursob	*Oxalis* spp	2b	Soluble oxalates
Spathiphyllum	*Spathiphyllum*	2a	Calcium oxalate crystals
Spindle tree	*Euonymous* spp	3	GI upset
Split leaf philodendron	*Philodendron* spp, *Monstera deliciosa*	2a	Calcium oxalate crystals
Squill	*Scilla, Urginea maritima*	1	Cardiac glycosides (p 222)
Star fruit	*Averrhoa carambola*	2b	Soluble oxalates; reports of acute hypocalcemia in renal failure patients
Star-of-Bethlehem[b]	*Ornithogalum* spp	1	Cardiac glycosides (p 222)
Star-of-Bethlehem[b]	*Hippobroma longiflora*	1	Lobeline
St. John's wort	*Hypericum perforatum*	1,3	Mild serotonin reuptake inhibitor (p 104) and MAO inhibitor (p 326)
Stinging nettles	*Urtica* spp	3	Dermatitis
Stink weed	*Datura stramonium*	1	Anticholinergic (p 97)
String of pearls/beads	*Senecio* spp	1	Hepatotoxic pyrrolizidine alkaloids

(*continued*)

TABLE II–52. PLANTS: ALPHABETICAL LIST (CONTINUED)

Common Name	Botanical Name	Toxic Group[a]	Remarks (see text and Table II–51)
Strychnine	*Strychnos nux-vomica*	1	Strychnine; seizures (p 429)
Sweet clover	*Melilotus* spp	1	Coumarins (p 459)
Sweet pea	*Lathyrus odoratus*	1	Neuropathy (lathyrism) after chronic use
Sweet William	*Dianthus barbatus*	3	GI upset, dermatitis
Swiss cheese plant	*Monstera deliciosa*	2a	Calcium oxalate crystals
Syrian rue	*Peganum harmala*	1	Hallucinogen
Tansy	*Tanacetum* spp	3	Dermatitis
Taro	*Alocasia macrorrhia*	2a	Calcium oxalate crystals
Taro	*Colocasia esculenta*	2a	Calcium oxalate crystals
Texas umbrella tree	*Melia azedarach*	1	Chinaberry
Thornapple	*Datura stramonium* and *inoxia*	1	Anticholinergic (p 97)
Tobacco (flowering tobacco)	*Nicotiana* spp	1	Nicotine (p 337)
Tobacco, wild; tobacco, Indian	*Lobelia inflata*	1	Lobeline (similar to nicotine, p 337)
Tonka bean	*Dipteryx odorata*	1	Coumarin glycosides (p 459)
Toyon (leaves)	*Heteromeles arbutifolia, Photinia arbutifolia*	1	Cyanogenic glycosides (p 208)
Tulip (bulb)	*Tulipa*	3	Dermatitis
Tung nut, tung tree	*Aleurites* spp	1,3	Euphorbiaceae
T'u-san-chi	*Gynura segetum*	1	Hepatotoxic pyrrolizidine alkaloids
Uva-ursi	*Arctostaphylos uvo-ursi*	1,3	Hydroquinone; berries edible
Valerian	*Valeriana officinalis*	1	Mild sedative, anxiolytic, hypnotic
Verbena	*Verbena officinalis and hastata*	3	Dermatitis
Virginia creeper	*Parthenocissus* spp	2b	Soluble oxalates
Walnut	*Juglans* spp	3	Dermatitis
Water hemlock	*Cicuta maculata*	1	Cicutoxin; seizures
Weeping fig (sap)	*Ficus benjamina*	3	Dermatitis
Weeping pagoda tree	*Saphora japonica*	1	Cytisine
Weeping tea tree	*Melaleuca leucadendron*	3	Dermatitis
Weeping willow	*Salix babylonica*	3	Dermatitis
White cedar[b]	*Melia azedarach*	1	Chinaberry; severe GI upset, seizures
White cedar[b]	*Hura crepitans*	3	GI upset, dermatitis
White cedar[b]	*Thuja occidentalis*	1	Abortifacient, stimulant
Wild calla	*Calla palustris*	2a	Calcium oxalates
Wild carrot[b]	*Daucus carota*	3	Dermatitis (psoralens)

(*continued*)

TABLE II–52. PLANTS: ALPHABETICAL LIST (CONTINUED)

Common Name	Botanical Name	Toxic Group[a]	Remarks (see text and Table II–51)
Wild carrot[b]	*Cicuta maculata*	1	Cicutoxin; seizures
Wild cassada	*Jatropha gossypifolia*	1	Euphorbiaceae
Wild cherry (chewed seeds)	*Prunus* spp	1	Cyanogenic glycosides
Wild coffee	*Polyscias guilfoyei*	3	Saponin
Wild cotton	*Asclepias syriaca*	1	Cardiac glycosides (p 222)
Wild cucumber	*Marah oreganus*	1,3	GI upset, cramping, shock, DIC, and death reported after drinking tea
Wild dagga	*Leonotis leonurus*	1	Mild hallucinogen, sedative
Wild fennel	*Nigella damascena*	3	Irritant, possible protoanemonin
Wild garlic	*Allium canadense*	3	GI upset, dermatitis
Wild hops	*Bryonia* spp	3	GI upset, dermatitis
Wild indigo, indigo weed	*Baptisia tinctora*	1	Cytisine
Wild iris	*Iris versicolor*	3	GI upset, dermatitis
Wild lemon	*pelatum*	1,3	Oil is keratolytic, irritant; podophyllotoxin is similar to colchicine (p 205)
Wild marjoram	*Origanum vulgare*	3	GI upset
Wild oats	*Arena fatua*	3	GI upset
Wild onion[b]	*Allium canadense*	3	GI upset, dermatitis
Wild onion[b]	*Zigadenus* spp	1	Veratrum alkaloids
Wild passion flower	*Passiflora incarnata*	1,3	Extract caused CNS depression, prolonged QT and ventricular tachycardia
Wild parsnip[b]	*Pastinaca sativa*	3	Dermatitis (psoralens)
Wild parsnip[b]	*Cicuta maculata*	1	Cicutoxin; seizures
Wild parsnip[b]	*Heracleum mantegazzianum*	3	Dermatitis
Wild parsnip[b]	*Angelica archangelica*	3	Dermatitis
Wild pepper	*Daphne mezereum*	3	Daphne
Wild rock rose	*Cistus incanus*	3	Dermatitis
Windflower	*Anemone*	1,3	Protoanemonin; dermatitis
Wisteria	*Wisteria*	3	GI upset
Witch hazel	*Hamamelis virginiana*	1	Tannin
Woodbind	*Parthenocissus* spp	2b	Soluble oxalates
Wood rose	*Ipomoea violacea, Merrermia tuberosa*	1	Seeds hallucinogenic
Wormwood, wormseed	*Artemisia absinthium*	1	Absinthe; possible CNS effects with large ingestion
Yarrow	*Achillea millefolium*	3	GI upset, dermatitis

(*continued*)

TABLE II–52. PLANTS: ALPHABETICAL LIST (CONTINUED)

Common Name	Botanical Name	Toxic Group[a]	Remarks (see text and Table II–51)
Yellow oleander	*Thevetia peruviana*	1	Cardiac glycosides (p 222)
Yerba buena	*Poliomintha incana* (not *Satureia douglasi,* which is not toxic)	1	Pennyroyal oil (p 176); hepatotoxicity, DIC, multiple-system failure
Yerba lechera	*Euphorbia* spp	1	Euphorbiaceae
Yerba mala	*Euphorbia* spp	1	Euphorbiaceae
Yerba mate	*Ilex paraguariensis*	1	Caffeine
Yesterday, today, and tomorrow	*Brunsfelsia australis*	1	Tremors, rigidity, hyperthermia in animals
Yew[b]	*Taxus* spp	1	Sodium and calcium channel blockade; AV block, wide QRS, hypotension
Yew, Japanese[b]	*Podocarpus macrophylla*	3	Dermatitis
Yohimbine	*Corynanthe yohimbe*	1	Central alpha-2-receptor blocker; hypertension, tachycardia. Purported aphrodisiac

[a]Toxic group (see text). 1, systemically active toxins; 2a, insoluble oxalate crystals; 2b, soluble oxalate salts; 3, skin or GI irritants.
[b]*Note:* common name similar to other plants that may have different toxicity.

C. Group 2b. Soluble oxalates may be absorbed into the circulation, where they precipitate with calcium. Acute hypocalcemia and multiple-organ injury, including renal tubular necrosis, may result (see "Oxalates," p 360).

D. Group 3. Skin or mucous membrane irritation may occur, although it is less severe than with Group 2 plants. Vomiting and diarrhea are common but usually mild to moderate and self-limited. Fluid and electrolyte imbalances caused by severe gastroenteritis are rare.

IV. Diagnosis usually is based on a history of exposure and the presence of plant material in vomitus. Identification of the plant is often difficult. Because common names sometimes refer to more than one plant, it is preferable to confirm the botanical name. If in doubt about the plant identification, take a cutting of the plant (not just a leaf or a berry) to a local nursery, florist, or college botany department.

A. Specific levels. Serum toxin levels are not available for most plant toxins. In selected cases, laboratory analyses for therapeutic drugs may be used (eg, digoxin assay for oleander glycosides, cyanide level for cyanogenic glycosides).

B. Other useful laboratory studies for patients with gastroenteritis include CBC, electrolytes, glucose, BUN, creatinine, and urinalysis. If hepatotoxicity is suspected, obtain liver aminotransferases and prothrombin time (PT/INR).

V. Treatment. Most ingestions cause no symptoms or only mild gastroenteritis. Patients recover quickly with supportive care.

A. Emergency and supportive measures

1. Maintain an open airway and assist ventilation if necessary (see pp 1–7). Administer supplemental oxygen.
2. Treat coma (p 18), seizures (p 23), arrhythmias (pp 10–15), and hypotension (p 15) if they occur.
3. Replace fluid losses caused by gastroenteritis with IV crystalloid solutions.

B. **Specific drugs and antidotes.** There are few effective antidotes. Refer to discussions elsewhere in Section II for further details.

C. **Decontamination** (p 50)

1. **Group 1 and Group 2b plants.** Administer activated charcoal orally if conditions are appropriate (see Table I–38, p 54). Gastric lavage is not necessary after small-to-moderate ingestions if activated charcoal can be given promptly. Gastric lavage may not be effective in removing larger plant parts. Whole-bowel irrigation (p 55) may be considered if large amounts of a toxic plant or plant parts were ingested and the patient arrives soon after the ingestion.

2. **Group 2a and Group 3 plants**

   a. Wash the affected areas with soap and water and give sips of water to drink.

   b. Administer ice cream, juice bars, pudding, or cold milk to soothe irritated oral mucous membranes after exposure to insoluble oxalate plants.

   c. Do ***not*** induce vomiting because of potential aggravation or irritant effects. Activated charcoal is not necessary.

D. **Enhanced elimination.** These procedures are generally not effective.

▶ POLYCHLORINATED BIPHENYLS (PCBs)

Timur S. Durrani, MD, MPH, MBA

Polychlorinated biphenyls (PCBs) are mixtures of up to 209 different chlorinated compounds that once were used widely as high-temperature insulators for transformers and other electric equipment. They were also found in carbonless copy papers, inks, paints, caulks, sealants and ceiling tiles. Many commercial PCB mixtures are known in the United States by the trade name Aroclor. Since 1974, all uses in the United States have been confined to closed systems. Most PCB poisonings are chronic occupational or environmental exposures, with delayed-onset symptoms the first indication that an exposure has occurred. In 1977, the US Environmental Protection Agency (EPA) banned further manufacturing of PCBs because they are suspected carcinogens and highly persistent in the environment. Exposure occurs through the consumption of meat, fish, and dairy because of biomagnification up the food chain, as well as by inhalation in contaminated indoor or outdoor environments. PCBs were widely used in building materials from 1950s to 1979, and remain present in buildings that were constructed or renovated during that period. Since many schools in use today were built or renovated during that era, they present a potential risk of exposure to children and staff.

I. **Mechanism of toxicity.** PCB metabolites may induce DNA strand breaks, resulting in cellular injury. PCBs are irritating to mucous membranes. When burned, PCBs may produce the more highly toxic polychlorinated dibenzodioxins (PCDDs) and polychlorinated dibenzofurans (PCDFs [p 224]). PCBs, and particularly the PCDD and PCDF contaminants, are mutagenic and teratogenic and are considered human carcinogens by the International Agency for Research on Cancer.

II. **Toxic dose.** PCBs are either oily liquids or solids that are colorless to light yellow. Some can exist as a vapor in air. PCBs have no known smell or taste. PCBs are well absorbed by all routes (skin, inhalation, and ingestion) and are widely distributed in fat; bioaccumulation occurs even with low-level exposure.

A. **Inhalation.** PCBs are mildly irritating to the skin at airborne levels of 0.1 mg/m^3 and very irritating at 10 mg/m^3. The ACGIH-recommended workplace limits (TLVTWA) are 0.5 mg/m^3 (for PCBs with 54% chlorine) and 1 mg/m^3 (for PCBs with 42% chlorine) as 8-hour time-weighted averages. The air level considered immediately dangerous to life or health (IDLH) for either type is 5 mg/m^3.

B. **Ingestion.** Acute toxicity after ingestion is unlikely; the oral 50% lethal dose (LD_{50}) is 1–10 g/kg.

III. Clinical presentation

A. **Acute PCB exposure** may cause skin, eye, nose, and throat irritation.

B. **Chronic exposure** may cause **chloracne** (cystic acneiform lesions predominantly found on the face, posterior neck, axillae, upper back, and abdomen); the onset usually occurs 6 weeks or longer after exposure. Skin pigmentation, porphyria, elevated hepatic transaminases, and thyroid hormone abnormalities may occur.

C. Epidemiologic studies suggest that PCB exposure is associated with decreased IQ and other neurobehavioral effects in newborns and children. Other effects include decreased birth weight and immune system effects in babies as a result of transplacental transmission or breastfeeding by mothers exposed to elevated levels of PCBs. Exposure to PCBs early in life has been shown in children to be associated with reductions of serum concentrations of antibodies against diphtheria and tetanus vaccinations. There is evidence that PCBs cause adverse estrogen activity in male neonates.

IV. Diagnosis usually is based on a history of exposure and the presence of chloracne or elevated hepatic transaminases.

A. **Specific levels.** PCB serum and fat levels are poorly correlated with health effects. Serum PCB concentrations are usually less than 20 mcg/L; higher levels may indicate exposure but not necessarily toxicity.

B. **Other useful laboratory studies** include BUN, creatinine, and liver enzymes.

V. Treatment

A. **Emergency and supportive measures**

1. Treat bronchospasm (p 8) if it occurs.
2. Monitor for elevated hepatic enzymes, chloracne, and nonspecific eye, GI, and neurologic symptoms.

B. **Specific drugs and antidotes.** There is no specific antidote.

C. **Decontamination** (p 50)

1. **Inhalation.** Remove the victim from exposure and give supplemental oxygen if available.
2. **Skin and eyes.** Remove contaminated clothing and wash exposed skin with soap and water. Irrigate exposed eyes with copious tepid water or saline.
3. **Ingestion.** Administer activated charcoal orally if conditions are appropriate (see Table I–38, p 54). Gastric lavage is not necessary after small-to-moderate ingestions if activated charcoal can be given promptly.

D. **Enhanced elimination.** There is no role for dialysis, hemoperfusion, or repeat-dose charcoal. Lipid-clearing drugs (eg, clofibrate and resins) have been suggested, but insufficient data exist to recommend them. Administration of the nonabsorbable fat substitute olestra has been described for dioxin poisoning (p 224), but human data are limited.

► PSEUDOEPHEDRINE, PHENYLEPHRINE, AND OTHER DECONGESTANTS

Neal L. Benowitz, MD

Pseudoephedrine and phenylephrine are sympathomimetic drugs that are widely available in nonprescription nasal decongestants and cold preparations. These remedies usually also contain antihistamines and cough suppressants. Nonprescription ephedrine-containing cough and cold preparations as well as ephedrine-containing dietary supplements were widely consumed until 2004, when their use was banned by the FDA because of the unacceptable risk for toxicity. **Ephedrine** and ephedra-containing herbal preparations (eg, *ma huang* and "herbal ecstasy"), often in combination with caffeine, were also used as alternatives to the amphetamine derivative "ecstasy" (p 81) or as adjuncts to body-building or weight loss programs. **Phenylpropanolamine** (PPA) had been marketed as a nonprescription decongestant and appetite suppressant for many years but was removed from the US market in 2000 because of an association with hemorrhagic stroke in women. The availability of nonprescription pseudoephedrine is limited in many states because it can be used to manufacture illicit methamphetamine. The FDA issued an advisory in 2008 recommending against the use of cough and cold medicines (which contain decongestants as well as antihistamines and/or dextromethorphan) to children younger than 2 years of age because of reports of serious and life-threatening side effects.

I. Mechanism of toxicity. All these agents stimulate the adrenergic system, with variable effects on alpha- and beta-adrenergic receptors, depending on the compound. Generally, these agents stimulate the CNS much less than do other phenylethylamines (see "Amphetamines," p 81).

A. PPA and phenylephrine are direct alpha-adrenergic agonists. In addition, PPA produces mild $beta_1$-adrenergic stimulation and acts in part indirectly by enhancing norepinephrine release.

B. Ephedrine and pseudoephedrine have both direct and indirect alpha- and beta-adrenergic activity but clinically produce more beta-adrenergic stimulation than does PPA or phenylephrine.

C. Pharmacokinetics. Peak effects occur within 1–3 hours, although absorption may be delayed with sustained-release products. These drugs have large volumes of distribution (eg, the Vd for PPA is 2.5–5 L/kg). Elimination half-lives are 3–7 hours (see also Table II–66, p 462).

II. Toxic dose. Table II–53 lists the usual therapeutic doses of each agent. Patients with autonomic insufficiency and those taking monoamine oxidase (MAO) inhibitors (p 326) may be extraordinarily sensitive to these and other sympathomimetic drugs, developing severe hypertension after ingestion of even subtherapeutic doses.

A. PPA, phenylephrine, and ephedrine have low toxic-to-therapeutic ratios. Toxicity often occurs after ingestion of just 2–3 times the therapeutic dose. Strokes and cardiac toxicity have been reported after therapeutic doses of ephedra and PPA.

B. Pseudoephedrine is less toxic, with symptoms occurring after four- to fivefold the usual therapeutic dose.

III. Clinical presentation. The time course of intoxication by these drugs is usually brief, with resolution within 4–6 hours (unless sustained-release preparations are involved). The major toxic effect of these drugs is **hypertension**, which may lead to headache, confusion, seizures, and intracranial hemorrhage.

A. Intracranial hemorrhage may occur in normal, healthy young persons after what appears to be only a modest elevation of blood pressure (ie, 170/110 mm Hg) and is often associated with focal neurologic deficits, coma, or seizures.

TABLE II–53. EPHEDRINE AND OTHER OTC DECONGESTANTS

Drug	Major Effects[a]	Usual Daily Adult Dose (mg)	Usual Daily Pediatric Dose (mg/kg)
Ephedrine	Beta, alpha	100–200	2–3
Phenylephrine	Alpha	40–60	0.5–1
Phenylpropanolamine[b]	Alpha	100–150	1–2
Pseudoephedrine	Beta, alpha	180–360	3–5

[a]Alpha, alpha-adrenergic receptor agonist; beta, beta-adrenergic receptor agonist.
[b]Removed from US market.

B. **Bradycardia or atrioventricular (AV) block** is common in patients with moderate-to-severe hypertension associated with PPA and phenylephrine owing to the baroreceptor reflex response to hypertension. The presence of drugs such as antihistamines and caffeine prevents reflex bradycardia and may enhance the hypertensive effects of PPA and phenylephrine.

C. **Myocardial infarction** and diffuse myocardial necrosis have been associated with ephedra use and PPA intoxication.

IV. **Diagnosis** usually is based on a history of ingestion of diet pills or decongestant medications and the presence of hypertension. Bradycardia or AV block suggests PPA or phenylephrine. Severe headache, focal neurologic deficits, or coma should raise the possibility of intracerebral hemorrhage.

A. **Specific levels.** Serum drug levels are not generally available and do not alter treatment. In high doses, these agents may produce positive results for amphetamines on urine drug abuse screening testing (see Table I–33, p 46) but can be distinguished on confirmatory testing.

B. **Other useful laboratory studies** include electrolytes, glucose, BUN, creatinine, creatine kinase (CK) with MB isoenzymes, cardiac troponin, 12-lead ECG and ECG monitoring, and CT head scan if intracranial hemorrhage is suspected.

V. **Treatment**

A. **Emergency and supportive measures**

1. Maintain an open airway and assist ventilation if necessary (pp 1–7). Administer supplemental oxygen.
2. Treat hypertension aggressively (see p 17 and Item B below). Treat seizures (p 23) and ventricular tachyarrhythmias (p 13) if they occur. Do ***not*** treat reflex bradycardia except indirectly by lowering blood pressure.
3. Monitor the vital signs and ECG for a minimum of 4–6 hours after exposure and longer if a sustained-release preparation has been ingested.

B. **Specific drugs and antidotes**

1. **Hypertension.** Treat hypertension if the diastolic pressure is higher than 100–105 mm Hg, especially in a patient with no prior history of hypertension. If there is CT or obvious clinical evidence of intracranial hemorrhage, lower the diastolic pressure cautiously to no lower than 90 mm Hg and consult a neurosurgeon immediately.
   a. Use a vasodilator such as **phentolamine** (p 605) or **nitroprusside** (p 593).
   b. ***Caution:*** Do not use beta blockers to treat hypertension without first giving a vasodilator; otherwise, paradoxical worsening of the hypertension may result.
   c. Many patients have moderate orthostatic variation in blood pressure; therefore, for immediate partial relief of severe hypertension, try placing the patient in an upright position.
2. **Arrhythmias**
   a. Tachyarrhythmias usually respond to low-dose **esmolol** (p 552) or **metoprolol.**
   b. Caution: Do ***not*** treat AV block or sinus bradycardia associated with hypertension; increasing the heart rate with atropine may abolish this reflex response that serves to limit hypertension, resulting in worsening hypertension.

C. **Decontamination** (p 50). Administer activated charcoal orally if conditions are appropriate (see Table I–38, p 54). Gastric lavage is not necessary after small-to-moderate ingestions if activated charcoal can be given promptly.

D. **Enhanced elimination.** Dialysis and hemoperfusion are not effective. Urinary acidification may enhance elimination of PPA, ephedrine, and pseudoephedrine but may also aggravate myoglobin deposition in the kidneys if the patient has rhabdomyolysis.

▶ PYRETHRINS AND PYRETHROIDS

Paul Khasigian, PharmD

Pyrethrins are naturally occurring insecticides derived from the chrysanthemum plant. Pyrethroids (Table II–54) are synthetically derived compounds. Acute human poisoning from exposure to these insecticides is rare; however, they can cause skin and upper airway irritation and hypersensitivity reactions. Piperonyl butoxide is added to these compounds to prolong their activity by inhibiting mixed oxidase enzymes in the liver that metabolize the pyrethrins. Common pyrethrin-containing pediculicides include A-200, Triple X, and RID.

I. **Mechanism of toxicity.** In insects, pyrethrins and pyrethroids rapidly cause death by paralyzing the nervous system through disruption of the membrane ion transport system in nerve axons, and pyrethroids prolong sodium influx and also may block inhibitory pathways. Mammals are generally able to metabolize these compounds rapidly and thereby render them harmless.

II. **Toxic dose.** The toxic oral dose in mammals is greater than 100–1,000 mg/kg, and the potentially lethal acute oral dose is 10–100 g. Pyrethrins are not well absorbed across the skin or from the GI tract. They have been used for many years as oral anthelminthic agents with minimum adverse effects other than mild GI upset.

  A. **Deltamethrin.** There is one report of seizures in a young woman who ingested 30 mL of 2.5% deltamethrin (750 mg). **Miraculous Insecticide Chalk** (illegally imported from China) contains up to 37.6 mg of deltamethrin per stick of chalk. Ingestion of a single stick of chalk is generally considered nontoxic.

  B. **Cypermethrin.** A 45-year-old man died after ingesting beans cooked in 10% cypermethrin.

III. **Clinical presentation.** Toxicity to humans is associated primarily with hypersensitivity reactions and direct irritant effects rather than with any pharmacologic property.

  A. **Anaphylactic** reactions including bronchospasm, oropharyngeal edema, and shock may occur in hypersensitive individuals.

  B. **Inhalation** of these compounds may precipitate wheezing in persons with asthma. An 11-year-old girl had a fatal asthma attack after applying a pyrethrin-containing shampoo to her dog. Inhalation or pulmonary aspiration may also cause a hypersensitivity pneumonitis.

  C. **Skin** exposure may cause burning, tingling, numbness, and erythema. The paresthesias are believed to result from a direct effect on cutaneous nerve endings.

  D. **Eyes.** Accidental eye exposure during scalp application of A-200 Pyrinate has caused corneal injury, including keratitis and denudation. The cause is uncertain but may be related to the surfactant (Triton-X) contained in the product.

  E. **Ingestion.** With large ingestions (200–500 mL of concentrated solution), the CNS may be affected, resulting in seizures, coma, or respiratory arrest.

IV. **Diagnosis** is based on a history of exposure. No characteristic clinical symptoms or laboratory tests are specific for identifying these compounds.

  A. **Specific levels.** These compounds are metabolized rapidly in the body, and methods for determining the parent compound are not routinely available.

TABLE II–54. PYRETHROIDS

Allethrin	Cypermethrin	Permethrin
Barthrin	Decamethrin	Phenothrin
Bioallethrin	Deltamethrin	Phthalthrin
Bioresmethrin	Dimethrin	Resmethrin
Cismethrin	Fenothrin	Supermethrin
Cyhalothrin	Fenvalerate	Tetramethrin
Cymethrin	Furamethrin	

B. Other useful laboratory studies include electrolytes, glucose, and arterial blood gases or oximetry.

V. Treatment

A. Emergency and supportive measures

1. Treat bronchospasm (p 8) and anaphylaxis (p 28) if they occur.
2. Observe patients with a history of large ingestions for at least 4–6 hours for any signs of CNS depression or seizures.

B. Specific drugs and antidotes. There is no specific antidote.

C. Decontamination (p 50)

1. **Inhalation.** Remove victims from exposure and give supplemental oxygen if needed.
2. **Skin.** Wash with copious soap and water. Topical application of vitamin E in vegetable oil was reported anecdotally to relieve paresthesias.
3. **Eyes.** Irrigate with copious water. After irrigation, perform a fluorescein examination and refer the victim to an ophthalmologist if there is evidence of corneal injury.
4. **Ingestion.** In the majority of cases, a subtoxic dose has been ingested and no decontamination is necessary. However, after a large ingestion of Chinese chalk or a concentrated solution, administer activated charcoal orally if conditions are appropriate (see Table I–38, p 54). Gastric lavage is not necessary after small-to-moderate ingestions if activated charcoal can be given promptly.

D. Enhanced elimination. These compounds are metabolized rapidly by the body, and extracorporeal methods of elimination would not be expected to enhance their elimination.

▶ QUINIDINE AND OTHER TYPE IA ANTIARRHYTHMIC DRUGS

Neal L. Benowitz, MD

Quinidine, procainamide (Pronestyl), and disopyramide (Norpace) are type Ia antiarrhythmic agents. These agents are used primarily for suppression of supraventricular arrhythmias. Disopyramide is also used to treat hypertrophic obstructive cardiomyopathy. Procainamide oral preparations are not available in the United States but are available in some other countries. All three agents have a low toxic-to-therapeutic ratio and may produce fatal intoxication (Table II–55). See the description of other antiarrhythmic agents on p 88.

I. Mechanism of toxicity

A. Type Ia agents depress the fast sodium-dependent channel, slowing phase zero of the cardiac action potential. At high concentrations, this results in reduced myocardial contractility and excitability and severe depression of cardiac

TABLE II–55. QUINIDINE AND TYPE IA ANTIARRHYTHMIC DRUGS

Drug	Serum Half-life (h)	Usual Adult Daily Dose (mg)	Therapeutic Serum Levels (mg/L)	Major Toxicity[a]
Disopyramide	4–10	400–800	2–4	B, V, H
Procainamide	4	1,000–4,000	4–10	B, V, H
NAPA[b]	5–7	N/A	15–25	H
Quinidine	6–8	1,000–2,000	2–4	S, B, V, H

[a]B, bradycardia; H, hypotension; S, seizures; V, ventricular tachycardia.
[b]NAPA, *N*-acetylprocainamide, an active metabolite of procainamide.

conduction velocity. Type Ia agents also inhibit the outward potassium channel, delaying repolarization, and resulting in a prolonged QT interval that may be associated with polymorphic ventricular tachycardia (torsade de pointes).

B. Quinidine and disopyramide also have anticholinergic activity; quinidine has alpha-adrenergic receptor–blocking activity, and procainamide has ganglionic and neuromuscular blocking activity.

C. Pharmacokinetics (see Table II–66, p 462)

II. Toxic dose. Acute adult ingestion of 1 g of quinidine, 5 g of procainamide, or 1 g of disopyramide and any ingestion in children should be considered potentially lethal.

III. Clinical presentation. The primary manifestations of toxicity involve the cardiovascular and central nervous systems.

A. Cardiotoxic effects of the type Ia agents include sinus bradycardia; sinus node arrest or asystole; PR-, QRS-, or QT-interval prolongation; sinus tachycardia (caused by anticholinergic effects); polymorphous ventricular tachycardia (torsade de pointes); and depressed myocardial contractility, which, along with alpha-adrenergic or ganglionic blockade, may result in hypotension and occasionally pulmonary edema. Anticholinergic effects may result in a rapid ventricular response with emergence of atrial fibrillation or flutter.

B. Central nervous system toxicity. Quinidine and disopyramide can cause anticholinergic effects such as dry mouth, dilated pupils, and delirium. All type Ia agents can produce seizures, coma, and respiratory arrest.

C. Other effects. Quinidine commonly causes nausea, vomiting, and diarrhea after acute ingestion and, especially with chronic doses, cinchonism (tinnitus, vertigo, deafness, and visual disturbances). Procainamide may cause GI upset and, with chronic therapy, a lupus-like syndrome. Anticholinergic effects of type Ia drugs can result in urinary retention and precipitation of acute glaucoma.

IV. Diagnosis is based on a history of exposure and typical cardiotoxic features such as QRS- and QT-interval prolongation, atrioventricular (AV) block, and polymorphous ventricular tachycardia.

A. Specific levels. Serum levels for each agent are generally available. Serious toxicity with these drugs usually occurs only with levels above the therapeutic range; however, some complications, such as QT prolongation and polymorphous ventricular tachycardia, may occur at therapeutic levels.

1. Methods for detecting quinidine may vary in specificity, with some also measuring metabolites and contaminants.
2. Procainamide has an active metabolite, *N*-acetylprocainamide (NAPA); with therapeutic procainamide dosing, NAPA levels can range from 15 to 25 mg/L.

B. Other useful laboratory studies include electrolytes, glucose, BUN, creatinine, arterial blood gases or oximetry, and ECG monitoring.

V. Treatment

A. Emergency and supportive measures

1. Maintain an open airway and assist ventilation if necessary (pp 1–7).
2. Treat hypotension (p 15), arrhythmias (pp 13–15), coma (p 18), and seizures (p 23) if they occur.
3. Treat recurrent ventricular tachycardia with magnesium, overdrive pacing and, if persistent, electrical cardioversion. Do ***not*** use other type Ia or Ic agents because they may worsen cardiac toxicity.
4. Mechanical support of the circulation (eg, cardiopulmonary bypass) may be useful in stabilizing patients with refractory shock, allowing time for the body to eliminate some of the drug.
5. Continuously monitor vital signs and ECG for a minimum of 6 hours and admit symptomatic patients until the ECG returns to normal.

B. Specific drugs and antidotes. Treat cardiotoxic effects such as wide QRS intervals and hypotension with **sodium bicarbonate** (p 520), 1–2 mEq/kg by rapid IV bolus, repeated every 5–10 minutes and as needed. Markedly impaired conduction or high-degree AV block unresponsive to bicarbonate therapy is an indication for insertion of a cardiac pacemaker.

C. **Decontamination** (p 50). Administer activated charcoal orally if conditions are appropriate (see Table I–38, p 54). Gastric lavage is not necessary after small-to-moderate ingestions if activated charcoal can be given promptly.

D. **Enhanced elimination** (p 56)

1. **Quinidine** has a very large volume of distribution, and therefore it is not effectively removed by dialysis. Acidification of the urine may enhance excretion, but this is not recommended because it may aggravate cardiac toxicity.
2. **Disopyramide, procainamide,** and NAPA have smaller volumes of distribution and are removed by dialysis.
3. The efficacy of repeat-dose activated charcoal has not been studied for the type Ia agents.

▶ QUININE

Michael A. Darracq, MD, MPH

Quinine is an optical isomer of quinidine, a class Ia sodium channel blocking antidysrhythmic drug, with which it shares similar pharmacologic effects. Quinine is the primary alkaloid found in the bark of the cinchona tree and was once widely used for the treatment of malaria and is still occasionally used for chloroquine-resistant cases. A 2006 FDA advisory warned against the use of quinine in the treatment of nocturnal muscle cramps. Quinine is found in tonic water and has been used to cut street heroin. It has also been used as an abortifacient.

I. **Mechanism of toxicity**

A. The mechanism of quinine toxicity is believed to be similar to that of quinidine (p 398); however, quinine is a much less potent cardiotoxin.

B. Quinine also has toxic effects on the retina that can result in blindness. At one time, vasoconstriction of retinal arterioles resulting in retinal ischemia was thought to be the cause of blindness; however, recent evidence indicates a direct toxic effect on photoreceptor and ganglion cells.

C. Inhibition of potassium channels may result in impaired hearing, tinnitus and vertigo and hypoglycemia.

D. Quinine has direct irritant effects on the gastrointestinal tract and stimulates CNS centers responsible for nausea and vomiting.

E. Hypersensitivity reactions include urticaria, photosensitivity dermatitis, cutaneous vasculitis, angioedema, and thrombocytopenia ("cocktail purpura").

F. **Pharmacokinetics** (see Table II–66, p 462)

II. **Toxic dose.** Quinine sulfate is available in capsules and tablets containing 130–325 mg. The minimum toxic dose is approximately 3–4 g in adults; 1 g has been fatal in a child.

III. **Clinical presentation.** Toxic effects involve the cardiovascular and central nervous systems, the eyes, and other organ systems.

A. **Mild intoxication** produces nausea, vomiting, and cinchonism (tinnitus, deafness, vertigo, headache, and visual disturbances).

B. **Severe intoxication** may cause ataxia, confusion, obtundation, convulsions, coma, and respiratory arrest. With massive intoxication, quinidine-like cardiotoxicity (hypotension, QRS- and QT-interval prolongation, atrioventricular [AV] block, and ventricular arrhythmias) may be fatal.

C. **Retinal toxicity** occurs 9–10 hours after ingestion and includes blurred vision, impaired color perception, constriction of visual fields, and blindness. The pupils are often fixed and dilated. Funduscopy may reveal retinal artery spasm, disc pallor, and macular edema. Although gradual recovery occurs, many patients are left with permanent visual impairment.

D. **Other toxic effects** of quinine include hypokalemia, hypoglycemia, hemolysis (in patients with glucose-6-phosphate dehydrogenase [G6PD] deficiency), and congenital malformations when used in pregnancy.

IV. **Diagnosis** is based on a history of ingestion and the presence of cinchonism and visual disturbances. Quinidine-like cardiotoxic effects may or may not be present.

A. **Specific levels.** Serum quinine levels can be measured by the same assay as for quinidine, as long as quinidine is not present. However, most hospital-based clinical laboratories no longer offer these assays. Plasma quinine levels above 10 mg/L have been associated with visual impairment; 87% of patients with levels above 20 mg/L reported blindness. Levels above 16 mg/L have been associated with cardiac toxicity.

B. **Other useful laboratory studies** include CBC, electrolytes, glucose, BUN, creatinine, arterial blood gases or oximetry, and ECG monitoring.

V. **Treatment**

A. **Emergency and supportive measures**

1. Maintain an open airway and assist ventilation if necessary (pp 1–7).
2. Treat coma (p 18), seizures (p 23), hypotension (p 15), and arrhythmias (pp 10–15) if they occur.
3. Avoid types Ia and Ic antiarrhythmic drugs; they may worsen cardiotoxicity.
4. Continuously monitor vital signs and the ECG for at least 6 hours after ingestion, and admit symptomatic patients to an intensive care unit.

B. **Specific drugs and antidotes**

1. Treat cardiotoxicity with **sodium bicarbonate** (p 520), 1–2 mEq/kg by rapid IV bolus.
2. Stellate ganglion block is no longer recommended for quinine-induced blindness, due to lack of evidence of efficacy and potential for serious complications.
3. Treat hypoglycemia with dextrose (p 36) and, if needed, octreotide (p 596).

C. **Decontamination** (p 50). Administer activated charcoal orally if conditions are appropriate (see Table I–38, p 54). Gastric lavage is not necessary after small-to-moderate ingestions if activated charcoal can be given promptly.

D. **Enhanced elimination.** Because of extensive tissue distribution (volume of distribution is 3 L/kg), dialysis and hemoperfusion procedures are ineffective. Acidification of the urine may slightly increase renal excretion but does not significantly alter the overall elimination rate and may aggravate cardiotoxicity.

▶ RADIATION (IONIZING)

Frederick Fung, MD, MS

Radiation poisoning is a rare but challenging condition. Dependence on nuclear energy and the expanded use of radioactive isotopes in industry and medicine have increased the possibility of accidental exposures. Ionizing radiation is generated from a variety of sources. **Particle-emitting** sources produce beta and alpha particles and neutrons. **Ionizing electromagnetic** radiation includes gamma rays and x-rays. In contrast, magnetic fields, microwaves, radiofrequency waves, and ultrasound are examples of **nonionizing** electromagnetic radiation.

Management of a radiation accident depends on whether the victim is contaminated or only irradiated. **Irradiated** victims pose no threat to health care providers and can be managed with no special precautions. In contrast, **contaminated** victims must be decontaminated to prevent the spread of radioactive materials to others and the environment.

A terrorist "**dirty bomb**" (dispersion bomb) will likely contain commonly acquired radioactive materials such as the following: americium (alpha emitter, found in smoke detectors and oil exploration equipment); cobalt (gamma emitter, used in food and mail irradiation); iridium (gamma emitter, used in cancer therapy); strontium (gamma emitter, used in medical treatment and power generation); and cesium (gamma emitter, used to sterilize medical equipment and for medical and industrial uses). Psychological effects (eg, panic) may overshadow medical concerns because significant acute radiation exposure by contamination is generally confined to the immediate blast area. Long-term exposure may increase the risk for cancer while adequate decontamination can be problematic, potentially making the blast area uninhabitable.

I. Mechanism of toxicity

A. Radiation impairs biological function by ionizing atoms and breaking chemical bonds. Consequently, the formation of highly reactive free radicals can damage cell walls, organelles, and DNA. Affected cells are either killed or inhibited in division. Cells with a high turnover rate (eg, bone marrow and epithelial coverings of skin, GI tract, and pulmonary system) are more sensitive to radiation. Lymphocytes are particularly sensitive.

B. Radiation causes a poorly understood inflammatory response and microvascular effects after moderately high doses (eg, 600 rad).

C. Radiation effects may be deterministic or stochastic. Deterministic effects are dose related and usually occur within an acute time frame (within a year). Stochastic effects have no known threshold and may occur after a latency period of years (eg, cancer).

II. Toxic dose

A. Gray (Gy) is the unit of radiation dose commonly referred to in exposures, whereas **Sievert (Sv)** is useful in describing dose-equivalent biological damage. For most exposures, these units can be considered interchangeable. The exception is alpha particle exposure (eg, plutonium), which causes greater double-stranded DNA damage and a higher Sievert compared with Gray.

B. Note: The International System of Units (SI units) has replaced the old "rad" and "rem" nomenclature. For conversion purposes, **1 gray (Gy) = 100 rad** and **1 sievert (Sv) = 100 rem**.

C. Toxicity thresholds

1. **Acute effects.** Exposure over 0.75 Gy (75 rad) causes nausea and vomiting. Exposure over 4 Gy (400 rad) is potentially lethal without medical intervention. Vomiting within 1–5 hours of exposure suggests an exposure of at least 6 Gy (600 rad). Brief exposure to 50 Gy (5,000 rad) or more usually causes death within minutes to hours.
2. **Carcinogenesis.** Radiation protection organizations have not agreed on a threshold dose for stochastic effects, such as cancer.

D. Recommended exposure limits

1. **Exposure to the general population.** The National Council on Radiation Protection (NCRP) recommends a maximum of 5 milliSieverts (500 millirem) per person per year. The background radiation at sea level is about 0.35 mSv (35 mrem) per year.
2. **Diagnostic x-rays.** The current US exposure standards are set at 50 mSv per year to the total body, gonads, or blood-forming organs and 750 mSv/y to the hands or feet. For comparison, a single chest radiograph results in radiation exposure to the patient of about 0.15 mSv (but only about 0.00006 mSv to nearby health care personnel at a distance of 160 cm). A CT scan exposes the head to about 2 mSv; an abdominal CT scan may expose that region to as much as 10–20 mSv.
3. **Radiation during pregnancy.** Guidelines vary but generally recommend a maximum exposure of no more than 0.5 mSv per month. Exposure to the ovaries and fetus from a routine abdominal (KUB) film may be as high as 1.5 mSv, whereas the dose from a chest radiograph is about 0.15 mSv.
4. **Exposure guidelines for emergency health care personnel.** To save a life, the NCRP recommends a maximum whole-body exposure of 500–750 mSv for a rescuer.

III. Clinical presentation

A. Acute radiation syndrome (ARS) consists of a constellation of symptoms and signs indicative of systemic radiation injury. It is described in four stages (prodrome, latency, manifest illness, and recovery). The onset and severity of each stage of radiation poisoning are determined largely by the dose.

1. The *prodromal* stage, from 0 to 48 hours, may include nausea, vomiting, abdominal cramps, and diarrhea. Severe exposures are associated with diaphoresis, disorientation, fever, ataxia, coma, shock, and death.
2. During the *latent* stage, symptoms may improve. The duration of this stage varies from hours to days, but it may be shorter or absent with massive exposures.
3. The *manifest illness* stage, from 1 to 60 days, is characterized by multiple-organ system involvement, particularly bone marrow suppression, which may lead to sepsis and death.
4. The *recovery* phase may be accompanied by hair loss, disfiguring burns, and scars.

B. Gastrointestinal system. Exposure to 1 Gy or more usually produces nausea, vomiting, abdominal cramps, and diarrhea within a few hours. After exposure to 6 Gy or more, loss of integrity of the GI mucosal layer results in denudation and severe necrotic gastroenteritis. The clinical picture may include marked dehydration, GI bleeding, and death within a few days. Doses of 15 Gy are believed to destroy GI stem cells completely.

C. Central nervous system. Acute exposures of several thousand rad may produce confusion and stupor, followed within minutes to hours by ataxia, convulsions, coma, and death. In animal models of massive exposure, a phenomenon known as "early transient incapacitation" occurs.

D. Bone marrow depression may be subclinical but apparent on a CBC after exposure to as little as 0.25 Gy. Immunocompromise usually follows exposure to more than 1 Gy.

1. Early neutropenia is caused by margination; the true nadir occurs at about 30 days or as soon as 14 days after severe exposure. Neutropenia is the most significant factor in septicemia.
2. Thrombocytopenia is usually not evident for 2 weeks or more after exposure.
3. The lymphocyte count is of great prognostic importance and usually reaches a nadir within 48 hours of severe exposure. A lymphocyte count of less than 300–500/mm^3 during this period indicates a poor prognosis, whereas 1,200/mm^3 or more suggests likely survival.

E. Other complications of high-dose acute radiation syndrome include multiple-organ system failure, veno-occlusive disease of the liver, interstitial pneumonitis, renal failure, tissue fibrosis, skin burns, and hair loss.

IV. Diagnosis depends on the history of exposure. The potential for contamination should be assessed by determining the type of radionuclide involved and the potential route(s) of exposure.

A. Specific levels

1. **Detection.** Depending on the circumstances, the presence of radionuclides may be verified by one or more of the following devices: survey meters with pancake or alpha probes, whole-body counts, chest counts, and nuclear medicine cameras.
2. **Biological specimens.** Nasopharyngeal and wound swabs, sputum, vomitus, skin wipes, wound bandages, and clothing articles (particularly shoes) may be collected for radionuclide analysis and counts. Collection of urine and feces for 24–72 hours may assist in the estimation of an internal dose. Serum levels of radioactive materials are not generally available or clinically useful.
3. **Other methods.** Chromosomal changes in lymphocytes are the most sensitive indication of exposures to as little as 0.1 Gy; DNA fragments, dicentric

rings, and deletions may be present. Exposure to 0.15 Gy may cause oligospermia, first seen about 45 days after the exposure.

B. **Other useful laboratory studies** include CBC (repeat every 6 hours), electrolytes, glucose, BUN, creatinine, and urinalysis. Immediately draw lymphocytes for human leukocyte antigen (HLA) typing in case bone marrow transplant is required later.

V. **Treatment.** The Radiation **Emergency Assistance Center and Training Site (REAC/TS)** provides incident response and consultation to physicians 24 hours a day, 7 days a week on managing the medical component of a radiation incident. The current website is **www.orise.orau.gov/reacts**. During regular office hours, call **1-865-576-3131,** or call **1-865-576-1005** after office hours or at any time for immediate assistance. REAC/TS is operated for the US Department of Energy (DOE) by the Oak Ridge Associated Universities (ORAU). Also contact the local or state agency responsible for radiation safety.

A. **Emergency and supportive measures.** Depending on the risk to the rescuers, treatment of serious medical problems takes precedence over radiologic concerns. If there is a potential for contamination of rescuers and equipment, appropriate radiation response protocols should be implemented, and rescuers should wear protective clothing and respirators. ***Note:*** If the exposure was to electromagnetic radiation only, the victim is not contaminating and does not pose a risk to any downstream personnel.

1. Maintain an open airway and assist ventilation if necessary (pp 1–7).
2. Treat coma (p 18) and seizures (p 23) if they occur.
3. Replace fluid losses from gastroenteritis with IV crystalloid solutions (p 15).
4. Treat leukopenia and resulting infections as needed. Immunosuppressed patients require reverse isolation and appropriate broad-spectrum antibiotic therapy. Bone marrow stimulants may help selected patients.

B. **Specific drugs and antidotes.** Chelating agents or pharmacologic blocking drugs may be useful in some cases of ingestion or inhalation of certain biologically active radioactive materials if they are given before or shortly after exposure (Table II–56). Contact REAC/TS (see above) for specific advice on the use of these agents.

C. Decontamination (p 50)

1. **Exposure to particle-emitting solids or liquids.** *The victim is potentially highly contaminating to rescuers, transport vehicles, and attending health personnel.*
   a. Remove victims from exposure, and if their condition permits, remove all contaminated clothing and wash the victims with soap and water.
   b. All clothing and cleansing water must be saved, evaluated for radioactivity, and disposed of properly.
   c. Rescuers should wear protective clothing and respiratory gear to avoid contamination. At the hospital, measures must be taken to prevent contamination of facilities and personnel (see Section IV, p 636).
   d. Induce vomiting or perform gastric lavage (p 52) if radioactive material has been ingested. Administer activated charcoal (p 54), although its effectiveness is unknown. Certain other adsorbent materials may also be effective (see Table II–56).
   e. Contact REAC/TS (see above) and the state radiologic health department for further advice. In some exposures, unusually aggressive steps may be needed (eg, lung lavage for significant inhalation of plutonium).
2. **Electromagnetic radiation exposure.** *The patient is not radioactive and does not pose a contamination threat.* There is no need for decontamination once the patient has been removed from the source of exposure unless electromagnetic radiation emitter fragments are embedded in body tissues.

D. **Enhanced elimination.** Chelating agents and forced diuresis may be useful for certain exposures (see Table II–56).

TABLE II–56. CHELATING AGENTS FOR SOME RADIATION EXPOSURES[a]

Radionuclide	Chelating or Blocking Agents
Americium 241	Ca-DTPA or Zn-DTPA (p 547): chelator. Dose: 1 g in 250 mL of D_5W IV over 30–60 minutes daily. Wound: Irrigate with 1 g of DTPA in 250 mL of water. EDTA (p 548) may also be effective if DTPA is not immediately available.
Cesium 137	Prussian blue (ferric hexacyanoferrate, p 620) adsorbs cesium in the GI tract and may also enhance elimination. Exposure burden establishes dose: at low exposure burden, 500 mg PO 6 times daily in 100–200 mL of water.
Cobalt 60	Limited evidence suggests possible use of Ca-DTPA or Zn-DTPA (p 547): chelator. Dose: 1 g in 250 mL of D_5W IV over 30–60 minutes daily. Wounds: Irrigate with 1 g of DTPA in 250 mL of water. EDTA (p 548) may also be tried if DTPA is not immediately available.
Iodine 131	Potassium iodide (p 566) dilutes radioactive iodine and blocks thyroid iodine uptake. Adult dose: 300 mg PO immediately, then 130 mg PO daily. Perchlorate, 200 mg PO, then 100 mg every 5 hours, has also been recommended.
Plutonium 239	Ca-DTPA or Zn-DTPA (p 547): chelator. Dose: 1 g in 250 mL of D_5W IV over 30–60 minutes daily. Wounds: Irrigate with 1 g of DTPA in 250 mL of water. EDTA (p 548) may also be effective if DTPA is not immediately available. Aluminum-containing antacids may bind plutonium in GI tract.
Strontium 90	Alginate or aluminum hydroxide–containing antacids may reduce intestinal absorption of strontium. Dose: 10 g PO, then 1 g 4 times daily PO. Barium sulfate may also reduce strontium absorption. Dose: 100 g in 250 mL of water PO. Calcium gluconate may dilute the effect of strontium. Dose: 2 g in 500 mL of water PO or IV. Ammonium chloride is a demineralizing agent. Dose: 3 g PO 3 times daily.
Tritium	Forced fluids, diuretics, (?) hemodialysis. Water dilutes tritium, enhances urinary excretion.
Uranium 233, 235, 238	Sodium bicarbonate forms a carbonate complex with the uranyl ion, which is then eliminated in the urine. Dose: 100 mEq in 500 mL of D_5W by slow, constant IV infusion. Aluminum-containing antacids may help prevent uranium absorption.

[a]Bhattacharyya MH, et al. Methods of treatment. *Radiat Prot Dosimetry* 1992;41(1):27–36; Ricks RC. *Hospital Emergency Department Management of Radiation Accidents*. Oak Ridge Associated Universities; 1984; Sugarman SL, et al. *The Medical Aspects of Radiation Incidents*. US Department of Energy and Oak Ridge Associated Universities; 2013.

► RODENTICIDES, MISCELLANEOUS

Kathryn H. Meier

Although intended to kill rodents, all rodenticides are potentially toxic to nontargeted mammals including humans. Many different compounds have been used to poison rodents throughout history, but in modern times governmental regulation has attempted to limit the most toxic substances in favor of new poisons with reduced environmental impact. Occasionally with today's global market access, foreign or banned formulations have been introduced into regulated markets and caused unexpected poisonings. There is no way to reliably identify a rodenticide based on its color, shape, or size, and mistakenly assuming that an unknown rodenticide is one of the commonly available products could lead to inappropriate treatment. Therefore, it is important to correctly identify the compound when determining an observation time and treatment plan.

I. Mechanism of toxicity. The mechanism of action and usual onset of action of the various rodenticides are described briefly in Table II–57.

TABLE II–57. MISCELLANEOUS RODENTICIDES[a,b]

Rodenticide	Mechanism of Toxicity	Estimated Toxic Dose	Clinical Presentation	Onset/Duration[a]	Antidote or Specific Treatment
Acetylcholinesterase inhibitors (Carbofuran severely restricted in the United States)	Cholinergic crisis (see Organophosphates, p 353)	Varies by product	Vomiting, diarrhea, salivation, sweating, bronchorrhea, fasciculations, muscle weakness	Depends on the specific compound	Atropine and pralidoxime (see p 512 and p 613)
ANTU	Covalent binding to pulmonary endothelial cells and hepatic microsomes leads to inflammation and cell damage.	Unknown	Sudden onset of white frothy and prolific bronchial secretions, pulmonary edema and hepatotoxicity. Used experimentally to induce acute lung injury in animals	Onset 1–4 h	No antidote. Ketamine and midazolam were protective in rat models. Glutathione depletion enhanced toxicity in rats
Arsenic (inorganic salts). Severely restricted in the United States	See Arsenic (p 140)	Varies with the form	Vomiting, watery diarrhea, rhabdomyolysis, cardiac and neurotoxicity	Onset minutes to hours	Consider chelation (see p 140)
Barium carbonate	Blocks potassium channels (p 152)	1–30 g	Vomiting, diarrhea, muscle weakness, profound hypokalemia, ventricular arrhythmias	Onset 10–60 min	Restore potassium levels. Oral magnesium sulfate to convert barium ions into insoluble barium sulfate
Bromethalin	Uncouples mitochondrial oxidative phosphorylation targeting the central nervous system leading to cerebral edema and myelin sheath abnormalities.	Unknown. Human death at 0.33 mg/kg	Based on animal and limited human data. Mild GI upset possible. CNS target symptoms: hyperexcitability, altered mental status, ataxia, tremor, seizures, coma, cerebral edema, increased intracranial pressure and paralysis	Dose-dependent onset in animal studies: high dose 2–36 h; lower dose 86 h latency. Time to peak 4 h, half-life 5, 6 days, Vd 0.7 L/kg	No antidote. Consider multi-dose activated charcoal to interrupt enterohepatic recirculation for the first 2–3 days unless intestinal ileus occurs
Chloralose	Unknown, possibly similar to other chloral sedative–hypnotics, but with additional unidentified neurostimulant action	Hypnotic oral dose 75 mg; severe toxicity ~20 mg/kg	Vomiting, bronchorrhea, metabolic acidosis, myoclonus or seizures, coma and respiratory depression. Potential irritation or burns	Duration ~24 h, possibly longer with higher doses	No antidote. Diazepam reported effective for myoclonus

Cholecalciferol (vitamin D_3)	Vitamin D analog causes severe hypercalcemia (see p 445)	4–5 mg/kg lethal in dogs	Nausea, vomiting, abdominal cramps, hypercalcemia. Toxicity more likely with chronic dosing compared with single ingestion	Onset delayed up to several days especially with repeated dosing	Symptomatic treatment for hypercalcemia
Coumarins (warfarin, "superwarfarins")	See p 459	Varies by product	Prolongs prothrombin time (INR) causing bleeding	Onset 1–2 days; can be prolonged	Vitamin K (see p 633)
Crimidine. No longer produced or sold in the United States	Vitamin B_6 antagonist: causes GABA deficiency leading to seizures	Less than 5 mg/kg	Limited human data. Vomiting, seizures and status epilepticus. Pulmonary edema reported	Onset 30–60 min. Duration possibly less than 1 day	IV pyridoxine (p 621) effective in dogs
Fluoroacetate (Compound 1080). Severely restricted in the United States	Metabolic poison interferes with Krebs cycle (see p 242)	Fatal dose 2–10 mg/kg	Vomiting, diarrhea, metabolic acidosis, shock, coma	Onset delayed up to several hours	No known antidote
Hydrogen sulfide	Metabolic toxin and irritant gas (see p 271)	600–800 ppm rapidly fatal	Rotten egg odor; eye and upper airway irritation; headache, nausea and vomiting; sudden collapse, seizures, coma	Rapid and sudden onset	Nitrites (p 592) of theoretical but unproven benefit
Norbromide	Unique calcium channel blocker capable of causing site-specific vascular effects in the rat that are not demonstrated in other animals	Unknown. Over 200 times more toxic to rats than other animals tested	Very limited data in humans; transient hypotension after oral 300 mg dose in one human report	Onset 1 h. Probably short-lived	No antidote known. Rats demonstrated hyperglycemia reversed by insulin
Organochlorines. No longer used in the United States	Lindane, endrin (see p 189)	Varies by product	Vomiting, tremor, confusion, seizures, coma	Onset within 30–60 min	No specific antidote
Phosphide, Aluminum or Zinc	Liberates phosphine gas which is a highly toxic mitochondrial poison (see p 372)	As little as 0.5 g aluminum phosphide or 4 g zinc fatal in humans	Vomiting, diarrhea, intractable hypotension, respiratory failure, coma; high mortality rate after suicidal ingestion	Onset of GI symptoms is rapid but cardiopulmonary effects may progress over hours	No known antidote

(*continued*)

TABLE II–57. MISCELLANEOUS RODENTICIDES[a,b] (CONTINUED)

Rodenticide	Mechanism of Toxicity	Estimated Toxic Dose	Clinical Presentation	Onset/Duration[a]	Antidote or Specific Treatment
Phosphorus (yellow or white)	Highly corrosive and toxic cellular poison (see p 373)	Fatal dose approx 1 mg/kg	Vomiting, abdominal pain, oral and gastric burns, "smoking stools", seizures, coma, shock, arrhythmias, hepatic and renal failure	Corrosive effects immediate, other effects may be delayed hours or days	No specific antidote
Pyriminil (Vacor). Banned in the United States	Nicotinamide disruption: inhibits NADH-ubiquinone reductase and mitochondrial respiration leading to pancreatic B islet cell death, and progressive polyneurotoxicity	Less than 5.6 mg/kg.	Transient hypoglycemia followed by diabetes mellitus. Delayed, progressive neuropathies: autonomic (orthostatic hypotension, dysphagia, and dystonia of bowel and bladder); peripheral (neurogenic myopathy, sensory and motor neuropathy); central (cortical and cerebellar dysfunction)	Onset dose dependent: high dose <7 h; smaller dose <48 h. Serious progressive symptoms evolve over weeks and are rarely reversible. Peak absorption 1–6 h	Nicotinamide given as early as possible followed by prolonged maintenance dosing
Red squill (*Drimia maritima*)	Major active toxicant is scilliroside, a bufadienolide cardiac glycoside	Unknown	Emesis, seizures, hyperkalemia, cardiotoxicity purportedly similar to digitalis (p 222)	Rapid onset of vomiting; cardiac effects may be delayed	Unknown if digoxin-specific antibodies are effective (p 542)
***Salmonella enteritidis*.**	"Ratin" no longer used in the United States or Europe because of public health threat of infection in humans	Unknown	Invasive enteric infection (salmonellosis)	Days	Treat as salmonella infection

Strychnine	Glycine inhibitor	As little as 16 mg fatal in an adult	Seizure-like tetanic muscle contractions, respiratory failure, rhabdomyolysis (see p 429)	Onset 15–30 min, duration 12–24 h	No specific antidote. Sedation and neuromuscular paralysis
Tetramine (Tetramethylene disulfotetramine). Banned worldwide since 1984 but still illegally produced, found in some Chinese rodenticides	$GABA_A$ antagonist	0.1 mg/kg oral and inhaled	Nausea, vomiting, dizziness, seizure, status epilepticus, and coma. Seizures very difficult to control	Onset appears dose dependent; 30 min is typical, but can be delayed 13 h. Seizures may occur later than other symptoms	Ketamine was successful in human case reports of status epilepticus; high-dose pyridoxine may also enhance effectiveness of benzodiazepines. DMPS effective in animals
Thallium. Banned in the United States	Generalized cellular poison (see p 433)	Minimum lethal dose probably 12–15 mg/kg, although as little as 200 mg has caused death	Vomiting, diarrhea, shock from fluid losses; delirium and seizures; followed by peripheral neuropathy, hair loss	Onset 12–14 h after ingestion	Prussian blue (see p 620)

[a]For most of these agents, onset/duration is based on animal studies; limited or no human data.
[b]Not all of these agents are available in the United States.

II. **Toxic dose.** See Table II–57.

III. **Clinical presentation.** The clinical manifestations of poisoning by each of the agents are described briefly in Table II–57.

IV. **Diagnosis** depends on the agent and may be very difficult if the identity of the product is unknown. For some agents, such as the superwarfarins (see Warfarin, p 459), prolongation of the PT/INR and onset of bleeding may be delayed by 1–3 days. The onset/duration for many of the listed products is an estimation based on acute human poisoning reports and mammalian poisoning studies when human data is lacking. Beware that for some substances the time of onset may be quicker with higher doses and slower with lower doses.

   A. **Specific levels** require special analytical testing not available in most hospitals. A commercial or university reference laboratory may be able to detect and quantify some agents. Consider contacting a poison control center (1-800-222-1222) for assistance to find a laboratory if needed.

   B. **Other useful laboratory studies.** Monitoring parameters are based on the clinical symptoms. For example, in the case of rodenticide-induced seizures, monitor glucose, venous or arterial blood gases, chemistry panel, lactate and CK and consider whether imaging, LP or continuous EEG monitoring are needed.

V. **Treatment**

   A. **Emergency and supportive measures** are outlined in Section I (pp 1–27).

   B. **Specific drugs and antidotes.** There are specific treatments for some but not all of the agents (see Table II–57).

   C. **Decontamination** (p 50) has not been well studied but should be considered if a patient with a substantial exposure presents before symptoms begin.

   D. **Enhanced elimination**

      1. **Bromethalin.** Because it undergoes enterohepatic recirculation and has a long half-life, multi-dose activated charcoal should be considered after significant bromethalin exposure.

      2. **Tetramine.** Enhanced elimination is unlikely to be effective, because of a large volume of distribution. Multiple rounds of charcoal hemoperfusion were claimed to have improved abnormal EEG findings, but recovered only a small fraction of ingested tetramine and did not change serum levels.

► SALICYLATES

Susan Kim-Katz, PharmD

Salicylates are used widely for their analgesic and anti-inflammatory properties. They are found in a variety of prescription and over-the-counter analgesics, cold preparations, topical keratolytic products (methyl salicylate), and even Pepto-Bismol (bismuth subsalicylate). Before the introduction of child-resistant containers, aspirin (acetylsalicylic acid) overdose was one of the leading causes of accidental death in children. Two distinct syndromes of intoxication may occur, depending on whether the exposure is **acute** or **chronic**.

I. **Mechanism of toxicity.** Salicylates have a variety of toxic effects.

   A. Central stimulation of the respiratory center results in hyperventilation, leading to respiratory alkalosis. Secondary consequences from hyperventilation include dehydration and compensatory metabolic acidosis.

   B. Intracellular effects include uncoupling of oxidative phosphorylation and interruption of glucose and fatty acid metabolism, which contribute to metabolic acidosis.

   C. The mechanism by which cerebral and pulmonary edema occurs is not known but may be related to an alteration in capillary integrity.

D. Salicylates alter platelet function and may also prolong the prothrombin time.

E. **Pharmacokinetics.** Salicylates are well absorbed from the stomach and small intestine. Large tablet masses and enteric-coated products may dramatically delay absorption (hours to days). The volume of distribution of salicylate is about 0.1–0.3 L/kg, but this can be increased by acidemia, which enhances movement of the drug into cells. Elimination is mostly by hepatic metabolism at therapeutic doses, but renal excretion becomes important with overdose. The elimination half-life is normally 2–4.5 hours but can be as long as 18–36 hours after overdose. Renal elimination is dependent on urine pH (see also Table II–66, p 462).

II. **Toxic dose.** The average therapeutic single dose of aspirin is 10 mg/kg, and the usual daily therapeutic dose is 40–60 mg/kg/d. Each tablet of aspirin contains 325–650 mg of acetylsalicylic acid. One teaspoon of concentrated **oil of wintergreen** contains 5 g of methyl salicylate, equivalent to about 7.5 g of aspirin. Each gram of bismuth subsalicylate (eg, Pepto-Bismol) contains 0.38 g of salicylate, equivalent to approximately 0.5 g of aspirin.

A. **Acute ingestion** of 150–200 mg/kg of aspirin will produce mild intoxication; severe intoxication is likely after acute ingestion of 300–500 mg/kg. Fatalities have been reported in children with ingestion of 5 mL or less of oil of wintergreen.

B. **Chronic intoxication** with aspirin may occur with ingestion of more than 100 mg/kg/d for 2 days or more.

III. **Clinical presentation.** Patients may become intoxicated after an acute accidental or suicidal overdose or as a result of chronic repeated overmedication for several days.

A. **Acute ingestion.** Vomiting occurs shortly after ingestion, followed by hyperpnea, tinnitus, and lethargy. Mixed respiratory alkalemia and metabolic acidosis are apparent when blood gases are determined. With severe intoxication, coma, seizures, hypoglycemia, hyperthermia, and pulmonary edema may occur. Death is caused by CNS failure and cardiovascular collapse.

B. **Chronic intoxication.** Victims are usually confused elderly persons who are taking salicylates therapeutically. The diagnosis is often overlooked because the presentation is nonspecific; confusion, dehydration, and metabolic acidosis are often attributed to sepsis, pneumonia, or gastroenteritis. However, morbidity and mortality rates are much higher than after an acute overdose. Cerebral and pulmonary edema is more common than with acute intoxication, and severe poisoning occurs at lower salicylate levels.

IV. **Diagnosis** is not difficult if there is a history of acute ingestion accompanied by typical signs and symptoms. In the absence of a history of overdose, diagnosis is suggested by the characteristic arterial blood gases, which reveal a mixed respiratory alkalemia and metabolic acidosis.

A. **Specific levels.** Obtain stat and serial serum salicylate concentrations. Systemic acidemia increases brain salicylate concentrations, worsening toxicity. Monitor serum pH frequently via arterial or venous blood gas determinations.

1. **Acute ingestion.** Serum salicylate levels greater than 90–100 mg/dL (900–1,000 mg/L, or 6.6–7.3 mmol/L) usually are associated with severe toxicity. Single determinations are ***not*** sufficient because of the possibility of prolonged or delayed absorption from sustained-release tablets or a tablet mass or bezoar (especially after massive ingestion). Obtain salicylate levels every 3–4 hours (or more frequently during the initial stages of an acute overdose) until the levels have peaked and are clearly declining.

2. **Chronic intoxication.** Symptoms correlate poorly with serum levels. Chronic therapeutic concentrations in arthritis patients range from 10 to 30 mg/dL (100 to 300 mg/L). A level greater than 60 mg/dL (600 mg/L, or 4.4 mmol/L) accompanied by acidosis and altered mental status is considered very serious.

B. Other useful laboratory studies include electrolytes (anion gap calculation), glucose, BUN, creatinine, prothrombin time, arterial or venous blood gases, and chest radiography.

V. Treatment

A. Emergency and supportive measures

1. Maintain an open airway and assist ventilation if necessary (pp 1–7). ***Warning:*** Ensure adequate ventilation to prevent respiratory acidosis and do not allow controlled mechanical ventilation to interfere with the patient's need for compensatory efforts to maintain the serum pH. Administer supplemental oxygen. Obtain serial arterial blood gases and chest radiographs to observe for pulmonary edema (more common with chronic or severe intoxication).
2. Treat coma (p 18), seizures (p 23), pulmonary edema (p 7), and hyperthermia (p 21) if they occur.
3. Treat metabolic acidosis with IV sodium bicarbonate (p 520). Do ***not*** allow the serum pH to fall below 7.4.
4. Replace fluid and electrolyte deficits caused by vomiting and hyperventilation with IV crystalloid solutions. Be cautious with fluid therapy because excessive fluid administration may contribute to pulmonary edema.
5. Administer supplemental glucose, and treat hypoglycemia (p 36) if it occurs. ***Note:*** Salicylate-poisoned patients may have low brain glucose levels despite normal measured serum glucose. It is prudent to routinely administer glucose-containing IV fluids.
6. Monitor asymptomatic patients for a minimum of 6 hours (longer if an enteric-coated preparation or a massive overdose has been ingested and there is suspicion of a tablet bezoar). Admit symptomatic patients to an intensive care unit.

B. Specific drugs and antidotes. There is no specific antidote for salicylate intoxication. **Sodium bicarbonate** is given frequently both to prevent acidemia and to promote salicylate elimination by the kidneys (see Item D below).

C. Decontamination (p 50). Decontamination is not necessary for patients with *chronic* intoxication.

1. Administer activated charcoal orally if conditions are appropriate (see Table I–38, p 54). Gastric lavage is not necessary after small-to-moderate ingestions if activated charcoal can be given promptly.
2. ***Note:*** With large ingestions of salicylate (eg, 30–60 g), very large doses of activated charcoal (300–600 g) are theoretically necessary to adsorb all the salicylate. In such cases, the charcoal can be given in several 25- to 50-g doses at 3- to 5-hour intervals. Whole-bowel irrigation (p 55) is recommended to help move the pills and charcoal through the intestinal tract.

D. Enhanced elimination (p 56)

1. **Urinary alkalinization** is effective in enhancing urinary excretion of salicylate, although it is often difficult to achieve in dehydrated or critically ill patients. The goal is to maintain a urine pH of 7.5 or higher.
   - **a.** Add 100 mEq of sodium bicarbonate to 1 L of 5% dextrose in quarter-normal saline and infuse intravenously at 200 mL/h (3–4 mL/kg/h). If the patient is dehydrated, start with a bolus of 10–20 mL/kg. Fluid and bicarbonate administration is potentially dangerous in patients at high risk for pulmonary edema (eg, chronic intoxication).
   - **b.** Unless renal failure is present, also add potassium, 30–40 mEq, to each liter of IV fluids (potassium depletion inhibits alkalinization). ***Caution:*** Watch for hyperkalemia in patients with poor urine output.
   - **c.** Alkalemia is not a contraindication to bicarbonate therapy in light of the fact that patients often have a significant base deficit despite the elevated serum pH.
2. **Hemodialysis** is very effective in rapidly removing salicylate and correcting acid–base and fluid abnormalities. Indications for urgent hemodialysis are as follows:

a. Patients with acute ingestion and serum levels higher than 90–100 mg/dL (900–1000 mg/L) with severe acidosis and other manifestations of intoxication.
b. Patients with chronic intoxication and serum levels higher than 60 mg/dL (600 mg/L) accompanied by acidosis, confusion, or lethargy, especially if they are elderly or debilitated or have renal insufficiency.
c. Any patient with severe acidemia and other manifestations of intoxication.

3. **Repeat-dose activated charcoal** therapy effectively reduces the serum salicylate half-life, but it is not as rapidly effective as dialysis, and frequent stooling may contribute to dehydration and electrolyte disturbances.
4. **Continuous venovenous hemodiafiltration** was reported to be effective in a few cases, but there is insufficient information about clearance rates to recommend this procedure.

► SCORPIONS

Richard F. Clark, MD

The order Scorpionida contains several families, genera, and species of scorpions. All have paired venom glands in a bulbous segment, called the telson, that is situated just anterior to a stinger on the end of the six terminal segments of the abdomen (often called a tail). The only systemically poisonous species in the United States is *Centruroides exilicauda* (formerly *C sculpturatus*), also known as the bark scorpion. The most serious envenomations usually are reported in children younger than 10 years of age. This scorpion is found primarily in the arid southwestern United States but has been found as a stowaway in cargo as far north as Michigan. Other dangerous scorpions are found in Mexico (*Centruroides* species), Brazil (*Tityus* species), India (*Buthus* species), the Middle East, and North Africa and the eastern Mediterranean (*Leiurus* and *Androctonus* species).

I. **Mechanism of toxicity.** The scorpion grasps its prey with its anterior pincers, arches its pseudoabdomen, and stabs with the stinger. Stings also result from stepping on the stinger. The venom of *C exilicauda* contains numerous digestive enzymes (eg, hyaluronidase and phospholipase) and several neurotoxins. These neurotoxins can cause alterations in sodium channel flow, resulting in excessive stimulation at neuromuscular junctions and the autonomic nervous system.

II. **Toxic dose.** Variable amounts of venom, from none to the complete contents of the telson, may be ejected through the stinger.

III. **Clinical presentation**

A. **Common scorpion stings.** Most stings result only in local, immediate burning pain. Some local tissue inflammation and occasionally local paresthesias may occur. Symptoms usually resolve within several hours. This is the typical scorpion sting most often seen in the United States.

B. **Dangerous scorpion stings.** In some victims, especially children younger than 10 years, systemic symptoms can occur after stings by *Centruroides* species, including weakness, restlessness, diaphoresis, diplopia, nystagmus, roving eye movements, hyperexcitability, muscle fasciculations, opisthotonus, priapism, salivation, slurred speech, hypertension, tachycardia, and rarely convulsions, paralysis, and respiratory arrest. Envenomations by *Tityus, Buthus, Androctonus,* and *Leiurus* species have caused pulmonary edema, cardiovascular collapse, and death, as well as coagulopathies, disseminated intravascular coagulation, pancreatitis, and renal failure with hemoglobinuria and jaundice. In nonfatal cases, recovery usually occurs within 12–36 hours.

IV. **Diagnosis.** The scorpion must have been seen by the patient or the clinician must recognize the symptoms. There is no readily available laboratory test to confirm scorpion envenomation. In the case of *Centruroides* stings, tapping on the sting site usually produces severe pain ("tap test").

A. **Specific levels.** Body fluid toxin levels are not available.

B. No other useful laboratory studies are needed for minor envenomations. For severe envenomations, obtain CBC, electrolytes, glucose, BUN, creatinine, and coagulation profile. In small children with severe symptoms, oximetry can be used to aid recognition of respiratory insufficiency.

V. **Treatment.** The majority of scorpion stings in the United States, including those by *Centruroides,* can be managed with symptomatic home care consisting of oral analgesics and cool compresses or intermittent ice packs.

A. **Emergency and supportive measures**

1. For severe envenomations, maintain an open airway and assist ventilation if necessary (pp 1–7). Administer supplemental oxygen. Atropine has been used successfully in some cases to dry the mouth and airway secretions.
2. Treat hypertension (p 17), tachycardia (p 12), and convulsions (p 23) if they occur.
3. Analgesics such as morphine and sedatives such as midazolam can be used as needed for severe pain and other neurologic abnormalities. Continuous infusions of midazolam have been used successfully in patients with severe *Centruroides* stings.
4. Clean the wound and provide tetanus prophylaxis if indicated.
5. Do ***not*** immerse the injured extremity in ice or hot water or perform local incision or suction.

B. **Specific drugs and antidotes.**

1. Antivenom (Centruroides scorpion Immune $F(ab)_2$ antivenom, see p 511) is now approved for the treatment of patients with *Centruroides* envenomation in the United States. Most patients in clinical trials of this antivenom were children, and use of the scorpion antivenom was found to be safe and effective in most cases. Due to the significant cost of this product, most clinicians reserve it for severe cases.
2. Specific antivenoms against other species may be available in other parts of the world but are not approved in the United States.

C. **Decontamination.** These procedures are not applicable.

D. **Enhanced elimination.** These procedures are not applicable.

▶ SEDATIVES–HYPNOTIC AGENTS

Ben T. Tsutaoka, PharmD

Sedative–hypnotic agents are used widely for the treatment of insomnia and anxiety. As a group, they are one of the most frequently prescribed medications. Barbiturates (p 150), benzodiazepines (p 156), antihistamines (p 110), skeletal muscle relaxants (p 419), antidepressants (pp 104 and 107), and anticholinergic agents (p 97) are discussed elsewhere in this book. This section and Table II–58 list some of the less commonly used hypnotic agents.

I. **Mechanism of toxicity.** The exact mechanism of action and the pharmacokinetics (see also Table II–66, p 462) vary for each agent. The major toxic effect that causes serious poisoning or death is CNS depression resulting in coma, respiratory arrest, and pulmonary aspiration of gastric contents.

II. **Toxic dose.** The toxic dose varies considerably between drugs and also depends largely on individual tolerance and the presence of other drugs, such as alcohol. For most of these drugs, ingestion of 3–5 times the usual hypnotic dose results in coma. However, co-ingestion of alcohol or other drugs may cause coma after smaller ingestions, whereas individuals who chronically use large doses of these drugs may tolerate much higher acute doses.

III. **Clinical presentation.** Overdose with many of these drugs may cause drowsiness, ataxia, nystagmus, stupor, coma, and respiratory arrest. Deep coma may

TABLE II–58. SEDATIVE–HYPNOTIC AGENTS[a]

Drug	Usual Adult Oral Hypnotic Dose (mg)	Approximate Lethal Dose (g)	Toxic Concentration (mg/L)	Usual Half-life[b] (h)
Buspirone	5–20	Unknown	—	2–4
Chloral hydrate	500–1,000	5–10	>20[c]	8–11[d]
Glutethimide	250–500	10–20	>10	10–12
Meprobamate	600–1,200	10–20	>60	10–11
Methaqualone	150–250	3–8	>5	20–60
Methyprylon	200–400	5–10	>10	7–11
Paraldehyde	5–10 mL	25 mL	>200	6–7
Ramelteon	8	Unknown	—	1–2.6
Suvorexant	5–20	Unknown	—	12
Tasimelteon	20	Unknown	—	1.3

[a]See also "Anticholinergics" (p 97), "Antihistamines" (p 110), "Barbiturates" (p 150), "Benzodiazepines" (p 156), and "Skeletal Muscle Relaxants" (p 419).
[b]Half-life in overdose may be considerably longer.
[c]Toxic concentration is measured as the metabolite trichloroethanol.
[d]Half-life of the metabolite trichloroethanol.

result in absent reflexes, fixed pupils, and depressed or absent electroencephalographic (EEG) activity. Hypothermia is common. Most of these agents also slow gastric motility and decrease muscle tone. Hypotension with a large overdose is caused primarily by depression of cardiac contractility and, to a lesser extent, loss of venous tone.

A. **Chloral hydrate** is metabolized to trichloroethanol, which also has CNS-depressant activity. In addition, trichloroethanol may sensitize the myocardium to the effects of catecholamines, resulting in cardiac arrhythmias.
B. **Buspirone** may cause nausea, vomiting, drowsiness, and miosis. There have been no reported deaths.
C. **Glutethimide** often produces mydriasis (dilated pupils) and other anticholinergic side effects, and patients may exhibit prolonged and cyclic or fluctuating coma. Glutethimide sometimes is taken in combination with codeine ("loads"), which may produce opioid effects.
D. **Meprobamate** has been reported to form tablet concretions in large overdoses, occasionally requiring surgical removal. Hypotension is more common with this agent than with other sedative–hypnotics. Meprobamate is the metabolite of the skeletal muscle relaxant carisoprodol (p 419).
E. **Methaqualone** is unusual among sedative–hypnotic agents in that it frequently causes muscular hypertonicity, clonus, and hyperreflexia. The skeletal muscle relaxant carisoprodol (p 419) also frequently causes increased muscle tone and myoclonus.
F. **Ramelteon and tasimelteon** are melatonin receptor agonists. They may cause mild CNS depression. There have been no reported deaths.
G. **Suvorexant** is an orexin receptor antagonist. It is expected to cause CNS depression. There have been no reported deaths.

IV. **Diagnosis** usually is based on a history of ingestion because clinical manifestations are fairly nonspecific. Hypothermia and deep coma may cause the patient to appear dead; thus, careful evaluation should precede the diagnosis of brain death. Chloral hydrate is radiopaque and may be visible on plain abdominal radiographs.
A. **Specific levels** and qualitative urine screening are usually available through commercial toxicology laboratories but are rarely of value in emergency management.

1. Drug levels do not always correlate with severity of intoxication, especially in patients who have tolerance to the drug or have also ingested other drugs or alcohol. In addition, early after ingestion, blood levels may not reflect brain concentrations.
2. Some agents (ie, chloral hydrate) have active metabolites whose levels may correlate better with the state of intoxication.

B. **Other useful laboratory studies** include electrolytes, glucose, serum ethanol, BUN, creatinine, arterial blood gases, ECG, and chest radiography.

V. **Treatment**

A. **Emergency and supportive measures**
1. Maintain an open airway and assist ventilation if necessary (pp 1–7). Administer supplemental oxygen.
2. Treat coma (p 18), hypothermia (p 20), hypotension (p 15), and pulmonary edema (p 7) if they occur.
3. Monitor patients for at least 6 hours after ingestion because delayed absorption may occur. Patients with **chloral hydrate** ingestion should be monitored for at least 18–24 hours because of the risk for cardiac arrhythmias. Tachyarrhythmias caused by myocardial sensitization may be treated with **propranolol** (p 617), 1–2 mg IV, or **esmolol** (p 552), 0.025–0.1 mg/kg/min IV.

B. **Specific drugs and antidotes.** None. Flumazenil is a specific antagonist of benzodiazepine receptors, but it is not effective for the drugs listed in this chapter.

C. **Decontamination** (p 50). Administer activated charcoal orally if conditions are appropriate (see Table I–38, p 54). Gastric lavage is not necessary after small-to-moderate ingestions if activated charcoal can be given promptly.

D. **Enhanced elimination.** Because of extensive tissue distribution, dialysis and hemoperfusion are not very effective for most of the drugs in this group.
1. Repeat-dose charcoal may enhance elimination of glutethimide (which undergoes enterohepatic recirculation) and meprobamate, although no studies have been performed to document clinical effectiveness.
2. Meprobamate has a relatively small volume of distribution (0.7 L/kg), and hemodialysis or continuous renal replacement therapy (CRRT) may be useful for deep coma complicated by intractable hypotension.

► SELENIUM

Richard J. Geller, MD, MPH

Selenium exists in four natural oxidation states (+6, +4, 0, and −2) and is found in several compounds capable of causing human poisoning, yet it is an essential trace element in the human diet. Table II–59 describes physical properties and toxic air concentrations or doses of common selenium compounds. Fatal acute selenium poisoning occurs most commonly from ingestion of selenious acid in gun bluing (coating) solutions. Other acute poisonings occur through the use of (often improperly formulated) dietary supplements as well as via exposure to industrial compounds. Illness caused by chronic exposure to selenium is uncommon but is seen in regions with high selenium content in food. Industries using selenium compounds include ceramics, electronics, glass, rubber, and metallurgy. Selenium dioxide is the most commonly used compound industrially. Selenium is produced largely as a by-product of copper refining.

I. **Mechanism of toxicity.** Precise cellular toxopathology is poorly understood. Animal studies implicate mechanisms involving the formation of superoxide and hydroxyl anions as well as hydrogen peroxide. Mechanistic knowledge makes no contribution to treatment currently. A garlic breath odor observed in various selenium poisonings is due to in vivo creation of dimethyl selenium.

TABLE II–59. SELENIUM COMPOUNDS

Compound (Synonyms)	Physical Properties	Toxic Dose or Air Concentration[a]
Elemental selenium CASRN 7782-49-2 (Se)	Amorphous or crystalline, red to gray solid	PEL 0.2 mg/m^3; IDLH 1 mg/m^3
Hydrogen selenide (selenium hydride) CASRN 7783-07-5 (H_2Se)	Odiferous colorless gas	PEL 0.05 ppm; IDLH 1 ppm
Sodium selenide CASRN 1313-85-5 (Na_2Se)	Red to white powder	PEL 0.2 mg/m^3 (as Se)
Selenious acid (hydrogen selenite) CASRN 7783-00-8 (H_2SeO_3)	White powder encountered as 2% solution in gun bluing	Ingestion of as little as 15 mL of a 2% solution was reportedly fatal in a child.
Sodium selenite (selenium trioxide) CASRN 10102-18-8 ($O_3Se.2Na$)	White powder	Mean lethal dose of selenite salts in dogs was 4 mg/kg. Human ingestion of 1–5 mg/kg caused moderate toxicity.
Selenium oxide (selenium dioxide) CASRN 7446-08-4 (O_2Se)	White crystal or powder	PEL 0.2 mg/m^3 (as Se)
Sodium selenate CASRN 13410-01-0 ($O_4Se.2Na$)	White crystals	PEL 0.2 mg/m^3 (as Se)
Selenic acid CASRN 7783-08-6 (H_2SeO_4)	White solid	PEL 0.2 mg/m^3 (as Se)
Selenium hexafluoride (selenium fluoride) CASRN 7783-79-1 (F_6Se)	Colorless gas	PEL 0.05 ppm; IDLH 2 ppm

[a]PEL, OSHA-regulated permissible exposure limit for occupational exposure as an 8-hour time-weighted average (TWA); IDLH, level considered immediately dangerous to life or health (NIOSH).

II. Toxic dose

A. Ingestion

1. **Acute overdose.** Rapidly fatal overdoses have occurred from ingestion of gun bluing solutions containing 2–9% selenious acid and 2–4% copper. Ingestion of 15 mL of gun bluing solution containing 4% selenious acid was fatal. The oral mean lethal dose (MLD) of selenite salts in the dog is about 4 mg/kg. Ingestion of 1–5 mg/kg sodium selenite in five adults caused moderate reversible toxicity. Survival after ingestion of 2,000 mg of selenium dioxide has been reported.
2. **Chronic ingestion.** Selenium is a component of more than 2 dozen essential proteins. The Food and Nutrition Board, Institute of Medicine recommended daily allowance (RDA) is 55 mcg. The Environmental Protection Agency (EPA) drinking water maximum contaminant level (MCL) is 0.05 mg/L (50 ppb). The EPA minimal risk level for selenium is 5 mcg/kg/d. Chronic ingestion of 850 mcg/d has been associated with toxicity.

B. Inhalation. The ACGIH-recommended threshold limit value (TLV) for occupational exposure to elemental selenium, as well as selenium compounds in general, has been set at 0.2 mg/m^3. The exposure levels considered immediately dangerous to life or health (IDLH) are listed in Table II–59.

III. Clinical presentation

A. Acute ingestion of selenious acid causes upper GI corrosive injury, vomiting and diarrhea, hypersalivation, and a garlic odor on the breath, with rapid deterioration of mental status and restlessness progressing to coma, hypotension from myocardial depression and decreased vascular resistance, respiratory insufficiency, and death. Suicidal ingestion of an unknown amount of **selenium dioxide** has been fatal. Ingestions of **sodium selenate** have produced gastroenteritis with garlic breath and T-wave inversion on the ECG. Five patients who ingested large amounts of **sodium selenite** developed vomiting, diarrhea, chills, and tremor but survived.

B. **Chronic ingestion of elemental selenium, sodium selenite, sodium selenate, or selenium dioxide** may cause pallor, stomach disorders, nervousness, metallic taste, and garlic breath.

C. **Acute inhalation of hydrogen selenide** produces dyspnea, abdominal cramps, and diarrhea. Inhalation of **selenium hexafluoride** produces severe corrosive injury and systemic toxicity from acids of selenium plus fluoride ion toxicity. **Selenium salt** inhalation causes dyspnea and skin and mucous membrane irritation.

IV. **Diagnosis** is difficult without a history of exposure. Acute severe gastroenteritis with garlic breath odor and hypotension may suggest selenious acid poisoning, but these findings are not specific.

A. **Specific levels** are not generally available. Various selenium compounds differ in toxic potential, yet selenium is usually determined as total selenium concentration. Selenium can be measured in the blood, hair, and urine. Following absorption, selenium slowly migrates into red blood cells, resulting in an elevated whole blood to plasma ratio. Plasma concentrations are preferred for assessing acute exposure; whole blood is preferred for chronic exposures.

1. On a normal diet, whole-blood selenium levels range from 0.1 to 0.2 mg/L. One patient with chronic intoxication after ingestion of 31 mg/d had a whole-blood selenium level of 0.53 mg/L.
2. Average hair levels are up to 0.5 ppm. The relationship between hair and tissue concentrations is not well understood. The utility of hair testing is complicated by the widespread use of selenium disulfide in shampoos.
3. Both whole-blood and urinary concentrations reflect dietary intake. Overexposure should be considered when blood selenium levels exceed 0.4 mg/L or urinary excretion exceeds 600–1,000 mcg/d.

B. **Other useful laboratory studies** include electrolytes, glucose, BUN, creatinine, liver aminotransferases, and ECG. After inhalation exposure, obtain arterial blood gases or oximetry and chest radiograph.

V. **Treatment**

A. **Emergency and supportive measures**

1. Maintain an open airway and assist ventilation if necessary (pp 1–7). Administer supplemental oxygen.
2. Treat coma (p 18), convulsions (p 23), bronchospasm (p 8), hypotension (p 15), and pulmonary edema (p 7) if they occur. Because hypotension is often multifactorial, evaluate and optimize volume status, peripheral vascular resistance, and myocardial contractility.
3. Observe for at least 6 hours after exposure.
4. After ingestion of selenious acid, consider endoscopy to rule out esophageal or gastric corrosive injury.

B. **Specific drugs and antidotes.** There is no specific antidote. The value of suggested therapies such as chelation, vitamin C, and *N*-acetylcysteine is not established.

C. **Decontamination** (p 50)

1. **Inhalation.** Immediately remove the victim from exposure and give supplemental oxygen if available.
2. **Skin and eyes.** Remove contaminated clothing and wash exposed skin with soap and copious water. Irrigate exposed eyes with copious tepid water or saline.

3. **Ingestion**
   a. Ingestion of elemental selenium or selenium salts does not usually benefit from GI decontamination. In light of the risk for severe corrosive GI injury, careful gastric lavage (using a soft nasogastric tube) plus activated charcoal may be of value for ingestions of selenious acid seen within 1 hour.

D. **Enhanced elimination.** There is no known role for any enhanced removal procedure.

▶ SKELETAL MUSCLE RELAXANTS

Susan Kim-Katz, PharmD

Drugs discussed in this chapter are centrally acting skeletal muscle relaxants that exert their effects indirectly. Dantrolene, a direct acting skeletal muscle relaxer, is described in Section III (p 537). The drugs commonly used as skeletal muscle relaxants are listed in Table II–60. Carisoprodol (Soma®) and baclofen (see also p 149) are often abused as recreational drugs.

I. **Mechanism of toxicity**
   A. **Central nervous system.** Most of these drugs cause generalized CNS depression.
      1. **Baclofen** (see also p 149) is an agonist at the GABA(B) receptor and can produce profound CNS and respiratory depression as well as paradoxical muscle hypertonicity and seizure-like activity.
      2. Spastic encephalopathy with increased muscle tone, hyperreflexia and myoclonus is common with **carisoprodol** overdose.
      3. **Cyclobenzaprine** and **orphenadrine** possess anticholinergic properties.
      4. Tizanidine, a centrally acting alpha$_2$ agonist, has effects similar to those of clonidine (p 197).
   B. **Cardiovascular effects.** Hypotension may occur after overdose. **Baclofen** has caused bradycardia in up to 30% of ingestions. **Orphenadrine** has sodium channel blocking effects similar to tricyclic antidepressants. Massive orphenadrine ingestions have caused supraventricular and ventricular tachycardia.
   C. **Pharmacokinetics** varies with the drug. Absorption may be delayed because of anticholinergic effects (see also Table II–66, p 462).

II. **Toxic dose.** The toxic dose varies considerably among drugs, depends largely on individual tolerance, and can be influenced by the presence of other drugs, such as ethanol. For most of these drugs, ingestion of more than 3–5 times the usual therapeutic dose may cause stupor or coma.

TABLE II–60. SKELETAL MUSCLE RELAXANTS

Drug	Usual Half-life (h)	Usual Daily Adult Dose (mg)
Baclofen	2.5–4	40–80
Carisoprodol[a]	1.5–8	800–1,600
Chlorzoxazone	1	1,500–3,000
Cyclobenzaprine	24–72	30–60
Metaxalone	2–3	2,400–3,200
Methocarbamol	1–2	4,000–4,500
Orphenadrine	14–16	200
Tizanidine	2.5	12–36

[a]Metabolized to meprobamate (p 414).

A. **Baclofen.** In adults, CNS depression, delirium, seizures, and hypertension occurred more frequently after ingestion of more than 200 mg. However, in children respiratory arrest was reported in a 22-month-old child who ingested 120 mg (10.9 mg/kg) and an estimated 60 mg of baclofen caused coma, flaccidity, hyporeflexia, bradycardia, and hypotension in a 3-year-old child.

B. **Carisoprodol.** Death was reported in a 4-year-old child who ingested approximately 3,500 mg, and a 2-year-old child who ingested two tablets (350 mg each) required intubation.

C. **Orphenadrine.** A 2-year-old child had seizures and tachycardia after ingesting 400 mg. In a series of 10 fatal cases, the mean amount ingested by 6 adults was 22 mg/kg and by 4 children was 72 mg/kg.

D. The lowest dose of **tizanidine** associated with coma in an adult was between 60 and 120 mg.

III. **Clinical presentation.** Onset of CNS depression usually is seen within 30–120 minutes of ingestion. Lethargy, slurred speech, ataxia, coma, and respiratory arrest may occur. Larger ingestions, especially when combined with alcohol, can produce unresponsive coma.

A. **Baclofen** overdose can cause profound coma, flaccid paralysis and absent brainstem reflexes lasting several days that may be mistaken for brain death. In addition to CNS and respiratory depression, baclofen overdose may cause seizures, bradycardia, hypotension or hypertension, and ECG abnormalities including first- and second-degree AV block and QTc prolongation. Nonconvulsive status epilepticus diagnosed by EEG, and prolonged delirium resulting in rhabdomyolysis have been reported. Hallucinations, seizures, and hyperthermia have occurred after abrupt **withdrawal** from baclofen, usually within 12–48 hours following discontinuation. While the withdrawal syndrome can occur from cessation of oral baclofen use, severe manifestations typically follow abruptly stopping intrathecal therapy.

B. **Carisoprodol** may cause paradoxical hyperreflexia, opisthotonus, and increased muscle tone.

C. **Cyclobenzaprine** and **orphenadrine** can produce anticholinergic findings such as tachycardia, dilated pupils, and delirium. Despite its structural similarity to tricyclic antidepressants, cyclobenzaprine has not been reported to cause quinidine-like cardiotoxicity, although it can cause hypotension. Status epilepticus, ventricular tachycardia, and asystolic arrest have been reported after **orphenadrine** overdose.

D. **Tizanidine** is similar to clonidine and can cause coma, profound hypotension, and bradycardia (p 197); in addition, sinoatrial (SA) and atrioventricular (AV) nodal dysfunction was reported after an overdose.

IV. **Diagnosis** usually is based on the history of ingestion and findings of CNS depression, often accompanied by muscle twitching or hyperreflexia. The differential diagnosis should include other sedative–hypnotic agents (p 414).

A. **Specific levels.** Many of these drugs can be detected on comprehensive urine toxicology screening. Quantitative drug levels do not always correlate with severity of intoxication, especially in patients who have tolerance to the drug or have also ingested other drugs or alcohol.

B. **Other useful laboratory studies** include electrolytes, glucose, serum ethanol, BUN, creatinine, arterial blood gases, and chest radiography.

V. **Treatment**

A. **Emergency and supportive measures**

1. Maintain an open airway and assist ventilation if necessary (pp 1–7). Administer supplemental oxygen.
2. Treat coma (p 18), hypothermia (p 20), hypotension (p 15), and pulmonary edema (p 7) if they occur. Hypotension usually responds promptly to supine position and IV fluids.

3. Monitor patients for at least 6 hours after ingestion because delayed absorption may occur.
4. The definitive treatment for baclofen withdrawal symptoms is reinstitution of baclofen therapy followed by a slow taper. Benzodiazepines can be helpful for the treatment of spasticity and CNS excitation.

B. **Specific drugs and antidotes.** There are no specific antidotes. Flumazenil (p 556) is a specific antagonist of benzodiazepine receptors and would not be expected to be beneficial for skeletal muscle relaxants, but it reportedly has been used successfully for chlorzoxazone and carisoprodol overdose. Although physostigmine may reverse the anticholinergic symptoms associated with cyclobenzaprine and orphenadrine overdose, it is not generally needed and may potentially cause seizures.

C. **Decontamination** (p 50). Administer activated charcoal orally if conditions are appropriate (see Table I–38, p 54). Gastric lavage is not necessary after small-to-moderate ingestions if activated charcoal can be given promptly.

D. **Enhanced elimination.** Because of extensive tissue distribution, dialysis, and hemoperfusion are not very effective for most of the drugs in this group. Hemodialysis may significantly enhance **baclofen** clearance, particularly for patients with impaired renal function. The elimination half-life of baclofen decreased from 15.7 to 3.1 hours before and during hemodialysis, respectively, in an adult with normal renal function.

► SMOKE INHALATION

Kent R. Olson, MD

Smoke inhalation commonly occurs in fire victims and is associated with high morbidity and mortality. In addition to thermal injury, burning organic and inorganic materials can produce a very large number of different toxins, leading to chemical injury to the respiratory tract as well as systemic effects from absorption of poisons through the lungs. "Smoke bombs" do not release true smoke but can be hazardous because of irritant components, particularly zinc chloride.

I. **Mechanism of toxicity.** Smoke is a complex mixture of gases, fumes, and suspended particles. Injury may result from the following:
   A. **Thermal damage** to the airway and tracheobronchial passages.
   B. **Irritant gases, vapors, and fumes** that can damage the upper and lower respiratory tract (p 255). Many common irritant substances are produced by thermal breakdown and combustion, including acrolein, hydrogen chloride, phosgene, and nitrogen oxides.
   C. **Asphyxia** due to consumption of oxygen by the fire and production of carbon dioxide and other gases.
   D. **Toxic systemic effects** of inhaled carbon monoxide, cyanide, and other systemic poisons. Cyanide is a common product of combustion of plastics, wool, and many other natural and synthetic polymers.

II. **Toxic dose.** The toxic dose varies depending on the intensity and duration of the exposure. Inhalation in a confined space with limited egress is typically associated with delivery of a greater toxic dose.

III. **Clinical presentation**
   A. **Thermal and irritant effects** include singed nasal hairs, carbonaceous material in the nose and pharynx, cough, wheezing, and dyspnea. Stridor is an ominous finding that suggests imminent airway compromise due to swelling in and around the larynx. Pulmonary edema, pneumonitis, and adult respiratory distress syndrome (ARDS) may occur. Inhalation of steam is strongly associated with deep thermal injury but is not complicated by systemic toxicity.
   B. **Asphyxia and systemic intoxicants** may cause dizziness, confusion, syncope, seizures, and coma. In addition, **carbon monoxide** poisoning (p 182),

cyanide poisoning (p 208), and **methemoglobinemia** (p 317) have been documented in victims of smoke inhalation.

IV. **Diagnosis** should be suspected in any patient brought from a fire, especially with facial burns, singed nasal hairs, carbonaceous deposits in the upper airways or in the sputum, or dyspnea.

A. **Specific levels.** Carboxyhemoglobin and methemoglobin levels can be measured with co-oximetry. Unfortunately, cyanide levels are not readily available with short turnaround times; thus, the diagnosis is usually based on clinical findings.

B. **Other useful laboratory studies** include arterial blood gases or oximetry, chest radiography, spirometry, or peak expiratory flow measurement. Arterial blood gases, pulse oximetry, and chest radiograph may reveal early evidence of chemical pneumonitis or pulmonary edema. However, arterial blood gases and conventional pulse oximetry are ***not*** reliable in patients with carbon monoxide poisoning or methemoglobinemia. (A newer pulse co-oximeter is capable of detecting carboxyhemoglobin and methemoglobin.)

V. **Treatment**

A. **Emergency and supportive measures**

1. Immediately assess the airway; hoarseness or stridor suggests laryngeal edema, which may necessitate direct laryngoscopy and endotracheal intubation if sufficient swelling is present (p 4). Assist ventilation if necessary (p 5).
2. Administer high-flow supplemental oxygen by tight-fitting non-rebreather mask (p 599).
3. Treat bronchospasm with aerosolized bronchodilators (p 8).
4. Treat pulmonary edema if it occurs (p 7).

B. **Specific drugs and antidotes**

1. **Carbon monoxide** poisoning. Provide 100% oxygen by mask or endotracheal tube. Consider hyperbaric oxygen (p 599).
2. **Cyanide** poisoning. Empiric antidotal therapy with **hydroxocobalamin** (p 563) is recommended for patients with altered mental status, hypotension, or acidosis. If hydroxocobalamin is not available, **sodium thiosulfate** (p 629) from the conventional cyanide antidote kit may also be effective. ***Note:*** Use of sodium nitrite is discouraged because it may cause hypotension and aggravate methemoglobinemia.
3. Treat **methemoglobinemia** with **methylene blue** (p 579).

C. **Decontamination** (p 50). Once the victim is removed from the smoke environment, further decontamination is not needed.

D. **Enhanced elimination.** Administer 100% oxygen and consider hyperbaric oxygen (p 599) for carbon monoxide poisoning.

▶ SNAKEBITE

Richard F. Clark, MD

Among the 14 families of snakes, five are poisonous (Table II–61). The annual incidence of snakebite in the United States is three to four bites per 100,000 population. Clinically significant morbidity occurs in fewer than 60% of cases, and only a few deaths are reported each year. Bites from rattlesnakes are the most common snake envenomation in the United States, and the victim is often a young intoxicated male who was attempting to handle or manipulate the snake. Snakes strike accurately to about one-third of their body length, with a maximum striking distance of a few feet.

I. **Mechanism of toxicity.** Snake venoms are complex mixtures of components that function to immobilize, kill, and pre-digest prey. In human victims, these substances produce local "digestive" or cytotoxic effects on tissues as well as hemotoxic, neurotoxic, and other systemic effects. The relative predominance of

TABLE II–61. POISONOUS SNAKES (SELECTED)

Families and Genera	Common Name	Comments
Colubridae		
Lampropeltis	King snake	Human envenomation difficult because of small mouth and small, fixed fangs in the rear of mouth. Larger African species may cause severe systemic coagulopathy.
Heterodon	Hognose	
Coluber	Racer	
Dispholidus	Boomslang	
Elapidae		
Micrurus	Coral snake	Fixed front fangs. Neurotoxicity usually predominates.
Naja	Cobra	
Bungarus	Krait	
Dendroaspis	Mamba	
Hydrophiinae	Sea snakes	Small, rear-located fangs. Envenomations are rare
Viperidae, subfamily Crotalinae		
Crotalus	Rattlesnake	Most common envenomation in the United States. Long, rotating fangs in front of mouth. Heat-sensing facial pits (hence the name "pit vipers").
Agkistrodon	Copperhead, cottonmouth	
Bothrops	Fer-de-lance	
Viperidae, subfamily Viperinae		
Bitis	Puff adder, gaboon viper	Long, rotating fangs in front of mouth, but no heat sensing facial pits.
Cerastes	Cleopatra's asp	
Echis	Saw-scaled viper	

cytotoxic, hemotoxic, and neurotoxic venom components depends on the species of the snake and on geographic and seasonal variables. This changing mix of components is the most likely reason why the clinical presentation of each rattlesnake envenomation is unique.

II. Toxic dose. The potency of the venom and the amount of venom injected vary considerably. About 20% of all snake strikes are "dry" bites in which no venom is injected.

III. Clinical presentation. The most common poisonous snake envenomations in the United States are from rattlesnakes (Viperidae, subfamily Crotalinae). Bites from common North American Elapidae (eg, coral snakes) and Colubridae (eg, king snakes) are also discussed here. For information about bites from other exotic snakes, contact a regional poison control center (1-800-222-1222) for a specific consultation.

A. Crotalinae. Fang marks may look like puncture wounds or lacerations, with the latter resulting from a glancing blow by the snake or a sudden movement by the victim. The fangs often penetrate only a few millimeters but occasionally enter deeper tissue spaces or blood vessels. Signs and symptoms of toxicity are almost always apparent within 8–12 hours of envenomation.

1. **Local effects.** Within minutes of envenomation, stinging, burning pain begins. Progressive swelling, erythema, petechiae, ecchymosis, and hemorrhagic blebs may develop over the next several hours. The limb may swell dramatically within the first few hours. Hypovolemic shock and rarely local compartment syndrome may occur secondary to fluid and blood sequestration in injured areas.
2. **Systemic effects** may include nausea and vomiting, weakness, muscle fasciculations, diaphoresis, perioral and peripheral paresthesias, a metallic taste, thrombocytopenia, and coagulopathy. Circulating vasodilator compounds may contribute to hypotension. Pulmonary edema and cardiovascular collapse have been reported, as well as allergic-type reactions to the venom

that may result in rapid airway compromise and severe hypotension. Coagulopathy may be delayed or recurrent after antivenom administration.

3. **Mojave rattlesnake** (*Crotalus scutulatus*) bites merit special consideration and caution because neurologic signs and symptoms of envenomation may be delayed, and there is often little swelling or evidence of tissue damage. The onset of muscle weakness, ptosis, and respiratory arrest has been reported to occur several hours after envenomation. Facial and laryngeal edema has also been reported.

B. **Elapidae.** Coral snake envenomation is rare because of the snake's small mouth and fangs. The largest and most venomous coral snakes in this country reside in the southeastern United States, where bites are more often severe when they occur.

1. **Local effects.** There is usually minimal swelling and inflammation initially around the fang marks. Local paresthesias may occur.
2. **Systemic effects.** Systemic symptoms usually occur within a few hours but may rarely be delayed 12 hours or more. Nausea and vomiting, confusion, diplopia, dysarthria, muscle fasciculations, generalized muscle weakness, and respiratory arrest may occur.

C. **Colubridae.** These small-mouthed, rear-fanged snakes must hang on to their victims and "chew" the venom into the skin before significant envenomation can occur.

1. **Local effects.** There is usually little local reaction other than mild pain and paresthesias, although swelling of the extremity may occur.
2. **Systemic effects.** The most serious effect of envenomation is systemic coagulopathy, which can be fatal but is rare in all but a few African colubrids.

D. **Exotic species.** "Collectors" are increasingly importing exotic snake species into the United States. In some states, such as Florida, laws have permitted this practice. The most commonly found exotic species, such as cobras and mambas, are elapids, but their bites may result in much larger venom injections than those of coral snakes. Symptoms may occur more rapidly and be more severe than those seen in coral snakebites, but the spectrum of toxicity may be similar. Neurologic signs and symptoms, progressing to respiratory arrest, may occur. In addition, local tissue damage with these species may be severe.

IV. **Diagnosis.** Correct diagnosis and treatment depend on proper identification of the offending snake, especially if more than one indigenous poisonous species or an exotic snake is involved.

A. Determine whether the bite was by an indigenous (wild) species or an exotic zoo animal or imported pet. (The owner of an illegal pet snake may be reluctant to admit this for fear of fines or confiscation.) Envenomation occurring during the fall and winter months (October–March) in cooler geographical regions, when snakes usually hibernate, is not likely to be caused by a wild species.

B. If the snake is available, attempt to have it identified. ***Caution:*** Accidental envenomation may occur even after the snake is dead.

C. **Specific levels.** These tests are not applicable.

D. **Other useful laboratory studies** include CBC, platelet count, prothrombin time (PT/INR), fibrin split products, fibrinogen, d-dimer, creatine kinase (CK), and urine dipstick for occult blood (positive with free myoglobin or hemoglobin). For severe envenomations with frank bleeding, hemolysis, or anticipated bleeding problems, obtain a blood type and screen early. If compromised respiratory function is suspected, closely monitor oximetry and arterial blood gases. Of these laboratory parameters, the platelet count and fibrinogen are most useful in predicting severity and need for treatment with antivenom. These coagulation studies may need to be repeated every 2–6 hours until stable.

V. **Treatment**

A. **Emergency and supportive measures.** Regardless of the species, prepare for both local and systemic manifestations. Monitor patients closely for at least

6–8 hours after a typical crotaline bite and for at least 12–24 hours after a *C. scutulatus* or an elapid bite. Treatment of all symptomatic bites should include consideration of antivenom. Other potential adjunct therapies are discussed in the following text.

1. **Local effects**
   a. **Monitor local swelling** at least hourly with measurements of limb girth and proximal extension of edema. Assess for the presence and extent of local ecchymosis and for compromised circulation.
   b. When indicated, obtain consultation with an experienced surgeon for the management of serious wound complications. Do not perform fasciotomy unless compartment syndrome is documented with tissue compartment pressure monitoring.
   c. Provide tetanus prophylaxis if needed.
   d. Wound infection rarely occurs after snakebite. Administer broad-spectrum antibiotics only if there are signs of infection.
2. **Systemic effects**
   a. **Monitor the victim for respiratory muscle weakness.** Maintain an open airway and assist ventilation if necessary (pp 1–7). Administer supplemental oxygen.
   b. Treat bleeding complications with antivenom, and if needed in severe cases, fresh-frozen plasma (see below). Treat hypotension with IV crystalloid fluids (p 15) and rhabdomyolysis (p 27) with fluids and sodium bicarbonate.

B. Specific drugs and antidotes. For patients with documented envenomation, be prepared to administer specific **antivenom.** Virtually all local and systemic manifestations of envenomation improve after sufficient antivenom administration. A notable exception is fasciculations after some rattlesnake envenomations, which may be refractory to antivenom. ***Caution:*** Life-threatening anaphylactic reactions may occur with administration of older, equine-derived IgG antivenom or foreign antivenom products, even after a negative skin test result. Life-threatening anaphylaxis is rare with newer Fab and $F(ab)_2$ antivenom products, and skin tests are seldom indicated.

1. For **rattlesnake** and other **Crotalinae** envenomations:
   a. Fang marks, limb swelling, ecchymosis, and severe pain at the bite site are considered minimal indications for **antivenom** (p 506). Progressive systemic manifestations such as muscle weakness and coagulopathy are indications for prompt and aggressive treatment. For a Mojave rattlesnake bite, the decision to administer antivenom is more difficult because there may initially be few local signs of toxicity.
   b. Administer the currently approved Fab antivenom for symptomatic Crotalinae bites in 4- to 6-vial increments until stabilization of swelling, defibrination, thrombocytopenia, and other systemic effects has occurred. A new $F(ab)_2$ antivenom product for crotaline envenomation has shown promise in early clinical trials in the United States but is not yet approved.
   c. Owing to renal clearance of both bound and unused Fab fragments, manifestations of toxicity (eg, thrombocytopenia) may recur after initial treatment in some Crotalinae envenomations. For this reason, it is recommended that all patients who required antivenom be reassessed by a health care provider 2–4 days after the last dose.
2. For **coral snake** envenomation, consult a regional poison control center (1-800-222-1222) or an experienced medical toxicologist to determine the advisability and availability of ***Micrurus fulvius*** **antivenin** (p 509). In general, if there is evidence of coagulopathy or neurologic toxicity, administer antivenom.
3. For **Colubridae** envenomations, there is no antivenom available.
4. For **other exotic snakes,** consult a regional poison control center (1-800-222-1222) for assistance in diagnosis, location of specific antivenom, and

indications for administration. Many herpetologists or snake enthusiasts in areas where exotic species are common may have private supplies of antivenom. Even expired supplies may be usable and effective in severe cases.

C. **Decontamination.** First aid measures are generally ineffective and may cause additional tissue damage.
   1. Remain calm, remove the victim to at least 20 ft from the snake, wash the area with soap and water, and remove any constricting clothing or jewelry. Apply ice sparingly to the site (excessive ice application or immersion in ice water can lead to frostbite and aggravate tissue damage).
   2. Loosely splint or immobilize the extremity near heart level or higher for comfort. *Do **not** apply a tourniquet.*
   3. Do ***not*** make cuts over the bite site.
   4. Use of external suction devices (ie, Sawyer extractor) is not recommended. These devices may delay transport to definitive medical care, have not been demonstrated to improve outcome, and may increase tissue damage. Mouth suction of the wound is also not advised.

D. **Enhanced elimination.** Dialysis, hemoperfusion, and charcoal administration are not applicable.

► SPIDERS

Jeffrey R. Suchard, MD

Many thousands of spider species are found worldwide, and nearly all possess venom glands connected to fangs in the large, paired jaw-like structures known as chelicerae. Fortunately, only a very few spider species have fangs long and tough enough to pierce human skin. In the United States, these spiders include ***Latrodectus*** (widow spider) and ***Loxosceles*** (brown spider) species, **tarantulas** (a common name given to several large spider species), and a few others.

Patient complaints of "spider bites" occur much more commonly than do actual spider bites. Unexplained skin lesions, especially those with a necrotic component, are often ascribed to spiders, especially the brown recluse spider. Health care providers should consider alternative etiologies in the absence of a convincing clinical history and presentation. Many alleged "spider bites" are actually infections, with community-acquired methicillin-resistant *Staphylococcus aureus* (MRSA) being a common etiology.

Latrodectus species (black widow spiders) are ubiquitous in the continental United States, and the female can cause serious envenomations with rare fatalities. Black widows construct their chaotic webs in dark places, often near human habitation in garages, wood piles, outdoor toilets, and patio furniture. The spider has a body size of 1–2 cm and is characteristically shiny black with a red to orange-red hourglass shape on the ventral abdomen. The brown widow spider (*L. geometricus*) has recently been introduced into southern California and has spread along the Gulf of Mexico coast from Florida to Texas. This spider has variegated tan, brown, and black markings, also with a reddish hourglass on the abdomen, and envenomations result in the same clinical effects as from black widows.

Loxosceles reclusa (the brown recluse spider) is found only in the central and southeastern United States (e.g., Missouri, Kansas, Arkansas, and Tennessee). Rare individual specimens have been found in other areas, but they represent stowaways on shipments from endemic areas. Other *Loxosceles* species may be found in the desert southwest, although they tend to cause less serious envenomations. The spider's nocturnal hunting habits and reclusive temperament result in infrequent contact with humans, and bites are generally defensive in nature. The spider is 1–3 cm in length and light to dark brown in color, with a characteristic violin- or fiddle-shaped marking on the dorsum of the cephalothorax.

Tarantulas rarely cause significant envenomation but can produce a painful bite because of their large size. Tarantulas also bear urticating hairs that they can flick at predators and that cause intense mucosal irritation. People who keep pet tarantulas have developed ocular inflammation (ophthalmia nodosa) when these hairs embed in their corneas, usually while they are cleaning their spiders' cages.

I. **Mechanism of toxicity.** Spiders use their hollow fangs (chelicerae) to inject their venoms, which contain various protein and polypeptide toxins that appear to be designed to induce rapid paralysis of their insect victims and aid in digestion.
   A. ***Latrodectus*** (widow) spider venom contains *alpha-latrotoxin,* which causes opening of nonspecific cation channels, leading to an increased influx of calcium and indiscriminate release of acetylcholine (at the motor endplate) and norepinephrine.
   B. ***Loxosceles*** (brown spider) venom contains a variety of digestive enzymes and sphingomyelinase D, which is cytotoxic and chemotactically attracts white blood cells to the bite site and also has a role in producing systemic symptoms such as hemolysis.

II. **Toxic dose.** Spider venoms are generally extremely potent toxins (far more potent than most snake venoms), but the delivered dose is extremely small. The size of the victim may be an important variable.

III. **Clinical presentation.** Manifestations of envenomation are quite different depending on the spider genus.
   A. ***Latrodectus*** (widow spider) bites may produce local signs ranging from mild erythema to a target lesion a few centimeters in size with a central puncture site, inner blanching, and an outer erythematous ring.
      1. The bite is often initially felt as an acute sting, but may go unnoticed. The site almost always becomes painful within 30–120 minutes. By 3–4 hours, painful cramping and muscle fasciculations occur in the involved extremity. This cramping progresses centripetally toward the chest, back, or abdomen and can produce board-like rigidity, weakness, dyspnea, headache, and paresthesias. Widow spider envenomation may mimic myocardial infarction or an acute surgical abdomen. Symptoms can wax and wane, and often persist for 12–72 hours.
      2. Additional common symptoms may include hypertension, regional diaphoresis, restlessness, nausea, vomiting, and tachycardia.
      3. Other, less common symptoms include leukocytosis, fever, delirium, arrhythmias, and paresthesias. Rarely, hypertensive crisis or respiratory arrest may occur after severe envenomation, mainly in very young or very old victims.
   B. ***Loxosceles*** bites are best known for causing slowly healing skin ulcers, a syndrome often called "cutaneous loxoscelism" or "necrotic arachnidism."
      1. Envenomation usually produces a painful burning sensation at the bite site within 10 minutes but can be delayed. Over the next 1–12 hours, a "bull's eye" lesion forms, consisting of a blanched ring enclosed by a ring of ecchymosis. The entire lesion can range from 1 to 5 cm in diameter. Over the next 24–72 hours, an indolent necrotic ulcer develops that may take several weeks to heal. However, in most cases, necrosis is limited and healing occurs rapidly.
      2. Systemic illness may occur in the first 24–48 hours and does not necessarily correlate with the severity of the ulcer. Systemic manifestations include fever, chills, malaise, nausea, and myalgias. Rarely, intravascular hemolysis and disseminated intravascular coagulopathy may occur.
   C. **Other spiders.** Bites from most other spider species are of minimal clinical consequence. Bites from a few species can cause mild-to-moderate systemic symptoms (myalgias, arthralgias, headache, nausea, vomiting). As with many arthropod bites, a self-limited local inflammatory reaction may occur, and any break in the skin may become secondarily infected. In addition to *Loxosceles* spiders, a few other species have been reported to cause necrotic skin

ulcers (eg, *Phidippus* spp and *Tegenaria agrestis*), but these associations are questionable.

IV. Diagnosis most commonly is based on the characteristic clinical presentation. Bite marks of all spiders but the tarantulas are usually too small to be easily visualized, and victims may not recall feeling the bite or seeing the spider. Spiders (especially the brown recluse) have bad reputations that far exceed their actual danger to humans, and patients may ascribe a wide variety of skin lesions and other problems to spider bites. Many other arthropods and insects also produce small puncture wounds, pain, itching, redness, swelling, and even necrotic ulcers. Arthropods that seek blood meals from mammals are more likely to bite humans than are spiders. Several other medical conditions can cause necrotic skin ulcers, including bacterial, viral, and fungal infections and vascular, dermatologic, and even factitious disorders. Thus, any prospective diagnosis of "brown recluse spider bite" requires careful scrutiny. Unless the patient gives a reliable eyewitness history, brings the offending animal for identification (not just any spider found around the home), or exhibits systemic manifestations clearly demonstrating spider envenomation, the evidence is circumstantial at best.

A. Specific levels. Serum toxin detection is used experimentally but is not commercially available.

B. Other useful laboratory studies.

1. ***Latrodectus.*** Electrolytes, calcium, glucose, CPK, and ECG (in cases with chest pain).
2. ***Loxosceles.*** CBC, BUN, and creatinine. If hemolysis is suspected, haptoglobin and urine dipstick for occult blood (positive with free hemoglobin) are useful; repeat daily for 1–2 days.

V. Treatment

A. Emergency and supportive measures

1. **General.**
   - **a.** Cleanse the wound and apply cool compresses or intermittent ice packs. Treat infection if it occurs.
   - **b.** Give tetanus prophylaxis if indicated.
2. ***Latrodectus* envenomation.**
   - **a.** Monitor victims for at least 6–8 hours. Because symptoms typically wax and wane, patients may appear to benefit from any therapy offered.
   - **b.** Maintain an open airway and assist ventilation if necessary (see pp 1–7), and treat severe hypertension (p 17) if it occurs.
3. ***Loxosceles* envenomation.**
   - **a.** Admit patients with systemic symptoms and monitor for hemolysis, renal failure, and other complications.
   - **b.** The usual approach to wound care in cases of necrotic arachnidism is watchful waiting. The majority of these lesions will heal with minimal intervention over the course of a few weeks. Standard wound care measures are indicated, and secondary infections should be treated with antibiotics if they occur. Surgical debridement and skin grafting may be indicated for large and/or very slowly healing wounds; however, prophylactic early surgical excision of the bite site is not recommended.

B. Specific drugs and antidotes.

1. **Latrodectus**
   - **a.** Most patients will benefit from opiate analgesics such as **morphine** (see p 583) and often are admitted for 24–48 hours for pain control in serious cases.
   - **b.** Muscle cramping has been treated with **intravenous calcium** (see p 526) or skeletal muscle relaxants such as methocarbamol. However, these therapies are often ineffective when used alone.
   - **c.** Antivenom (see p 508) is rapidly effective but infrequently used because symptomatic therapy is often adequate and because of the small risk of

anaphylaxis. It is indicated for seriously ill, elderly, or pediatric patients who do not respond to conventional therapy for hypertension, muscle cramping, or respiratory distress and for pregnant victims threatening premature labor. Widow spider antivenom is more routinely used in some other countries, including Australia and Mexico. The perceived risk of anaphylaxis may be overestimated in the United States. A $F(ab)_2$ fragment antivenom, which may pose an even lower risk of anaphylaxis, is undergoing clinical trials.

2. **Loxosceles.** Therapy for necrotic arachnidism has been difficult to evaluate because of the inherent difficulty of accurate diagnosis.
   - **a.** Dapsone has shown some promise in reducing the severity of necrotic ulcers in anecdotal case reports but has not been effective in controlled animal models.
   - **b.** Steroids usually are not recommended.
   - **c.** There is no commercially available antivenom in the United States.
   - **d.** Hyperbaric oxygen has been proposed for significant necrotic ulcers, but results from animal studies are equivocal, and insufficient data exist to recommend its use.

C. Decontamination. These measures are not applicable. There is no proven value in early excision of *Loxosceles* bite sites to prevent necrotic ulcer formation.

D. Enhanced elimination. These procedures are not applicable.

► STRYCHNINE

Sean Patrick Nordt, MD, PharmD

Strychnine is an alkaloid derived from the seeds of the tree *Strychnos nux-vomica.* Brucine, a similar but weaker alkaloid, comes from the same seeds. Strychnine can be found in other plants (eg, Saint Ignatius bean *Strychnos ignatii,* Snakewood *Lignum colubrinum*). It is odorless and colorless, with a bitter taste. At one time, strychnine was an ingredient in a variety of over-the-counter tonics and laxatives, and was used clinically in the treatment of cardiac arrest and snake envenomation, and as an analeptic. Although strychnine is no longer found in pharmaceuticals; it is still available as a pesticide and rodenticide. It is also sometimes found as an adulterant in illicit drugs (eg, cocaine, heroin).

I. Mechanism of toxicity

A. Strychnine competitively antagonizes glycine, an inhibitory neurotransmitter released by postsynaptic inhibitory neurons in the spinal cord. Strychnine binds to the chloride ion channel, causing increased neuronal excitability and exaggerated reflex arcs. This results in generalized seizure-like contraction of skeletal muscles. Simultaneous contraction of opposing flexor and extensor muscles causes severe muscle injury, with rhabdomyolysis, myoglobinuria, and, in some cases, acute renal failure.

B. Pharmacokinetics. Strychnine is absorbed rapidly after ingestion or nasal inhalation and distributed rapidly into the tissues. It has low plasma protein binding and a large volume of distribution (Vd estimated at 13 L/kg in one case report). Strychnine is metabolized by the hepatic cytochrome P450 microsome system to a major metabolite, strychnine *N*-oxide, by first-order kinetics. Elimination is predominantly extrarenal, with an elimination half-life of about 10–16 hours (see also Table II–66, p 462).

II. Toxic dose. A toxic threshold dose is difficult to establish. The potentially fatal dose is approximately 50–100 mg (1 mg/kg), although death was reported in an adult who had ingested 16 mg. Signs of toxicity can occur rapidly, and because management decisions should be based on clinical findings rather than the reported amount ingested, any dose of strychnine should be considered potentially life-threatening.

III. Clinical presentation. Signs and symptoms usually develop within 15–30 minutes of ingestion and may last up to 12–24 hours.

A. Muscular stiffness and painful cramps precede generalized muscle contractions, extensor muscle spasms, and opisthotonus. The face may be drawn into a forced grimace (*risus sardonicus,* "sardonic grin"). Muscle contractions are intermittent and easily triggered by emotional, auditory, or minimal physical stimuli. Repeated and prolonged muscle contractions often result in hypoxia, hypoventilation, hyperthermia, rhabdomyolysis, myoglobinuria, and renal failure.

B. Muscle spasms may resemble the tonic phase of a grand mal seizure, but strychnine does not cause true convulsions, as its target area is the spinal cord, not the brain. The patient is usually awake and painfully aware of the contractions, described as "conscious seizures." Profound metabolic acidosis from increased lactic acid production is common.

C. Victims may also experience hyperacusis, hyperalgesia, and increased visual stimulation. Sudden noises or other sensory input may trigger muscle contractions. Rarely, anterior tibial compartment syndrome can be seen.

D. Death usually is caused by respiratory arrest that results from intense contraction of the respiratory muscles. Death may also be secondary to hyperthermia or rhabdomyolysis and renal failure.

IV. Diagnosis is based on a history of ingestion (eg, rodenticide or recent IV drug abuse) and the presence of seizure-like generalized muscle contractions, often accompanied by hyperthermia, lactic acidosis, and rhabdomyolysis (with myoglobinuria and elevated creatine kinase [CK]). In the differential diagnosis (see Table I–16, p 28), consider other causes of generalized muscle rigidity, such as tetanus (p 432), *Latrodectus* envenomation (p 426), and neuroleptic malignant syndrome (p 21).

A. Specific levels. Strychnine can be measured in the gastric fluid, urine, or blood by various analytic techniques, such as HPLC, GC/MS, and LC/MS. The toxic serum concentration is reported to be 1 mg/L, although blood levels do not correlate well with the severity of toxicity. Mortality has been reported with levels of 0.29–61 mg/L.

B. Other useful laboratory studies include electrolytes, BUN, creatinine, hepatic aminotransferases, CK, arterial blood gases or oximetry, and urine test for occult blood (positive in the presence of urine myoglobinuria).

V. Treatment

A. Emergency and supportive measures

1. Maintain an open airway and assist ventilation if necessary (pp 1–7).
2. Treat hyperthermia (p 21), metabolic acidosis (p 35), and rhabdomyolysis (p 27) if they occur.
3. Limit external stimuli such as noise, light, and touch.
4. **Treat muscle spasms** aggressively.
   - **a.** Administer **diazepam** (p 516), 0.1–0.2 mg/kg IV, **lorazepam,** 0.05–0.1 mg/kg IV, or **midazolam,** 0.05– 0.1 mg/Kg IV, to patients with mild muscle contractions. Give **morphine** (p 583) for pain relief. ***Note:*** These agents may impair respiratory drive.
   - **b.** In more severe cases, use **rocuronium,** 0.6–1 mg/kg, or another nondepolarizing neuromuscular blocker (eg, vecuronium, pancuronium [p 586]) to produce complete neuromuscular paralysis. Depolarizing agents (eg, succinylcholine) should be avoided due to potential unknown presence of hyperkalemia. ***Caution:*** Neuromuscular paralysis will cause respiratory arrest; patients will need endotracheal intubation and assisted ventilation.

B. Specific drugs and antidotes. There is no specific antidote.

C. Decontamination (p 50). Administer activated charcoal orally or by nasogastric tube if conditions are appropriate (see Table I–38, p 54). Do ***not*** induce vomiting because of the risk for aggravating muscle spasms. Gastric lavage is not necessary after small-to-moderate ingestions if activated charcoal can be given promptly.

D. Enhanced elimination. Symptoms usually abate within several hours and can be managed effectively with intensive supportive care. Hemodialysis and hemoperfusion have not been beneficial for enhancing the clearance of strychnine. The use of repeat-dose activated charcoal has not been studied.

▶ SULFUR DIOXIDE

John R. Balmes, MD

Sulfur dioxide is a colorless, nonflammable gas formed by the burning of materials that contain sulfur. It is a major air pollutant from automobiles, smelters, and plants that burn soft coal or oils with a high sulfur content. It is soluble in water to form sulfurous acid, which may be oxidized to sulfuric acid; both are components of acid rain. Occupational exposures to sulfur dioxide occur in ore and metal refining, chemical manufacturing, and wood pulp treatment and in its use as a disinfectant, refrigerant, and dried-food preservative.

I. **Mechanism of toxicity.** Sulfur dioxide is an irritant because it rapidly forms sulfurous acid on contact with moist mucous membranes. Most effects occur in the upper respiratory tract because 90% of inhaled sulfur dioxide is deposited rapidly there, but with very large exposures, sufficient gas reaches the lower airways to cause chemical pneumonitis and pulmonary edema.

II. **Toxic dose.** The sharp odor or taste of sulfur dioxide is noticed at 1–5 ppm. Throat and conjunctival irritation begins at 8–12 ppm and is severe at 50 ppm. The ACGIH-recommended workplace permissible limit (TLV) is 0.25 ppm (0.65 mg/m^3) as a short-term exposure limit (STEL). The NIOSH-recommended 8-hour time-weighted average is 2 ppm, and its recommended STEL is 5 ppm (13 mg/m^3); the air level considered immediately dangerous to life or health (IDLH) is 100 ppm. Persons with asthma may experience bronchospasm with brief exposure to 0.5–1 ppm.

III. **Clinical presentation**
   - A. **Acute exposure** causes burning of the eyes, nose, and throat; lacrimation; and cough. Laryngospasm may occur. Wheezing may be seen in normal subjects as well as persons with asthma. Chemical bronchitis is not uncommon. With a very high-level exposure, chemical pneumonitis and noncardiogenic pulmonary edema may occur.
   - B. **Asthma and chronic bronchitis** may be exacerbated.
   - C. **Sulfhemoglobinemia** resulting from absorption of sulfur has been reported.
   - D. **Frostbite** injury to the skin may occur from exposure to liquid sulfur dioxide.

IV. **Diagnosis** is based on a history of exposure and the presence of airway and mucous membrane irritation. Symptoms usually occur rapidly after exposure.
   - A. **Specific levels.** Blood levels are not available.
   - B. **Other useful laboratory studies** include arterial blood gases or oximetry, chest radiography, and spirometry or peak expiratory flow rate.

V. **Treatment**
   - A. **Emergency and supportive measures**
     1. Remain alert for progressive upper airway edema or obstruction and be prepared to intubate the trachea and assist ventilation if necessary (pp 1–7).
     2. Administer humidified oxygen, treat wheezing with bronchodilators (p 8), and observe the victim for at least 4–6 hours for the development of pulmonary edema (p 7).
   - B. **Specific drugs and antidotes.** There is no specific antidote.
   - C. **Decontamination**
     1. **Inhalation.** Remove the victim from exposure and give supplemental oxygen if available.
     2. **Skin and eyes.** Wash exposed skin and eyes with copious tepid water or saline. Treat frostbite injury as for thermal burns.
   - D. **Enhanced elimination.** There is no role for these procedures.

▶ TETANUS

Joshua B. Radke, MD

Tetanus is a rare disease in developed countries. The incidence of tetanus ranges from 10,000 to 1 million cases per year globally, with only 50–100 of those cases occurring in the United States. Success in prevention of tetanus is largely due to vaccination programs. In developed countries, tetanus is most commonly seen in older persons, recent immigrants, and IV drug users who have not maintained adequate tetanus immunization. Tetanus is caused by an exotoxin produced by *Clostridium tetani,* an anaerobic, spore-forming, gram-positive rod found widely in soil and in the GI tract.

I. **Mechanism of toxicity.** The toxin tetanospasmin is produced in wounds by *C. tetani* under anaerobic conditions. The toxin travels by retrograde axonal transport through peripheral motor nerves to synapses in the CNS. There, it inhibits the release of the presynaptic inhibitory neurotransmitters gamma-aminobutyric acid (GABA) and glycine. The loss of inhibitory transmission results in intense muscle spasms.

II. **Toxic dose.** Tetanospasmin is an extremely potent toxin. Fatal tetanus can result from a minor puncture wound in a susceptible individual.

III. **Clinical presentation.** The incubation period between the initial wound and the development of symptoms averages 1–2 weeks (range, 2–56 days). The wound is not apparent in about 5% of cases. Wound cultures are positive for *C. tetani* only about one-third of the time. There are several different clinical forms of tetanus; generalized, localized, cephalic, and neonatal.

   A. Generalized tetanus is the most common form of tetanus. The most common initial complaint is pain and stiffness of the jaw, progressing to trismus, *risus sardonicus* ("sardonic grin"), and opisthotonus over several days. Uncontrollable and painful reflex spasms involving all muscle groups are precipitated by minimal stimulation and can result in fractures, rhabdomyolysis, hyperpyrexia, and asphyxia. The patient remains awake during the spasms, which may persist for days or weeks.

      1. A syndrome of sympathetic hyperactivity often accompanies generalized tetanus, with hypertension, tachycardia, arrhythmias, and diaphoresis that may alternate with hypotension and bradycardia.

   B. Localized tetanus occurs when circulating anti-toxin prevents systemic spread of the toxin. This causes similar painful muscle contractions, but only in the region of the wound.

   C. Cephalic tetanus has been associated with head wounds and involves only the cranial nerves. CN VII is the most commonly affected, though any cranial nerve with motor function can be affected.

   D. Neonatal tetanus can occur as a result of inadequate maternal immunity or poor hygiene, especially around the necrotic umbilical stump.

IV. **Diagnosis** is based on the finding of characteristic muscle spasms in an awake person with a wound and an inadequate immunization history. Strychnine poisoning produces identical muscle spasms and should be considered in the differential diagnosis. Other considerations include hypocalcemia, neuroleptic malignant syndrome, seizures, stiff-man syndrome, and dystonic reactions.

   A. **Specific levels.** There are no specific toxin assays. A serum antibody level of 0.1 IU/mL or greater suggests prior immunity and makes the diagnosis less likely.

   B. **Other useful laboratory studies** include electrolytes, glucose, calcium, BUN, creatinine, creatine kinase (CK), and urine dipstick for occult blood (positive with myoglobinuria).

V. **Treatment**

   A. **Emergency and supportive measures**

      1. Maintain an open airway and assist ventilation if necessary (pp 1–7).

      2. Treat hyperthermia (p 21), arrhythmias (pp 10–15), metabolic acidosis (p 35), and rhabdomyolysis (p 27) if they occur.

      3. Limit external stimuli such as noise, light, and touch.

4. Antibiotics. Both **penicillin** and **metronidazole** have efficacy against *C. tetani*. Metronidazole is likely a better option, as high doses of penicillin may potentiate the action of tetanospasmin through GABA-A inhibition. Dosing for metronidazole is 500 mg (7.5 mg/kg for infants) IV or PO, every 6 hours, for 10 days.
5. **Treat muscle spasms** aggressively. Initiate therapy with benzodiazepines in mild to moderate cases, progressing to neuromuscular paralytics in severe cases.
   a. Administer **diazepam** (p 516), 0.1–0.2 mg/kg IV, or **midazolam,** 0.05–0.1 mg/kg IV, to patients with mild muscle contractions. Give **morphine** for pain relief. ***Note:*** These agents may impair respiratory drive.
   b. In more severe cases, use a non-depolarizing neuromuscular blocker (p 586) such as **rocuronium** (0.6–1.0 mg/kg bolus followed by 0.01 mg/kg/min) or **vecuronium** (0.08–0.1 mg/kg bolus followed by 0.01–0.02 mg/kg every 10–20 minutes) to produce complete neuromuscular paralysis. ***Caution:*** Neuromuscular paralysis will cause respiratory arrest; patients will need endotracheal intubation and assisted ventilation.

B. **Specific drugs and antidotes**
1. **Human tetanus immune globulin** (HTIg), 500 IU administered IM, will neutralize circulating toxin but has no effect on toxin that has already bound to neurons. HTIg should be given as early as possible to a patient with suspected tetanus, or in a patient with an incomplete immunization history and a tetanus-prone wound. Use of HTIg has not decreased mortality from tetanus, but may decrease the severity and duration of disease.
2. **Magnesium** (p 577) has been demonstrated to decrease the dose of medications needed for sedation and cardiac instability.
3. Beta blockers such as **labetalol** (p 571) or **esmolol** (p 552) can be used to treat the tachycardia and hypertension related to sympathetic hyperactivity.
4. **Prevention** can be ensured by an adequate immunization series with tetanus toxoid in childhood and repeated boosters at 10-year intervals. Surviving tetanus may not protect against future exposures because the small amount of toxin required to cause disease is inadequate to confer immunity.

C. **Decontamination.** Thoroughly irrigate and debride the wound, including removal of any foreign bodies.

D. **Enhanced elimination.** There is no role for these procedures.

▶ THALLIUM

Thomas J. Ferguson, MD, PhD

Thallium is a soft metal that quickly oxidizes upon exposure to air. It is a minor constituent in a variety of ores. Thallium salts are used in the manufacture of jewelry, semiconductors, and optic devices. Thallium no longer is used in the United States as a depilatory or rodenticide because of its high human toxicity.

I. **Mechanism of toxicity.** The mechanism of thallium toxicity is not known. It appears to affect a variety of enzyme systems, resulting in generalized cellular poisoning. Thallium metabolism has some similarities to that of potassium, and it may inhibit potassium flux across biologic membranes by binding to Na^+/K^+-ATP transport enzymes.

II. **Toxic dose.** The minimum lethal dose of thallium salts is probably 12–15 mg/kg, although toxicity varies widely with the compound, and there have been reports of death after adult ingestions of as little as 200 mg. The more water-soluble salts (eg, thallous acetate and thallic chloride) are slightly more toxic than the less soluble forms (thallic oxide and thallous iodide). Some thallium salts are well absorbed across intact skin.

III. **Clinical presentation.** Symptoms do not occur immediately but are typically delayed for 12–14 hours after ingestion.

A. **Acute effects** include abdominal pain, nausea, vomiting, and diarrhea (sometimes with hemorrhage). Shock may result from massive fluid or blood loss. Within 2–3 days, delirium, seizures, respiratory failure, and death may occur.

B. **Chronic effects** include painful peripheral neuropathy, myopathy, chorea, stomatitis, and ophthalmoplegia. Hair loss and nail dystrophy (Mees lines) may appear after 2–4 weeks.

IV. **Diagnosis.** Thallotoxicosis should be considered when gastroenteritis and painful paresthesia are followed by alopecia.

A. **Specific levels.** Urinary thallium is normally less than 0.8 mcg/L. Concentrations higher than 20 mcg/L provide evidence of excessive exposure and may be associated with subclinical toxicity during workplace exposures. Blood thallium levels are not considered reliable measures of exposure except after large exposures. Hair levels are of limited value, used mainly in documenting past exposure and in forensic cases.

B. **Other useful laboratory studies** include CBC, electrolytes, glucose, BUN, creatinine, and hepatic aminotransferases. Because thallium is radiopaque, plain abdominal radiographs may be useful after acute ingestion.

V. **Treatment**

A. **Emergency and supportive measures**

1. Maintain an open airway and assist ventilation if necessary (pp 1–7).
2. Treat seizures (p 23) and coma (p 18) if they occur.
3. Treat gastroenteritis with aggressive IV replacement of fluids (and blood if needed). Use pressors only if shock does not respond to fluid therapy (p 15).

B. **Specific drugs and antidotes.** There is currently no recommended specific treatment in the United States.

1. **Prussian blue** (ferric ferrocyanide, Radiogardase; p 620) is the mainstay of therapy in Europe and received FDA approval for use in the United States in 2003. This compound has a crystal lattice structure that binds thallium ions and interrupts enterohepatic recycling. Insoluble Prussian blue (Radiogardase) is available as 500-mg tablets, and the recommended adult dose is 3 g orally 3 times per day. Prussian blue appears to be nontoxic at these doses. In the United States, Prussian blue should be available through pharmaceutical suppliers, and an emergency supply may be available through Oak Ridge Associated Universities at 1-865-576-1005, the Radiation Emergency Assistance Center/Training Site (REAC/TS) 24-hour phone line. Radiogardase is manufactured by HEYL Chemisch-pharmazeutische Fabrik GmbH & Co KG in Berlin, Germany.
2. **Activated charcoal** is readily available and has been shown to bind thallium in vitro. Multiple-dose charcoal is recommended because thallium apparently undergoes enterohepatic recirculation. In one study, charcoal was shown to be superior to Prussian blue in eliminating thallium.
3. **BAL** (p 514) and other chelators have been tried with varying success. Penicillamine and diethyldithiocarbamate should be avoided because studies have suggested that they contribute to redistribution of thallium to the brain.

C. **Decontamination** (p 50). Administer activated charcoal orally if conditions are appropriate (see Table I–38, p 54). Ipecac-induced vomiting may be useful for initial treatment at the scene (eg, children at home) if it can be given within a few minutes of exposure. Consider gastric lavage for large recent ingestions.

D. **Enhanced elimination.** Repeat-dose activated charcoal (p 59) may enhance fecal elimination by binding thallium secreted into the gut lumen or via the biliary system, interrupting enterohepatic or enteroenteric recirculation. Forced diuresis, routine dialysis, and hemoperfusion are of no proven benefit. However, thallium is not highly protein bound and there may be some benefit with for hemodialysis early after acute ingestion; a nephrology workgroup 2012 strongly encouraged extracorporeal removal in severe poisonings (serum thallium >1 mg/L) within the first 24–48 hours of ingestion.

▶ THEOPHYLLINE

Kent R. Olson, MD

Theophylline is a methylxanthine that once was used widely for the treatment of asthma. Intravenous infusions of aminophylline, the ethylenediamine salt of theophylline, are sometimes used to treat bronchospasm, congestive heart failure, and neonatal apnea. Theophylline most commonly is used orally in sustained-release preparations (Theo-Dur, Slo-Phyllin, Theo-24, and many others).

I. **Mechanism of toxicity**

A. The exact mechanism of toxicity is not known. Theophylline is an antagonist of adenosine receptors, and it inhibits phosphodiesterase at high levels, increasing intracellular cyclic adenosine monophosphate (cAMP). It also is known to release endogenous catecholamines at therapeutic concentrations.

B. **Pharmacokinetics.** Absorption may be delayed with sustained-release preparations. The volume of distribution is approximately 0.5 L/kg. The normal elimination half-life is 4–6 hours; this may be doubled by illnesses (eg, liver disease, congestive heart failure, influenza) or interacting drugs (eg, erythromycin, cimetidine) that slow hepatic metabolism and may increase to as much as 20 hours after overdose (see also Table II–66, p 462).

II. **Toxic dose.** An acute single dose of 8–10 mg/kg can raise the serum level by up to 15–20 mg/L, depending on the rate of absorption. Acute oral overdose of more than 50 mg/kg may potentially result in a level above 100 mg/L and severe toxicity.

III. **Clinical presentation.** Two distinct syndromes of intoxication may occur, depending on whether the exposure is **acute** or **chronic.**

A. **Acute single overdose** is usually a result of a suicide attempt or accidental childhood ingestion but also may be caused by accidental or iatrogenic misuse (therapeutic overdose).

1. Usual manifestations include vomiting (sometimes hematemesis), tremor, anxiety, and tachycardia. Metabolic effects include pronounced hypokalemia, hypophosphatemia, hyperglycemia, and metabolic acidosis.
2. With serum levels above 90–100 mg/L, hypotension, ventricular arrhythmias, and seizures are common; status epilepticus is frequently resistant to anticonvulsant drugs.
3. Seizures and other manifestations of severe toxicity may be delayed 12–16 hours or more after ingestion, in part owing to delayed absorption of drug from sustained-release preparations.

B. **Chronic intoxication** occurs when excessive doses are administered repeatedly over 24 hours or longer or when intercurrent illness or an interacting drug interferes with the hepatic metabolism of theophylline. The usual victims are very young infants and elderly patients, especially those with chronic obstructive lung disease.

1. Vomiting may occur but is not as common as in acute overdose. Tachycardia is common, but hypotension is rare. Metabolic effects such as hypokalemia and hyperglycemia do not occur.
2. Seizures may occur with lower serum levels (eg, 40–60 mg/L) and have been reported with levels as low as 20 mg/L.

IV. **Diagnosis** is based on a history of ingestion or the presence of tremor, tachycardia, and other manifestations in a patient known to be on theophylline. Hypokalemia strongly suggests an acute overdose rather than chronic intoxication.

A. **Specific levels.** Serum theophylline levels are essential for diagnosis and determination of emergency treatment. After acute oral overdose, obtain repeated levels every 2–4 hours; single determinations are not sufficient because continued absorption from sustained-release preparations may result in peak levels 12–16 hours or longer after ingestion.

1. Levels of less than 80–100 mg/L after acute overdose usually are not associated with severe symptoms, such as seizures and ventricular arrhythmias.

2. However, with chronic intoxication, severe toxicity may occur with levels of 40–60 mg/L. ***Note:*** Acute caffeine overdose (p 169) will cause a similar clinical picture and produce falsely elevated theophylline concentrations with some older commercial immunoassays (check with the clinical laboratory).

B. Other useful laboratory studies include electrolytes, glucose, BUN, creatinine, hepatic function tests, and ECG monitoring.

V. Treatment

A. Emergency and supportive measures

1. Maintain an open airway and assist ventilation if necessary (pp 1–7).
2. Treat seizures (p 23), arrhythmias (pp 12–15), and hypotension (p 15) if they occur. Tachyarrhythmias and hypotension are best treated with a beta-adrenergic agent (see Item B below).
3. Hypokalemia is caused by intracellular movement of potassium and does not reflect a significant total body deficit; it usually resolves spontaneously without aggressive treatment.
4. Monitor vital signs, ECG, and serial theophylline levels for at least 16–18 hours after a significant oral overdose.

B. Specific drugs and antidotes. Hypotension, tachycardia, and ventricular arrhythmias are caused primarily by excessive beta-adrenergic stimulation. Treat with low-dose **propranolol** (p 617), 0.01–0.03 mg/kg IV, or **esmolol** (p 552), 0.025–0.05 mg/kg/min. Use beta blockers cautiously in patients with a prior history of asthma or wheezing.

C. Decontamination (p 50). Administer activated charcoal orally if conditions are appropriate (see Table I–38, p 54). Gastric lavage is not necessary after small-to-moderate ingestions if activated charcoal can be given promptly. Consider the use of repeated doses of activated charcoal and whole-bowel irrigation after a large ingestion of a sustained-release formulation.

D. Enhanced elimination (p 56). Theophylline has a small volume of distribution (0.5 L/kg) and is efficiently removed by hemodialysis, charcoal hemoperfusion, or repeat-dose activated charcoal. Although it is protein bound at therapeutic concentrations, the free fraction dominates at higher levels.

1. **Hemodialysis** should be performed if the patient is in status epilepticus or if the serum theophylline concentration is greater than 100 mg/L.
2. **Repeat-dose activated charcoal** (p 59) is not as effective but may be used for stable patients with levels below 100 mg/L.

▶ THYROID HORMONE

F. Lee Cantrell, PharmD

Thyroid hormone is available in the synthetic forms liothyronine (triiodothyronine, or T_3), levothyroxine (tetraiodothyronine, or T_4), and liotrix (both T_3 and T_4) and as natural desiccated animal thyroid (containing both T_3 and T_4). Dosage equivalents are listed in Table II–62. Despite concern about the potentially life-threatening manifestations of thyrotoxicosis, serious toxicity rarely occurs after acute thyroid hormone ingestion.

I. Mechanism of toxicity. Excessive thyroid hormone potentiates adrenergic activity in the cardiovascular, GI, and nervous systems. The effects of T_3 overdose are manifested within the first 6 hours after ingestion. In contrast, symptoms of T_4 overdose may be delayed 2–5 days after ingestion while metabolic conversion to T_3 occurs.

TABLE II–62. THYROID HORMONE: DOSE EQUIVALENTS

Desiccated animal thyroid	65 mg (1 grain)
Thyroxine (T_4, levothyroxine)	0.1 mg (100 mcg)
Triiodothyronine (T_3, liothyronine)	0.025 mg (25 mcg)

II. Toxic dose

A. An acute ingestion of more than 5 mg of **levothyroxine** (T_4) or 0.75 mg of **triiodothyronine** (T_3) is considered potentially toxic. An adult has survived an ingestion of 48 g of unspecified thyroid tablets; a 15-month-old child had moderate symptoms after ingesting 1.5 g of desiccated thyroid.

B. Euthyroid adults and children appear to have a high tolerance to the effects of an acute overdose. Patients with pre-existing cardiac disease and those with chronic overmedication have a lower threshold of toxicity. Sudden deaths have been reported after chronic thyroid hormone abuse in healthy adults.

C. Pharmacokinetics (see Table II–66, p 462)

III. Clinical presentation. The effects of an acute T_4 overdose may not be evident for several days because of a delay in the metabolism of T_4 to the more active T_3.

A. Mild-to-moderate intoxication may cause sinus tachycardia, elevated temperature, flushing, diarrhea, vomiting, headache, anxiety, agitation, psychosis, and confusion.

B. Severe toxicity may include supraventricular tachycardia, hyperthermia, and hypertension. There are case reports of seizures after acute overdose.

IV. Diagnosis is based on a history of ingestion and signs and symptoms of increased sympathetic activity.

A. Specific levels. Serum T_4, T_3 and thyroid-stimulating hormone (TSH) concentrations are difficult to interpret early after acute ingestion, but may be of use in confirming the diagnosis in symptomatic patients.

B. Other useful laboratory studies include electrolytes, glucose, BUN, creatinine, and ECG monitoring.

V. Treatment

A. Emergency and supportive measures

1. Maintain an open airway and assist ventilation if necessary (pp 1–7).
2. Treat seizures (p 23), hyperthermia (p 21), and arrhythmias (pp 10–15) if they occur.
3. Repeated evaluation over several days is recommended after large T_4 or combined ingestions because serious symptoms may be delayed.
4. Significant morbidity is unlikely and most patients recover with simple supportive care.

B. Specific drugs and antidotes

1. Treat serious tachyarrhythmias with **propranolol** (p 617), 0.01–0.1 mg/kg IV repeated every 2–5 minutes to the desired effect, or **esmolol** (p 552), 0.025–0.1 mg/kg/min IV. Simple sinus tachycardia may be treated with oral propranolol, 0.1–0.5 mg/kg every 4–6 hours.

C. Decontamination (p 50). Administer activated charcoal orally if conditions are appropriate (see Table I–38, p 54). Gastric lavage is not necessary after small-to-moderate ingestions if activated charcoal can be given promptly.

D. Enhanced elimination. Diuresis and hemodialysis are not useful because thyroid hormones are extensively protein bound. Treatment with charcoal hemoperfusion, plasmapheresis, and exchange transfusion has been employed but did not appear to influence clinical outcome.

▶ TOLUENE AND XYLENE

Paul D. Blanc, MD, MSPH

Toluene (methylbenzene, methylbenzol, phenylmethane, toluol) and xylene (dimethylbenzene, methyltoluene, and xylol) are common aromatic solvents found as additives in glues, inks, dyes, lacquers, varnishes, paints, paint removers, pesticides, cleaners, and de-greasers and as inherent constituents of gasoline. Xylene occurs in three isomers (meta-, ortho-, and para-), and commercial grade xylene contains a mixture of these with the meta-isomer predominant. Toluene and xylene are both clear, colorless liquids with a sweet, pungent odor that is detectable at low air concentrations. They are less dense than water and highly volatile, readily producing flammable and toxic concentrations at room temperature. The vapor is heavier than air and may accumulate in low-lying areas. Toluene is sometimes intentionally abused by inhaling lacquer thinner, paints, glues, and other commercial products to induce a "sniffer's high."

I. Mechanism of toxicity

A. Toluene and xylene cause generalized CNS depression. Like other aromatic hydrocarbons, they may sensitize the myocardium to the arrhythmogenic effects of catecholamines. They are mild mucous membrane irritants that can affect the eyes and the respiratory and GI tracts.

B. Pulmonary aspiration may cause a hydrocarbon pneumonitis (p 266).

C. Chronic overexposure can lead to degenerative CNS disease as well as other target end-organ effects.

D. Kinetics. Symptoms of CNS toxicity are apparent rapidly after inhalation of high concentrations and 30–60 minutes after ingestion. Pulmonary effects may not appear for up to 6 hours after exposure. Toluene and xylene are each metabolized by multiple hepatic cytochrome P450 enzymes leading to predictable metabolites including hippuric acid (toluene) and methylhippuric acid (xylene). Cresols are a minor metabolite of toluene.

II. Toxic dose

A. Ingestion. As little as 15–20 mL of toluene is reported to cause serious toxicity. A 60-mL dose was fatal in a male adult, with death occurring within 30 minutes.

B. Inhalation. The recommended workplace limits for toluene are 20 ppm (ACGIH TLV-TWA, with a "skin" notation for absorption), 10 ppm (California OSHA PEL-TWA, also "skin") and 200 ppm (Federal OSHA PEL-TWA) and for xylene 100 ppm (ACGIH TLV-TWA and California and Federal OSHA PELs). The air levels considered immediately dangerous to life or health (IDLH, NIOSH) are 500 ppm for toluene and 900 ppm for xylene. Death has been reported after exposure to toluene at 1,800–2,000 ppm for 1 hour. The EPA reference concentration (RfC) is 5 mg/m^3 for toluene and 0.1 mg/m^3 for xylene, which is an estimate of the air level for the general population (including sensitive subgroups) that is likely to be without risk for deleterious effects over lifetime exposure.

C. Prolonged **dermal exposure** may cause chemical burns in additional to systemic absorption effects. Both toluene and xylene are well absorbed across the skin.

III. Clinical presentation. Toxicity may be the result of ingestion, pulmonary aspiration, skin absorption, or inhalation.

A. Acute inhalation (or heavy skin absorption) can be irritating to the respiratory tract and produce euphoria, dizziness, headache, nausea, and weakness. Exposure to high concentrations may cause delirium, coma, pulmonary edema, respiratory arrest, although most victims regain consciousness rapidly after they are removed from exposure. Arrhythmias may result from cardiac sensitization. Massive exposures can cause pulmonary edema and ventilatory failure.

B. Chronic inhalation of toluene may cause permanent CNS impairment, including tremors; ataxia; brainstem, cerebellar, and cerebral atrophy; and cognitive and neurobehavioral abnormalities. Other neurotoxic end-organ adverse effects of toluene include hearing and color vision impairment. Renal tubular acidosis is another important manifestation of chronic toluene toxicity. Chronic xylene exposure also has CNS neurotoxic potential as well as potential adverse renal, hepatic, and bone marrow effects.

C. Ingestion of toluene or xylene may cause vomiting and diarrhea. If pulmonary aspiration occurs, chemical pneumonitis may result. Systemic absorption may lead to CNS depression.

D. Reproductive effects. Toluene is an established experimental and human reproductive hazard. Although reproductive toxicity from xylene is less firmly established, both solvents cross the placenta and are excreted in breast milk.

IV. Diagnosis of acute toxicity is based on a history of exposure and typical CNS manifestations, such as euphoria or "drunkenness." After acute ingestion, pulmonary aspiration is suggested by coughing, choking, tachypnea, or wheezing and is confirmed by chest radiography. Chronic past toxicity may be more difficult to establish beyond an exposure history and consistent end-organ effects without another likely cause.

A. Specific levels. In acute symptomatic exposures, toluene or xylene may be detectable in blood drawn with a gas-tight syringe, but usually only for a few hours. The metabolites hippuric acid, *o*-cresol (toluene), and methylhippuric acid (xylene) are excreted in the urine and can be used to monitor exposure. Urine levels may correlate poorly with systemic effects.

B. Other useful laboratory studies may include CBC, electrolytes, glucose, BUN, creatinine, liver aminotransferases, creatine kinase (CK), blood gas assessment (to assess acidosis), and urinalysis. Chest radiographs and oxygenation assessment are recommended for severe inhalation or if pulmonary aspiration is suspected.

V. Treatment

A. Emergency and supportive measures

1. **Inhalational exposure.** Maintain an open airway and assist ventilation if necessary (pp 1–7). Administer supplemental oxygen and monitor oxygenation.
   - **a.** If the patient is coughing or dyspneic, consider aspiration pneumonia. Treat for hydrocarbon pneumonia (p 266).
   - **b.** If the patient remains asymptomatic after a 6-hour observation, chemical pneumonia is unlikely, and further observation or chest radiography is not needed.
2. Treat coma (p 18), arrhythmias (pp 13–15), and bronchospasm (p 8) if they occur. ***Caution:*** Epinephrine and other sympathomimetic amines may provoke or aggravate cardiac arrhythmias. Tachyarrhythmias may be treated with **propranolol** (p 617), 1–2 mg IV, or **esmolol** (p 552), 0.025–0.1 mg/kg/min IV.

B. Specific drugs and antidotes. There is no specific antidote.

C. Decontamination. Patients exposed only to solvent vapor who have no skin or eye irritation do not need decontamination. However, victims whose clothing or skin is contaminated with liquid can secondarily contaminate response personnel by direct contact or through off-gassing vapor.

1. **Inhalation**. Remove the victim from exposure and give supplemental oxygen if available.
2. **Skin and eyes.** Remove contaminated clothing and wash exposed skin with soap and water. Flush exposed or irritated eyes with plain water or saline.
3. **Ingestion.** Consider activated charcoal orally if conditions are appropriate (see Table I–38, p 54), or removal via nasogastric tube if a very large, recent ingestion.

D. Enhanced elimination. There is no role for enhanced elimination.

▶ TRICHLOROETHANE, TRICHLOROETHYLENE, AND TETRACHLOROETHYLENE

Dennis Shusterman, MD, MPH

Trichloroethane and trichloroethylene are organic solvents that have historically been used as ingredients in many products, including typewriter correction fluid ("Wite-Out"), color film cleaners, insecticides, spot removers, fabric-cleaning solutions, adhesives, and paint removers. They have also been used extensively in industry as degreasers. Trichloroethane is available in two isomeric forms, 1,1,2-trichloroethane and 1,1,1-trichloroethane, with the latter (also known as methyl chloroform) being the more common. Tetrachloroethylene (perchloroethylene) is another related solvent that is widely used in the dry cleaning industry, although some regulatory agencies, such as the California Air Resources Board, have mandated its gradual phase-out for this application. Similarly, recognition of the stratospheric ozone depletion potential of 1,1,1-trichloroethane has resulted in the substitution of other chemicals for most applications.

I. Mechanism of toxicity

A. These solvents act as respiratory and CNS depressants and skin and mucous membrane irritants. As a result of their high lipid solubility and CNS penetration, they have rapid anesthetic action, and both trichloroethylene and trichloroethane were used for this purpose medically until the advent of safer agents. Peak blood levels occur within minutes of inhalation exposure or 1–2 hours after ingestion. Their proposed mechanism of action includes neuronal calcium channel blockade and gamma-aminobutyric acid (GABA) stimulation.

B. Trichloroethane, trichloroethylene, their metabolite trichloroethanol, and tetrachloroethylene may sensitize the myocardium to the arrhythmogenic effects of catecholamines.

C. Trichloroethylene or a metabolite may act to inhibit acetaldehyde dehydrogenase, blocking the metabolism of ethanol and causing "degreaser's flush."

D. Carcinogenicity.

1. In 2014, the International Agency for Research on Cancer (IARC) upgraded its classification of **trichloroethylene** from probable human carcinogen (Group 2A) to carcinogenic in humans (Group 1), based on sufficient evidence for kidney cancer and suggestive evidence for non-Hodgkin lymphoma and liver cancer. IARC continues to classify **tetrachloroethylene** as having limited evidence as a human bladder carcinogen, but showing sufficient evidence in animals (Group 2A). The US National Toxicology Program (NTP) classifies both trichloroethylene and tetrachloroethylene as "Reasonably Anticipated to be Human Carcinogens."

2. Both **1,1,1-** and **1,1,2-trichloroethane** are listed by IARC as "not classifiable as to carcinogenicity in humans" (Group 3), and neither has been systematically evaluated by the NTP.

II. Toxic dose

A. Trichloroethane. The acute lethal oral dose to humans is reportedly between 0.5 and 5 mL/kg. The recommended workplace limits (ACGIH TLV-TWA) in air for the 1,1,1-trichloroethane and 1,1,2-trichloroethane isomers are 350 and 10 ppm, respectively, and the air levels considered immediately dangerous to life or health (IDLH) are 700 and 100 ppm, respectively. Anesthetic levels are in the range of 10,000–26,000 ppm. The odor is detectable by a majority of people at 500 ppm, but olfactory fatigue commonly occurs.

B. Trichloroethylene. The acute lethal oral dose is reported to be approximately 3–5 mL/kg. The recommended workplace limit (ACGIH TLV-TWA) is 10 ppm (269 mg/m^3), and the air level considered immediately dangerous to life or health (IDLH) is 1,000 ppm.

C. Tetrachloroethylene. The recommended workplace limit (ACGIH TLV-TWA) is 25 ppm (170 mg/m^3), and the air level considered immediately dangerous to life or health (IDLH) is 150 ppm.

III. Clinical presentation. Toxicity may be a result of inhalation, skin contact, or ingestion.

A. Inhalation or ingestion may cause nausea, euphoria, headache, ataxia, dizziness, agitation, confusion, and lethargy and, if intoxication is significant, respiratory arrest, seizures, and coma. Hypotension and cardiac dysrhythmias may occur. Inhalational exposure may result in cough, dyspnea, and bronchospasm. With severe overdose, renal and hepatic injury may be apparent 1–2 days after exposure.

B. Local effects of exposure to liquid or vapors include irritation of the eyes, nose, and throat. Prolonged skin contact can cause a defatting dermatitis and, in the case of trichloroethane and tetrachloroethylene, may result in scleroderma-like skin changes.

C. **Ingestion** can produce GI irritation associated with nausea, vomiting, diarrhea, and abdominal pain. Aspiration into the tracheobronchial tree may result in hydrocarbon pneumonitis (p 266).

D. **Degreaser's flush.** Workers exposed to trichloroethylene vapors may have a transient flushing and orthostatic hypotension if they ingest alcohol, owing to a disulfiram-like effect (see "Disulfiram," p 226).

E. **Other.** Numerous case reports link high-level trichloroethylene exposures with the development of cranial neuropathies. Sporadic cases of optic neuritis have also been reported after trichloroethylene or tetrachloroethylene exposure. Several studies link occupational exposures to tetrachloroethylene (and environmental exposures to trichloroethane) to the occurrence of spontaneous abortion. Based on exposure modeling, tetrachloroethylene is likely to be present in breast milk.

IV. **Diagnosis** is based on a history of exposure and typical symptoms.

A. **Specific levels**

1. Although all three solvents can be measured in expired air, blood, and urine, levels are not routinely rapidly available and are not needed for emergency evaluation or treatment. Confirmation of exposure to trichloroethane may be possible by detecting the metabolite trichloroethanol in the blood or urine. Hospital laboratory methods are not usually sensitive to these amounts.
2. Breath analysis is becoming more widely used for workplace exposure control, and serial measurements may allow estimation of the amount absorbed.

B. **Other useful laboratory studies** include electrolytes, glucose, BUN, creatinine, liver transaminases, arterial blood gases, chest radiography, and ECG monitoring.

V. **Treatment**

A. **Emergency and supportive measures**

1. Maintain an open airway and assist ventilation if necessary (pp 1–7). Administer supplemental oxygen and treat hydrocarbon aspiration pneumonitis (p 266) if it occurs.
2. Treat seizures (p 23), coma (p 18), and dysrhythmias (pp 10–15) if they occur. ***Caution:*** Avoid the use of epinephrine or other sympathomimetic amines because of the risk for inducing or aggravating cardiac dysrhythmias. Tachyarrhythmias caused by myocardial sensitization may be treated with **propranolol** (p 617), 1–2 mg IV, or **esmolol** (p 552), 0.025–0.1 mg/kg/min IV.
3. Monitor for a minimum of 4–6 hours after significant exposure.

B. **Specific drugs and antidotes.** There is no specific antidote.

C. **Decontamination** (p 50)

1. **Inhalation.** Remove the victim from exposure and administer supplemental oxygen, if available.
2. **Skin and eyes.** Remove contaminated clothing and wash exposed skin with soap and water. Irrigate exposed eyes with copious tepid water or saline.
3. **Ingestion.** Do ***not*** give activated charcoal or induce vomiting because of the danger of rapid absorption and abrupt onset of seizures or coma. Consider removal by nasogastric tube only if the ingestion was very large and recent (<30 minutes). The efficacy of activated charcoal is unknown.

D. **Enhanced elimination.** These procedures are not effective or necessary.

▶ VALPROIC ACID

Thomas E. Kearney, PharmD

Valproic acid (Depakene or Depakote [divalproex sodium]) is a structurally unique anticonvulsant. It is used for the treatment of absence seizures, partial complex seizures, and generalized seizure disorders and is a secondary agent for refractory status epilepticus. It is also used commonly for the prophylaxis and treatment of acute manic episodes and other affective disorders, chronic pain syndromes, and migraine prophylaxis.

I. Mechanism of toxicity

A. Valproic acid is a low–molecular-weight (144.21) branched-chain carboxylic acid (pKa = 4.8) that increases levels of the inhibitory neurotransmitter gamma-aminobutyric acid (GABA) and prolongs the recovery of inactivated sodium channels. These properties may be responsible for its action as a general CNS depressant. Valproic acid also alters fatty acid metabolism, with impairment of mitochondrial beta-oxidation and disruption of the urea cycle, and can cause hyperammonemia, hepatotoxicity, metabolic perturbations, pancreatitis, cerebral edema, and bone marrow depression. Some of these effects may be associated with carnitine deficiency.

B. Pharmacokinetics

1. Valproic acid is rapidly and completely absorbed from the GI tract. There is a delay in the absorption with the preparation Depakote (divalproex sodium) because of its delayed-release formulation as well as the intestinal conversion of divalproex to two molecules of valproic acid.

2. At therapeutic levels, valproic acid is highly protein bound (80–95%) and confined primarily to the extracellular space, with a small (0.1–0.5 L/kg) volume of distribution (Vd). In overdose and at levels exceeding 90 mg/L, saturation of protein-binding sites occurs, resulting in a greater circulating free fraction of valproic acid and a larger Vd.

3. Valproic acid is metabolized predominantly by the liver and may undergo some degree of enterohepatic recirculation. The elimination half-life is 5–20 hours (average, 10.6 hours). In overdose, the half-life may be prolonged to as long as 30 hours (there are case reports of up to 60 hours, but this may have been due to delayed absorption). A level exceeding 1,000 mg/L may not drop into the therapeutic range for at least 3 days. In addition, active metabolites (eg, the neurotoxic 2-en-valproic acid and the hepatotoxic 4-en-valproic acid) produced via beta-oxidation and omega-oxidation pathways may contribute to prolonged or delayed toxicity.

II. Toxic dose. The usual daily dose for adults is 1.2–1.5 g to achieve therapeutic serum levels of 50–150 mg/L, and the suggested maximum daily dose is 60 mg/kg. Acute ingestions exceeding 200 mg/kg are associated with a high risk for significant CNS depression, and ingestions exceeding 400 mg/kg are associated with coma, respiratory depression, cerebral edema, and hemodynamic instability. The lowest published fatal dose is 15 g (750 mg/kg) in a 20-month-old child, but adult patients have survived after ingestions of 75 g.

III. Clinical presentation

A. Acute overdose

1. Acute ingestion commonly causes GI upset, variable CNS depression (confusion, disorientation, obtundation, and coma with respiratory failure), and occasionally hypotension with tachycardia and a prolonged QT interval. The pupils may be miotic, and the presentation may mimic that of an opiate poisoning. Cardiorespiratory arrest has been associated with severe intoxication, and the morbidity and mortality from valproic acid poisoning seem to be related primarily to hypoxia and refractory hypotension.

2. Paradoxical seizures may occur in patients with a pre-existing seizure disorder.

3. Transient rises of transaminase levels have been observed without evidence of liver toxicity. Hyperammonemia with encephalopathy has been observed with therapeutic levels and in overdose without other evidence of hepatic dysfunction. Hyperammonemia may also be associated with a higher risk for cerebral edema.

4. At very high serum levels (>1,000 mg/L) after large ingestions, other metabolic and electrolyte abnormalities may be observed, including an increased anion gap acidosis, hypocalcemia, and hypernatremia.

5. Other complications or late sequelae (days after ingestion) associated with severe intoxication may include myelosuppression, optic nerve atrophy, cerebral edema, noncardiogenic pulmonary edema, anuria, and hemorrhagic pancreatitis.

B. **Adverse effects of chronic valproic acid therapy** include hepatic failure (high-risk patients are younger than 2 years of age, are receiving multiple anticonvulsants, or have other long-term neurologic complications) and weight gain. Hepatitis is not dose related and usually is not seen after an acute overdose. Pancreatitis usually is considered a non–dose-related effect but has been reported with acute fatal overdoses. Alopecia, red cell aplasia, thrombocytopenia, and neutropenia have been associated with both acute and chronic valproic acid intoxication.

C. **Use in pregnancy. FDA Categories D & X (for migraine).** Valproic acid is a known **human teratogen.**

IV. **Diagnosis** is based on the history of exposure and typical findings of CNS depression and metabolic disturbances. The differential diagnosis is broad and includes most CNS depressants. Encephalopathy and hyperammonemia may mimic Reye syndrome.

A. **Specific levels.** Obtain a stat serum valproic acid level. Serial valproic acid level determinations should be obtained, particularly after ingestion of divalproex-containing preparations (Depakote), because of the potential for delayed absorption. Peak levels have been reported up to 18 hours after Depakote overdose and can be reached even later after ingestion of the extended-release formulation, Depakote ER.

1. In general, serum levels exceeding 450 mg/L are associated with drowsiness or obtundation, and levels greater than 850 mg/L are associated with coma, respiratory depression, and metabolic perturbations. However, there appears to be poor correlation of serum levels with outcome. Moreover, assays may or may not include metabolites.

2. Death from acute valproic acid poisoning has been associated with peak levels ranging from 106 to 2,728 mg/L, but survival was reported in a patient with a peak level of 2,120 mg/L.

B. **Other useful laboratory studies** include electrolytes, glucose, BUN, creatinine, calcium, ammonia (***note:*** use oxalate/gray-top blood tube to prevent false elevation of ammonia due to in vitro amino acid breakdown), liver aminotransferases, bilirubin, prothrombin time, lipase or amylase, serum osmolality and osmol gap (see p 33; serum levels $>$1,500 mg/L may increase the osmol gap by $\geq$10 mOsm/L), arterial blood gases or oximetry, ECG monitoring, and CBC. Valproic acid may cause a false-positive urine ketone determination.

V. **Treatment**

A. **Emergency and supportive measures**

1. Maintain an open airway and assist ventilation if needed (pp 1–7). Administer supplemental oxygen.

2. Treat coma (p 18), hypotension (p 15), and seizures (p 23) if they occur. There are anecdotal reports of the use of corticosteroids, hyperventilation, barbiturates, and osmotic agents to treat cerebral edema.

3. Treat acidosis, hypocalcemia, and hypernatremia if they are severe and symptomatic.

4. Monitor patients for at least 6 hours after ingestion and for up to 12 hours after ingestion of Depakote (divalproex sodium) because of the potential for delayed absorption.

B. **Specific drugs and antidotes.** There is no specific antidote. Naloxone (p 584) has been reported to increase arousal, but inconsistently, with the greatest success in patients with serum valproic acid levels of 185–190 mg/L. L-Carnitine (p 528) has been used to treat valproic acid–induced hyperammonemia and hepatotoxicity. Although data on clinical outcomes are not conclusive, it appears to have a safe adverse reaction profile.

C. **Decontamination** (p 50)

1. Administer activated charcoal orally if conditions are appropriate (see Table I–38, p 54). Gastric lavage is not necessary after small-to-moderate ingestions if activated charcoal can be given promptly.
2. Moderately large ingestions (eg, >10 g) theoretically require extra doses of activated charcoal to maintain the desired charcoal-to-drug ratio of 10:1. The charcoal is not given all at once but in repeated 25- to 50-g quantities over the first 12–24 hours.
3. The addition of **whole-bowel irrigation** (p 55) may be helpful in large ingestions of sustained-release products such as divalproex (Depakote or Depakote ER).

D. **Enhanced elimination** (p 56). Although valproic acid is highly protein bound at therapeutic serum levels, saturation of protein binding in overdose (binding decreases to as low as 15% at levels exceeding 1,000 mg/L) makes valproic acid amenable to enhanced removal methods. These procedures should be considered in patients with high serum levels (eg, >850 mg/L) associated with severe intoxication (eg, coma, respiratory failure, hyperammonemia, hemodynamic instability).

1. **Hemodialysis and hemoperfusion.** Hemodialysis may result in a 4- to 10-fold decrease in elimination half-life in overdose patients and is the method of choice. Dialysis also corrects metabolic disturbances, removes valproic acid metabolites and ammonia, and is associated with a rise in free carnitine levels. It is uncertain if use of high-efficiency and/or high-flux dialyzers is more advantageous. Charcoal hemoperfusion (alone and in series with hemodialysis) has also been used with clearances similar to those observed with hemodialysis and is subject to column saturation. However, the availability of hemoperfusion columns may be limited.
2. **Continuous renal replacement therapy (CRRT),** such as continuous arteriovenous hemofiltration (CAVH), continuous venovenous hemofiltration (CVVH), and continuous venovenous hemodiafiltration (CVVHDF), is sometimes preferred for hemodynamically unstable patients but achieves lower reported clearances.
3. **Repeat-dose activated charcoal.** Theoretically, repeated doses of charcoal may enhance clearance by interrupting enterohepatic recirculation, but no controlled data exist to confirm or quantify this effect. Another benefit is enhanced GI decontamination after a large or massive ingestion because single doses of charcoal are inadequate to adsorb all ingested drug.

▶ VASODILATORS

Jeffrey Fay, PharmD

A variety of vasodilators and alpha receptor blockers are used in clinical medicine. Nonselective alpha-adrenergic blocking agents (eg, phenoxybenzamine, phentolamine, and tolazoline) have been used in clinical practice since the 1940s. The first selective $alpha_1$ blocker, prazosin, was introduced in the early 1970s; doxazosin, indoramin, terazosin, trimazosin, urapidil, and tamsulosin are newer $alpha_1$-selective agents. Minoxidil, hydralazine, and diazoxide are directly acting peripheral vasodilators. Fenoldopam is a dopamine-1 receptor agonist approved for short-term management of severe hypertension. Nesiritide is a recombinant peptide that is used for the intravenous treatment of acutely decompensated congestive heart failure. Sildenafil, tadalafil, vardenafil, and avenafil are used in the treatment of male erectile dysfunction. Nitroprusside (p 342) and nitrates (p 339) are discussed elsewhere.

I. **Mechanism of toxicity.** All these drugs dilate peripheral arterioles to lower blood pressure. A reflex sympathetic response often results in tachycardia and occasionally cardiac arrhythmias. Prazosin and other, newer, alpha$_1$-specific agents are associated with little or no reflex tachycardia; however, postural hypotension is common, especially in patients with hypovolemia.

II. Toxic dose. The minimum toxic or lethal doses of these drugs have not been established. Fatalities have been reported with indoramin overdose and excessive IV doses of phentolamine.

- **A. Indoramin.** A 43-year-old woman died 6 hours after ingesting 2.5 g; CNS stimulation and seizures were also reported.
- **B. Prazosin.** A young man developed priapism 24 hours after an overdose of 150 mg. A 19-year-old man became hypotensive after taking 200 mg and recovered within 36 hours. Two elderly men who ingested 40–120 mg were found comatose with Cheyne–Stokes breathing and recovered after 15–18 hours.
- **C. Minoxidil.** Two adults developed profound hypotension (with tachycardia) that required pressor support after 1.3- and 3-g ingestions of topical minoxidil solutions.
- **D. Sildenafil** is generally well tolerated in accidental pediatric ingestions.
- **E. Pharmacokinetics** (see Table II–66, p 462)

III. Clinical presentation. Acute overdose may cause headache, nausea, dizziness, weakness, syncope, orthostatic hypotension, warm flushed skin, and palpitations. Lethargy and ataxia may occur in children. Severe hypotension may result in cerebral and myocardial ischemia and acute renal failure. First-time users of alpha$_1$ blockers may experience syncope after therapeutic dosing.

IV. Diagnosis is based on a history of exposure and the presence of orthostatic hypotension, which may or may not be accompanied by reflex tachycardia.

- **A. Specific levels.** Blood levels of these drugs are not routinely available or clinically useful.
- **B. Other useful laboratory studies** include electrolytes, glucose, BUN, creatinine, and ECG monitoring.

V. Treatment

- **A. Emergency and supportive measures**
  1. Maintain an open airway and assist ventilation if necessary (pp 1–7).
  2. Hypotension usually responds to supine positioning and IV crystalloid fluids. Occasionally, pressor therapy is needed (p 16).
- **B. Specific drugs and antidotes.** There is no specific antidote.
- **C. Decontamination** (p 50). Administer activated charcoal orally if conditions are appropriate (see Table I–38, p 54). Gastric lavage is not necessary after small-to-moderate ingestions if activated charcoal can be given promptly.
- **D. Enhanced elimination.** There is no clinical experience with extracorporeal drug removal for these agents. Terazosin and doxazosin are long acting and are eliminated 60% in feces; thus, repeat-dose activated charcoal may enhance their elimination.

▶ VITAMINS

Joyce Go, PharmD

Acute toxicity is unlikely after ingestion of vitamin products that do not contain iron (for situations in which iron is present, see p 277). Vitamins A and D may cause toxicity, but only after chronic use. Serious toxicity has been reported in individuals attempting to mask urine drug screens by ingesting large quantities of niacin.

I. Mechanism of toxicity

- **A. Vitamin A.** The mechanism by which excessive amounts of vitamin A produce increased intracranial pressure is not known.
- **B. Vitamin C.** Chronic excessive use and large IV doses can produce increased levels of the metabolite oxalic acid. Urinary acidification promotes calcium oxalate crystal formation, which can result in nephropathy or acute renal failure.

C. **Vitamin D.** Chronic ingestion of excessive amounts of vitamin D enhances calcium absorption and produces hypercalcemia.

D. **Niacin.** The most common adverse effects of niacin are cutaneous flushing and pruritus mediated by prostaglandin release.

E. **Pyridoxine.** Chronic overdose may alter neuronal conduction, resulting in paresthesias and muscular incoordination.

II. **Toxic dose**

A. **Vitamin A.** Acute ingestion of more than 12,000 IU/kg is considered toxic. Chronic ingestion of more than 25,000 IU/d for 2–3 weeks may produce toxicity.

B. **Vitamin C.** Acute intravenous doses of more than 1.5 g and chronic ingestion of more than 4 g/d have produced nephropathy.

C. **Vitamin D.** Acute ingestion is highly unlikely to produce toxicity. In children, chronic ingestion of more than 5,000 IU/d for several weeks may result in toxicity (adults >25,000 IU/d).

D. **Niacin.** Acute ingestion of more than 100 mg may cause a dermal flushing reaction. Immediate-release products are more likely to cause flushing than are the timed-release preparations. Ingestion of 2.5 g produced nausea, vomiting, dizziness, hypoglycemia followed by hyperglycemia, and coagulopathy.

E. **Pyridoxine.** Chronic ingestion of 2–5 g/d for several months has resulted in neuropathy.

III. **Clinical presentation.** Most acute overdoses of multivitamins are associated with nausea, vomiting, and diarrhea.

A. Chronic **vitamin A** toxicity is characterized by dry, peeling skin; alopecia; and signs of increased intracranial pressure (headache, altered mental status, and blurred vision [pseudotumor cerebri]). Bulging fontanelles have been described in infants. Liver injury may cause jaundice and ascites.

B. **Vitamin C.** Calcium oxalate crystals may cause acute renal failure or chronic nephropathy. Hemolysis can occur in patients with G6PD deficiency and iron overload in patients with history of hemochromatosis.

C. Chronic excessive use of **vitamin D** resulting in levels greater than 940 ng/mL has been associated with hypercalcemia, leading to weakness, altered mental status, nausea, vomiting, constipation, polyuria, polydipsia, renal tubular injury, musculoskeletal pains, weight loss, occasionally cardiac arrhythmias, and tumoral calcinosis around joints and in the vasculature). However, a level as low as 106 ng/mL was associated with hypercalcemia, hypertension, vomiting, constipation, and lethargy in a 2-year-old child who received 2,400,000 IU vitamin D over 4 days.

D. Chronic excessive use of **vitamin E** can cause nausea, headaches, and weakness.

E. **Vitamin K** can cause hemolysis in newborns (particularly if they are G6PD deficient).

F. Acute ingestion of **niacin**, but not niacinamide (nicotinamide), may produce unpleasant, dramatic cutaneous flushing and pruritus that may last for a few hours. Intentional ingestion of large amounts in an attempt to produce a negative urine drug screen has caused nausea, vomiting, abdominal pain, palpitations, dizziness, and hypoglycemia, followed by persistent hyperglycemia, anion gap metabolic acidosis, hypotension, and coagulopathy. Chronic excessive use (particularly of the sustained-release form) has been associated with hepatitis.

G. Chronic excessive **pyridoxine** use may result in peripheral neuropathy.

H. Large doses of **B vitamins** may intensify the yellow color of urine, and **riboflavin** may produce yellow perspiration.

IV. **Diagnosis** of vitamin overdose usually is based on a history of ingestion. Cutaneous flushing and pruritus suggest a niacin reaction but may be caused by other histaminergic agents.

A. **Specific levels.** Serum vitamin A (retinol) or carotenoid assays may assist in the diagnosis of hypervitaminosis A. Levels of 25-hydroxy vitamins D_2 and

D_3 are useful in assessing excessive intake and the form of the supplement taken, and are increasingly available through clinical laboratories.

B. **Other useful laboratory studies** include CBC, electrolytes, glucose, BUN, calcium, creatinine, liver aminotransferases, and urinalysis.

V. **Treatment**

A. **Emergency and supportive measures**

1. Treat fluid losses caused by gastroenteritis with IV crystalloid solutions (p 16).
2. Treat vitamin A-induced elevated intracranial pressure and vitamin D–induced hypercalcemia if they occur.
3. Nonsteroidal anti-inflammatory agents may prevent or alleviate prostaglandin-mediated niacin flushing or pruritus.

B. **Specific drugs and antidotes.** There is no specific antidote.

C. **Decontamination** (p 50). Usually, gut decontamination is unnecessary unless a toxic dose of vitamin A or D has been ingested or the product contains a toxic amount of iron.

D. **Enhanced elimination.** Forced diuresis, dialysis, and hemoperfusion are of no clinical benefit.

▶ WARFARE AGENTS—BIOLOGICAL

Timur S. Durrani, MD, MPH, MBA

Biological weapons have been used since antiquity, with documented cases dating back to the 6th century BC, when the Assyrians poisoned wells with ergots. In the late 1930s and early 1940s, the Japanese Army (Unit 731) experimented on prisoners of war in Manchuria with biological agents that are thought to have resulted in at least 10,000 deaths. Although in 1972 over 100 nations signed the Biological Weapons Convention, both the former Soviet Union and Iraq have admitted to the production of biological weapons, and many other countries are suspected of continuing their programs. Today, bioweapons are considered the cheapest and easiest weapons of mass destruction to produce.

The US government groups bioterrorism agents into three categories: A, B and C. **Category A** includes organisms or toxins that pose the highest risk to the public and national security because they can be easily spread or transmitted from person to person; result in high death rates and have the potential for major public health impact; might cause public panic and social disruption; and require special action for public health preparedness. **Category B** agents are the second highest priority: they are moderately easy to spread; result in moderate illness rates and low death rates; and require specific enhancements of CDC's laboratory capacity and enhanced disease monitoring. **Category C** agents are the third highest priority and include emerging pathogens that could be engineered for mass spread in the future because they are easily available; easily produced and spread; and have potential for high morbidity and mortality rates and major health impact. See http://emergency.cdc.gov/bioterrorism/overview.asp.

Category A agents (see the following text and Table II–63) include *Bacillus anthracis* (anthrax), *Yersinia pestis* (plague), *Clostridium botulinum* toxin (botulism), *Variola major* (smallpox), and *Francisella tularensis* (tularemia), and viral hemorrhagic fevers. All these agents can be weaponized easily for aerial dispersion.

The effect of a biological weapon on a population was demonstrated in an attack on the east coast of the United States in September 2001. Anthrax spores were delivered through the mail and resulted in 11 cases of inhalational anthrax and 12 cases of the cutaneous form of the disease. Even on that small scale, the effect on the public health system was enormous, and an estimated 32,000 people received prophylactic antibiotic therapy.

TABLE II–63. BIOLOGICAL WARFARE AGENTS (SELECTED)

Agent	Mode of Transmission	Latency Period	Clinical Effects
Anthrax	Spores can be inhaled or ingested or cross the skin. **No person-to-person transmission**, so patient isolation not required. Lethal dose estimated to be 2,500–50,000 spores.	Typically 1–7 days, but can be as long as 60 days	*Inhaled:* fever, malaise; dyspnea, nonproductive cough, hemorrhagic **mediastinitis**; shock. *Ingested:* nausea, vomiting, abdominal pain, hematemesis or hematochezia, sepsis. *Cutaneous:* painless red macule or papule enlarging over days into ulcer, leading to eschar; adenopathy; untreated may lead to sepsis. *Treatment:* ciprofloxacin, other antibiotics (see text); anthrax vaccine, anthrax immunoglobulin.
Plague	Inhalation of aerosolized bacteria or inoculation via flea bite or wound. **Victims are contagious via respiratory droplets**. Toxic dose 100–500 organisms.	1–6 days	After aerosol attack, most victims would develop pulmonary form: malaise, high fever, chills, headache; nausea, vomiting, abdominal pain; dyspnea, pneumonia, respiratory failure; sepsis and multiple-organ failure. Black, necrotic skin lesions can result from hematogenous spread. Skin buboes otherwise unlikely unless bacteria inoculated through skin (eg, flea bite, wound). *Treatment:* tetracyclines, aminoglycosides, other antibiotics (see text); vaccine not available.
Smallpox	Virus transmitted in clothing, on exposed skin, as aerosol. **Victims most contagious from start of exanthem**. Toxic dose 100–500 organisms.	7–17 days	Fever, chills, malaise, headache, and vomiting, followed 2–3 days later by maculopapular rash starting on the face and oral mucosa and spreading to trunk and legs. Pustular vesicles are usually in the same stage of development (unlike those of chickenpox). Death in about 30% from generalized toxemia. *Treatment:* vaccinia vaccine, immune globulin (see text).
Tularemia	Inhalation of aerosolized bacteria, ingestion, or inoculation via tick or mosquito bite. Skin and clothing contaminated. **Person-to-person transmission not reported**. Toxic dose 10–50 organisms if inhaled.	3–5 days (range, 1–4 days)	*Inhalation:* fever, chills, sore throat, fatigue, myalgias, nonproductive cough, hilar lymphadenopathy, pneumonia with hemoptysis and respiratory failure. *Skin:* ulcer, painful regional adenopathy, fever, chills, headache, malaise. *Treatment:* doxycycline, aminoglycosides, fluoroquinolones (see text); investigational vaccine.

Viral hemorrhagic fevers	Variety of routes, including insect or arthropod bites, handling contaminated tissues, and person-to-person transmission.	Variable (up to 2–3 weeks)	Ebola virus, Marburg virus, arenavirus, hantavirus, several others; severe multiple-system febrile illness with shock, delirium, seizures, coma, and diffuse bleeding into skin, internal organs, and body orifices. *Treatment:* None. Isolate victims, provide supportive care.
Botulinum toxins	Toxin aerosolized or added to food or water. Exposed surfaces may be contaminated with toxin. **Toxic dose 0.01 mcg/kg for inhalation and 70 mcg for ingestion.**	Hours to a few days	See p 163. Symmetric, descending flaccid paralysis with initial bulbar palsies (ptosis, diplopia, dysarthria, dysphagia) progressing to diaphragmatic muscle weakness and respiratory arrest; dry mouth and blurred vision due to toxin blockade of muscarinic receptors. Toxin cannot penetrate intact skin but is absorbed across mucous membranes or wounds. *Treatment:* botulinum antitoxin (p 522).
Ricin	Derived from castor bean (*Ricinus communis*); may be delivered as a powder or dissolved in water and may be inhaled, ingested, or injected.	Onset within 4–6 hours; death usually within 3–4 days	Nausea, vomiting, abdominal pain, and diarrhea, often bloody. Not well absorbed orally. Severe toxicity, such as cardiovascular collapse, rhabdomyolysis, renal failure, and death, more likely after injection. Lethal dose by injection estimated to be 5–20 mcg/kg. Inhalation may cause congestion, wheezing, pneumonitis. *Treatment:* Supportive. Not contagious, no need to isolate victims. Prophylactic immunization with ricin toxoid and passive postexposure treatment with antiricin antibody have been reported in animals.
Staphylococcal enterotoxin B	Enterotoxin produced by *Staphylococcus aureus*; may be inhaled or ingested.	Onset as early as 3–4 hours; duration, 3–4 days	Fever, chills, myalgia, cough, dyspnea, headache, nausea, vomiting; usual onset of symptoms 8–12 hours after exposure. *Treatment:* Supportive. Victims are not contagious, do not need isolation. Vaccine and immunotherapy effective in animals.
T-2 mycotoxin	Yellow, sticky liquid aerosol or dust (alleged “yellow rain” in 1970s) is poorly soluble in water.	Minutes to hours	Highly toxic trichothecene toxin can cause burning skin discomfort; nausea, vomiting, and diarrhea, sometimes bloody; weakness, dizziness, and difficulty walking; chest pain and cough; gingival bleeding and hematemesis; hypotension; skin vesicles and bullae, ecchymosis, and necrosis. Eye exposure causes pain, tearing, redness. Leukopenia, granulocytopenia, and thrombocytopenia reported *Treatment:* Supportive. Rapid skin decontamination with copious water, soap; consider using military skin decontamination kit.

I. **Mechanism of toxicity**

A. **Anthrax** spores penetrate the body's defenses by inhalation into terminal alveoli or by penetration of exposed skin or the GI mucosa. They then are ingested by macrophages and transported to lymph nodes, where germination occurs (this may take up to 60 days). The bacteria multiply and produce two toxins: "lethal factor" and "edema factor." Lethal factor produces local necrosis and toxemia by stimulating the release of tumor necrosis factor and interleukin 1-beta from macrophages.

B. **Plague** bacteria (*Y. pestis*) penetrate the body's defenses either by inhalation into terminal alveoli or by the bite of an infected flea. Dissemination occurs through lymphatics, where the bacteria multiply, leading to lymph node necrosis. Bacteremia, septicemia, and endotoxemia result in shock, coagulopathy, and coma. Historically, plague is famous as the "Black Death" of the 14th and 15th centuries, which killed 20–30 million people in Europe.

C. **Botulinum toxins** are one of the most potent toxins known, with microgram quantities potentially lethal to an adult. Botulinum toxin (p 163) cannot penetrate intact skin but can be absorbed through wounds or across mucosal surfaces. Once absorbed, the toxins are carried to presynaptic nerve endings at neuromuscular junctions and cholinergic synapses, where they bind irreversibly, impairing the release of acetylcholine.

D. **Smallpox** virus particles reach the lower respiratory tract, cross the mucosa, and travel to lymph nodes, where they replicate and cause a viremia that leads to further spread and multiplication in the spleen, bone marrow, and lymph nodes. A secondary viremia occurs, and the virus spreads to the dermis and oral mucosa. Death results from the toxemia associated with circulating immune complexes and soluble variola antigens.

E. **Tularemia.** *F. tularensis* bacteria usually cause infection by exposure to bodily fluids of infected animals or through the bites of ticks or mosquitoes. Aerosolized bacteria can also be inhaled. An initial focal, suppurative necrosis is followed by bacterial multiplication within macrophages and dissemination to lymph nodes, lungs, spleen, liver, and kidneys. In the lungs, the lesions progress to pneumonic consolidation and granuloma formation and can result in chronic interstitial fibrosis.

II. **Toxic doses** are variable but generally extremely small. As few as 10–50 *F. tularensis* organisms may cause tularemia, and less than 100 mcg of botulinum toxin can result in botulism.

III. **Clinical presentation** (see Table II–63 and the Centers for Disease Control website on biological and chemical terrorism at http://emergency.cdc.gov/bioterrorism)

A. **Anthrax** may present in three different forms: inhalational, cutaneous, and GI. Inhalational anthrax is extremely rare, and any case should raise the suspicion of a biological attack. Cutaneous anthrax typically follows exposure to infected animals and is the most common form, with over 2,000 cases reported annually. GI anthrax is rare and follows the ingestion of contaminated meat.

B. **Plague.** Although plague traditionally is spread through infected fleas, biological weapons programs have attempted to increase its potential by developing techniques to aerosolize it. Depending on the mode of transmission, there are two forms of plague: bubonic and pneumonic. The *bubonic* form would be seen after dissemination of the bacteria through infected fleas into a population (this was investigated by the Japanese in the 1930s in Manchuria). After an aerosolized release, the predominant form would be *pneumonic*.

C. **Botulism** poisoning is described in more detail on p 163. Patients may present with blurred vision, ptosis, difficulty swallowing or speaking, and dry mouth, with progressive muscle weakness leading to flaccid paralysis and respiratory arrest within 24 hours. Because the toxins act irreversibly, recovery may take months.

D. **Smallpox** infection causes generalized malaise and fever due to viremia, followed by a characteristic diffuse pustular rash in which most of the lesions are in the same stage of development.

E. **Tularemia.** After inhalation, victims may develop nonspecific symptoms resembling those of any respiratory illness, including fever, nonproductive cough, headache, myalgias, sore throat, fatigue, and weight loss. Skin inoculation causes an ulcer, painful regional lymphadenopathy, fever, chills, headache, and malaise.

IV. **Diagnosis.** Recognition of a bioweapon attack most likely will be made retrospectively, based on epidemiologic investigations. Specific indicators might include patients presenting with exotic or nonendemic infections, clusters of a particular disease, and infected animals in the region where an outbreak is occurring. A historical example is the downwind pattern of disease and proximity of animal deaths that helped prove that the anthrax outbreak in Sverdlovsk (in the former Soviet Union) in 1979 was caused by the release of anthrax spores from a biological weapons plant.

A. **Anthrax**

1. Obtain a Gram stain and culture of vesicle fluid and blood. Rapid diagnostic tests (enzyme-linked immunosorbent assay [ELISA], polymerase chain reaction [PCR]) are available at national reference laboratories.
2. Chest radiograph may reveal widened mediastinum and pleural effusions. Chest CT may reveal mediastinal lymphadenopathy.

B. **Plague**

1. Obtain a Gram stain of blood, cerebrospinal fluid, lymph node aspirate, or sputum. Other diagnostic tests include direct fluorescent antibody testing and PCR for antigen detection.
2. Chest radiograph may reveal patchy or consolidated bilateral opacities.

C. **Botulism** (see also p 163)

1. The toxin may be present on nasal mucous membranes and be detected by ELISA for 24 hours after inhalation. Refrigerated samples of serum, stool, or gastric aspirate can be sent to the CDC or specialized public health laboratories that can run a mouse bioassay.
2. Electromyography (EMG) may reveal normal nerve conduction velocity; normal sensory nerve function; a pattern of brief, small-amplitude motor potentials; and, most distinctively, an incremental response to repetitive stimulation, often seen only at 50 Hz.

D. **Smallpox** virus can be isolated from the blood and scabs and can be seen under light microscopy as Guarnieri bodies or by electron microscopy. Cell culture and PCR may also be employed.

E. **Tularemia**

1. Obtain blood and sputum cultures. *F. tularensis* may be identified by direct examination of secretions, exudates, or biopsy specimens with the use of direct fluorescent antibody or immunohistochemical stains. Serology may confirm the diagnosis retrospectively.
2. Chest radiograph may reveal evidence of opacities with pleural effusions that are consistent with pneumonia.

V. **Treatment.** Contact the **Centers for Disease Control and Prevention (CDC) 24-hour emergency response hotline at 1-770-488-7100** for assistance with diagnosis and management.

A. **Emergency and supportive measures.**

1. Provide supportive care. Treat hypotension (p 15) with IV fluids and vasopressors and respiratory failure (p 5) with assisted ventilation.
2. **Isolate** patients with suspected plague, smallpox, or viral hemorrhagic fevers, who may be highly contagious. Patient isolation is not needed for suspected anthrax, botulism, or tularemia because person-to-person transmission is not likely. However, health care workers should always use universal precautions.

B. Specific drugs and antidotes

1. **Antibiotics** are indicated for suspected anthrax, plague, or tularemia. All three bacteria are generally susceptible to fluoroquinolones, tetracyclines, and aminoglycosides. The following drugs and doses often are recommended as *initial empiric treatment,* pending results of culture and sensitivity testing (see also *MMWR.* 2001;50(42):909–919, which is available on the Internet at http://www.cdc.gov/mmwr/preview/mmwrhtml/mm5042a1.htm).
   a. **Ciprofloxacin,** 400 mg IV every 12 hours (children: 20–30 mg/kg/d up to 1 g/d).
   b. **Doxycycline,** 100 mg orally or IV every 12 hours (children 45 kg: 2.2 mg/kg). ***Note:*** Doxycycline may discolor teeth in children younger than 8 years of age.
   c. **Gentamicin,** 5 mg/kg IM or IV once daily, or streptomycin.
   d. Antibiotics should be continued for 60 days in patients with anthrax infection. **Postexposure antibiotic prophylaxis** is recommended after exposure to anthrax, plague, and tularemia.
   e. Antibiotics are ***not*** indicated for ingested or inhaled botulism; aminoglycosides can make muscle weakness worse (p 163).
2. **Vaccines.** Anthrax and smallpox vaccines can be used before exposure and also for postexposure prophylaxis. Vaccines are not currently available for plague, tularemia, and viral hemorrhagic fevers.
3. **Antitoxins**
   a. **Botulism.** A heptavalent antitoxin (H-BAT; see p 522) for botulism is an equine-derived antibody that covers toxin types A, B, C, D, E, F, and G. It is accessible only through the CDC.
   b. **Anthrax Immune Globulin** (Anthrasil™) is purified human immune globulin G (IgG) containing polyclonal antibodies that bind the protective antigen component of *Bacillus anthracis* lethal and edema toxins. **Raxibacumab** is a human IgG_1 gamma monoclonal antibody directed at the protective antigen of *B. anthracis.* **Obiltoxaximab** (Anthim™) is a chimeric IgG_1 kappa monoclonal antibody directed at the protective antigen of *B. anthracis.*
   c. **Vaccinia Immune Globulin** (VIG-IV) is a purified human immunoglobulin G (IgG) with trace amounts of IgA and IgM. It is derived from adult human plasma collected from donors who received booster immunizations with the smallpox vaccine. VIG-IV contains high titers of antivaccinia antibodies.

C. Decontamination. ***Note:*** The clothing and skin of exposed individuals may be contaminated with spores, toxin, or bacteria. Rescuers and health care providers should take precautions to avoid secondary contamination.

1. Remove all potentially contaminated clothing and wash the patient thoroughly with soap and water.
2. Dilute bleach (0.5%) and ammonia are effective for cleaning surfaces possibly contaminated with viruses and bacteria.
3. All clothing should be cleaned with hot water and bleach.

D. Enhanced elimination. These procedures are not relevant.

► WARFARE AGENTS—CHEMICAL

Richard F. Clark, MD

Chemical warfare has a long history that may have reached its zenith during World War I with the battlefield use of chlorine, phosgene, and mustard gases. More recently, Iraq used chemical agents in its war with Iran and against its own Kurdish population. In 1995, Aum Shinrikyo, a terrorist cult, released the nerve agent sarin in the Tokyo subway system during rush hour. It is also alleged that nerve agents were used in Syria.

Chemical warfare agents are divided into groups largely on the basis of their mechanism of toxicity (Table II–64): nerve agents, vesicants or blister agents, blood agents or cyanides, choking agents, and incapacitating agents. Presenting symptoms and the clinical circumstances may help identify the agent and lead to effective treatment as well as proper decontamination.

I. Mechanism of toxicity

A. Nerve agents include GA (tabun), GB (sarin), GD (soman), GF, and VX. These potent organophosphorus agents cause inhibition of acetylcholinesterase and subsequent excessive muscarinic and nicotinic stimulation (p 353).

B. Vesicants (blister agents). Nitrogen and sulfur mustards are hypothesized to act by alkylating cellular DNA and depleting glutathione, leading to lipid peroxidation by oxygen free radicals; lewisite combines with thiol moieties in many enzymes and also contains trivalent arsenic.

C. Choking agents include chlorine and lacrimator agents. These gases and mists are highly irritating to mucous membranes. In addition, some may combine with the moisture in the respiratory tract to form free radicals that lead to lipid peroxidation of cell walls. Phosgene causes less acute irritation but may lead to delayed pulmonary injury due to deeper pulmonary inspiration (p 371).

D. Cyanides (blood agents) include cyanide, hydrogen cyanide, and cyanogen chloride (p 208). These compounds have high affinity for metalloenzymes such as cytochrome aa3, thus inhibiting cellular respiration and leading to a metabolic acidosis.

E. Incapacitating agents. A variety of agents have been considered, including strong antimuscarinic compounds such as BZ and scopolamine (see "Anticholinergics," p 97), stimulants such as amphetamines and cocaine, hallucinogens such as LSD (p 297), and CNS depressants such as opioids (p 350). A form of fentanyl gas mixed with an inhalational anesthetic may have been used by Russian authorities in 2002 in an attempt to free hostages being held in a Moscow theater.

II. Toxic doses vary widely and also depend on the physical properties of the agents as well as the route and duration of exposure. Apart from the mechanism of toxicity of the chemical weapon, the following are important for consideration:

A. Physical state of the chemical. Agents delivered as aerosols and in large droplets generally have more persistence and can accumulate on surfaces. Gases tend to disperse, whereas vaporized forms of liquids may reliquefy in a cooler environment, leading to the potential for delayed dermal exposure. The use of high–molecular-weight thickeners to decrease evaporation of substances has been shown to increase agent persistence.

B. Volatility. Highly volatile agents (eg, hydrogen cyanide) vaporize rapidly and can be easily inhaled, whereas chemicals with low volatility (eg, VX) can remain in the environment for long periods.

C. Environmental factors. The presence of wind and rain can reduce the effectiveness of chemical weapon delivery by increasing dispersion and dilution. Cold weather may reduce vapor formation but increase the persistence of the liquid form of some agents. Gases and vapors heavier than air may accumulate in low-lying areas.

D. Agent decomposition (see Table II–64). Some warfare agents produce toxic by-products when exposed to acidic environments. GA may produce hydrogen cyanide and carbon monoxide. GB and GD produce hydrogen fluoride under acidic conditions. Lewisite is corrosive to steel and in nonalkaline conditions may decompose to trisodium arsenate. VX forms the toxic product EA2192 when it undergoes alkaline hydrolysis.

III. Clinical presentation

A. Nerve agents are potent cholinesterase-inhibiting organophosphorus compounds (p 353). Symptoms of muscarinic and nicotinic overstimulation include abdominal pain, vomiting, diarrhea, excessive salivation and sweating,

TABLE II–64. CHEMICAL WARFARE AGENTS (SELECTED)

	Appearance	Vapor Pressure and Saturated Air Concentration (at 25°C)	Persistence in Soil	Toxic Doses (for 70-kg Man)	Comments (see text for additional clinical description)
Nerve agents (cholinesterase inhibitors; see text and p 353)					
Tabun (GA)	Colorless to brown liquid with fairly fruity odor	0.07 mm Hg 610 mg/m^3 Low volatility	1–1.5 d	LC_{50} 400 $mg\text{-}min/m^3$ LD_{50} skin 1 g	Rapid onset; aging half-time 13–14 h.
Sarin (GB)	Colorless, odorless liquid	2.9 mm Hg 22,000 mg/m^3 Highly volatile	2–24 h	LC_{50} 100 $mg\text{-}min/m^3$ LD_{50} skin 1.7 g	Rapid onset; aging half-time 3–5 h.
Soman (GD)	Colorless liquid with fruity or camphor odor	0.4 mm Hg 3,060 mg/m^3 Moderately volatile	Relatively persistent	LC_{50} 50 $mg\text{-}min/m^3$ LD_{50} skin 350 mg	Rapid onset; aging half-time 2–6 min.
VX	Colorless to straw-colored odorless liquid	0.0007 mm Hg 10.5 mg/m^3 Very low volatility	2–6 d	LC_{50} 10 $mg\text{-}min/m^3$ LD_{50} skin 10 mg	Rapid onset; aging half-time 48 h.
Vesicants					
Sulfur mustard (HD)	Pale yellow to dark brown liquid	0.011 mm Hg 600 mg/m^3 Low volatility	2 wk-3 y	LC_{50} 1,500 $mg\text{-}min/m^3$ LD_{50} 100 mg/kg	Pain onset hours after exposure; fluid-filled blisters.
Phosgene oxime (CX)	Colorless crystalline solid or liquid with intensely irritating odor	11.2 mm Hg 1,800 mg/m^3 Moderately volatile	2 h	LC_{50} 3,200 $mg\text{-}min/m^3$ LD_{50} unknown	Immediate pain, tissue damage within seconds; solid wheal formation.
Lewisite (L)	Colorless to amber or brown oily liquid with geranium odor	0.58 mm Hg 4,480 mg/m^3 Volatile	Days	LC_{50} 1,200 $mg\text{-}min/m^3$ LD_{50} 40.50 mg/kg	Immediate pain, tissue damage in seconds to minutes; fluid-filled blisters.

Riot control agents (lacrimators)					
CS (chloroben-zylidene malonitrile)	White crystalline powder with pungent pepper odor	0.00034 mm Hg 0.71 mg/m^3 Very low volatility	Variable	LC_{50} 60,000 mg-min/m^3 Incapacitating dose: IC_{50} 3–5 mg-min/m^3	Rapidly severe eye pain and blepharospasm; skin tingling or burning sensation; duration 30–60 min after removal from exposure.
CN (mace, chloroace-tophenone)	Solid or powder with fragrant apple blossom odor	0.0054 mm Hg 34.3 mg/m^3 Low volatility	Short	LC_{50} 7–14,000 mg-min/m^3 Incapacitating dose: IC_{50} 20–40 mg-min/m^3	
DM (diphenylamine arsine)	Yellow-green odorless crystalline substance	4.5 × 10–11 mm Hg Insignificant Virtually nonvolatile	Persistent	LC_{50} 11–35,000 mg-min/m^3 Incapacitating dose: IC_{50} 22–150 mg-min/m^3 Nausea and vomiting: 370 mg-min/m^3	Delayed onset (minutes); irritation, uncontrollable coughing and sneezing; vomiting and diarrhea can last hours.
Cyanides (p 208)					
Hydrogen cyanide (AC)	Gas with odor of bitter almonds or peach kernels	630 mm Hg 1,100,000 mg/m^3 Gas lighter than air	$<$1h	LC_{50} 2,500–5,000 mg-min/m^3 LD_{50} skin 100 mg/kg	Rapidly acting gaseous cyanide.
Cyanogen chloride (CK)	Colorless gas or liquid	1,230 mm Hg 2,600,000 mg/m^3 Gas density heavier than that of air	Not persistent	LC_{50} 11,000 mg-min/m^3	Irritating to eyes and lungs, can cause delayed pulmonary edema.
Incapacitating agents (see text)					

Sources: *Medical Management of Chemical Casualties Handbook.* Chemical Casualty Care Office, Medical Research Institute of Chemical Defense, US Army Aberdeen Proving Ground, 1995; and *Textbook of Military Medicine: Medical Aspects of Chemical and Biological Warfare.* US Army, 1997. Available free on the Internet after registration at https://ccc.apgea.army.mil/products/handbooks/books.htm.

bronchospasm, copious pulmonary secretions, muscle fasciculations and weakness, and respiratory arrest. Seizures, bradycardia, or tachycardia may be present. Severe dehydration can result from volume loss caused by sweating, vomiting, and diarrhea.

B. **Vesicants (blister agents).** The timing of onset of symptoms depends on the agent, route, and degree of exposure.
   1. Skin blistering is the major cause of morbidity and can lead to severe tissue damage.
   2. Ocular exposure causes tearing, itching, and burning and can lead to severe corneal damage, chronic conjunctivitis, and keratitis. Permanent blindness usually does not occur.
   3. Pulmonary effects include cough and dyspnea, chemical pneumonitis, and chronic bronchitis.

C. **Choking agents** can cause varying degrees of mucous membrane irritation, cough, wheezing, and chemical pneumonitis. Phosgene exposure may also present with delayed pulmonary edema that can be severe and sometimes lethal.

D. **Cyanides** cause dizziness, dyspnea, confusion, agitation, and weakness, with progressive obtundation and even coma. Seizures and hypotension followed by cardiovascular collapse may occur rapidly. The effects of these agents tend to be all or nothing in a gas exposure, so if patients survive the initial insult, they can be expected to recover.

E. **Incapacitating agents.** The clinical features depend on the agent (see Item I.E above).
   1. **Antimuscarinics.** As little as 1.5 mg of scopolamine can cause delirium, poor coordination, stupor, tachycardia, and blurred vision. BZ (3-quinuclidinyl benzilate, or QNB) is about three times more potent than scopolamine. Other signs include dry mouth, flushed skin, and dilated pupils.
   2. **LSD** and similar hallucinogens cause dilated pupils, tachycardia, CNS stimulation, and varying degrees of emotional and perceptual distortion.
   3. **CNS stimulants** can cause acute psychosis, paranoia, tachycardia, sweating, and seizures.
   4. **CNS depressants** generally cause somnolence and depressed respiratory drive (with apnea possible).

IV. **Diagnosis** is based mainly on symptoms as well as the setting in which the exposure occurred.

A. **Specific levels**
   1. **Nerve agents.** Plasma and red blood cell cholinesterase activity is depressed, but interpretation may be difficult because of wide inter-individual variability and broad normal ranges (p 353).
   2. **Pulmonary agents and vesicants.** There are no specific blood or urine levels that will assist in diagnosis or management.
   3. **Cyanides.** Cyanide levels will be elevated, but rapid testing is not widely available. Suspect cyanide poisoning if a patient has severe metabolic acidosis, especially if mixed venous oxygen saturation is greater than 90%.

B. **Other laboratory tests** include CBC, electrolytes, glucose, BUN, creatinine, arterial blood gases, amylase/lipase and liver transaminases, chest radiography, and ECG monitoring. In addition, obtain serum lactate and mixed venous oxygen saturation if cyanide poisoning is suspected (p 208).

C. **Methods of detection.** The military has developed various devices to detect commonly known chemical warfare agents encountered in liquid or vapor forms. These devices include individual soldier detection systems such as **M8** and **M9 paper**, which identify persistent and nonpersistent nerve or blister agents. These tests are sensitive but not specific. More sophisticated chemical agent detector kits, such as the **M256** and **M256A1 kits**, which can identify a larger number of liquids or vapors, are also available. Systems that monitor air concentrations of various agents also have been used, such as the US military's CAM (Chemical Agent Monitor), ICAM (Improved Chemical Agent Monitor), and ACADA (Automatic Chemical Agent Detector/Alarm). Complexity and portability vary widely among detection methods: M9 paper may simply indicate that an agent is present, whereas the Chemical Biological Mass Spectrometer Block II analyzes air samples with a mass spectrometer. Further development of such systems is under way in both the private and governmental/military sectors.

V. Treatment. For expert assistance in management of chemical agent exposures and to access pharmaceutical antidote stockpiles that may be needed, contact your local or state health agency or a local poison control center (1-800-222-1222). In addition, if an act of terrorism is suspected, contact the Federal Bureau of Investigation (FBI).

A. Emergency and supportive measures. ***Caution:*** Rescuers and health care providers should take measures to prevent direct contact with the skin or clothing of contaminated victims because secondary contamination and serious illness may result (see Section IV, p 636).

1. Maintain an open airway and assist ventilation if necessary (pp 1–7). Administer supplemental oxygen. Monitor patients closely; airway injury may result in abrupt obstruction and asphyxia. Muscle weakness caused by nerve agents may cause abrupt respiratory arrest. Delayed pulmonary edema may follow exposure to less soluble gases such as phosgene (p 371).
2. Treat hypotension (p 15), seizures (p 23), and coma (p 18) if they occur.

B. Specific drugs and antidotes

1. **Nerve agents** (p 353)
   - **a. Atropine.** Give 0.5–2 mg IV initially (p 512) and repeat the dose as needed. Initial doses may also be given IM. The most clinically important indication for continued atropine administration is persistent wheezing or bronchorrhea. ***Note:*** Atropine will reverse muscarinic but not nicotinic (muscle weakness) effects.
   - **b. Pralidoxime** (2-PAM, Protopam [p 613]) is a specific antidote for organophosphorus agents. It should be given immediately (to potentially improve muscular weakness and fasciculations) as a 1- to 2-g initial bolus dose (20–40 mg/kg in children) IV over 5–10 minutes, followed by a continuous infusion. It is most effective if started early, before irreversible phosphorylation of cholinesterase, but may still be effective if given later. Initial doses can be given by the IM route if IV access is not immediately available. ***Note:*** Oximes such as HI-6, obidoxime, and P2S may be available in other countries for cholinesterase regeneration. The availability of these agents in the United States is currently very limited.
   - **c. Benzodiazepines.** Anticonvulsant therapy may be beneficial even before the onset of seizures and should be considered as soon as exposure is recognized. The initial diazepam dose is 5–10 mg IV in adult patients (0.1–0.3 mg/kg in children), while the dose of lorazepam is 1–2 mg IM or IV in adults (0.05–0.1 mg/kg in children). See p 516.
2. **Vesicants.** Treat primarily as a chemical burn (p 186).
   - **a.** British anti-lewisite (BAL [p 514]), a chelating agent used in the treatment of arsenic, mercury, and lead poisoning, originally was developed for the treatment of lewisite exposures. Topical BAL has been recommended for eye and skin exposure to lewisite; however, preparations for ocular and dermal use are not widely available.
   - **b.** Sulfur donors such as sodium thiosulfate have shown promise in animal models of mustard exposures when given before or just after an exposure. The role of this antidote in human exposures is not clear.
3. **Choking agents.** Treatment is mainly symptomatic, with the use of bronchodilators as needed for wheezing. Hypoxia should be treated with humidified oxygen, but caution should be exercised in treating severe chlorine or

phosgene exposure because excessive oxygen administration may worsen the lipid peroxidation caused by oxygen free radicals. Steroids may be indicated for patients with underlying reactive airways disease.

4. **Cyanides** (p 208). **Hydroxocobalamin** (Cyanokit [p 563]) chelates cyanide to form cyanocobalamin (vitamin B_{12}), which is then renally excreted. The initial dose is 5 g (2 vials) given IV over 15 minutes. The pediatric dose is 70 mg/kg. If hydroxocobalamin is not available, the older **cyanide antidote package** (Nithiodote and others) can be used instead. It consists of sodium **nitrite** (p 592), which produces cyanide-scavenging methemoglobinemia, and sodium **thiosulfate** (p 629), which accelerates the conversion of cyanide to thiocyanate. Amyl nitrite may also be included in older kits.
5. **Incapacitating agents**
   a. Antimuscarinic delirium may respond to physostigmine (p 609).
   b. Stimulant toxicity and bad reactions to hallucinogens may respond to lorazepam, diazepam, and other benzodiazepines (p 516).
   c. Treat suspected opioid toxicity with naloxone (p 584).

C. **Decontamination.** ***Note:*** Rescuers should wear appropriate chemical-protective clothing, as some agents can penetrate clothing and latex gloves. Butyl chemical-protective gloves should be worn, especially in the presence of mustard agents. Preferably, a well-trained hazardous materials team should perform initial decontamination before transport to a health care facility (see Section IV, pp 640-642). Decontamination of exposed equipment and materials may also be necessary but can be difficult because agents may persist or even polymerize on surfaces. Currently, the primary methods of decontamination are physical removal and chemical deactivation of the agent. Gases and vapors in general do not require any further decontamination other than simple physical removal of the victim from the toxic environment. Off-gassing is unlikely to cause a problem unless the victim was thoroughly soaked with a volatile liquid.

1. **Physical removal** involves removal of clothing, dry removal of gross contamination, and flushing of exposed skin and eyes with copious amounts of water. The **M291 kit** employed by the US military for individual decontamination on the battlefield uses ion-exchange resins and adsorbents to enhance physical removal of chemical agents before dilution and chemical deactivation. It consists of a carrying pouch that contains six individual pads impregnated with a resin-based powder. The **M258A1 kit** contains two types of packets for removal of liquid chemical agents, one for the G-type nerve agents (Packet 1) and the other for nerve agent VX and liquid mustard (Packet 2).
2. **Chemical deactivation of chemical agents.** Nerve agents typically contain phosphorus groups and are subject to deactivation by hydrolysis, whereas mustard and VX contain sulfur moieties subject to deactivation via oxidation reactions. Various chemical means of promoting these reactions have been used.
   a. **Oxidation.** Dilute sodium or calcium hypochlorite (0.5%) can oxidize susceptible chemicals. This alkaline solution is useful for both organophosphorus compounds and mustard agents. ***Caution:*** *Dilute hypochlorite solutions should* ***not*** *be used for ocular decontamination or for irrigation of wounds involving the peritoneal cavity, brain, or spinal cord.* A 5% hypochlorite solution is used for equipment.
   b. **Hydrolysis.** Alkaline hydrolysis of phosphorus-containing nerve agents is an effective means of decontamination of personnel exposed to these agents (VX, tabun, sarin, soman). Dilute hypochlorite is slightly alkaline. The simple use of water with soap to wash an area may also cause slow hydrolysis.

D. **Enhanced elimination.** There is no role for these procedures in managing illness caused by chemical warfare agents.

► WARFARIN AND SUPERWARFARINS

Ilene B. Anderson, PharmD

Dicumarol and other natural anticoagulants are found in sweet clover. Coumarin derivatives are used both therapeutically and as rodenticides. Warfarin (Coumadin) is used widely as a therapeutic anticoagulant but is no longer popular as a rodenticide because of rodent resistance. The most common anticoagulant rodenticides available today contain long-acting "**superwarfarins**" such as brodifacoum, diphacinone, bromadiolone, chlorophacinone, difenacoum, pindone, and valone, which have profound and prolonged anticoagulant effects. Other rodenticides are described elsewhere (see p 405).

I. Mechanism of toxicity.

A. All these compounds inhibit vitamin K 2,3-epoxide reductase and vitamin K quinone reductase, two enzymes responsible for the conversion of vitamin K to its active form, necessary cofactors in the hepatic synthesis of coagulation factors II, VII, IX, and X. Only the synthesis of new factors is affected, and the anticoagulant effect is delayed until currently circulating factors have been degraded.

B. Overdose during **pregnancy** has caused fetal hemorrhage, spontaneous miscarriage, and still birth. Major congenital malformations, fetal warfarin syndrome, and spontaneous miscarriage may occur with chronic use during pregnancy.

C. Pharmacokinetics.

1. Warfarin. The mean half-life of oral warfarin is approximately 40 hours. The onset of the anticoagulant effect may be apparent within 15–20 hours. Peak effects usually are not observed for 2–3 days because of the long half-lives of factors IX and X (24–60 hours). The duration of anticoagulant effect after a single dose of **warfarin** is normally about 5 days. (See also Table II–66, p 462.)

2. Superwarfarins. The onset of anticoagulation after superwarfarin ingestion may not be evident for up to 2 days after ingestion and may continue to produce significant anticoagulation for weeks to months after a single ingestion.

II. Toxic dose. The toxic dose is highly variable.

A. Generally, a single small ingestion of **warfarin** (eg, 10–20 mg) will not cause serious intoxication (most warfarin-based rodenticides contain 0.05% warfarin). In contrast, chronic or repeated ingestion of even small amounts (eg, 2 mg/d) can produce significant anticoagulation. Patients with hepatic dysfunction, malnutrition, or a bleeding diathesis are at greater risk.

B. Superwarfarins are estimated to be 100 times as potent as warfarin. The minimum toxic dose is unclear. Single, intentional adult poisonings have resulted in life-threatening and prolonged anticoagulation. In contrast, single, accidental pediatric ingestions are unlikely to result in clinical anticoagulation although minor elevation in coagulation studies and rare cases of anticoagulation have been reported. In contrast, repeated small superwarfarin ingestions have resulted in prolonged anticoagulation in both children and adults.

C. Multiple **drug interactions** are known to alter the anticoagulant effect of warfarin (see Table II–65 for selected examples of drug–drug interactions with warfarin).

III. Clinical presentation. Excessive anticoagulation may cause ecchymoses, subconjunctival hemorrhage, bleeding gums, or evidence of internal hemorrhage (eg, hematemesis, melena, hematochezia, menorrhagia, or hematuria). The most immediately life-threatening complications are massive GI bleeding and intracranial hemorrhage. With superwarfarin ingestions prolonged INR and risk of bleeding may persist for several weeks to months.

IV. Diagnosis is based on the history and evidence of anticoagulant effects. It is important to identify the exact product ingested to ascertain whether a superwarfarin is involved.

A. Specific levels. Brodifacoum levels are available through some commercial laboratories and may be useful in making the diagnosis and determining the end point for vitamin K therapy. Levels of less than 4–10 ng/mL are not expected to interfere with coagulation.

TABLE II–65. WARFARIN INTERACTIONS (SELECTED EXAMPLES)

Increased Anticoagulant Effect	Decreased Anticoagulant Effect
Acetaminophen	Antibiotics
Allopurinol	Azathioprine
Amiodarone	Barbiturates
Anabolic/androgenic steroids	Carbamazepine
Antibiotics/Antifungals	Cholestyramine
Anticoagulant/antiplatelet drugs	Glutethimide
Capecitabine	Green Tea
Chloral hydrate	Nafcillin
Cimetidine	Oral contraceptives
Disulfiram	Phenytoin
Ginkgo biloba	Rifampin
Mirtazapine	St. John's wort
Nonsteroidal anti-inflammatory agents	Vitamin K containing foods
Quinidine	
Salicylates	
Selective serotonin reuptake inhibitors	
Sulfonamides	

Note: This list represents *only a small sample* of drugs that may interfere with the pharmacokinetics and anticoagulant action of warfarin. For a more complete list, consult a drug information reference.

1. Anticoagulant effect is best quantified by baseline and daily repeated measurement of the **prothrombin time** (PT/INR), which may not be elevated for 1 day (warfarin) or 2 days (superwarfarins) after ingestion. A normal PT/INR at 24 hours (warfarin) or 48 hours (superwarfarin) rules out significant ingestion.
2. Blood levels of clotting factors II, VII, IX, and X will be decreased.

B. **Other useful laboratory studies** include CBC and blood type and cross-match. The partial thromboplastin time, thrombin time, fibrinogen, and platelet count may be useful in ruling out other causes of bleeding.

V. **Treatment.** The approach to treatment depends on several variables including the measured PT/INR, presence and severity of bleeding, any underlying medical condition requiring anticoagulation, the type of anticoagulant involved (warfarin or superwarfarin), and fluid status of the patient.

A. **Emergency and supportive measures.** If significant bleeding occurs, be prepared to treat shock with transfusions of whole blood and/or fresh-frozen plasma (FFP) and obtain immediate neurosurgical consultation if intracranial bleeding is suspected.

1. Take care not to precipitate hemorrhage in severely anticoagulated patients; prevent falls and other trauma. If possible, avoid the use of nasogastric or endotracheal tubes or central IV lines.
2. Hold further anticoagulant doses.
3. Avoid drugs that may enhance bleeding or decrease metabolism of the anticoagulant (see Table II–65 for selected examples. For a more complete list of drug interactions, consult a drug information reference).

B. **Specific drugs and antidotes.**

1. **Four-factor prothrombin complex concentrate** (4F-PCC, containing II, VII, IX, X, see p 534) is the preferred agent in conjunction with Vitamin K_1 for cases of life-threatening bleeding.)
2. **Fresh-frozen plasma (FFP)** is preferred over whole blood because it contains higher concentrations of clotting factors. FFP and whole blood should be used cautiously in patients with volume overload.

3. **Vitamin K_1** (phytonadione [p 633]) but ***not*** **vitamin K_3** (menadione) effectively restores the production of clotting factors. It should be given if there is evidence of significant anticoagulation. ***Note:*** If vitamin K_1 is given prophylactically after an acute ingestion, the 48-hour PT/INR cannot be used to determine the severity of the overdose, and it is suggested that the patient be monitored for a minimum of 5 days after the last vitamin K_1 dose. ***Caution:*** Vitamin K–mediated reversal of anticoagulation may be dangerous for patients who require constant anticoagulation (eg, those with prosthetic heart valves). However, when vitamin K is indicated in these patients, heparin may be used for maintenance anticoagulation.
   a. **Oral vitamin K_1** (p 633). Doses of up to 800 mg daily have been required to maintain a satisfactory INR. Vitamin K can also be administered subcutaneously or IV, but the IV route is not recommended because of the risk for anaphylaxis, and the subcutaneous route is considered only when the oral route is not feasible.
   b. Because vitamin K will not begin to restore clotting factors for 6 or more hours (peak effect, 24 hours), patients with active hemorrhage may require immediate replacement of active clotting factors, such **as 4F-PCC, fresh-frozen plasma, or fresh whole blood**.
   c. **Prolonged dosing** of vitamin K may be required for several weeks to months in patients who have ingested a long-acting superwarfarin product. Blood levels of clotting factors (II, VII, IX, and X) may be useful in evaluating when vitamin K may be safely tapered following superwarfarin poisonings.
   d. **Three Factor Prothrombin Complex Concentrate** ([3F-PCC] II, IX, X) in conjunction with factor VIIa and vitamin K_1 (see page 534).
   e. **Recombinant activated factor VIIa** (Novoseven) may also be used as an alternative or adjunct to 3F-PCC, FFP and vitamin K_1 (see page 534).

C. **Decontamination** (p 50). Administer activated charcoal orally if conditions are appropriate (see Table I–38, p 54). Gastric lavage is not necessary after small to moderate ingestions if activated charcoal can be given promptly and should be avoided in a person with prior anticoagulation.

D. **Enhanced elimination.** There is no role for enhanced elimination procedures.

TABLE II–66. PHARMACOKINETIC DATA[a] (Table compiled by Ilene B. Anderson, PharmD, with the assistance of Gilberto Araya-Rodríguez.)

Drug	Onset (h)	Peak (h)	Half-life (h)	Active Metabolite	Half-life of Active Metabolite (h)	Vd (L/kg)	Protein Binding (%)	Comments
Abacavir		Rapid	1.54 ± 0.63			0.86 ± 0.15	50	Metabolism by alcohol dehydrogenase
Acarbose						0.32	Negligible	
Acebutolol	1–3	2–3	3–6	Yes	8–13	3	10–26	
Acetaminophen	0.5	0.5–2	1–3			0.8–1	10–30	
Acetaminophen ER		0.5–3						
Acetazolamide	1–1.5	1–4	4–8			0.2	70–90	90% renal excretion. Half-life 26 h in end-stage renal failure
Acetazolamide ER	2	3–6						
Acetohexamide	2	4	1.3	Yes			65–90	
Acrivastine	Rapid	1–2	1.5–3.5	Yes			50	
Acyclovir		1.5–2	2.5–3.3			0.66–0.8	9–33	
Adefovir		1.75	5.83–9.13			0.317–0.467	<4	
Alatrofloxacin			9.4–12.7	Yes		1.2–1.4	76	
Albiglutide		3–5 days	5 days			11 liters		
Albuterol	0.25–0.5	1–4	5–7.2			2	10	
Albuterol ER		6	9.3					
Alfuzosin	1.5	3–4	3–10			3.2	82–90	
Alfuzosin ER		8	10					
Alogliptin		1–3	21			417 liters	20	
Alprazolam	Intermediate	1–2	6.3–26.9			0.9–1.2	80	
Alprazolam SR		5–11						

Alprenolol	0.5	2–4	2–3	Yes	1	3–6	80	
Amantadine	1–4	1–4	7–37			4–8	60–70	
Amikacin		1	2–3			0.25–0.34	0–11	
Amiloride	2	3–10	21–144			5	23	
Amiodarone			50 days	Yes	61 days	1.3–66	95	
Amitriptyline	1–2	4	9–25	Yes	18–35	6–10	95	Metabolized to nortriptyline
Amlodipine		6–9	30–50			21	95	
Amobarbital	<1	2	10–40			0.9–1.4	59	
Amoxapine		1–2	8–30	Yes	30	0.9–1.2	90	
Amoxicillin		1–2	1.3			0.41	20	
Amoxicillin ER		3.1						
Amphetamine	0.5–1	1–3	7–14	Yes		3.5–6	20	Route-dependent kinetics
Amphetamine ER		7						
Ampicillin		1	1.5			0.28	18	
Amprenavir		1–2	7.1–10.6			430 liters	90	
Anisotropine		5–6						
Apixaban	Rapid	1–3	8–15			21 liters	87	CYP3A4 metabolism; 25–27% renal excretion
Aprobarbital	<1	12	14–34				20–55	
Aripiprazole		3–5	75–146	Yes	94	4.9	99	

[a]Data provided are based on therapeutic dosing, not overdose. Variability in pharmacokinetics, even in therapeutic doses, occur for a variety of reasons including age, phenotype, renal and hepatic function, gastrointestinal absorption, drug–drug interaction, urine pH, etc. In general, after overdose of immediate-release and especially ER/SR formulations, the peak effect is delayed and the half-life and duration of effect are prolonged. Changes may occur in the volume of distribution and the percentage protein-bound. Kinetics may vary depending on the formulation.
h, hours; min, minutes; L, liters; kg, kilogram; CR, controlled-release formulation; DR, delayed-release formulation; EC, enteric-coated formulation; ER, XR, extended-release formulation; IM, intramuscular; IV, intravenous; MR, modified-release formulation; PR, prolonged-release formulation; SR, sustained-release formulation; SL, sublingual; SQ, subcutaneous.
The apparent volume of distribution (Vd) is reported in liters per kilogram (L/kg) unless the entry specifically states liters.

(continued)

TABLE II–66. PHARMACOKINETIC DATA[a] (CONTINUED)

Drug	Onset (h)	Peak (h)	Half-life (h)	Active Metabolite	Half-life of Active Metabolite (h)	Vd (L/kg)	Protein Binding (%)	Comments
Articaine			1–2					
Asenapine (SL)		0.5–1.5	24			20–25	95	Only available sublingual (SL). Bioavailability SL 35%; Oral <2%.
Aspirin	0.4	1–2	2–4.5	Yes	2–3	0.1–0.3	50–80	Dose-dependent kinetics
Aspirin SR		1–12						
Astemizole		1–4	20–24	Yes	10–12 days	250	97	
Atazanavir		2.5	6.5–7.9				86	Fecal elimination primarily
Atenolol	2–3	2–4	4–10			50–75 liters	5	
Atomoxetine		1–2	3–4			250 liters	98	
Atropine	Rapid	Rapid	2–4			2	5–23	
Azatidine		3–4	9					
Azelastine		2–3	22	Yes	54	14.5	88	
Azide	1 min							Duration 0.25 h
Azithromycin	2–3	2.4–4	68		70	23–31	7–50	
Azithromycin ER		5			59			
Bacitracin		1–2 IM						Renal elimination
Baclofen	0.5–1	2–3	2.5–4			1–2.5	30–36	
Bedaquiline		5	5.5 months	Yes	5.5 months	164 liters	>99.9	Fecal elimination primarily
Benazepril		2–6	0.6	Yes	22	0.7	97	Vd for active metabolite
Bendroflumethiazide	2	4	3–4					
Benzphetamine		3–4	6–12	Yes	4–14			Metabolized to amphetamine/ methamphetamine

Benzthiazide	2	4–6						
Benztropine	1–2	4–6	4–6.5					
Bepridil	2–3		24	Yes		8	99	
Betaxolol	2–3	2–6	12–22			5–13	55	
Biperiden		1.5	18–24			24		
Bisoprolol		3	8–12			3	30	
Boceprevir		2	3.4			772 liters	75	Extensive metabolism to inactive metabolites
Bretylium	<0.1	1–2	5–14			5.9	5	
Bromazepam		1–4	8–30	Yes		0.9		
Bromfenac	0.5	1–3	1–2			0.15	99	
Bromocriptine		1.4	6–50			1–3	90–96	
Brompheniramine	0.5	2–5	25			12		
Buclizine		3	15					
Bumetanide	0.5–1	1–2	2			13–25	95	
Bupivacaine	<0.1	0.5–1	2–5			0.4–1	82–96	
Buprenorphine (SL)	1.7	1.6–2.5	31–35	Yes	34	97–187 liters	96	Long duration (24–48 h) with risk of delayed apnea.
Buprenorphine Transdermal Patch	11–21	60–80	22–36	Yes	34	430 liters	96	
Bupropion		2	16	Yes	20–24	20–47	84	

[a]Data provided are based on therapeutic dosing, not overdose. Variability in pharmacokinetics, even in therapeutic doses, occur for a variety of reasons including age, phenotype, renal and hepatic function, gastrointestinal absorption, drug–drug interaction, urine pH, etc. In general, after overdose of immediate-release and especially ER/SR formulations, the peak effect is delayed and the half-life and duration of effect are prolonged. Changes may occur in the volume of distribution and the percentage protein-bound. Kinetics may vary depending on the formulation.
h, hours; min, minutes; L, liters; kg, kilogram; CR, controlled-release formulation; DR, delayed-release formulation; EC, enteric-coated formulation; ER, XR, extended-release formulation; IM, intramuscular; IV, intravenous; MR, modified-release formulation; PR, prolonged-release formulation; SR, sustained-release formulation; SL, sublingual; SQ, subcutaneous.
The apparent volume of distribution (Vd) is reported in liters per kilogram (L/kg) unless the entry specifically states liters.

(*continued*)

TABLE II–66. PHARMACOKINETIC DATA[a] (CONTINUED)

Drug	Onset (h)	Peak (h)	Half-life (h)	Active Metabolite	Half-life of Active Metabolite (h)	Vd (L/kg)	Protein Binding (%)	Comments
Bupropion PR		2.5–3			20–37			
Buspirone		0.67–1.5	2–4	Yes	2	5.3	95	
Butabarbital	<1	0.5–1.5	35–50				26	
Butalbital		1–2	35			0.8	26	
Butanediol (BD)				Yes				Metabolized to GHB
Butorphanol	<0.2	0.5–1.0	5–6			7–8	83	
Caffeine	0.25–0.75	0.5–2	3–10	Yes	2–16	0.7–0.8	36	Half-life prolonged in infants
Canagliflozin		1–2	10.6–13.1			119 liters	99	
Candesartan	2–4	3–4	9			0.13	>99	
Captopril	0.5	0.5–1.5	1.9			0.7	25–30	
Carbamazepine		6–24	5–55	Yes	5–10	1.4–3	75–78	
Carbamazepine ER, XR		3–24	35–40					
Carbenicillin		1	1.0–1.5			0.18	50	
Carbinoxamine			10–20			0.25	0	
Carisoprodol	0.5	1–4	1.5–8	Yes	10–11			Metabolized to meprobamate
Carprofen		1–3	4–10				99	
Carteolol	1	3–6	6	Yes	8–12		25–30	
Carvedilol	1–1.5	4–7	6–10	Yes		1.5–2.0	98–99	
Carvedilol ER		5	7–10			115 liters		
Cefaclor		0.75–1	0.6–0.9			0.36	60–85	
Cefamandole		0.2 IV, 0.5–2 IM	0.5 IV, 1 IM			0.145	56–78	

Cefazolin			1.5–2			0.14	60–80	
Cefditoren pivoxil		1.5–3	1.2–2				90	
Cefepime (IV)		1.4–1.6	2			18	20	
Cefmetazole			1.2				65	
Cefoperazone			1.5–2.5			0.15	82–93	
Cefotetan		<0.5 IV, 1–3 IM	3–4.6			0.14	88–90	
Ceftriaxone		0.5	4.3–4.6			5.78–13.5	85–95	Extensive bile excretion
Celecoxib		2–3	11			4–8	97	
Cephaloridine		0.5	0.8					
Cephalothin		0.5		Yes		0.24	65–79	70% renally eliminated unchanged
Cetirizine	Rapid	1	8			0.5	98	
Chloral hydrate	0.5–1	0.25–0.5	0.07	Yes	8–11	0.6–1.6	35–41	Vd for trichloroethanol, the active metabolite
Chloramphenicol		1	4			0.57–1.55	60	
Chlordiazepoxide	Intermediate	0.5–4	5–30	Yes	18–96	0.3	96	
Chloroprocaine			1.5–6 min					
Chloroquine		2	2 months	Yes	35–67 days	150–250	55	
Chlorothiazide	2	4	1–2			0.2	95	
Chlorphenesin		2	3.5			1.27		
Chlorpheniramine	0.5–2	2–6	10–43			4–12	70	
Chlorpromazine	0.5–1	2–4	8–30	Yes	4–12	12–30	90–99	

[a]Data provided are based on therapeutic dosing, not overdose. Variability in pharmacokinetics, even in therapeutic doses, occur for a variety of reasons including age, phenotype, renal and hepatic function, gastrointestinal absorption, drug–drug interaction, urine pH, etc. In general, after overdose of immediate-release and especially ER/SR formulations, the peak effect is delayed and the half-life and duration of effect are prolonged. Changes may occur in the volume of distribution and the percentage protein-bound. Kinetics may vary depending on the formulation.
h, hours; min, minutes; L, liters; kg, kilogram; CR, controlled-release formulation; DR, delayed-release formulation; EC, enteric-coated formulation; ER, XR, extended-release formulation; IM, intramuscular; IV, intravenous; MR, modified-release formulation; PR, prolonged-release formulation; SR, sustained-release formulation; SL, sublingual; SQ, subcutaneous.
The apparent volume of distribution (Vd) is reported in liters per kilogram (L/kg) unless the entry specifically states liters.

(*continued*)

TABLE II–66. PHARMACOKINETIC DATA[a] (CONTINUED)

Drug	Onset (h)	Peak (h)	Half-life (h)	Active Metabolite	Half-life of Active Metabolite (h)	Vd (L/kg)	Protein Binding (%)	Comments
Chlorpropamide	1	3–6	25–48			0.13–0.23	60–90	
Chlorprothixene	1.5–2	2.5–3	8–12	Yes	20–40	10–25		
Chlorthalidone	2–3	2–6	40–65			3.9	75	
Chlorzoxazone	1	1–2	1					
Cidofovir			2.5	Yes	17	0.41–0.54	<6	
Cinnarizine		2–4	3–6					
Ciprofloxacin		1–2	4			2	20–40	
Ciprofloxacin XR		1–4	5–32					
Citalopram		4	35	Yes		12	80	CYP3A4 and CYP2C19 metabolism; CYP2C19 poor metabolizers have higher levels
Clarithromycin		2–4	3–4	Yes	5–9	2.7–4.4	42–80	
Clarithromycin MR			5.3	Yes	7.7		41–70	Saturable protein binding. Prolonged half-life at higher doses.
Clemastine	Rapid	3–5	21			13		
Clenbuterol	0.5	2–3	25–39				89–98	
Clidinium	1		2–20					
Clindamycin		0.75	2.4–3	Yes		1	>90	
Clobazam		0.5–4	10–50	Yes	30–82	1	80–90	
Clomipramine		3–4	20–40	Yes	54–77	10–20	97	
Clonazepam	Intermediate	1–4	18–50			3.2	85	
Clonidine	0.5–1	2–4	5–13			3–5.5	20–40	

Clorazepate	Fast	1–2	2.3	Yes	40–120	0.2–1.3	97–98	
Clozapine		2	8–13			0.5–3	97	
Cocaine		0.5	1–2.5	Yes	4–5	2–2.7	10	Route-dependent kinetics
Codeine	0.5–1	0.5–1.0	2–4	Yes	2–4	3.5	20	
Codeine SR		1.1–2.3	2.6					
Colchicine		0.5–1	4.4–31			2	30–50	Symptoms delayed 2–12 h in overdose
Cyclizine	0.5	2	7–24	Yes	20			
Cyclobenzaprine	1	3–4	24–72				93	
Cyclobenzaprine ER		6	32–33					
Cyproheptadine	2–3	6–9	16					
Dabigatran etexilate	Rapid	1–3	12–17			50–70 liters	35	Prodrug converted to dabigatran; 80% renal elimination; bioavailability <7% but nearly doubles if pellets taken without the capsule shell.
Dalbavancin (IV)			346				93	
Dalteparin (SQ)	<2	2–4	3–5			0.4–0.6	Low	
Dapagliflozin		2	12.9			118 liters	91	
Dapsone	2–4	4–8	30 (10–50)	Yes		1.5	70–90	
Daptomycin			8–9			0.092–0.12	90–95	
Dasabuvir		4–5	5.5–6			396 liters	99.5	Extensive metabolism to inactive metabolites

[a]Data provided are based on therapeutic dosing, not overdose. Variability in pharmacokinetics, even in therapeutic doses, occur for a variety of reasons including age, phenotype, renal and hepatic function, gastrointestinal absorption, drug–drug interaction, urine pH, etc. In general, after overdose of immediate-release and especially ER/SR formulations, the peak effect is delayed and the half-life and duration of effect are prolonged. Changes may occur in the volume of distribution and the percentage protein-bound. Kinetics may vary depending on the formulation.
h, hours; min, minutes; L, liters; kg, kilogram; CR, controlled-release formulation; DR, delayed-release formulation; EC, enteric-coated formulation; ER, XR, extended-release formulation; IM, intramuscular; IV, intravenous; MR, modified-release formulation; PR, prolonged-release formulation; SR, sustained-release formulation; SL, sublingual; SQ, subcutaneous.
The apparent volume of distribution (Vd) is reported in liters per kilogram (L/kg) unless the entry specifically states liters.

(*continued*)

TABLE II–66. PHARMACOKINETIC DATA[a] (CONTINUED)

Drug	Onset (h)	Peak (h)	Half-life (h)	Active Metabolite	Half-life of Active Metabolite (h)	Vd (L/kg)	Protein Binding (%)	Comments
Delavirdine		1	2–11			2.7	98	
Darifenacin		7	3–4			163–276 liters	98	
Darifenacin ER		7	14–16			163 liters	98	
Darunavir		2.5–4	15				95	Metabolized by CYP3A
Demeclocycline			10–17			1–2	40–80	
Desipramine		3–6	12–24	Yes	22	22–60	80	
Desloratadine	1	3	27	Yes	25–30	10–30	82	
Desvenlafaxine		7.5	10–11			3.4	30	
Dexbrompheniramine		5	22					
Dexchlorpheniramine	0.5–1	2	20–24				72	Half-life in children 10–12h
Dexfenfluramine	1.5–8	1.5–8.0	17–20	Yes	32	12	36	
Dextroamphetamine	1–1.5	1–3	10–12			6	15–34	Half-life dependent on urinary pH
Dextroamphetamine SR		3–8	7–24					Half-life dependent on urinary pH
Dextromethorphan	<0.5	2–2.5	3–38	Yes	3.4–5.6	5–6	55	Half-life phenotype-dependent
Dextromethorphan CR		7		Yes				
Diazepam	Very fast	0.5–2	20–80	Yes	40–120	1.1	98	
Diazoxide	1	3–5	24				90	
Dichlorphenamide	1	2–4						
Diclofenac	0.2	1–3	2	Yes	1–3	0.1–0.5	99	
Diclofenac SR		4	1–2	Yes	1–3		99.7	
Dicyclomine	1–2	1.5	2–10			3.7		

Didanosine		0.25–1.5	1.5±0.4			0.86–1.3	<5	Intracellular half-life = 8–40h
Didanosine EC, DR		2	1.5±0.4					
Diethylpropion		2	2.5–6	Yes	6			
Diflunisal	1	2–3	8–12			0.1	99	
Digitoxin	2–4	10	5–8 days	Yes	30–50	0.5	95	
Digoxin	1–2	6–12	30–50	Yes		5–10	25	
Dihydroergotamine	0.5	0.5–3	2–4	Yes		15	90	Vasospasm may last for weeks
Diltiazem	1	2–4	4–6	Yes	11	5.3	77–93	
Diltiazem ER		10–14	5–8				80–85	
Dimenhydrinate	<0.5							
Dimethindene	0.5	2	5.9–6.3			1.3–4.3	90	
Dimethindene SR			11					
Diphenhydramine	<0.5	2–4	2.4–9.3			4–6.9	80–85	
Diphenoxylate	1	2–4	2.5	Yes	3–14	3.8		
Dirithromycin		4	44 (16–55)			504–1,041 liters	15–30	
Disopyramide	0.5–3		4–10			0.6–1.3	35–95	
Disopyramide ER		5	12				50–65	
Disulfiram	3–12	8–12	7–8	Yes	9–22		96	
Dofetilide		2–3	10	?		3	60–70	

[a]Data provided are based on therapeutic dosing, not overdose. Variability in pharmacokinetics, even in therapeutic doses, occur for a variety of reasons including age, phenotype, renal and hepatic function, gastrointestinal absorption, drug–drug interaction, urine pH, etc. In general, after overdose of immediate-release and especially ER/SR formulations, the peak effect is delayed and the half-life and duration of effect are prolonged. Changes may occur in the volume of distribution and the percentage protein-bound. Kinetics may vary depending on the formulation.

h, hours; min, minutes; L, liters; kg, kilogram; CR, controlled-release formulation; DR, delayed-release formulation; EC, enteric-coated formulation; ER, XR, extended-release formulation; IM, intramuscular; IV, intravenous; MR, modified-release formulation; PR, prolonged-release formulation; SR, sustained-release formulation; SL, sublingual; SQ, subcutaneous.

The apparent volume of distribution (Vd) is reported in liters per kilogram (L/kg) unless the entry specifically states liters.

(*continued*)

TABLE II–66. PHARMACOKINETIC DATA[a] (CONTINUED)

Drug	Onset (h)	Peak (h)	Half-life (h)	Active Metabolite	Half-life of Active Metabolite (h)	Vd (L/kg)	Protein Binding (%)	Comments
Dolutegravir		2–3	14			17.4	98.9	Extensive metabolism to inactive metabolites
Doripenem		1	1			16.8	8.1	
Doxazosin	4–8	2–5	8–22			1–3.4	98–99	
Doxazosin PR		8–9	22					
Doxepin		2	8–15	Yes	28–52	9–33	80	
Doxycycline		2	15–24			0.75	82–93	
Doxycycline MR		3	21					
Doxylamine	0.5	2–3	10			2.7		
Dronabinol	0.5–1	2–4	20–30	Yes	4–36	10	90–99	Half-life longer in chronic users
Dronedarone		3–6	13–19	Yes		20	>98	
Droperidol (IV, IM)	Rapid	0.5 IV, 0.5–1 IM	2			0.6–2	85–90	
Duloxetine		4–6	8–17			17–26	90	
Duloxetine DR		6	12.1			23.4	96	Half-life longer with hepatic impairment
Edoxaban	Rapid	1–3	9–11				50	35–50% renal elimination
Efavirenz		3–5	40–76			4–8	99	
Elvitegravir		4	13				98–99	Extensive metabolism to inactive metabolites
Emtricitabine	Rapid	1–2	10				<4	Renal elimination primarily
Enalapril	1	1	1.3	Yes	35–38	1–2.4	50–60	
Encainide		1	2–11	Yes	11–24	2.7–4.3	70–85	Kinetics dependent on phenotype

Enfuvirtide		4	3.2–4.4		5.5 ± 1.1	92	
Enoxaparin (SQ)	<0.5	3–5	3–6		4.3–6 liters	Low	
Entecavir		0.5–1.5	128–149		Extensive	13	Vd > total body water
Ephedrine	0.25–1	2.4	3–6		2.6–3.1		Half-life prolonged in alkaline urine
Eprosartan		1–2	5–9		308 liters	98	
Ergonovine	<1	2–3					In overdose, vasospasm may last for weeks
Ergotamine		1–3	3–12		1.8		In overdose, vasospasm may last for weeks
Ertapenem		2.3 (IM)	4		0.12–0.16	85–95	Half-life 2.5 h in children 3 months–12 years old
Erythromycin		1	1.4		0.6–1.4	75–90	
Escitalopram		3–6	22–32		1,330 liters	56	
Esmolol	<1 min IV	5 min IV	9 min IV		3.4	55	
Estazolam	Fast	2	8–28			93	
Eszopiclone		1.6	6		1.1–1.7	52–59	
Etravirine		2.5–4	20–60			99.9	
Ethacrynic acid	0.5	2	2–4	Yes			
Ethambutol			4				
Ethchlorvynol	0.5	1–2	10–20		2–4	35–50	

[a]Data provided are based on therapeutic dosing, not overdose. Variability in pharmacokinetics, even in therapeutic doses, occur for a variety of reasons including age, phenotype, renal and hepatic function, gastrointestinal absorption, drug–drug interaction, urine pH, etc. In general, after overdose of immediate-release and especially ER/SR formulations, the peak effect is delayed and the half-life and duration of effect are prolonged. Changes may occur in the volume of distribution and the percentage protein-bound. Kinetics may vary depending on the formulation.
h, hours; min, minutes; L, liters; kg, kilogram; CR, controlled-release formulation; DR, delayed-release formulation; EC, enteric-coated formulation; ER, XR, extended-release formulation; IM, intramuscular; IV, intravenous; MR, modified-release formulation; PR, prolonged-release formulation; SR, sustained-release formulation; SL, sublingual; SQ, subcutaneous.
The apparent volume of distribution (Vd) is reported in liters per kilogram (L/kg) unless the entry specifically states liters.

(*continued*)

TABLE II–66. PHARMACOKINETIC DATA[a] (CONTINUED)

Drug	Onset (h)	Peak (h)	Half-life (h)	Active Metabolite	Half-life of Active Metabolite (h)	Vd (L/kg)	Protein Binding (%)	Comments
Ethionamide		1	1.7–2.2			74–113 liters	30	
Etidocaine	<0.1	0.25–0.5	1.5			1.9	96	
Etodolac	0.5	1–2	7			0.36	99	
Etodolac ER or PR		6–8	8.4			0.57	≥99	
Exenatide (Byetta)		2	2.4			0.064		Kinetics are for subcutaneous route. Duration 6–8 h
Exenatide ER (Bydureon)		Biphasic: 2 weeks, then 6–7 weeks						Duration 10 weeks
Ezogabine		0.5–2	7–11	Yes	7–11	2–3	80	
Famciclovir		0.5–0.9	2–2.3	Yes	2–2.3	0.91–1.25	<20	Prodrug metabolized to penciclovir
Famotidine	1.5	1–3.5	2.6–4			0.82–2	10–28	
Felbamate			20–23			0.67–0.83	23	
Felodipine	2–5	2–4	11–16			9.7	99	
Felodipine PR		3–5	25			10	99	
Fenfluramine	1–2	2–4	10–30	Yes		12–16	12–16	
Fenoldopam	0.25	0.5–2	0.16			0.6		
Fenoprofen	0.5	2	3				99	
Fentanyl	<0.25	<0.5	1–5			4	80	
Fesoterodine		5		Yes	4–7	169 liters	50	Prodrug rapidly metabolized; peak reflects metabolite
Fexofenadine	Rapid	2–3	14			12	60–70	

Fidaxomicin		1–5	12	Yes	8.2–14.2			
Finasteride		1–2	3–13	Yes		0.6–1.4	90	
Flavoxate	1	1.5		Yes				
Flecainide		3	14–15			9	40–68	
Flunarizine		2–4	18–23 days			43.2	>90	
Flunitrazepam	0.33	<4	9–30			3.3–5.5	78	
Fluoride	<1.0	0.5–1.0	2–9			0.5–0.7		
Fluoxetine		6–8	1–3 days	Yes	4–16 days	1,000–7,200 liters	94.5	Enteric coating delays absorption 1–2 h; Half-life dependent on phenotype
Fluphenazine	<1	1–3	12–19	Yes		1–21	99	
Flurazepam	<0.75	0.5–1	2–3	Yes	47–100	3.4	97	
Fluvoxamine		5	15			25	77	
Fluvoxamine CR			16.3			25	80	Inactive or weakly active metabolites
Fosamprenavir		Rapid		Yes (amprenavir)	7.1–10.6	4.7–8.6	90	Rapidly hydrolyzed in gut to amprenavir
Foscarnet			3.3–4			0.41–0.52	14–17	Active tubular secretion
Fosfomycin		1.5–3	12			1.5–2.4	< 3	Half-life increases in renal insufficiency
Fosinopril	1	3–4	<1	Yes	11.5–12	10 liters	89–99	

[a]Data provided are based on therapeutic dosing, not overdose. Variability in pharmacokinetics, even in therapeutic doses, occur for a variety of reasons including age, phenotype, renal and hepatic function, gastrointestinal absorption, drug–drug interaction, urine pH, etc. In general, after overdose of immediate-release and especially ER/SR formulations, the peak effect is delayed and the half-life and duration of effect are prolonged. Changes may occur in the volume of distribution and the percentage protein-bound. Kinetics may vary depending on the formulation.
h, hours; min, minutes; L, liters; kg, kilogram; CR, controlled-release formulation; DR, delayed-release formulation; EC, enteric-coated formulation; ER, XR, extended-release formulation; IM, intramuscular; IV, intravenous; MR, modified-release formulation; PR, prolonged-release formulation; SR, sustained-release formulation; SL, sublingual; SQ, subcutaneous.
The apparent volume of distribution (Vd) is reported in liters per kilogram (L/kg) unless the entry specifically states liters.

(*continued*)

TABLE II–66. PHARMACOKINETIC DATA[a] (CONTINUED)

Drug	Onset (h)	Peak (h)	Half-life (h)	Active Metabolite	Half-life of Active Metabolite (h)	Vd (L/kg)	Protein Binding (%)	Comments
Fosphenytoin				Yes	7–60	4.3–10.8	>95	Converted to phenytoin within 0.25 h
Furosemide	0.5	1–2	1			0.11	99	
Gabapentin		1–3	5–7			0.8	<3	
Gamma-butyro-lactone (GBL)	0.33 h			Yes	<1			Metabolized to GHB
Gamma-hydroxy-butyrate (GHB)	0.25	<1	<1			0.4	0	Zero-order kinetics
Ganciclovir		1.8 (3 with food)	4 oral 3.5 IV			0.57–0.84	1–2	
Gatifloxacin		1–2	7–14			1.5–2.0	20	>80% excreted unchanged
Gemifloxacin		0.5–2	7			1.7–12.1	60–70	
Gentamicin		0.5	2			0.25	<10	
Glimepiride	2–3	2.9	5–9	Yes	3	0.1–0.13	>99	
Glipizide	0.5	1–3	2–4			0.07–0.16	98–99	Duration <24 h. Prolonged hypoglycemia in overdose
Glipizide ER	2–3	6–12	2–5			0.11	97–99	Duration 45 h. Prolonged hypoglycemia in overdose
Glutethimide	0.5	1–6	10–12			2.7	35–59	
Glyburide [micronized form]	0.5	4 [2–3]	5–10	Yes		0.3	99	Prolonged hypoglycemia in overdose
Glycopyrrolate		0.5–5	0.5–2			0.6		
Grepafloxacin		2–5	11.5–19.9			5.07–8.11	50	
Guanabenz	1	2–5	6–14			7.4–13.4	90	

Guanfacine	2	1–4	12–24			6.3	72	
Guanfacine ER		4–8	14–22					
Haloperidol	1	2–6	13–35	Yes		18–30	>90	
Heparin (IV;SC), unfractionated	Immediate IV 0.33–1 SC	2 min IV 4h SC	1–2.5			0.6	high	
Heroin		0.2	1–2	Yes	2–4	25	40	Rapidly hydrolyzed to morphine
Hydralazine	<0.5	0.5–1	3–5	Yes	2	1.6	88–90	
Hydrazoic acid	Rapid							Duration 0.25 h
Hydrochlorothiazide	2	4	2.5			0.83	64	
Hydrocodone		1–2	3–4	Yes	1.5–4	3–5	6–8	
Hydroflumethiazide	2	4	2–17			3.49		
Hydromorphone	0.5	1	1–4			1.6–4.2	<30	
Hydromorphone ER	6	12–16	8–15					
Hydroxychloroquine			40 days	Yes		580–815	45	
Hydroxyzine	<0.5	2–4	20–25	Yes	8	19		
Hyoscyamine	0.5	0.5–1	3–5				50	
Hyoscyamine SR	0.3–0.5	2.5	5–9					
Ibuprofen	0.5	1–2	2–4			0.12–0.2	90–99	
Ibutilide			2–12	Yes		11	40	
Iloperidone		2–4	10–30	Yes		1,340–2,800 liters	95	

[a]Data provided are based on therapeutic dosing, not overdose. Variability in pharmacokinetics, even in therapeutic doses, occur for a variety of reasons including age, phenotype, renal and hepatic function, gastrointestinal absorption, drug–drug interaction, urine pH, etc. In general, after overdose of immediate-release and especially ER/SR formulations, the peak effect is delayed and the half-life and duration of effect are prolonged. Changes may occur in the volume of distribution and the percentage protein-bound. Kinetics may vary depending on the formulation.
h, hours; min, minutes; L, liters; kg, kilogram; CR, controlled-release formulation; DR, delayed-release formulation; EC, enteric-coated formulation; ER, XR, extended-release formulation; IM, intramuscular; IV, intravenous; MR, modified-release formulation; PR, prolonged-release formulation; SR, sustained-release formulation; SL, sublingual; SQ, subcutaneous.
The apparent volume of distribution (Vd) is reported in liters per kilogram (L/kg) unless the entry specifically states liters.

(continued)

TABLE II–66. PHARMACOKINETIC DATA[a] (CONTINUED)

Drug	Onset (h)	Peak (h)	Half-life (h)	Active Metabolite	Half-life of Active Metabolite (h)	Vd (L/kg)	Protein Binding (%)	Comments
Imipenem/cilastatin		0.33	1/1				20/40	Kinetics are listed for both agents
Imipramine		1–2	11–25	Yes	12–24	10–20	70–90	Metabolized to desipramine
Indapamide	1–2	2–3	14–18			0.3–0.4	75	
Indinavir		0.8	1.8			2.5–3.1	60	
Indomethacin	0.5	1–2	3–11			0.3–0.9	99	
Indomethacin SR		6.2	3–11				>90	
Indoramin		1–2	1–2			7.4	72–92	
Insulin, aspart (Novolog)	0.25	1–3						Duration 3–5 h
Insulin, detemir (Levemir)	1	6–8						Duration 20 h
Insulin, glargine (Lantus)	1.5	Sustained effect						Duration 22–24 h
Insulin, glulisine (Apidra)	0.3	0.6–1						Duration 5 h
Insulin, isophane (NPH)	1–2	8–12						Duration 18–24 h
Insulin, lispro (Humalog)	0.25	0.5–1.5						Duration 6–8 h
Insulin, protamine zinc (PZI)	4–8	14–20						Duration 36 h
Insulin, rapid zinc (semilente)	0.5	4–7						Duration 12–16 h
Insulin, extended zinc (ultralente)	4–8	16–18						Duration 36 h
Insulin, zinc (lente)	1–2	8–12						Duration 18–24 h
Insulin, regular	0.5–1	2–3						Duration 8–12 h

Insulin, regular Inhaled (Afrezza)		0.9						Duration 3 h
Ipratropium		1.5–3	2–3.8					
Irbesartan	2	1.5–2	11–15			0.6–1.5	90	
Isoniazid	<1	1–2	0.5–4			0.6–0.7	0–10	
Isopropanol	<1	<1	2.5–8	Yes	17–27	0.6	<10	
Isosorbide dinitrate	<0.2	<0.5–1	1–4	Yes	4–5	6.3–8.9	28	
Isosorbide dinitrate PR		5–11		Yes	5.4			
Isosorbide mononitrate	<1	0.5–2	6–7			0.7	<4	
Isosorbide mononitrate PR		3.1–4.5	6.5			0.6		
Isradipine	1–2	2–3	8			3	95–97	
Isradipine CR,ER	2	7–18						
Kanamycin		1	2–3			0.19	0–3	
Ketamine	<1 min (IV)		2–4	Yes		2–4	27	Duration 0.5–2 h
Ketoprofen		1–2	2–4			0.1	99	High fat meal delays peak. Prolonged half-life in elderly.
Ketoprofen ER		6–8	8					High fat meal delays peak. Prolonged half-life in elderly.
Ketorolac		1	4–6			0.15–0.3	99	
Labetalol	1–2	2–4	6–8			5–9	50	

[a]Data provided are based on therapeutic dosing, not overdose. Variability in pharmacokinetics, even in therapeutic doses, occur for a variety of reasons including age, phenotype, renal and hepatic function, gastrointestinal absorption, drug–drug interaction, urine pH, etc. In general, after overdose of immediate-release and especially ER/SR formulations, the peak effect is delayed and the half-life and duration of effect are prolonged. Changes may occur in the volume of distribution and the percentage protein-bound. Kinetics may vary depending on the formulation.

h, hours; min, minutes; L, liters; kg, kilogram; CR, controlled-release formulation; DR, delayed-release formulation; EC, enteric-coated formulation; ER, XR, extended-release formulation; IM, intramuscular; IV, intravenous; MR, modified-release formulation; PR, prolonged-release formulation; SR, sustained-release formulation; SL, sublingual; SQ, subcutaneous.

The apparent volume of distribution (Vd) is reported in liters per kilogram (L/kg) unless the entry specifically states liters.

(*continued*)

TABLE II–66. PHARMACOKINETIC DATA[a] (CONTINUED)

Drug	Onset (h)	Peak (h)	Half-life (h)	Active Metabolite	Half-life of Active Metabolite (h)	Vd (L/kg)	Protein Binding (%)	Comments
Lacosamide			13					
Lamivudine			5–7			0.9–1.7	<36	70% renal elimination
Lamotrigine		1.4–4.8	22–36			0.9–1.3	55	Peak, half-life vary with age and concomitant anticonvulsant medications.
Lamotrigine ER,XR		4–11						Peak, half-life vary with age and concomitant anticonvulsant medications.
Ledipasvir		4–4.5	47				>99.8	
Levetiracetam	1	1	6–8			0.7	<10	Half-life prolonged in elderly and renal impairment
Levetiracetam ER,XR			7					Half-life prolonged in elderly and renal impairment
Levobunolol		3	5–6	Yes	7	5.5		
Levobupivacaine			1–3					
Levocetirizine		0.9	8–9			0.4	91–92	
Levofloxacin		1–2	6–8			74–112 liters	24–38	
Levomilnacipran ER		6–8	12			387–473 liters	22	
Levothyroxine (T_4)	48–120	10–20 days	6–7 days	Yes	2 days	8.7–9.7 liters	99	
L–Hyoscyamine	0.5	0.5–1	3–12				50	
Lidocaine			1.2			0.8–1.3	40–80	Half-life 2 h with epinephrine
Linagliptin		1.5	> 100			1,110 liters	75–99	
Lincomycin		2–4	4.4–6.4			64–105 liters	28–86	
Linezolid		1–2	4.5–5.5			0.44–0.79	31	

Liothyronine (T_3)	2–4	2–3 days	16–49			41–45 liters		
Liraglutide		8–12	10–14			13 liters	>98%	
Lisinopril	1	6–8	12			1.6	Minimal	
Lithium carbonate		2–6	14–30			0.7–1.4	0	Half-life prolonged in elderly and renal impairment
Lithium carbonate PR		2–12	18–36					Half-life prolonged in elderly and renal impairment
Lomefloxacin		0.8–1.4	8			1.8–2.5	10–21	
Loperamide	0.5–3	3–5	9–14				97	
Lopinavir		4–6	5–6			0.92–1.86	98–99	
Loratadine	1–3	3–5	12–15	Yes	28	40–200	97	
Lorazepam	Intermediate	2–4	10–20			1–1.3	85	
Losartan		1	2	Yes	6–9	0.21–0.69	98	
Loxapine	0.5	1–2	5–14	Yes	8–30			
Lurasidone		1–3	18	Yes	7.5–10	6,173 liters	99	Vd is for active metabolite
Lysergic acid (LSD)	0.5–2	1–2	3			0.27	80	
Magnesium	1–3	1–2	4–5			0.5	34	
Maprotiline		8–16	21–50	Yes		18–22	90	
Maraviroc		0.5–4	14–18			194 liters	76	Metabolized by CYP3A
Mazindol	0.5–1	2	10	Yes	5.2 days			
Meclizine	1–2		6					

[a]Data provided are based on therapeutic dosing, not overdose. Variability in pharmacokinetics, even in therapeutic doses, occur for a variety of reasons including age, phenotype, renal and hepatic function, gastrointestinal absorption, drug–drug interaction, urine pH, etc. In general, after overdose of immediate-release and especially ER/SR formulations, the peak effect is delayed and the half-life and duration of effect are prolonged. Changes may occur in the volume of distribution and the percentage protein-bound. Kinetics may vary depending on the formulation.
h, hours; min, minutes; L, liters; kg, kilogram; CR, controlled-release formulation; DR, delayed-release formulation; EC, enteric-coated formulation; ER, XR, extended-release formulation; IM, intramuscular; IV, intravenous; MR, modified-release formulation; PR, prolonged-release formulation; SR, sustained-release formulation; SL, sublingual; SQ, subcutaneous.
The apparent volume of distribution (Vd) is reported in liters per kilogram (L/kg) unless the entry specifically states liters.

(*continued*)

TABLE II–66. PHARMACOKINETIC DATA[a] (CONTINUED)

Drug	Onset (h)	Peak (h)	Half-life (h)	Active Metabolite	Half-life of Active Metabolite (h)	Vd (L/kg)	Protein Binding (%)	Comments
Meclofenamate		0.5–2	1–3	Yes	2.4	0.3	99	
Mefenamic acid		2–4	2			1.06	99	
Mefloquine		6–24	20 days			13–29	98	
Melatonin	0.5	0.5–2	0.5–1			35 liters		
Meloxicam	1.5	5–6; 2nd peak at 12–14 h	15–20			0.13–0.23	99.4	2nd peak suggests GI recirculation
Meperidine	<1	1–2	2–5	Yes	15–30	3.7–4.2	55–75	
Mephobarbital	0.5–2		10–70	Yes	80–120	2.6	40–60	Metabolized to phenobarbital
Meprobamate	<1	1–3	10–11			0.75	20	
Meropenem		1	1				2	
Mesoridazine		4–6	5–15	Yes		3–6	75–91	
Metaldehyde	1–3		27					De-polymerizes to acetaldehyde
Metaproterenol	0.5	2–4	3–7			6	10	
Metaxalone	1	3	2–3			800 liters		
Metformin		2	2.5–6			80 liters	Negligible	
Metformin ER		4–8						
Methadone	0.5–1.0	2–4	20–30			3.6	80	
Methamphetamine		1–3	4–15	Yes	7–24	3.5–5	10–20	Half-life prolonged in alkaline urine
Methaqualone		1–2	20–60			2.4–6.4	80	
Methazolamide	2–4	6–8	14				55	
Methicillin		1	0.5			0.43	28–49	
Methocarbamol	0.5	1–2	1–2			0.4–0.6		

Methohexital	<0.2 IV	<0.1	3–5			1–2.6	83	
Methotrexate		1–2	3–15			0.5–1	50	Longer half-life with higher doses
Methscopolamine	1							
Methyclothiazide	1–2	6						
Methyldopa	3–6	6–9	2–14	Yes		0.24	10	Prodrug
Methylenedioxy-methampheta-mine (MDMA)	0.3–1		5–9	Yes		5–8	65	
Methylergonovine	<0.5	1–3	2–5			0.17–0.34		
Methylphenidate		1–3	2–7	Yes	4	12–33	15	
Methylphenidate SR		1.3–8.6	1.3–7.7			6–13	10–33	
Methyprylon	0.75	1–2	7–11	Yes		0.6–1.5	60	
Methysergide		1–3	1	Yes	3–4	0.8–1.0	84	In overdose, vasospasm may last for weeks
Metolazone	1	2	6–20			1.6	95	
Metoprolol	1	1.5–2	3–7			5.6	12	
Metoprolol CR, SR		4–5	1–9					
Metronidazole		1–2	6–14	Yes	10	0.25–0.85	<20	
Metronidazole ER		4.6–6.8	7.4–8.7					
Mexiletine		2–3	10–12			5–7	50–70	
Mezlocillin		0.5	0.8–1.1			0.14–0.26	16–42	

[a]Data provided are based on therapeutic dosing, not overdose. Variability in pharmacokinetics, even in therapeutic doses, occur for a variety of reasons including age, phenotype, renal and hepatic function, gastrointestinal absorption, drug–drug interaction, urine pH, etc. In general, after overdose of immediate-release and especially ER/SR formulations, the peak effect is delayed and the half-life and duration of effect are prolonged. Changes may occur in the volume of distribution and the percentage protein-bound. Kinetics may vary depending on the formulation.

h, hours; min, minutes; L, liters; kg, kilogram; CR, controlled-release formulation; DR, delayed-release formulation; EC, enteric-coated formulation; ER, XR, extended-release formulation; IM, intramuscular; IV, intravenous; MR, modified-release formulation; PR, prolonged-release formulation; SR, sustained-release formulation; SL, sublingual; SQ, subcutaneous.

The apparent volume of distribution (Vd) is reported in liters per kilogram (L/kg) unless the entry specifically states liters.

(*continued*)

TABLE II–66. PHARMACOKINETIC DATA[a] (CONTINUED)

Drug	Onset (h)	Peak (h)	Half-life (h)	Active Metabolite	Half-life of Active Metabolite (h)	Vd (L/kg)	Protein Binding (%)	Comments
Mibefradil	1–2	2–6	17–25			130–190 liters	99	
Midazolam	<5 min IV	0.2–2.7	2.2–6.8	Yes	2–7	1–3	97	
Miglitol		2–3	2			0.18	<4	
Milnacipram		2–4	6–8			400 liters	13	Half-life increases in renal and hepatic impairment
Minocycline		1–4	11–26			1–2	55–75	
Minocycline ER		3.5–4						
Minoxidil	1	2–8	3–4	Yes		2.8–3.3	Minimal	
Mirtazapine		1.5–2	20–40	Yes	25	107 liters	85	
Moclobemide		1–2	2–4.6	Yes		1.2	50	
Modafinil		2–4	7.5–15			0.85	60	
Moexipril	1	1.5–6	1	Yes	2–10	183 liters	50–70	
Molindone		1.5						
Montelukast	3	2–4	3–6			0.1–0.15	99	
Moricizine	2	0.5–2	1.5–3.5	Yes	3	8–11	95	
Morphine	<1	1	2–4.5	Yes		1–6	20–36	
Morphine CR, ER, SR		3–12	15	Yes				ER, CR may release drug for 24–48h
Moxalactam		<0.25 IV	2–2.5			0.18–44	36–52	
Moxifloxacin		1.5–3	12			1.7–2.7	30–50	
Nabumetone		4–12	24	Yes	24–39	5.3–7.5	99	
Nadolol	3–4	4	10–24			2	30	

Nafcillin		1	1			1.1	84–90	
Nalbuphine	<0.2 IV	0.5–1.0	5			3.8–8.1		
Nalidixic acid		2–4	1.1–2.5				93	
Naloxone	2 min IV	0.25–0.5 IV	0.5–1.5			3.6	54	Duration 1–4 h
Naltrexone		1	4–10	Yes	4–13	3	20	Duration 24–72 h
Naproxen		2–4	12–17			0.16	99	
Naproxen DR		4						
Nateglinide	0.25	1–2	1.5–3	Yes			97–99	
Nebivolol		0.5–6	12–19	Yes	12–19	695–2,755 liters	98	Metabolism and half-life differ with phenotype.
Nefazodone		0.5–2	3	Yes	2–33	0.2–0.9	99	
Nelfinavir		2–4	3–5			2–7		
Nevirapine		4	25–45			1.2	60	
Nevirapine ER		24						
Niacin	<1	3–4		Yes				
Niacin ER		4–5	0.9	Yes		4.3		
Nicardipine	0.5	0.5–2	8			8.3	>95	
Nicardipine SR	0.5	1–4	8.6				>95%	
Nicotine			2			3	5–20	Kinetics vary with formulation; half-life is urine pH-dependent

[a]Data provided are based on therapeutic dosing, not overdose. Variability in pharmacokinetics, even in therapeutic doses, occur for a variety of reasons including age, phenotype, renal and hepatic function, gastrointestinal absorption, drug–drug interaction, urine pH, etc. In general, after overdose of immediate-release and especially ER/SR formulations, the peak effect is delayed and the half-life and duration of effect are prolonged. Changes may occur in the volume of distribution and the percentage protein-bound. Kinetics may vary depending on the formulation.
h, hours; min, minutes; L, liters; kg, kilogram; CR, controlled-release formulation; DR, delayed-release formulation; EC, enteric-coated formulation; ER, XR, extended-release formulation; IM, intramuscular; IV, intravenous; MR, modified-release formulation; PR, prolonged-release formulation; SR, sustained-release formulation; SL, sublingual; SQ, subcutaneous.
The apparent volume of distribution (Vd) is reported in liters per kilogram (L/kg) unless the entry specifically states liters.

(*continued*)

TABLE II–66. PHARMACOKINETIC DATA[a] (CONTINUED)

Drug	Onset (h)	Peak (h)	Half-life (h)	Active Metabolite	Half-life of Active Metabolite (h)	Vd (L/kg)	Protein Binding (%)	Comments
Nifedipine	0.5	1	2–5			0.8–2.2	95	
Nifedipine ER		1.5–6	6–11				92–98	
Nisoldipine		1–3	4	Yes		4–5	99	
Nisoldipine ER		4–14.3	9.4–18					
Nitrendipine	1–2	2	2–20			6	98	
Nitrofurantoin			0.3			0.8	25–60	
Nitrofurantoin ER, PR		1–2	0.3–1				25–60	
Nitroprusside	1 min IV	1 min IV	3–11 min					
Norfloxacin		1	3–4				10–15	
Nortriptyline		7	18–35	Yes		15–27	93	
Ofloxacin		1–2	6.1–9.7			1.8–3.3	32	
Olanzapine		6	21–54	Yes	59	1,000 liters	93	
Ombitasvir/Paritaprevir/ Ritonavir		4–5	Ombitasvir 21–25 Paritaprev 5.5			Ombitasvir 50.1 liters Paritaprevir 16.7 liters	Ombitasivir 99.9 Paritaprevir 97–98.6	Extensive metabolism to inactive metabolites
Oritavancin (IV)			245			87.6 liters	85	
Orphenadrine		2–4	14–16				20	
Oseltamir phosphate			1–3	Yes	6–10	23–26 liters	3	Prodrug converted to oseltamir carboxylate
Oxaprozin		2–4	42–50			0.16–0.24	99	
Oxazepam	Slow	2–4	5–20			0.4–0.8	87	
Oxcarbazepine		1–3	1–5	Yes	7–20	0.8		Vd for active metabolite

Oxybutynin	0.5–1	1–3	1–12	Yes	4–10	2.7		
Oxybutynin ER		13	13	Yes			99	
Oxycodone	<0.5	1	2–5	Yes	7.3–9.4	1.8–3.7	45	
Oxycodone CR		3	4.5–8	Yes	7.3–9.4			
Oxymetazoline	<0.5		5–8					
Oxymorphone	0.5–1		7–11	Yes	7.3–18	3.08 ± 1.14	10–12	
Oxymorphone ER		1–2	0.5–22.1	Yes			10–12	Drug continues to be released 24 h after use
Oxyphenbutazone			27–64				90	
Oxyphencyclimine		4	13					
Oxprenolol	2	3	1–3			1.2	70–80	
Oxprenolol SR	2.5–6	4–12						
Paliperidone		24	23			487 liters	74	
Paliperidone ER		24	23			487 liters	74	
Paraldehyde	<0.3	0.5–1	6–7			0.9–1.7		
Paroxetine		3–8	21			8.7	95	
Paroxetine ER		6–10	15–20					
Pemoline		2–4	9–14			0.2–0.6	40–50	
Penbutolol	1–3	1.5–3	17–26	Yes	9–54	32–42 liters	80–98	
Penciclovir			2–2.3			1.5	<20	Parent drug is famciclovir

[a]Data provided are based on therapeutic dosing, not overdose. Variability in pharmacokinetics, even in therapeutic doses, occur for a variety of reasons including age, phenotype, renal and hepatic function, gastrointestinal absorption, drug–drug interaction, urine pH, etc. In general, after overdose of immediate-release and especially ER/SR formulations, the peak effect is delayed and the half-life and duration of effect are prolonged. Changes may occur in the volume of distribution and the percentage protein-bound. Kinetics may vary depending on the formulation.
h, hours; min, minutes; L, liters; kg, kilogram; CR, controlled-release formulation; DR, delayed-release formulation; EC, enteric-coated formulation; ER, XR, extended-release formulation; IM, intramuscular; IV, intravenous; MR, modified-release formulation; PR, prolonged-release formulation; SR, sustained-release formulation; SL, sublingual; SQ, subcutaneous.
The apparent volume of distribution (Vd) is reported in liters per kilogram (L/kg) unless the entry specifically states liters.

(continued)

TABLE II–66. PHARMACOKINETIC DATA[a] (CONTINUED)

Drug	Onset (h)	Peak (h)	Half-life (h)	Active Metabolite	Half-life of Active Metabolite (h)	Vd (L/kg)	Protein Binding (%)	Comments
Penicillin		1	0.5				60–80	
Pentazocine	<0.5	1–2	2–3			4.4–8.0	65	
Pentobarbital	0.25	0.5–2	15–50			0.65–1	45–70	
Peramivir		0.25–0.5	20			12.5 liters	<30%	
Perampanel		0.5–2.5	105				95–96	
Pergolide		1–2	27	Yes			90	
Perindopril	1.5	1	0.8–1	Yes	3–120	0.22	60	
Perphenazine		3–6	8–12	Yes		10–35		
Phenazepam		4	15–60	Yes		4.7–6 liters		
Phencyclidine	<0.1	0.5	1 (30–100 in adipose)	Yes		6	65	Duration 11 h–4 days
Phendimetrazine	1	1–3	5–12.5	Yes	8		15	
Phendimetrazine SR		1–2	2–4	Yes	8			
Pheniramine		1–2.5	16–19			2		
Phenmetrazine		2–5	8					
Phenobarbital	<0.1	0.5–2	80–120			0.5–1	20–50	
Phenoxybenzamine	1 (IV)		24					
Phentermine		3–4.4	7–24			3–4		Half-life is urine pH dependent
Phentermine ER, MR			25					Delayed absorption and peak with ER, MR. Half-life is urine pH dependent
Phentolamine	1 min (IV)		19 min				<72	

Phenylbutazone		2–3	50–100	Yes	27–64	0.14	98	
Phenylephrine	0.25 IV		2–3			5		
Phenylpropanolamine	0.25–1	5.5	3–7			2.5–4.4		
Phenyltoloxamine	1	2–3						
Phenytoin		1.5–3	7–60			0.5–0.8	>90	Zero-order kinetics; half-life increases as levels rise
Phenytoin ER		4–12	7–42					
Pimozide		6–8	55–66					
Pindolol	1–3	2	3–4			1.2–2	40–60	
Pioglitazone		2–4	3–7	Yes	16–24	0.63	>99	
Piperacillin		0.5	0.6–1.2			0.29	22	
Piroxicam		0.5	45–50			0.13	99	
Polymyxin B			4.3–6					
Polymixin E (colistin)			2–3					
Pramlintide		0.3–0.5	0.5–0.8			56 liters	60	Duration 3h
Prazosin	2–4	2–4	2–4	Yes		0.6–1.7	95	
Pregabalin	0.5	1.5	6–9			0.5	0	
Primaquine		1–2	3–8	Yes	22–30	269 ± 121 liters		Accumulation with chronic use
Primidone			3.3–12	Yes	29–120	0.4–1.0	20–30	Metabolized to PEMA/ phenobarbital

[a]Data provided are based on therapeutic dosing, not overdose. Variability in pharmacokinetics, even in therapeutic doses, occur for a variety of reasons including age, phenotype, renal and hepatic function, gastrointestinal absorption, drug–drug interaction, urine pH, etc. In general, after overdose of immediate-release and especially ER/SR formulations, the peak effect is delayed and the half-life and duration of effect are prolonged. Changes may occur in the volume of distribution and the percentage protein-bound. Kinetics may vary depending on the formulation.
h, hours; min, minutes; L, liters; kg, kilogram; CR, controlled-release formulation; DR, delayed-release formulation; EC, enteric-coated formulation; ER, XR, extended-release formulation; IM, intramuscular; IV, intravenous; MR, modified-release formulation; PR, prolonged-release formulation; SR, sustained-release formulation; SL, sublingual; SQ, subcutaneous.
The apparent volume of distribution (Vd) is reported in liters per kilogram (L/kg) unless the entry specifically states liters.

(continued)

TABLE II–66. PHARMACOKINETIC DATA[a] (CONTINUED)

Drug	Onset (h)	Peak (h)	Half-life (h)	Active Metabolite	Half-life of Active Metabolite (h)	Vd (L/kg)	Protein Binding (%)	Comments
Procaine			7–8 min					
Procainamide	1–2.5	1–2	4	Yes	5–7	1.5–2.5	15	
Procarbazine		1	0.2 IV					
Prochlorperazine	0.5	2–4	7–23	Yes		12–18		
Procyclidine		1–2	7–16			1.1		
Promethazine	0.5	2–3	7–16			171	93	
Propafenone		2–3	2–10			1.9–3	77–97	
Propafenone ER, SR		3–8						
Propantheline	<1	6	1–9					
Propoxyphene	0.5–1.0	2–3	6–12	Yes	30–36	12–26		
Propranolol	1–2	2–4	2–6	Yes	5–7.5	6	93	
Propranolol ER		6	10–20			4	90	
Protriptyline		25	54–92			22	92	
Pseudoephedrine	0.5	3	5–8			2.5–3	20	
Pseudoephedrine ER		8	15					
Pyrazinamide		2	9–10				10	
Pyridoxine	<1	1–2	15–20 days	Yes				
Pyridoxine DR		2.6–5	<0.5	Yes	46–86			
Pyrilamine	0.25–1		1.5–2.3					
Pyrimethamine		0.5	2–6			96	87	
Quazepam		2	39	Yes	70–75	5–8.6	>95	

Quetiapine		1.5	6–7	Yes	12	6–14	83	
Quetiapine ER		6	7	Yes	12	6–14	83	
Quinacrine		1–3	5 days			620		
Quinapril	1	0.5–2	0.8	Yes	2		97	
Quinidine	0.5	1–3	6–8	Yes		2–3	70–90	
Quinidine ER		3–5	3–8	Yes	12	2–3	70–88	
Quinine		1–3	8–14			1.2–1.7	80	
Raltegravir		3	9				83	
Ramelteon		0.5–1.5	1–2.6	Yes	2–5	73.6 liters	82	
Ramipril	2	0.7–2	1–5	Yes	13–17		73	
Repaglinide	0.5	1–1.5	1–1.5			0.44	98	
Ribavirin		1–1.7	298			2,825 liters		
Rifabutin		2–4	36	Yes		7.8–10.8		
Rifampin		2–4	1.5–5	Yes		1.6	89	
Rifapentine		3–10	13	Yes	10–16	61–79	97.7	
Rilpivirine		4–5	50				99.7	Extensive metabolism to inactive metabolites
Risperidone		1–2	20–30	Yes	21–30	1–2	90	Clearance decreases in renal impairment.
Risperidone ER			3–6 days	Yes		1–2	90	Clearance decreases in renal impairment.

[a]Data provided are based on therapeutic dosing, not overdose. Variability in pharmacokinetics, even in therapeutic doses, occur for a variety of reasons including age, phenotype, renal and hepatic function, gastrointestinal absorption, drug–drug interaction, urine pH, etc. In general, after overdose of immediate-release and especially ER/SR formulations, the peak effect is delayed and the half-life and duration of effect are prolonged. Changes may occur in the volume of distribution and the percentage protein-bound. Kinetics may vary depending on the formulation.

h, hours; min, minutes; L, liters; kg, kilogram; CR, controlled-release formulation; DR, delayed-release formulation; EC, enteric-coated formulation; ER, XR, extended-release formulation; IM, intramuscular; IV, intravenous; MR, modified-release formulation; PR, prolonged-release formulation; SR, sustained-release formulation; SL, sublingual; SQ, subcutaneous.

The apparent volume of distribution (Vd) is reported in liters per kilogram (L/kg) unless the entry specifically states liters.

(*continued*)

TABLE II–66. PHARMACOKINETIC DATA[a] (CONTINUED)

Drug	Onset (h)	Peak (h)	Half-life (h)	Active Metabolite	Half-life of Active Metabolite (h)	Vd (L/kg)	Protein Binding (%)	Comments
Ritodrine		1	1–2	Yes	15	0.7	32	
Ritonavir		2–4	2–4					Excreted renally and in feces
Rivaroxaban	Rapid	2–4	5–9			50 liters	92–95%	Half-life 11–13 h in elderly; food increases bioavailability; CYP3A4 and CYP2J2 metabolism; 35% renal elimination
Rofecoxib		2–3	17			86–91 liters	87	
Rosiglitazone		1–3.5	3–4			0.25	99.8	
Saquinavir						700 liters	90	Interaction with garlic
Saxagliptin		2	2.5	Yes	3.1		Negligible	
Scopolamine	0.5	1	3			1.5		
Secobarbital	0.25	1–6	15–40			1.5–1.9	45–70	
Selegiline	0.5–1	0.5–2	0.3–1.2	Yes	7–20		94	
Sertraline		4–8	28	Yes	60–100	20	99	
Simeprevir		4–6	10–13				>99.9	
Sitagliptin		1–4	12.4			198 liters	38	
Sofosbuvir		1.8–1	0.4	Yes	27		61–65 (parent; minimal (metabolite)	>90% metabolized to active metabolite
Solifenacin succinate		3–8	45–68	Yes		600 liters	98	
Sotalol	1–2	2–3	7–18			1.6–2.4	<5	
Sparfloxacin		0.4–6	16–30			3.1–4.7	45	
Spectinomycin		1	1.2–2.8					

Spironolactone	24	24–48	2	Yes	16.5		95	
Stavudine		1	1.44 PO, 1.15 IV			0.5–0.73	Negligible	Active tubular secretion
Streptomycin		1	2.5					
Strychnine	0.5		10–16			13		Vd based on only one case report
Sulfamethoxazole			9–12			0.21	70	
Sulindac		2	7–16	Yes	16		98	
Sumatriptan	0.5	2–2.5	2–3.1			2.4–2.7	14–21	
Suvorexant		2	12			49 liters	>99	
Tamsulosin	4–8	4–8	9–13			0.2	94–99	
Tamsulosin ER, MR		6	19					
Tapentadol	0.5–1	1.25	4			442–638 liters	20	Metabolized by glucuronic acid conjugation.
Tapentadol ER		3–6	5					
Tasimelteon		0.5–3	1.3			56–126 liters	90	
Tazobactam (IV)	0.5		1–1.2			18.2 liters	30	Half-life increases in elderly, hepatic and renal disease
Tedizolid		2.5–3.5	12	Yes		67–80 liters	70–90	
Telaprevir		4–5	9–11			252 liters	69–76	Extensive metabolism to weakly active metabolite
Telavancin			6.5–9.5			122–168 liters	90	

[a]Data provided are based on therapeutic dosing, not overdose. Variability in pharmacokinetics, even in therapeutic doses, occur for a variety of reasons including age, phenotype, renal and hepatic function, gastrointestinal absorption, drug–drug interaction, urine pH, etc. In general, after overdose of immediate-release and especially ER/SR formulations, the peak effect is delayed and the half-life and duration of effect are prolonged. Changes may occur in the volume of distribution and the percentage protein-bound. Kinetics may vary depending on the formulation.
h, hours; min, minutes; L, liters; kg, kilogram; CR, controlled-release formulation; DR, delayed-release formulation; EC, enteric-coated formulation; ER, XR, extended-release formulation; IM, intramuscular; IV, intravenous; MR, modified-release formulation; PR, prolonged-release formulation; SR, sustained-release formulation; SL, sublingual; SQ, subcutaneous.
The apparent volume of distribution (Vd) is reported in liters per kilogram (L/kg) unless the entry specifically states liters.

(*continued*)

TABLE II–66. PHARMACOKINETIC DATA[a] (CONTINUED)

Drug	Onset (h)	Peak (h)	Half-life (h)	Active Metabolite	Half-life of Active Metabolite (h)	Vd (L/kg)	Protein Binding (%)	Comments
Telbivudine		2	15					Vd is > total body water
Telmisartan	3	0.5–1	24			500 liters	99.5	
Temazepam	Intermediate	1.2–1.6	3.5–18.4			0.6–1.3	96	
Tenofovir		1	17			1.2–1.3	7.2	Active tubular secretion
Terazosin		1–2	9–12			25–30 liters	90–94	
Terbutaline	0.5–1	3	4–16			1.5	15	
Terfenadine	1–2	2–4	6–8.5	Yes	8.5		97	
Tetracaine			5–10 min					
Tetracycline			6–12			1–2	65	
Tetrahydrozoline	0.25–1		1.2–4					
Theophylline	0.5–1	1–2	4–6			0.5	40	
Theophylline ER		6–9	5.3–13.4					
Thiopental	<0.1	<0.1	8–10			1.4–6.7	72–86	
Thioridazine		1–2	10–36	Yes	1–2	18	96	
Thiothixene	1–2	1–3	34					
Thyroid, desiccated	2 days	8–10 days	2–7 days	Yes	2 days		99	
Tiagabine	Rapid	1	7–9				96	
Ticarcillin		0.5	1–1.2			0.22	45	
Tigecycline			37–67					
Timolol		0.5–3	2–4			1.5	<10	
Tinidazole		0.9–2.3	12–14			50 liters	12	
Tinzaparin (SQ)	2–3	4–5	3–4			3.1–5 liters	Low	

Tipranavir		2	5.5			7.7–10.2	>99.9	Fecal elimination primarily
Tizanidine		1.5	2.5			2.4	30	
Tobramycin		0.5	2–2.5				0–3	
Tocainide		1–2	11–15			2–4	10–22	
Tolazamide	1	4–6	7	Yes				
Tolazoline			3–10			1.61		
Tolbutamide	1	5–8	4.5–6.5				80–99	
Tolmetin		1	1			0.13	99	
Tolterodine	Rapid	1	2–3	Yes	3	0.9–1.6	96	
Tolterodine ER, XR		2–6	6–10	Yes	10	1.6		
Topiramate	Rapid	1.8–4.3	21			0.6–0.8	13–17	
Torsemide	0.5–1	1–4	2–4			0.14	97	
Tramadol	1	2–3	6–7.5	Yes	7.5	2.6–2.9	20	
Tramadol ER		4.8–17	7.9	Yes	8.8			Half-life increases in hepatic and renal impairment
Trandolapril		0.5–2	0.6–1.6	Yes	16–24	18 liters	80	
Tranylcypromine		0.7–3.5	1.5–3.5	Yes		3		
Trazodone		0.5–2	3–9	Yes		1.3	90–95	
Triamterene	2–4	2–8	1.5–2	Yes	3	2.5	65	
Triazolam	Fast	1–2	1.5–5.5			0.7–1.5	78–89	

[a]Data provided are based on therapeutic dosing, not overdose. Variability in pharmacokinetics, even in therapeutic doses, occur for a variety of reasons including age, phenotype, renal and hepatic function, gastrointestinal absorption, drug–drug interaction, urine pH, etc. In general, after overdose of immediate-release and especially ER/SR formulations, the peak effect is delayed and the half-life and duration of effect are prolonged. Changes may occur in the volume of distribution and the percentage protein-bound. Kinetics may vary depending on the formulation.
h, hours; min, minutes; L, liters; kg, kilogram; CR, controlled-release formulation; DR, delayed-release formulation; EC, enteric-coated formulation; ER, XR, extended-release formulation; IM, intramuscular; IV, intravenous; MR, modified-release formulation; PR, prolonged-release formulation; SR, sustained-release formulation; SL, sublingual; SQ, subcutaneous.
The apparent volume of distribution (Vd) is reported in liters per kilogram (L/kg) unless the entry specifically states liters.

(continued)

TABLE II–66. PHARMACOKINETIC DATA[a] (CONTINUED)

Drug	Onset (h)	Peak (h)	Half-life (h)	Active Metabolite	Half-life of Active Metabolite (h)	Vd (L/kg)	Protein Binding (%)	Comments
Trichlormethiazide	2	4	2–7					
Trifluoperazine		2–5	5–18	Yes			90–99	
Trihexyphenidyl	1	2–3	3.3–4.1					
Trimazosin	1	1	2.7	Yes			99	
Trimeprazine		3.5–4.5	4–8					
Trimethobenzamide	0.5	1	1			0.5		
Trimethoprim		1–4	8–11				44	
Trimipramine		2	15–30	Yes		31	95	
Tripelennamine	0.5	2–3	3–5			9–12		
Triprolidine		1.5–2.5	3–5					
Trospium chloride		5–6	15–21			395 liters	50–85	
Trospium chloride ER		3–7.5	36					
Trovafloxacin		1–2	9.1–12.7	Yes		1.2–1.4	76	
Urapidil	<0.4		5	Yes	12.5	0.4–0.77	75–80	
Valacyclovir		0.5		Yes	2.5–3.3			Prodrug, converted to acyclovir
Valdecoxib		3	8–11	Yes		86 liters	98	
Valganciclovir		2		Yes	4	0.57–0.84	1–2	Prodrug converted to ganciclovir
Valproic acid		1–4	9–16	Yes		0.1–0.5	80–95	
Valproic acid (Divalproex)		4–8	9–16	Yes		0.1–0.5	80–95	
Valproic acid (Divalproex ER)		4–17	5–17	Yes		0.1–0.5	80–95	

Valproic acid DR		2	6–17	Yes		0.1–0.5	80–95	
Valproic acid ER		4–17	8–20	Yes		0.1–0.5	80–95	
Valsartan	2	2–4	6			17 liters	95	
Vancomycin		1	4–6			0.3–0.7	55	
Venlafaxine		1–2	5	Yes	11	6–7	30	
Venlafaxine ER		5.5	5		11		27–30	Half-life increases with renal impairment
Verapamil	0.5–2	6–8	2–8	Yes	10–19	4.7	83–92	
Verapamil ER		4–11	9			1.8–6.7		
Vidarabine				Yes	2.4–3.3		20–30	
Vigabatrin	Rapid	2	4–8			0.8	Negligible	
Warfarin	24–72	3–7 days	36–72	Yes	20–90	0.15	99	
Zalcitabine			1–3			0.534		Renal excretion primarily
Zaleplon	1.5	1	1			1.4	45–75	
Zanamivir		1–2	2.5–5.1				<10	
Zidovudine (AZT)		0.5–1.5	0.5–1.5			1.6	34–38	
Ziprasidone		4.5	4–10			1.5–2.3	>99	
Zolpidem	1	1.6	1.4–4.5			0.54	92.5	
Zolpidem CR		1.5–2	1.6–4.1					Peak delayed with food 2–4h
Zonisamide		2–6	50–68			1.45	40	

[a]Data provided are based on therapeutic dosing, not overdose. Variability in pharmacokinetics, even in therapeutic doses, occur for a variety of reasons including age, phenotype, renal and hepatic function, gastrointestinal absorption, drug–drug interaction, urine pH, etc. In general, after overdose of immediate-release and especially ER/SR formulations, the peak effect is delayed and the half-life and duration of effect are prolonged. Changes may occur in the volume of distribution and the percentage protein-bound. Kinetics may vary depending on the formulation.
h, hours; min, minutes; L, liters; kg, kilogram; CR, controlled-release formulation; DR, delayed-release formulation; EC, enteric-coated formulation; ER, XR, extended-release formulation; IM, intramuscular; IV, intravenous; MR, modified-release formulation; PR, prolonged-release formulation; SR, sustained-release formulation; SL, sublingual; SQ, subcutaneous.
The apparent volume of distribution (Vd) is reported in liters per kilogram (L/kg) unless the entry specifically states liters.

SECTION III. **Therapeutic Drugs and Antidotes**

▶ INTRODUCTION

Thomas E. Kearney, PharmD

This section provides detailed descriptions of antidotes and other therapeutic agents used in the management of a poisoned patient. For each agent, a summary is provided of its pharmacologic effects, clinical indications, adverse effects and contraindications, use in pregnancy, dosage, available formulations, and recommended minimum stocking levels for the hospital pharmacy (for availability within 60 minutes) and emergency department (for immediate availability).

I. **Use of antidotes in pregnancy.** It is always prudent to avoid or minimize drug exposure during pregnancy, and physicians are often reluctant to use an antidote for fear of fetal harm. This reluctance, however, must be tempered with a case-by-case risk-benefit analysis of the use of the particular therapeutic agent. An acute drug overdose or poisoning during pregnancy may threaten the life of the mother as well as the life of the fetus, and the antidote or therapeutic agent, despite unknown or questionable effects on the fetus, may have a lifesaving benefit. The inherent toxicity and large body burden of the drug or toxic chemical involved in the poisoning may far exceed those of the therapeutic agent or antidote.

For most of the agents discussed in this section, little or no information is available about their use in pregnant patients. The **Food and Drug Administration (FDA)** established five categories (A, B, C, D, and X) of required labeling to indicate the potential for teratogenicity (Table III–1). The distinction between categories depends mainly on the amount and reliability of animal and human data and the risk-benefit assessment for the use of a specific agent. This has led to confusion, with the misbelief that risk increases in a predictable way from Category A to Category X. Note that the categorization may also be based on

TABLE III–1. FDA PREGNANCY CATEGORIES FOR TERATOGENIC EFFECTS

FDA Pregnancy Category	Definition
A	Adequate and well-controlled studies in pregnant women have failed to demonstrate a risk to the fetus in the first trimester, and there is no evidence of a risk later in pregnancy. The possibility of fetal harm appears remote.
B	Either (1) animal reproduction studies have failed to demonstrate any adverse effect (other than a decrease in fertility) but there are no adequate and well-controlled studies in pregnant women or (2) animal studies that have shown an adverse effect that has not been confirmed by adequate and well-controlled studies in pregnant women. The possibility of fetal harm is probably remote.
C	Either (1) animal reproduction studies have shown an adverse effect on the fetus and there are no adequate and well-controlled human studies or (2) there are no animal or human studies. The drug should be given only if the potential benefit outweighs the potential risk to the fetus.
D	There is positive evidence of human fetal risk based on adverse reaction data from investigational or marketing experience or human studies, but the potential risks may be acceptable in light of potential benefits (eg, use in a life-threatening situation for which safer drugs are ineffective or unavailable).
X	Studies in animals or humans have demonstrated fetal abnormalities, there is positive evidence of fetal risk based on human experience, or both, and the risk of using the drug in a pregnant patient outweighs any possible benefit. The drug in contraindicated in women who are or may become pregnant.

From *Code of Federal Regulations*, title 21, section 201.57 (revised April 1, 2010). Cite: 21 CFR §201.57.

anticipated chronic or repeated use and may not be relevant to a single use or brief antidotal treatment. ***Note:*** In 2015, the Pregnancy and Lactation Labeling Final Rule went into effect, which will replace the former FDA A-X pregnancy categories with narrative sections to include Pregnancy and Lactation with subsections addressing risk summary, clinical considerations, and data.

II. Hospital stocking. The hospital pharmacy should maintain a medical staff–approved stock of antidotes and other emergency drugs. Surveys of hospitals consistently have demonstrated inadequate stocks of antidotes. Many antidotes are used only infrequently, have a short shelf life, or are expensive. There have also been disruptions and delays in the supply of antidotes from manufacturers as well as discontinuation of some products (eg, multiple-dose glucagon). The optimal and most cost-effective case management of poisonings, however, requires having adequate supplies of antidotes readily available. Fortunately, only a minimal acquisition and maintenance cost is required to stock many of these drugs adequately. Other cost reduction strategies may include employment of an institutional approval and utilization review process (eg, requiring local poison center approval for the use of selected costly antidotes), arrangements with suppliers to replace expired and unused antidotes (note that some manufacturers have such a policy), redistribution of soon-to-expire antidotes, and consignment (the hospital has possession of the antidote, but it is owned by the supplier who can charge at the time of usage). In addition, some antidotes (eg, DMPS [dimercaptopropanesulfonic acid]) may be available only through compounding pharmacies; therefore, they may not be listed by wholesalers, and additional diligence is needed to ensure the purity of the product (because the drug may be supplied by multiple foreign sources and require extemporaneous preparation).

A. The basis for our **suggested minimum stocking level** is a combination of factors: the highest total dose of a drug generally given during an 8-hour and a 24-hour period as quoted in the literature, the manufacturer's maximum recommended or tolerated daily dose, and an estimation of these quantities for a 100-kg adult. It is recommended that some antidotes be immediately available and stocked in the emergency department while others be accessible through the hospital pharmacy and available within 60 minutes on a 24-hour basis.

B. Larger quantities of a drug may be needed in unusual situations (eg, chemical terrorism), particularly if multiple patients are treated simultaneously or for extended periods. There may also be regional variations and risks (eg, endemic poisonous snakes, industrial chemical facilities, agricultural pesticide use) that need to be factored into stocking strategies. Hospitals in close proximity may wish to explore the practicality of sharing or pooling stocks but should carefully consider the logistics of such arrangements (eg, transferring stocks after hours or on weekends). Hospitals should be linked with regional emergency response plans for hazardous (and nuclear/biological/chemical terrorism) materials, mass casualty incidents, and the mobilization of local and national antidote stockpiles (i.e., Strategic National Stockpile).

▶ ACETYLCYSTEINE (*N*-ACETYLCYSTEINE [NAC])

Thomas E. Kearney, PharmD

I. Pharmacology. Acetylcysteine (*N*-acetylcysteine [NAC]) is a mucolytic agent that acts as a sulfhydryl group donor, substituting for the usual sulfhydryl donor of the liver, glutathione. It rapidly binds (detoxifies) the highly reactive electrophilic intermediates of metabolism, or it may enhance the reduction of the toxic intermediate, NAPQI, to the parent, acetaminophen. It is most effective in preventing acetaminophen-induced liver injury when given early in the course of intoxication (within 8–10 hours), but it may also be of benefit in reducing the severity of acetaminophen and non–acetaminophen-induced liver injury by several proposed mechanisms (improved blood flow and oxygen delivery, modified cytokine production, free radical or oxygen scavenging), even when given after 24 hours. This proposed role of NAC as a glutathione precursor, direct sulfhydryl binding agent, and antioxidant has also been the basis for its investigational use for poisonings from agents that are associated with a free radical or oxidative stress mechanism of toxicity or that bind to sulfhydryl groups. This mechanism coupled with improved renal hemodynamics may prevent contrast-induced nephropathy and provide a rescue from cisplatin and ifosfamide-induced nephrotoxicity. It may be used empirically when the severity of ingestion is unknown or serum concentrations of the ingested drug are not immediately available.

II. Indications

A. Acetaminophen overdose.

B. Case reports of or investigational use in carbon tetrachloride, chloroform, acrylonitrile, doxorubicin, arsenic, gold, amanitin mushroom, carbon monoxide, chromium, cyanide, nitrofurantoin, paraquat, and methyl mercury poisoning.

C. Pennyroyal oil and clove oil poisoning (case reports). The mechanism of hepatic injury by pennyroyal oil and clove oil is similar to that of acetaminophen, and empiric use of NAC seems justified for any significant pennyroyal oil or clove oil ingestion.

D. Cisplatin or ifosfamide-induced nephrotoxicity and prevention of contrast-induced nephropathy.

E. Pyroglutamic aciduria (5-oxoprolinuria).

F. Non–acetaminophen-induced liver failure.

III. Contraindications. Known acute hypersensitivity or IgE-mediated anaphylaxis (rare). Anaphylactoid reactions, although similar in clinical effects, may be prevented or ameliorated, as discussed below.

IV. Adverse effects

A. Acetylcysteine typically causes nausea and vomiting when given **orally.** If the dose is vomited, it should be repeated. The dose calculation and proper dilution (to 5%) should be verified (this effect may be dose- and concentration-dependent). Use of a gastric tube, slower rate of administration, and strong antiemetic agent (eg, metoclopramide [p 581], ondansetron [p 597]) may be necessary.

B. Rapid **intravenous** administration can cause flushing, rash, angioedema, hypotension, and bronchospasm (anaphylactoid reaction). Death (status epilepticus, intracranial hypertension) was reported in a 30-month-old child who accidentally received a massive dose intravenously (2,450 mg/kg over 6 hours, 45 minutes), and fatal bronchospasm occurred in an adult with severe asthma.

1. Reactions may be reduced by giving the loading dose slowly (over at least 60 minutes) in a dilute (3–4%) solution and by exercising extra caution in patients with asthma (carefully titrate with more dilute solutions and slower infusion rates; pretreat with antihistamines).

2. An additional risk factor for anaphylactoid reaction may be low serum levels of acetaminophen, whereas high levels may be protective against reactions.

3. If an anaphylactoid reaction occurs, stop the infusion immediately and treat with diphenhydramine (p 544) if urticaria, angioedema, or both are present and with epinephrine (p 551) for more serious reactions (shock, bronchoconstriction). Once symptoms have resolved, the infusion may be recommenced at a slower rate (by further dilution and given over at least 1 hour).

C. ***Note:*** Dilutional hyponatremia and seizures developed in a 3-year-old after IV administration from excess free water (see Item VI.C.2 below for precautions regarding pediatric dilution).

D. Use in pregnancy. FDA Category B (see Table III–1). There is no evidence of teratogenicity. Use of this drug to treat acetaminophen overdose is considered beneficial to both mother and developing fetus. However, maternal hypotension

TABLE III–2. DILUTION GUIDELINES FOR ORAL ADMINISTRATION OF *N*-ACETYLCYSTEINE (NAC)

	Volume of NAC (mL/kg)	Approximate Volume of Soda/Juice Needed to Make 5% Solution (mL/kg)
Loading dose (140 mg/kg)		
With 20% NAC (200 mg/mL) solution	0.7	2
With 10% NAC (100 mg/mL) solution	1.4	1.4
Maintenance dose (70 mg/kg)		
With 20% NAC (200 mg/mL) solution	0.35	1
With 10% NAC (100 mg/mL) solution	0.7	0.7

or hypoxia due to a serious anaphylactoid reaction from IV administration may harm the fetus.

V. Drug or laboratory interactions

A. Activated charcoal adsorbs acetylcysteine and may interfere with its systemic absorption. When both are given orally together, data suggest that peak acetylcysteine levels are decreased by about 30% and that the time to reach peak level may be delayed. However, these effects are not considered clinically important.

B. NAC can produce a false-positive test for ketones in the urine.

C. NAC can prolong the measured prothrombin time (by 0.2–3.9 seconds) and INR.

VI. Dosage and method of administration

A. Oral loading dose. Give 140 mg/kg of the 10% (1.4 mL/kg) or 20% (0.7 mL/kg) solution diluted in juice or soda to enhance palatability. Dilute the loading dose of 10% NAC with 1.4 mL/kg of juice or soda (for 20% NAC dilute with 2 mL/kg of juice/soda). Oral dilution guidelines are presented in Table III–2.

B. Maintenance oral dose

1. Give 70 mg/kg (as a 5% solution) every 4 hours. Dilute the maintenance dose of 10% NAC (0.7 mL/kg) with 0.7 mL/kg of juice or soda (for 20% NAC, dilute 0.35 mL/kg with 1 mL/kg of juice/soda). Oral dilution guidelines are presented in Table III–2.
2. Duration of treatment. The conventional protocol for treatment of acetaminophen poisoning in the United States calls for 17 doses of oral NAC given over 72 hours. However, based on the success of shorter intravenous protocols in Canada and Europe, we use a 20-hour oral regimen (70 mg/kg every 4 hours for a total of five doses) for uncomplicated poisonings treated within 8 hours of ingestion. At the end of the 20-hour regimen, if there is any detectable acetaminophen or elevation of hepatic aminotransferases, we continue giving NAC at 70 mg/kg every 4 hours until evidence of toxicity is resolved.

C. An **intravenous** preparation (Acetadote, Cumberland Pharmaceuticals) was approved in 2004 by the US FDA and is indicated if the patient is unable to tolerate the oral formulation because of vomiting, ileus, intestinal obstruction, or other GI problems.

1. The package insert recommends the following 21-hour regimen for uncomplicated poisonings treated within 8 hours (in adults): a loading dose of 150 mg/kg (maximum dose, 15 g) in 200 mL of 5% dextrose in water (D_5W) over 60 minutes, followed by 50 mg/kg in 500 mL of D_5W over 4 hours and then 100 mg/kg in 1,000 mL of D_5W over 16 hours. For patients weighing more than 100 kg, the loading dose should be no more than 15 g. Guidelines and precautions for IV Acetadote administration are presented in Table III–3.

TABLE III–3. DILUTION GUIDELINES FOR INTRAVENOUS ADMINISTRATION OF ACETADOTE

	Dose of Acetadote (20% Solution = 200 mg/mL)	Volume of Diluent (D_5W)[a] Needed	Duration of Infusion
Loading dose (150 mg/kg)	0.75 mL/kg[b]	3 mL/kg (children <20 kg) 100 mL (children 20–40 kg) 200 mL (adults)	Over at least 45–60 minutes recommended to reduce risk for anaphylactoid reactions.
First maintenance dose (50 mg/kg)	0.25 mL/kg	7 mL/kg (children <20 kg) 250 mL (children 20–40 kg) 500 mL (adults)	Over 4 hours.
Second maintenance dose (100 mg/kg)	0.5 mL/kg	14 mL/kg (children <20 kg) 500 mL (children 20–40 kg) 1,000 mL (adults)	Over 16 hours.

[a]Manufacturer indicates that NAC is also stable in 0.45% normal saline at room temperature for 24 hours.
[b]Manufacturer suggests the following for patients weighing more than 100 kg: loading dose = 15 g (75 mL of Acetadote); 4-hour maintenance dose = 5 g (25 mL of Acetadote); 16-hour maintenance dose = 10 g (50 mL of Acetadote).

a. If there is evidence of hepatic toxicity or remaining acetaminophen in the serum at the end of the infusion, continue giving the 16-hour NAC maintenance dose regimen (6.25 mg/kg/h) until toxic effects resolve (i.e., liver function tests are clearly improving) and there is no detectable acetaminophen in the patient's serum.

b. The standard IV dosing regimen may be insufficient in situations that involve massive ingested amounts (eg, >400–600 mg/kg) or coingestants that delay systemic absorption (eg, anticholinergic agents or opioids), resulting in persistently high or delayed peak serum acetaminophen levels.

i. For **massive ingestions**, consider following the IV loading dose of NAC with an infusion of 17.5 mg/kg/h or 70 mg/kg every 4 hours (equivalent to the oral dose regimen) until the acetaminophen level is no longer detectable.

ii. For **persistent elevation** of acetaminophen levels due to prolonged or delayed absorption, continue the maintenance infusion until the level is no longer detectable.

iii. It is advisable to seek consultation from a regional poison center (1-800-222-1222) or medical toxicologist for guidance.

2. Pediatric patients should have an alternate dilution volume or a saline-containing solution to avoid overhydration and hyponatremia (see Table III–3 for IV Acetadote administration guidelines and precautions).

3. Many patients can be switched to an oral regimen after the first one to two IV doses if vomiting has ceased.

4. If Acetadote is not available, then the oral preparation may be administered by the IV route (with use of an in-line micropore filter).

Contact a medical toxicologist or regional poison center (1-800-222-1222) for advice, and see Section VII below for preparation and administration.

D. Dosage during hemodialysis. The clearance of acetylcysteine may be doubled during hemodialysis. It has been recommended to double the dose of NAC during hemodialysis by increasing the infusion rate of the maintenance dose administered during hemodialysis (eg, if on second 4-hour bag increase to 25 mg/kg/h or if during third 16-hour bag increase to 12.5 mg/kg/h) and administer an additional half loading dose of 75 mg/kg if hemodialysis exceeds 6 hours.

E. Dosage for the prevention of radiographic contrast-induced nephropathy.

1. There are several dosage regimens and it is uncertain which one is optimal.
   a. Option 1: Give 600–1,200 mg of NAC orally twice on the day before and twice on the day of the procedure (total of four doses over 2 days).
   b. Option 2: Give IV NAC 150 mg/kg over 30 minutes just before administration of contrast agent, followed by 50 mg/kg over 4 hours after administration of the contrast agent.
   c. Option 3: A mixed regimen of 500–600 mg NAC intravenously, followed by 600–1,200 mg orally twice daily.
2. These regimens are coupled with IV hydration with either normal saline at 1 mL/kg/h for 12 hours before and after the procedure or use of 154 mEq/L of sodium bicarbonate in 5% dextrose at 3 mL/kg/h for 1 hour immediately before the administration of the contrast agent, then 1 mL/kg/h during and 6 hours after administration of the contrast agent.

VII. Formulations

A. Oral. The usual formulation is as a 10% (100-mg/mL) or 20% (200-mg/mL) solution, supplied as an inhaled mucolytic agent (Mucomyst, or generic substitute). This form is available through most hospital pharmacies or respiratory therapy departments. The preparation is ***not*** FDA-approved for parenteral use. In rare circumstances, when intravenous administration of this preparation is required and Acetadote is not available, dilute the loading dose to a 3–4% solution (in D_5W), use a micropore (0.22-micron) filter, and administer over 45–60 minutes. To make a 4% solution, dilute the loading dose of 10% NAC (1.4 mL/kg = 140 mg/kg) with 2.1 mL/kg of D_5W (for 20% NAC dilute 0.7 mL/kg with 2.8 mL/kg of D_5W).

B. The intravenous formulation (Acetadote) is available as a 20% solution in 30-mL (200-mg/mL) vials in a carton of four vials. ***Note:*** Special precautions are needed to avoid accidental overdose or overdilution with D_5W in pediatric patients (see Table III–3 for IV Acetadote administration guidelines and precautions).

C. Suggested minimum stocking levels for the treatment of a 100-kg adult for the first 8 hours and 24 hours:

1. Oral, *first 8 hours*: 28 g or five vials (30 mL each) of 20% (oral) solution; first 24 hours: 56 g or 10 vials (30 mL each) of 20% (oral) solution.
2. **IV,** *first 8 hours*: 24 g or one carton of four vials (30 mL each) of 20% (IV) solution; *first 24 hours:* 30 g or five vials (30 mL each) of 20% (IV) solution.

   We suggest that both preparations be stocked and that the oral solution be used preferentially in most cases.

▶ ANTIPSYCHOTIC DRUGS (HALOPERIDOL, DROPERIDOL, OLANZAPINE, AND ZIPRASIDONE)

Thomas E. Kearney, PharmD

I. Pharmacology

A. Haloperidol and droperidol are butyrophenone neuroleptic drugs, often referred to as "first-generation" or "typical" antipsychotics, that are useful for the management of acutely agitated psychotic patients and as antiemetics. They have strong central antidopaminergic activity and weak anticholinergic and anti–alpha-adrenergic effects.

B. Olanzapine and ziprasidone are second-generation or "atypical" antipsychotic agents. They have weaker and more selective antidopaminergic activity and a higher ratio of serotonin-to-dopamine antagonism. This provides less risk for extrapyramidal side effects. However, olanzapine has greater anticholinergic effects, and both have greater antihistaminic and anti–alpha-adrenergic effects. Therefore, they have a greater propensity to cause sedation and orthostatic hypotension.

C. Pharmacokinetics. Haloperidol is well absorbed from the GI tract and by the intramuscular route. Droperidol is available only for parenteral use and is also well absorbed by the intramuscular route. Droperidol has a more predictable and rapid onset of 3–10 minutes, and both have peak pharmacologic effects that occur within 30–40 minutes of an intramuscular injection. Both drugs are metabolized principally by the liver. The serum half-life for haloperidol is 12–24 hours. Olanzapine and ziprasidone are well absorbed from the GI tract and by the intramuscular route. Olanzapine IM results in rapid absorption, with peak levels occurring within 15–45 minutes, whereas ziprasidone IM has peak levels occurring at approximately 30–60 minutes. Both drugs are metabolized principally by the liver. The serum half-life for olanzapine is 20–54 hours, and for ziprasidone, it is 2–5 hours.

II. Indications

A. Haloperidol is used for the management of acute agitated functional psychosis or extreme agitation induced by stimulants or hallucinogenic drugs, especially when drug-induced agitation has not responded to a benzodiazepine.

B. Droperidol has a more rapid onset and greater efficacy for agitation and is also useful for drug- or toxin-induced nausea and vomiting, but its role in routine therapy is uncertain because of reports of deaths and a "black box" warning about QT prolongation (see Item IV. D below). Therefore, other antiemetic drugs (eg, metoclopramide [p 581] and ondansetron [p 597]) should be considered as first-line drugs to control persistent nausea and vomiting.

C. Olanzapine and ziprasidone by the intramuscular (IM) route are approved for the management of acute agitation associated with schizophrenia, in addition to bipolar mania for olanzapine. Both have been used for the management of acute undifferentiated agitation of either psychiatric or organic (eg, drug-induced) origin. They may have comparable efficacy to haloperidol when administered by the IM route to treat acute agitation.

D. ***Note:*** **Benzodiazepines** are the usual first-line therapy for stimulant (eg, cocaine or amphetamine) intoxications and alcohol withdrawal syndromes. Combining an antipsychotic with a benzodiazepine may shorten the time to sedation for the treatment of acute agitation.

E. Nonbenzodiazepine sedatives (either **propofol** [p 613] or **dexmedetomidine** [p 540]) are often the preferred agents for sedation in mechanically ventilated adult ICU patients.

III. Contraindications

A. Severe CNS depression in the absence of airway and ventilatory control.

B. Severe parkinsonism.

C. Known hypersensitivity to the individual agent. Droperidol is structurally similar to haloperidol. Olanzapine is a thienobenzodiazepine and similar to clozapine. Ziprasidone has a unique chemical structure, a benzisothiazolyl piperazine.

D. Prolonged QTc interval. Before droperidol administration, a 12-lead ECG is recommended.

IV. Adverse effects

A. Haloperidol and droperidol produce less sedation and less hypotension than the atypical agents but are associated with a higher incidence of extrapyramidal side effects.

B. Rigidity, diaphoresis, and hyperpyrexia may be a manifestation of neuroleptic malignant syndrome (p 21) induced by haloperidol, droperidol, and other neuroleptic or antipsychotic agents.

C. Antipsychotic agents may lower the seizure threshold and should be used with caution in patients with known seizure disorder or those who have ingested a convulsant drug.

D. Large doses of haloperidol can prolong the QT interval and cause torsade de pointes (p 14). The FDA has added a **black box warning** for droperidol that QT prolongation and torsade de pointes have occurred at or below recommended doses. Ziprasidone may have a greater capacity to cause prolongation of the QT interval than does olanzapine. Risk factors for torsade de pointes arrhythmias may include bradycardia, hypokalemia, hypomagnesemia, congenital long-QT syndrome, and concomitant use of other drugs that cause QT prolongation.

E. All antipsychotic drugs may cause orthostatic hypotension and tachycardia. The atypicals have a greater propensity than do haloperidol and droperidol.

F. Some oral haloperidol tablets contain tartrazine dye, which may precipitate allergic reactions in susceptible patients.

G. The FDA has issued a **black box warning** for olanzapine and ziprasidone concerning increased mortality in geriatric patients with dementia-related psychosis.

H. The FDA has issued a black box warning for olanzapine concerning postinjection delirium/sedation syndrome. This has been associated with the use of the extended-release preparation for IM administration (Zyprexa Relprevv). Use of this product is restricted through the Zyprexa Relprevv Patient Care Program.

I. Atypical antipsychotics have been associated with hyperglycemia, ketoacidosis, hyperosmolar coma, and death.

J. Ziprasidone should be used with caution in patients with renal impairment because the excipient (cyclodextrin) in the IM preparation is cleared renally.

K. Olanzapine has anticholinergic effects and can cause tachycardia, dry mouth, and constipation.

L. Use in pregnancy. FDA Category C (indeterminate). These drugs are teratogenic and fetotoxic in animals and cross the placenta. Their safety in human pregnancy has not been established (p 498).

V. Drug or laboratory interactions

A. Antipsychotics can potentiate CNS-depressant effects of opioids, antidepressants, phenothiazines, ethanol, barbiturates, and other sedatives.

B. Combined therapy with lithium may increase the risk for neuroleptic malignant syndrome (p 21).

C. Combined therapy with agents that cause prolongation of the QT interval may increase the risk for a torsade de pointes arrhythmia.

VI. Dosage and method of administration

A. Oral. Give 2–5 mg of haloperidol PO; repeat once if necessary; usual daily dose is 3–5 mg 2–3 times (children older than 3 years: 0.05–0.15 mg/kg/d or 0.5 mg in two to three divided doses). **Olanzapine** is available as a rapidly disintegrating oral tablet; 10 mg has been used in adults to control agitation in patients with acute psychiatric disorders.

B. Parenteral. ***Caution:*** Monitor the QT interval continuously and treat torsade de pointes if it occurs (p 14).

1. **Haloperidol.** Give 2–5 mg of haloperidol IM; may repeat once after 20–30 minutes and hourly if necessary (children older than 3 years: same dosing as orally). Haloperidol is not approved for intravenous use in the United States, but that route has been used widely and is apparently safe (except with the decanoate salt formulation, which is a depo product for monthly deep IM injections only).
2. **Droperidol.** Usual adult dose for delirium is 5 mg IM, and sedative dose is 2.5–5.0 mg IM (initial maximum dose of 2.5 mg, with additional 1.25-mg doses titrated to desired effect). For antiemetic effects, usually given for 30–60 minutes as a premedication, 2.5–10 mg (children: 0.088–0.165 mg/kg) slowly IV or IM. ***Note:*** See warnings described above; use alternative antiemetics as first-line therapy.

3. **Olanzapine.** Usual adult dose for acute agitation is 2.5–10 mg IM (with additional 10-mg doses titrated at least 2 hours from the first dose and 4 hours from the second dose to the desired effect, up to a maximum daily dose of 30 mg). These higher doses are associated with a higher risk for orthostatic hypotension. Use lower dose (2.5–5 mg) in patients at risk for hypotensive reactions. Safety and efficacy in children are unknown.
4. **Ziprasidone.** Usual adult dose for acute agitation is 10–20 mg IM (with additional 10-mg doses titrated every 2 hours or 20-mg doses every 4 hours, up to a maximum daily dose of 40 mg). Safety and efficacy in children are unknown.

VII. Formulations

A. Haloperidol

1. **Oral.** Haloperidol (Haldol), 0.5-, 1-, 2-, 5-, 10-, and 20-mg tablets; 2-mg (as lactate)/mL concentrate in 15 and 120 mL; and 5- and 10-mL unit dose.
2. **Parenteral.** Haloperidol (Haldol), 5 mg (as lactate)/mL, 1-mL ampules, syringes, and vials, and 2-, 2.5-, and 10-mL vials. ***Note:*** Avoid use of the decanoate salt for acute agitation; it is a depo product for monthly deep IM injections only.

B. Droperidol (Inapsine, others), 2.5 mg/mL, 1- and 2-mL ampules or vials.

C. Olanzapine (Zyprexa IntraMuscular, various), injection, powder for solution 10-mg vial. Reconstitute with 2.1 mL of sterile water for a 5-mg/mL solution. ***Note:*** Avoid use of Zyprexa Relprevv, the extended-release powder for suspension.

D. Ziprasidone (Geodon for Injection), lyophilized powder for solution 20-mg vial. Reconstitute with 1.2 mL of sterile water for a 20-mg/mL solution.

E. Suggested minimum stocking levels to treat a 100-kg adult for the first 8 hours and 24 hours:

1. **Haloperidol,** *first 8 hours:* 10 mg or two vials of haloperidol (5 mg/mL, 10 mL each); *first 24 hours:* 30 mg or six vials of haloperidol (5 mg/mL, 10 mL each).
2. **Droperidol,** *first 8 hours:* 15 mg or three vials of droperidol (2.5 mg/mL, 2 mL each); *first 24 hours:* 45 mg or six vials of droperidol (2.5 mg/mL, 2 mL each).
3. **Olanzapine,** *first 8 hours:* 30 mg or three vials of olanzapine (10 mg each); *first 24 hours:* 30 mg or three vials of olanzapine (10 mg each).
4. **Ziprasidone,** *first 8 hours:* 40 mg or two vials of ziprasidone (20 mg each); *first 24 hours:* 40 mg or two vials of ziprasidone (20 mg each).

▶ ANTIVENOM, CROTALINAE (RATTLESNAKE)

Richard F. Clark, MD

I. **Pharmacology.** The older equine-based product, Antivenom Crotalinae Polyvalent (Wyeth-Ayerst), is no longer produced in the United States and it has been replaced by the ovine-based Crotalinae polyvalent immune Fab (CroFab, Protherics).

To produce this antivenom, sheep are hyperimmunized with pooled venom from four North American snakes: *Crotalus adamanteus, Crotalus atrox, Crotalus scutulatus, and Agkistrodon piscivorus.* Papain is added to the pooled serum product collected from the donor animals to cleave the immunogenic Fc fragment from the IgG antibody. The result is an affinity-purified Fab fragment antivenom. After administration, the antivenom is distributed widely throughout the body, binding to venom.

II. **Indications.** Antivenom is used for the treatment of signs and symptoms of envenomation by Crotalinae species (Table III–4 and p 422).

III. **Contraindications.** Known hypersensitivity to sheep or sheep serum, or to papain or papayas.

TABLE III–4. INITIAL DOSE OF CROTALINAE ANTIVENOM

Severity of Envenomation	Initial Dose (No. of Vials): Antivenom Crotalinae Polyvalent (Wyeth)	Initial Dose (No. of Vials): CroFab (Protherics)
None or minimal	None	None
Mild (local pain and swelling)	5	4
Moderate (proximal progression of swelling, ecchymosis, mild systemic symptoms)	10	4–6
Severe (hypotension, rapidly progressive swelling and ecchymosis, coagulopathy)	15	6–12

IV. Adverse effects

A. Immediate hypersensitivity reactions (including life-threatening anaphylaxis) are rare but may occur, even in patients with no history of animal serum sensitivity. Skin testing is ***not*** indicated with CroFab.

B. Mild flushing and wheezing is rare but can occur within the first 30 minutes of intravenous administration and often will decrease after the rate of infusion has been slowed.

C. Delayed hypersensitivity (serum sickness) used to occur in many patients who received the whole-IgG equine antivenom. CroFab administration can also lead to delayed hypersensitivity reactions, but these are rare.

D. Use in pregnancy. FDA Category C (indeterminate; see Table III–1). There are no data on teratogenicity. Anaphylactic reaction resulting in shock or hypoxemia in the mother could conceivably adversely affect the fetus. However, severe snake envenomation of the mother should be treated aggressively to limit venom effects that could affect the fetus or placenta.

V. Drug or laboratory interactions. There are no known interactions.

VI. Dosage and method of administration. The initial dose is based on the severity of symptoms, not on body weight (see Table III–4). Children may require doses as large as or larger than those for adults. The end point of antivenom therapy is the reversal of systemic manifestations (eg, shock, coagulopathy, and paresthesias) and the halting of progressive edema and improvement in pain. In some severe cases, large quantities of antivenom may be required (eg, 4-6 vials every hour), and laboratory blood clotting parameters may be refractory to even large doses. However, most cases can at least be stabilized with aggressive antivenom therapy. Antivenom may be effective even if given up to several days after envenomation.

A. Treat all patients in an intensive care or monitored setting.

B. Before antivenom administration, insert at least one and preferably two secure intravenous lines.

C. Reconstitute each lyophilized vial of CroFab antivenom with the 10 mL of diluent provided or sterile saline and gently swirl to solubilize the material. Avoid shaking, which may destroy the immunoglobulins (as indicated by foam formation). Further dilution with normal saline may facilitate solubilization. Reconstituted product should be used within 4 hours.

D. Administer antivenom by the intravenous route only. Start slowly, increasing the rate as tolerated. The infusion of 4–6 vials of CroFab should be completed over 60 minutes, but the infusion rate may be increased or decreased as tolerated and clinically indicated.

E. If there is an inadequate response to the initial dose, give an additional 4–6 vials of CroFab over 60 minutes. Repeat in four- to six-vial increments per hour until the progression of symptoms is halted and stabilization attained.

F. Recurrence of symptoms of envenomation may occur in patients treated with CroFab owing to the shorter half-life within the body of the Fab molecule.

1. Recurrence after CroFab usually manifests 12–36 hours after stabilization has been achieved with the initial dosing and can be seen in 30% or more cases in some regions. Repeating laboratory tests and observing for progression or recurrence of swelling are, therefore, recommended for 24–48 hours or more after the last antivenom infusion.
2. As an alternative to help prevent recurrence, the CroFab package insert suggests for severe envenomations to consider two-vial dosing every 6 hours for three additional doses after stabilization, but in our experience, these extra doses are often not effective in preventing recurrent effects of envenomation.
3. Case reports have also suggested using a continuous low-dose infusion of 2–4 vials of CroFab per day for several days in severe cases of recurrence, but clinical trials of this regimen are lacking.

VII. Formulations

A. Crotalinae polyvalent immune Fab (CroFab). Each box contains 2 vials of CroFab.

Supplies can be located by a regional poison center (1-800-222-1222).

B. Suggested minimum stocking levels to treat a 100-kg adult for the first 8 hours and 24 hours: **Crotalinae polyvalent immune Fab (CroFab)**, *first 8 hours: 18 vials; first 24 hours:* 36 vials.

▶ ANTIVENOM, *LATRODECTUS MACTANS* (BLACK WIDOW SPIDER)

Richard F. Clark, MD

I. Pharmacology. To produce the antivenom, horses are hyperimmunized with *Latrodectus mactans* (black widow spider) venom. The lyophilized protein product from pooled equine sera contains whole-IgG antibodies specific to certain venom fractions as well as residual serum proteins such as albumin and globulins. After intravenous administration, the antivenom distributes widely throughout the body, where it binds to and neutralizes venom. A new $F(ab)_2$ antivenom for black widow spider envenomation has been developed but is not yet approved for use in the United States. The new product may be safer than the presently approved whole-IgG product.

II. Indications

A. Black widow envenomation–induced severe hypertension or muscle pain or cramping that is not alleviated by muscle relaxants, analgesics, or sedation; consider particularly in patients at the extremes of age (ie, younger than 1 year or older than 65 years).

B. Black widow envenomation in **pregnancy** may cause abdominal muscle spasms severe enough to threaten spontaneous abortion or early onset of labor.

III. Contraindications. Known hypersensitivity to horse serum.

IV. Adverse effects

A. Immediate hypersensitivity may rarely occur, including life-threatening anaphylaxis.

B. Delayed-onset serum sickness may occur after 7–14 days but is rare owing to the small volume of antivenom used in most cases.

C. Use in pregnancy. FDA Category C (indeterminate). There are no data on teratogenicity. An anaphylactic reaction resulting in shock or hypoxemia in the mother could conceivably affect the fetus adversely (see Table III–1).

V. Drug or laboratory interactions. No known interactions.

VI. Dosage and method of administration. In most cases, one vial of antivenom is sufficient to treat black widow envenomation in adults or children. The antivenom is dosed on the basis of symptoms, not on patient weight.

A. Treat all patients in a monitored setting, such as an emergency department.

B. Before a skin test or antivenom administration, insert at least one and preferably two secure intravenous lines.

C. Perform a skin test for horse serum sensitivity by using a 1:10 dilution of antivenom (some experts prefer this method) or the sample of horse serum provided in the antivenom kit (according to package instructions). Do not perform the skin test unless signs of envenomation are present and imminent antivenom therapy is anticipated. If the skin test is positive, reconsider the need for antivenom as opposed to supportive care, but do ***not*** abandon antivenom therapy if it is needed. Even if the skin test is negative, anaphylaxis may still occur unpredictably in rare cases.

D. If antivenom is used in a patient with horse serum sensitivity, pretreat with intravenous diphenhydramine (p 544) and ranitidine or another H_2 blocker (p 532) and have ready at the bedside a preloaded syringe containing epinephrine (1:10,000 for intravenous use) in case of anaphylaxis. Dilute the antivenom 1:10 to 1:1,000 and administer it very slowly in these cases.

E. Reconstitute the lyophilized product to 2.5 mL with the supplied diluent, using gentle swirling for 15–30 minutes to avoid shaking and destroying the immunoglobulins (as indicated by the formation of foam).

F. Dilute this solution to a total volume of 10–50 mL with normal saline.

G. Administer the diluted antivenom slowly over 15–30 minutes. One or two vials are sufficient in most cases.

VII. Formulations

A. Lyophilized antivenom (*L. mactans*), 6,000 units, contains 1:10,000 thimerosal as a preservative. ***Note:*** Product is also listed as antivenin (*L. mactans*).

B. Suggested minimum stocking levels to treat a 100-kg adult for the first 8 hours and 24 hours: **antivenom (*L. mactans*)**, *first 8 hours:* one vial; *first 24 hours:* one vial. ***Note:*** Merck is the manufacturer of the only approved black widow spider antivenom in the United States, and the company has suspended production of the product. Inventories are now quite low, and Merck, in cooperation with the FDA, has extended the expiration date on some lots of this product. Emergency supplies are available for symptomatic patients by contacting the Merck National Service Center at 1-800-672-6372.

▶ ANTIVENOM, *MICRURUS FULVIUS* (CORAL SNAKE), AND EXOTIC ANTIVENOMS

Richard F. Clark, MD

I. Pharmacology

A. To produce the antivenom for North American **coral snake** bites, horses are hyperimmunized with venom from *Micrurus fulvius,* the eastern coral snake. The lyophilized protein preparation from pooled equine sera contains IgG antibodies to venom fractions as well as residual serum proteins. Administered intravenously, the antibodies distribute widely throughout the body, where they bind the target venom.

B. Exotic antivenoms. Companies outside the United States produce a variety of antivenoms for exotic snakebites. Most of these products are used to treat snakebites by elapids because this family of snakes causes the most severe envenomations worldwide. Many of these are still whole-antibody products derived from horses. A few are produced as Fab fragments, or the slightly larger $F(ab)_2$ molecule (cleaved with pepsin instead of papain). In both of these cases, the Fc is removed from the solution. Many foreign antivenom products are polyvalent, a mixture of antivenoms for several species.

II. Indications

A. Envenomation by the eastern coral snake (*M. fulvius*) or the Texas coral snake (*M. fulvius tenere*).

B. *May not be effective* for envenomation by the western, Arizona, or Sonora coral snake (*Micrurus euryxanthus*), but symptomatic bites by these small western US elapids are very rare.

III. Contraindications. Known hypersensitivity to *Micrurus* antivenom or to horse serum is a relative contraindication; if a patient with significant envenomation needs the antivenom, it should be given with caution. Antivenoms produced outside the United States may be made from horse or sheep serum.

IV. Adverse effects

A. Immediate hypersensitivity, including life-threatening anaphylaxis, may occur even after a negative skin test for horse serum sensitivity.

B. Delayed hypersensitivity (serum sickness) may occur 1–3 weeks after whole-antibody antivenom administration, with the incidence and severity depending on the total quantity of antivenom administered.

C. Use in pregnancy. FDA Category C (indeterminate). There are no data on teratogenicity. Anaphylactic reactions resulting in shock or hypoxemia in expectant mothers could conceivably affect the fetus adversely. This should be weighed against the potential detrimental effect of the venom on both the placenta and the fetus (see Table III–1).

D. Exotic antivenoms. All whole-antibody preparations carry the same risk for immediate and delayed allergy.

V. Drug or laboratory interactions. There are no known interactions.

VI. Dosage and method of administration. Generally, the recommended initial dose of *Micrurus* antivenom is three to five vials. The drug is most effective if given before the onset of signs or symptoms of envenomation. An additional three to five vials may be given, depending on the severity of neurologic manifestations but not on body weight (children may require doses as large as or even larger than those for adults).

The recommended dose of exotic snake antivenom will vary. With other elapids, such as cobras, the antivenom is also more effective if given early in the course of the envenomation.

A. Treat all patients in an intensive care unit setting.

B. Before a skin test or antivenom administration, insert at least one and preferably two secure intravenous lines.

C. Perform a skin test for horse serum sensitivity, using a 1:10 dilution of antivenom (some experts prefer this method) or the sample of horse serum provided in the antivenom kit (according to package instructions). If the skin test is positive, reconsider the need for antivenom as opposed to supportive care, but do not abandon antivenom therapy if it is needed. Even if the skin test is negative, anaphylaxis may occur unpredictably.

Antivenoms to exotic species may not contain skin-testing solutions. A small amount (0.1 mL) of antivenom can be used as a skin test for these preparations, or this step may be omitted. Fab and $F(ab)_2$ antivenom preparations generally do not require skin testing before administration.

D. If antivenom is used in a patient with a positive skin test, pretreat with intravenous diphenhydramine (p 544) and ranitidine or another H_2 blocker (p 532) and have ready at the bedside a preloaded syringe containing epinephrine (1:10,000 for intravenous use) in case of anaphylaxis. Dilute the antivenom 1:10–1:1,000 and administer very slowly in these cases.

E. Reconstitute the lyophilized *Micrurus* antivenom with 10 mL of the diluent supplied, gently swirling for 10–30 minutes. Avoid shaking the preparation because this may destroy the immunoglobulins (as indicated by the formation of foam). Dilution with 50–200 mL of saline may aid solubilization.

F. Administer the antivenom intravenously over 15–30 minutes per vial.

G. Exotic elapids. Envenomation by exotic elapids, such as cobras, mambas, and all the poisonous snakes of Australia, would be expected to produce a degree of neurotoxicity the same as or worse than that seen in envenomation from coral snakes from the United States, and antivenom administration is required as soon as possible. It is conceivable that bites from snakes within the same family could respond to antivenom made from venom of another snake in that family. Therefore, if type-specific antivenom is not available for a severe snakebite, same-family antivenom may be substituted with some possible efficacy. Regional poison centers (1-800-222-1222) may be able to assist in obtaining exotic antivenoms from collectors or zoos.

VII. Formulations

A. Antivenom (*M. fulvius*) vial of lyophilized powder with 0.25% phenol and 0.005% thimerosal as preservatives. ***Note:*** This product is also listed as antivenin (*M. fulvius*).

B. Suggested minimum stocking levels to treat a 100-kg adult for the first 8 hours and 24 hours: **antivenom (*M. fulvius*)**, *first 8 hours:* five vials; *first 24 hours:* 10 vials. ***Note:*** The production of *Micrurus* antivenom has ceased in the United States. Stocks remain in some geographic locations where coral snakes are most common, but supplies will likely be scarce or run out in the future. No alternative foreign antivenom is currently available as a substitute, but clinical trials are underway that may result in new products. As a temporizing measure, the US Food and Drug Administration (FDA) has tested expiring lots of remaining vials of *Micrurus* antivenom and found that they are active beyond their expiration date. The FDA has therefore extended the expiration date on many remaining supplies of *Micrurus* antivenom.

▶ ANTIVENOM, *CENTRUROIDES* (SCORPION) IMMUNE F(ab')$_2$ (EQUINE)

Richard F. Clark, MD

I. Pharmacology. To produce the antivenom, horses are hyperimmunized with venom from four species of *Centruroides* scorpions (*C. noxius*, *C.l. limpidus*, *C.l. tecomanus*, and *C.s. suffuses*). The equine scorpion antibodies are cleaved with pepsin to form F(ab')$_2$ fragments. After intravenous administration, the antivenom distributes widely throughout the body, where it binds to venom.

II. Indications. Clinical signs of serious *Centruroides* scorpion envenomation, such as loss of muscle control, severe pain, roving or abnormal eye movements, slurred speech, respiratory distress, excessive salivation, frothing at the mouth, and vomiting.

III. Contraindications. Although the package insert does not list any contraindications, known hypersensitivity to horse serum or horses may predispose patients to anaphylaxis after administration of equine-derived antivenom.

IV. Adverse effects

A. Immediate hypersensitivity may rarely occur, including life-threatening anaphylaxis.

B. Delayed-onset serum sickness may occur but is less likely than with whole-IgG antivenoms.

C. The most commonly reported adverse effects include vomiting, fever, rash, and itching. Each vial of the scorpion antivenom contains a small amount of cresol, and localized reactions and myalgias have occurred with the use of cresol as an excipient.

D. **Use in pregnancy.** FDA Category C (indeterminate). There are no data on teratogenicity. An anaphylactic reaction resulting in shock or hypoxemia in the mother could conceivably affect the fetus adversely (see Table III–1, p 498).

V. **Drug or laboratory interactions.** No known interactions.

VI. **Dosage and method of administration.** The starting dose of *Centruroides* scorpion antivenom is three vials. Dose is based on symptoms, not on patient weight. If additional doses of antivenom are required, they should be administered one vial at a time.

A. Treat all patients in an emergency department or intensive care setting.

B. No skin testing is required before scorpion antivenom administration.

C. If antivenom is used in a patient with known or suspected horse serum sensitivity, it may be helpful to pretreat with intravenous diphenhydramine (p 544) and ranitidine or another H_2 blocker (p 532) and have ready at the bedside a preloaded syringe containing epinephrine (1:10,000 for intravenous use) in case of anaphylaxis.

D. Reconstitute each vial of the lyophilized product with 5 mL of normal saline, using gentle swirling to avoid shaking and destroying the immunoglobulins (as indicated by the formation of foam).

E. Dilute the starting dose of three vials to a total volume of 50 mL with normal saline.

F. Administer the diluted antivenom intravenously over 10 minutes. When needed, administer additional doses one vial at a time at 30–60 minute intervals. Three vials are sufficient in most cases.

VII. **Formulations**

A. Lyophilized antivenom (*Centruroides*), each vial contains no more than 120 mg of protein (>85% $F(ab)_2$, <7% Fab, and <5% intact immunoglobulin); sodium chloride, sucrose, and glycine are used as stabilizers, and trace amounts of cresol, pepsin, borates, and sulfates may be present from the production process.

B. **Suggested minimum stocking levels** to treat a 100-kg adult for the first 8 hours and 24 hours: *Centruroides (Scorpion) Immune $F(ab)_2$ (Equine), first 8 hours:* three vials; *first 24 hours:* three vials.

▶ ATROPINE AND GLYCOPYRROLATE

Richard J. Geller, MD, MPH

I. **Pharmacology.** Atropine and glycopyrrolate competitively block the action of acetylcholine at muscarinic receptors. Desired therapeutic effects for treating poisoning include decreased secretions from salivary and other glands, decreased bronchorrhea and wheezing, decreased intestinal secretion and peristalsis, increased heart rate, and enhanced atrioventricular conduction.

A. **Atropine** is a naturally occurring tertiary amine that crosses the blood–brain barrier and has significant structural and functional similarity to scopolamine, homatropine, and ipratropium. The elimination half-life of atropine is 2–4 hours (longer in children), with approximately 50% excreted unchanged in urine.

B. **Glycopyrrolate** is a synthetic quaternary amine that crosses the blood–brain barrier poorly and is less likely than atropine to cause altered mental status or tachycardia. It has approximately twice the potency of atropine. Glycopyrrolate is excreted unchanged primarily in the bile and the urine.

C. ***Note:*** These drugs do ***not*** reverse the effects of excess acetylcholine at nicotinic receptors of the neuromuscular junctions, ganglia of the parasympathetic and sympathetic nervous system, and CNS.

II. **Indications**

A. Correction of bronchorrhea and excessive oral and GI tract secretions associated with cholinesterase inhibitor (eg, organophosphorus and carbamate insecticide) intoxication. Glycopyrrolate may be especially useful in managing peripheral muscarinic symptoms in cholinesterase inhibitor poisoning. Although glycopyrrolate will not reverse CNS toxicity associated with cholinesterase inhibitor poisoning, it also will not cause the CNS side effects seen with large doses of atropine, which are difficult to distinguish from the toxic effects of cholinesterase inhibitors.

B. Acceleration of the rate of sinus node firing and atrioventricular (AV) nodal conduction velocity in the presence of drug-induced AV conduction impairment (eg, caused by cardiac glycosides, beta-adrenergic blocking agents, calcium channel antagonists, organophosphorus or carbamate insecticides, or physostigmine).

C. Reversal of central (by atropine) and peripheral (by atropine and glycopyrrolate) muscarinic symptoms in patients with intoxication by *Clitocybe* or *Inocybe* mushroom species.

D. When either neostigmine or pyridostigmine is used to reverse nondepolarizing neuromuscular blockade, glycopyrrolate is the preferred agent to block unwanted muscarinic effects (see "Neuromuscular Blockers," p 586).

III. Contraindications. All these contraindications are relative, and in some clinical situations benefit exceeds possible harm.

A. Patients with hypertension, tachyarrhythmias, thyrotoxicosis, congestive heart failure, coronary artery disease, valvular heart disease, or other illnesses, who might not tolerate a rapid heart rate. ***Note:*** Patients with cholinesterase inhibitor poisoning are often tachycardic, but antimuscarinics may still be given because they can improve oxygenation, thereby reducing catecholamine release associated with hypoxia; glycopyrrolate may be less likely than atropine to cause excessive tachycardia.

B. Angle-closure glaucoma, in which papillary dilation may increase intraocular pressure (may be used safely if the patient is being treated with a miotic agent).

C. Partial or complete obstructive uropathy.

D. Myasthenia gravis.

E. Obstructive diseases of the GI tract, severe ulcerative colitis, bacterial infections of the GI tract.

IV. Adverse effects

A. Adverse effects include dry mouth, blurred vision, cycloplegia and mydriasis, palpitations, tachycardia, aggravation of angina, congestive heart failure (CHF), and constipation. Urinary retention is common, and a Foley catheter may be needed. Duration of effects may be prolonged (several hours). Additionally, CNS antimuscarinic toxicity (delirium) may occur with the large doses of atropine needed to treat cholinesterase inhibitor poisoning.

B. Atropine doses of less than 0.5 mg (in adults) and those administered by very slow intravenous push may result in paradoxical slowing of the heart rate.

C. Use in pregnancy. Atropine is classified as FDA Category C (indeterminate). It readily crosses the placenta. However, this does not preclude its acute, short-term use for a seriously symptomatic patient (p 498). Glycopyrrolate is classified as FDA Category B and crosses the placenta poorly.

V. Drug or laboratory interactions

A. Atropinization may occur more rapidly if atropine and pralidoxime are given concurrently to patients with cholinesterase inhibitor poisoning.

B. Atropine and glycopyrrolate have an additive effect with other antimuscarinic and antihistaminic compounds.

C. Slowing of GI motility may delay absorption of orally ingested materials.

VI. Dosage and method of administration

A. Cholinesterase inhibitor poisoning (eg, organophosphorus or carbamate insecticides, "nerve agents")

1. Atropine. For adults, begin with 1–5 mg IV; for children, give 0.02 mg/kg IV. (The drug may also be given via the intratracheal route; dilute the dose in normal saline to a total volume of 1–2 mL.) Double the dose every 5 minutes until satisfactory atropinization is achieved (mainly decreased bronchial secretions and wheezing). Severely poisoned patients may require very large doses (eg, up to 100 mg over a few hours). In mass casualty situations, atropine can be given IM. It may also be administered by ophthalmic and inhalation routes for reversal of topical effects from gas or mist exposures.

2. **Glycopyrrolate.** Initial IV dose for adults is 0.5–2 mg (children: 0.025 mg/kg). As with atropine, the dose may be doubled every 5 minutes until satisfactory antimuscarinic effects have been achieved.
3. **Other agents.** If a mass casualty situation depletes the local supply of atropine and glycopyrrolate, other muscarinic receptor antagonist agents, such as scopolamine (tertiary) and ipratropium (quaternary), may be considered.
4. **Therapeutic end points.** The goal of therapy is the drying of bronchial secretions (this end point may be reached prematurely if the patient is dehydrated) and reversal of wheezing and significant bradycardia.

B. **Drug-induced bradycardia.** Atropine is usually the drug of choice in this circumstance. For adults, give 0.5–1 mg IV; for children and adolescents, give 0.02 mg/kg IV up to a maximum of 0.5 and 1 mg, respectively. Repeat as needed. Note that 3 mg is a fully vagolytic dose in adults. If a response is not achieved after the administration of 3 mg, the patient is unlikely to benefit from further treatment unless bradycardia is caused by excessive muscarinic effects (eg, carbamate or organophosphorus poisoning).

VII. **Formulations**

A. **Parenteral.** Atropine sulfate injection is available as 0.05-, 0.1-, 0.4-, 0.5-, and 1-mg/mL solutions and is packaged in 0.5- to 10-mL syringes, 0.5- to 1-mL ampules, and 1- to 30-mL vials. (Atropine is stockpiled by the Strategic National Stockpile [SNS] program as 20-mL vials of the 0.4-mg/mL solution and combined [2 mg per dose] with pralidoxime [600 mg per dose] in the Mark 1 auto-injector kits.) Use preservative-free formulations when massive doses are required. Glycopyrrolate injection (Robinul, others), 0.2 mg/mL in 1-, 2-, 5-, and 20-mL vials (some with 0.9% benzyl alcohol).

B. **Suggested minimum stocking levels** to treat a 100-kg adult for the first 8 hours and 24 hours:

1. **Atropine sulfate,** *first 8 hours*: 100 mg or 13 vials of atropine (0.4 mg/mL, 20 mL each); *first 24 hours*: 200 mg or 26 vials of atropine (0.4 mg/mL, 20 mL each).
2. **Glycopyrrolate,** *first 8 hours*: 52 mg or 13 vials of glycopyrrolate (0.2 mg/mL, 20 mL each); *first 24 hours:* 100 mg or 25 vials of glycopyrrolate (0.2 mg/mL, 20 mL each).

► BAL (DIMERCAPROL)

Michael J. Kosnett, MD, MPH

I. **Pharmacology.** BAL (British anti-lewisite; dimercaprol; 2,3-dimercaptopropanol) is a dithiol chelating agent that is used in the treatment of poisoning by the heavy metals arsenic, mercury, lead, and gold. Because the vicinal thiol groups are unstable in aqueous solution, the drug is supplied as a 10% solution (100 mg/mL) in peanut oil that also contains 20% (200 mg/mL) benzyl benzoate. It is administered by deep IM injection. Most of the drug is absorbed within 1 hour and undergoes widespread distribution to most tissues. BAL, or its in vivo biotransformation product(s), is believed to form complexes with selected toxic metals, thereby minimizing the reaction of the metals with endogenous ligands and increasing their excretion in urine. In a study of humans treated with BAL after exposure to arsenicals, peak urinary arsenic excretion occurred in 2–4 hours and then declined rapidly.

II. Indications

A. Acute inorganic **arsenic** poisoning. Limited data suggest that it may also be useful in the early stages of arsine poisoning (ie, during the first 24 hours).

B. Mercury poisoning (except with monoalkyl mercury). BAL is most effective in preventing renal damage if it is administered within 4 hours after acute ingestion of inorganic mercury salts; its value in averting or treating the acute or chronic neurologic effects of elemental mercury vapor is unknown.

C. Lead poisoning (except with alkyl lead compounds). BAL has been used concomitantly with calcium EDTA (p 548) in the treatment of pediatric lead encephalopathy, in which the joint regimen was associated with an accelerated decline in blood lead levels and increased urinary lead excretion. ***Note:*** BAL is not for use as a single-drug regimen in lead poisoning.

D. Gold. BAL has been associated with an increase in urinary gold excretion and clinical improvement in patients treated for adverse dermatologic, hematologic, or neurologic complications of pharmaceutical gold preparations.

III. Contraindications

A. Because BAL is dispensed in peanut oil, avoid use in patients with peanut allergy.

B. Use with caution in patients who have hepatic and renal impairment. A few reports suggest that dimercaprol or its metabolites are dialyzable and that BAL increases the dialysis clearance of mercury in patients with renal failure.

C. BAL has caused hemolysis in patients with glucose-6-phosphate dehydrogenase (G6PD) deficiency.

D. Because BAL is given by IM injection, use with caution in patients with thrombocytopenia or coagulopathies.

IV. Adverse effects

A. Local pain at injection site, sterile or pyogenic abscess formation.

B. Dose-related hypertension, with or without tachycardia. Onset, 15–30 minutes; duration, 2 hours. Use with caution in hypertensive patients.

C. Other adverse symptoms. Nausea and vomiting; headache; burning sensations in the eyes, lips, mouth, and throat, sometimes accompanied by lacrimation, rhinorrhea, or salivation; myalgias; paresthesias; fever (particularly in children); a sensation of constriction in the chest; and generalized anxiety. Central nervous system depression and seizures have occurred in overdose.

D. Use in pregnancy. FDA Category C (indeterminate [p 498]). High doses of BAL are teratogenic and embryotoxic in mice. The safety of BAL in human pregnancy is not established, although it has been used in a pregnant patient who had Wilson disease without apparent harm. It should be used in pregnancy only for life-threatening acute intoxication.

E. Redistribution of metals to the brain. Despite its capacity to increase survival in acutely poisoned animals, BAL has been associated with redistribution of mercury and arsenic into the brain. Avoid use in chronic elemental mercury poisoning or alkyl (eg, methyl) mercury poisoning, in which the brain is a key target organ.

V. Drug or laboratory interactions

A. Because a toxic complex with iron may be formed, avoid concurrent iron replacement therapy.

B. BAL may abruptly terminate gold therapy–induced remission of rheumatoid arthritis.

VI. Dosage and method of administration (adults and children)

A. Arsenic, mercury, and gold poisoning. Give BAL, 3-mg/kg deep intramuscular injection every 4–6 hours for 2 days, then every 12 hours for up to 7–10 days if the patient remains symptomatic and/or metal levels remain highly elevated. In patients with severe arsenic or mercury poisoning, an initial dose of up to 5 mg/kg may be used. Consider changing to oral succimer (p 624) or oral unithiol (p 630) once the patient is stable and able to absorb an oral formulation. ***Note:*** Intravenous unithiol has a more favorable therapeutic index than BAL does and may be a preferable alternative in the treatment of acute arsenic or mercury intoxication.

B. **Lead encephalopathy** (only in conjunction with calcium EDTA therapy [p 548]). For acute pediatric lead encephalopathy, some clinicians initiate treatment with BAL, 3–4 mg/kg IM (75 mg/m^2), followed in 4 hours by concomitant use of calcium EDTA and BAL, 3–4 mg/kg (75 mg/m^2) every 4–6 hours for up to 3 days.

C. **Arsine poisoning** (p 144). Consider the use of BAL, 3 mg/kg IM every 4–6 hours for 1 day, if it can be begun within 24 hours of the onset of arsine poisoning.

D. **Lewisite burns to the eye.** Create a 5% solution of BAL by diluting the 10% ampule 1:1 in vegetable oil and *immediately* apply to the surface of the eye and conjunctivae. Parenteral treatment may also be necessary to treat systemic effects (p 452).

VII. **Formulations**

A. **Parenteral** (for deep IM injection only; must ***not*** be given IV). BAL in oil, 100-mg/mL, 3-mL ampules.

B. **Suggested minimum stocking levels** to treat a 100-kg adult for the first 8 and 24 hours: **BAL**, *first 8 hours:* 600 mg or two ampules (100 mg/mL, 3 mL each); *first 24 hours:* 1,800 mg or six ampules (100 mg/mL, 3 mL each).

▶ BENZODIAZEPINES (DIAZEPAM, LORAZEPAM, AND MIDAZOLAM)

Thomas E. Kearney, PharmD

I. **Pharmacology**

A. Benzodiazepines potentiate inhibitory gamma-aminobutyric acid (GABA) neuronal activity in the CNS. Pharmacologic effects include reduction of anxiety, suppression of seizure activity, CNS depression (possible respiratory arrest when benzodiazepines are given rapidly intravenously), and inhibition of spinal afferent pathways to produce skeletal muscle relaxation.

B. Benzodiazepines interact with other receptors outside the CNS, especially in the heart. Diazepam has been reported to antagonize the cardiotoxic effect of chloroquine (the mechanism is unknown, but diazepam may compete with chloroquine for fixation sites on cardiac cells).

C. Benzodiazepines generally have little effect on the autonomic nervous system or cardiovascular system. However, enhancement of GABA neurotransmission may blunt sympathetic discharge (and lower blood pressure elevation associated with sympathomimetic intoxications). Additionally, diazepam may have an effect on choline transport and acetylcholine turnover in the CNS, which may be part of the basis for its beneficial effect in victims of nerve agent poisoning (eg, sarin, VX).

D. **Pharmacokinetics.** All these agents are well absorbed orally, but diazepam is not well absorbed intramuscularly. The drugs are eliminated by hepatic metabolism, with serum elimination half-lives of 1–50 hours. The duration of CNS effects is determined by the rate of drug redistribution from the brain to peripheral tissues. Active metabolites further extend the duration of effect of diazepam.

1. **Diazepam.** Onset of action is fast after intravenous injection but slow to intermediate after oral or rectal administration. The half-life is longer than 24 hours, although anticonvulsant effects and sedation are often shorter as a result of redistribution from the CNS.
2. **Lorazepam.** Onset is intermediate after intramuscular dosing. The elimination half-life is 10–20 hours, and owing to slower CNS redistribution, its anticonvulsant effects are generally longer than those of diazepam.
3. **Midazolam.** Onset is rapid after intramuscular or intravenous injection and intermediate after nasal application or ingestion. The half-life is 1.5–3 hours,

and the duration of effects is very short owing to rapid redistribution from the brain. However, sedation may persist for 10 hours or longer after prolonged infusions as a result of saturation of peripheral sites and slowed redistribution.

II. Indications

A. **Anxiety and agitation.** Benzodiazepines often are used for the treatment of anxiety or agitation (eg, caused by sympathomimetic, anticholinergic, cannabinoid, or hallucinogenic drug, plant, or venom intoxications). ***Note:*** physostigmine (p 609) is a more selective antidote for anticholingeric-induced agitated delirium.

B. **Convulsions.** All three drugs can be used for the treatment of acute seizure activity or status epilepticus resulting from idiopathic epilepsy or convulsant drug or toxin overdose. Midazolam and lorazepam have the advantage of rapid absorption after intramuscular injection. Also, the duration of anticonvulsant action of lorazepam is longer than that of the other two agents.

C. **Hypertension and tachycardia.** These drugs can be used for the initial treatment of sympathomimetically induced hypertension and tachycardia.

D. **Muscle relaxant.** These drugs can be used for relaxation of excessive muscle rigidity and contractions (eg, as in strychnine poisoning or black widow spider envenomation, or in rigidity syndromes with hyperthermia, dyskinesias, or tetanus).

E. **Chloroquine poisoning**. Diazepam may antagonize cardiotoxicity.

F. **Alcohol or sedative–hypnotic withdrawal**. Diazepam and lorazepam are used to abate symptoms and signs of alcohol and hypnotic–sedative withdrawal (eg, anxiety, tremor, and seizures).

G. **Conscious sedation**. Midazolam is used to induce sedation and amnesia during brief procedures and in conjunction with neuromuscular paralysis for endotracheal intubation.

H. **Nerve agents.** These drugs can be used for the treatment of agitation, muscle fasciculations, and seizures associated with nerve agent poisoning (p 452). They may have an additive or synergistic effect with other nerve agent antidotes (2-PAM, atropine).

III. Contraindications. Do not use in patients with a known sensitivity to benzodiazepines.

IV. Adverse effects

A. Central nervous system–depressant effects may interfere with evaluation of neurologic function. They also may cause a paradoxical reaction (restlessness, agitation) in less than 1% of patients (adults and children). Flumazenil (p 556) has been used successfully to manage this effect.

B. Excessive or rapid intravenous administration may cause respiratory arrest.

C. The drug may precipitate or worsen hepatic encephalopathy.

D. Rapid or large-volume IV administration may cause cardiotoxicity similar to that seen with phenytoin (p 608) because of the diluent propylene glycol. Continuous infusions with this vehicle may also result in hyperlactatemia, increased osmolar gap, and renal dysfunction. Infusions of lorazepam (1 mL of injection solution contains 0.8 mL or 834 mg of propylene glycol) exceeding 4 mg/h or with cumulative 24-hour doses exceeding 100 mg are associated with potentially toxic serum propylene glycol levels ($>$25 mg/dL). Several products also contain up to 2% benzyl alcohol as a preservative.

E. **Use in pregnancy.** FDA Category D. All these drugs readily cross the placenta. However, this does not preclude their acute, short-term use for a seriously symptomatic patient (p 498).

V. Drug or laboratory interactions

A. Benzodiazepines will potentiate the CNS-depressant effects of opioids, ethanol, and other sedative–hypnotic and depressant drugs.

B. **Flumazenil** (p 556) will reverse the effects of benzodiazepines and may trigger an acute abstinence syndrome in patients who use the drugs chronically.

Patients who have received flumazenil will have an unpredictable but reduced or absent response to benzodiazepines.

C. Diazepam may produce a false-positive glucose reaction with Clinistix and Diastix test strips.

VI. Dosage and method of administration

A. Anxiety or agitation, muscle spasm or hyperactivity, hypertension

1. **Diazepam.** Give 2–10 mg (children aged 30 days to 5 years: 1–2 mg) IV initially (no faster than 5 mg/min in adults; administer over 3 minutes in children), depending on severity (tetanus requires higher doses); may repeat every 1–4 hours as needed. The oral dose is 2–10 mg (geriatric patients: lower doses, not to exceed 2.5 mg and given at less frequent intervals; children older than 6 months: 1–2.5 mg). Doses should be adjusted according to tolerance and response. ***Caution:*** Do ***not*** give intramuscularly because of erratic absorption and pain on injection. Use lorazepam or midazolam if IM administration is necessary.
2. **Lorazepam.** Give 1–2 mg (children: 0.04 mg/kg) IV, not to exceed 2 mg/min or 0.05 mg/kg IM (maximum, 4 mg). The usual adult oral dose is 2–6 mg daily.
3. **Midazolam.** Give 0.05 mg/kg (up to 0.35 mg/kg for anesthesia induction) IV over 20–30 seconds (usual adult dose: varies from 1 mg to a maximum of 5 mg given in increments of 2.5 mg every 2 minutes; geriatric patients: lower dose with maximum at 3.5 mg) or 0.07–0.1 mg/kg IM. Repeat after 10–20 minutes if needed. Continuous infusions have also been used to maintain effect with initial rates of 0.02–0.1 mg/kg/h (usual adult dose: 1–7 mg/h; children: 1–2 mcg/kg/min) that are then titrated to effect. ***Caution:*** There have been several reports of respiratory arrest and hypotension after rapid intravenous injection, especially when midazolam was given in combination with opioids. Prolonged continuous infusion may lead to persistent sedation after the drug is discontinued because midazolam accumulates in tissues.

B. Convulsions. ***Note:*** If convulsions persist after initial doses of benzodiazepines, consider alternative anticonvulsant drugs such as phenobarbital (p 604), pentobarbital (p 602), and propofol (p 613), and give pyridoxine (p 621) for isoniazid or hydrazine-containing mushroom intoxications. Also, see "Seizures" (p 23).

1. **Diazepam.** Give 5–10 mg IV, not to exceed 5 mg/min, every 5–10 minutes (children 5 years of age or older: 1–2 mg; children younger than 5 years: 0.2–0.5 mg) to a maximum total of 30 mg (adults) or 10 mg (older children) or 5 mg (young children). If no IV access, may give rectally (adults and children older than 12 years: 0.2 mg/kg; children 6–11 years: 0.3 mg/kg; children 2–5 years: 0.5 mg/kg).
2. **Lorazepam.** Give 1–2 mg (neonates: 0.05–0.1 mg/kg; older children: 0.04 mg/kg) IV, not to exceed 2 mg/min; repeat if needed after 5–10 minutes. Usual dose for status epilepticus is up to 4 mg slow IV push over 2 minutes (dilute with an equal volume of saline). If seizure recurs, repeat dose after 10–15 minutes. The drug can also be given IM (0.05 mg/kg; maximum, 4 mg), with onset of effects after 6–10 minutes.
3. **Midazolam.** Give 0.05 mg/kg (up to 0.2 mg/kg for refractory status epilepticus) IV over 20–30 seconds or 0.1–0.2 mg/kg IM; this may be repeated if needed after 5–10 minutes or maintained with a continuous infusion (see "***Note***" above). The drug is absorbed rapidly after IM injection and can be used when IV access is not readily available. Other available routes of administration in children include intranasal (0.2–0.5 mg/kg) and buccal (0.3 mg/kg or 10 mg in older children and adolescents).

C. Chloroquine and hydroxychloroquine intoxication. There is reported improvement of cardiotoxicity with **high-dose** administration of **diazepam** at 1–2 mg/kg IV (infuse over 30 minutes), followed by an infusion of 1–2 mg/kg/24 h.

Caution: This probably will cause apnea; the patient must be intubated, and ventilation must be controlled.

D. Alcohol withdrawal syndrome

1. **Diazepam.** Administer 5–10 mg IV initially, then 5 mg every 10 minutes until the patient is calm. Large doses may be required to sedate patients with severe withdrawal. The oral dose is 10–20 mg initially, repeated every 1–2 hours until the patient is calm.
2. **Lorazepam.** Administer 1–2 mg IV initially, then 1 mg every 10 minutes until the patient is calm. Large doses by intermittent IV bolus or with high rates of administration by continuous infusion may be required to sedate patients in severe withdrawal. (***Caution:*** Multiple-dose vials may contain diluents and preservatives such as propylene glycol and benzyl alcohol, which can be toxic in high doses; see Item IV.D above.) The usual oral dose is 2–4 mg, repeated every 1–2 hours until the patient is calm.

VII. Formulations

A. Parenteral

1. **Diazepam** (Valium, others): 5-mg/mL solution; 2-mL prefilled syringes; 1-, 2-, and 10-mL vials. A 10-mg IM auto-injector (ComboPen) is available for nerve agent poisoning; see "***Caution***" above.
2. **Lorazepam** (Ativan, others): 2- and 4-mg/mL solutions; 1 mL in 2-mL syringe for dilution; 1-mL vial and 10-mL multiple-dose vials.
3. **Midazolam** (Versed, others): 1- and 5-mg/mL solutions; 1-, 2-, 5-, and 10-mL vials; 2-mg/2 mL and 10-mg/2 mL in 2-mL prefilled syringes.

B. Oral

1. **Diazepam** (Valium, Diazepam Intensol 5 mg/mL concentrate, others): 2-, 5-, and 10-mg tablets; 1-mg/mL oral solution in 5-mL cup and 5-mg/ mL oral concentrate in 30-mL bottle.
2. **Lorazepam** (Ativan, others): 0.5-, 1-, and 2-mg tablets; 2-mg/mL oral concentrate in 30-mL bottle.
3. **Midazolam** (Midazolam HCL): 2-mg/mL oral syrup in 118-mL bottle.

C. Rectal

1. **Diazepam** (Diastat, Diastat AcuDial, others): 2.5-, and 10-mg rectal gel/jelly (pediatrics); 20-mg rectal gel/jelly (adults).

D. Suggested minimum stocking levels to treat a 100-kg adult for the first 8 hours and 24 hours:

1. **Diazepam**, *first 8 hours:* 200 mg or four vials of diazepam (5 mg/mL, 10 mL each); *first 24 hours:* 400 mg or eight vials of diazepam (5 mg/mL, 10 mL each).
2. **Lorazepam**, *first 8 hours:* 8 mg or two vials of lorazepam (4 mg/mL, 1 mL each); *first 24 hours:* 24 mg or one vial of lorazepam (2 mg/mL, 10 mL each) and one vial (4 mg/mL, 1 mL each).
3. **Midazolam**, *first 8 hours:* 50 mg or two vials of midazolam (5 mg/mL, 5 mL each); *first 24 hours:* 130 mg or two vials of midazolam (5 mg/mL, 10 mL each) and three vials (5 mg/mL, 2 mL each).

► BENZTROPINE

Thomas E. Kearney, PharmD

I. Pharmacology. Benztropine is an antimuscarinic agent with pharmacologic activity similar to that of atropine. The drug also exhibits antihistaminic properties. Benztropine is used for the treatment of parkinsonism and the control of extrapyramidal side effects associated with neuroleptic drug use.

II. Indications. Benztropine is an alternative in adults to diphenhydramine (the drug of choice for children) for the treatment of acute dystonic reactions associated with neuroleptic drugs or metoclopramide. It has a longer duration of action than does diphenhydramine and is administered twice daily. ***Note:*** It is not effective for tardive dyskinesia, nor neuroleptic malignant syndrome (p 21).

III. Contraindications

A. Angle-closure glaucoma.

B. Obstructive uropathy (prostatic hypertrophy).

C. Myasthenia gravis.

D. Not recommended for children younger than 3 years by the manufacturer; alternatively, use diphenhydramine (p 544) or consider benztropine if the patient is unresponsive or hypersensitive to diphenhydramine and is experiencing a severe or life-threatening situation (eg, dystonic laryngeal or pharyngeal spasms).

E. Tardive dyskinesia.

F. Known hypersensitivity.

IV. Adverse effects

A. Adverse effects include sedation, confusion, blurred vision, tachycardia, urinary hesitancy or retention, intestinal ileus, flushing, dry mouth, and hyperpyrexia. Adverse effects are minimal after single doses.

B. Use in pregnancy. Not categorized by FDA. Safe use not established. However, this does not preclude its acute, short-term use for a seriously symptomatic patient (p 498).

V. Drug or laboratory interactions

A. Benztropine has additive effects with other drugs that exhibit antimuscarinic properties (eg, antihistamines, phenothiazines, cyclic antidepressants, and disopyramide).

B. Slowing of GI motility may delay or inhibit absorption of certain drugs.

VI. Dosage and method of administration

A. Parenteral. Give 1–2 mg IV or IM (children 3 years of age: 0.02 mg/kg and 1 mg maximum). May repeat dose in 15 minutes if the patient is unresponsive.

B. Oral. Give 1–2 mg PO every 12 hours (children 3 years old: 0.02 mg/kg and 1 mg maximum) for 2–3 days to prevent recurrence of symptoms. Maximum recommended dose for adults is 6 mg/d.

VII. Formulations

A. Parenteral. Benztropine mesylate (Cogentin, generic), 1-mg/mL, 2-mL ampules and vials.

B. Oral. Benztropine mesylate (Generic), 0.5-, 1-, and 2-mg tablets.

C. Suggested minimum stocking levels to treat a 100-kg adult for the first 8 hours and 24 hours: **benztropine**, *first 8 hours:* 4 mg or two ampules of benztropine (1 mg/mL, 2 mL each); *first 24 hours:* 6 mg or three ampules of benztropine (1 mg/mL, 2 mL each).

▶ BICARBONATE, SODIUM

Thomas E. Kearney, PharmD

I. Pharmacology

A. Sodium bicarbonate is a buffering agent that reacts with hydrogen ions to correct acidemia and produce alkalemia. Urinary alkalinization from renally excreted bicarbonate ions enhances the renal elimination of certain acidic drugs.

B. It also may help prevent renal tubular damage from deposition of myoglobin in patients with rhabdomyolysis; precipitation (by enhancing solubility) of methotrexate; and dissociation of BAL-metal complex; and it may prevent contrast-induced nephropathy (by slowing free radical production). In addition, maintenance of a normal or high serum pH may prevent intracellular distribution of weak acids such as salicylate.

C. The sodium ion load and alkalemia produced by hypertonic sodium bicarbonate reverse the sodium channel–dependent membrane-depressant ("quinidine-like") effects of several drugs (eg, tricyclic antidepressants, type Ia and type Ic antiarrhythmic agents, propranolol, propoxyphene, cocaine, diphenhydramine).

D. Alkalinization causes an intracellular shift of potassium and is used for the acute treatment of hyperkalemia.

E. Sodium bicarbonate given orally or by gastric lavage forms an insoluble salt with iron and theoretically may help prevent absorption of ingested iron tablets (unproven).

F. Neutralization of acidic substances to prevent caustic injury usually is not recommended because of the potential for an exothermic reaction, generation of gas, and lack of evidence that tissue injury is minimized. Nebulized sodium bicarbonate has been used to neutralize the hydrochloric acid formed on mucosal surfaces from chlorine gas exposures (efficacy uncertain).

G. Early animal studies and human case series of organophosphate (OP) poisonings in regions lacking sufficient access to traditional antidotes (oximes, atropine) have suggested beneficial outcomes from high-dose IV bicarbonate therapy (5 mEq/kg over 60 minutes, then 5–6 mEq/kg/d). The authors of those studies theorize that alkalinization may enhance degradation or elimination of OPs, improve tissue perfusion with volume expansion, and enhance the efficacy of 2-PAM. Systematic reviews of human trials have failed to show differences in mortality but have demonstrated a trend toward improved outcomes (lower atropine requirements and shorter length of hospital stay).

II. Indications

A. Severe metabolic acidosis resulting from intoxication by methanol, ethylene glycol, or salicylates or from excessive lactic acid production (eg, resulting from status epilepticus or shock, mitochondrial toxins or chemical asphyxiants, cyanide, carbon monoxide, metformin).

B. To produce urinary alkalinization, enhance elimination of certain acidic drugs (salicylate, phenobarbital, chlorpropamide, chlorophenoxy herbicide 2,4-D [dichlorophenoxyacetic acid]). ***Note:*** Although enhanced elimination may be achieved, it is uncertain whether clinical outcomes are improved with this therapy.

C. To prevent nephrotoxicity resulting from the renal deposition of myoglobin after severe rhabdomyolysis; the precipitation of methotrexate; dissociation of BAL-metal complex; and to prevent contrast-induced nephropathy.

D. Also recommended for internal contamination of uranium from radiation emergencies to prevent acute tubular necrosis (see "Radiation," p 401).

E. Cardiotoxicity with impaired ventricular depolarization (as evidenced by a prolonged QRS interval) caused by tricyclic antidepressants, type Ia or type Ic antiarrhythmics, and other membrane-depressant drugs. ***Note:*** Not effective for dysrhythmias associated with abnormal repolarization (prolonged QT interval and torsade de pointes). Wide-complex dysrhythmias associated with yew berries (*Taxus spp*) and bupropion intoxications may not be responsive to sodium bicarbonate (mechanism of toxicity may not be related to sodium channel blockade).

III. Contraindications. The following contraindications are relative:

A. Significant metabolic or respiratory alkalemia or hypernatremia.

B. Severe pulmonary edema associated with volume overload.

C. Intolerance to sodium load (renal failure, CHF).

IV. Adverse effects

A. Excessive alkalemia: impaired oxygen release from hemoglobin, hypocalcemic tetany, paradoxical intracellular acidosis (from elevated PCO_2 concentrations), and hypokalemia.

B. Hypernatremia and hyperosmolality. Caution is necessary with rapid infusion of hypertonic solutions in neonates and young children.

C. Aggravation of CHF and pulmonary edema.
D. Extravasation leading to tissue inflammation and necrosis (product is hypertonic).
E. May exacerbate QT prolongation and associated dysrhythmias (eg, torsade de pointes) as a result of electrolyte shifts (hypokalemia).
F. **Use in pregnancy.** FDA Category C (indeterminate). However, this does not preclude its acute, short-term use for a seriously symptomatic patient (p 498).

V. **Drug or laboratory interactions.** Do not mix with other parenteral drugs because of the possibility of drug inactivation or precipitation.

VI. **Dosage and method of administration (adults and children)**
A. **Metabolic acidemia.** Give 0.5- to 1-mEq/kg IV bolus; repeat as needed to correct serum pH to at least 7.2. For salicylates, methanol, or ethylene glycol, raise the pH to at least 7.4–7.5.
B. **Urinary alkalinization.** Give 44–100 mEq in 1 L of 5% dextrose in 0.25% normal saline or 88–150 mEq in 1 L of 5% dextrose at 2–3 mL/kg/h (adults: 150– 200 mL/h). Check urine pH frequently and adjust flow rate to maintain urine pH level at 7–8. ***Note:*** Hypokalemia and fluid depletion prevent effective urinary alkalinization; add 20–40 mEq of potassium to each liter unless renal failure is present. Prevent excessive systemic alkalemia (keep blood pH <7.55) and hypernatremia. Monitor urine pH and serum electrolytes hourly. Prevent fluid overload with ongoing evaluation of intake, output, and retention volumes.
C. **Cardiotoxic (sodium channel blocker) drug intoxication.** Give 1- to 2-mEq/kg IV bolus over 1–2 minutes; repeat as needed to improve cardiotoxic manifestations (eg, prolonged QRS interval, wide-complex tachycardia, hypotension) and maintain serum pH at 7.45–7.55. There is no evidence that constant infusions are as effective as boluses given as needed.

VII. **Formulations**
A. Several products are available, ranging from 4.2% (0.5 mEq/mL, preferred for neonates and young children) to 7.5% (0.89 mEq/mL) to 8.4% (1 mEq/mL) in volumes of 10–500 mL. The most commonly used formulation available in most emergency "crash carts" is 8.4% ("hypertonic") sodium bicarbonate, 1 mEq/mL, in 50-mL ampules or prefilled syringes.
B. **Suggested minimum stocking levels** to treat a 100-kg adult for the first 8 hours and 24 hours: **bicarbonate, sodium**, *first 8 hours:* 63 g (750 mEq) or 750 mL of 8.4% sodium bicarbonate solution; *first 24 hours:* 84 g (1,000 mEq) or 1 L of 8.4% sodium bicarbonate solution.

► BOTULISM ANTITOXIN

Raymond Y. Ho, PharmD

I. **Pharmacology.** Botulism antitoxin contains equine polyclonal antibody fragments directed against the botulinum neurotoxins produced by the various strains of *Clostridium botulinum*. It provides passive immunization by binding to free circulating botulinum neurotoxins.
A. **Botulism antitoxin heptavalent (BAT)** has replaced the bivalent (A, B) and monovalent (E) forms of the antitoxin. BAT contains equine-derived antibody fragments that bind botulinum neurotoxin serotypes A, B, C, D, E, F, and G. It is composed of F(ab')2 and F(ab')2-related immunoglobulin. The investigational pentavalent botulism toxoid vaccine for laboratory workers has been discontinued and is no longer recommended by the CDC.
B. A human-derived botulism immune globulin (IgG antibodies), **BabyBIG**, is approved for the treatment of infant botulism caused by toxins A and B and has demonstrated significant reduction in the length of hospitalization associated with infant botulism.

C. The antitoxins bind and inactivate only freely circulating botulinum neurotoxins; they do ***not*** remove toxin that is already bound to nerve terminals. Because antitoxin will not reverse established paralysis once it occurs, it must be administered before paralysis sets in. Treatment within 24 hours of the onset of symptoms may shorten the course of intoxication and prevent progression to total paralysis.

II. Indications

A. BAT heptavalent is indicated for the treatment of symptomatic botulism (see p 163) following documented or suspected exposure to botulinum neurotoxin serotypes A, B, C, D, E, F, or G.

B. Human-derived **BabyBIG** immune globulins used for the treatment of infant botulism.

III. Contraindications

A. Equine-derived antibodies (BAT). No absolute contraindications. Administration of this product to a patient with known or suspected hypersensitivity to botulinum antitoxin or horse serum requires extreme caution and skin sensitivity testing (See dosage section).

B. Human-derived immune globulin. BabyBIG should not be given to patients with a prior history of severe reaction to human immunoglobulin products. Baby-BIG contains trace amounts of IgA. Individuals with selective IgA deficiency may develop anaphylactic reactions to subsequently administered blood products with IgA.

IV. Adverse effects

A. Equine-derived antibodies. Immediate hypersensitivity reactions (anaphylaxis) resulting from the equine source of antibodies. Prepare for monitoring and management of allergic reactions (See dosage section). Monitor for delayed allergic reactions (serum sickness), which may occur 10 to 21 days after administration.

B. Human-derived immune globulin. Mild transient erythematous rashes of the face and trunk have been reported commonly. Infusion rate–related reactions ranging from mild flushing to severe anaphylaxis may occur. Flulike symptoms similar to those seen with the use of other immune globulin intravenous products have been observed.

C. Use in pregnancy. There are no data on teratogenicity. Anaphylactic reaction resulting in shock or hypoxemia in the mother could conceivably affect the fetus adversely.

V. Drug or laboratory interactions. BAT heptavalent contains maltose and can produce falsely elevated glucose readings with some testing systems; use of glucose-specific testing is advised. Human-derived immune globulin (BabyBIG) preparations contain antibodies that may interfere with the immune response to live vaccines such as those for polio, measles, mumps, and rubella. Vaccination with live virus vaccines should be delayed until approximately 3 months or more after administration of BabyBIG.

VI. Dosage and method of administration

A. BAT heptavalent. Consider skin sensitivity testing for patients with suspected horse serum sensitivity (See VI.A.4. below). In patients at risk for hypersensitivity reactions, begin BAT administration at lowest rate achievable. Otherwise, administer by slow IV infusion after 1:10 dilution in normal saline as follows:

1. **Adult.** Total dose is 1 vial. Start at a rate of 0.5 mL/min for 30 minutes. If tolerating infusion, double the rate every 30 minutes to a maximum of 2 mL/min.
2. **Pediatric** (1 year to <17 years). Give 20–100% of the adult dose by weight (see below). Start at 0.01 mL/kg/min not to exceed 0.5 mL/min for 30 minutes. If tolerating infusion, increase to a maximum of 0.03 mL/kg/min, not to exceed 2 mL/min. *Percentage of adult dose by weight:* 10–14 kg = 20%, 15–19 kg = 30%, 20–24 kg = 40%, 25–29 kg = 50%, 30–34 kg = 60%, 35–39 kg = 65%, 40–44 kg = 70%, 45–49 kg = 75%, 50–54 kg = 80%, ≥55 kg = 100%.

3. **Infant** (<1 year). Give 10% of the adult dose regardless of body weight. Start at 0.01 mL/kg/min for 30 minutes. If tolerating infusion, increase to 0.01 mL/kg/min every 30 minutes to a maximum of 0.03 mL/kg/min.
4. **Skin test** for patients at risk of anaphylaxis due to suspected horse serum sensitivity. Dilute BAT in saline (1:1,000) and inject 0.02 mL intradermally on the volar surface of the forearm. Perform a concurrent positive (histamine) and negative (saline) control test. A positive test is a wheal with surrounding erythema at least 3 mm larger than the control test; read at 15–20 minutes. The histamine control must be positive for valid interpretation. If a hypersensitivity reaction occurs, discontinue BAT administration immediately, maintain airway, treat hypotension with IV fluids, and administer epinephrine and diphenhydramine depending on the severity of the reaction (see p 28).

B. BabyBIG. In cases of infant botulism, the recommended dosage is 1 mL/kg (50 mg/kg) as a single intravenous infusion as soon as a clinical diagnosis of infant botulism is made. BabyBIG should be administered at 0.5 mL/kg/h (25 mg/kg/h). The rate may be increased to 1.0 mL/kg/h (50 mg/kg/h) if no untoward reaction occurs 15 minutes after the initial infusion rate. The half-life of injected BabyBIG is approximately 28 days in infants, and a single intravenous infusion is expected to provide a protective level of neutralizing antibodies for 6 months.

VII. Formulations

A. Parenteral.

1. Each vial (either a 20- or 50-mL size) of **BAT heptavalent**, regardless of size or fill volume, contains a minimum antitoxin potency of 4,500 U of serotype A, 3,300 U of serotype B, 3,000 U of serotype C, 600 U of serotype D, 5,100 U of serotype E, 3,000 U of serotype F, and 600 U of serotype G. To obtain BAT heptavalent, healthcare providers should first contact their local or state health department for reporting and to facilitate access to the antitoxin. Additional emergency consultation is available 24/7 from the botulism duty officer via the CDC Emergency Operations Center at 1-770-488-7100.
2. **BabyBIG** (human) is supplied in a single-dose vial containing approximately 100 mg ± 20 mg lyophilized immunoglobulin for reconstitution with 2 mL of Sterile Water for Injection USP. Reconstituted BabyBIG should be used within 2 hours. To obtain or determine the availability of BabyBIG for suspected infant botulism, contact the Infant Botulism Treatment and Prevention Program (IBTPP) at 1-510-231-7600. More information is available at www.infantbotulism.org.

B. Suggested minimum stocking levels. Not relevant; available only through federal or state health department (see above).

► BROMOCRIPTINE

Thomas E. Kearney, PharmD

I. **Pharmacology.** Bromocriptine mesylate is a semisynthetic derivative of the ergopeptide group of ergot alkaloids with dopaminergic agonist effects. It also has minor alpha-adrenergic antagonist properties. The dopaminergic effects account for its inhibition of prolactin secretion and its beneficial effects in the treatment of parkinsonism, acromegaly, neuroleptic malignant syndrome (NMS [p 21]), and cocaine craving as well as its adverse effect profile and drug interactions. A key limitation is the inability to administer bromocriptine by the parenteral route coupled with poor bioavailability (only about 6% of an oral dose is absorbed). In addition, the onset of therapeutic effects (eg, alleviation of muscle rigidity, hypertension, and hyperthermia) in the treatment of NMS may take several hours to days.

II. Indications

A. Treatment of NMS caused by neuroleptic drugs (eg, haloperidol and other antipsychotics) or levodopa withdrawal. ***Note:*** If the patient has significant hyperthermia (eg, rectal or core temperature ≥40°C [104°F]), bromocriptine should be considered secondary and adjunctive therapy to immediate measures such as neuromuscular paralysis and aggressive external cooling. Its efficacy to treat NMS is uncertain, and there is concern that it could worsen other types of hyperthermia (eg, malignant hyperthermia, heat stroke) owing to activation of dopamine and 5-HT_{2A} receptors.

B. Bromocriptine has been used experimentally to alleviate craving for cocaine. However, a Cochrane database review (2003) concluded that current research does not support the use of dopamine agonists for the treatment of cocaine dependence. ***Caution:*** There is one case report of a severe adverse reaction (hypertension, seizures, and blindness) when bromocriptine was used in a cocaine abuser during the postpartum period.

C. ***Note:*** Bromocriptine is ***not*** considered appropriate first-line therapy for acute drug-induced extrapyramidal or parkinsonian symptoms (p 26).

III. Contraindications

A. Uncontrolled hypertension or toxemia of pregnancy.

B. Known hypersensitivity to the drug.

C. A relative contraindication is a history of angina, myocardial infarction, stroke, vasospastic disorders (eg, Raynaud disease), or bipolar affective disorder. In addition, there is no published experience in children younger than 7 years. Children may achieve higher blood levels and require lower doses.

IV. Adverse effects. Most adverse effects are dose-related and of minor clinical consequence; some are unpredictable.

A. The most common side effect is nausea. Epigastric pain, dyspepsia, and diarrhea also have been reported.

B. Hypotension (usually transient) and syncope may occur at the initiation of treatment, and hypertension may occur later. Other cardiovascular effects include dysrhythmias (with high doses), exacerbation of angina and vasospastic disorders such as Raynaud disease, and intravascular thrombosis resulting in acute myocardial infarction (one case report).

C. Nervous system side effects vary considerably and include headache, drowsiness, fatigue, hallucinations, mania, psychosis, agitation, seizures, and cerebrovascular accident. Multiple interrelated risk factors include dose, concurrent drug therapy, and preexisting medical and psychiatric disorders.

D. Rare effects include pulmonary toxicity (infiltrates, pleural effusion, and thickening) and myopia with long-term, high-dose treatment (months). There has been one case of retroperitoneal fibrosis.

E. Use in pregnancy. FDA Category B (p 498). This drug has been used therapeutically during the last trimester of pregnancy for the treatment of a pituitary tumor. It has been shown to inhibit fetal prolactin secretion, and it may precipitate premature labor and inhibit lactation in the mother.

V. Drug or laboratory interactions

A. Bromocriptine may accentuate hypotension in patients receiving antihypertensive drugs.

B. Theoretically, this drug may have additive effects with other ergot alkaloids, and its potential to cause peripheral vasospasm may be exacerbated by propranolol.

C. Bromocriptine may reduce ethanol tolerance.

D. There has been one case report of apparent serotonin syndrome (p 21) in a patient with Parkinson's disease who received levodopa and carbidopa.

VI. Dosage and method of administration for NMS. In adults, administer 2.5–10 mg orally or by gastric tube 3–4 times daily (average adult dose, 5 mg every 8 hours). The pediatric dose is unknown (one case report of 0.08 mg/kg every 8 hours in a

7-year-old; the tablets were mixed in a 2.5-mg/10 mL slurry and given by feeding tube). Use small, frequent doses to minimize nausea.

A. A therapeutic response usually is achieved with total daily doses of 5–30 mg (maximum daily dose for the treatment of NMS, 45 mg).

B. Continue treatment for 7–10 days after control of rigidity and fever, then slowly taper the dose over 3 days (to prevent recurrence). Several days of therapy may be required for complete reversal of NMS.

VII. Formulations

A. Oral. Bromocriptine mesylate (Parlodel, others), 0.8-mg tablets, 2.5-mg scored (SnapTabs) tablets, and 5-mg capsules.

B. Suggested minimum stocking levels to treat a 100-kg adult for the first 8 hours and 24 hours: **bromocriptine mesylate**, *first 8 hours:* 15 mg or three capsules (5 mg each); *first 24 hours:* 30 mg or six capsules (5 mg each).

► CALCIUM

Janna H. Villano, MD and Binh T. Ly, MD

I. Pharmacology

A. Calcium is a cation that is necessary for the normal functioning of a variety of enzymes and organ systems, including muscle and nerve tissue. Hypocalcemia, or a blockade of the effects of calcium, may cause muscle cramps, tetany, and ventricular fibrillation. Antagonism of calcium-dependent channels results in hypotension, bradycardia, and atrioventricular (AV) block.

B. Calcium ions rapidly bind to fluoride ions, abolishing their toxic effects.

C. Calcium can reverse the negative inotropic effects of calcium antagonists; however, depressed automaticity and AV nodal conduction velocity and vasodilation caused by these agents may not respond to calcium administration.

D. Calcium stabilizes cardiac cell membranes in hyperkalemic states.

E. Calcium is a physiologic antagonist to the effects of hypermagnesemia.

II. Indications

A. Symptomatic hypocalcemia resulting from intoxication by fluoride, oxalate, or the intravenous anticoagulant citrate.

B. Hydrofluoric acid exposure (p 269).

C. Hypotension in the setting of calcium channel antagonist (eg, verapamil) toxicity (p 172).

D. Severe hyperkalemia with cardiac manifestations.

E. Symptomatic hypermagnesemia.

III. Contraindications

A. Hypercalcemia except in the setting of calcium channel antagonist poisoning, in which hypercalcemia may be desirable.

B. Older textbooks list digoxin poisoning as a contraindication, but this warning is not supported by animal studies or human case reports.

C. ***Note:*** Calcium *chloride* salt should *not* be used for intradermal, subcutaneous, or intra-arterial injection because it is highly concentrated and may result in further tissue damage. When given intravenously, use a central line or a secure, freely-flowing large peripheral venous line.

IV. Adverse effects

A. Tissue irritation, particularly with calcium chloride salt; extravasation may cause local irritation or necrosis.

B. Hypercalcemia, especially in patients with diminished renal function.

C. Hypotension, bradycardia, syncope, and cardiac dysrhythmias caused by rapid intravenous administration.

D. Neuromuscular weakness.

E. Constipation caused by orally administered calcium salts.

F. **Use in pregnancy.** FDA Category C (indeterminate). This does not preclude its acute, short-term use for a seriously symptomatic patient (p 498).

V. **Drug or laboratory interactions**

A. Inotropic and dysrhythmogenic effects of digoxin and other cardiac glycosides may be potentiated by calcium, but this interaction appears largely theoretical, and animal studies have failed to demonstrate harm when calcium is used to treat severe hyperkalemia.

B. A precipitate will form with solutions containing soluble salts of carbonates, phosphates, or sulfates, and with sodium bicarbonate and various antibiotics.

VI. **Dosage and method of administration.** ***Note:*** A 10% solution of calcium chloride contains three times the amount of calcium ions per milliliter that a 10% solution of calcium gluconate contains. (A 10% solution of calcium chloride contains 27.2 mg/mL of elemental calcium; a 10% solution of calcium gluconate contains 9 mg/mL of elemental calcium.)

A. **Oral fluoride ingestion.** Administer calcium-containing antacid (calcium carbonate) orally to complex fluoride ions.

B. **Symptomatic hypocalcemia, hyperkalemia**. Give 20–30 mL (2–3 g) of 10% calcium gluconate (children: 0.3–0.4 mL/kg), or 5–10 mL (0.5–1 g) of 10% calcium chloride (children: 0.1–0.2 mL/kg), slowly IV over 5–10 minutes. Repeat as needed every 10–20 minutes.

C. **Calcium antagonist poisoning.** May start with doses as described above. Typically, give an initial IV dose of 30 mL (3 g) of 10% calcium gluconate (children: 0.6 mL/kg or 60 mg/kg), or 10 mL (1 g) of 10% calcium chloride (children: 0.2 mL/kg or 20 mg/kg). *High-dose calcium* therapy has been reported to be effective in some cases of severe calcium channel blocker overdose. Corrected calcium concentrations of approximately 1.5–2 times normal have correlated with improved cardiac function. In the setting of calcium channel antagonist overdose, as much as 30 g of calcium gluconate has been given over 10 hours, resulting in a serum calcium concentration of 23.8 mg/dL, which was tolerated without adverse effect. However, not all patients will tolerate extreme elevations in serum calcium concentrations. Administer calcium as multiple boluses (eg, 3 g of calcium gluconate or 1 g of calcium chloride every 10–20 minutes) or as a continuous infusion (eg, 0.6–1.5 mL/kg/h (60–150 mg/kg/h) of 10% calcium gluconate, or 0.2–0.5 mL/kg/h (20–50 mg/kg/h) of 10% calcium chloride, since bolus dosing briefly increases only ionized calcium levels. Serum calcium concentrations should be measured every 1–2 hours during therapy with high-dose calcium.

D. **Dermal hydrofluoric acid exposure.** For any exposure involving the hand or fingers, obtain immediate consultation from an experienced hand surgeon or medical toxicologist. Regardless of the specific therapy chosen, systemic opioid analgesics should be strongly considered as adjunctive therapy.

1. **Topical.** Calcium concentrations for topical therapy have ranged from 2.5 to 33%; the optimal concentration has not been determined. In many industrial settings, a commercially available 2.5% calcium gluconate gel (Calgonate) is kept at the work site for rapid treatment of occupational exposures. A 2.5% gel can also be prepared in the emergency department by combining 1 g of calcium gluconate per 40 g (approximately 40 mL) of water-soluble base material (eg, Surgilube, K-Y Jelly). A 32.5% gel can be made by compounding a slurry of ten 650-mg calcium carbonate tablets in 20 mL of water-soluble lubricant. For exposures involving the hand or fingers, place the gel in a large surgical latex glove to serve as an occlusive dressing to maximize skin contact. Topical calcium gluconate treatment is much more effective if applied within 3 hours of the injury.

2. For **subcutaneous** injection (when topical treatment fails to relieve pain), inject 5–10% calcium gluconate (***not*** chloride) SC intralesionally and

perifocally (0.5–1 mL/cm^2 of affected skin), using a 27-gauge or smaller needle. This can be repeated two to three times at 1- to 2-hour intervals if pain is not relieved. No more than 0.5 mL should be injected into each digit.

3. **Bier block technique**
   a. Establish distal IV access in the affected extremity (eg, dorsum of the hand).
   b. Exsanguinate the extremity by elevation for 5 minutes. Alternatively, an Esmarch bandage may be used by wrapping from the distal to the proximal extremity.
   c. Inflate a blood pressure cuff to just above systolic blood pressure. The arm can then be lowered or the bandage removed.
   d. With the cuff kept inflated, infuse 25–50 mL of a 2% calcium gluconate solution (10 mL of 10% calcium gluconate diluted with 40 mL of D_5W) into the empty veins.
   e. After 20–25 minutes, slowly release the cuff over 3–5 minutes.
   f. Repeat if pain persists or use the intra-arterial infusion.
4. For **intra-arterial** administration, dilute 10 mL of 10% calcium gluconate with 50 mL of D_5W and infuse over 4 hours through either the brachial or the radial artery catheter. The patient should be monitored closely over the next 4–6 hours, and if pain recurs, a second infusion should be given. Some authors have reported 48–72 hours of continuous infusion.

E. **Other sites of hydrofluoric acid exposure**
   1. **Nebulized** 2.5% calcium gluconate has been reported for cases of inhalational hydrofluoric acid exposure. Inhalational exposure should be considered with dermal exposures of more than 5% of the total body surface area. Add 1.5 mL of 10% calcium gluconate to 4.5 mL of sterile water to make a 2.5% solution.
   2. **Ocular** administration of 1% calcium gluconate solutions every 4–6 hours has been used for 24–48 hours but is of unproven efficacy compared with irrigation with saline or water. Higher concentrations of calcium gluconate may worsen corrosive injury to ocular structures. Ophthalmology consultation should be obtained.

VII. **Formulations**
   A. **Oral.** Calcium carbonate, suspension, tablets, or chewable tablets, 300–800 mg.
   B. **Parenteral.** Calcium gluconate (10%), 10 mL (1 g contains 4.5 mEq of calcium); calcium chloride (10%), 10 mL (1 g contains 13.6 mEq).
   C. **Topical.** Calcium gluconate gel (2.5%) in 25- and 30-g tubes, but none of these commercially available formulations has been approved by the FDA.
   D. **Suggested minimum stocking levels** to treat a 100-kg adult for the first 8 hours and 24 hours:
      1. **Calcium chloride**, *first 8 hours:* 10 g or 10 vials (1 g each) of 10% calcium chloride; *first 24 hours:* 10 g or 10 vials (1 g each) of 10% calcium chloride.
      2. **Calcium gluconate**, *first 8 hours:* 30 g or 30 vials (1 g each) of 10% calcium gluconate; *first 24 hours:* 30 g or 30 vials (1 g each) of 10% calcium gluconate.

▶ CARNITINE (LEVOCARNITINE)

Derrick Lung, MD, MPH

I. **Pharmacology**
   A. Levocarnitine (L-carnitine) is an endogenous carboxylic acid that facilitates transport of long-chain fatty acids into mitochondria for beta-oxidation and prevents intracellular accumulation of toxic acyl-CoA. L-Carnitine is ubiquitous in diets rich in meats and dairy products and is also synthesized

in the body from the amino acids lysine and methionine. Although dietary deficiencies are rare, hypocarnitinemia can result from certain medical conditions and inborn errors of metabolism, and it may develop in patients receiving multiple anticonvulsant medications. It is hypothesized that valproic acid (VPA [p 441]) causes carnitine deficiency, resulting in mitochondrial dysfunction. The resultant impaired beta-oxidation favors production of toxic VPA metabolites via microsomal oxidation. These metabolites are implicated in hepatotoxicity and urea cycle disruption, causing hyperammonemia. Supplementation with L-carnitine has been shown to be beneficial in both the prevention and the treatment of hyperammonemia associated with VPA therapy, and it may improve the outcome in cases of VPA-induced hepatotoxicity and encephalopathy.

B. L-Carnitine is also sold as a dietary supplement with a wide range of unproven claims ranging from improved sperm motility to prevention of Alzheimer disease. It is postulated that carnitine supplementation enhances fat utilization during exercise, thereby improving endurance and promoting weight loss. However, published studies have failed to show that supraphysiologic doses of L-carnitine have any benefit in well-nourished individuals. Because the FDA does not regulate dietary supplements, the safety of L-carnitine supplements cannot be guaranteed (see "Herbal and Alternative Products," p 261).

II. Indications

A. Hyperammonemia, encephalopathy, and hepatotoxicity related to VPA therapy or overdose

B. Low plasma-free carnitine concentrations (reference range, 19–60 mcmol/L) or total carnitine (reference range, 30–73 mcmol/L) in patients taking valproic acid.

C. Primary or secondary carnitine deficiency.

D. Infants and children younger than 2 years receiving VPA as part of a regimen of multiple anticonvulsant drugs.

III. Contraindications. None known.

IV. Adverse effects

A. Dose- and duration-related nausea, vomiting, and diarrhea, and a fishy body odor.

B. Tachydysrhythmias, hypertension, and hypotension associated with IV administration were reported during FDA postmarketing surveillance, although they appear to be rare.

C. Seizures were reported during FDA postmarketing surveillance in five patients but due to underlying seizure disorders or concurrent use of other medications, no direct link could be established.

D. Use in pregnancy. FDA Category B (p 498). No adequate studies have been conducted in pregnant women. It is not known whether this drug is secreted in human breast milk.

V. Drug or laboratory interactions. None known.

VI. Dosage and method of administration

A. Severe valproate-induced hepatotoxicity, hyperammonemia, encephalopathy, or acute valproic acid overdose. Early intervention with IV carnitine has been associated with better outcomes. Intravenous administration is preferred because of poor oral bioavailability (5–15%). Optimal dosing is unknown, but a common approach is a loading dose of 100 mg/kg (by IV infusion over 15–30 minutes or slow bolus injection over 2–3 minutes), followed by a maintenance dose of 50 mg/kg (up to a maximum of 3 g per dose) every 8 hours. Therapy can continue until clinical improvement occurs and/or ammonia levels decrease. Up to 4 days of carnitine therapy has been required in case reports.

B. **Drug-induced carnitine deficiency and asymptomatic hyperammonemia.** Give 100 mg/kg/d orally in divided doses for up to 3 g/d in adults and 2 g/d in children.

VII. **Formulations**

A. **Oral.** Levocarnitine (Carnitor, L-Carnitine), 330- and 500-mg tablets, 250-mg capsules, and oral solution (1 g/10 mL) in 118-mL multiple-use containers.

B. **Parenteral.** Levocarnitine (Carnitor, others), injection of single-dose (200 mg/mL) 5-mL vials and ampules containing a total of 1 g of L-carnitine per vial or ampule.

C. **Suggested minimum stocking levels** to treat a severely ill 100-kg adult for the first 8 hours and 24 hours: **levocarnitine**, *first 8 hours:* 10 g or 10 vials (1 g each); *first 24 hours:* 19 g or 19 vials (1 g each).

▶ CHARCOAL, ACTIVATED

Thomas E. Kearney, PharmD

I. **Pharmacology.** Activated charcoal, by virtue of its large surface area, adsorbs many drugs and toxins. Highly ionic salts (eg, iron, lithium, and cyanide) and small polar molecules (eg, alcohols) are poorly adsorbed. Repeated oral doses of activated charcoal can increase the rate of elimination of some drugs that have a small volume of distribution and that undergo enterogastric or enterohepatic recirculation (eg, digitoxin) or diffuse into the GI lumen from the intestinal circulation (eg, phenobarbital and theophylline). See also discussion in Section I, p 53. Coadministration with cathartics is of unproven benefit and is associated with risks (see p 54).

II. **Indications**

A. Activated charcoal is often used orally after an ingestion to limit drug or toxin absorption, although there is debate concerning its routine use. It is most likely to be useful if given within 1 hour of an ingestion, but effectiveness is subject to numerous variables (eg, charcoal-to-substance ratio, contact time, pH, substance solubility, and whether ingested drug is likely to persist in the stomach or upper small intestine).

B. Repeated doses of activated charcoal may be indicated to enhance elimination of some drugs if (1) more rapid elimination will benefit the patient and (2) more aggressive means of removal (eg, hemodialysis) are not immediately indicated or available (p 59).

C. Repeated doses of activated charcoal may be useful when the quantity of drug or toxin ingested is greater than one-tenth of the usual charcoal dose (eg, an aspirin ingestion of >6–10 g) or when surface contact with the drug is hindered (eg, pharmacobezoars and wrapped or packaged drugs).

III. **Contraindications**

A. Gastrointestinal ileus or obstruction may prevent the administration of more than one or two doses. Patients at risk for gastrointestinal perforation or hemorrhage (recent surgery) should not receive activated charcoal.

B. Acid or alkali ingestions, unless other drugs have also been ingested (charcoal makes endoscopic evaluation more difficult).

C. Use of charcoal-sorbitol mixtures should be avoided in children (risk for hypernatremia and dehydration from excessive sorbitol).

D. Obtunded patients at risk for aspiration of charcoal (unless airway is protected).

IV. **Adverse effects**

A. Pneumonitis and bronchiolitis obliterans have been reported after pulmonary aspiration of gastric contents containing activated charcoal.

B. Constipation (may be prevented by coadministration of a cathartic, although this is not routinely advised).

C. Diarrhea, dehydration, hypermagnesemia, and hypernatremia resulting from coadministered cathartics, especially with repeated doses of charcoal and cathartics or even after a single large dose of a premixed sorbitol-containing charcoal product.

D. Intestinal bezoar with obstruction (in particular with multiple doses given to patients who have impaired bowel motility).

E. Corneal abrasions have occurred when activated charcoal was spilled in the eyes.

F. Use in pregnancy. Activated charcoal is not systemically absorbed. Diarrhea resulting in shock or hypernatremia in the mother could conceivably affect the fetus adversely.

V. Drug or laboratory interactions

A. Activated charcoal may reduce, prevent, or delay the absorption of orally administered antidotes or other drugs (eg, acetylcysteine).

B. The adsorptive capacity of activated charcoal may be diminished by the concurrent ingestion of ice cream, milk, or sugar syrup; the clinical significance is unknown but is probably minor.

C. Repeated doses of charcoal may enhance the elimination of some necessary therapeutic drugs (eg, anticonvulsants).

VI. Dosage and method of administration

A. Initial dose

1. Administer activated charcoal, 1 g/kg (adult dose: 50–100 g; child younger than 5 years: 0.5–1 g/kg or 10–25 g) orally or via gastric tube, or if the quantity of toxin ingested is known, at least 10 times the amount of ingested toxin by weight. For massive overdoses (eg, 60–100 g of aspirin), this may need to be given in divided doses over 1–2 days.

2. Palatability may be improved by mixing with flavored drinks (cola) and, for children, placing in an opaque, covered cup and having them use a straw.

3. The airway should be protected in obtunded patients to help prevent aspiration of activated charcoal.

B. Repeat-dose charcoal

1. Administer activated charcoal, 15–30 g (0.25–0.5 g/kg) every 2–4 hours or hourly (adults: average rate of 12.5 g/h; children: rate of 0.2 g/kg/h) orally or by gastric tube. (The optimal regimen and dose are unknown, but more frequent dosing or continuous gastric infusion may be advantageous.)

2. Consider adding a small dose of cathartic with every second or third charcoal dose (benefit is unproven). Do ***not*** use a cathartic with every activated charcoal dose. Continuous whole-bowel irrigation (p 55) can be substituted for episodic cathartics.

3. End points for repeat-dose charcoal therapy include clinical improvement and declining serum drug level; the usual empiric duration is 24–48 hours.

C. For patients with nausea or vomiting, administer antiemetics (metoclopramide [p 581] or ondansetron [p 597]) and consider giving the charcoal by gastric tube.

VII. Formulations

A. There are a variety of formulations and a large number of brands of activated charcoal. It is available as a powder, pellets, granules, a liquid aqueous suspension (preferable), and a liquid suspension in sorbitol or propylene glycol. ***Note:*** The use of charcoal-containing tablets or capsules is not appropriate for the management of poisonings.

B. Suggested minimum stocking levels to treat a 100-kg adult for the first 8 hours and 24 hours: **activated charcoal**, *first 8 hours:* 200 g or four bottles containing 50 g of activated charcoal each; *first 24 hours*: 300 g or six bottles containing 50 g of activated charcoal each. Preferred stock is the plain aqueous suspension.

▶ CIMETIDINE AND OTHER H_2 BLOCKERS

Thomas E. Kearney, PharmD

I. **Pharmacology.** Cimetidine, ranitidine, famotidine, and nizatidine are selective competitive inhibitors of histamine on H_2 receptors. These receptors modulate smooth muscle, vascular tone, and gastric secretions and may be involved in clinical effects associated with anaphylactic and anaphylactoid reactions as well as ingestion of histamine or histamine-like substances (eg, scombroid fish poisoning). Cimetidine, as an inhibitor of cytochrome P450 enzymes, has been proposed or studied in animals as an agent to block the production of toxic intermediate metabolites (eg, acetaminophen, carbon tetrachloride, halothane, *Amanita* mushroom poisoning, dapsone), but this has not been shown to be beneficial for human poisonings or toxicity with the possible exception of patients on chronic dapsone therapy (see "Indications"). Cimetidine is also an inhibitor of alcohol dehydrogenase (see "Drug or Laboratory Interactions") and has been suggested for use in patients with an atypical aldehyde dehydrogenase enzyme to minimize a disulfiram reaction ("Oriental flushing") to acute alcohol ingestion.

II. **Indications**

A. Adjunctive with H_1 blockers such as diphenhydramine (p 544) in the management and prophylactic treatment of anaphylactic and anaphylactoid reactions (see chapters on various antivenoms, pp 506–511).

B. Adjunctive with H_1 blockers such as diphenhydramine (p 544) in the management of scombroid fish poisoning (p 246).

C. **Ranitidine** has been used to reduce vomiting associated with theophylline poisoning. Because cimetidine may interfere with hepatic elimination of theophylline, it should not be used.

D. **Cimetidine** has been used to decrease methemoglobin levels by inhibiting oxidative metabolite formation and thereby improve tolerance for patients on chronic dapsone therapy.

III. **Contraindications.** Known hypersensitivity to H_2 blockers.

IV. **Adverse effects**

A. Headache, drowsiness, fatigue, and dizziness have been reported but are usually mild.

B. Confusion, agitation, hallucinations, and even seizures have been reported with cimetidine use in the elderly, the severely ill, and patients with renal failure. A case was reported of a dystonic reaction after IV cimetidine administration.

C. A reversible, dose-dependent rise in serum alanine aminotransferase activity has been reported with nizatidine, a related agent. Hepatitis has also occurred with ranitidine.

D. Cardiac dysrhythmias (bradycardia, tachycardia) and hypotension have been associated with rapid IV bolus of cimetidine and ranitidine (rare). ***Note:*** Maximum infusion rates provided on Table III–5.

E. Severe delayed hypersensitivity after high oral doses of cimetidine (case report).

F. Preparations containing the preservative benzyl alcohol have been associated with "gasping syndrome" in premature infants.

G. **Use in pregnancy.** FDA Category B (p 498). Fetal harm is extremely unlikely.

V. **Drug or laboratory interactions**

A. Cimetidine, and to a lesser extent ranitidine, reduces hepatic clearance and prolongs the elimination half-life of several drugs as a result of inhibition of cytochrome P450 activity and reduction of hepatic blood flow. Examples of drugs affected include phenytoin, theophylline, phenobarbital, cyclosporine, morphine, lidocaine, calcium channel blockers, tricyclic antidepressants, and warfarin.

B. Cimetidine, ranitidine, and nizatidine inhibit gastric mucosal alcohol dehydrogenase and, therefore, increase the systemic absorption of ethyl alcohol.

C. Increased gastric pH may inhibit the absorption of some pH-dependent drugs, such as ketoconazole, ferrous salts, and tetracyclines.

TABLE III–5. CIMETIDINE, FAMOTIDINE, NIZATIDINE, AND RANITIDINE

Drug	Route	Dose[a]
Cimetidine	PO	300 mg every 6–8 hours or 400 mg every 12 hours (maximum, 2,400 mg/d). Children: 10 mg/kg (maximum, 300 mg), then 5–10 mg/kg every 6–8 hours up to 20–40 mg/kg/d.
	IV, IM	300 mg IV or IM every 6–8 hours. For IV administration, dilute in normal saline to a total volume of 20 mL and give over 5 minutes or longer. May give by continuous IV infusion at initial rate of 25–50 mg/h and titrate to effect (mean rates of 160 mg/h reported; maximum 2,400 mg/d). Children: 10 mg/kg (maximum, 300 mg), then 5–10 mg/kg every 6–8 hours up to 20–40 mg/kg/d.
Famotidine	PO	20–40 mg once or twice daily (as much as 160 mg every 6 hours has been used). Children: 0.5 mg/kg/dose once to twice daily (maximum 40 mg twice daily).
	IV	20 mg IV every 12 hours (dilute in normal saline to a total volume of 5–10 mL)and give at a rate of 10 mg/min or less over at least 2 minutes). Children: 0.25–0.5 mg/kg/dose (maximum dose, 20 mg) once to twice daily.
Nizatidine	PO	150 mg once to twice daily (or 300 mg once daily).
Ranitidine	PO	150 mg twice daily (up to 6 g/d has been used). Children: 2–4 mg/kg once to twice daily (maximum dose, 300 mg/d).
	IV, IM	50 mg IV or IM every 6–8 hours. For IV use, dilute in normal saline or 5% dextrose to a total volume of 20 mL and inject over 5 minutes or longer. May give by continuous IV infusion at the rate of 6.25 mg/h and titrate to effect (rates as high as 220 mg/h reported). Children: 12.5–50 mg (0.5–1 mg/kg) every 6–8 hours up to 2–4 mg/kg/d (maximum, 200 mg/d).

[a]May need to reduce dose in patients with renal insufficiency.

VI. Dosage and method of administration. In general, there are no clinically proven advantages of any one of the H_2 blockers, although cimetidine is more likely to be associated with drug–drug interactions. The lowest-strength dosage forms are available over the counter, and several oral dosage form options (chewable tablets, oral solutions) may enhance palatability. Oral and parenteral doses are presented in Table III–5.

VII. Formulations

A. Cimetidine (Tagamet, others)

1. **Oral.** 200-, 300-, 400-, and 800-mg tablets; 300-mg/5 mL oral solution (contains parabens and propylene glycol).
2. **Parenteral.** 150 mg/mL in 2- and 8-mL vials (Tagamet preparation has 0.5% phenol, others may contain 9 mg/mL of benzyl alcohol); premixed 300 mg in 50 mL of saline (6 mg/mL).

B. Famotidine (Pepcid, Pepcid AC, Pepcid RPD)

1. **Oral.** 10-, 20-, and 40-mg tablets; 10-mg chewable tablets and gelcaps; 20- and 40-mg disintegrating tablets; 40-mg/5 mL oral suspension (powder to be reconstituted).
2. **Parenteral.** 10 mg/mL in 1- and 2-mL single-dose and 4-, 20-, and 50-mL multiple-dose vials (may contain mannitol or benzyl alcohol); premixed 20 mg in 50 mL of saline.

C. Ranitidine (Zantac, others)

1. **Oral.** 75-, 150-, and 300-mg tablets and capsules; 15 mg/mL in 10 mL of syrup (may contain alcohol and parabens); 25- and 150-mg effervescent tablets.
2. **Parenteral.** 1.0 mg/mL in 50-mL container; 25 mg/mL in 2- and 6-mL vials (with phenol).

D. **Nizatidine (Axid, others)**
   1. **Oral.** 75-mg tablets and 150- and 300-mg capsules; 15-mg/mL oral solution (with parabens) in 480-mL container.
   2. **Parenteral.** Not available in this dosage form.

E. **Suggested minimum stocking levels** to treat a 100-kg adult for the first 8 hours and 24 hours (all are parenteral dose form):
   1. **Cimetidine,** *first 8 hours:* 600 mg or two vials (150 mg/mL, 2 mL each); *first 24 hours:* 1,200 mg or one vial (150 mg/mL, 8 mL each).
   2. **Famotidine,** *first 8 hours:* 20 mg or one vial (10 mg/mL, 2 mL each); *first 24 hours:* 40 mg or one vial (10 mg/mL, 4-mL multiple-dose vial).
   3. **Ranitidine,** *first 8 hours:* 100 mg or two vials (25 mg/mL, 2 mL each); *first 24 hours:* 250 mg or two vials (25 mg/mL, 6 mL each).

► CLOTTING FACTOR REPLACEMENT PRODUCTS

Ann Arens, MD and Curtis Geier, PharmD

I. **Pharmacology**

Prothrombin complex concentrates (PCCs) and activated prothrombin complex concentrate (APCC) are derived from pooled human plasma, and, depending on the preparation, contain differing amounts of the human clotting factors II, VII, IX, X, and proteins C and S.

   A. **Three-factor PCCs** include factors II, IX, and X without appreciable amounts of factor VII.
   B. **Four-factor PCC** products include factors II, VII, IX, and X as well as protein Cs and S.
   C. **APCC,** also known as Factor Eight Inhibitor Bypassing Activity (FEIBA® NF), contains factors II, IX, X, and activated factor VII.
   D. **Recombinant factor VIIa** (rFVIIa, NovoSeven RT®) is structurally similar to human plasma-derived factor VII but is cultured in animal cells and contains only activated factor VII without appreciable amounts of other clotting factors.
   E. All preparations are given only intravenously and are immediately bioavailable. Their distribution is limited to the vascular space; they are likely removed from circulation by the hepatic reticuloendothial system, similar to endogenous coagulation factors.

II. **Indications**
   A. Reversal of life-, limb-, or sight-threatening bleeding (eg, intracranial hemorrhage, massive GI bleed, life-threatening traumatic injury, compartment syndrome, retinal hemorrhage) in patients with acquired deficiencies of clotting factors associated with the use of vitamin K antagonists (eg, warfarin), direct thrombin inhibitors (eg, dabigatran), or factor Xa inhibitors (eg, rivaroxaban, apixaban, or edoxaban).

III. **Contraindications**
   A. Previous anaphylaxis to PCC, APCC, or rFVIIa, or any of their components.
   B. Patients with a history of anaphylaxis to heparin, or history of heparin-induced thrombocytopenia (HIT), should not be given the Bebulin® VH, Octaplex®, Beriplex® PN, or KCentra®. These products contain small amounts of heparin. ***Note:*** Activated PCC (FEIBA® NF), rFVIIa (NovoSeven RT®), and Profilnine® SD DO NOT contain heparin.
   C. NovoSeven® should not be given to patients with known hypersensitivity to mouse, hamster, or bovine proteins.
   D. Octaplex® is contraindicated in patients with IgA deficiency and known anti-IgA antibodies.
   E. Prothrombin complex concentrates increase the risk of thromboembolic events when given to patients with disseminated intravascular coagulation (DIC), myocardial infarction, and pulmonary embolism and should not be given to patients with these acute conditions.

F. The risks of anaphylaxis, HIT, and thromboembolic events must be weighed against the benefits of anticoagulant reversal depending on the individual patient situation.

G. Recombinant factor VIIa should NOT be given concurrently with PCC because of a significant increased risk of thrombotic events. ***Note:*** Fresh frozen plasma has been successfully given after rFVIIa administration.

IV. Adverse effects

A. Black box warning.

1. **KCentra®.** Serious venous and arterial thromboembolic complications have been reported in clinical trials and postmarketing surveillance.
2. **FEIBA® NF.** Thrombotic and thromboembolic events have been reported in postmarketing surveillance particularly in high doses or in patients with underlying risk factors for thrombosis.
3. **NovoSeven RT®.** Serious venous and arterial thrombotic events have been reported.

B. Other. Mild adverse effects include headache, nausea, vomiting, diarrhea, abdominal pain, dyspnea, hypertension, pain at the injection site, pyrexia, and dizziness/somnolence.

1. Octaplex® has been associated with a transient mild transaminitis.
2. Reported effects of FEIBA® include dysgeusia and hypoesthesia.
3. NovoSeven RT® use has been associated with hemorrhage, edema, and rash.

C. Infection. While products are screened for viral infections, PCC and APCC are derived from human plasma and thus carry the risk of communicable disease. Octaplex® has been associated with seroconversion of Parvovirus B19 titers (3 of 90 patients enrolled in clinical trials).

D. Use in pregnancy. FDA Category C. No sufficient human studies exist to determine the safety of PCC, APCC, or rVIIa in pregnancy. Pregnant women receiving PCC or APCC should be advised of the risk of possible communicable infections.

V. Drug or laboratory interactions. No clear laboratory interactions have been identified. However, three- and four-factor PCCs contain small amounts of heparin, and this should be taken into account when interpreting coagulation studies.

VI. Dosage and method of administration

A. PCCs and APCC. See Table III–6 for reversal of vitamin K antagonists based upon initial INR. See Table III–7 for reversal of direct thrombin inhibitors and factor Xa inhibitors.

TABLE III–6. DOSES FOR REVERSAL OF VITAMIN K ANTAGONISTS (eg, WARFARIN, "SUPERWARFARINS") BASED ON INR

	INR 2.0–2.4	INR 2.5–2.9	INR 3.0–3.4	INR 3.5–3.9	INR 4.0–5.9	INR ≥6	Maximum Dose
Four-factor PCCs[a]							
Octaplex®	22.5 U/kg	32.5 U/kg	40 U/kg	47.5 U/kg	47.5 U/kg	47.5 U/kg	3,000 U
Beriplex®	25 U/kg	25 U/kg	25 U/kg	25 U/kg	35 U/kg	50 U/kg	5,000 U
KCentra®	25 U/kg	25 U/kg	25 U/kg	25 U/kg	35 U/kg	50 U/kg	5,000 U
Three-factor PCCs[a]							
Profilnine®	50 U/kg	50 U/kg	50 U/kg	50 U/kg	50 U/kg	50 U/kg	50 U/kg
Bebulin®	50 U/kg	50 U/kg	50 U/kg	50 U/kg	50 U/kg	50 U/kg	50 U/kg

[a]Four-factor PCC is the preferred agent; if unavailable, then give three-factor PCC with 10–15 mL/kg of fresh-frozen plasma (FFP). If unable to give PPC or FFP, consider recombinant factor VIIa (rFVIIa) in a single dose of 1,200 mcg. All patients should receive one dose of vitamin K unless contraindicated (see p 633).

TABLE III–7. DOSES OF CLOTTING FACTOR COMPLEXES FOR REVERSAL OF NEWER ORAL ANTICOAGULANTS[a]

	Dose	Maximum Dose
Activated PCC[b]		
FEIBA®	25–100 U/kg	100 U/kg in a single dose
Four-factor PCCs[c]		
Octaplex®	50 U/kg	3,000 U
Beriplex®	50 U/kg	5,000 U
KCentra®	50 U/kg	5,000 U
Three-factor PCCs		
Profilnine®	50 U/kg	50 U/kg
Bebulin®	50 U/kg	50 U/kg

[a]Specific reversal agents have been developed for dabigatran (idarucizumab, Praxbind®) and the factor Xa inhibitors (andexanet alfa), and if available, these should be given first.
[b]APCC is the preferred clotting factor complex for direct thrombin inhibitors (eg, dabigatran). If not available, give a four-factor PCC. If neither of these is available, give a three-factor PCC with 10–15 mL/kg of fresh-frozen plasma (FFP). Consider recombinant factor VIIa (rFVIIa) if unable to give PPC or FFP.
[c]Four-factor PCC is the preferred clotting factor complex for factor Xa inhibitors. If not available, give a three-factor PCC with FFP. If neither of these is available, give FFP alone. Consider recombinant factor VIIa (rFVIIa) if unable to give PPC or FFP.

B. Recombinant factor VIIa (Novoseven RT®). There is no consensus on the dosing of rVIIa for the reversal of vitamin K antagonists, direct thrombin inhibitors, or factor Xa inhibitors. A single dose of 1,200 mcg has been recommended for reversal of vitamin K antagonists, while a dose of 90 mcg/kg has been recommended for reversal of dabigatran.

VII. Formulations

A. All formulations are for intravenous use only, are lyophilized, and must be reconstituted with sterile diluent to listed concentrations. Strengths of three- and four-factor PCCs are given as factor IX potency.

1. **Profilnine® SD.** Factor IX (FIX) complex. Contains factors II, IX, X, and a very small amount of factor VII. It DOES NOT contain heparin. Supplied in vials with nominal potencies of 500 IU/5 mL, 1,000 IU/10 mL, or 1,500 IU/10 mL.
2. **Bebulin® VH.** Factor IX complex. Contains factors II, IX, X, very low amounts of factor VII, and small amounts of heparin (less than 0.15 IU heparin per IU of FIX). Supplied in vials of 200–1200 IU/20 mL.
3. **Octaplex®.** Human prothrombin complex. Contains factors II, VII, IX, X, proteins C and S, and heparin (80–310 IU/20 mL vial; 160–620 IU/40 mL vial). Supplied in vials of 500 IU/20 mL and 1000 IU/40 mL..
4. **Beriplex® P/N.** Human prothrombin complex. Contains factors II, VII, IX, X, Proteins C and S, heparin, human albumin, and human antithrombin III. Supplied in vials with nominal potencies of 250 IU/10 mL, 500 IU/20 mL, and 1,000 IU/40 mL.
5. **Kcentra®.** Human PCC. Contain factors II, VII, IX, X, proteins C and S, and 8–30 IU heparin/vial. Supplied in vials with nominal potencies of 500 IU/20 mL and 1,000 IU/40 mL.
6. **FEIBA® NF.** Anti-inhibitor coagulant complex. Contains factors II, IX, X, activated factor VII, 1–6 units of factor VIII coagulant antigen per mL. FEIBA DOES NOT contain heparin. Supplied in vials with nominal factor VIII inhibitor bypass activity potencies of 500 IU/20 mL, 1,000 IU/20 mL, and 2,500 IU/50 mL.

7. **NovoSeven RT®.** Recombinant coagulation factor VIIa. Supplied in vials of 1 mg, 2 mg, 5 mg, and 8 mg of rFVIIa.

B. **Suggested minimum stocking levels** for the treatment of a 100-kg adult for the first 8 hours and 24 hours depend upon the individual PCC.
1. Three- and four-factor PCCs have only been recommended as single doses for reversal and should be stocked at the maximum doses (see Tables III–6 and III–7).
2. FEIBA® has a maximum dose of 20,000 U in 100-kg adult over a 24-hour period.
3. Recombinant VIIa does not have a reported maximum dose. The suggested minimum stocking level for a 100-kg adult is 9,000 mcg.

▶ CYPROHEPTADINE

F. Lee Cantrell, PharmD

I. **Pharmacology.** Cyproheptadine is a first-generation histamine 1 (H_1) blocker with nonspecific serotonin (5-HT) antagonism. The administration of cyproheptadine to patients with serotonin syndrome appears to antagonize excessive stimulation of 5-HT_{1A} and 5-HT_2 receptors, resulting in improvements in clinical symptoms (based on anecdotal case reports).

II. **Indications. Cyproheptadine** may be beneficial in alleviating mild to moderate symptoms in cases of suspected serotonin syndrome (p 21).

III. **Contraindications**
A. Known hypersensitivity to cyproheptadine.
B. Angle-closure glaucoma.
C. Stenosing peptic ulcer.
D. Symptomatic prostatic hypertrophy.
E. Bladder neck obstruction.
F. Pyloroduodenal obstruction.

IV. **Adverse effects**
A. Transient mydriasis and urinary retention may result from anticholinergic properties.
B. **Use in pregnancy.** FDA Category B (p 498). Unlikely to cause harm with short-term therapy.

V. **Drug or laboratory interactions.** Additive anticholinergic effects when given with other antimuscarinic drugs.

VI. **Dosage and method of administration (adults and children):** The initial dose is 4–12 mg orally, followed by 4 mg every 1–4 hours as needed until symptoms resolve or a maximum daily dose of 32 mg is reached (children: 0.25 mg/kg/d divided every 6 hours with a maximum of 12 mg/d).

VII. **Formulations**
A. **Oral.** Cyproheptadine hydrochloride (Periactin, others), 4-mg tablets, 2-mg/5 mL syrup.
B. **Suggested minimum stocking levels** to treat a 100-kg adult for the first 8 hours and 24 hours: **cyproheptadine hydrochloride**, *first 8 hours:* 32 mg or eight tablets (4 mg each); *first 24 hours:* 32 mg or eight tablets (4 mg each).

▶ DANTROLENE

Thomas E. Kearney, PharmD

I. **Pharmacology.** Dantrolene relaxes skeletal muscle by inhibiting the release of calcium from the sarcoplasmic reticulum, thereby reducing actin–myosin contractile activity. Dantrolene can help control hyperthermia that results from excessive muscle hyperactivity, particularly when hyperthermia is caused by a defect within the muscle cells (eg, malignant hyperthermia). Dantrolene is not a substitute for other temperature-controlling measures (eg, sponging and fanning).

II. Indications

A. The primary indication for dantrolene is malignant hyperthermia (p 21).

B. Dantrolene may be useful in treating hyperthermia and rhabdomyolysis caused by drug-induced muscular hyperactivity that is not controlled by usual cooling measures or neuromuscular paralysis.

1. There are a number of case reports suggesting benefit for the management of several conditions associated with muscle hyperactivity or rigidity, including neuroleptic malignant syndrome (NMS); monoamine oxidase (MAO) inhibitor–induced hyperthermia; serotonin toxicity; methylenedioxymethamphetamine (MDMA) overdose; dinitrophenol-induced hyperthermia; muscle rigidity from baclofen withdrawal; hypertonicity from carbon monoxide poisoning; tetanus; thyroid storm; and black widow spider envenomation. It should be noted that a meta-analysis of NMS case reports found that dantrolene use was associated with higher mortality than supportive care alone.

C. Theoretically, dantrolene is not expected to be effective for hyperthermia caused by conditions other than muscular hyperactivity, such as increased metabolic rate (eg, salicylate or dinitrophenol poisoning); impaired heat dissipation (eg, anticholinergic syndrome); and environmental exposure (heat stroke).

III. Contraindications. No absolute contraindications exist. Patients with muscular weakness or respiratory impairment must be observed closely for possible respiratory arrest.

IV. Adverse effects

A. Muscle weakness, which may aggravate respiratory depression.

B. Drowsiness, fatigue, dizziness, photosensitivity, and diarrhea.

C. Black box warning. Potential for fatal hepatotoxicity (hypersensitivity hepatitis) reported after chronic therapy. May also be dose-related (more common with 800 mg/d). Transaminases are elevated in about 10% of patients treated with dantrolene.

D. Intravenous administration has been associated with pulmonary edema (mannitol may contribute), phlebitis (avoid extravasation), and urticaria.

E. Use in pregnancy. FDA Category C (indeterminate). This does not preclude acute, short-term use of dantrolene for a seriously symptomatic patient (p 498).

V. Drug or laboratory interactions

A. Dantrolene may have additive CNS-depressant effects with sedative and hypnotic drugs.

B. Dantrolene and verapamil coadministration is associated with hyperkalemia and hypotension (case report).

C. Each 20-mg vial of Dantrium contains 3 g of mannitol; this should be taken into consideration, as it may have additive effects with any mannitol given to treat rhabdomyolysis. Use only sterile water (without bacteriostatic agent) to reconstitute. Incompatible with D_5W and NS.

VI. Dosage and method of administration (adults and children)

A. Initial dose. Give a minimum of 1 mg/kg and up to 2.5 mg/kg rapidly IV through a secure, free-flowing peripheral or central line; this may be repeated as needed every 5–15 minutes to a cumulative total dose of 10 mg/kg (up to 30 mg/kg has been used). Satisfactory response usually is achieved with an average total dose of 2.5 mg/kg.

B. Postcrisis maintenance. To prevent recurrence of hyperthermia, administer 1–2 mg/kg intravenously or orally (up to 100 mg maximum) 4 times a day for 1–3 days. Daily dose not to exceed 400 mg (see black box warning). For prevention (patients at risk for malignant hyperthermia), give orally 1–2 days before surgery (with the last dose given 3–4 hours before surgery), or give IV at 2.5 mg/kg infused over at least 1 minute (Ryanodex) or 1 hour (Dantrium) 1 ¼ hours (75 minutes) before anesthesia.

VII. Formulations

A. Parenteral. Dantrolene sodium (Dantrium), 20 mg of lyophilized powder for reconstitution (after reconstitution, protect from light and use within 6 hours to ensure maximal activity). Each 20-mg vial contains 3 g of mannitol (see "Adverse effects" and "Drug or laboratory interactions") and should be reconstituted with 60 mL of sterile water (prewarmed water will decrease time for dissolution and need to shake until clear).

New product: Intravenous suspension of dantrolene sodium (Ryanodex), 250 mg per 20-mL vial for reconstitution with 5 mL of nonbacteriostatic sterile water (after reconstitution, protect from light and use within 6 hours to ensure maximal activity). Each vial contains 125 mg of mannitol. Need to shake well until a uniform orange colored suspension is achieved. Rapidly dissolves within 1 minute and one vial is equivalent to 12.5 vials of other products.

B. Oral. Dantrolene sodium (Dantrium, others) in 25-, 50-, and 100-mg capsules.

C. Suggested minimum stocking levels to treat a 100-kg adult for the first 8 hours and 24 hours: **dantrolene sodium**, *first 8 hours:* 1,000 mg or 50 vials (20 mg each) or four vials (250 mg each) of Ryanodex; *first 24 hours:* 1,300 mg or 56 vials (20 mg each) or five vials (250 mg each) of Ryanodex.

▶ DEFEROXAMINE

F. Lee Cantrell, PharmD

I. Pharmacology. Deferoxamine is a specific chelating agent for iron. It binds free iron and, to some extent, loosely bound iron (eg, from ferritin or hemosiderin). Iron bound to hemoglobin, transferrin, cytochrome enzymes, and all other sites is not affected. The red iron-deferoxamine (ferrioxamine) complex is water-soluble and excreted renally; it may impart an orange–pink (*vin rosé*) color to the urine. One hundred milligrams of deferoxamine is capable of binding 8.5 mg of elemental iron and 4.1 mg of aluminum in vitro. Deferoxamine and both the aluminoxamine and ferrioxamine complexes are dialyzable. The basic science literature supports the use of the drug, but clinical evidence of efficacy and safety is lacking.

II. Indications

A. Deferoxamine is used to treat iron intoxication (p 277) when the serum iron is greater than 450–500 mcg/dL or when clinical signs of significant iron intoxication exist (eg, shock, acidosis, severe gastroenteritis, or numerous radiopaque tablets visible in the GI tract by radiography).

B. Deferoxamine sometimes is used as a "test dose" to determine the presence of free iron by observing the characteristic *vin rosé* color in the urine; however, a change in urine color is not a reliable indicator.

C. Deferoxamine has also been used for the treatment of aluminum toxicity in patients with renal failure.

III. Contraindications. No absolute contraindications to deferoxamine use exist in patients with serious iron poisoning. The drug should be used with caution in patients who have a known sensitivity to deferoxamine and patients with renal failure/anuria who are not undergoing hemodialysis.

IV. Adverse effects

- **A.** Hypotension or an anaphylactoid-type reaction may occur from very rapid intravenous administration; this can be avoided by limiting the rate of administration to 15 mg/kg/h.
- **B.** Local pain, induration, and sterile abscess formation may occur at intramuscular injection sites. Large intramuscular injections may also cause hypotension.
- **C.** The ferrioxamine complex may itself cause hypotension and may accumulate in patients with renal impairment; hemodialysis may be necessary to remove the ferrioxamine complex.
- **D.** Deferoxamine, as a siderophore, promotes the growth of certain bacteria, such as *Yersinia enterocolitica,* and may predispose patients to *Yersinia* sepsis.
- **E.** Infusions exceeding 24 hours have been associated with pulmonary complications (acute respiratory distress syndrome).
- **F. Use in pregnancy.** FDA Category C (indeterminate). Although deferoxamine is a teratogen in animals, it has relatively poor placental transfer, and there is no evidence that short-term treatment is harmful in human pregnancy (p 498). More importantly, failure to treat serious acute iron intoxications may result in maternal and fetal morbidity or death.

V. Drug or laboratory interactions. Deferoxamine may interfere with determinations of serum iron (falsely low) and total iron-binding capacity (falsely high). It may chelate and remove aluminum from the body.

VI. Dosage and method of administration

- **A.** The intravenous route is preferred in all cases. In children or adults, give deferoxamine at an infusion rate starting at 5 mg/kg/h and increasing over 15 minutes as tolerated to a rate generally not to exceed 15 mg/kg/h to minimize risk of hypotension (although rates of up to 40–50 mg/kg/h have been used in patients with massive iron intoxication). This correlates to a binding of 1.3 mg/kg/h when administered at 15 mg/kg/h. The maximum cumulative daily dose generally should not exceed 6 g (doses of up to 16 g have been tolerated). The end points of therapy include the absence of *vin rosé*–colored urine, a serum iron level of less than 350 mcg/dL, and resolution of clinical signs of intoxication.
- **B.** Oral complexation is ***not*** recommended.
- **C.** Intramuscular injection is ***not*** recommended. If the patient is symptomatic, use the intravenous route. If the patient is not symptomatic but serious toxicity is expected to occur, intravenous access is essential (eg, for fluid boluses), and intravenous dosing provides more reliable administration.

VII. Formulations

- **A. Parenteral.** Deferoxamine mesylate (Desferal, and others), vials containing 500 mg and 2 g of lyophilized powder.
- **B. Suggested minimum stocking levels** to treat a 100-kg adult for the first 8 hours and 24 hours: **deferoxamine mesylate**, *first 8 hours:* 12 g or six vials (2 g each); *first 24 hours:* 36 g or 18 vials (2 g each).

▶ DEXMEDETOMIDINE

Mark Sutter, MD

I. Pharmacology

- **A.** Dexmedetomidine is a potent alpha-2- adrenergic receptor agonist. It shares structural and functional similarities with clonidine; however, the alpha-2/alpha-1 specificity ratio is eight times higher for dexmedetomidine. In addition, dexmedetomidine has more affinity for the alpha-2 A and C receptor subtypes, making it more effective than clonidine for sedation and analgesia. It can provide sedation with limited effects on respiratory depression. The sympatholytic effects are mediated via neuronal presynaptic alpha-2 receptors that provide negative feedback to reduce synaptic transmission.

B. When given as an intravenous loading dose, followed by continuous infusion, the onset of action is 5–15 minutes and peak concentrations are achieved within 1 hour.

C. The drug is rapidly distributed in a two-compartment model to a steady-state volume of distribution (Vd) of 118–152 L. Dexmedetomidine is 94% protein bound and has a distributional half-life of approximately 6 minutes following IV bolus and an elimination half-life of 2–2.67 hours.

D. Dexmedetomidine undergoes complete biotransformation to inactive metabolites via N-glucuronidation, N-methylation, and hydroxylation via CYP P450 2D6.

II. Indications

A. Dexmedetomidine is FDA approved for sedation in mechanically intubated patients not to exceed 24 hours in adults. It is also approved for use in nonintubated adults prior to and/or during surgical and other procedures. There is no FDA-approved indication in pediatrics despite its wide use.

B. Specific clinical conditions where it has been used include sedation for critically ill patients; sedation for minimally invasive procedures; premedication for surgery; opioid, benzodiazepine, and ethanol withdrawal states; fentanyl- or sufentanil-induced cough; and postanesthetic shivering. It may have potential neuroprotective use in neurological surgery due to its stable hemodynamics.

III. Contraindications

A. No specific contraindications exist. However, dose reductions are recommended in patients with impaired liver function and patients older than 65 years. Caution is also advised in patients with advanced heart block and/or severe ventricular dysfunction.

IV. Adverse effects

A. Bradycardia and hypotension are the most common dose-dependent and clinically important adverse effects. Hypotension may be preceded by a brief phase of hypertension lasting 5–10 minutes.

B. Most adverse effects occur during or shortly after the loading dose and may be minimized by slowing or omitting the loading dose. More pronounced effects may occur in patients older than 65 years and those with diabetes mellitus, advanced heart block, chronic hypertension, hypovolemia, and/or ventricular dysfunction.

C. There are postmarketing reports of other cardiovascular (atrial fibrillation, AV block, ventricular arrhythmias), CNS (agitation, confusion, delirium, convulsions), and respiratory (apnea, bronchospasm, pulmonary congestion) adverse effects.

D. Abrupt cessation of dexmedetomidine infusion has resulted in a rebound tachycardia and hypertension. Other drug withdrawal symptoms including nausea, vomiting, and agitation have been reported.

E. Prolonged administration (>24 hours) may lead to tolerance (tachyphylaxis), requiring higher doses.

F. Use in pregnancy. FDA Category C. No human data exist for use in labor or in breast-feeding mothers.

V. Drug or laboratory interactions

A. Use caution when administering dexmedetomidine with other drugs known to cause bradycardia or hypotension.

B. Despite the high protein binding of dexmedetomidine, no significant displacement of warfarin, phenytoin, digoxin, theophylline or propranolol was evident when studied.

VI. Dosage and Method of administration

A. Give a **loading dose** of 1 mcg/kg (children: 0.25–1 mcg/kg) IV over 10 minutes (procedural sedation: 0.5 mcg/kg), followed by **continuous infusion** of 0.2–0.7 mcg/kg/h for a maximum of 24 hours.

1. ***Note.*** Most adverse effects occur during or shortly after the loading dose (see adverse section described previously).
2. Exact dosage must be individualized and titrated to clinical effect.
3. Reduce dose in patients older than 65 years or with hepatic impairment.

B. **Intranasal** dose for procedural or preoperative sedation is 1 mcg/kg (children: 1–2 mcg/kg) administered bilaterally (one half in each nostril).

C. **Intramuscular** doses of 0.5–1.5 mcg/kg (children: 1–4.5 mcg/kg) have been used as adjunct therapy 1 hour prior to surgery.

VII. **Formulations**

A. Parenteral. Dexmedetomidine hydrochloride (Precedex), 100 mcg/mL in 2-mL vials, and 200 mcg/50 mL and 400 mcg/100 mL in 0.9% sodium chloride in glass bottles. ***Note.*** When supplied in 100 mcg/mL concentration in 2-mL vials, reconstitute with the addition of 48 mL of 0.9% saline to form a concentration of 4 mcg/mL.

B. **Suggested minimum stocking level** for the treatment of a 100-kg adult for the first 8 and 24 hours: Dexmedetomidine hydrochloride, *first 8 hours*: 800 mcg or four vials (100 mcg/mL, 2 mL each); *first 24 hours*: 2,000 mcg or 10 vials (100 mcg/mL, 2 mL each).

▶ DIGOXIN-SPECIFIC ANTIBODIES

Thomas E. Kearney, PharmD

I. **Pharmacology.** Digoxin-specific antibodies are produced in immunized sheep and have a high binding affinity for digoxin and, to a lesser extent, digitoxin and other cardiac glycosides. The Fab fragments used to treat poisoning are derived by cleaving the whole antibodies. Once the digoxin-Fab complex is formed, the digoxin molecule is no longer pharmacologically active. The complex enters the circulation, is renally eliminated and cleared by the reticuloendothelial system, and has a half-life of 14–20 hours (may increase 10-fold with renal impairment). Reversal of signs of digitalis intoxication usually occurs within 30–60 minutes of administration (average initial response, 19 minutes), with complete reversal varying up to 24 hours (average, 88 minutes).

II. **Indications.** Digoxin-specific antibodies are used for life-threatening arrhythmias, hyperkalemia (≥5 mEq/L), or hemodynamic instability caused by acute and chronic cardiac glycoside intoxication (p 222). Treatment should be based on elevated levels that are at steady state (or are postdistributional) as well as the presence of significant symptoms (eg, hyperkalemia, ventricular arrhythmias, bradyarrhythmias, and hypotension).

III. **Contraindications.** No contraindications are known. Caution is warranted in patients with known sensitivity to ovine (sheep) products; a skin test for hypersensitivity may be performed in such patients, with the use of diluted reconstituted drug. There are no reports of hypersensitivity reactions in patients who have received the drug more than once (although this is a theoretical risk). Product may contain traces of papain; therefore, caution is advised in patients with allergies to papain, chymopapain, papaya extracts, and the pineapple enzyme bromelain.

IV. **Adverse effects**

A. Monitor the patient for potential hypersensitivity reactions and serum sickness. A dose- and rate-related (anaphylactoid) reaction may occur with rapid IV administration.

B. In patients with renal insufficiency and impaired clearance of the digitalis-Fab complex, a delayed rebound of free serum digoxin levels may occur for up to 130 hours.

C. Removal of the inotropic effect of digitalis may exacerbate preexisting heart failure.

D. With removal of the digitalis effect, patients with preexisting atrial fibrillation may develop an accelerated ventricular response.

E. Removal of the digitalis effect may reactivate sodium-potassium-ATPase and shift potassium into cells, causing a drop in the serum potassium level.

TABLE III–8. APPROXIMATE DIGOXIN-FAB DOSE IF AMOUNT INGESTED IS KNOWN

Tablets Ingested (0.125-mg Size)	Tablets Ingested (0.25-mg Size)	Approximate Dose Absorbed (mg)	Recommended Dose (No. of Vials)
5	2.5	0.5	1
10	5	1	2
20	10	2	4
50	25	5	10
100	50	10	20

F. Use in pregnancy. FDA Category C (indeterminate). This does not preclude its acute, short-term use for a seriously symptomatic patient (p 498).

V. Drug or laboratory interactions

A. Digoxin-specific Fab fragments will bind other cardiac glycosides, including digitoxin, ouabain, oleander glycosides, and possibly glycosides in lily of the valley, *Strophanthus,* squill, and toad venom (*Bufo* species cardenolides).

B. The digoxin-Fab complex cross-reacts with the antibody commonly used in quantitative immunoassay techniques. This results in falsely high serum concentrations of digoxin owing to measurement of the inactive Fab complex (total serum digoxin levels may increase 10- to 21-fold). However, some assays and procedures may measure free digoxin levels, which may be useful for patients with renal impairment (to monitor a rebound in free serum digoxin levels after administration of Fab fragments).

VI. Dosage and method of administration. Each vial of either digoxin–immune Fab product binds 0.5 mg of digoxin.

A. Complete neutralization/equimolar dosing; known level or amount ingested. Estimation of the dose of Fab is based on the body burden of digitalis. This may be calculated if the approximate amount ingested is known (Table III–8) or if the steady-state (postdistributional) serum drug concentration is known (Table III–9). The steady-state serum drug concentration should be determined at least 12–16 hours after the last dose. ***Note:* Use of the ingested digoxin dose calculation will generally overestimate the Fab dose requirement.** Also, calculation of the digoxin body burden is based on an estimated volume of distribution of 5–6 L/kg; however, the Vd may be as high as 10 L/kg. If the patient fails to respond to the initial treatment, the dose may have to be increased by an additional 50%.

B. Empiric dosing (unknown level and severe toxicity). If the amount ingested or the postdistributional level is not known and the patient has life-threatening dysrhythmias, dosing may have to be empiric. The manufacturer recommends that 20 (10 for children) and six vials be given empirically for acute and chronic

TABLE III–9. APPROXIMATE DIGOXIN-FAB DOSE BASED ON SERUM CONCENTRATION AT STEADY STATE (AFTER EQUILIBRATION)

Digoxin[a]: $\text{Number of digoxin} - \text{Fab vials} = \dfrac{\text{Serum digoxin (ng/mL)} \times \text{body weight (kg)}}{100}$

Digitoxin: $\text{Number of digoxin} - \text{Fab vials} = \dfrac{\text{Serum digoxin (ng/mL)} \times \text{body weight (kg)}}{1{,}000}$

[a]This calculation provides a quick estimate of the number of vials needed but can underestimate the actual need because of variations in the volume of distribution (5–7 L/kg). Be prepared to increase the dose by 50% if the clinical response to the initial dose is not satisfactory.

overdoses, respectively. However, average dose requirements are 10 vials for acute and 1–3 vials for chronic digoxin intoxication.

C. **Titration dosing.** Theoretically, Fab may be used to neutralize a *portion* of the digoxin body burden to reverse toxicity but maintain therapeutic benefits. Many patients will respond to one-half or less of the calculated neutralizing dose based on body burden. The Fab dose can be estimated by subtracting the desired digoxin level from the measured postdistributional level before the calculation is completed. Alternately, if the patient is hemodynamically stable, the drug can be given empirically, 1–2 vials at a time, with titration to clinical effect. A proposed strategy has been to infuse the initial or loading dose over 30–60 minutes and then allow 1 hour after the end of the infusion period to assess the need for additional doses. This may optimize binding and reduce wastage of the antidote. However, partial dosing has been associated with recurrences of symptoms in some digoxin-poisoned patients.

D. Reconstitute the drug with 4 mL of Sterile Water for Injection USP and administer intravenously over at least 30 minutes. The reconstituted product may be added to 0.9% sodium chloride. ***Note:*** Longer infusion periods (1–7 hours) or constant infusions have been suggested to optimize binding of digoxin to the antibodies. The drug may also be given as a rapid bolus for immediately life-threatening arrhythmias.

VII. Formulations

A. **Parenteral.** DigiFab, 40 mg of lyophilized digoxin-specific Fab fragments per vial. ***Note:*** Digibind was discontinued in 2011.

B. **Suggested minimum stocking levels** to treat a 100-kg adult for the first 8 hours and 24 hours: **digoxin-specific Fab fragments**, *first 8 hours:* 15 vials of either product; *first 24 hours:* 20 vials of either product.

▶ DIPHENHYDRAMINE

Thomas E. Kearney, PharmD

I. **Pharmacology.** Diphenhydramine is an antihistamine with anticholinergic, **antitussive**, antiemetic, and local anesthetic properties. The antihistaminic property affords relief from itching and minor irritation caused by plant-induced dermatitis and insect bites, and when used as pretreatment, it provides partial protection against anaphylaxis caused by animal serum–derived antivenoms or antitoxins. Drug-induced extrapyramidal symptoms respond to the anticholinergic effect of diphenhydramine. The effects of diphenhydramine are maximal at 1 hour after intravenous injection and last up to 7 hours. The drug is eliminated by hepatic metabolism, with a serum half-life of 3–7 hours.

II. Indications

A. Relief of symptoms caused by excessive histamine effect (eg, ingestion of scombroid-contaminated fish or niacin and rapid intravenous administration of acetylcysteine). Diphenhydramine may be combined with cimetidine or another histamine 2 (H_2) receptor blocker (p 532).

B. Pretreatment before administration of animal serum–derived antivenoms or antitoxins, especially in patients with a history of hypersensitivity or with a positive skin test. Diphenhydramine can be combined with cimetidine or another H_2 receptor blocker.

C. Neuroleptic drug–induced extrapyramidal symptoms and priapism (one case report).

D. Pruritus caused by poison oak, poison ivy, or minor insect bites.

III. Contraindications

A. Angle-closure glaucoma.

B. Prostatic hypertrophy with obstructive uropathy.

C. Concurrent therapy with monoamine oxidase inhibitors.

IV. Adverse effects

A. Sedation, drowsiness, and ataxia may occur. Paradoxical excitation is possible in small children.

B. Excessive doses may cause flushing, tachycardia, blurred vision, delirium, toxic psychosis, urinary retention, and respiratory depression.

C. Some preparations may contain sulfite preservatives, which can cause allergic-type reactions in susceptible persons.

D. Diphenhydramine may exacerbate dyskinetic movement disorders as a result of increased dopamine (eg, amphetamine or cocaine intoxication) or decreased cholinergic effects in the CNS.

E. Extravasation from an IV dose of 500 mg into arm soft tissue resulted in a chronic regional pain syndrome (case report). Local necrosis from subcutaneous route.

F. Use in pregnancy. FDA Category B (p 498). Fetal harm is extremely unlikely.

V. Drug or laboratory interactions

A. Additive sedative effect with opioids, ethanol, and other sedatives.

B. Additive anticholinergic effect with other antimuscarinic drugs.

VI. Dosage and method of administration

A. Pruritus. Give 25–50 mg PO every 4–6 hours (children: 5 mg/kg/d in divided doses; usual oral doses for ages 6–12 years are 12.5–25 mg every 4–6 hours, and for ages 2–6 years, they are 6.25 mg every 4–6 hours); maximum daily dose: 37.5 mg (children aged 2–6 years), 150 mg (children aged 6–12 years), and 300 mg (adults). The drug may also be applied topically, although systemic absorption and toxicity have been reported, especially when it is used on large areas with blistered or broken skin.

B. Pretreatment before antivenom administration. Give 50 mg (children: 0.5–1 mg/kg) IV; if possible, it should be given at least 15–20 minutes before antivenom use. Rate of IV administration should not exceed 25 mg/min.

C. Drug-induced extrapyramidal symptoms. Give 50 mg (children: 0.5–1 mg/kg) IV (at a rate not to exceed 25 mg/min) or deep IM; if there is no response within 30–60 minutes, repeat dose to a maximum of 100 mg (adults). Provide oral maintenance therapy, 25–50 mg (children: 0.5–1 mg/kg; usual oral dose if <9 kg, 6.25–12.5 mg, and if >9 kg, 12.5–25 mg) every 4–6 hours for 2–3 days to prevent recurrence; maximum daily dose: 300 mg (children) and 400 mg (adults).

VII. Formulations

A. Oral. Diphenhydramine hydrochloride (Benadryl, others), 25- and 50-mg tablets and capsules, 12.5- and 25-mg chewable tablets and disintegrating strips; elixir, syrup, and oral solution, 12.5 mg/5 mL; suspension, 25 mg/5 mL.

B. Parenteral. Diphenhydramine hydrochloride (Benadryl, others), 50 mg/mL in 1-mL cartridges, ampules, Steri-Vials, and syringes, and in 10-mL Steri-Vials (may contain benzethonium chloride).

C. Suggested minimum stocking levels to treat a 100-kg adult for the first 8 hours and 24 hours: **diphenhydramine (parenteral)**, *first 8 hours*: 150 mg or three ampules (50 mg/mL, 1 mL each); *first 24 hours*: 400 mg or eight ampules (50 mg/mL, 1 mL each).

► DOPAMINE

Alicia B. Minns, MD

I. Pharmacology. Dopamine is an endogenous catecholamine and the immediate metabolic precursor of norepinephrine. It stimulates alpha- and beta-adrenergic receptors directly and indirectly. In addition, it acts on specific dopaminergic receptors. Its relative activity at these various receptors is dose-related. At low doses

(1–5 mcg/kg/min), dopamine causes vasodilation of renal vascular beds thereby increasing renal blood flow and urine output. At intermediate doses (5–10 mcg/kg/min), dopamine stimulates beta-1 activity (increased heart rate and contractility) in addition to increasing renal and mesenteric blood flow through dopaminergic agonist activity. At high infusion rates (10–20 mcg/kg/min), alpha-adrenergic stimulation predominates, resulting in increased peripheral vascular resistance. Dopamine is not effective orally. After IV administration, its onset of action occurs within 5 minutes, and the duration of effect is less than 10 minutes. The plasma half-life is about 2 minutes.

II. Indications

A. Dopamine is used to increase blood pressure, cardiac output, and urine flow in patients with shock who have not responded to intravenous fluid challenge, correction of hypothermia, or reversal of acidosis.

B. Low-dose infusion is most effective for hypotension caused by venodilation or reduced cardiac contractility; high-dose dopamine is indicated for shock resulting from decreased peripheral arterial resistance.

III. Contraindications

A. Tachyarrhythmias or ventricular fibrillation. Electrolyte imbalances should be corrected prior to use to minimize the risk of dysrhythmias.

B. Uncorrected hypovolemia.

C. Pheochromocytoma.

D. High-dose infusion is relatively contraindicated in the presence of peripheral arterial occlusive disease with thrombosis and in patients with ergot poisoning. It should also be used with caution in patients with active or recent myocardial infarction.

IV. Adverse effects

A. Severe hypertension, which may result in intracranial hemorrhage, pulmonary edema, or myocardial necrosis.

B. Aggravation of tissue ischemia, resulting in gangrene (with high-dose infusion).

C. Ventricular arrhythmias, especially in patients intoxicated by halogenated or aromatic hydrocarbon solvents or anesthetics.

D. Tissue necrosis after extravasation (see Item VI. A below for the treatment of extravasation).

E. Anaphylactoid reaction induced by sulfite preservatives in sensitive patients.

F. **Use in pregnancy.** FDA Category C (indeterminate). There may be a dose-related effect on uterine blood flow. This does not preclude its acute, short-term use for a seriously symptomatic patient (p 498).

V. Drug or laboratory interactions

A. Enhanced pressor response may occur in the presence of cocaine and cyclic antidepressants owing to inhibition of neuronal reuptake.

B. Enhanced pressor response may occur in patients taking monoamine oxidase inhibitors owing to inhibition of neuronal metabolic degradation.

C. Chloral hydrate and halogenated hydrocarbon anesthetics may enhance the arrhythmogenic effect of dopamine owing to sensitization of the myocardium to the effects of catecholamines.

D. Alpha- and beta-blocking agents antagonize the adrenergic effects of dopamine; haloperidol and other dopamine antagonists may antagonize the dopaminergic effects.

E. There may be a reduced pressor response in patients with depleted neuronal stores of catecholamines (eg, chronic disulfiram or reserpine use).

VI. Dosage and method of administration (adults and children)

A. **Avoid extravasation.** ***Caution:*** The intravenous infusion must be free-flowing, and the infused vein should be observed frequently for the signs of subcutaneous infiltration (pallor, coldness, and induration). If extravasation occurs, immediately infiltrate the affected area with phentolamine (p 605), 5–10 mg in 10–15 mL of normal saline (children: 0.1–0.2 mg/kg; maximum, 10 mg total) via a fine (25–27-gauge) hypodermic needle; improvement is evidenced by hyperemia and return to normal temperature. Topical nitrates and infiltration of terbutaline have also been reported to be successful for the treatment of extravasation involving other catecholamines.

B. For **predominantly inotropic effects**, begin with 1 mcg/kg/min and increase infusion rate as needed to 5–10 mcg/kg/min.

C. For **predominantly vasopressor effects**, infuse 10–20 mcg/kg/min and increase as needed. Doses greater than 20–30 mcg/kg/min may increase the risk of tachydysrhythmias. Doses greater than 50 mcg/kg/min may result in severe peripheral vasoconstriction and gangrene.

VII. Formulations

A. Dopamine hydrochloride (Intropin and others), as a concentrate for admixture to intravenous solutions (40, 80, and 160 mg/mL in 5-mL ampules, 5- and 10-mL vials or syringes, and 20-mL vials) or a premixed parenteral product for injection (0.8, 1.6, and 3.2 mg/mL in 5% dextrose). All contain sodium bisulfite as a preservative.

B. Suggested minimum stocking levels to treat a 100-kg adult for the first 8 hours and 24 hours: **dopamine hydrochloride**, *first 8 hours:* 800 mg or one vial (160 mg/mL, 5 mL each); *first 24 hours:* 2,400 mg or three vials (160 mg/mL, 5 mL each).

▶ DTPA (DIETHYLENETRIAMINEPENTAACETATE)

Tanya Mamantov, MD

I. Pharmacology. Diethylenetriaminepentaacetate (Zn-DTPA and Ca-DTPA) is a chelating agent that is used in exposures to the transuranic elements plutonium, americium, and curium. DTPA is used as a salt of calcium or zinc and forms a chelate that is excreted in the urine. DTPA has a plasma half-life of 20–60 minutes and is distributed in the extracellular space. It has a small amount of protein binding and does not undergo significant metabolism or tissue accumulation. Ca-DTPA resulted in a 10-fold higher rate of elimination of plutonium compared with Zn-DTPA, so this salt is preferred in initial patient management if available.

II. Indications. Internal contamination with plutonium, americium, or curium. It has also been used for the treatment of internal contamination with californium and berkelium.

III. Contraindications

A. Known hypersensitivity to the agent.

B. DTPA should not be used in uranium or neptunium exposures because it may increase bone deposition of these elements.

C. Ca-DTPA should not be used in patients with renal failure, nephrotic syndrome, or bone marrow suppression, or in those who are pregnant.

IV. Adverse effects

A. Nausea, vomiting, and diarrhea.

B. Fever, chills, myalgias, headache, metallic taste, dermatitis.

C. Life-threatening side effects are distinctly uncommon, with no serious toxicity in human subjects after 4,500 administrations of Ca-DTPA and 1,000 administrations of Zn-DTPA.

D. Use in pregnancy. FDA Category D (Ca-DTPA) and Category C (Zn-DTPA); Zn-DTPA may be used in pregnancy, although fetal risks are not completely known (p 498).

V. Drug or laboratory interactions

A. There are no major known drug interactions.

B. There does not appear to be a decrement of body trace elements associated with the use of DTPA.

VI. Dosage and method of administration

A. Upon known exposure, usual therapy would involve Ca-DTPA or Zn-DTPA given in a 1-g dose as soon as possible. This may be given IV over 3–5 minutes in an undiluted form or may be diluted in 100–250 mL of normal saline, lactated Ringer's solution, or 5% dextrose in water. Administration time should not exceed 2 hours. Initial dose for pediatric patients is 14 mg/kg, not to exceed 1 g.

B. It is preferable to give Ca-DTPA for the initial dose because it is more effective than Zn-DTPA during the first 24 hours. After 24 hours, Zn-DTPA and Ca-DTPA are equally effective. If Ca-DTPA is not available or is contraindicated in a patient, the same dose of Zn-DTPA may be substituted. The FDA advises that Zn-DTPA is preferred for maintenance therapy because it is associated with smaller losses of essential minerals.

C. After the initial dose of Ca-DTPA, repeat doses of 1 g of Ca-DTPA or Zn-DTPA should be based on suspected level of internal contamination. Starting at the time of exposure, collect urine and fecal samples for bioassay to guide further treatment after the initial dose. The doses may be continued (usually 2–3 times per week) until the excretion rate of the transuranic is not increased by chelation administration (duration may vary from days to years). For long-term use, Ca-DTPA should be given with supplemental zinc therapy due to endogenous metal depletion.

D. Intramuscular dosing generally is not recommended owing to significant pain with injection.

E. Pregnant women should be treated only with Zn-DTPA.

F. Nebulization in a 1:1 dilution is safe and effective for persons contaminated only via inhalation. The intravenous route should be used if multiple routes of internal contamination occurred or the route is unknown.

VII. Formulations

A. Parenteral or nebulization. Pentetate Calcium Trisodium Injection (Ca-DTPA), Pentetate Zinc Trisodium Injection (Zn-DTPA). One gram in 5 mL of diluent (200 mg/mL) packaged in single-use clear glass ampules. This is provided in boxes of 10 ampules for each salt (Ca-DTPA and Zn-DTPA) by Geritex.

B. Suggested minimum stocking levels to treat a 100-kg adult for the first 8 hours and 24 hours:

1. **Pentetate Calcium Trisodium,** *first 8 hours:* 1 g or one ampule (200 mg/mL, 5 mL each); *first 24 hours:* 1 g or one ampule (200 mg/mL, 5 mL each).
2. **Pentetate Zinc Trisodium,** *first 8 hours:* 1 g or one ampule (200 mg/mL, 5 mL each); *first 24 hours:* 1 g or one ampule (200 mg/mL, 5 mL each).

It is advisable to stock both Ca-DTPA and Zn-DTPA. DTPA is kept in the Strategic National Stockpile (SNS) at the Centers for Disease Control and Prevention (CDC). The Radiation Emergency Assistance Center/Training Site (REAC/TS) can be contacted for information on obtaining DTPA and its recommended dosing via telephone at 1-865-576-3131 (If during nonbusiness hours and in an emergency, will be referred to the Oakridge Operations Office at 1-865-576-1005) or on the Internet at www.orau.gov/reacts.

▶ EDTA, CALCIUM (CALCIUM DISODIUM EDTA, CALCIUM DISODIUM EDETATE, CALCIUM DISODIUM VERSENATE)

Michael J. Kosnett, MD, MPH

I. Pharmacology. Calcium EDTA (ethylenediaminetetraacetate) has been used as a chelating agent to enhance elimination of certain toxic metals, principally lead. The elimination of endogenous metals, including zinc, manganese, iron, and copper, may also occur to a lesser extent. The plasma half-life of the drug is

20–60 minutes, and 50% of the injected dose is excreted in urine within 1 hour. Increased urinary excretion of lead begins within 1 hour of EDTA administration and is followed by a decrease in whole-blood lead concentration over the course of treatment. Calcium EDTA mobilizes lead from soft tissues and from a fraction of the larger lead stores present in bone. In persons with a high body lead burden, cessation of EDTA chelation often is followed by an upward rebound in blood lead levels as bone stores equilibrate with lower soft-tissue levels. ***Note:*** Calcium EDTA should ***not*** be confused with sodium EDTA (edetate disodium), which occasionally is used to treat life-threatening severe hypercalcemia.

II. Indications

A. Calcium EDTA has been used to decrease blood lead concentrations and increase urinary lead excretion in individuals with symptomatic lead intoxication and in asymptomatic persons with high blood lead levels. Although clinical experience associates calcium EDTA chelation with relief of symptoms (particularly lead colic) and decreased mortality, controlled clinical trials demonstrating therapeutic efficacy are lacking, and treatment recommendations have been largely empiric.

B. Calcium EDTA may have possible utility in poisoning by zinc, manganese, and certain heavy radioisotopes.

III. Contraindications. Because calcium EDTA increases renal excretion of lead, anuria is a relative contraindication. Accumulation of EDTA increases the risk for nephropathy, especially in volume-depleted patients. In patients with moderate renal insufficiency, reduce the dose in relative proportion to the deficit in creatinine clearance. The use of EDTA in conjunction with high-flux hemodialysis or hemofiltration has been reported in patients with renal failure.

IV. Adverse effects

A. Nephrotoxicity (eg, acute tubular necrosis, proteinuria, and hematuria) may be minimized by adequate hydration, establishment of adequate urine flow, avoidance of excessive doses, and limitation of continuous administration to 5 days or fewer. Laboratory assessment of renal function should be performed daily during the treatment for severe intoxication and after the second and fifth days in other cases.

B. Black box warning. In individuals with lead encephalopathy, rapid or high-volume infusions may exacerbate increased intracranial pressure. In such cases, it is preferable to use lower volumes of more concentrated solutions for intravenous infusions. Alternatively, intramuscular injection may be considered.

C. Local pain may occur at intramuscular injection sites. Lidocaine (1 mL of 1% lidocaine per 1 mL of EDTA concentrate) may be added to intramuscular injections to decrease discomfort.

D. Inadvertent use of sodium EDTA (edetate disodium) may cause serious **hypocalcemia**.

E. Calcium EDTA may result in short-term zinc depletion, which has uncertain clinical significance.

F. Use in pregnancy. The safety of calcium EDTA in human pregnancy has not been established, although uncomplicated use late in pregnancy has been reported. Fetal malformations with high doses have been noted in animal studies, possibly as a consequence of zinc depletion. If severe lead poisoning necessitates use during pregnancy, maternal zinc supplementation should be considered.

V. Drug or laboratory interactions. Intravenous infusions may be incompatible with 10% dextrose solutions, amphotericin, or hydralazine.

VI. Dosage and method of administration for lead poisoning (adults and children). ***Note:*** Administration of EDTA should never be a substitute for removal from lead exposure. In adults, the federal OSHA lead standard requires removal from occupational lead exposure of any worker with a single blood lead concentration in excess of 60 mcg/dL or an average of three successive values in excess of 50 mcg/dL. (However, recent declines in background lead levels and concern about adverse health effects of lower-level exposure support removal at even lower levels.) ***Prophylactic chelation,*** defined as the routine use of chelation to prevent elevated blood lead concentrations or to lower blood lead levels below the standard in asymptomatic workers, **is *not* permitted.** Consult the local or state health department or OSHA (see Table IV–3, p 652) for more detailed information.

A. Lead poisoning with encephalopathy, acute lead colic, or blood lead levels greater than 150 mcg/dL

1. **Adults:** 2–4 g (or 30–50 mg/kg) IV per 24 hours as a continuous infusion (diluted to 2–4 mg/mL in normal saline or 5% dextrose). Courses of treatment should not exceed 5 days.
2. **Children:** 1,000–1,500 mg/m^2 per 24 hours as a continuous IV infusion (diluted to 2–4 mg/mL in normal saline or 5% dextrose). Some clinicians advocate that treatment of patients with lead encephalopathy, particularly children, be initiated along with a single dose of BAL (dimercaprol [p 514]), followed 4 hours later by the concomitant administration of BAL and calcium EDTA. BAL is discontinued after 3 days; EDTA may be continued for up to 5 days consecutively.

B. Symptomatic lead poisoning without encephalopathy or colic. Administer calcium EDTA at an adult dose of 2–4 g (or 30–50 mg/kg) IV per 24 hours or at a pediatric dose of 1,000–1,500 mg/m^2/d (approximately 20–30 mg/kg as a continuous IV infusion, diluted to 2–4 mg/mL) for 3–5 days.

C. Although intravenous administration is preferable, the daily dose (see above) may be administered by deep intramuscular injection in two or three divided doses (every 8–12 hours).

D. Because EDTA enhances urinary lead excretion, provide adequate fluids to maintain urine flow (optimally 1–2 mL/kg/h). However, avoid overhydration, which may aggravate cerebral edema.

E. Treatment courses should be separated by a minimum of 2 days, and an interval of 2 weeks or more may be indicated to assess the extent of posttreatment rebound in blood lead levels. An additional course of calcium EDTA treatment may be considered on the basis of posttreatment blood lead concentrations and the persistence or recurrence of symptoms.

F. Consider changing to oral succimer (p 624) or oral unithiol (p 630) after 3–5 days of calcium EDTA treatment provided that encephalopathy or colic has resolved, the blood lead level has fallen to less than 100 mcg/dL, and the patient is able to absorb an oral formulation.

G. Single-dose EDTA chelation lead mobilization tests have been advocated by some clinicians to evaluate body lead burden or assess the need for a full course of treatment in patients with moderately elevated blood lead levels, but the value and necessity of these tests are controversial.

H. Oral EDTA therapy is *not* recommended for prevention or treatment of lead poisoning because it may *increase* the absorption of lead from the GI tract.

I. Use in renal failure. For patients with severe lead intoxication and renal failure, a recommended protocol is to administer 1 g of calcium EDTA in 250-cc normal saline intravenously over 1 hour, followed immediately by 4 hours of hemodialysis using a high flux dialysis membrane, such as the F160.

VII. Formulations

A. Parenteral. Calcium disodium edetate (Versenate), 200 mg/mL, 5-mL ampules. For intravenous infusion, dilute to 2–4 mg/mL in normal saline or 5% dextrose solution. ***Note:*** Lower cost pharmaceutical grade calcium disodium EDTA bulk powder may be obtained by hospital pharmacies for the preparation of compounded intravenous solutions.

B. Suggested minimum stocking levels to treat a 100-kg adult for the first 8 hours and 24 hours: **calcium disodium edetate**, *first 8 hours:* 1 g or one ampule (200 mg/mL, 5 mL each); *first 24 hours:* 3 g or three ampules (200 mg/mL, 5 mL each).

▶ EPINEPHRINE

Alicia B. Minns, MD

I. **Pharmacology.** Epinephrine is an endogenous catecholamine with alpha- and beta-adrenergic agonist properties that is used primarily in emergency situations to treat anaphylaxis or cardiac arrest. Beneficial effects include inhibition of histamine release from mast cells and basophils, bronchodilation, positive inotropic effects, and peripheral vasoconstriction. Epinephrine is not active after oral administration. Subcutaneous injection produces effects within 5–10 minutes, with peak effects at 20 minutes. Intravenous or inhalational administration produces much more rapid onset. Epinephrine is inactivated rapidly in the body, with an elimination half-life of 2 minutes.

II. **Indications**
   - **A.** Anaphylaxis and anaphylactoid reactions.
   - **B.** Epinephrine occasionally is used for hypotension resulting from overdose with beta-blockers, calcium antagonists, and other cardiac-depressant drugs.
   - **C.** Asystole/pulseless arrest, pulseless ventricular tachycardia/ventricular fibrillation.
   - **D.** Symptomatic bradycardia unresponsive to atropine or pacing.

III. **Contraindications.** There are no absolute contraindications in a life-threatening situation. Epinephrine is relatively contraindicated in patients with organic heart disease, peripheral arterial occlusive vascular disease with thrombosis, or ergot poisoning, narrow-angle glaucoma, general anesthesia with halogenated hydrocarbons, and in situations in which vasopressors may be contraindicated such as thyrotoxicosis.

IV. **Adverse effects**
   - **A.** Anxiety, restlessness, tremor, and headache.
   - **B.** Severe hypertension, which may result in intracranial hemorrhage, pulmonary edema, or myocardial necrosis or infarction.
   - **C.** Other cardiovascular effects such as chest pain, palpitations, tachycardia, ectopy, and ventricular dysrhythmias.
   - **D.** Use with caution in patients intoxicated by halogenated or aromatic hydrocarbon solvents and anesthetics because these agents may sensitize the myocardium to the arrhythmogenic effects of epinephrine.
   - **E.** Tissue necrosis after extravasation or intra-arterial injection.
   - **F.** Aggravation of tissue ischemia, resulting in gangrene.
   - **G.** Anaphylactoid reaction, which may occur owing to the bisulfite preservative in patients with sulfite hypersensitivity.
   - **H.** Hypokalemia, hypophosphatemia, hyperglycemia, and leukocytosis may occur owing to the beta-adrenergic effects of epinephrine.
   - **I. Use in pregnancy.** FDA Category C (indeterminate). Epinephrine is teratogenic in animals, crosses the placenta, can cause placental ischemia, and may suppress uterine contractions, but these effects do not preclude its acute, short-term use for a seriously symptomatic patient (p 498).

V. **Drug or laboratory interactions**
   - **A.** An enhanced arrhythmogenic effect may occur when epinephrine is given to patients with chloral hydrate overdose or anesthetized with halogenated general anesthetics.
   - **B.** Use in patients taking propranolol and other nonselective beta-blockers may produce severe hypertension owing to blockade of beta$_2$-mediated vasodilation, resulting in unopposed alpha-mediated vasoconstriction.
   - **C.** Cocaine and cyclic antidepressants may enhance stimulant effects owing to inhibition of neuronal epinephrine reuptake.
   - **D.** Monoamine oxidase inhibitors may enhance pressor effects because of decreased neuronal epinephrine metabolism.
   - **E.** Digitalis intoxication may enhance the arrhythmogenicity of epinephrine.

VI. Dosage and method of administration

A. *Caution:* Avoid extravasation. The intravenous infusion must be free-flowing, and the infused vein should be observed frequently for signs of subcutaneous infiltration (pallor, coldness, or induration).

1. If extravasation occurs, immediately infiltrate the affected area with phentolamine (p 605), 5–10 mg in 10–15 mL of normal saline (children: 0.1–0.2 mg/kg; maximum, 10 mg total) via a fine (25–27-gauge) hypodermic needle; improvement is evidenced by hyperemia and return to normal temperature.

2. Alternatively, topical application of nitroglycerin 2% paste and infiltration of terbutaline have been reported to be successful.

B. Mild-to-moderate allergic reaction. Give 0.2–0.5 mg IM (children: 0.01 mg/kg of the 1-mg/mL solution; maximum, 0.5 mg). May be repeated after 5–15 minutes if needed.

C. Severe anaphylaxis. Give 0.05–0.1 mg IV (0.5–1 mL of the 0.1-mg/mL solution) every 5–10 minutes (children: 0.01 mg/kg; maximum, 0.1 mg) or an IV infusion at 1–4 mcg/min. If intravenous access is not available, the endotracheal route may be used; give 0.5 mg (5 mL of the 0.1-mg/mL solution) down the endotracheal tube.

D. Hypotension. Infuse at 0.5–1 mcg/min; titrate upward every 5 minutes as necessary. If the patient has refractory hypotension and is on a beta-adrenergic–blocking drug, consider glucagon (p 559).

VII. Formulations

A. Parenteral. Epinephrine hydrochloride (Adrenalin, EpiPen, Twinjet, Auvi-Q, others), 0.1 mg/mL in 10-mL prefilled syringes; 0.5 mg/mL (0.15 mg) in 0.3-mL single-dose auto-injectors; and 1 mg/mL in 1-mL ampules and vials, 30-mL vials, and 0.3-mL (0.3 mg) single-dose auto-injectors. Most preparations contain sodium bisulfite or sodium metabisulfite as a preservative.

B. Suggested minimum stocking levels to treat a 100-kg adult for the first 8 hours and 24 hours: **epinephrine hydrochloride**, *first 8 hours:* 4.0 mg or four ampules (1 mg/mL, 1 mL each); *first 24 hours:* 12.0 mg or 12 ampules (1 mg/mL, 1 mL each).

► ESMOLOL

Thomas E. Kearney, PharmD

I. Pharmacology. Esmolol is a short-acting, IV, cardioselective beta-adrenergic blocker with no intrinsic sympathomimetic or membrane-depressant activity. In usual therapeutic doses, it causes little or no bronchospasm in patients with asthma. Esmolol produces peak effects within 6–10 minutes of administration of an intravenous bolus. It is hydrolyzed rapidly by red blood cell esterases, with an elimination half-life of 9 minutes; therapeutic and adverse effects disappear within 30 minutes after the infusion is discontinued.

II. Indications

A. Rapid control of supraventricular and ventricular tachyarrhythmias and hypertension, especially if caused by excessive sympathomimetic activity (eg, stimulant drugs, hyperthyroid state).

B. Reversal of hypotension and tachycardia caused by excessive beta-adrenergic activity resulting from theophylline or caffeine overdose.

C. Control of ventricular tachyarrhythmias caused by excessive myocardial catecholamine sensitivity (eg, chloral hydrate and chlorinated hydrocarbon solvents).

III. Contraindications

A. Contraindications include hypotension, bradycardia, and congestive heart failure secondary to intrinsic cardiac disease or cardiac-depressant effects of drugs and toxins (eg, cyclic antidepressants and barbiturates).

B. Hypertension caused by alpha-adrenergic or generalized stimulant drugs (eg, cocaine, amphetamines), unless esmolol is coadministered with a vasodilator (eg, nitroprusside or phentolamine). Paradoxic hypertension may result from an unopposed alpha effect, although it is less likely than that associated with the use of a nonspecific beta-adrenergic blocker (propranolol).

IV. Adverse effects

A. Hypotension, bradycardia, and cardiac arrest may occur, especially in patients with intrinsic cardiac disease or cardiac-depressant drug overdose.

B. Bronchospasm may occur in patients with asthma or chronic bronchospasm, but it is less likely than with propranolol or other nonselective beta-blockers and is rapidly reversible after the infusion is discontinued.

C. Esmolol may mask physiologic responses to hypoglycemia (tremor, tachycardia, and glycogenolysis) and, therefore, should be used with caution in patients with diabetes.

D. Avoid extravasation. Infusion site reactions include irritation as well as necrosis and thrombophlebitis.

E. Use in pregnancy. FDA Category C (indeterminate). This does not preclude its short-term use for a seriously symptomatic patient (p 498). High-dose infusion may contribute to placental ischemia.

V. Drug or laboratory interactions

A. Esmolol may transiently increase the serum digoxin level by 10–20%, but the clinical significance of this is unknown.

B. Esmolol may increase the risk of hypotension, bradycardia, AV conduction impairment if used concurrently with calcium channel antagonists, sympatholytics (clonidine), or amiodarone.

C. Recovery from succinylcholine-induced neuromuscular blockade may be delayed slightly (5–10 minutes). Similarly, esmolol metabolism may be inhibited by anticholinesterase agents (eg, organophosphates).

D. Esmolol is not compatible with sodium bicarbonate solutions.

VI. Dosage and method of administration

A. Dilute before intravenous injection to a final concentration of 10 mg/mL with 5% dextrose, lactated Ringer injection, or saline solutions.

B. Give as an intravenous infusion, starting at 0.025–0.05 mg/kg/min and increasing as needed up to 0.2 mg/kg/min (average dose, 0.1 mg/kg/min). Steady-state concentrations are reached approximately 30 minutes after each infusion adjustment. A loading dose of 0.5–1.0 mg/kg should be given over 30 seconds to 1 minute if more rapid onset of clinical effects (5–10 minutes) is desired.

C. Infusion rates greater than 0.2 mg/kg/min are likely to produce excessive hypotension. At rates greater than 0.3 mg/kg/min, the beta-blocking effects lose their $beta_1$ selectivity.

VII. Formulations

A. Parenteral. Esmolol hydrochloride (Brevibloc, others), 2.5 g in 10-mL ampules (250 mg/mL), 100 mg in 10-mL vials (10 mg/mL), and 20 mg/mL (double strength) in 5-mL vials and 100-mL bags.

B. Suggested minimum stocking levels to treat a 100-kg adult for the first 8 hours and 24 hours: **esmolol hydrochloride**, *first 8 hours:* 5.0 g or two ampules (250 mg/mL, 10 mL each); *first 24 hours:* 15.0 g or six ampules (250 mg/mL, 10 mL each).

▶ ETHANOL

Thomas E. Kearney, PharmD

I. Pharmacology. Ethanol (ethyl alcohol) acts as a competitive substrate for the enzyme alcohol dehydrogenase, preventing the formation of toxic metabolites from methanol or ethylene glycol. A serum ethanol concentration of 100 mg/dL, or at least a 1:4 molar ratio of ethanol to toxic alcohol/glycol, effectively saturates alcohol dehydrogenase and prevents further methanol and ethylene glycol metabolism (see also "Fomepizole [4-Methylpyrazole, 4-MP]," p 558). Ethanol is well absorbed from the GI tract when given orally, but the onset is more rapid and predictable when it is given intravenously. The elimination of ethanol is zero order; the average rate of decline is 15 mg/dL/h. However, this is highly variable and will be influenced by prior chronic use of alcohol, recruitment of alternate metabolic pathways, and concomitant hemodialysis (eg, to remove methanol or ethylene glycol).

II. Indications. Suspected **methanol** (methyl alcohol [p 314]) or **ethylene glycol** (p 234) poisoning with the following:

A. A suggestive history of ingestion of a toxic dose but no available blood concentration measurements;

B. Metabolic acidosis and an unexplained elevated osmol gap (p 33); or

C. A serum methanol or ethylene glycol concentration of 20 mg/dL or higher.

D. ***Note:*** Since the introduction of fomepizole (4-methylpyrazole [p 558]), a potent inhibitor of alcohol dehydrogenase, most patients with ethylene glycol or methanol poisoning probably will be treated with this drug instead of ethanol, particularly in cases involving small children, patients taking disulfiram, patients with pancreatitis, and hospitals lacking laboratory support to perform rapid ethanol levels (for monitoring treatment). Ethanol is more difficult to dose, requires more monitoring, and has a greater risk of adverse effects. Studies suggest that despite the higher acquisition costs for fomepizole, it may be more cost-effective than ethanol.

E. Other substances that are metabolized by alcohol dehydrogenase to toxic metabolites include propylene glycol, diethylene glycol, triethylene glycol, glycol ethers (eg, ethylene glycol ethyl ether, ethylene glycol butyl ether), and 1,4-butanediol. The criteria for ethanol therapy and evidence for improved outcomes are lacking for these substances.

III. Contraindications. Use of interacting drugs, which may cause disulfiram-type reaction (see Item V. B below).

IV. Adverse effects

A. Nausea, vomiting, and gastritis may occur with oral administration. Ethanol may also exacerbate pancreatitis.

B. Inebriation, sedation, and hypoglycemia (particularly in children and malnourished adults) may occur.

C. Intravenous use sometimes is associated with local phlebitis (especially with ethanol solutions 10%). Hyponatremia may result from large doses of sodium-free intravenous solutions.

D. Acute flushing, palpitations, and postural hypotension may occur in patients with atypical aldehyde dehydrogenase enzyme (up to 50–80% of Japanese, Chinese, and Korean individuals).

E. Use in pregnancy. FDA Category C (indeterminate). Ethanol crosses the placenta. Chronic overuse in pregnancy is associated with birth defects (fetal alcohol syndrome). The drug reduces uterine contractions and may slow or stop labor. However, these effects do not preclude its acute, short-term use for a seriously symptomatic patient (p 498).

V. Drug or laboratory interactions

A. Ethanol potentiates the effect of CNS-depressant drugs and hypoglycemic agents.

B. Disulfiram reaction (p 226), including flushing, palpitations, and postural hypotension, may occur in patients taking disulfiram as well as a variety of other medications (eg, metronidazole, furazolidone, procarbazine, chlorpropamide, some cephalosporins, and *Coprinus* mushrooms). In such cases, fomepizole is the recommended alternative to ethanol treatment.

C. Drugs or chemicals metabolized by alcohol dehydrogenase (eg, chloral hydrate, isopropyl alcohol) also have impaired elimination. Fomepizole inhibits the metabolism of ethanol, and vice versa.

TABLE III–10. ETHANOL DOSING (ADULTS AND CHILDREN)

Dose	Intravenous[a] 5%	Intravenous[a] 10%	Oral[b] 20% (40 Proof)
Loading[c]	20 mL/kg	10 mL/kg	5 mL/kg
Maintenance[d]	2.5–4 mL/kg/h	1.25–2 mL/kg/h	0.5–1 mL/kg/h
Maintenance during hemodialysis[d]	4.5–8 mL/kg/h	2.25–4 mL/kg/h	1-1.7 mL/kg/h

[a]% is mL ethanol/100 mL (v/v). Infuse intravenous loading dose over 20–60 minutes as tolerated. For slower rates, add 1 mL/kg to the loading dose to account for ethanol metabolism during the infusion.
[b]% is mL ethanol/100 mL (v/v). Dilute to an ethanol concentration of 20% or less and administer orally or by nasogastric tube.
[c]If the patient's serum ethanol level is greater than zero, reduce the loading dose in a proportional manner. Multiply the calculated loading dose by the following factor:

$$\frac{100 - [\text{Patient's serum ethanol level in mg/dL}]}{100}$$

[d]Doses may vary according to the individual. Persons with chronic alcoholism have a higher rate of ethanol elimination, and maintenance doses should be adjusted to maintain an ethanol level of approximately 100–150 mg/dL.

VI. Dosage and method of administration. See Table III–10. Ethanol may be given orally or intravenously (see Formulations, below). The desired serum concentration is approximately 100 mg/dL (20 mmol/L).

A. Loading dose. Give approximately 800 mg/kg as a loading dose, unless the patient already has an elevated ethanol level, in which case the loading dose should be reduced by a proportional amount (see Table III–10 footnote).

B. Maintenance dose. Administer approximately 100–150 mg/kg/h (give the larger dose to persons with chronic alcoholism). Obtain serum ethanol levels after the loading dose and frequently during maintenance therapy to ensure a concentration of 100 mg/dL (eg, every 1–2 hours until goal achieved or after a change in the infusion rate, then every 2–4 hours during the maintenance dosing).

C. Dosing during hemodialysis. Increase the maintenance infusion rate to 175–350 mg/kg/h (use the larger dose for persons with chronic alcoholism) during hemodialysis to offset the increased rate of ethanol elimination. Alternatively, ethanol may be added to the dialysate.

VII. Formulations. ***Note:*** Ethanol formulations in % are normally expressed as volume of ethanol per volume of solution (v/v) instead of weight per volume (w/v). The specific gravity of ethanol (0.789 g/mL) is less than that of water (1 g/mL); to convert mL/dL to g/dL, multiply by 0.789. A 10% ethanol solution is preferred for IV administration (to minimize fluid load, but it may require central venous access in children); a solution of 20% (usually diluted with juice for better palatability and absorption) is preferred for oral administration.

A. Oral. Pharmaceutical-grade ethanol (70%, 95%, 96% v/v USP). Mix with juice and dilute to a final ethanol concentration of 20% (v/v).

1. ***Note:*** Commercial liquor may be used orally if pharmaceutical-grade ethanol is not available. To convert "proof" to percent ethanol by volume, divide by 2.

B. Parenteral. Dehydrated (anhydrous) alcohol (98% v/v ethyl alcohol, preservative-free) injection solution, 5-mL vials and 1- and 5-mL ampules. To prepare a 10% v/v ethanol solution, add 55 mL of sterile ethanol USP (98% ethanol) to 500 mL of 5% dextrose in water.

C. Suggested minimum stocking levels to treat a 100-kg adult for the first 8 hours and 24 hours: **ethanol parenteral solution**, *first 8 hours:* 22 (5 mL) vials or ampules; *first 24 hours*: 44 (5 mL) vials or ampules.

▶ FLUMAZENIL

Raymond Y. Ho, PharmD

I. **Pharmacology.** Flumazenil (Romazicon) is an imidazobenzodiazepine derivative that competitively inhibits the activity of CNS benzodiazepine receptors and antagonizes the CNS effects of benzodiazepines. It has no demonstrable benzodiazepine agonist activity and no significant toxicity, even in high doses. It has no effect on other GABAergic drugs (eg, barbiturates), opioids, or alcohol intoxication. Flumazenil has poor oral bioavailability (16%) owing to high first-pass effect, and it is most effective when administered parenterally. After intravenous administration, the onset of benzodiazepine reversal occurs within 1–2 minutes, with 80% response reached within 3 minutes; reversal peaks at 6–10 minutes and lasts for 1–5 hours depending on the dose of flumazenil and the degree of preexisting benzodiazepine effect. Flumazenil is eliminated by hepatic metabolism and has a terminal half-life of approximately 1 hour (41–79 minutes). Hepatic dysfunction can significantly reduce normal flumazenil clearance.

II. **Indications**

A. Rapid reversal of benzodiazepine overdose–induced coma and respiratory depression, both as a diagnostic aid and as a potential substitute for endotracheal intubation. **Routine use of flumazenil in patients with coma of unknown etiology or with possible mixed drug overdose is not recommended**, especially in high-risk patients (see Adverse Effects, below). Lowest-risk patients include those with a known iatrogenic exposure, toddlers with an ingestion, and patients with a paradoxical response (characterized by agitation or excitement and excessive movement or restlessness) to a therapeutic dose of a benzodiazepine when reversal of effect is desired.

B. Postoperative or postprocedure reversal of benzodiazepine sedation.

C. Flumazenil may also reverse CNS depression from certain nonbenzodiazepine sedatives and hypnotics (eg, zolpidem [Ambien], zaleplon [Sonata], and eszopiclone [Lunesta]).

D. Flumazenil may have significant transient effect in patients with hepatic encephalopathy but no impact on recovery or survival.

III. **Contraindications**

A. Known hypersensitivity to flumazenil or benzodiazepines.

B. Suspected serious tricyclic antidepressant or other proconvulsant overdose.

C. Benzodiazepine use for control of a potentially life-threatening condition (eg, status epilepticus or increased intracranial pressure).

IV. **Adverse effects**

A. Anxiety, agitation, headache, dizziness, nausea, vomiting, tremor, and transient facial flushing.

B. **Black box warning.** Rapid reversal of benzodiazepine effect in high-tolerance patients, such as those with benzodiazepine addiction or chronic use, especially if they have a history of seizures, may result in an acute withdrawal state, including hyperexcitability, tachycardia, and seizures.

C. **Black box warning.** Seizures may be unmasked in patients with a serious tricyclic antidepressant or other proconvulsant overdose due to loss of protective effect of benzodiazepines.

D. Flumazenil has precipitated arrhythmias in a patient with mixed benzodiazepine and chloral hydrate overdose.

E. Other risks include re-sedation and aspiration.

F. **Use in pregnancy.** FDA Category C (indeterminate). This does not preclude its acute, short-term use for a seriously symptomatic patient (p 498).

V. **Drug or laboratory interactions.** No known interactions. Flumazenil does not appear to alter the kinetics of benzodiazepines or other drugs.

VI. **Dosage and method of administration**

A. **Benzodiazepine overdose.** Titrate the dose until the desired response is achieved.

1. Administer 0.2 mg IV over 30 seconds (pediatric dose is not established; start with 0.01 mg/kg and see dosing information below for pediatric reversal of conscious sedation). If there is no response, give 0.3 mg. If there still is no response, give 0.5 mg and repeat every 30 seconds if needed to a total maximum dose of 3 mg (1 mg in children) within 1 hour.
2. Because effects last only 1–5 hours, continue to monitor the patient closely for resedation. If multiple repeated doses are needed, consider a continuous infusion (0.2–1 mg/h).

B. Reversal of conscious sedation or anesthetic doses of benzodiazepine. Dose of 0.2 mg given intravenously is usually sufficient and may be repeated, with titration up to 1 mg. In pediatric patients 1 year of age or older, administer 0.01 mg/kg (up to 0.2 mg) IV over 15 seconds. If there is no response, the previous dose may be repeated at 60-second intervals to a maximum total dose of 0.05 mg/kg or 1 mg. (***Note:*** Successful reversal of midazolam sedation in pediatric patients via rectal administration has been described in the literature; this may be an alternative route of administration for a pediatric patient with poor or no IV access.)

VII. Formulations

A. Parenteral. Flumazenil (Romazicon, generic), 0.1 mg/mL, 5- and 10-mL vials with parabens and EDTA. Flumazenil is compatible with 5% dextrose in water, lactated Ringer's solution, and normal saline solution.

B. Suggested minimum stocking levels to treat a 100-kg adult for the first 8 hours and 24 hours: **flumazenil**, *first 8 hours:* 6 mg or six vials (0.1 mg/mL, 10 mL each); *first 24 hours:* 12 mg or 12 vials (0.1 mg/mL, 10 mL each).

▶ FOLIC ACID

F. Lee Cantrell, PharmD

I. Pharmacology. Folic acid is a B-complex vitamin that is essential for protein synthesis and erythropoiesis. In addition, the administration of folate to patients with methanol poisoning may enhance the conversion of the toxic metabolite formic acid to carbon dioxide and water, based on studies in folate-deficient primates. ***Note:*** Folic acid requires metabolic activation and may not be effective for the treatment of acute poisoning by dihydrofolate reductase inhibitors (eg, methotrexate and trimethoprim). Leucovorin (p 572) is the proper agent in these situations.

II. Indications. Adjunctive treatment for methanol poisoning and possibly ethylene glycol poisoning.

III. Contraindications. No known contraindications.

IV. Adverse effects

A. Rare allergic reactions have been reported after intravenous administration.

B. Use in pregnancy. FDA Category A (p 498). Folic acid is a recommended supplement.

V. Drug or laboratory interactions. This agent may decrease phenytoin levels by enhancing its metabolism.

VI. Dosage and method of administration. The dose required for methanol (or ethylene glycol) poisoning is not established, although 1–2 mg/kg (typical doses are 50–70 mg IV) every 4–6 hours has been recommended. Folic acid should be readministered following hemodialysis as it is readily removed by the procedure.

VII. Formulations

A. Parenteral. Sodium folate 5 mg/mL, 10-mL vials.

B. Suggested minimum stocking levels to treat a 100-kg adult for the first 8 hours and 24 hours: **folate sodium**, *first 8 hours:* 100–200 mg or 2–4 vials (5 mg/mL, 10 mL each); *first 24 hours:* 300–600 mg or 6–12 vials (5 mg/mL, 10 mL each).

► FOMEPIZOLE (4-METHYLPYRAZOLE, 4-MP)

Thomas E. Kearney, PharmD

I. Pharmacology

A. Fomepizole (4-methylpyrazole) is a potent competitive inhibitor of alcohol dehydrogenase, the first enzyme in the metabolism of ethanol and other alcohols. Fomepizole can prevent the formation of toxic metabolites after methanol or ethylene glycol ingestion. Furthermore, early treatment with fomepizole for ethylene glycol or methanol poisoning (before the appearance of a significant acidosis) may obviate the need for dialysis. Since the introduction of fomepizole, most patients with ethylene glycol or methanol poisoning probably will be treated with this drug instead of ethanol, particularly in cases involving small children, patients taking disulfiram, patients with altered consciousness and ingestion of multiple substances, patients with pancreatitis or active liver disease, and hospitals lacking laboratory support to perform rapid ethanol levels (for monitoring treatment). Economic models have suggested that fomepizole may be more cost-effective than ethanol despite the high acquisition cost of fomepizole.

B. Fomepizole is eliminated mainly via zero-order kinetics, but cytochrome P-450 metabolism can undergo autoinduction within 2–3 days. The drug is dialyzable. It is well absorbed and has been used successfully with PO administration but is not approved for this route in the United States.

II. Indications are suspected or confirmed **methanol** (methyl alcohol [p 314]) or **ethylene glycol** (p 234) poisoning with one or more of the following:

A. A reliable history of ingestion of a toxic dose but no available blood concentration measurements (when used empirically, allows a 12-hour "window" after one dose to assess the patient);

B. Metabolic acidosis and an unexplained elevated osmol gap (p 33); or

C. Serum methanol or ethylene glycol concentration of 20 mg/dL or higher.

D. Other substances that are metabolized by alcohol dehydrogenase to toxic metabolites include propylene glycol, diethylene glycol, triethylene glycol, glycol ethers (eg, ethylene glycol ethyl ether, ethylene glycol butyl ether), and 1,4-butanediol. The criteria for fomepizole therapy and evidence for improved outcomes are lacking for all these substances. However, case reports of poisonings from some of these other glycols (eg, propylene glycol, diethylene glycol) have suggested benefit when fomepizole therapy is coupled with dialysis to remove the potentially toxic parent compound and concomitantly prevent the formation of toxic metabolites.

E. Disulfiram reaction (or risk for): to halt progression or the production of acetaldehyde, assuming that ethanol is still present (based on case reports).

III. Contraindications. History of allergy to the drug or to other pyrazoles.

IV. Adverse effects

A. Venous irritation and phlebosclerosis after intravenous injection of the undiluted product.

B. Headache, nausea, and dizziness are the most commonly reported side effects. Less common effects are vomiting, tachycardia, hypotension, feeling of inebriation, rash, fever, and eosinophilia.

C. Transient non–dose-dependent elevation of hepatic transaminases has been reported after multiple doses.

D. Although safety and effectiveness in children have not been established by the manufacturer, fomepizole has been used successfully and reported for pediatric poisonings (in children as young as 8 months).

E. Use in pregnancy. FDA Category C (indeterminate). Has been used in pregnant patients without immediate adverse effects on the mother or the fetus (p 498).

V. Drug or laboratory interactions

A. Drugs or chemicals metabolized by alcohol dehydrogenase (eg, chloral hydrate, ethanol, isopropyl alcohol) will also have impaired elimination. Fomepizole inhibits the metabolism of ethanol, and vice versa.

B. Drugs or chemicals metabolized by cytochrome P-450 enzymes may compete with fomepizole for elimination. Also, induction of cytochrome P-450 activity by these drugs or by fomepizole may alter metabolism.

VI. Dosage and method of administration. ***Note:*** The interval between the initial dose and subsequent maintenance doses, 12 hours, provides an opportunity to confirm the diagnosis with laboratory testing.

A. Initial dose. Give a loading dose of 15 mg/kg (up to 1.5 g). Dilute in at least 100 mL of normal saline or 5% dextrose and infuse intravenously slowly over 30 minutes to avoid venous irritation and thrombophlebitis. (Oral administration may be considered for patients lacking IV access.) Patients weighing more than 100 kg may receive a loading dose of 1,500 mg (one vial) to avoid wastage from opening a second vial of fomepizole. However, it is unknown whether sufficient enzyme blockade will be achieved in all patients, and additional doses are recommended if there is evidence of a worsening acidosis before the next maintenance dose 12 hours later. ***Note:*** The drug may solidify at room temperature and should be inspected visually before administration. If there is any evidence of solidification, hold the vial under a stream of warm water or roll between the hands.

B. Maintenance therapy. Give 10 mg/kg every 12 hours for four doses (or 48 hours), then increase to 15 mg/kg (to offset increased metabolism resulting from autoinduction) until methanol or ethylene glycol serum levels are below 20 mg/dL.

C. Adjustment for hemodialysis. To offset loss of fomepizole during dialysis, administer one additional dose of fomepizole at the beginning of dialysis (if 6 hours or more has elapsed since the last dose). Dosing of fomepizole at the completion of dialysis: if less than 1 hour since the last dose, do not give another dose; if 1–3 hours has elapsed since last dose, then give 50% of the next scheduled dose; if greater than 3 hours since last dose, administer another full dose at the completion of dialysis, then continue with usual dosing every 12 hours thereafter. (***Note:*** With newer, high-flux hemodialysis equipment, fomepizole half-life averages 1.7 hours, compared with 3 hours with standard dialysis.)

VII. Formulations

A. Parenteral. Fomepizole (Antizol, Paladin Labs; generic, X-Gen Pharmaceuticals), 1 g/mL in 1.5-mL vials, prepackaged in tray packs containing four vials.

B. Suggested minimum stocking levels to treat a 100-kg adult for the first 8 hours and 24 hours: **fomepizole**, *first 8 hours:* 1.5 g or one vial of either product; *first 24 hours:* 6.0 g or four vials of either product. ***Note:*** Manufacturers will replace free of charge or provide a credit for any expired vials of fomepizole if they are in the original packaging and returned within 12 months of the expiration date.

► GLUCAGON

Thomas E. Kearney, PharmD

I. Pharmacology. Glucagon is a polypeptide hormone that stimulates the formation of adenyl cyclase, which in turn increases the intracellular concentration of cyclic adenosine monophosphate (cAMP). This results in enhanced glycogenolysis and an elevated serum glucose concentration, vascular smooth-muscle relaxation, and positive inotropic, chronotropic, and dromotropic effects. These effects occur independently of beta-adrenergic stimulation (glucagon has a separate receptor on the myocardium) and seem to be most effective at increasing the heart rate. Glucagon may also increase arachidonic acid levels in cardiac tissue via an active metabolite, mini-glucagon. Arachidonic acid improves cardiac contractility owing to its effects on calcium. Glucagon is destroyed in the GI tract and must be given parenterally. After intravenous administration, effects are seen within 1–2 minutes and persist for 10–20 minutes. The serum half-life is about 3–10 minutes. ***Note:*** Glucagon usually is not considered first-line therapy for hypoglycemia because of its slow onset of action and reliance on glycogen stores. Instead, use glucose (p 562) if it is available.

II. Indications

A. Hypotension, bradycardia, or conduction impairment caused by beta-adrenergic blocker intoxication (p 158). Also consider in patients with hypotension associated with anaphylactic or anaphylactoid reactions who may be on beta-adrenergic–blocking agents.

B. Possibly effective for severe cardiac depression caused by intoxication with calcium antagonists, tricyclic antidepressants, quinidine, or other types Ia and Ic antiarrhythmic drugs. Because of the benign side-effect profile of glucagon, consider its early empiric use in any patient with myocardial depression (bradycardia, hypotension, or low cardiac output) who does not respond rapidly to usual measures.

C. To facilitate passage of obstructed gastric foreign bodies (eg, drug packets) through the pylorus into the intestine (based on a case report).

III. Contraindications. Known hypersensitivity to the drug (rare) or pheochromocytoma (stimulates the release of catecholamines and may result in severe hypertension) or insulinoma (indirectly stimulates release of insulin and may result in hypoglycemia).

IV. Adverse effects

A. Hyperglycemia (usually transient), hypokalemia.

B. Nausea and vomiting are dose-dependent (especially if >1 mg is administered) and caused by delayed gastric emptying and hypotonicity.

C. Use in **pregnancy.** FDA Category B. Fetal harm is extremely unlikely (p 498).

V. Drug or laboratory interactions. Concurrent administration of epinephrine potentiates and prolongs the hyperglycemic and cardiovascular effects of glucagon. It is unknown whether glucagon interferes with the effectiveness of insulin and glucose therapy for severe calcium antagonist poisoning. Note that glucagon stimulates endogenous insulin secretion.

VI. Dosage and method of administration.

A. Initial dose. Give 3–10 mg IV (may also titrate with 0.05-mg/kg boluses) over 1–2 minutes and repeat every 3–5 minutes until response (usually a cumulative total of 10 mg, but up to 30 mg has been given).

B. Maintenance infusion. Infuse 1–5 mg/h (children: 0.15 mg/kg IV, or titrate with 0.05 mg/kg every 3 minutes, followed by 0.05–0.1 mg/kg/h). Alternatively, determine the total dose required to achieve the initial response and give this amount every hour. Infusions of up to 10 mg/h have been used for adults. ***Note:*** Tachyphylaxis may occur with prolonged infusions (case report with infusion duration >24 hours).

C. For very large doses, consider using sterile water or D_5W to reconstitute the powder rather than the glycerine-containing diluent provided with the drug (eg, add 4 mg of glucagon to 50 mL D_5W for continuous infusion).

VII. Formulations. ***Note:*** Glucagon is no longer available in 10-mg vials; instead, the 1-mg kits must be used at a considerably higher cost to attain adequate dosing for the management of poisonings.

A. Parenteral. Glucagon Emergency (or Diagnostic) Kit, 1 unit (approximately 1 mg, with 1-mL syringe for diluent with glycerine), and GlucaGen (glucagon hydrochloride) Diagnostic Kit or HypoKit (1 mg with 1 mL of sterile water for diluent in a vial or syringe). Also available as a 10-pack (10 x 1 mg vials), but does not contain syringe or diluent. ***Note:*** Should be used immediately after reconstitution and discard any unused drug.

B. Suggested minimum stocking levels to treat a 100-kg adult for the first 8 hours and 24 hours: **glucagon hydrochloride**, *first 8 hours:* 90 mg or 90 kits (1 unit each); *first 24 hours:* 250 mg or 250 kits (1 unit each).

▶ GLUCARPIDASE

Hallam Gugelmann, MD, MPH

I. **Pharmacology.** Glucarpidase (carboxypeptidase G_2, $CPDG_2$) is a recombinant form of carboxypeptidase G_2, which rapidly hydrolyzes the carboxyl-terminal glutamate residue of folate and folate analogues such as methotrexate. Methotrexate is inactivated producing the nontoxic metabolites 4-deoxy- 4-diamino-N^{10}-methylpteroic acid (DAMPA) and glutamic acid, resulting in a ≥97% reduction of methotrexate levels within 15 minutes, independent of renal clearance. Because of its large molecular size, it distributes primarily in the intravascular space and does not cross the blood–brain barrier or cell membranes, and it does not inactivate methotrexate in the gut lumen. Its half-life ranges from 5.6 hours to 8.2 hours (renal impairment).

II. **Indications**

A. Glucarpidase is indicated for the adjunctive treatment of toxic plasma methotrexate (see p 319) concentrations in the setting of impaired renal clearance or persistent toxic levels. It should be used in conjunction with leucovorin rescue (with staggered dosing; see V. B. below) and supportive care (IV hydration and urinary alkalinization).

B. Unlabeled uses include intrathecal administration for inadvertent intrathecal methotrexate overdose.

III. **Contraindications.** None are listed by the manufacturer.

IV. **Adverse effects**

A. Immunologic: Antibody development (21%) is of uncertain clinical importance but may impact effectiveness of repeat dosing (see dosing and method of administration below).

B. Allergic: Severe allergic reactions have been reported in postmarketing surveillance. Typically, less severe reactions occur including a burning sensation, flushing, nausea, vomiting, headache, and hypotension.

C. **Use in pregnancy.** FDA Category C (see Table III–1, p 498). There are no well-controlled studies in pregnant animal or human subjects with this drug.

V. **Drug or laboratory interactions**

A. The inactive hydrolysis product of methotrexate, DAMPA, may interfere with methotrexate immunoassays, resulting in overestimation of methotrexate concentrations in samples collected within 48 hours of glucarpidase administration. Chromatographic methotrexate assays are accurate during this time frame.

B. Leucovorin is also a substrate for glucarpidase, and the manufacturer advises against administration of leucovorin within 2 hours before or after administration of glucarpidase.

VI. **Dosage and method of administration (adults and children)**

A. **Toxic methotrexate levels.** Give 50 units/kg infused by IV bolus over 5 minutes. Reconstitute powder for injection by adding 1 mL of sterile 0.9% sodium chloride for injection. A second dose may be considered 24–48 hours later if there is evidence of persistent toxic methotrexate levels. However, administration of a second dose has not been shown to provide benefit.

B. **Acute intrathecal overdose.** Give 2,000 units, reconstituted in sterile 0.9% sodium chloride, as soon as possible after methotrexate overdose, administered over 5 minutes via ventriculostomy, lumbar route, ventriculostomy, or Ommaya reservoir.

VII. **Formulations**

A. Parenteral and intrathecal. Lyophilized powder 1,000 units per vial, stable in normal saline.

B. Suggested minimum stocking levels: Glucarpidase is distributed as Voraxaze® through ASD Healthcare; procurement information is available at 1-855-7-VORAXAZE (1-855-786-7292). Certain pharmacy wholesalers in the United States are capable of shipping glucarpidase for overnight delivery; additional information at http://www.btgplc.com/products/specialty-pharmaceuticals/voraxaze.

▶ GLUCOSE (DEXTROSE)

Thomas E. Kearney, PharmD

I. **Pharmacology.** Glucose is an essential carbohydrate that is used as a substrate for energy production within the body. Although many organs use fatty acids as an alternative energy source, the brain is totally dependent on glucose as its major energy source; thus, hypoglycemia may cause serious brain injury rapidly. Dextrose administered with insulin shifts potassium intracellularly and maintains euglycemia for the treatment of calcium antagonist and beta-adrenergic blocker poisoning (hyperinsulinemia–euglycemia [HIE] therapy).

II. **Indications**
   A. Hypoglycemia.
   B. Empiric therapy for patients with stupor, coma, or seizures who may have unsuspected hypoglycemia.
   C. Use with an insulin infusion for severe calcium antagonist poisoning, beta-blocker poisoning, and hyperkalemia.

III. **Contraindications.** No absolute contraindications for empiric treatment of comatose patients with possible hypoglycemia. However, hyperglycemia and (possibly) recent ischemic brain injury may be aggravated by excessive glucose administration.

IV. **Adverse effects**
   A. Hyperglycemia and serum hyperosmolality.
   B. Local phlebitis and cellulitis after extravasation (occurs with concentrations $\geq$10%) from the intravenous injection site.
   C. Administration of a large glucose load may precipitate acute Wernicke–Korsakoff syndrome in thiamine-depleted patients. For this reason, thiamine (p 628) is given routinely along with glucose to alcoholic or malnourished patients.
   D. Administration of large volumes of sodium-free dextrose solutions may contribute to fluid overload, hyponatremia, hypokalemia, and mild hypophosphatemia.
   E. **Use in pregnancy.** FDA Category C (indeterminate). This does not preclude its acute, short-term use for a seriously symptomatic patient (p 498).

V. **Drug or laboratory interactions.** No known interactions.

VI. **Dosage and method of administration**
   A. As empiric therapy for coma, give 50–100 mL of 50% dextrose (equivalent to 25–50 g of glucose) slowly (eg, about 3 mL/min) via a secure intravenous line (children: 2–4 mL/kg of 25% dextrose, or 5–10 mL/kg of 10% dextrose; do ***not*** use 50% dextrose in children). Dextrose can also be given by intraosseous route in concentrations that range from 10% (neonates), 25% (children) to 50% (adolescents).
   B. Persistent hypoglycemia (eg, resulting from poisoning by sulfonylurea agent) may require repeated boluses of 25% (for children) or 50% dextrose and infusion of 5–10% dextrose, titrated as needed. Consider the use of octreotide (p 596) in such situations. ***Note:*** Glucose can stimulate endogenous insulin secretion, which may exacerbate a hyperinsulinemia (resulting in wide fluctuations of blood glucose levels during treatment of sulfonylurea poisonings).
   C. **Hyperinsulinemia–euglycemia** therapy usually requires an initial dextrose bolus of 25 g (50 mL of 50% dextrose) or 0.5 g/kg (children, 0.25 g/kg given in a 10–25% dextrose solution) unless the patient's initial blood glucose is already >200 mg/dL, followed by a dextrose infusion at an initial rate of 0.1–0.5 g/kg/h using a 5–10% dextrose solution to maintain the glucose in

a normal range while insulin (p 564) is infused. Adjust the rate and dextrose concentration (if >10% dextrose solution, administer via a central line) and supplement with dextrose boluses as needed.

VII. Formulations

A. Parenteral. Dextrose (*d*-glucose) injection 50%, 50-mL ampules, vials, and prefilled injector; 25% dextrose, 10-mL syringes; various solutions of 2.5–70% dextrose, some in combination with saline or other crystalloids.

B. Suggested minimum stocking levels to treat a 100-kg adult for the first 8 hours and 24 hours: **dextrose**, *first 8 hours:* 450 g or six prefilled injectors (50%) and three bottles or bags (10%, 1 L each); *first 24 hours:* 1,250 g or six prefilled injectors (50%) and 11 bottles or bags (10%, 1 L each).

▶ HYDROXOCOBALAMIN

Kathryn H. Meier, PharmD

I. Pharmacology. Hydroxocobalamin is an analog of vitamin B_{12} that is used for the treatment of vitamin B_{12} deficiency syndromes in small doses and as an antidote for human cyanide poisoning in large doses. Hydroxocobalamin rapidly exchanges its hydroxyl group with free cyanide to produce nontoxic, stable cyanocobalamin. Since the molar binding ratio of hydroxocobalamin to cyanide is 1:1, 5 g of hydroxocobalamin will neutralize 97 mg of cyanide. Independent of its cyanide binding, hydroxocobalamin scavenges nitric oxide, a mediator of vasodilation. When administered to patients with cyanide poisoning, it rapidly improves the heart rate, systolic blood pressure, and acidemia. In humans, outcome is best when hydroxocobalamin is administered before cardiopulmonary arrest occurs. In normal individuals given 5- and 10-g hydroxocobalamin doses, the plasma half-life values for cobalamin compounds average 26 and 31 hours, respectively. Oral absorption is poor; absorption by intranasal route provides only small nontherapeutic doses for cyanide poisoning; large fluid volumes (200 mL) required for each 5 g dose preclude IM use; and intraosseous administration is under investigation.

II. Indications

A. Treatment of acute cyanide poisoning or symptomatic patients suspected to be at high risk for cyanide poisoning (eg, smoke inhalation victims [p 421]).

B. Prophylaxis or treatment of cyanide poisoning during nitroprusside infusion has been proposed.

III. Contraindications. Use caution when managing patients with known hypersensitivity to hydroxocobalamin or cyanocobalamin and consider alternative treatments.

IV. Adverse effects

A. Adverse reactions in healthy volunteers include chromaturia (red-colored urine) in 100%, erythema in 94–100%, rash in 20–44%, high blood pressure in 18–28%, nausea in 6–11%, headache in 6–33%, decreased lymphocyte percentage in 8–17%, and infusion site reaction in 6–39%. Although red-colored body fluids usually normalize within 2–7 days, erythema can last up to 2 weeks and chromaturia up to 35 days. A self-limiting acneiform rash may occur 7–28 days after infusion.

B. Allergic reactions have not been reported with acute intravenous therapy for cyanide poisoning. However, allergic reactions have been reported in patients using chronic IM therapy and in healthy volunteers unexposed to cyanide who were given IV hydroxocobalamin while participating in clinical safety trials.

C. Use in pregnancy. FDA Category C. The acute, short-term use of hydroxocobalamin for a seriously symptomatic, cyanide-poisoned patient (p 498) is not precluded in pregnancy and is preferred over nitrite administration. Cobalamin compounds cross the placenta and have been detected in human newborn urine samples.

V. Drug or laboratory interactions

A. Coloration of bodily fluids caused by cobalamins can interfere with colorimetric laboratory tests for periods ranging from 12 to 48 hours for blood and serum and up to 8 days for urine. Sampling and storing specimens before antidote administration is recommended, if possible. Test interferences are variable depending on which brand of analyzer is used. Test results that are commonly affected include:

1. ***Falsely decreased*** ALT and amylase.
2. ***Falsely increased*** AST, serum creatinine, glucose, alkaline phosphatase, albumin, total protein, bilirubin, triglycerides, cholesterol, hemoglobin, MCH, MCHC, basophils, and most urine chemistry parameters.
3. ***Unpredictable effects*** for carbon monoxide, lactate, CK, CKMB, and PT/INR.
4. Currently, interference has ***not*** been documented in serum tests for Na, K, Cl, Ca, BUN, and GGT (gamma-glutamyltransferase).

B. Hydroxocobalamin has been reported to falsely trigger the automated blood leak detector in some hemodialysis machines, causing them to shut off.

C. Administration of hydroxocobalamin should be via a separate IV line from other medications. To date, chemical or physical incompatibility has been documented for diazepam, dobutamine, dopamine, fentanyl, nitroglyerin, pentobarbital, propofol, thiopental, sodium thiosulfate, sodium nitrate, and ascorbic acid.

VI. Dosage and method of administration

A. Acute cyanide poisoning. Give 5 g (children: 70 mg/kg) by IV infusion over 15 minutes; for severe cases, a second 5-g dose may be infused over 15 minutes to 2 hours if needed.

B. Prophylaxis during nitroprusside infusion: Administer 25 mg/h IV.

VII. Formulations

A. Parenteral

1. Cyanokit consists of one 250-mL glass vial containing 5 g of freeze-dried hydroxocobalamin. Hydroxocobalamin should be reconstituted with 200 mL of sterile 0.9% sodium chloride in a gentle rocking motion for a final concentration of 25 mg/mL; the solution is stable for about 6 hours. If normal saline is not available, then lactated Ringer's or 5% dextrose injection fluids may be used. Cyanokit is designed for field use and available in Europe from Merck Santé SAS, France, and in the United States through Meridian Medical Technologies.
2. Hydroxocobalamin is also available in a 1-mg/mL concentration for IM use in treating vitamin B_{12} deficiency, but the quantity of active drug in the 10- and 30-mL vials is not sufficient to treat cyanide poisoning. Moreover, these formulations may contain the preservative parabens.

B. Suggested minimum stocking levels to treat a 100-kg adult for the first 8 hours and 24 hours: **hydroxocobalamin**, *first 8 hours:* 10 g or two Cyanokits; *first 24 hours:* 10 g or two Cyanokits. ***Note:*** Smoke inhalation often involves several victims exposed to cyanide gas, which can require multiple kits. Stocking levels should be based on the historical number of severely poisoned patients brought to the hospital after a smoke inhalation episode.

▶ INSULIN

Kathleen Birnbaum, PharmD[1]

I. Pharmacology

A. Insulin, a hormone secreted by the beta cells of the pancreas, promotes cellular uptake of glucose into skeletal and cardiac muscles and adipose tissue. Insulin shifts potassium intracellularly.

[1]The author and editors acknowledge the valuable advice provided by Kristin Engebretsen, PharmD, in the revision of this chapter.

B. There are several mechanisms by which high-dose insulin (hyperinsulinemia–euglycemia [HIE]) therapy may improve cardiac output:

1. In calcium antagonist and beta-adrenergic blocker overdose, myocardial metabolism shifts from free fatty acid to carbohydrate metabolism; insulin increases myocardial uptake of glucose, lactate, and oxygen.
2. High-dose insulin increases calcium-dependent inotropic effects.
3. High-dose insulin enhances nitric oxide synthase activity, which dilates coronary, pulmonary and systemic blood vessels, leading to improved cellular perfusion.

C. Human regular insulin is biosynthetically prepared with recombinant DNA technology. The onset of action to decrease blood glucose for regular insulin is 30 minutes to 1 hour, and the duration of action is 5–8 hours. The onset of action for high-dose insulin is not known but is frequently stated to be 15–45 minutes. The serum half-life of regular insulin at normal doses is 4–5 minutes after IV administration.

II. Indications

A. Hyperglycemia and diabetic ketoacidosis.

B. Severe hyperkalemia (p 39).

C. Administration with dextrose for hypotension induced by calcium antagonists (p 172) and beta-adrenergic blockers (p 158). Improved hemodynamics have been reported in case reports of patients with calcium antagonist toxicity and beta-adrenergic blocker overdose.

III. Contraindications.

Known hypersensitivity to the drug (less frequent with human insulin than with animal-derived insulin).

IV. Adverse effects

A. Hypoglycemia.

B. Hypokalemia.

C. Lipohypertrophy or lipoatrophy at injection site (more common with repeated use).

D. Fluid overload and hyponatremia with high-dose insulin infusion. Consider using concentrated solutions of insulin and dextrose, given via a central line.

E. Use in pregnancy. FDA Category B (p 498). Human insulin does not cross the placental barrier.

V. Drug or laboratory interactions

A. Hypoglycemia may be potentiated by ethanol, sulfonylureas, and salicylates.

B. Corticosteroids (by decreasing peripheral insulin resistance and promoting gluconeogenesis), glucagon (by enhanced glycogenolysis), and epinephrine (via beta-adrenergic effects) may antagonize the effects of insulin.

VI. Dosage and method of administration

A. Hyperglycemia. Administer regular insulin 5–10 U IV initially, followed by infusion of 5–10 U/h, while monitoring the effect on serum glucose levels (children: 0.1 U/kg initially, then 0.1 U/kg/h).

B. Hyperkalemia. Administer regular insulin 0.1 U/kg IV with 50 mL of 50% dextrose (children: 0.1 U/kg insulin with 2 mL/kg of 25% dextrose).

C. Hypotension from calcium antagonists and beta-adrenergic blockers unresponsive to conventional therapy (hyperinsulinemia-euglycemia therapy):

1. **Bolus** of regular human insulin 1 U/kg IV. If blood glucose is below 200 mg/dL, give 50 mL (25 g) of 50% dextrose IV (children: 0.25 g/kg of 25% dextrose).
2. **Continuous infusion.** Wide variations in insulin dose and duration have been reported. Doses as high as 10 U/kg/h have been administered. The most commonly recommended infusion rate is 1–10 U/kg/h. Start at 1 U/kg/h and increase by 1–2 U/kg/h every 10 minutes as needed to maintain satisfactory perfusion of vascular beds. Because of the vasodilation associated with HIE therapy, do not make dose adjustments based on the blood pressure alone.
3. Insulin solutions are often made by diluting 500 U of regular human insulin in 500 mL of 0.9% saline (insulin concentration, 1 U/mL). However, to avoid

fluid overload, a **concentrated insulin** infusion of 10 U/mL (10,000 U of regular human insulin in 1 L of 0.9% saline) or greater may be used.

4. **Maintain euglycemia** with boluses and infusions of dextrose as needed. D10W may be given by peripheral IV line if no central line is available. Typically, at insulin doses greater than 5–10 U/kg/h, more concentrated dextrose solutions given via central line will be needed to maintain euglycemia and avoid fluid overload.
5. **Monitoring**
   a. Measure blood **glucose** at least every 10 minutes while titrating the insulin infusion upward or downward, until blood glucose has remained in the 100–200 mg/dL range for several hours; glucose testing may be decreased to every 30 minutes. Blood glucose monitoring should be continued for at least 24 hours after the HIE infusion has been discontinued.
   b. Monitor **potassium** hourly initially, then at least every 4–6 hours after HIE infusion and the patient's potassium level has stabilized. Replete potassium as needed to maintain potassium above 3.0 mEq/L (goal 2.7–3.2). Magnesium and phosphorus levels may also fluctuate.
6. **Onset of effect** of HIE is not known but is frequently stated to be 15–45 minutes.
7. **Duration of therapy.** Duration of insulin–dextrose treatment has varied from a single insulin bolus to infusions lasting 6 hours to days. Average insulin infusion duration is 24–31 hours.
8. ***Note:*** There are currently no studies illustrating the best way to decrease HIE therapy. Once hemodynamic parameters have stabilized, the infusion may be gradually tapered and discontinued.

VII. **Formulations**

A. **Parenteral.** Human regular insulin (Humulin R, Novolin R), 100 U/mL, 10-mL vials. Only human regular insulin can be administered intravenously.

B. **Suggested minimum stocking levels** to treat a 100-kg adult for the first 8 and 24 hours: **regular insulin**, *first 8 hours:* 1,000 U or one vial (100 U/mL, 10 mL each); *first 24 hours:* 3,000 U or three vials (100 U/mL, 10 mL each).

▶ IODIDE (POTASSIUM IODIDE, KI)

Freda Rowley, PharmD

I. **Pharmacology.** Iodine 131 is a product of fission reactions and likely to be a major form of internal radioactive contamination after a major nuclear reactor accident or weapon detonation. Potassium iodide (KI) blocks thyroid gland uptake of the radioactive isotopes of iodine by both diluting the radioactive iodine and "filling" the gland with nontoxic iodine. The radioactive molecules are subsequently excreted in the urine.

For optimal protection, KI should be administered before or at the time of exposure to radioactive iodines but will have protective effects if initiated up to 4 hours after exposure. Daily administration is indicated until the risk for exposure to radioactive iodines no longer exists.

II. **Indications.** Potassium iodide is indicated for prevention of uptake of radioactive isotopes of iodine by the thyroid gland. The highest risk groups for radioiodine-induced thyroid cancer include infants, children, and pregnant and nursing females. The lowest risk group is persons older than 40 years. ***Note:*** KI should be used only when and if directed by federal, state, or local public health officials.

III. **Contraindications**

A. Known iodine allergy. Persons with the rare disorders of dermatitis herpetiformis and hypocomplemententemic vasculitis are at increased risk for sensitivity.

B. Patients who have heart disease accompanied by nodular thyroid disease should not take KI.

C. Patients with multinodular goiter, Graves' disease, and autoimmune thyroiditis should be treated with caution, especially if dosing exceeds a few days.

IV. Adverse effects

A. Gastrointestinal upset, diarrhea, burning of throat, metallic taste in mouth, sore gums, and rarely inflammation of the salivary glands. These effects become more common as duration of therapy and dose increase.

B. Allergic reactions ranging from skin rashes to respiratory distress may occur, although life-threatening reactions are very uncommon.

C. Iodine-induced thyrotoxicosis, hypothyroidism, and goiter may occur, but incidence is less than 2%, even if therapy is used for longer durations.

D. A bluish skin discoloration involving the sweat glands may occur after large doses of iodine-containing products.

E. Use in pregnancy. FDA Category D. KI crosses the placenta and can suppress thyroid function in the fetus. The FDA recommends that pregnant women avoid repeated dosing unless other protective measures are not available. Risk is minimal with short-term use (<10 days) and when given long before term.

F. Use in neonates. Increased risk for hypothyroidism in infants, especially in neonates less than 1 month of age. Thyroid function tests should be monitored in neonates given more than a single dose of KI.

G. Use in breast-feeding. KI and radioiodines both pass into breast milk, and lactating mothers should be cautioned to not breast-feed infants unless no other alternative is available.

V. Drug or laboratory interactions

A. Synergistic hypothyroid activity with lithium.

B. Thyroid-stimulating hormone (TSH) and free thyroxine (T_4) monitoring of thyroid function is reliable in the setting of standard dosing of KI. Recommended in all neonates treated with KI.

C. Risk for hyperkalemia with prolonged use along with other potassium supplements and potassium-sparing medications (eg, spironolactone). However, the daily dose of potassium from KI is only 3–4 mEq.

VI. Dosage and method of administration

A. There are various dosing guidelines, including those recommended by the US Food and Drug Administration (FDA) and the World Health Organization (WHO). Public health officials should decide on the regimen they will use in a specific situation. A guidance document from the CDC is available at emergency.cdc.gov/radiation/ki.asp.

B. A single dose provides 24 hours of protection. Once-a-day dosing is recommended.

C. Dose by age group:

1. Adults older than 18 years: 130 mg orally once a day.
2. Adolescents and children (3–18 years): 65 mg daily. (Adolescents weighing 150 lb or more should be given the adult dose of 130 mg.)
3. Infants (1 month–3 years): 32 mg daily.
4. Neonates (0–1 month): 16 mg one-time dose with protective measures (evacuation, avoiding breast milk and local cow's milk) put in place.

D. Duration of therapy may be from 1 day to many weeks, depending on public health recommendations. Prolonged prophylaxis may be required for protection from radioactive iodine–contaminated produce and milk. The study of childhood thyroid cancers following Chernobyl suggests that continued dosing long after the initial accident may result in decreased cellular proliferation and reduced risk for thyroid cancer.

VII. Formulations

A. Oral (Iosat, ThyroSafe). Scored tablets (130 and 65 mg) of potassium iodide. ThyroShield 65 mg/mL potassium iodide oral solution.

B. Potassium iodide oral solution can be made from crushed KI tablets for use in children and adults unable to swallow tablets. Crush a 130-mg tablet and mix with four teaspoons (20 mL) of water until dissolved, then add four teaspoons (20 mL) of chocolate milk, orange juice, soda, or baby formula. This results in a solution containing 3.25 mg/mL. Plain water or low-fat milk may not adequately mask the salty, unpleasant taste of KI tablets. The solution will keep for up to 7 days in the refrigerator. The FDA recommends that the solution be prepared weekly and the unused portion discarded.

C. Suggested minimum stocking levels to treat a 100-kg adult for the first 24 hours: **potassium iodide**, *first 24 hours*: 130 mg or one tablet (130 mg each).

▶ ISOPROTERENOL

Thomas E. Kearney, PharmD

I. Pharmacology. Isoproterenol is a catecholamine-like drug that stimulates beta-adrenergic receptors ($beta_1$ and $beta_2$). Its pharmacologic properties include positive inotropic and chronotropic cardiac effects, peripheral vasodilation, and bronchodilation. Isoproterenol is not absorbed orally and shows variable and erratic absorption from sublingual and rectal sites. The effects of the drug are terminated rapidly by tissue uptake and metabolism; effects persist only a few minutes after intravenous injection.

II. Indications

A. Severe bradycardia or conduction block resulting in hemodynamically significant hypotension (p 9). ***Note:*** After beta-blocker overdose, even exceedingly high doses of isoproterenol may not overcome the pharmacologic blockade of beta-receptors, and glucagon (p 559) is the preferred agent.

B. To increase heart rate and thereby abolish polymorphous ventricular tachycardia (torsade de pointes) associated with QT-interval prolongation (p 14).

C. To relieve bronchospasm (although $beta_2$-selective drugs such as albuterol are preferred).

III. Contraindications

A. Do not use isoproterenol for ventricular fibrillation or ventricular tachycardia (other than torsade de pointes).

B. Use with extreme caution in the presence of halogenated or aromatic hydrocarbon solvents or anesthetics or chloral hydrate.

IV. Adverse effects

A. Increased myocardial oxygen demand may result in angina pectoris or acute myocardial infarction.

B. Peripheral $beta_2$-adrenergic–mediated vasodilation may worsen hypotension.

C. The drug may precipitate ventricular arrhythmias.

D. Sulfite preservative in some parenteral preparations may cause hypersensitivity reactions.

E. Hypokalemia may occur secondary to $beta_2$-adrenergic–mediated intracellular potassium shift.

F. Use in pregnancy. FDA Category C (indeterminate). This does not preclude its acute, short-term use for a seriously symptomatic patient (p 498). However, it may cause fetal ischemia and also can reduce or stop uterine contractions.

V. Drug or laboratory interactions

A. Additive beta-adrenergic stimulation occurs in the presence of other sympathomimetic drugs, theophylline, and glucagon.

B. Administration in the presence of cyclopropane, halogenated anesthetics, or other halogenated or aromatic hydrocarbons may enhance the risk for ventricular arrhythmias because of sensitization of the myocardium to the arrhythmogenic effects of catecholamines.

C. Digitalis-intoxicated patients are more prone to develop ventricular arrhythmias when isoproterenol is administered.

D. Beta-blockers may interfere with the action of isoproterenol by competitive blockade at beta-adrenergic receptors.

VI. Dosage and method of administration

A. For intravenous infusion, use a solution containing 4 mcg/mL (dilute 5 mL of 1:5,000 solution in 250 mL of D_5W,); begin with an infusion at 0.5–1 mcg/min (children: 0.1 mcg/kg/min) and increase as needed for desired effect or as tolerated (determined by monitoring for arrhythmias). Usual dosage range is 2–10 mcg/min. For emergency treatment, the infusion rate may start at 5 mcg/min. The usual upper dose is 20 mcg/min (1.5 mcg/kg/min in children), but as much as 200 mcg/min has been given in adults with propranolol overdose. Preparations will degrade (and turn dark) with exposure to light, air, or heat.

B. For IV bolus, the usual adult dose is 20–60 mcg (1–3 mL of a 1:50,000 solution) and repeat bolus doses of 10–200 mcg. Make a solution of 1:50,000 (20 mcg/mL) by diluting 1 mL of the 1:5,000 solution to a volume of 10 mL with normal saline or D_5W.

VII. Formulations

A. Parenteral. Isoproterenol hydrochloride (Isuprel, others), 200 mcg/mL (1:5,000) in 1- and 5-mL ampules, which may contain sodium bisulfite or sodium metabisulfite as a preservative.

B. Suggested minimum stocking levels to treat a 100-kg adult for the first 8 hours and 24 hours: **isoproterenol hydrochloride**, *first 8 hours:* 10,000 mcg or 10 ampules (1:5,000, 5 mL each); *first 24 hours*: 30,000 mcg or 30 ampules (1:5,000, 5 mL each).

► KETAMINE

Patil Armenian, MD

I. Pharmacology. Ketamine, an arylcylohexylamine dissociative anesthetic agent similar to phencyclidine (PCP), is widely used as an induction agent for rapid sequence intubation (RSI) and in pediatric procedural sedation. It is a racemic mixture, and the S isomer is more potent with a shorter duration of action. The analgesic and dissociative effects are mediated through N-methyl-d-aspartate (NMDA) receptor antagonism. Sympathomimetic effects are mediated through inhibition of reuptake of dopamine, norepinephrine, and serotonin in the brain; these effects may contribute to its cardiovascular side effects as well as potential therapeutic benefit for patients with depression. Additionally, ketamine binds to mu-, delta-, sigma-, and kappa-opioid receptors contributing to its analgesic effects. Other pharmacologic effects mediated via epigenetic modulation and expression of microRNA, inflammatory mediators, and nitric oxide synthase may mediate its sustained therapeutic effects for the management of psychiatric and mood disorders, anti-inflammatory actions, and treatment of status asthmaticus. Ketamine is well absorbed via the intramuscular route and is metabolized in the liver to an active metabolite norketamine. It has poor oral (16%) and variable intranasal (25–50%) bioavailability. The relatively high lipid solubility and low protein binding facilitate rapid uptake into the brain with a rapid onset of action, which may occur 30 seconds after intravenous administration and 3 minutes after intramuscular administration and lasting up to 10 and 25 minutes, respectively. The serum half-life is 2–3 hours.

II. Indications

A. Induction agent for rapid sequence intubation (RSI). Ketamine may be used to facilitate sedation for endotracheal intubation, especially in trauma patients and hypotensive patients.

B. **Procedural sedation.** Ketamine can produce sedation and amnesia with minimal respiratory depression.

C. **Analgesia.** Low-dose ketamine has been used alone or with opioids for analgesia in emergency department, postoperative, and cancer-associated pain.

D. **Agitation.** Ketamine may be used as a sedating agent, either alone or in combination with midazolam, although this use has not been thoroughly studied in emergency department patients.

E. Other potential indications include postanesthetic shivering, complex regional pain syndrome, status asthmaticus, depression and mood disorders, suicidal ideation, refractory status epilepticus, and opioid and alcohol withdrawal.

III. Contraindications

A. Known hypersensitivity to the drug.

B. Do not use in infants younger than 3 months due to propensity for airway adverse events.

C. Use with caution in patients with high blood pressure or when elevation of blood pressure is unwanted.

D. Use with caution if ketamine-induced increased intraocular pressure could cause acute complications (eg, in a patient with a ruptured orbit).

IV. Adverse effects

A. Emergence reactions (dreamlike states, vivid imagery, hallucinations) or recovery agitation has been reported with variable incidence, ranging from 0% to 36%. Premedication with intravenous midazolam (p 516) minimizes this risk.

B. Laryngotracheal spasm is rare, occurring in 0.3% of children. The effect is temporary and usually responsive to bag-valve-mask ventilation.

C. Transient apnea or respiratory depression is also rare, occurring in 0.8% of children and less so in adults. It is more common with rapid IV infusions and prevented by slow IV administration over at least 60 seconds.

D. Hypertension; hypersalivation; emesis (7–26%); muscular hypertonicity; random, purposeless movements; clonus; and hiccupping may occur.

E. Ketamine is a potential drug of abuse. Long-term users may develop cystitis or bladder problems and a decline in mental health (cognitive impairments, psychotomimetic effects).

F. **Use in pregnancy.** This drug has not been categorized by the FDA. Therefore, safe use in pregnancy has not been established.

V. Drug or laboratory interactions

A. Ketamine will potentiate the CNS-depressant effects of opioids, ethanol, benzodiazepines, sedative-hypnotics, and other sedating drugs.

B. Although structurally similar to phencyclidine (PCP), it does not cross-react with any of the commercially available urine drug-testing assays.

VI. Dosage and method of administration

A. **Induction agent for RSI.** Give 2 mg/kg IV or 4–5 mg/kg IM along with a neuromuscular blocking agent. The IV route is preferable in patients requiring RSI.

B. **Procedural sedation.** Give 4–5 mg/kg IM or 1.5–2 mg/kg IV in children. Give 4 mg/kg IM or 1 mg/kg IV in adults. Administer intravenous doses over 30–60 seconds since more rapid administration may result in respiratory depression or apnea. A single loading dose is preferred to initiating the sedation with titration. If sedation is inadequate after 5–10 minutes, additional half to full doses may be given. Intravenous midazolam (0.03 mg/kg) may minimize the risk of emergence reactions in adults.

C. **Analgesia.** Give 0.1–0.6 mg/kg IV alone or as an adjunct to opioid analgesia.

D. **Agitation.** Give 4 mg/kg IM or 1 mg/kg IV to agitated, combative adults. Initiate cardiopulmonary monitoring after ketamine administration. If sedation is inadequate after 5–10 minutes, additional half doses may be given.

VII. Formulations

A. **Ketamine hydrochloride** (Ketalar, others), 10-, 50-, and 100-mg base/mL stocked in 10- and 20-mL vials. To prepare a dilute solution containing ketamine

1 mg/mL or 0.1% solution, transfer 10 mL (50 mg/mL) or 5 mL (100 mg/mL) to 500 mL of dextrose 5% injection or sodium chloride 0.9% injection and mix well. For patients with fluid restrictions, use 250 mL of diluent to achieve a 2 mg/mL solution.

B. The **suggested minimum stocking level** to treat a 70-kg adult for the first 24 hours is one vial (50 mg/mL, 10-mL vial).

▶ LABETALOL

Thomas E. Kearney, PharmD

I. Pharmacology. Labetalol is a mixed alpha- and beta-adrenergic antagonist; after intravenous administration, the nonselective beta-antagonist properties are approximately sevenfold greater than the alpha1 antagonist activity. Hemodynamic effects generally include decreases in heart rate, blood pressure, and systemic vascular resistance. Atrioventricular conduction velocity may be decreased. After intravenous injection, hypotensive effects are maximal within 10–15 minutes and persist for about 2–4 hours. The drug is eliminated by hepatic metabolism and has a half-life of 5–6 hours.

II. Indications. Labetalol may be used to treat hypertension accompanied by tachycardia associated with stimulant drug overdose (eg, cocaine or amphetamines) and clonidine withdrawal. ***Note:*** Hypertension with bradycardia suggests excessive alpha-mediated vasoconstriction (pp 17, 394); in this case, a pure alpha blocker such as phentolamine (p 605) is preferable because the reversal of $beta_2$-mediated vasodilation may worsen hypertension. In addition, it may have an unpredictable effect on coronary vascular tone; other agents, such as nitroglycerin, may be preferable for stimulant-induced coronary vasoconstriction.

III. Contraindications

A. Asthma.

B. Congestive heart failure.

C. Atrioventricular block.

D. Known hypersensitivity to the drug.

IV. Adverse effects

A. Paradoxical hypertension may result when labetalol is used in the presence of stimulant intoxicants that have strong mixed alpha- and beta-adrenergic agonist properties (eg, cocaine, amphetamines) and in patients with pheochromocytoma owing to the relatively weak alpha-antagonist properties of labetalol compared with its beta-blocking ability. (***Note:*** This has been reported with propranolol but not with labetalol.)

B. Orthostatic hypotension and negative inotropic effects may occur.

C. Dyspnea and bronchospasm may result, particularly in patients with asthma.

D. Nausea, abdominal pain, diarrhea, tremors, dizziness, and lethargy have been reported.

E. Labetalol may mask physiologic responses to hypoglycemia (tremor, tachycardia, and glycogenolysis) and, therefore, should be used with caution in patients with diabetes.

F. Use in pregnancy. FDA Category C (indeterminate). This does not preclude its acute, short-term use for a seriously symptomatic patient (p 498).

V. Drug or laboratory interactions

A. Additive blood pressure lowering with other antihypertensive agents, halothane, calcium channel antagonists, or nitroglycerin.

B. Cimetidine increases the oral bioavailability of labetalol.

C. Labetalol is incompatible with 5% sodium bicarbonate injection (forms a precipitate).

D. Labetalol may cause false-positive elevation of urinary catecholamine levels and can produce a false-positive test for amphetamines on urine drug screening.

VI. **Dosage and method of administration**

A. **Adult.** Give 20-mg slow (over 2 minutes) IV bolus initially; repeat with 40–80-mg doses at 10-minute intervals until blood pressure is controlled or a cumulative dose of 300 mg is achieved (most patients will respond to a total dose of 50–200 mg). Alternatively, administer a constant infusion of 0.5–2 mg/min (adjust rate) until blood pressure is controlled or a 300-mg cumulative dose is reached. After this, give oral labetalol starting at 100 mg twice daily.

B. **Children (off-label dosing).** Initial dose of 0.2–1 mg/kg is given intravenously over 2 minutes (maximum dose, 40 mg). May repeat every 10 minutes as needed.

VII. **Formulations**

A. **Parenteral.** Labetalol hydrochloride (Normodyne, Trandate, others), 5 mg/mL, 20- and 40-mL multiple-dose vials (with EDTA and parabens as preservatives), and 4-and 8-mL prefilled syringes.

B. **Oral.** Labetalol hydrochloride (Normodyne, Trandate, others), 100-, 200-, and 300-mg tablets.

C. **Suggested minimum stocking levels** to treat a 100-kg adult for the first 8 hours and 24 hours: **labetalol hydrochloride**, *first 8 hours:* 300 mg or three vials (5 mg/mL, 20 mL each); *first 24 hours:* 400 mg or two vials (5 mg/mL, 40 mL each).

▶ LEUCOVORIN CALCIUM

Kathy Birnbaum, PharmD

I. **Pharmacology.** Leucovorin (folinic acid or citrovorum factor) is a metabolically functional form of folic acid. Unlike folic acid, leucovorin does not require reduction by dihydrofolate reductase, and, therefore, it can participate directly in the one-carbon transfer reactions necessary for purine biosynthesis and cellular DNA and RNA production. In animal models of methanol intoxication, replacement of a deficiency of leucovorin and folic acid can reduce morbidity and mortality because these agents catalyze the oxidation of the highly toxic metabolite formic acid to nontoxic products. However, there is no evidence that their administration in the absence of a deficiency is effective.

II. **Indications**

A. **Folic acid antagonists (eg, methotrexate, trimethoprim, and pyrimethamine).** ***Note:*** Leucovorin treatment is essential because cells are incapable of using folic acid owing to inhibition of dihydrofolate reductase.

B. **Methanol poisoning.** Leucovorin is the preferred form of folic acid to enhance the breakdown of formic acid; if leucovorin is not available, then use folic acid.

III. **Contraindications.** No known contraindications.

IV. **Adverse effects**

A. Allergic reactions as a result of prior sensitization have been reported.

B. Hypercalcemia from the calcium salt may occur (limit infusion rate to 160 mg/min in adults).

C. **Use in pregnancy.** FDA Category C (indeterminate). This does not preclude its acute, short-term use in a seriously symptomatic patient (p 498).

V. **Drug or laboratory interactions.** Leucovorin bypasses the antifolate effect of methotrexate.

VI. **Dosage and method of administration**

A. **Methotrexate poisoning.** ***Note:*** Efficacy depends on early administration. Leucovorin should be given within 1 hour of poisoning, if possible; do not wait for methotrexate levels to initiate therapy. The drug should be given intravenously. The most effective dose and duration of treatment are uncertain.

1. **Methotrexate level unknown.** Administer intravenously a dose equal to or greater than the dose of methotrexate. Leucovorin doses typically range from 10 to 25 mg/m^2 every 6 hours, but doses of up to 1,000 mg/m^2 have

been used. Most serious cases are treated with 100 mg/m^2 (or about 150 mg in an average-size adult) IV over 15–30 minutes, followed by 10 mg/m^2 (or ~15 mg) IV every 6 hours for at least 3 days, or until the serum methotrexate level falls below 0.01 mcmol/L or is undetectable.

2. **Elevated methotrexate level or elevated serum creatinine**
   a. If the 24-hour serum creatinine increases 50% in the first 24 hours after methotrexate or if the 24-hour methotrexate level exceeds 5 mcmol/L or if the 48-hour methotrexate level exceeds 0.9 mcmol/L, increase the leucovorin dose to 100 mg/m^2 intravenously every 3 hours until the methotrexate level is less than 0.01 mcmol/L or is undetectable.
   b. If the 24-hour serum creatinine increases 100% in the first 24 hours after methotrexate or if the 24-hour methotrexate level reaches or exceeds 50 mcmol/L or if the 48-hour methotrexate level reaches or exceeds 5 mcmol/L, increase the leucovorin dose to 150 mg intravenously every 3 hours until the methotrexate level is less than 1 mcmol/L. Then give a dose of 15 mg intravenously every 3 hours until the methotrexate level is less than 0.01 mcmol/L or is undetectable.

B. **Other folic acid antagonists.** Administer 5–15 mg/d IM, IV, or PO for 5–7 days.

C. **Methanol poisoning.** For adults and children, give 1 mg/kg (up to 50–70 mg) IV every 4 hours for one to two doses. Oral folic acid is given thereafter at the same dose every 4–6 hours until resolution of symptoms and adequate elimination of methanol from the body (usually 2 days).

VII. **Formulations**

A. **Parenteral.** Leucovorin calcium (folinic acid, citrovorum factor), 10-mg/mL vials; 50-, 100-, 200-, and 350-mg powders for reconstitution. Use sterile water rather than diluent with benzyl alcohol.

B. **Oral.** Leucovorin calcium (various), 5-, 15-, and 25-mg tablets.

C. **Suggested minimum stocking levels** to treat a 100-kg adult for the first 8 hours and 24 hours: **leucovorin calcium**, *first 8 hours:* 300 mg or three vials (100 mg each); *first 24 hours:* 300 mg or three vials (100 mg each).

▶ LIDOCAINE

Thomas E. Kearney, PharmD

I. **Pharmacology**

A. Lidocaine is a local anesthetic and a type Ib antiarrhythmic agent. It inhibits fast sodium channels and depresses automaticity within the His-Purkinje system and the ventricles but has a variable effect and may shorten the effective refractory period and action potential duration. Conduction within ischemic myocardial areas is depressed, abolishing reentrant circuits. Unlike quinidine and related drugs, lidocaine exerts a minimal effect on the automaticity of the sinoatrial node and on conduction through the AV node, and it does not decrease myocardial contractility or blood pressure in usual doses. It also has rapid "on-off" binding to sodium channels (to allow reactivation of the channel) and competes with other sodium channel blockers (that are slow to release and block the channel throughout the cardiac cycle). This may account for its antiarrhythmic effect with poisonings from other sodium channel blockers (type 1a antiarrhythmics, tricyclic antidepressants).

B. The oral bioavailability of lidocaine is poor owing to extensive first-pass hepatic metabolism (although systemic poisoning is possible from ingestion). After intravenous administration of a single dose, the onset of action is within 60–90 seconds and the duration of effect is 10–20 minutes. The elimination half-life of lidocaine is approximately 1.5–2 hours; active metabolites have elimination half-lives of 2–10 hours. Lidocaine clearance declines with continuous infusions, which may be attributable to its metabolite monoethylglycinexylidide (MEGX). Drug accumulation may occur in patients with congestive heart failure or with liver or renal disease.

II. **Indications.** Lidocaine is used for the control of ventricular arrhythmias arising from poisoning by a variety of cardioactive drugs and toxins (eg, digoxin, cyclic antidepressants, stimulants, and theophylline). Patients with atrial arrhythmias usually do not respond to this drug.

III. **Contraindications**

A. The presence of nodal or ventricular rhythms in the setting of third-degree AV or intraventricular block. These are usually reflex escape rhythms that may provide lifesaving cardiac output, and abolishing them may result in asystole.

B. Hypersensitivity to lidocaine or other amide-type local anesthetics (rare).

IV. **Adverse effects**

A. Excessive doses produce dizziness, confusion, agitation, and seizures.

B. Conduction defects, bradycardia, and hypotension may occur in patients with extremely high serum concentrations or in those with underlying conduction disease.

C. **Use in pregnancy.** FDA Category B. Fetal harm is extremely unlikely (p 498).

V. **Drug or laboratory interactions**

A. Cimetidine and propranolol may decrease the hepatic clearance of lidocaine.

B. Lidocaine may produce additive effects with other local anesthetics. In severe cocaine intoxication, lidocaine theoretically may cause additive neuronal depression.

VI. **Dosage and method of administration (adults and children)**

A. Administer 1- to 1.5-mg/kg (usual adult dose: 50–100 mg; children: 1 mg/kg) IV bolus at a rate of 25–50 mg/min, followed by infusion of 1–4 mg/min (20–50 mcg/kg/min) to maintain serum concentrations of 1.5–5 mg/L. Can also be administered by intraosseous infusion.

B. If significant ectopy persists after the initial bolus, repeat doses of 0.5 mg/kg IV can be given if needed at 5- to 10-minute intervals (to a maximum 300-mg or 3-mg/kg total dose in any 1-hour period; children may be given repeated 1-mg/kg doses every 5–10 minutes to a maximum of 5 mg/kg or up to 100 mg).

C. In patients with congestive heart failure or liver disease, use half the recommended maintenance infusion dose.

VII. **Formulations**

A. **Parenteral.** Lidocaine hydrochloride for cardiac arrhythmias (Xylocaine, others), direct IV: 0.5% (5 mg/mL), 1% (10 mg/mL), 1.5% (15 mg/mL), 2% (20 mg/mL), and 4% (40 mg/mL) in 5-mL prefilled syringes, 2- to 50-mL ampules, and single-dose and multiple-dose vials; 4%, 10%, and 20% in 1- and 2-g single-dose vials or additive syringes for preparing intravenous infusions; 0.4% (in 250 and 500 mL) and 0.8% (in 250 and 500 mL) in D_5W solutions prepared for infusions; and 5% in 7.5% dextrose in 2-mL ampules. ***Note:*** Some contain methylparabens and sodium metabisulfite as preservatives.

B. **Suggested minimum stocking levels** to treat a 100-kg adult for the first 8 hours and 24 hours: **lidocaine hydrochloride**, *first 8 hours:* 2.3 g or three prefilled 100-mg syringes and two 1-g vials for infusions; *first 24 hours:* 6.3 g or three prefilled 100-mg syringes and six 1-g vials for infusions.

▶ LIPID EMULSION

Thomas E. Kearney, PharmD

I. **Pharmacology.** Intravenous lipid emulsion (ILE) therapy is one of the newest treatments touted for cardiovascular toxicity from fat-soluble drugs. It was first used in resuscitations from local anesthetic toxicity, particularly bupivacaine. Some animal studies have demonstrated dramatic benefits, including resuscitation from cardiac arrest, severe hypotension, and bradycardia induced by cardiotoxic drugs, but others had variable results. Anecdotal human case reports suggest that ILE might be effective for reversal of cardiovascular or neurological toxicity in some cases of local anesthetic and other poisonings but is less or not effective in others and may be subject to reporting bias in favor of positive results. Effectiveness in controlled studies with animal models has been inconsistent with human case experiences.

A. The mechanisms for the efficacy of ILE are uncertain and several of the following have been proposed:

1. The "lipid sink" theory—ILE may sequester lipid-soluble drugs within the intravascular compartment, making less of the drug available for tissue toxicity.
2. ILE may provide extra fatty acids to cardiac myocyte mitochondria for a heart unable to use its usual energy supply when stressed.
3. Long-chain fatty acids may activate calcium channels in myocytes, augmenting further release of intracellular calcium and resulting in improved contractility.
4. Medium- and long-chain fatty acids stimulate a rise of cytosolic calcium in pancreatic cells, causing release of insulin, which in turn may improve cardiac performance in shock.
5. ILE may reverse nitric oxide–induced vasodilation by inhibition of endothelial nitric oxide synthase.

B. The infused fat particles behave like natural chylomicrons. Circulating triglycerides are quickly hydrolyzed by intravascular lipoprotein lipase, releasing free fatty acids. These fatty acids are taken up by Kupfer cells in the liver as well as the reticuloendothelial system. With large infusions, free fatty acids are also taken up by skeletal muscle and subcutaneous tissue. Any free fatty acids that enter tissues can be stored or transported into the mitochondria, where they undergo beta-oxidation.

II. Indications

A. The initial use of ILE for overdose was based on case reports of return of spontaneous circulation in patients with overdose of local anesthetic drugs, including bupivacaine and mepivacaine.

B. Human case reports of a variety of other poisonings (tricyclic antidepressants, calcium channel blockers, beta-blockers, GABA agonists, antiarrhythmics, anticonvulsants, pesticides, diphenhydramine, sedative hypnotics, cocaine, and others) have demonstrated mixed results.

C. In patients who are hemodynamically unstable from overdoses with fat-soluble xenobiotics, when more conventional resuscitative interventions have failed, consider ILE as adjunctive therapy for refractory hypotension. This should be reserved for life-threatening situations and not considered a standard of care.

III. Contraindications

A. Allergy to soy or egg products.

B. Black box warning. Neonates: Deaths have occurred in preterm infants owing to intravenous lipid accumulation in the lungs as a result of impaired clearance and elimination of the drug.

C. Relative contraindications include pulmonary disease, pancreatitis, and fat metabolism disorders.

1. ILE given too quickly in large amounts to patients with lung disease, particularly ARDS, can temporarily impair proper oxygenation.
2. Pancreatitis has resulted after repeated doses, and ILE infusion may exacerbate existing pancreatitis.
3. The manufacturer states that abnormal fat metabolism, hyperlipidemia, and lipid nephrosis are all contraindications to the administration of ILE.

IV. Adverse effects

A. Fat emboli syndrome. Excessive infusion of lipid emulsion may transiently increase pulmonary vascular resistance and decrease pulmonary gas diffusion, especially in patients with underlying pulmonary disease. However, 10-fold dosing errors, with infusions approaching 10 mL/kg/h for several hours, have not resulted in untoward effects. Animal studies suggest 70 mL/kg infused over 30 minutes as a best approximation of a 50% lethal dose (LD_{50}) in rats.

B. There is a potential for pancreatitis or exacerbation of preexisting disease.

C. Phlebitis, macroscopic hematuria, and transient rises in amylase levels have been noted in case reports.

D. Use in pregnancy. Owing to lack of data, the FDA has assigned ILE to Pregnancy Category C (p 498) for all trimesters. However, parenteral lipid products have been used in pregnant women for nutrition without untoward effects.

V. Drug or laboratory interactions

A. Mixing of ILE with calcium can cause flocculation, and, therefore, simultaneous administration should be avoided.

B. Immediately after very high infusions of ILE, tests of hemoglobin, hematocrit, white blood cell count, platelet count, electrolytes, glucose, hepatic transaminases, creatinine, creatine kinase, and coagulation studies are uninterpretable for several hours. There are also problems with co-oximetry for blood gases: oxygen saturation may not be measureable, and methemoglobin may be falsely elevated.

C. Higher doses of vasopressors (epinephrine or vasopressin) impaired the efficacy of ILE in animal studies.

VI. Dosage and method of administration

A. Initial bolus. Typical starting dose in adults is 100 mL (or 1.5 mL/kg of lean body mass) of a 20% intravenous LE suspension given over 2–3 minutes. In children, start with 1.5 mL/kg. If there is minimal or no response initially, the bolus can be repeated twice at 5-minute intervals.

B. Infusion. Continuous infusions can be given after the initial bolus at 0.25–0.5 mL/kg/min for 30–60 minutes. A maximum dose of 10–12 mL/kg over the first 30–60 minutes has been recommended and is the total dose in most case reports with successful results.

C. *Note:* The optimal dose and duration of therapy of ILE are uncertain. A patient's condition can deteriorate after initial improvement because the duration of benefit from ILE therapy may be shorter than the effects of the cardiotoxic drug.

VII. Formulations

A. Lipid emulsion therapy is readily available in most hospitals for hyperalimentation.

1. **Intralipid** consists mainly of soybean oil (20%) and egg yolk phospholipids (1.2%) emulsified in glycerin and water. The result is a mixture of medium- and long-chain triglycerides containing the free fatty acids linoleate, oleate, palmitate, linolenate, and stearate. Intralipid 20% is available in convenient 100-mL bags.
2. An alternate formulation, **Liposyn III**, also comes in a 20% formulation with soybean oil (20%) and egg yolk phospholipids (1.2%) available in 200-mL bags.
3. Other preparations include **Clinolipid 20%** with 16% olive oil and 4% soybean and egg yolk phospholipids (1.2%) but available only in 1,000-mL bags. **Nutrilipid 20%** with soybean oil (20%) and egg yolk phospholipids (1.2%) is available in 250-mL bags.
4. ***Note:*** **Intralipid** comes in a 30% formulation and **Liposyn III** in a 10% formulation, but it is unknown whether these are comparable in efficacy and safety to the 20% formulation. Also, it is unknown whether **Intralipid** and **Liposyn III** are equally efficacious products. It is believed that lipid emulsions with long-chain fatty acids may have an advantage in binding capacity.

B. Suggested minimum stocking levels to treat a 100-kg adult for the first 8 hours and 24 hours: **Intralipid 20%**, *first 8 hours:* 3,300 mL or three bags (100 mL each) plus six bags (500 mL each); *first 24 hours:* 3,300 mL or three bags (100 mL each) plus six bags (500 mL each).

▶ MAGNESIUM

R. David West, PharmD

I. Pharmacology

A. Magnesium is the fourth most common cation in the body and the second most abundant intracellular cation after potassium. Magnesium plays an essential role as an enzymatic cofactor in a number of biochemical pathways, including energy production from adenosine triphosphate (ATP).

B. Magnesium is a cofactor and has a direct effect on the Na^+/K^+-ATPase pump in both cardiac and nerve tissues. It may facilitate the influx of K^+ and stabilize myocardial membrane potentials leading to correction of dispersed ventricular repolarizations. Further, magnesium has some calcium-blocking activity and may indirectly antagonize digoxin at the myocardial Na^+/K^+-ATPase pump.

C. Magnesium modifies skeletal and smooth-muscle contractility. Infusions can cause vasodilation, hypotension, and bronchodilation. It can reduce or abolish seizures of toxemia.

D. Magnesium is primarily an intracellular ion, and only 1% is in the extracellular fluid. A low serum Mg level ($<$1.2 mg/dL) may indicate a net body deficit of 5,000 mg or more.

E. Hypomagnesemia can be associated with a number of acute or chronic disease processes (malabsorption, pancreatitis, diabetic ketoacidosis). It may result from chronic diuretic use, cisplatin administration, or alcoholism. It is a potentially serious, life-threatening consequence of hydrofluoric acid and ammonium bifluoride poisoning.

II. Indications

A. Replacement therapy for patients with hypomagnesemia.

B. Torsade de pointes ventricular tachycardia (p 14).

C. Other arrhythmias suspected to be related to hypomagnesemia. Magnesium may be helpful in selected patients with cardiac glycoside toxicity but is not a substitute for digoxin-specific Fab fragments.

D. Prevention of torsade de pointes ventricular tachycardia in cases of medication or toxin-induced QTc prolongation.

E. Barium ingestions (p 152). Magnesium sulfate can be used orally to convert soluble barium to insoluble, nonabsorbable barium sulfate if given early.

F. Magnesium may have a role in the treatment of cardiac arrhythmias associated with aluminum and zinc phosphide intoxications.

III. Contraindications

A. Magnesium should be administered cautiously in patients with renal impairment to avoid the potential for serious hypermagnesemia.

B. Heart block and bradycardia.

IV. Adverse effects

A. Flushing, sweating, hypothermia.

B. Depression of deep tendon reflexes, flaccid paralysis, respiratory paralysis.

C. Depression of cardiac function, hypotension, bradycardia, general circulatory collapse (in particular with rapid administration).

D. Gastrointestinal upset and diarrhea with oral administration.

E. Use in pregnancy. FDA Category A. Magnesium sulfate is used commonly as an agent for premature labor (p 498).

V. Drug or laboratory interactions

A. General CNS depressants. Additive effects may occur when CNS depressants are combined with magnesium infusions.

B. Neuromuscular blocking agents. Concomitant administration of magnesium with neuromuscular blocking agents may enhance and prolong their effect. Dose adjustment may be needed to avoid prolonged respiratory depression.

VI. Dosage and method of administration (adults and children)

A. Magnesium can be given orally, IV, or by IM injection. When it is given parenterally, the IV route is preferred and the sulfate salt generally is used.

B. Magnesium dosing is highly empiric and guided by both the clinical response and the estimated total body deficit of Mg based on serum levels.

C. Adults: Give 1 g (8.12 mEq) every 6 hours IV for four doses. For severe hypomagnesemia, doses as high as 1 mEq/kg/24 h or 8–12 g/d in divided doses have been used. Magnesium sulfate can be diluted in 50–100 mL of D_5W or NS and infused over 5–60 minutes. **Children:** Give 25–50 mg/kg per dose IV for three to four doses. Maximum single dose should not exceed 2,000 mg (16 mEq). Higher doses of 100 mg/kg per dose IV have also been employed.

D. For treatment of **life-threatening arrhythmias** (ventricular tachycardia or fibrillation associated with hypomagnesemia) in adults, give 1–2 g (children, 25–50 mg/kg up to 2 g) IV or IO over 1–2 minutes (if pulseless) or over 5–60 minutes (in a patient with a pulse), diluted in 50–100 mL of D_5W or NS. A second dose can be given if the ventricular arrhythmia recurs. A common regimen for adults is 2 g IV over 20 minutes.

E. For soluble barium ingestions, magnesium sulfate can be given to form insoluble, poorly absorbed barium sulfate. Adults should receive 30 g orally or by lavage, and children 250 mg/kg. Magnesium sulfate should not be given IV in these cases.

VII. Formulations

A. Parenteral. Magnesium sulfate vials, 50% (4.06 mEq/mL, 500 mg/mL) in volumes of 2, 10, 20, and 50 mL in which 2 mL is equivalent to 1 g or 8.12 mEq. Also available in 10% (0.8 mEq/mL) and 12.5% (1 mEq/mL) solutions in 20- and 50-mL ampules and vials as well as large-volume premixed bags. Magnesium chloride injection is also available but used less commonly.

B. Oral. A large number of oral dosage forms are available, formulated in both immediate- and sustained-release formulations.

C. Suggested minimum stocking levels to treat a 100-kg adult for the first 8 hours and 24 hours: **magnesium sulfate**, *first 8 hours:* 4 g or four vials (500 mg/mL, 2 mL each); *first 24 hours:* 12 g or 12 vials (500 mg/mL, 2 mL each).

▶ MANNITOL

Gary W. Everson, PharmD

I. Pharmacology

A. Mannitol is an osmotically active solute diuretic. Mannitol inhibits water reabsorption at the loop of Henle and the proximal tubule. The increase in urine output usually is accompanied by an increase in solute excretion. In addition, mannitol transiently increases serum osmolality and decreases cerebrospinal fluid (CSF) pressure by creating an osmotic gradient between brain tissue and the vascular compartment. Water moves across this gradient into the blood vessels, lowering the CSF pressure and decreasing intracranial pressure.

B. Mannitol may reverse the effects of ciguatoxin by inhibiting ciguatoxin-induced opening of sodium channels. In addition, it is possible that mannitol may decrease neuronal edema, act as a scavenger of ciguatoxin-generated free radicals, and reduce cellular excitability. Mannitol may also increase the dissociation of ciguatoxin from its binding sites on cell membranes.

C. In the past, mannitol was used to induce "forced diuresis" for some poisonings (eg, phenobarbital, salicylate) to enhance their renal elimination, but this use has been abandoned because of lack of efficacy and potential risks of cerebral and pulmonary edema.

II. Indications

A. Proposed as a treatment for neurologic and neurosensory manifestations caused by ciguatera poisoning (p 246). However, a double-blind, randomized study found that mannitol was not superior to normal saline in relieving signs or symptoms of ciguatera fish poisoning.

B. Possible adjunctive agent in treating severe vitamin A toxicity associated with increased intracranial pressure (pseudotumor cerebri).

C. Sometimes used as an adjunct to fluid therapy for acute oliguria resulting from massive rhabdomyolysis (p 27).

III. Contraindications

A. Severe dehydration.

B. Acute intracranial bleeding.

C. Pulmonary edema.

D. Congestive heart failure.

E. Anuria associated with severe renal disease.

IV. Adverse effects

A. Mannitol may cause excessive expansion of the intravascular space when administered in high concentrations at a rapid rate. This may result in congestive heart failure and pulmonary edema.

B. Mannitol causes movement of intracellular water to the extracellular space and can produce both transient hyperosmolality and hyponatremia. Generalized electrolyte disturbances may also be seen.

C. Oliguric or anuric renal failure has occurred in patients receiving mannitol. Low-dose mannitol appears to result in renal vasodilating effects, whereas high doses (>200 g/d) may produce renal vasoconstriction.

D. Use in pregnancy. FDA Category C (indeterminate). This does not preclude its acute, short-term use in a seriously symptomatic patient (p 498).

V. Drug or laboratory interactions. Diuresis may result in decreased potassium and magnesium levels, which may increase the risk for QT prolongation in patients taking drugs such as sotalol and droperidol.

VI. Dosage and method of administration

A. Ciguatera poisoning. Recommended dose is 0.5–1.0 g/kg administered IV over 30–45 minutes. Reportedly most effective when given within 24–72 hours of onset of symptoms or exposure, but case reports describe alleged benefit up to several weeks after exposure. Ciguatera poisoning may be accompanied by dehydration, which must be treated with intravenous fluids before the administration of mannitol.

B. Vitamin A–induced pseudotumor cerebri. Give 0.25–1 g/kg intravenously.

VII. Formulations

A. Parenteral. Mannitol 10% (500 mL, 1,000 mL); 15% (150 mL, 500 mL); 20% (250 mL, 500 mL); 25% (50-mL vials and syringes).

B. Suggested minimum stocking levels to treat a 100-kg adult for the first 8 hours and 24 hours: mannitol, *first 8 hours:* 100 g or one bottle (20% mannitol, 500 mL each); *first 24 hours:* 100 g or one bottle (20% mannitol, 500 mL each).

▶ METHYLENE BLUE

Fabian Garza, PharmD and Thomas E. Kearney, PharmD

I. Pharmacology

A. Methylene blue is a thiazine dye that increases the conversion of methemoglobin to hemoglobin. Methylene blue is reduced via methemoglobin reductase and nicotinamide adenosine dinucleotide phosphate (NADPH) to leukomethylene blue, which in turn reduces methemoglobin. Glucose-6-phospate dehydrogenase (G6PD) is essential for the generation of NADPH and is thus essential for the function of methylene blue as an antidote. Therapeutic effect is seen within 30 minutes. Methemoglobin is excreted in bile and urine, which may turn blue or green.

B. Methylene blue has been used to treat ifosfamide-induced encephalopathy, but the exact pathophysiologic mechanisms responsible are not known. Methylene blue may reverse the neurotoxic effects of the ifosfamide metabolites.

C. Methylene blue, as a guanylate cyclase inhibitor, reduces cyclic guanosine monophosphate (cGMP) production and nitric oxide (NO) stimulation. Excessive NO activity may contribute to refractory vasodilatory shock associated with sepsis, vasoplegia following cardiac surgery, anaphylactic shock, and metformin and amlodipine toxicity. Methylene blue has been used to improve hemodynamics in each of these circumstances.

D. Methylene blue is an MAO-A inhibitor and has been responsible for the precipitation of a serotonin syndrome in patients treated with selective serotonin reuptake inhibitors (SSRIs) when used for cardiac and parathyroid surgery.

II. Indications

A. Methylene blue is used to treat methemoglobinemia (p 317) if the patient has symptoms or signs of hypoxemia (eg, dyspnea, confusion, or chest pain) or a methemoglobin level higher than 30%. ***Note:*** Methylene blue is not effective for sulfhemoglobinemia.

B. Methylene blue has been used to reverse and prevent ifosfamide-related encephalopathy.

C. Has been used as an adjunctive therapy to improve hemodynamics in patients with refractory vasodilator shock due to sepsis, anaphylaxis, and metformin and calcium channel blocker toxicity (case report of amlodipine-induced shock).

III. Contraindications

A. G6PD deficiency. Treatment with methylene blue is ineffective for reversal of methemoglobinemia and may cause hemolysis.

B. Severe renal failure.

C. Known hypersensitivity to methylene blue.

D. Methemoglobin reductase deficiency.

E. Reversal of nitrite-induced methemoglobinemia for the treatment of cyanide poisoning.

F. Adult respiratory distress syndrome in vasodilator shock.

IV. Adverse effects

A. Gastrointestinal upset, headache, and dizziness may occur.

B. Excessive doses of methylene blue (≥7 mg/kg) can actually cause methemoglobinemia by directly oxidizing hemoglobin. Doses higher than 15 mg/kg are associated with hemolysis, particularly in neonates. May also dye secretions and mucous membranes and interfere with clinical findings of cyanosis.

C. Long-term administration may result in marked anemia.

D. Extravasation may result in local tissue necrosis.

E. **Use in pregnancy.** FDA Category X (fetal abnormalities demonstrated when used in amniocentesis). This does not preclude its acute, short-term use for a seriously symptomatic patient (p 498).

V. Drug or laboratory interactions

A. **Serotonin syndrome** is a potential risk when methylene blue is administered with other serotoninergic drugs owing to its inhibition of MAO-A.

B. The intravenous preparation should not be mixed with other drugs.

C. Transiently false-positive methemoglobin levels of about 15% are produced by doses of methylene blue of 2 mg/kg. Methylene blue may also alter pulse oximeter readings.

VI. Dosage and method of administration (adults and children)

A. Methemoglobinemia

1. Administer 1–2 mg/kg (0.1–0.2 mL/kg of 1% solution) IV slowly over 5 minutes. May be repeated in 30–60 minutes.
2. Simultaneous administration of dextrose may be warranted to provide adequate NAD and NADPH cofactors.

3. If no response after two doses, do not repeat dosing; consider G6PD deficiency or methemoglobin reductase deficiency.
4. Patients with continued production of methemoglobin from a long-acting oxidant stress (eg, dapsone) may require repeated dosing every 6–8 hours for 2–3 days. Alternatively, give as a continuous IV infusion of 0.10–0.25 mg/kg/h (compatible with normal saline and dilute to a concentration of 0.05%).
5. Flush IV line with 15–30 mL of normal saline to reduce incidence of local pain.

B. **Ifosfamide encephalopathy**
1. **Prophylaxis.** Administer 50 mg PO or IV (slowly over 5 minutes) every 6–8 hours while the patient is receiving ifosfamide.
2. **Treatment.** Administer 50 mg IV (slowly over 5 minutes) every 4–6 hours until symptoms resolve.

C. **Vasodilator shock.** Reported dosing is 1–2 mg/kg IV (slowly over 5 minutes) for persistent hypotension despite vasopressor administration. This was followed with a continuous IV infusion of 1 mg/kg/h in a case of amlodipine toxicity.

VII. **Formulations**
A. **Parenteral.** Methylene blue injection 1% (10 mg/mL).
B. **Suggested minimum stocking levels** to treat a 100-kg adult for the first 8 hours and 24 hours: **methylene blue,** *first 8 hours:* 400 mg or four ampules (10 mg/mL, 10 mL each); *first 24 hours:* 600 mg or six ampules (10 mg/mL, 10 mL each).

▶ METOCLOPRAMIDE

Justin C. Lewis, PharmD

I. **Pharmacology.** Metoclopramide is a dopamine antagonist with antiemetic activity at the chemoreceptor trigger zone. It also accelerates GI motility and facilitates gastric emptying. The onset of effect is 1–3 minutes after intravenous administration, and therapeutic effects persist for 1–2 hours after a single dose regardless of route. The drug is excreted primarily by the kidneys. The elimination half-life is about 5–6 hours but may be as long as 14.8 hours in patients with renal insufficiency and 15.4 hours in patients with cirrhosis.

II. **Indications**
A. Metoclopramide is used to prevent and control persistent nausea and vomiting, particularly when vomiting can compromise the ability to administer activated charcoal (eg, treatment of theophylline poisoning) or another oral antidotal therapy (eg, acetylcysteine for acetaminophen poisoning).
B. Theoretic (unproven) use to stimulate bowel activity in patients with ileus who require repeat-dose activated charcoal or whole-bowel irrigation.

III. **Contraindications**
A. Known hypersensitivity to the drug; possible cross-sensitivity with procainamide.
B. Mechanical bowel obstruction, active gastrointestinal hemorrhage, or intestinal perforation.
C. Pheochromocytoma (metoclopramide may cause hypertensive crisis by enhancing tumor catecholamine secretion).
D. Patients with seizure disorders (the frequency and severity of seizures may be increased).
E. Patients receiving other drugs that are likely to cause extrapyramidal reactions (consider using selective 5-HT3 receptor antagonists as alternatives in these patients).

IV. **Adverse effects**
A. Sedation, restlessness, fatigue, and diarrhea may occur.

B. Extrapyramidal reactions may result, particularly with high-dose treatment. Pediatric patients and adults younger than 30 years appear to be more susceptible. These reactions may be treated or prevented with diphenhydramine (p 544).

C. Parenteral formulations that contain sulfite preservatives may precipitate bronchospasm in susceptible individuals.

D. Use in pregnancy. FDA Category B. Not likely to cause harm when used as short-term therapy (p 496).

V. Drug or laboratory interactions

A. Additive sedation in the presence of other CNS depressants.

B. Due to an increased risk for extrapyramidal reactions in the presence of other dopamine antagonist agents (eg, haloperidol and other antipsychotic agents), concurrent use is contraindicated.

C. In one study involving hypertensive patients, metoclopramide enhanced the release of catecholamines. As a result, the manufacturer advises cautious use in hypertensive patients and suggests that the drug should not be used in patients taking monoamine oxidase inhibitors.

D. Agitation, diaphoresis, and extrapyramidal movement disorder were reported in two patients taking selective serotonin reuptake inhibitors (sertraline, venlafaxine) who received IV metoclopramide.

E. The drug may enhance the absorption of ingested drugs by promoting gastric emptying.

F. Anticholinergic agents may inhibit bowel motility effects.

G. Numerous IV incompatibilities: calcium gluconate, sodium bicarbonate, cimetidine, furosemide, and many antibiotic agents (eg, ampicillin, chloramphenicol, erythromycin, penicillin G potassium, tetracycline).

VI. Dosage and method of administration

A. Low-dose therapy. Effective for *mild* nausea and vomiting. Give 10–20 mg IM, orally, sublingually, or slowly IV (children: 0.1 mg/kg per dose). Doses of 10 mg or less can be given by IV push undiluted over 1–2 minutes.

B. High-dose therapy. For control of *severe or persistent* vomiting. For adults and children, give a 1- to 2-mg/kg IV infusion over 15 minutes in 50 mL of saline or dextrose. May be repeated every 2 to 4 hours; maximum five doses per day.

1. Metoclopramide is most effective if given before emesis or 30 minutes before administration of a nausea-inducing drug (eg, glucagon, acetylcysteine).
2. If no response to initial dose, may give additional 2 mg/kg and repeat every 2–3 hours up to maximum daily dose of 10 mg/kg/d (five total doses of 2 mg/kg).
3. Pretreatment with 50 mg (children: 1 mg/kg) of diphenhydramine (p 544) helps prevent extrapyramidal reactions.
4. Dosing adjustment in patients with reduced creatinine clearance (CrCL):
   - **a.** CrCL 40–50 mL/min: Administer 75% of dose.
   - **b.** CrCL 10–40 mL/min: Administer 50% of dose.
   - **c.** CrCL <10 mL/min: Administer 25–50% of dose.

VII. Formulations

A. Parenteral. Metoclopramide hydrochloride (Reglan, generic); 5 mg/mL (2-mL vials). Also available in preservative-free 5 mg/mL (2-mL vials).

B. Oral. Metoclopramide hydrochloride (Reglan, generic); 5 mg, 10 mg. Oral solution (generic) 5 mg/5mL (10 mL, 473 mL); orally dispersible tablets (Metozolv ODT) are available in five, 10-mg tablets.

C. Suggested minimum stocking levels to treat a 100-kg adult for the first 8 hours and 24 hours: **metoclopramide**, *first 8 hours:* 750 mg or 75 vials (5 mg/mL, 2 mL each); *first 24 hours:* 1,000 mg or 100 vials (5 mg/mL, 2 mL each).

▶ MORPHINE

Thomas E. Kearney, PharmD

I. Pharmacology. Morphine is the principal alkaloid of opium and a potent analgesic and sedative agent. In addition, it decreases venous tone and systemic vascular resistance, resulting in reduced preload and afterload. Morphine is absorbed variably from the GI tract and usually is used parenterally. After intravenous injection, peak analgesia is attained within 20 minutes and usually lasts 3–5 hours. Morphine is eliminated by hepatic metabolism, with a serum half-life of about 3 hours; however, the clearance of morphine is slowed and the duration of effect is prolonged in patients with renal failure resulting from accumulation of the active metabolite morphine-6-glucuronide.

II. Indications

- **A.** Severe pain associated with black widow spider envenomation, rattlesnake envenomation, and other bites or stings.
- **B.** Pain caused by corrosive injury to the eyes, skin, or GI tract.
- **C.** Pulmonary edema resulting from congestive heart failure. Chemically induced noncardiogenic pulmonary edema is ***not*** an indication for morphine therapy.

III. Contraindications

- **A.** Known hypersensitivity to morphine.
- **B.** Respiratory or CNS depression with impending respiratory failure unless the patient is already intubated or equipment is available and trained personnel are standing by for intervention if necessary with intubation or the reversal agent naloxone (p 584).
- **C.** Suspected head injury. Morphine may obscure or cause exaggerated CNS depression.

IV. Adverse effects

- **A.** Respiratory and CNS depression may result in respiratory arrest. Depressant effects may be prolonged in patients with liver disease and chronic renal failure. Risk factors or comorbidities increasing risk for morphine-induced respiratory depression include naive user lacking tolerance, hypothyroidism, morbid obesity, and sleep apnea syndrome. ***Note:*** Tidal volume may be depressed without perceptible changes in respiratory rate, and these effects are influenced by external stimuli (eg, noise, manipulation).
- **B.** Hypotension may occur owing to decreased systemic vascular resistance and venous tone.
- **C.** Nausea, vomiting, and constipation may occur.
- **D.** Bradycardia, wheezing, flushing, pruritus, urticaria, and other histamine-like effects may occur.
- **E.** Sulfite preservative in some parenteral preparations may cause hypersensitivity reactions.
- **F. Use in pregnancy.** FDA Category C (indeterminate). This does not preclude its acute, short-term use in a seriously symptomatic patient (p 498).

V. Drug or laboratory interactions

- **A.** Additive depressant effects with other opioid agonists, ethanol and other sedative–hypnotic agents, tranquilizers, MAO inhibitors, and antidepressants.
- **B.** Naloxone and naltrexone will antagonize the analgesic actions of morphine and may precipitate a withdrawal syndrome in morphine-dependent patients.
- **C.** Morphine is physically incompatible with solutions containing a variety of drugs, including aminophylline, phenytoin, phenobarbital, and sodium bicarbonate.

VI. Dosage and method of administration

- **A.** Morphine may be injected subcutaneously, intramuscularly, or intravenously. The oral and rectal routes produce erratic absorption and are not recommended for use in acutely ill patients.

B. The usual initial adult dose is 2–10 mg IV (may dilute with 4–5 mL of sterile water and give slowly over 4–5 minutes as well as titrate in small increments, 1–4 mg, every 5 minutes) or 10–15 mg SC or IM, with maintenance analgesic doses of 5–20 mg every 4 hours. The usual pediatric dose is 0.05–0.1 mg/kg administered very slowly IV up to a maximum single dose of 10 mg, or 0.1–0.2 mg/kg SC or IM up to a maximum of 15 mg.

1. ***Note:*** The dosage range may vary, and risk factors for respiratory depression should be carefully considered. In particular, exercise caution in morbidly obese patients and children.
2. Remember that peak analgesic (and toxic) effects may be delayed (by an average of 20 minutes with IV administration), and naloxone should be immediately accessible if respiratory depression occurs.

VII. Formulations

A. Parenteral. Morphine sulfate for injection; variety of available concentrations from 0.5 to 50 mg/mL. ***Note:*** Some preparations contain sulfites as a preservative.

B. Suggested minimum stocking levels to treat a 100-kg adult for the first 8 hours and 24 hours: **morphine sulfate**, *first 8 hours:* 50 mg or 10 ampules (0.5 mg/mL, 10 mL each); *first 24 hours:* 150 mg or 30 ampules (0.5 mg/mL, 10 mL each).

▶ NALOXONE

Joyce Go, PharmD

I. Pharmacology. Naloxone is a synthetic N-allyl derivative with pure opioid antagonist activity that **competitively** blocks mu-, kappa-, and delta-opiate receptors within the CNS. It has no opioid agonist properties and can be given safely in large doses without producing respiratory or CNS depression. Take-home naloxone programs are being developed in which opiate users and their families are supplied naloxone for use on the scene in case of accidental overdose. The most common routes of administration for this purpose are intranasal and intramuscular or subcutaneous by autoinjector or syringe.

A. Naloxone undergoes extensive first-pass metabolism and is not effective orally but may be given by intravenous, intramuscular, subcutaneous, nebulized, intranasal, and intraosseous routes. After intravenous administration, opioid antagonism occurs within 1–2 minutes and persists for approximately 30–120 minutes. The plasma half-life ranges from 30 to 81 minutes. Table III–11 is a comparison of the routes of administration for naloxone.

B. Nalmefene is a pure opioid antagonist that has been used to treat acute opioid intoxication. It has a longer elimination half-life and duration of action than naloxone. However, its production was discontinued in 2008 and is no longer available in the United States.

C. Naltrexone is another potent competitive opioid antagonist that is active orally and used to prevent recidivism in patients detoxified after opioid abuse. It has also been used to reduce craving for alcohol. It is ***not*** used for the acute reversal of opioid intoxication.

II. Indications

A. Reversal of acute opioid intoxication manifested by coma, respiratory depression, or hypotension.

B. Empiric therapy for stupor or coma suspected to be caused by opioid overdose.

C. Anecdotal reports suggest that high-dose naloxone may partially reverse the CNS and respiratory depression associated with clonidine (p 197), ethanol (p 231), benzodiazepine (p 156), or valproic acid (p 441) overdoses, although these effects are inconsistent.

TABLE III–11. COMPARISON OF ROUTES OF ADMINISTRATION OF NALOXONE

Route	Advantages	Disadvantages
Intravenous	Rapid onset and best predictable dose and bioavailability	Requires IV access; higher likelihood of precipitating withdrawal in opioid-dependent patient.
Intramuscular/ subcutaneous	Delivery via syringe or autoinjector (with electronic voice to guide use); option for take-home naloxone program	Slower onset; systemic absorption depends on blood flow at injection site and may be erratic.
Intranasal	Delivery via mucosal atomizer device and circumvents needle; option for take-home naloxone program; onset is comparable to IM	Slower onset; systemic absorption depends on blood flow at nasal mucosal surface and open nasal passage (may be limited if topical vasoconstrictor used prior to administration, eg, snorting cocaine or use of nasal decongestant, or presence of epistaxis); requires assembly.
Nebulized/ endotracheal		Unpredictable dose delivered and more variable in hypoventilating patient. Least desirable for ED management.

III. Contraindications. Do not use in patients with a known hypersensitivity to naloxone or nalmefene (may have cross-sensitivity).

IV. Adverse effects. Human studies have documented an excellent safety record for naloxone.

- **A.** Use in opiate-dependent patients may precipitate acute withdrawal syndrome. Neonates of addicted mothers may have more severe withdrawal symptoms, including seizures. Aggressive use of opiate antagonists in so-called rapid opioid detoxification (ROD) and ultra-rapid opioid detoxification (UROD) has been associated with marked increases in plasma corticotropin, cortisol, and catecholamine levels and in sympathetic activity; pulmonary edema; acute renal failure; ventricular bigeminy; psychosis; delirium; and death.
- **B.** Pulmonary edema or ventricular fibrillation occasionally has occurred shortly after naloxone administration in opioid-intoxicated patients. Pulmonary edema has also been associated with postanesthetic use of naloxone, especially when catecholamines and large fluid volumes have been administered.
- **C.** Reversing the sedative effects of an opioid may amplify the toxic effects of other drugs. For example, agitation, hypertension, and ventricular irritability have occurred after naloxone administration to persons high on a "speedball" (heroin plus cocaine or methamphetamine).
- **D.** There has been one case report of hypertension after naloxone administration in a patient with clonidine overdose. Hypertension has been associated with postoperative use of naloxone. Use caution in patients with cardiovascular risk factors, especially patients with a previous history of uncontrolled hypertension.
- **E. Use in pregnancy.** FDA Category B (p 498). Naloxone may produce an acute opioid withdrawal syndrome in both mother and fetus and may precipitate labor in an opioid-dependent mother.

V. Drug or laboratory interactions. Naloxone antagonizes the analgesic effect of opioids. Naloxone does not give a positive urine screen for opiates.

VI. Dosage and method of administration for suspected opioid-induced coma.

A. Adults

1. **Initial dose.** Administer 0.4–2 mg IV; repeat at 2- to 3-minute intervals until desired response is achieved. Titrate carefully in opioid-dependent patients (start at 0.04 mg).

a. The total dose required to reverse the effects of the opioid is highly variable and dependent on the concentration and receptor affinity of the opioid. Some drugs (eg, propoxyphene, diphenoxylate-atropine [Lomotil], buprenorphine, pentazocine, and the fentanyl derivatives) do not respond to usual doses of naloxone. However, if no response is achieved by a total dose of 10–15 mg, the diagnosis of opioid overdose should be questioned.

b. ***Caution:*** Resedation can occur when the naloxone wears off in 1–2 hours. Repeated doses of naloxone may be required to maintain reversal of the effects of opioids with prolonged elimination half-lives (eg, methadone) or sustained-release formulations; they may also be required when packets or vials have been ingested.

2. **Continuous infusion.** Give 0.4–0.8 mg/h in normal saline or 5% dextrose, titrated to clinical effect. Another method is to estimate two-thirds of the initial dose needed to awaken the patient and give that amount each hour. The manufacturer recommends diluting 2 mg of naloxone in 500 mL of fluid, resulting in a concentration of 4 mcg/mL. However, in fluid-restricted individuals, concentrations of up to 40 mcg/mL have been used without any reported problems.

B. **Pediatric dosing**

1. **Total reversal required** (narcotic toxicity secondary to overdose): Give 0.1 mg/kg (maximum dose: 2 mg) IV every 2 minutes as needed until desired response is achieved.
2. **Total reversal not required** (eg, reversal of respiratory depression associated with therapeutic use): 0.001–0.005 mg/kg IV; titrate to desired effect.
3. **Maintain reversal:** 0.002–0.16 mg/kg/h IV infusion.

C. ***Note:*** Although naloxone can be given by the intramuscular or subcutaneous route, absorption is erratic and incomplete. Naloxone is not effective orally. The nebulized and intranasal routes have been successfully used in prehospital and emergency department settings when IV access is unavailable. However, its onset is delayed compared to the IV route.

VII. **Formulations**

A. **Naloxone** hydrochloride (Narcan), 0.4 mg/mL (1-mL or 10-mL vials), 1 mg/mL (2-mL prefilled syringe), or 0.4 mg/0.4 mL autoinjector (Evzio).

B. **Intranasal naloxone.** Naloxone 1 mg/mL (2 mL) in a needleless prefilled syringe or Mucosal Atomization Device (MAD).

C. **Suggested minimum stocking levels** to treat a 100-kg adult for the first 8 hours and 24 hours: **Naloxone hydrochloride**, *first 8 hours*: 20 mg or five vials (0.4 mg/mL, 10 mL each); *first 24 hours*: 40 mg or 10 vials (0.4 mg/mL, 10 mL each). Note that take-home naloxone kits should contain two doses of naloxone and delivery devices.

▶ NEUROMUSCULAR BLOCKERS

Sam Jackson, MD, MBA

I. **Pharmacology**

A. Neuromuscular blocking agents produce skeletal muscle paralysis by inhibiting the action of acetylcholine at the neuromuscular junction (NMJ). **Depolarizing agents** (succinylcholine; Table III–12) depolarize the motor end plate and block recovery; transient muscle fasciculations occur with the initial depolarization. **Nondepolarizing agents** (atracurium, pancuronium, and others; see Table III–12) competitively block the action of acetylcholine at the motor end plate, preventing depolarization. Therefore, with nondepolarizing agents, no initial muscle fasciculations occur and a flaccid paralysis is produced.

TABLE III–12. SELECTED NEUROMUSCULAR BLOCKERS

Drug	Onset (minutes)	Duration (minutes)[a]	Dose (All Intravenous)
Depolarizing			
Succinylcholine	0.5–1	2–3	0.6 mg/kg[b] (children: 1 mg/kg[c]) over 10–20 seconds; repeat as needed.
Nondepolarizing			
Atracurium	3–5	20–45	0.4–0.5 mg/kg (children <2 years: 0.3–0.4 mg/kg).
Cisatracurium	1.5–2	55–61	0.15–0.2 mg/kg (children 2–12 years: 0.1 mg/kg), then 1–3 mcg/kg/min to maintain blockade.
Doxacurium	5–7	56–160	0.05–0.08 mg/kg (children: 0.03–0.05 mg/kg), then 0.005–0.01 mg/kg every 30–45 minutes to maintain blockade (children may require more frequent dosing).
Mivacurium	2–4	13–23	0.15–0.25 mg/kg (children: 0.2 mg/kg), then 0.1 mg/kg every 15 minutes or by continuous infusion; start with 0.01 mg/kg/min and maintain with average adult dose of 0.006–0.007 mg/kg/min (children: 0.014 mg/kg/min).
Pancuronium	2–3	35–45	0.06–0.1 mg/kg; then 0.01–0.02 mg/kg every 20–40 minutes as needed to maintain blockade.
Pipecuronium	3–5	17–175	0.05–0.1 mg/kg (adjust for renal function); then 0.01–0.015 mg/kg every 17–175 minutes (children may be less sensitive and require more frequent dosing).
Rocuronium	0.5–3	22–94	0.6–1 mg/kg; then 0.01 mg/kg/min to maintain blockade.
Vecuronium	1–2	25–40	For children older than 1 year and adults: 0.08–0.1-mg/kg bolus, then 0.01–0.02 mg/kg every 10–20 minutes to maintain blockade.

[a]For most agents, onset and duration are dose- and age-dependent. With succinylcholine or mivacurium, effects may be prolonged in patients who have a genetic plasma cholinesterase deficiency or organophosphate intoxication.
[b]To prevent fasciculations, administer a small dose of a nondepolarizing agent (eg, pancuronium, 0.01 mg/kg) 2–3 minutes before succinylcholine.
[c]Pretreat children with atropine at 0.005–0.01 mg/kg to prevent bradycardia or atrioventricular block.

B. The neuromuscular blockers produce complete muscle paralysis with no depression of CNS function (they are positively charged and water-soluble compounds that do not cross the brain–blood barrier rapidly). Thus, **patients who are conscious will remain awake but be unable to move, and patients with status epilepticus may continue to have seizure activity despite paralysis**. Furthermore, the neuromuscular blockers **do not relieve pain or anxiety** and have no sedative or amnestic effects.

C. Succinylcholine produces the most rapid onset of neuromuscular blockade. After intravenous administration, total paralysis ensues within 30–60 seconds and lasts 10–20 minutes. It is hydrolyzed rapidly by pseudocholinesterase, an enzyme present in the vascular compartment but not at the NMJ. Therefore, a relatively small fraction of the administered dose reaches the site of action, and diffusion from the NMJ back into the intravascular space determines metabolism. Larger (1.5 mg/kg IV based on *total body weight* in adults) rather than smaller doses should be used to achieve optimal paralysis during rapid-sequence intubation (RSI).

D. Rocuronium, a nondepolarizing agent, also has a rapid onset of effect when used at an RSI dose of 1 mg/kg IV (based on *ideal body weight*) in adults. However, the duration of the blockade (20–90 minutes) is considerably longer than that of succinylcholine. **Sugammadex**, a specific and rapid reversal agent for rocuronium and vecuronium, has recently received FDA approval for use in adult patients undergoing surgery. The utility of this agent in the patient who requires emergent intubation is not clear.

The onset and duration of several other neuromuscular blockers are described in Table III–12.

II. Indications

A. Neuromuscular blockers are used to abolish excessive muscular activity, rigidity, or peripheral seizure activity when continued muscle activity may produce or aggravate rhabdomyolysis, mechanical injury, or hyperthermia. Their primary indication is to improve the view of the larynx and other relevant anatomy during endotracheal intubation (see II. B, below). They are also employed when excessive muscular movement may place the patient (or others) at risk for injury.

1. Drug overdoses involving stimulants (eg, amphetamines, cocaine, phencyclidine, monoamine oxidase inhibitors) or strychnine.
2. Tetanus. Nondepolarizing agents should be chosen because infection with *Clostridium* species can predispose patients to pathologic hyperkalemia induced by the use of succinylcholine.
3. Hyperthermia associated with muscle rigidity or hyperactivity (eg, status epilepticus, neuroleptic malignant syndrome, or serotonin syndrome [p 21]). ***Note:*** In susceptible patients, malignant hyperthermia (p 21) can be triggered by succinylcholine (see discussion under "adverse effects").
4. In intubated patients, partial or complete neuromuscular blockade may facilitate improved patient-ventilator synchrony and enhanced gas exchange and lower the risk for barotrauma.
5. Suspected or verified cervical spine injury, or any setting in which there is increased intracranial pressure (eg, intracranial hemorrhage, hepatic encephalopathy). ***Note:*** Succinylcholine can cause an increase in intracranial pressure, and in this setting, agents intended to blunt the increase may be administered before administration of the paralytic drug (see V. C, below).
6. Paralytic agents can also be used to treat acute laryngospasm.

B. Although they are not always needed for orotracheal intubation, neuromuscular blockers can provide prompt paralysis, offering the intubator a superior view of laryngeal structures to facilitate accurate placement of the endotracheal tube. The preferred agents for this purpose, succinylcholine and rocuronium, are characterized by a rapid onset and minimal cardiovascular effects when used in appropriate doses.

III. Contraindications

A. Lack of preparedness or inability to intubate the trachea and ventilate the patient after total paralysis ensues. Proper equipment and trained personnel must be assembled before the drug is given.

B. Known or family history of malignant hyperthermia is an absolute contraindication to the use of succinylcholine.

C. Known hypersensitivity or anaphylactic reaction to the agent or its preservative. Succinylcholine and rocuronium are implicated most commonly, but anaphylaxis has been reported with other agents. "Gasping baby" syndrome is caused by benzyl alcohol (a common preservative) in newborn infants, all of whom lack the capacity to fully metabolize the preservative. This entity is dose-dependent and is not a hypersensitivity reaction. Preservative-free preparations are now available for pediatric use.

D. Known history of or high risk for succinylcholine-induced hyperkalemia. Diseases that predispose patients to succinylcholine-induced hyperkalemia include the inherited myopathies (eg, Duchenne muscular dystrophy) and the progressive neuromuscular disorders (multiple sclerosis and amyotrophic lateral sclerosis; see Item IV. D below).

IV. Adverse effects

A. Complete paralysis results in **respiratory depression** and apnea. The **intubating healthcare provider must be prepared to provide adequate and sustained ventilation and oxygenation in paralyzed patients.**

B. Succinylcholine can stimulate vagal nerves, resulting in sinus bradycardia and AV block. Infants, who are particularly sensitive to vagotonic effects, can experience significant bradycardia with the first dose of succinylcholine, but in older children or adults, bradycardia is more often seen with repeated doses. In either case, this effect can be mitigated with atropine pretreatment (0.02 mg/kg IV). In infants younger than 12 months, pretreatment with atropine or another vagolytic such as glycopyrrolate is recommended. In high doses, succinylcholine can cause catecholamine release, resulting in hypertension and tachycardia.

C. Muscle fasciculations seen with succinylcholine (but not with nondepolarizing agents) may cause increased intracranial, intraocular, and intragastric pressure. A defasciculating dose of a nondepolaring neuromuscular blocking agent can be administered before the succinylcholine. Many authors have abandoned this recommendation, however, arguing that the need for prompt control of the airway supersedes the small clinical risk associated with increased ICP.

D. Mild **rhabdomyolysis** and myoglobinuria may also be observed owing to muscular activity associated with fasciculations, especially in children. There is an association between muscle fasciculations and postoperative myalgia, but this is controversial and not well characterized.

E. Black Box warning for succinylcholine (hyperkalemia). Risk of cardiac arrest from hyperkalemic rhabdomyolysis. Succinylcholine often causes a transient rise in serum potassium of approximately 0.5 mEq/L in a "typical" patient. This relatively modest increase is distinct from the pathologic increase in serum potassium of up to 5–10 mEq/L that can occur in clinical situations featuring postjunctional acetylcholine receptor upregulation or rhabdomyolysis.

1. Although the process begins within hours of the triggering event, receptor upregulation can become clinically relevant about 3–5 days after denervation (eg, spinal cord injury or stroke), burns, radiation and crush injuries, and infection by *Clostridium botulinum* and *C. tetani*. Receptor upregulation can also occur in the setting of prolonged neuromuscular blockade, especially when it is coupled with another trigger, such as lengthy immobilization or burn injury. Hyperkalemia has been reported after burn injury to only a single limb (8% body surface area).
2. Patients with a disease characterized by chronic denervation, such as an inherited myopathy (eg, Duchenne or Becker muscular dystrophy), Guillain–Barre syndrome, multiple sclerosis, or amyotrophic lateral sclerosis, are always at risk for pathologic hyperkalemia if exposed to succinylcholine. Succinylcholine carries a black box warning issued by the FDA for pediatric use, reflecting **the small but nontrivial danger of its use in the setting of undiagnosed inherited skeletal myopathy in children** (primarily boys 8 years of age or younger).
3. It is unclear whether preexisting mild hyperkalemia (eg, from acute renal failure or diabetic ketoacidosis) represents a significant clinical risk with the use of succinylcholine.
4. **A nondepolarizing agent** such as rocuronium should be employed in patients with electrocardiographic changes consistent with hyperkalemia or in chronic renal failure patients who have missed dialysis appointments.

F. Many **benzylisoquinolines** (eg, cisatracurium, mivacurium, atracurium, and especially tubocurarine) can cause histamine release, resulting in hypotension and bronchospasm. These effects can be mitigated by slow infusion. Tubocurarine is unique in that it also blocks nicotinic acetylcholine receptors at the sympathetic ganglia, preventing the reflex tachycardia that usually accompanies vasodilation. Cisatracurium and atracurium may be preferred in the setting of hepatic and/or renal disease because they are both eliminated primarily by Hoffman degradation. Seizure activity in animals has been noted with high doses of atracurium when the metabolite, laudanosine, accumulates to high levels. The relevance of this phenomenon in humans is unknown, however.

G. **Aminosteroids.** Bronchospasm occurs at a rate of 5–10% with rapacuronium (which was withdrawn from the United States market by the manufacturer for this reason). The vagal blockade associated with rapacuronium and pancuronium can cause tachycardia, hypertension, and increased myocardial oxygen consumption. In contrast, rocuronium and vecuronium are associated with minimal cardiovascular side effects. Patients with renal or hepatic insufficiency may experience prolonged neuromuscular blockade with vecuronium, which is partially metabolized by the liver to an active metabolite that is dependent on renal elimination.

H. **Neuromuscular blockade can be potentiated by** acidosis, hypokalemia, hypocalcemia, and hypermagnesemia. Prior administration of certain agents (eg, aminoglycosides, propranolol, calcium channel blockers) may increase the potency of neuromuscular blocking agents. Theophylline, glucocorticoids, and carbamazepine can antagonize nondepolarizing neuromuscular blockade. The relevance of these interactions in the RSI setting is likely to be minimal, however.

I. **Prolonged effects** may occur after succinylcholine or mivacurium use in patients who have genetic variants of plasma pseudocholinesterase or liver disease, or who have recently used cocaine (which is metabolized by plasma pseudocholinesterases). About 1 in 3,500 whites are homozygous for a defective pseudocholinesterase gene, which may lead to markedly prolonged paralysis after administration of succinylcholine (3–8 hours). Some genetic groups may have a higher incidence of variant genes.

J. **Prolonged effects** may also occur in patients with neuromuscular disease (eg, myasthenia gravis, Eaton–Lambert syndrome).

K. **Prolonged use** of neuromuscular blockade has been associated **with critical illness myopathy**, also known as acute quadriplegic myopathy syndrome and other names. The strongest risk factors seem to be concomitant use of intravenous glucocorticoids. The etiology may be related to chemical denervation, which is usually reversible. Daily "holiday" periods from neuromuscular blockade are a potential mitigation strategy but discontinuation of intravenous glucocorticoids should be the primary goal to avoid this complication.

L. Patients with certain genetic abnormalities that affect the cellular physiology of calcium in skeletal muscle are susceptible to malignant hyperthermia after exposure to succinylcholine. **Malignant hyperthermia** is a life-threatening condition that requires immediate treatment with the antidote **dantrolene** (p 537). Tachycardia is usually the first sign; other features can include trismus, autonomic instability, muscular rigidity, hypo- or hypercalcemia, rhabdomyolysis and myoglobinemia, hyperkalemia, altered mental status, and a severe lactic acidosis. Hyperthermia is a late finding and an ominous sign.

M. **Trismus or masseter spasm.** Succinylcholine increases the muscular tone of the masseter muscle, especially in children undergoing concurrent anesthesia with halothane anesthetics. Usually, this effect is transient. Very rarely, trismus—in which the teeth are clamped shut, preventing visualization of the laryngeal structures—may develop. In this situation, administration of a nondepolarizing agent may facilitate intubation, but the intubator should be prepared to establish an alternative airway. Because increased muscular tone is a prominent feature of malignant hyperthermia, this diagnosis should also be entertained in patients with trismus.

N. Use in pregnancy. FDA Category C (indeterminate). This does not preclude their acute, short-term use in a seriously ill patient (p 498).

V. Drug or laboratory interactions

A. Actions of the nondepolarizing agents are potentiated by volatile anesthetics and inhibited or reversed by anticholinesterase agents (eg, neostigmine, physostigmine, and carbamate and organophosphate insecticides). **Sugammadex** is a recently approved rapid reversal agent for rocuronium and vecuronium.

B. Organophosphate or carbamate (p 353) insecticide intoxication may potentiate or prolong the effect of succinylcholine.

C. Numerous drugs may potentiate neuromuscular blockade. These include calcium antagonists, dantrolene, aminoglycoside antibiotics, propranolol, membrane-stabilizing drugs (eg, quinidine), magnesium, lithium, and thiazide diuretics.

D. Anticonvulsants (carbamazepine and phenytoin) and theophylline may delay the onset and shorten the duration of action of some nondepolarizing agents. Carbamazepine has additive effects, and reduction of the neuromuscular blocker dose may be required.

E. Dysrhythmias are possible with myocardial sensitizers (eg, halothane) and sympathetic stimulating agents (eg, pancuronium).

VI. Dosage and method of administration (see Table III–12).

VII. Formulations

A. Succinylcholine chloride (Anectine and Quelicin), 20 and 100 mg/mL in 10-mL vials (may contain parabens and benzyl alcohol). **Suggested minimum stocking levels** to treat a 100-kg adult for the first 8 hours and 24 hours: *first 8 hours:* 200 mg or one (10-mL) vial (20 mg/mL); *first 24 hours:* 500 mg or one (10-mL) vial (50 mg/mL).

B. Atracurium besylate (Tracrium, others), 10 mg/mL in 5-mL single-dose and 10-mL multiple-dose vials (10-mL vials contain benzyl alcohol, other preservative free). **Suggested minimum stocking levels** to treat a 100-kg adult for the first 8 hours and 24 hours: *first 8 hours:* 200 mg or two (10-mL) multiple-dose vials (10 mg/mL); *first 24 hours:* 400 mg or four (10-mL) multiple-dose vials (10 mg/mL).

C. Cisatracurium besylate (Nimbex, others), 2 mg/mL in 5- and 10-mL vials; 10 mg/mL in 20-mL vials (with benzyl alcohol). **Suggested minimum stocking levels** to treat a 100-kg adult for the first 8 hours and 24 hours: *first 8 hours:* 200 mg or one (20-mL) vial (10 mg/mL); *first 24 hours:* 300 mg or one (20-mL) vial (10 mg/mL) and one 10-mL vial (10 mg/mL).

D. Mivacurium chloride (Mivacron), 0.5 mg/mL and 2 mg/mL in 5- and 10-mL single-use vials. **Suggested minimum stocking levels** to treat a 100-kg adult for the first 8 hours and 24 hours: *first 8 hours:* 80 mg or four (10-mL) vials (2 mg/mL); *first 24 hours:* 240 mg or 12 (10-mL) vials (2 mg/mL).

E. Pancuronium bromide (Pavulon, others), 1 and 2 mg/mL in 2-, 5-, and 10-mL vials, ampules (some with benzyl alcohol), and syringes. **Suggested minimum stocking** levels to treat a 100-kg adult for the first 8 hours and 24 hours: *first 8 hours:* 80 mg or eight (5-mL) vials (2 mg/mL); *first 24 hours:* 140 mg or 14 (5-mL) vials (2 mg/mL).

F. Rocuronium bromide (Zemuron, others), 10 mg/mL in 5- and 10-mL vials. **Suggested minimum stocking levels** to treat a 100-kg adult for the first 8 hours and 24 hours: *first 8 hours:* 800 mg or eight (10-mL) vials (10 mg/mL); *first 24 hours:* 1,400 mg or 14 (10-mL) vials (10 mg/mL).

G. Vecuronium bromide (Norcuron, others), 10- and 20-mg vials of lyophilized powder for reconstitution (Norcuron contains mannitol, and diluent may contain benzyl alcohol). **Suggested minimum stocking levels** to treat a 100-kg adult for the first 8 hours and 24 hours: *first 8 hours:* 60 mg or three (20-mg) vials; *first 24 hours:* 100 mg or five (20-mg) vials.

► NITRITE, SODIUM, AND AMYL

Ben Tsutaoka, PharmD

I. **Pharmacology.** Sodium nitrite injectable solution and amyl nitrite crushable ampules for inhalation are components of the cyanide antidote package. The value of nitrites as an antidote to cyanide poisoning is twofold: They oxidize hemoglobin to methemoglobin, which binds free cyanide, and they may enhance endothelial cyanide detoxification by producing vasodilation. Inhalation of an ampule of amyl nitrite produces a methemoglobin level of about 5%. Intravenous administration of a single 300-mg dose of sodium nitrite in adults is anticipated to produce a methemoglobin level of about 15–20%.

II. **Indications**

- A. Symptomatic cyanide poisoning (p 208). Nitrites are not usually used for empiric treatment unless cyanide is suspected very strongly, and they are not recommended for smoke inhalation victims.
- B. Nitrites are possibly effective for hydrogen sulfide poisoning if given within 30 minutes of exposure (p 271).

III. **Contraindications**

- A. Significant preexisting methemoglobinemia (>40%).
- B. Severe hypotension is a relative contraindication because it may be worsened by nitrites.
- C. Administration to patients with concurrent carbon monoxide poisoning is a relative contraindication; generation of methemoglobin may further compromise oxygen transport to the tissues. Hydroxocobalamin (p 563) has supplanted nitrites for smoke inhalation victims (patients often have mixed carbon monoxide and cyanide poisoning) in countries where it is available.

IV. **Adverse effects**

- A. Headache, facial flushing, dizziness, nausea, vomiting, tachycardia, and sweating may occur. These side effects may be masked by the symptoms of cyanide poisoning.
- B. Rapid intravenous administration may result in hypotension.
- C. Excessive and potentially fatal methemoglobinemia may result.
- D. **Use in pregnancy.** No assigned FDA category. These agents may compromise blood flow and oxygen delivery to the fetus and may induce fetal methemoglobinemia. Fetal hemoglobin is more sensitive to the oxidant effects of nitrites. However, this does not preclude their acute, short-term use for a seriously symptomatic patient (p 498).

V. **Drug or laboratory interactions**

- A. Hypotension may be exacerbated by the concurrent presence of alcohol or other vasodilators or any antihypertensive agent.
- B. Methylene blue should not be administered to a cyanide-poisoned patient because it may reverse nitrite-induced methemoglobinemia and theoretically result in the release of free cyanide ions. However, it may be considered when severe and life-threatening excessive methemoglobinemia is present.
- C. Binding of methemoglobin to cyanide (cyanomethemoglobin) may lower the measured free methemoglobin level.

VI. **Dosage and method of administration**

- A. **Amyl nitrite crushable ampules.** Crush one to two ampules in gauze, cloth, or a sponge and place under the nose of the victim, who should inhale deeply for 30 seconds. Rest for 30 seconds, then repeat. Each ampule lasts about 2–3 minutes. If the victim is receiving respiratory support, place the ampules in the face mask or port access to the endotracheal tube. Stop ampule use when administering intravenous sodium nitrite.
- B. **Sodium nitrite parenteral**
  1. **Adults.** Administer 300 mg of sodium nitrite (10 mL of 3% solution) IV over 3–5 minutes.

TABLE III–13. PEDIATRIC DOSING OF SODIUM NITRITE BASED ON HEMOGLOBIN CONCENTRATION

Hemoglobin (g/dL)	Initial Dose (mg/kg)	Initial Dose of 3% Sodium Nitrite (mL/kg)
7	5.8	0.19
8	6.6	0.22
9	7.5	0.25
10	8.3	0.27
11	9.1	0.3
12	10	0.33
13	10.8	0.36
14	11.6	0.39

2. **Children.** Give 5.8–11.6 mg/kg to a maximum of 300 mg. Pediatric dosing should be based on the hemoglobin concentration if it is known (Table III–13). If anemia is suspected or hypotension is present, start with the lower dose, dilute in 50–100 mL of saline, and give over at least 5 minutes.
3. Oxidation of hemoglobin to methemoglobin occurs within 30 minutes. If no response to treatment occurs within 30 minutes, an additional half-size dose of intravenous sodium nitrite may be given.

VII. Formulations

A. Amyl nitrite inhalant, packaged in 0.3-mL crushable ampules, 12 per box. It is no longer a component of the conventional cyanide antidote kit (Nithiodote®).

B. Sodium nitrite parenteral. A component of the cyanide antidote kit (Nithiodote®), 300 mg in 10 mL of sterile water (3%), one vial per kit.

C. Suggested minimum stocking level to treat a 100-kg adult for the first 8 hours and 24 hours are two Nithiodote® **kits,** containing two 300-mg vials of sodium nitrite or the equivalent as a separate stock (which is a less expensive option) plus one box of amyl nitrite inhalant ampules. Suggested for hospitals to prepare for multiple patients: two cyanide antidote kits for small hospitals, six kits for major **medical centers** (one kit should be kept in the emergency department). ***Note:*** Consider stocking the hydroxocobalamin antidote kit (Cyanokit®) as an alternative antidote for cyanide poisoning.

▶ NITROPRUSSIDE

Thomas E. Kearney, PharmD

I. Pharmacology. Nitroprusside is an ultra–short-acting, titratable parenteral hypotensive agent that acts by directly relaxing vascular smooth muscle as a nitric oxide donor. Both arterial dilation and venous dilation occur; the effect is more marked in patients with hypertension. A small increase in heart rate may be observed in hypertensive patients. Intravenous administration produces a nearly immediate onset of action, with a duration of effect of 1–10 minutes. Resistance may occur with high renin activity. Nitroprusside is metabolized rapidly, with a serum half-life of about 1–2 minutes. Cyanide is produced during metabolism and is converted to the less toxic thiocyanate. Thiocyanate has a half-life of 2–3 days and accumulates in patients with renal insufficiency.

II. Indications

A. Rapid control of severe hypertension (eg, in patients with stimulant intoxication or monoamine oxidase inhibitor toxicity).

B. Arterial vasodilation in patients with ergot-induced peripheral arterial spasm.

III. Contraindications

A. Compensatory hypertension—for example, in patients with increased intracranial pressure (eg, hemorrhage or mass lesion) or patients with coarctation of the aorta. If nitroprusside is required in such patients, use with extreme caution.

B. Use with caution in patients with hepatic insufficiency because cyanide metabolism may be impaired.

IV. Adverse effects

A. Nausea, vomiting, headache, and sweating may be caused by excessively rapid lowering of blood pressure.

B. Cyanide toxicity, manifested by altered mental status and metabolic (lactic) acidosis, may occur with rapid high-dose infusion (10–15 mcg/kg/min) for periods of 1 hour or longer. Patients with depleted thiosulfate stores (eg, malnourished) may have elevated cyanide levels at lower infusion rates. Continuous intravenous infusion of hydroxocobalamin, 25 mg/h (p 563), or thiosulfate (p 629) has been used to limit cyanide toxicity. If severe cyanide toxicity occurs, discontinue the nitroprusside infusion and consider antidotal doses of thiosulfate and sodium nitrite (p 592) or high-dose hydroxocobalamin (p 563).

C. Thiocyanate intoxication, manifested by disorientation, delirium, muscle twitching, and psychosis, may occur with prolonged high-dose nitroprusside infusions (usually ≥3 mcg/kg/min for ≥48 hours), particularly in patients with renal insufficiency (may occur at rates as low as 1 mcg/kg/min). Thiocyanate production is also enhanced by coadministration of sodium thiosulfate. Monitor thiocyanate levels if the nitroprusside infusion lasts more than 1–2 days; toxicity is associated with thiocyanate levels of 50 mg/L or greater. Usually treat by lowering the infusion rate or discontinuing the use of nitroprusside. Thiocyanate is removed effectively by hemodialysis.

D. Rebound hypertension may be observed after sudden discontinuance.

E. Methemoglobinemia may be observed in patients receiving more than 10 mg/kg but is typically not severe.

F. Use in pregnancy. FDA Category C (indeterminate [p 498]). It may cross the placenta and may affect uterine blood flow; however, it has been used successfully in pregnant women.

V. Drug or laboratory interactions. A hypotensive effect is potentiated by other antihypertensive agents and inhalational anesthetics.

VI. Dosage and method of administration

A. Use only in an emergency or intensive care setting with the capability of frequent or continuous blood pressure monitoring.

B. Dilute the 50-mg vial (2 mL, 25 mg/mL) of sodium nitroprusside with 5% dextrose to a volume of 250, 500, or 1,000 mL to achieve a concentration of 200, 100, or 50 mcg/mL, respectively. Protect the solution from light to avoid photodegradation (as evidenced by a color change) by covering the bottle and tubing with paper or aluminum foil.

C. Start with an intravenous infusion rate of 0.3 mcg/kg/min; use a controlled infusion device and titrate to desired effect. The average dose is 3 mcg/kg/min in children and adults (range, 0.5–10 mcg/kg/min).

1. The maximum rate should not exceed 10 mcg/kg/min to avoid the risk for acute cyanide toxicity. If there is no response after 10 minutes at the maximum rate, discontinue the infusion and use an alternative vasodilator (eg, phentolamine [p 605]).
2. Sodium thiosulfate (p 629) has been added in a ratio of 10-mg thiosulfate to 1-mg nitroprusside to reduce or prevent cyanide toxicity.

VII. Formulations

A. Parenteral. Nitroprusside sodium (Nitropress and others), amber-colored single-dose 2-mL vial containing 50 mg (25 mg/mL). ***Note:*** Boxed warning that this concentrated intravenous solution **must be diluted** before administration (see dosage and administration).

B. Suggested minimum stocking levels to treat a 100-kg adult for the first 8 hours and 24 hours: **nitroprusside sodium**, *first 8 hours:* 400 mg or eight vials (50 mg each); *first 24 hours:* 1,200 mg or 24 vials (50 mg each).

▶ NOREPINEPHRINE

Alicia B. Minns, MD

I. Pharmacology. Norepinephrine, an endogenous catecholamine, is a potent $alpha_1$-adrenergic receptor agonist with some $beta_1$-adrenergic receptor activity. It is used primarily as a vasopressor to increase systemic vascular resistance and venous return to the heart. It also may increase heart rate and cardiac contractility because of its $beta_1$ effects. Norepinephrine is not effective orally and is absorbed erratically after subcutaneous injection. After intravenous administration, the onset of action is nearly immediate, and the duration of effect is 1–2 minutes after the infusion is discontinued.

II. Indications. Norepinephrine is used to increase blood pressure and cardiac output in patients with shock caused by venodilation, low systemic vascular resistance, or both. Hypovolemia, depressed myocardial contractility, hypothermia, and electrolyte imbalance should be corrected first or concurrently.

III. Contraindications

- **A.** Uncorrected hypovolemia.
- **B.** Norepinephrine is relatively contraindicated in patients who have mesenteric or peripheral arterial occlusive vascular disease with thrombosis, or ergot poisoning (p 229).
- **C.** Use with caution in patients intoxicated with chloral hydrate or halogenated or aromatic hydrocarbon solvents or anesthetics.

IV. Adverse effects

- **A.** Severe hypertension, which may result in intracranial hemorrhage, pulmonary edema, or myocardial necrosis.
- **B.** Reflex bradycardia.
- **C.** Ventricular dysrhythmias.
- **D.** Aggravation of tissue ischemia, resulting in gangrene.
- **E.** Tissue necrosis after extravasation.
- **F.** Anxiety, restlessness, tremor, and headache.
- **G.** Anaphylaxis induced by sulfite preservatives in sensitive patients. Use with extreme caution in patients with known hypersensitivity to sulfite preservatives.
- **H.** Increased cardiac irritability due to myocardial sensitization of catecholamines in the setting of exposures to halogenated hydrocarbons, such as certain anesthetics, solvents, and medications.
- **I. Use in pregnancy.** FDA category C. This drug crosses the placenta; it can cause placental ischemia and reduce uterine contractions.

V. Drug or laboratory interactions

- **A.** Enhanced vasopressor response may occur in the presence of cocaine and cyclic antidepressants (owing to inhibition of neuronal reuptake) or with other vasoactive drugs (eg, dihydroergotamine).
- **B.** Enhanced vasopressor response may occur in patients taking monoamine oxidase inhibitors or COMT inhibitors owing to inhibition of neuronal metabolic degradation.
- **C.** Alpha- and beta-blocking agents may antagonize the adrenergic effects of norepinephrine.
- **D.** Anticholinergic drugs may block reflex bradycardia, which normally occurs in response to norepinephrine-induced hypertension, enhancing the hypertensive response.

E. Chloral hydrate overdose, cyclopropane, and halogenated or aromatic hydrocarbon solvents and anesthetics may enhance myocardial sensitivity to the arrhythmogenic effects of norepinephrine.

VI. Dosage and method of administration

A. *Black box warning:* Avoid extravasation. The intravenous infusion must be free-flowing, and the infused vein should be observed frequently for signs of infiltration (pallor, coldness, or induration).

1. If extravasation occurs, immediately infiltrate the affected area with phentolamine (p 605), 5–10 mg in 10–15 mL of normal saline (children: 0.1–0.2 mg/kg; maximum, 10 mg), via a fine (25–27-gauge) hypodermic needle; improvement is evidenced by hyperemia and return to normal temperature.
2. Alternatively, nitroglycerin topical 2% ointment can be applied to the affected area. Infiltration of terbutaline has been reportedly successful; 1 mg diluted in 10 mL of normal saline for a large extravasation site or 1 mg diluted in 1-mL normal saline for a small site.

B. Intravenous infusion. Initial dose 8–12 mcg/min with a usual maintenance range of 2–4 mcg/min; dose range varies depending on clinical situation (children: 1–2 mcg/min or 0.05–0.1 mcg/kg/min) and increases as needed every 5–10 minutes.

VII. Formulations. Norepinephrine bitartrate is oxidized rapidly on exposure to air; it must be kept in its airtight ampule until immediately before use. If the solution appears brown or contains a precipitate, do not use it. The stock solution must be diluted in 5% dextrose or 5% dextrose–saline for infusion; usually, a 4-mg ampule is added to 1 L of fluid to provide 4 mcg/mL of solution. Avoid administration through an IV line containing any alkaline solution, or inactivation of norepinephrine may occur.

A. Parenteral. Norepinephrine bitartrate (Levophed, generic), 1 mg/mL, 4-mL ampule. Contains sodium bisulfite as a preservative.

B. Suggested minimum stocking levels to treat a 100-kg adult for the first 8 hours and 24 hours: **norepinephrine bitartrate**, *first 8 hours*: 8.0 mg or two ampules (1 mg/mL, 4 mL each); *first 24 hours*: 24.0 mg or six ampules (1 mg/mL, 4 mL each).

▶ OCTREOTIDE

Thomas E. Kearney, PharmD

I. Pharmacology

A. Octreotide is a synthetic polypeptide and a long-acting analog of somatostatin. It significantly antagonizes pancreatic insulin release and is useful for the management of hypoglycemia resulting from xenobiotic-induced endogenous secretion of insulin.

B. Octreotide also suppresses pancreatic function, gastric acid secretion, and biliary and GI tract motility.

C. As a polypeptide, it is bioavailable only by parenteral administration (intravenously or subcutaneously). Approximately 30% of octreotide is excreted unchanged in the urine, and it has an elimination half-life of 1.7 hours. Its half-life may be increased in patients with renal dysfunction and in the elderly.

II. Indications. Oral sulfonylurea hypoglycemic overdose (p 217) or quinine-induced hypoglycemia (p 400) when serum glucose concentrations cannot be maintained with an intravenous 5% dextrose infusion. It may also be considered a first-line agent along with dextrose because it can reduce glucose requirements and prevent rebound hypoglycemia in patients with sulfonylurea poisoning. It is not used in the management of exogenous insulin poisoning, where it has a theoretic disadvantage of blocking beneficial counterregulatory reactions (prevents glucagon and growth hormone secretion) to hypoglycemia.

III. Contraindications. Hypersensitivity to the drug (anaphylactic shock has occurred).

IV. Adverse effects. In general, the drug is well tolerated. Patients may experience pain or burning at the injection site. For the most part, the adverse-effect profile is based on long-term therapy for other disease states.

- **A.** The suppressive effects on the biliary tract may lead to significant gallbladder disease (cholelithiasis) and pancreatitis.
- **B.** Gastrointestinal effects (diarrhea, nausea, discomfort) may occur in 5–10% of users. Headache, dizziness, and fatigue have also been observed.
- **C.** Cardiac effects may include bradycardia, conduction abnormalities (QT prolongation), hypertension, and exacerbation of congestive heart failure. These effects have been observed primarily in patients treated for acromegaly.
- **D. Use in pregnancy.** FDA Category B. Not likely to cause harm with short-term therapy (p 498).

V. Drug or laboratory interactions

- **A.** Octreotide may inhibit the absorption of dietary fats and cyclosporine.
- **B.** The drug depresses vitamin B_{12} levels and can lead to abnormal Schilling test results.

VI. Dosage and method of administration

- **A. Oral sulfonylurea overdose.** Give 50–100 mcg (children: 1–1.25 mcg/kg) by subcutaneous or intravenous injection every 6–12 hours as needed. Some patients with sulfonylurea poisoning may require more frequent (every 4 hours) and higher doses and several days of therapy. Continuous infusions of up to 50–125 mcg/h have been used. Some children have been successfully treated with a 2–2.5-mcg/kg IV dose, followed by a 2-mcg/kg/h infusion. Most patients require approximately 24 hours of therapy and typically do not experience recurrent hypoglycemia upon discontinuation of octreotide (although hypoglycemia has recurred 30 hours after a glipizide exposure). Monitor for recurrent hypoglycemia for 24 hours after termination of octreotide therapy.
- **B. Quinine-induced hypoglycemia.** A dose of 50 mcg/h has been used in adult patients who are being treated with quinine for malaria.
- **C.** Subcutaneous injection sites should be rotated.
- **D.** For IV administration, dilute in 50 mL of normal saline or 5% dextrose and infuse over 15–30 minutes. Alternatively, the dose may be given as an IV push over 3 minutes.
- **E.** ***Note:*** Optimal dosage regimen is not known. For other indications, the dosage range for children is 2–40 mcg/kg/d, and daily doses of up to 1,500 mcg are used in adults (120 mg has been infused over 8 hours without severe adverse effects).

VII. Formulations

- **A. Parenteral.** Octreotide acetate (Sandostatin, generic), 0.05, 0.1, and 0.5 mg/mL in 1-mL ampules, vials, and syringes; 0.2 and 1 mg/mL in 5-mL multiple-dose vials (with phenol preservative). ***Note:*** Avoid use of the long-acting agent Sandostatin LAR Depot. This product is for once-a-month dosing in patients with acromegaly.
- **B. Suggested minimum stocking levels** to treat a 100-kg adult for the first 8 hours and 24 hours: **octreotide acetate**, *first 8 hours*: 200 mcg or two (1-mL) ampules or vials (0.1 mg/mL); *first 24 hours*: 1,000 mcg or one (5-mL) multiple-dose vial (0.2 mg/mL).

▶ ONDANSETRON

Joanne M. Goralka, PharmD

I. Pharmacology. Ondansetron is a selective serotonin (5-HT_3) receptor antagonist with antiemetic activity due to its actions on serotonin receptors located peripherally on vagal nerve terminals and centrally in the chemoreceptor trigger zone. The mean peak plasma level occurred at 10 minutes after a 4-mg IV injection and

1.7–2.2 hours after an oral 8-mg dose given to normal adult volunteers. The drug is metabolized extensively in the liver via hydroxylation, followed by glucuronide or sulfate conjugation. Ondansetron is a substrate for human hepatic cytochrome P-450 enzymes, primarily CYP3A4, and to a lesser extent CYP1A2, CYP2D6. The mean elimination half-life in adults is 3.1–6.2 hours, increasing to as long as 20 hours in patients with severe liver disease.

II. Indications

A. FDA-approved for the prevention of nausea and vomiting associated with cancer chemotherapy, radiation therapy, and in the postoperative period.

B. Ondansetron is used to treat intractable nausea and vomiting, particularly when the ability to administer activated charcoal or antidotal therapy (eg, *N*-acetylcysteine) is compromised. These are not FDA-approved indications.

III. Contraindications/Warnings

A. Hypersensitivity to ondansetron or any component of the formulation. Hypersensitivity reactions, including anaphylaxis and bronchospasm, have also been reported in patients who have experienced hypersensitivity to other selective 5-HT_3 receptor antagonists.

B. The concomitant use of apomorphine with ondansetron is contraindicated on the basis of reports of profound hypotension and loss of consciousness.

C. Concurrent use of ondansetron and other medications known to cause prolonged QT interval increases the risk for torsades de pointes

D. ECG monitoring is recommended in patients with electrolyte abnormalities, (eg, hypokalemia or hypomagnesemia), congestive heart failure, or bradydysrhythmias.

E. Avoid in patients with congenital long QT syndrome.

F. Patients with phenylketonuria should be informed that Zofran ODT orally disintegrating tablets contain phenylalanine (a component of aspartame). Use with caution in patients with phenylketonuria.

G. Ondansetron is metabolized by hepatic cytochrome P-450 enzymes CYP3A4, CYP2D6, CYP1A2, and inducers or inhibitors of these enzymes may change the clearance and half-life of ondansetron.

IV. Adverse effects

A. Rare cases of immediate hypersensitivity reactions including anaphylactic reactions, angioedema, bronchospasm, cardiopulmonary arrest, hypotension, and laryngeal edema have been reported. Also, delayed hypersensitivity reactions, Stevens–Johnson syndrome and toxic epidermal necrolysis, have been reported.

B. Dose-dependent QT interval prolongation and dysrhythmias. Postmarketing cardiovascular events reported have included: torsade de pointes, ventricular and supraventricular tachycardia, PVCs, atrial fibrillation, bradycardia, second-degree heart block, and QT/QTc interval prolongation. Risk factors included IV administration of ondansetron, concomitant use of another QT interval prolonging medication, and preexisting cardiac disease or disorders associated with electrolyte abnormalities (eg, hypokalemia, hypomagnesemia).

C. Anxiety, headache, drowsiness, fatigue, fever, dizziness, paresthesias, and migraine headaches. Rare cases of grand mal seizure.

D. Rare reports consistent with, but not diagnostic of, extrapyramidal reactions. Oculogyric crisis, appearing either alone or with other dystonic reactions.

E. Hepatic necrosis and increased liver enzymes associated with IV administration and concomitant hepatotoxic medications. Do not exceed a total daily dose of 8 mg in patients with severe liver disease.

F. Diarrhea, constipation, and xerostomia.

G. Injection site reactions (pain, redness), pruritus, and rash.

H. Cases of transient blindness, predominantly during IV administration, have been reported.

I. Use in pregnancy. FDA Category B (p 498).

V. Drug or laboratory interactions

A. Ondansetron and the other selective 5-HT_3 antagonists have been associated with dose-dependent ECG changes, including increases in PR, QRS, and QT intervals. See sections III and IV, previously.

B. Numerous IV incompatibilities, including aminophylline, sodium bicarbonate, furosemide, lorazepam, dexamethasone, methylprednisolone, sodium succinate, and thiopental. Ondansetron should not be mixed with alkaline solutions because a precipitate may form.

C. Serotonin syndrome has been described following the concomitant use of 5-HT_3 receptor antagonists and other serotonergic drugs, including selective serotonin reuptake inhibitors (SSRIs) and serotonin/norepinephrine reuptake inhibitors (SNRIs).

VI. Dosage and method of administration

A. Antiemetic for chemotherapy- and radiotherapy-induced nausea and vomiting. Ondansetron is most effective for prophylaxis when given at least 30 minutes before its antiemetic properties are needed (eg, prior to administration of chemotherapy).

1. Adults: Give 0.15 mg/kg (maximum single dose of 16 mg) IV in 50 mL of normal saline or 5% dextrose infused over 15 minutes. This may be repeated twice at 4-hour intervals. ***Note:*** The 32-mg single IV dose is no longer FDA approved due to an increased risk of QT interval prolongation, which can lead to torsade de pointes.

2. Children: Give 0.15 mg/kg (maximum of 16 mg) (6 months to 18 years) IV over 15 minutes. This may be repeated twice at 4-hour intervals.

B. Antiemetic for postoperative-induced nausea and vomiting.

1. Adults. Give 4 mg IV over at least 30 seconds but preferably over 2–5 minutes. It may also be administered by IM route as a single injection.

2. Pediatric patients (1 month through 12 years): Give 0.1 mg/kg/dose for patients 40 kg or less and 4 mg for patients greater than 40 kg. Administer IV dose over at least 30 seconds and preferably over 2–5 minutes.

VII. Formulations

A. Parenteral. Ondansetron hydrochloride (Zofran), 2 mg/mL in 2-mL single-dose vials and 20-mL multiple-dose vials.

B. Suggested minimum stocking levels to treat a 100-kg adult for the first 8 hours and 24 hours: **ondansetron hydrochloride**, *first 8 hours:* 32 mg or eight (2-mL) vials (2 mg/mL); *first 24 hours:* 45 mg or one (20-mL) multiple-dose vial (2 mg/mL) plus two (2-mL) vials (2 mg/mL).

▶ OXYGEN AND HYPERBARIC OXYGEN

Kent R. Olson, MD

I. Pharmacology. Oxygen is a necessary oxidant to drive biochemical reactions. Room air contains 21% oxygen. Hyperbaric oxygen (HBO), which is 100% oxygen delivered to the patient in a pressurized chamber at 2–3 atm of pressure, may be beneficial for patients with severe carbon monoxide (CO) poisoning. It can hasten the reversal of CO binding to hemoglobin and intracellular myoglobin and provide oxygen independently of hemoglobin, and it may have protective actions in reducing postischemic brain damage. Randomized controlled studies have reported conflicting outcomes with HBO treatment, but there may be a marginal benefit in preventing subtle neuropsychiatric sequelae.

II. Indications

A. Supplemental oxygen is indicated when normal oxygenation is impaired because of pulmonary injury, which may result from aspiration (chemical pneumonitis) or inhalation of toxic gases. The PO_2 should be maintained at 70–80 mm Hg or higher if possible.

B. Supplemental oxygen usually is given empirically to patients with altered mental status or suspected hypoxemia.

C. Oxygen (100%) is indicated for patients with carbon monoxide poisoning to increase the conversion of carboxyhemoglobin and carboxymyoglobin to hemoglobin and myoglobin, respectively, and to increase the oxygen saturation of the plasma and subsequent delivery to tissues.

D. Hyperbaric oxygen may be beneficial for patients with severe carbon monoxide poisoning, although the clinical evidence is mixed. Potential indications include history of a loss of consciousness, metabolic acidosis, age more than 36 years, pregnancy, carboxyhemoglobin level greater than 25%, and cerebellar dysfunction (eg, ataxia; see Table II–20, p 184).

E. Hyperbaric oxygen has also been advocated for the treatment of poisoning with carbon tetrachloride, cyanide, and hydrogen sulfide and for severe methemoglobinemia, but the experimental and clinical evidence is scanty.

III. Contraindications

A. In **paraquat** poisoning, oxygen may contribute to lung injury. In fact, slightly *hypoxic* environments (10–12% oxygen) have been advocated to reduce the risk for pulmonary fibrosis from paraquat (see p 361).

B. Relative contraindications to hyperbaric oxygen therapy include a history of recent middle ear or thoracic surgery, untreated pneumothorax, seizure disorder, and severe sinusitis.

IV. Adverse effects. ***Caution:*** Oxygen is extremely flammable.

A. Prolonged high concentrations of oxygen are associated with pulmonary alveolar tissue damage. In general, the fraction of inspired oxygen (FIO_2) should not be maintained at greater than 80% for more than 24 hours.

B. Oxygen therapy may increase the risk for retrolental fibroplasia in neonates.

C. Administration of oxygen at high concentrations to patients with severe chronic obstructive pulmonary disease and chronic carbon dioxide retention who are dependent on hypoxemia to provide a drive to breathe may result in respiratory arrest.

D. Hyperbaric oxygen treatment can cause hyperoxic seizures, aural trauma (ruptured tympanic membrane), and acute anxiety resulting from claustrophobia. Seizures are more likely at higher atmospheric pressures (eg, $\geq$3 atm).

E. Oxygen may potentiate toxicity via enhanced generation of free radicals with some chemotherapeutic agents (eg, bleomycin, Adriamycin, and daunorubicin).

F. Use in pregnancy. No known adverse effects.

V. Drug or laboratory interactions. None known.

VI. Dosage and method of administration

A. Supplemental oxygen. Provide supplemental oxygen to maintain a PO_2 of at least 70–80 mm Hg. If a PO_2 above 50 mm Hg cannot be maintained with an FIO_2 of at least 60%, consider positive end-expiratory pressure or continuous positive airway pressure.

B. Carbon monoxide poisoning. Provide 100% oxygen by tight-fitting mask or via endotracheal tube. Consider **hyperbaric oxygen therapy** if the patient has serious poisoning (see "Indications" above) and can be treated within 6 hours of the exposure. Consult with a poison center (1-800-222-1222) or a hyperbaric specialist to determine the location of the nearest HBO facility. Usually, three HBO treatments at 2.5–3 atm are recommended over a 24-hour period.

VII. Formulations

A. Nasal cannula. Provides 24–40% oxygen, depending on the flow rate and patient's breathing pattern.

B. Ventimask. Provides variable inspired oxygen concentrations from 24 to 40%.

C. **Nonrebreathing reservoir mask.** Provides inspired oxygen concentrations of 60–90%.

D. **Hyperbaric oxygen.** One hundred percent oxygen can be delivered at a pressure of 2–3 atm.

▶ PENICILLAMINE

Thomas E. Kearney, PharmD

I. **Pharmacology.** Penicillamine is a derivative of penicillin that has no antimicrobial activity but effectively chelates some heavy metals, such as lead, mercury, and copper. It has been used as adjunctive therapy after initial treatment with calcium EDTA (p 548) or BAL (dimercaprol [p 514]), although it largely has been replaced by the oral chelator succimer (DMSA [p 624]) because of its poor safety profile. Penicillamine is well absorbed orally, and the penicillamine–metal complex is eliminated in the urine. No parenteral form is available.

II. **Indications**

A. Penicillamine may be used to treat heavy metal poisoning caused by lead or mercury, although oral succimer (p 624) is preferable, as it may result in greater metal excretion with fewer adverse effects. Unithiol (p 630) may be an alternative to succimer for lead or mercury poisoning.

B. For copper poisoning (p 206) and treatment of Wilson disease to remove copper deposits in tissues.

C. Penicillamine has also been used for arsenic, bismuth, and nickel poisoning, but it is not the agent of choice owing to its toxicity.

III. **Contraindications**

A. Penicillin allergy is a contraindication (penicillamine products may be contaminated with penicillin).

B. Renal insufficiency is a relative contraindication because the complex is eliminated only through the urine.

C. Concomitant administration with other hematopoiesis-depressant drugs (eg, gold salts, immunosuppressants, antimalarial agents, and phenylbutazone) is not recommended.

D. Cadmium poisoning. Penicillamine may increase renal levels of cadmium and the potential for nephrotoxicity.

IV. **Adverse effects. Black box warning:** Due to high incidence of and fatalities associated with penicillamine-induced adverse effects, therapy must be closely monitored and patients warned to promptly report symptoms suggesting toxicity.

A. Hypersensitivity reactions: rash, pruritus, drug fever, hematuria, antinuclear antibodies, Goodpasture's syndrome, exfoliative dermatitis, thyroiditis, and proteinuria.

B. Bone marrow suppression and blood dyscrasias: Leukopenia, thrombocytopenia, hemolytic anemia, sideroblastic anemia, aplastic anemia, and agranulocytosis.

C. Hepatitis and pancreatitis.

D. Neurologic: Tinnitus, optic neuritis, peripheral motor and sensory neuropathy, and myasthenia gravis.

E. Gastrointestinal: Anorexia, nausea, vomiting, epigastric pain, and impairment of taste.

F. Pulmonary: Obliterative bronchiolitis, bronchial asthma, alveolitis, pulmonary hemorrhage, interstitial pneumonitis, and pulmonary fibrosis.

G. The requirement for pyridoxine is increased, and the patient may require daily supplementation (p 621).

H. **Use in pregnancy.** FDA Category D (p 498). Birth defects have been associated with use during pregnancy.

V. **Drug or laboratory interactions**
   A. Penicillamine may potentiate the hematopoiesis-depressant effects of drugs such as gold salts, immunosuppressants, antimalarial agents, and phenylbutazone.
   B. Several drugs (eg, antacids and ferrous sulfate) and food can reduce GI absorption of penicillamine substantially.
   C. Penicillamine may produce a false-positive test for ketones in the urine.

VI. **Dosage and method of administration**
   A. Penicillamine should be taken on an empty stomach at least 1 hour before or at least 2 hours after meals and at bedtime. For patients with difficulty swallowing, penicillamine may be extemporaneously prepared as a suspension (see formulations) or be administered in 15–30 mL of chilled pureed fruit or fruit juice within 5 minutes of administration.
   B. The usual dose is 1–1.5 g/d (children: 20–30 mg/kg/d), administered in three or four divided doses. Initiating treatment at 25% of this dose and gradually increasing to the full dose over 2–3 weeks may minimize adverse reactions. Therefore, use a starting dose of 250 mg/d (children: 10 mg/kg/d), then increase to 500 mg/d (15 mg/kg) during week 2 and to the full dose by week 3. The maximum adult daily dose is 2 g (up to 4 g for treatment of cystinuria). In children with mild to moderate lead poisoning, a lower dose of 15 mg/kg/d has been shown to lower blood levels while minimizing adverse effects.
   C. Weekly measurement of urinary and blood concentrations of the intoxicating metal is indicated to assess the need for continued therapy. Treatment for as long as 3 months has been tolerated.

VII. **Formulations.** ***Note:*** Although the chemical derivative *N*-acetylpenicillamine may demonstrate better CNS and peripheral nerve penetration, it is not currently available in the United States.
   A. **Oral.** Penicillamine (Cuprimine, Depen), 125- and 250-mg capsules, 250-mg titratable tablets.
   B. **Oral suspension.** May extemporaneously compound a 50 mg/mL suspension from capsules. Mix sixty 250-mg capsules with 3-g carboxymethylcellulose, 150-g sucrose, 300-mg citric acid, and parabens (methylparaben 120 mg, propylparaben 12 mg). Add propylene glycol in a sufficient quantity to make 100 mL, then add purified water to make a total volume of 300 mL. May add cherry flavoring and label to shake well and refrigerate (stable for 30 days).
   C. **Suggested minimum stocking levels** to treat a 100-kg adult for the first 8 hours and 24 hours: **penicillamine,** *first 8 hours*: 500 mg or two titratable tablets (250 mg each); *first 24 hours*: 1,500 mg or six titratable tablets (250 mg each).

▶ PENTOBARBITAL

Thomas E. Kearney, PharmD

I. **Pharmacology.** Pentobarbital is a short-acting barbiturate with anticonvulsant as well as sedative-hypnotic properties. It is used as a third-line drug in the treatment of status epilepticus. It also may reduce intracranial pressure in patients with cerebral edema by inducing vasoconstriction. After intravenous administration of a single dose, the onset of effect occurs within about 1 minute and lasts about 15 minutes. After intramuscular administration, the onset of effect is slower (10–15 minutes). Pentobarbital demonstrates a biphasic elimination pattern; the half-life of the initial phase is 4 hours, and the terminal phase half-life is 35–50 hours. Effects are prolonged after termination of a continuous infusion.

II. **Indications**
   A. Pentobarbital is used for the management of status epilepticus that is unresponsive to conventional anticonvulsant therapy (eg, diazepam, phenytoin, or

phenobarbital). If the use of pentobarbital for seizure control is considered, consultation with a neurologist is recommended.

B. Pentobarbital is used to manage elevated intracranial pressure in conjunction with other agents.

C. It may be used therapeutically or diagnostically for patients with suspected alcohol or sedative–hypnotic drug withdrawal syndrome.

D. It has been used to manage stimulant-induced agitation and sympathomimetic symptoms refractory to benzodiazepines.

III. Contraindications

A. Known sensitivity to the drug.

B. Manifest or latent porphyria.

IV. Adverse effects

A. Central nervous system depression, coma, and respiratory arrest may occur, especially with rapid bolus or excessive doses.

B. Hypotension may result, especially with rapid intravenous infusion (>50 mg/min). This may be caused by the drug itself or the propylene glycol diluent.

C. Laryngospasm and bronchospasm have been reported after rapid intravenous injection, although the mechanism is unknown.

D. Parenteral solutions are highly alkaline, and precautions need to be taken to avoid extravasation. Intra-arterial infusions may cause vasospasms and gangrene. Subcutaneous administration may cause necrosis and is not recommended.

E. Use in pregnancy. FDA Category D (possible fetal risk). Pentobarbital readily crosses the placenta, and chronic use may cause hemorrhagic disease of the newborn (owing to vitamin K deficiency) or neonatal dependency and withdrawal syndrome. However, these potential effects do not preclude its acute, short-term use in a seriously symptomatic patient (p 498).

V. Drug or laboratory interactions

A. Pentobarbital has additive CNS and respiratory depression effects with other barbiturates as well as with sedative and opioid drugs.

B. Hepatic enzyme induction generally is not encountered with acute pentobarbital overdose, although it may occur within 24–48 hours.

C. Clearance may be enhanced by hemoperfusion, so that supplemental doses are required during the procedure.

VI. Dosage and method of administration

A. Intermittent intravenous bolus. Give 100 mg IV slowly over at least 2 minutes; repeat as needed at 2-minute intervals to a maximum dose of 300–500 mg (children: 1–3 mg/kg IV, repeated as needed to a maximum total of 5–6 mg/kg or 150–200 mg).

B. Intramuscular. Inject 150–200 mg (children: 2–6 mg/kg IM, not to exceed 100 mg) into a large muscle mass (preferably the upper outer quadrant of the gluteus maximus). No more than 5 mL should be administered at an injection site.

C. Continuous intravenous infusion. ***Note:*** Monitor blood pressure and provide airway and ventilatory support as needed.

1. **Low-dose regimen:** Administer a loading dose of 5–6 mg/kg IV over 1 hour (not to exceed 50 mg/min; children: 1 mg/kg/min), followed by a maintenance infusion of 0.5–3 mg/kg/h titrated to the desired effect.
2. **For treatment of refractory status epilepticus,** give a loading dose of 5–15 mg/kg by IV infusion over 1–2 hours (may give an additional 5–10 mg/kg bolus), followed by a maintenance infusion of 0.5–5 mg/kg/h. If breakthrough seizures occur, administer an additional 5 mg/kg bolus and increase the infusion rate by 0.5–1 mg/kg/h every 12 hours. ***Note:*** allow a period of at least 24-48 hours of seizure control before withdrawing the continuous infusion.
3. **For barbiturate coma in severe head trauma with elevated intracranial pressure**, give a loading dose of 10 mg/kg by IV infusion over 30 minutes,

followed by 5 mg/kg bolus every hour for three doses, followed by a maintenance infusion of 1 mg/kg/h and may increase to 2–5 mg/kg/h to maintain burst suppression on EEG (burst suppression usually occurs with a serum pentobarbital concentration of 25–40 mcg/mL).

D. Oral. For treatment of barbiturate or other sedative–drug withdrawal syndrome, give 200 mg orally, repeated every hour until signs of mild intoxication appear (eg, slurred speech, drowsiness, and nystagmus). Most patients respond to 600 mg or less. Repeat the total initial dose every 6 hours as needed. Phenobarbital is an alternative (see below).

VII. Formulations

A. Parenteral. Pentobarbital sodium (Nembutal and others), 50 mg/mL in 1- and 2-mL tubes and vials and in 20- and 50-mL vials. ***Note:*** Solutions are alkaline and contain propylene glycol.

B. Oral. Capsules (30, 50, and 100 mg) and suppositories (30, 60, 120, and 200 mg). Also available as an elixir equivalent to 18.5 mg/5 mL.

C. Suggested minimum stocking levels to treat a 100-kg adult for the first 8 hours and 24 hours: **pentobarbital sodium**, *first 8 hours:* 1,000 mg or one (20-mL) vial (50 mg/mL); *first 24 hours:* 3,000 mg or three (20-mL) vials (50 mg/mL).

▶ PHENOBARBITAL

Thomas E. Kearney, PharmD

I. Pharmacology. Phenobarbital is a barbiturate commonly used as an anticonvulsant. Because of the delay in onset of the therapeutic effect of phenobarbital, diazepam (p 516) is usually the initial agent for parenteral anticonvulsant therapy. After an oral dose of phenobarbital, peak brain concentrations are achieved within 10–15 hours. Onset of effect after intravenous administration usually occurs within 5 minutes, although peak effects may take up to 30 minutes. Therapeutic plasma levels are 15–35 mg/L. The drug is eliminated by metabolism and renal excretion, and the elimination half-life is 48–100 hours.

II. Indications

A. Control of tonic–clonic seizures and status epilepticus, generally as a second- or third-line agent after diazepam or phenytoin has been tried. ***Note:*** For treatment of drug-induced seizures, especially seizures caused by theophylline, phenobarbital is preferred over phenytoin.

B. Management of withdrawal from ethanol and other sedative–hypnotic drugs.

III. Contraindications

A. Known sensitivity to barbiturates.

B. Manifest or latent porphyria.

IV. Adverse effects

A. Central nervous system depression, coma, and respiratory arrest may result, especially with rapid bolus or excessive doses.

B. Hypotension may result from rapid intravenous administration. This can be prevented by limiting the rate of administration to less than 50 mg/min (children: 1 mg/kg/min). Hypotension may be due to the drug itself or to the diluent propylene glycol.

C. Parenteral solutions are highly alkaline, and precautions need to be taken to avoid extravasation. Intra-arterial infusions may cause vasospasms and gangrene. Subcutaneous administration may cause necrosis and is not recommended.

D. Use in pregnancy. FDA Category D (possible fetal risk). Phenobarbital readily crosses the placenta, and chronic use may cause hemorrhagic disease of the newborn (owing to vitamin K deficiency) or neonatal dependency and withdrawal syndrome. However, these potential effects do not preclude its acute, short-term use in a seriously symptomatic patient (p 498).

V. Drug or laboratory interactions

A. Phenobarbital has additive CNS and respiratory depression effects with other sedative drugs.

B. Hepatic enzyme induction with chronic use, although this is ***not*** encountered with acute phenobarbital dosing.

C. Extracorporeal removal techniques (eg, hemodialysis, hemoperfusion, and repeat-dose–activated charcoal [p 56]) may enhance the clearance of phenobarbital, so that supplemental dosing may be required to maintain therapeutic levels.

VI. Dosage and method of administration

A. Parenteral. Administer slowly intravenously (rate: ≤50 mg/min; children: ≤1 mg/kg/min) until seizures are controlled or the loading dose of 10–15 mg/kg is achieved. For status epilepticus, give 20 mg/kg IV over 10–15 minutes, not to exceed 100 mg/min (as much as 30 mg/kg has been required in the first 24 hours to treat status epilepticus in children). Slow the infusion rate if hypotension develops. Intermittent infusions of 2 mg/kg every 5–15 minutes may diminish the risk for respiratory depression or hypotension. For acute alcohol withdrawal, regimens have included 60–130 mg every 15–30 minutes until signs of mild intoxication or a single IV dose of 10 mg/kg (in 100-mL saline) infused over 30 minutes. For sedation, the average dose is 100–320 mg up to a maximum of 600 mg/d.

1. If intravenous access is not immediately available, phenobarbital may be given intramuscularly; the initial dose in adults and children is 3–5 mg/kg IM (average adult dose 100–320 mg). Maximum volume of single IM injection is 5 mL.

2. It may also be given by the intraosseous route.

B. Oral. For treatment of barbiturate or sedative drug withdrawal, give 60–120 mg orally and repeat every hour until signs of mild intoxication appear (eg, slurred speech, drowsiness, and nystagmus).

VII. Formulations

A. Parenteral. Phenobarbital sodium (Luminal and others), 30, 60, 65, and 130 mg/mL in 1-mL Tubex syringes, vials, and ampules. ***Note:*** Solutions are alkaline and contain propylene glycol.

B. Oral. 15-, 16.2-, 30-, 32.4-, 60-, 64.8-, 97.2-, and 100-mg tablets; 16-mg capsule; also elixir and solution (15 and 20 mg/5 mL).

C. Suggested minimum stocking levels to treat a 100-kg adult for the first 8 hours and 24 hours: **phenobarbital sodium**, *first 8 hours*: 2,000 mg or 16 (1-mL) ampules (130 mg each); *first 24 hours*: 2,000 mg or 16 (1-mL) ampules (130 mg each).

▶ PHENTOLAMINE

Thomas E. Kearney, PharmD

I. Pharmacology. Phentolamine is a competitive presynaptic and postsynaptic alpha-adrenergic receptor blocker that produces peripheral vasodilation. By acting on both venous and arterial vessels, it decreases total peripheral resistance and venous return. It also may stimulate beta-adrenergic receptors, causing cardiac stimulation. Phentolamine has a rapid onset of action (usually 2 minutes) and a short duration of effect (approximately 15–20 minutes).

II. Indications

A. Hypertensive crisis associated with stimulant drug overdose (eg, amphetamines, cocaine, or ephedrine). Also an adjunct for cocaine-induced acute coronary syndrome to reverse coronary artery vasoconstriction.

- **B.** Hypertensive crisis resulting from interaction between monoamine oxidase inhibitors and tyramine or other sympathomimetic amines.
- **C.** Hypertensive crisis associated with sudden withdrawal of sympatholytic antihypertensive drugs (eg, clonidine).
- **D.** Extravasation of vasoconstrictive agents (eg, epinephrine, norepinephrine, and dopamine).

III. Contraindications. Use with extreme caution in patients who have intracranial hemorrhage or ischemic stroke; excessive lowering of blood pressure may aggravate brain injury.

IV. Adverse effects

- **A.** Hypotension and tachycardia may occur from excessive doses.
- **B.** Anginal chest pain and cardiac arrhythmias may occur.
- **C.** Slow intravenous infusion (≤0.3 mg/min) may result in transiently increased blood pressure caused by stimulation of beta-adrenergic receptors.
- **D. Use in pregnancy.** FDA Category C. Phentolamine was used to manage pheochromocytoma during a delivery, with no adverse effects to the newborn attributable to the drug (p 498).

V. Drug or laboratory interactions. Additive or synergistic effects may occur with other antihypertensive agents, especially other alpha-adrenergic antagonists (eg, prazosin, terazosin).

VI. Dosage and method of administration

- **A. Parenteral.** Give 1–5 mg IV (children: 0.02–0.1 mg/kg up to a maximum of 2.5 mg) as a bolus; repeat at 5- to 10-minute intervals as needed to lower blood pressure to a desired level (usually 90–100 mm Hg diastolic in adults and 70–80 mm Hg diastolic in children, but this may vary with the clinical situation). Dose range for adults with pheochromocytoma is up to 20–30 mg. Once hypertension is controlled, repeat every 2–4 hours as needed.
- **B. Catecholamine extravasation.** Infiltrate 5–10 mg in 10–15 mL of normal saline (children: 0.1–0.2 mg/kg; maximum, 10 mg) into an affected area with a fine (25–27-gauge) hypodermic needle; improvement is evidenced by hyperemia and return to normal temperature.

VII. Formulations

- **A. Parenteral.** Phentolamine mesylate, 5 mg in 2-mL vials (lyophilized powder with mannitol). Reconstitute with 1 mL of sterile water and then use immediately (not to be stored).
- **B. Suggested minimum stocking levels** to treat a 100-kg adult for the first 8 hours and 24 hours: **phentolamine mesylate**, *first 8 hours:* 40 mg or eight vials (5 mg each); *first 24 hours*: 100 mg or 20 vials (5 mg each).

▶ PHENYLEPHRINE

Thomas E. Kearney, PharmD

I. Pharmacology. Phenylephrine directly and preferentially stimulates $alpha_1$-adrenergic receptors, although at higher doses it may also stimulate $alpha_2$- and $beta_1$-adrenergic receptors. It is a potent vasoconstrictor with little inotropic or chronotropic effect. Thus, in poisonings it is used primarily as a vasopressor to increase systemic vascular resistance. The onset of action following intravenous administration is immediate, and the effect persists for 15–30 minutes after infusion has stopped.

II. Indications. Phenylephrine is used to increase blood pressure in patients with hypotension caused by vasodilation or low systemic vascular resistance. Phenylephrine may be particularly useful in patients with tachycardia or dysrhythmia that might otherwise be exacerbated by the use of beta-adrenergic agents. Volume resuscitation should be done before or during administration of phenylephrine.

III. Contraindications

- **A.** Uncorrected hypovolemia.
- **B.** Relatively contraindicated in patients with peripheral vascular disease accompanied by severe localized ischemia or thrombosis.
- **C.** Use with caution in patients with bradycardia or hyperthyroidism.

IV. Adverse effects

- **A.** Hypertension.
- **B.** Decreased cardiac output.
- **C.** Reflex bradycardia.
- **D.** Decreased renal perfusion and reduced urine output.
- **E.** Decreased tissue perfusion, resulting in necrosis and/or lactic acidosis.
- **F.** Tissue necrosis after extravasation.
- **G.** Anxiety, restlessness, tremor, and headache.
- **H.** Anaphylaxis induced by bisulfite preservatives in patients with hypersensitivity to sulfites.
- **I. Use in pregnancy.** FDA Category C (indeterminate). This does not preclude its short-term use for a seriously symptomatic patient (p 498).

V. Drug or laboratory interactions

- **A.** Enhanced pressor response may occur in the presence of atomoxetine, cocaine, or cyclic antidepressants owing to inhibition of neuronal norepinephrine reuptake.
- **B.** Enhanced pressor response may occur in patients taking monoamine oxidase inhibitors owing to increased norepinephrine stores in the nerve endings.
- **C.** Propranolol and other $beta_2$-adrenergic blockers may increase blood pressure owing to unopposed alpha-adrenergic stimulation.
- **D.** Chloral hydrate overdose, cyclopropane, and halogenated or aromatic hydrocarbon solvents and anesthetics may enhance myocardial sensitivity to the arrhythmogenic effects of phenylephrine. Risk may be with high doses of phenylephrine.

VI. Dosage and method of administration

- **A. *Caution*: Avoid extravasation.** The intravenous infusion must be free-flowing, and the infused vein should be observed frequently for signs of infiltration (pallor, coldness, or induration).
  1. If extravasation occurs, immediately infiltrate the affected area with phentolamine (p 605), 5–10 mg in 10–15 mL of normal saline (children: 0.1–0.2 mg/kg; maximum, 10 mg) via a fine (25–27-gauge) hypodermic needle; improvement is evidenced by hyperemia and return to normal temperature.
  2. Alternatively, topical application of nitroglycerin paste and infiltration of terbutaline have been reported successful.
- **B. Intravenous Dose.** Start at 0.5 mcg/kg/min and titrate upward to desired effect. Usual dose range is 0.5–2 mcg/kg/min.

VII. Formulations. Phenylephrine HCl solution must be protected from light and should not be used if it appears brown or contains a precipitate.

- **A.** For **continuous IV infusion**, stock solution of 10 mg (1 mL of 1% solution) should be added to 250 or 500 mL of 5% dextrose or normal saline to provide a 40 mcg/mL and 20 mcg/mL solution, respectively. Some institutions have also used concentrations of 60, 100, 160, and 200 mcg/mL. Note that stability information may not be available at all of these concentrations.
- **B. Parenteral formulations.** Phenylephrine hydrochloride (Neo-Synephrine, others), 1% (10 mg/mL), 1-, 5-, and 10-mL vials and 1-mL ampule. Also comes as a compounded product with 50 mg in 500-mL 5% dextrose (100 mcg/mL) and 10 mg in 250 mL in normal saline (40 mcg/mL). Contains sodium metabisulfite as a preservative.

C. **Suggested minimum stocking levels** to treat a 100-kg adult for the first 8 hours and 24 hours: **phenylephrine hydrochloride,** *first 8 hours:* 40 mg or four 1-mL vials (10 mg/mL); *first 24 hours*: 100 mg or ten 1-mL vials (10 mg/mL).

▶ PHENYTOIN AND FOSPHENYTOIN

Justin C. Lewis, PharmD

I. **Pharmacology.** The neuronal membrane–stabilizing actions of phenytoin through sodium channel blockade make this drug popular for sustained control of acute and chronic seizure disorders and useful for certain cardiac arrhythmias. Because of the relatively slow onset of anticonvulsant action, phenytoin usually is administered after diazepam. At serum concentrations considered therapeutic for seizure control, phenytoin acts similarly to lidocaine to reduce ventricular premature depolarization and suppress ventricular tachycardia. After intravenous administration, peak therapeutic effects are attained within 1 hour. The therapeutic serum concentration for seizure control is 10–20 mg/L. Elimination is nonlinear, with an apparent half-life averaging 22 hours. **Fosphenytoin**, a prodrug of phenytoin for intravenous use, is converted to phenytoin after injection, with a conversion half-life of 8–32 minutes.

II. **Indications**

A. Control of generalized tonic–clonic seizures or status epilepticus. However, benzodiazepines (p 516) and phenobarbital (p 604) are more effective for treating drug-induced seizures.

B. Control of cardiac arrhythmias, particularly those associated with digitalis intoxication.

III. **Contraindications.** Known hypersensitivity to phenytoin or other hydantoins.

IV. **Adverse effects**

A. Rapid intravenous administration of phenytoin (>50 mg/min in adults or 1 mg/kg/min in children) may produce hypotension, AV block, and cardiovascular collapse, probably owing to the propylene glycol diluent. Fosphenytoin is readily soluble and does not contain propylene glycol, and, therefore, a hypotensive response is not expected. However, a few cases of bradycardia and asystole have been reported after very large IV doses of fosphenytoin.

B. Extravasation of phenytoin may result in local tissue necrosis and sloughing. Phenytoin may induce the "purple glove" syndrome (edema, discoloration, and pain) after peripheral IV administration. This can occur hours after infusion, in the absence of clinical signs of extravasation, and can lead to limb ischemia and necrosis from a compartment syndrome. Elderly patients receiving large multiple doses are at risk; other risk factors include use of small IV catheters, high infusion rates, and use of the same catheter site for two or more IV push doses. Extravasation problems have not been observed with fosphenytoin.

C. Drowsiness, ataxia, nystagmus, and nausea may occur.

D. **Use in pregnancy.** FDA category D. Congenital malformations (fetal hydantoin syndrome) and hemorrhagic disease of the newborn have occurred with chronic use. However, this does not preclude acute, short-term use in a seriously symptomatic patient (p 498).

V. **Drug or laboratory interactions**

A. The various drug interactions associated with chronic phenytoin dosing (ie, accelerated metabolism of other drugs) are not applicable to its acute emergency use.

B. Extracorporeal removal methods (eg, hemoperfusion and repeat-dose activated charcoal) will enhance phenytoin clearance. Supplemental dosing may be required during such procedures to maintain therapeutic levels.

VI. Dosage and method of administration

A. Parenteral

1. **Phenytoin.** Administer a loading dose of 15–20 mg/kg IV slowly at a rate not to exceed 50 mg/min.
   - **a.** Highly sensitive patients (elderly, patients with preexisting cardiovascular conditions) should receive phenytoin more slowly (20 mg/min), and children at 1 mg/kg/min.
   - **b.** Phenytoin may be diluted in 50–150 mL of normal saline with the use of an in-line 0.22–0.5 micron filter. Further **dilution to 5 mg/mL may help reduce the risk of purple glove syndrome.**
   - **c.** Phenytoin has been administered via the intraosseous route in children. Do ***not*** administer by the intramuscular route.
2. **Fosphenytoin.** Dose is based on the phenytoin equivalent: 750 mg of fosphenytoin is equivalent to 500 mg of phenytoin. (For example, the equivalent of a loading dose of 1 g of phenytoin would be a loading dose of 1.5 g of fosphenytoin.) Dilute twofold to 10-fold in 5% dextrose or normal saline and administer at a rate no faster than 225 mg/min.

B. Maintenance oral phenytoin dose. Give 5 mg/kg/d as a single oral dose of capsules or twice daily for other dosage forms and in children. Monitor serum phenytoin levels.

VII. Formulations

A. Parenteral. Phenytoin sodium, 50 mg/mL, 2- and 5-mL ampules and vials. Fosphenytoin sodium (Cerebyx), 150 mg (equivalent to 100 mg of phenytoin) in 2-mL vials or 750 mg (equivalent to 500 mg of phenytoin) in 10-mL vials.

B. Oral. Phenytoin sodium (Dilantin and others), 30-mg, 100-mg, 200-mg, and 300-mg capsules. 50-mg chewable tablets. 125 mg/5 mL oral suspension.

C. Suggested minimum stocking levels to treat a 100-kg adult for the first 8 hours and 24 hours:

1. **Phenytoin sodium,** *first 8 hours*: 2 g or eight vials (50 mg/mL, 5 mL each); *first 24 hours:* 2 g or eight vials (50 mg/mL, 5 mL each).
2. **Fosphenytoin sodium,** *first 8 hours:* 3 g or four vials (75 mg/mL, 10 mL each); *first 24 hours:* 3 g or four vials (75 mg/mL, 10 mL each).

► PHYSOSTIGMINE AND NEOSTIGMINE

Thomas E. Kearney, PharmD

I. Pharmacology. Physostigmine and neostigmine are carbamates and reversible inhibitors of acetylcholinesterase, the enzyme that degrades acetylcholine. They increase concentrations of acetylcholine, causing stimulation of both muscarinic and nicotinic receptors. Physostigmine may also have a direct action on the acetylcholine receptor. The tertiary amine structure of physostigmine allows it to penetrate the blood–brain barrier and exert central cholinergic effects as well. Neostigmine, a quaternary ammonium compound, is unable to penetrate the CNS. Owing to cholinergic stimulation of the reticular activating system of the brainstem, physostigmine has nonspecific analeptic (arousal) effects. After parenteral administration of physostigmine, the onset of action is within 3–8 minutes and the duration of effect is usually 30–90 minutes. The average elimination half-life is 22 minutes (range 12–40). Neostigmine has a slower onset of 7–11 minutes and a longer duration of effect of 60–120 minutes.

II. Indications

A. Physostigmine is used for the management of severe anticholinergic syndrome (agitated delirium, urinary retention, severe sinus tachycardia, or hyperthermia with absent sweating) from antimuscarinic agents (eg, benztropine, atropine, jimson weed [Datura], diphenhydramine). The typical indication is for reversal of agitated delirium in patients requiring physical and/or chemical restraints. For a discussion of anticholinergic toxicity, see p 97. Although there are anecdotal case reports of the use of physostigmine to treat delirium and coma associated with gamma-hydroxybutyrate (GHB), baclofen, and several atypical antipsychotic (olanzapine, clozapine, quetiapine) agents, its safety and efficacy are uncertain with these intoxications.

B. Physostigmine is sometimes used diagnostically to differentiate functional psychosis from anticholinergic delirium.

C. Neostigmine is used primarily to reverse the effect of nondepolarizing neuromuscular blocking agents.

III. Contraindications

A. Serious tricyclic antidepressant overdose. Physostigmine may worsen cardiac conduction disturbances, cause bradyarrhythmias or asystole, and aggravate or precipitate seizures.

B. Do ***not*** use physostigmine concurrently with depolarizing neuromuscular blockers (eg, succinylcholine).

C. Known hypersensitivity to agent or preservative (eg, benzyl alcohol, bisulfite).

D. Relative contraindications may include bronchospastic disease or asthma, peripheral vascular disease, intestinal and bladder blockade, parkinsonian syndrome, and cardiac conduction defects (AV block).

IV. Adverse effects

A. Bradycardia, heart block, and asystole.

B. Seizures (particularly with rapid administration or excessive dose of physostigmine).

C. Nausea, vomiting, hypersalivation, and diarrhea.

D. Bronchorrhea and bronchospasm (caution required in patients with asthma).

E. Fasciculations and muscle weakness.

F. Use in pregnancy. FDA Category C (p 498). Transient weakness has been noted in neonates whose mothers were treated with physostigmine for myasthenia gravis.

V. Drug or laboratory interactions

A. May potentiate agents metabolized by the cholinesterase enzyme (eg, depolarizing neuromuscular blocking agents—succinylcholine, cocaine, esmolol), cholinesterase inhibitors (eg, organophosphate and carbamate insecticides), and other cholinergic agents (eg, pilocarpine).

B. They may inhibit or reverse the actions of nondepolarizing neuromuscular blocking agents (eg, pancuronium, vecuronium). Neostigmine is used therapeutically for this purpose.

C. They may have additive depressant effects on cardiac conduction in patients with cyclic antidepressant, beta-adrenergic antagonist, or calcium antagonist overdoses.

D. Physostigmine, through its nonspecific analeptic effects, may induce arousal in patients with GHB, opioid, benzodiazepine, or sedative–hypnotic intoxication, or with ketamine- or propofol-induced sedation.

VI. Dosage and method of administration. ***Note:*** The patient should be on a cardiac monitor in case of bradyarrhythmia.

A. Physostigmine

1. Adult dose. Give 0.5–1 mg IV slowly (diluted in 10 mL of D_5W or normal saline) over 2–5 minutes, carefully observing for improvement or side effects (especially bradycardia or heart block). If there is no effect, give additional 0.5-mg doses at 10- to 15-minute intervals up to a maximum total dose of 2 mg over the first hour (delirium reversal is usually achieved with an initial total dose of $\leq$2 mg). If larger doses are needed, consult with a medical toxicologist.

2. **The pediatric dose** is 0.01 mg/kg (not to exceed 0.5 mg) repeated as needed up to a maximum dose of 0.04 mg/kg (not to exceed a total dose of 2 mg for the first hour).
3. **Atropine** (p 512) should be kept nearby to reverse excessive muscarinic stimulation (adults: 1–4 mg; children: 1 mg).
4. Do ***not*** administer physostigmine intramuscularly.
5. Doses may need to be repeated every 30–60 minutes owing to the short duration of action of physostigmine.

B. Neostigmine (parenteral). Give 0.5- to 2-mg slow IV push (children: 0.025–0.08 mg/kg per dose) and repeat as required (total dose rarely exceeds 5 mg). Premedicate with glycopyrrolate (0.2 mg/mg of neostigmine; usual adult dose: 0.2–0.6 mg; children: 0.004–0.02 mg/kg) or atropine (0.4 mg/mg of neostigmine; usual adult dose: 0.6–1.2 mg; children: 0.01–0.04 mg/kg) several minutes before or simultaneously with neostigmine to prevent muscarinic effects (bradycardia, secretions).

VII. Formulations

A. Parenteral. Physostigmine salicylate (generic), 1 mg/mL in 2-mL ampules (contains benzyl alcohol and bisulfite). Neostigmine methylsulfate (Bloxiverz, others), 0.5 mg/mL, 1 mg/mL, in 10-mL multidose vials (contains phenol or parabens) and 5 mg/5 mL in prefilled syringe.

B. Suggested minimum stocking levels to treat a 100-kg adult for the first 8 hours and 24 hours:

1. **Physostigmine salicylate,** *first 8 hours:* 4 mg or two ampules (1 mg/mL, 2 mL each); *first 24 hours:* 20 mg or 10 ampules (1 mg/mL, 2 mL each).
2. **Neostigmine methylsulfate,** *first 8 hours:* 5 mg or one 10-mL vial of 0.5 mg/mL; *first 24 hours:* 5 mg or one 10-mL vial of 0.5 mg/mL.

▶ POTASSIUM

Justin C. Lewis, PharmD

I. Pharmacology. Potassium is the primary intracellular cation, which is essential for the maintenance of acid–base balance; intracellular tonicity; transmission of nerve impulses; contraction of cardiac, skeletal, and smooth muscle; and maintenance of normal renal function (and ability to alkalinize urine). Potassium also acts as an activator in many enzyme reactions and participates in many physiological processes such as carbohydrate metabolism, protein synthesis, and gastric secretion. Potassium is critical in regulating nerve conduction and muscle contraction, especially in the heart. A variety of toxins cause alterations in serum potassium levels (see Table I–27, p 39).

II. Indications

A. For treatment or prevention of hypokalemia (see p 39).

B. Supplement to bicarbonate therapy (see p 520) for alkalinization of urine.

III. Contraindications

A. Potassium should be administered cautiously in patients with renal impairment or impairment of renal excretion of potassium (ACE inhibitor toxicity and hypoaldosteronism, potassium-sparing diuretics) to avoid the potential for serious hyperkalemia.

B. Potassium should be administered cautiously in patients with impairment of intracellular transport of potassium (due to inhibition of Na-K ATPase pump with cardiac glycosides or inhibition of beta-adrenergic transport with beta-blockers). Administration of potassium may lead to large incremental rises in serum levels.

C. Potassium should be administered cautiously in patients with intracellular spillage of potassium (rhabdomyolysis, hemolysis).

D. Potassium should be administered cautiously in patients with severe acute dehydration.

IV. **Adverse effects.** Hyperkalemia is the most serious adverse reaction (see p 39).

A. Nausea, vomiting, abdominal pain, and diarrhea with oral administration.

B. **Parenteral administration**. ***Note:*** DO NOT use undiluted injectable potassium preparations: direct injection can be lethal if given too rapidly; pain at the injection site and phlebitis may occur, especially during infusion of solutions containing greater than 30 mEq/L.

C. **Use in pregnancy.** FDA Category C (indeterminate) (see p 498).

V. **Drug or laboratory interactions**

A. Drug interactions, see Contraindications, above.

B. Numerous IV incompatibilities: mannitol, diazepam, dobutamine, ergotamine, fat emulsion, nitroprusside, ondansetron, phenytoin, penicillin G sodium, promethazine, streptomycin.

C. Serum potassium levels may be fictitiously elevated if the blood sample is hemolyzed.

VI. **Dosage and method of administration (adults and children).** The dose depends on the serum potassium level and severity of symptoms. Potassium depletion resulting in a 1-mEq/L decrease in serum potassium level may require as much as 100–200 mEq to restore body stores in an adult. However, this does not apply to conditions where the level is low because of an intracellular shift of potassium (eg, methylxanthine or beta-adrenergic agonist toxicity).

A. For parenteral administration, potassium must be diluted (see Adverse effects, above).

B. The usual daily **adult maintenance dose** is 40–80 mEq (children: 2–3 mEq/kg or 40 mEq/m^2).

C. **For a serum potassium of 3.0 mEq/L or higher**, the oral route is the preferred method of repletion.

D. **Intravenous dosing.** ***Note:*** Continuous cardiac monitoring with frequent laboratory monitoring is recommended during administration of IV potassium (especially for rates >0.5 mEq/kg/h). Adjust the volume of fluid to the patient's body size.

1. **For a serum potassium between 2.5 mEq/L and 3.0 mEq/L**, the maximum IV infusion rate of potassium is 10 mEq/h, the maximum concentration is 40 mEq/L, and the maximum dose is 200 mEq per 24 hours.
2. **For a serum potassium less than 2.5 mEq/L**, the maximum infusion rate of potassium in adults is 40 mEq/h, although infusions of 50 mEq/h have been used for short periods of time. The maximum concentration is 80 mEq/L, and maximum dose is 400 mEq per 24 hours.
3. **For pediatric patients,** the recommended dose is 0.5–1 mEq/kg/dose (maximum of 30 mEq per dose) to infuse at 0.3–0.5 mEq/kg/h.

VII. **Formulations**

A. **Potassium acetate** injection: 2 mEq/mL in 20-, 50-, and 100-mL vials; 4 mEq/mL in 50-mL vials.

B. **Potassium chloride** for injection concentrate: 2 mEq/mL in 250 and 500 mL; 10 mEq in 5-, 10-, 50-, and 100-mL vials and 5-mL additive syringes; 20 mEq in 10- and 20-mL vials, 10-mL additive syringes, and 10-mL ampules; 30 mEq in 15-, 20-, 30-, and 100-mL vials and 20-mL additive syringes; 40 mEq in 20-, 30-, 50-, and 100-mL vials, 20-mL ampules, and 20-mL additive syringes; 60 mEq in 30-mL vials; and 90 mEq in 30-mL vials.

C. The **suggested minimum stocking level** to treat a 70-kg adult for the first 24 hours is 500 mEq.

▶ PRALIDOXIME (2-PAM) AND OTHER OXIMES

Richard J. Geller, MD, MPH

I. Pharmacology. Although antimuscarinic agents (atropine and glycopyrrolate) are the most important therapy of cholinesterase inhibitor poisoning, they affect only muscarinic receptors and create no clinical effects at the four sites enervated by nicotinic receptors. Oximes reverse acetylcholinesterase (AChE) inhibition (thus reversing cholinergic excess at both muscarinic *and* nicotinic receptors) by reactivating the phosphorylated AChE and protecting the enzyme from further inhibition. Several recent reviews have called into question the efficacy of oximes and pointed out the lack of randomized trials supporting their utility and safety. However, they are the only agents available capable of reactivating AChE and reversing the excess acetylcholine at the nicotinic receptors of the (1) neuromuscular junction (reversing skeletal muscle weakness and fasciculations), (2) parasympathetic and (3) sympathetic ganglia, and at (4) CNS nicotinic receptors (reversing agitation, confusion, coma, and central respiratory failure). Although this effect is most pronounced with organophosphorus (OP) insecticides, positive clinical results have been seen with carbamate (CBM) insecticides that have nicotinic toxicity and variably with cholinesterase inhibitors formulated as "nerve gas" chemical weapons.

- **A.** Pralidoxime chloride (2-PAM) is the only oxime currently approved for use in the United States. Oximes differ in their effectiveness against specific agents, recommended doses, and side effect profiles. Oximes commonly used in other countries include obidoxime, trimedoxime, and HI-6.
- **B.** Oximes are more effective when given before AChE has been bound irreversibly ("aged") by the organophosphate. The rate of aging varies considerably with each OP compound. For dimethyl compounds (eg, dichlorvos, malathion), the aging half-life is approximately 3.7 hours, whereas for diethyl compounds (eg, diazinon, parathion), the aging half-life is approximately 33 hours. For some chemical warfare agents, aging may occur within several minutes (soman phosphorylated AChE aging half-life is about 2–6 minutes). However, late therapy with 2-PAM may still be appropriate even several days after exposure, for example, in patients poisoned by highly fat-soluble compounds (eg, fenthion, demeton) that can be released from tissue stores over days, causing continuous or recurrent intoxication.
- **C.** "Nerve" agents prepared as chemical warfare weapons, such as sarin, soman, tabun, and VX, are mechanistically similar to AChE-inhibiting insecticides. However, they are far more potent and are responsive only to certain oximes. Pralidoxime is not effective against tabun, for example, but HI-6 has been found to be. Current oxime research seeking drugs with broader activity against nerve agents is evaluating HI-6, K027, K048, K074, and K075.
- **D.** Inadequate dosing of 2-PAM may be linked to the "intermediate syndrome," which is characterized by prolonged muscle weakness.
- **E.** Peak plasma concentrations are reached within 5–15 minutes after intravenous 2-PAM administration. Pralidoxime is eliminated by renal excretion and hepatic metabolism, with a half-life of 0.8–2.7 hours.

II. Indications

- **A.** Oximes are used to treat poisonings caused by cholinesterase inhibitor insecticides and nerve agents, including OPs, mixtures of OP and CBM insecticides, and pure CBM insecticides. Pralidoxime has low toxicity, is able to reverse nicotinic as well as muscarinic effects, and may reduce atropine requirements. For these reasons, pralidoxime should be considered early and empirically for suspected cholinesterase inhibitor poisoning, particularly in the context of muscle fasciculation or weakness.
- **B.** With carbamate (CBM) poisoning, cholinesterase inhibition spontaneously resolves without "aging" of the enzyme. As a result, many references state that pralidoxime is not needed for CBM poisoning. However, spontaneous

reversal of enzyme inhibition may take up to 30 hours, and case reports suggest that pralidoxime is effective in human CBM poisoning. Data suggesting increased toxicity of pralidoxime in carbaryl (Sevin) poisoning are based on limited animal studies, and the results are not applicable to humans.

III. Contraindications

A. Use in patients with myasthenia gravis may precipitate a myasthenic crisis.

B. Use with caution and in reduced doses in patients with renal impairment.

IV. Adverse effects

A. Nausea, headache, dizziness, drowsiness, diplopia, and hyperventilation may occur.

B. Rapid intravenous administration may result in tachycardia, hypertension, laryngospasm, muscle rigidity, and transient neuromuscular blockade. Hypertension is reversible with drug cessation or by administration of a vasodilator (eg, sodium nitroprusside [p 593]).

C. Use in pregnancy. FDA Category C (indeterminate). This does not preclude its acute, short-term use in a seriously symptomatic patient (see p 498).

V. Drug or laboratory interactions. Reversal of muscarinic blockade may occur more quickly when atropine (or glycopyrrolate) and pralidoxime are administered concurrently.

VI. Dosage and method of administration. Start pralidoxime at the earliest possible time (before AChE aging occurs) and via the intravenous route (to rapidly achieve predictable serum levels). Intermittent intramuscular or subcutaneous administration is possible, if circumstances dictate, but may result in wide fluctuation in serum levels and erratic clinical effects. Pralidoxime has a short elimination half-life, so the loading dose should be followed by a continuous infusion. However, no standard continuous infusion rate has been established, and rates cited below should be considered as guidelines to be modified by clinical response (ie, relief of muscle fasciculations and muscle weakness).

A. Adult intravenous dosing. A typical loading dose is 1,000–2,000 mg in 100 mL of saline infused over 15–30 minutes. Repeat the initial dose after 1 hour if muscle weakness or fasciculations are not relieved. This is followed by a continuous infusion of 1% pralidoxime in saline (eg, 1 g in 100 mL). The manufacturer cites continuous infusion rates of 400–600 mg/h, and rates as high as 8–10 mg/kg/h have been utilized. (The World Health Organization recommends a bolus dose of 2 g, followed by a continuous infusion of 8–10 mg/kg/h.)

B. Pediatric intravenous dosing (for patients aged 16 years and younger). A typical loading dose is 30 mg/kg (range 20–50 mg/kg), not to exceed 2,000 mg, as a 1% solution in saline, infused over 15–30 minutes. Repeat the initial dose after 1 hour if muscle weakness or fasciculations are not relieved. This is followed by a continuous infusion of 1% pralidoxime in saline. The manufacturer cites continuous pediatric infusion rates of 10–20 mg/kg/h.

C. Immediate field treatment of suspected nerve agent poisoning is by intramuscular injection. The dose is 600 mg IM for mild to moderate symptoms and up to 1,800 mg for severe poisonings. The Mark I autoinjector kit contains 600-mg pralidoxime plus 2-mg atropine and is designed for self-administration.

D. Duration of therapy. Despite earlier recommendations that pralidoxime should be given for only 24 hours, therapy may have to be continued for several days, particularly when long-acting, lipid-soluble organophosphates are involved. Gradually reduce the dose and carefully observe the patient for signs of recurrent fasciculations, muscle weakness, or other signs of toxicity. ***Note:*** Pralidoxime may accumulate in patients with renal insufficiency.

VII. Formulations

A. Parenteral. Pralidoxime chloride (2-PAM, Protopam), 1 g with 20-mL sterile water.

B. The **suggested minimum stocking level** to treat a 70-kg adult for the first 24 hours is 18 × 1 g (20 mL) vials. ***Note:*** In agricultural areas or urbanized regions preparing for possible accidental or terrorist release of a large amount of cholinesterase inhibitor agent, much larger stockpiling may be appropriate. Pralidoxime is stockpiled by the Strategic National Stockpile (SNS) program as Mark I autoinjector kits and 1-g vials of pralidoxime chloride.

▶ PROPOFOL

Joanne M. Goralka, PharmD

I. Pharmacology

A. Propofol (2,6-diisopropylphenol) is a sedative–hypnotic–anesthetic agent in a class of alkyl phenol compounds. It is an oil at room temperature, highly lipid-soluble, and administered as an emulsion. It is also an antioxidant, anticonvulsant, and anti-inflammatory agent, reduces intracranial pressure, and has bronchodilator properties. The proposed site of action of propofol is at the GABA(A) receptor, where it activates the chloride channel. There may also be some action at the glutamate and glycine receptor sites. Propofol is considered an antagonist at the *N*-methyl-D-aspartate (NMDA) receptor. It is also an inhibitor of cytochrome P-450 enzymes.

B. Intravenous injection of a therapeutic dose of propofol induces hypnosis within approximately 40 seconds.

C. It is highly protein bound (97–99%), with a volume of distribution of approximately 60 L/kg after a continuous 10-day infusion. Propofol has a high clearance rate estimated at 1.6–3.4 L/min in 70-kg adults. This clearance rate exceeds hepatic blood flow and suggests extrahepatic metabolism.

D. Propofol is metabolized rapidly in the liver by conjugation to glucuronide and sulfate intermediates that are water-soluble and inactive. This occurs predominantly via oxidation by cytochrome P-450 (CYP) enzyme 2B6. Cytochrome P-450 isoforms 2A6, 2C9, 2C19, 2D6, 2E1, 3A4, and 1A2 are also involved in the metabolism of propofol to a lesser extent. There is minimal enterohepatic circulation, and less than 1% is excreted unchanged.

II. Indications

A. Induction and maintenance of general anesthesia in adults and children aged 3 years and older. Can be used for maintenance in children aged 2 months and older.

B. Monitored sedation in adults during procedures.

C. Monitored sedation in intubated, mechanically ventilated adult patients.

D. Propofol has also been used as an adjunct anesthetic agent in the management of refractory withdrawal syndromes associated with alcohol or other sedative–hypnotics (eg, GHB and barbiturates) and in the treatment of status epilepticus. (These are not FDA-approved indications.)

III. Contraindications

A. Hypersensitivity to propofol or any of its components. Contraindicated in patients with allergies to eggs, egg products, soybeans, and soy products. The labeling on the Europe-manufactured product (Fresenius Propoven 1%) includes peanut hypersensitivity as a contraindication owing to concerns regarding potential peanut oil and soybean oil cross-reactivity.

B. Formulations vary and may contain benzyl alcohol, sodium benzoate, disodium edetate, or sodium metabisulfite. Consult individual product labeling for specific excipient information.

IV. Adverse effects

A. Pain at the injection site can occur (use larger veins or premedicate with lidocaine).

B. Anaphylaxis, apnea, hypotension, bradycardia, supraventricular tachydysrhythmias, conduction disturbances, cough, bronchospasm, rash, pruritus, and hyperlipidemia may occur.

C. Anesthetic doses require respiratory support. Avoid rapid bolus doses because of the higher risk for hypotension, bradycardia, apnea, and airway obstruction.

D. Anesthetic doses may be associated with myoclonus, posturing, and seizure-like movement phenomena (jerking, thrashing). Seizures have been noted when patients were weaned from propofol.

E. **Propofol infusion syndrome** is a serious and life-threatening condition characterized by severe metabolic acidosis, hyperkalemia, lipemia, renal failure, rhabdomyolysis, hepatomegaly, cardiac arrhythmias, and myocardial failure. Risk factors include patients with decreased oxygen delivery to tissues, serious neurological injury, sepsis, high dosages of vasoconstrictors, steroids, inotropes, and prolonged high-dose propofol infusions (>5 mg/kg/h for >48 hours). This syndrome has also been reported following large-dose, short-term infusion of propofol during surgical anesthesia.

F. Acute pancreatitis with single or prolonged use can occur. Hyperlipidemia can also occur after prolonged use.

G. Use with caution in patients who have a history of seizures. When propofol is administered to a patient with epilepsy, there is a risk for seizures during the recovery phase.

H. Propofol vials can still support the growth of microorganisms despite the addition of additives to inhibit their rate of growth. Strictly adhere to product labeling recommendations for handling and administering propofol.

I. Decreased zinc levels can occur during prolonged therapy (>5 days) or in patients with a predisposition to zinc deficiency, such as those with burns, diarrhea, or sepsis, when formulations containing disodium edetate (a strong chelator of trace minerals) are used.

J. There have been reports of the abuse of propofol, which have resulted in fatalities and other injuries.

K. Urine may be discolored green or dark green.

L. **Use in pregnancy.** FDA Category B. Propofol crosses the placenta and may be associated with neonatal CNS depression (p 498).

V. Drug or laboratory interactions

A. An additive effect with other CNS depressants may result in lower propofol dose requirements if propofol is given concomitantly. Through its inhibition of cytochrome P-450 enzymes, propofol may increase levels of substrate drugs including midazolam, diazepam, and opiates such as sufentanil and alfentanil, causing respiratory depression, bradycardia, and hypotension.

B. Propofol levels may be increased by lidocaine, bupivacaine, and halothane, producing an increased hypnotic effect.

C. Concurrent use with succinylcholine may result in bradycardia.

VI. Dosage and method of administration. Propofol currently is administered as an intravenous medication only, and the dose must be individualized and titrated (see Table III–14).

VII. Formulations

A. Parenteral

1. US-manufactured propofol (Diprivan) 1% (10 mg/mL) emulsion and APP Propofol (1%) Injectable Emulsion, USP. Contain propofol (1%), soybean oil (100 mg/mL), glycerol (22.5 mg/mL), egg lecithin (12 mg/mL), and disodium edetate (0.005%), with sodium hydroxide to adjust the pH to 7–8.5. Diprivan is available in 20-, 50-, and 100-mL single patient infusion vials. ***Note:*** Diprivan (1%) and APP Propofol (1%) are provided as ready-to-use preparations, but if dilution is necessary, use only D5W and do not dilute to concentrations of less than 2 mg/mL. In diluted form, it has been shown to be more stable when in contact with glass than with plastic.

TABLE III–14. DOSING GUIDELINES FOR PROPOFOL

Indication	Doses[a,b,c] (All Intravenous)	
	Initial Dose	Maintenance Dose (mg/kg/h)
Sedation		
Patient undergoing procedural sedation	0.3–0.75 mg/kg over 3–5 min	1.5–3
Intubated patient in ICU	Start with 0.3 mg/kg/h; titrate in small increments every 5–10 min to effect.	0.3–3
Status epilepticus	1–2 mg/kg	1.2–12

[a]Dose rates vary and should be titrated to desired clinical effect.
[b]Some institutions avoid use in children younger than 16 years and have put limits on maximum infusion rates and duration (eg, not to exceed 4 mg/kg/h for 24–48 hours, not to be used beyond 72 hours, or not more than 9 mg/kg/h for 2–4 hours) to prevent propofol infusion syndrome.
[c]In elderly, debilitated, or neurosurgical patients, use 80% of usual adult dose.

2. Europe-manufactured propofol 1% (Fresenius Propoven 1%) emulsion for injection or infusion. Excipients include soybean oil, refined medium-chain triglycerides, purified egg phosphatides, glycerol, oleic acid, sodium hydroxide, and water for injection. Not FDA-approved but was imported in agreement with the FDA as a temporary supplemental supply. Differs from FDA-approved propofol 1% (Diprivan 1%) in that it does not contain any preservatives and has a combination of medium-chain and long-chain triglycerides. Some vial sizes do not contain spikes or stopcocks.
3. There may be formulation-specific variations. Formulations may contain benzyl alcohol, sodium benzoate, edetate disodium, sulfites, or other excipients/preservatives.
4. Generic versions of Diprivan (propofol 1%) have been approved by the FDA.

B. **Suggested minimum stocking levels** to treat a 100-kg adult for the first 8 hours and 24 hours: **propofol**, *first 8 hours:* 10 g or ten 100-mL vials (10 mg/mL) for general anesthesia; *first 24 hours:* 20 g or twenty 100-mL vials (10 mg/mL) for maintenance of sedation.

▶ PROPRANOLOL

Thomas E. Kearney, PharmD

I. **Pharmacology.** Propranolol is a nonselective beta-adrenergic blocker that acts on beta$_1$-receptors in the myocardium and beta$_2$-receptors in the lung, vascular smooth muscle, and kidney. Within the myocardium, propranolol depresses the heart rate, conduction velocity, myocardial contractility, and automaticity. Although propranolol is effective orally, for toxicologic emergencies, it usually is administered by the intravenous route. After intravenous injection, the onset of action is nearly immediate and the duration of effect is 10 minutes to 2 hours, depending on the cumulative dose. The drug is eliminated by hepatic metabolism, with a half-life of about 2–3 hours. Propranolol also has antagonistic properties at the serotonin (5-HT$_{1A}$) receptor and has been used to treat serotonin syndrome with mixed success (anecdotal case reports).

II. **Indications**

A. To control excessive sinus tachycardia or ventricular arrhythmias caused by catecholamine excess (eg, theophylline or caffeine), sympathomimetic drug intoxication (eg, amphetamines, pseudoephedrine, or cocaine), excessive myocardial sensitivity (eg, chloral hydrate, Freons, or chlorinated and other hydrocarbons), or thyrotoxicosis.

B. To control hypertension in patients with excessive beta$_1$-mediated increases in heart rate and contractility; used in conjunction with a vasodilator (eg, phentolamine) in patients with mixed alpha-and beta-adrenergic hyperstimulation.

C. To raise diastolic blood pressure in patients with hypotension caused by excessive beta$_2$-mediated vasodilation (eg, theophylline or metaproterenol).

D. May ameliorate or reduce beta-adrenergic–mediated electrolyte and other metabolic abnormalities (eg, hypokalemia, hyperglycemia, and lactic acidosis).

E. Serotonin syndrome (p 21).

III. Contraindications

A. Use with extreme caution in patients with asthma, congestive heart failure, sinus node dysfunction, or another cardiac conduction disease and in those receiving calcium antagonists and other cardiac-depressant drugs.

B. Do not use as a single therapy for hypertension resulting from sympathomimetic overdose. Propranolol produces peripheral vascular beta-blockade, which may abolish beta$_2$-mediated vasodilation and allow unopposed alpha-mediated vasoconstriction, resulting in paradoxical worsening of hypertension; coronary artery constriction may cause or exacerbate acute coronary syndrome.

IV. Adverse effects

A. Bradycardia and sinus and atrioventricular block.

B. Hypotension and congestive heart failure.

C. Bronchospasm in patients with asthma or bronchospastic chronic obstructive pulmonary disease. ***Note:*** Propranolol (in *small* intravenous doses) has been used successfully in patients with asthma overdosed on theophylline or beta$_2$ agonists without precipitating bronchospasm.

D. Use in pregnancy. FDA Category C (first trimester) and Category D (second and third trimesters). Propranolol may cross the placenta, and neonates delivered within 3 days of administration of this drug may have persistent beta-adrenergic blockade. However, this does not preclude its acute, short-term use in a seriously symptomatic patient (p 498).

V. Drug or laboratory interactions

A. Propranolol may allow unopposed alpha-adrenergic stimulation in patients with mixed adrenergic stimulation (eg, epinephrine surge in patients with acute hypoglycemia, pheochromocytoma, or cocaine or amphetamine intoxication), resulting in severe hypertension or end-organ ischemia.

B. Propranolol has an additive hypotensive effect with other antihypertensive agents.

C. This drug may potentiate competitive neuromuscular blockers (p 586).

D. Propranolol has additive depressant effects on cardiac conduction and contractility when given with calcium antagonists.

E. Cimetidine reduces hepatic clearance of propranolol.

F. Propranolol may worsen vasoconstriction caused by ergot alkaloids.

VI. Dosage and method of administration

A. Parenteral. Give 0.5–3 mg slowly IV not to exceed 1 mg/min (children: 0.01–0.1 mg/kg slowly IV over 5 minutes; maximum, 1 mg per dose) while monitoring heart rate and blood pressure; dose may be repeated as needed after 5–10 minutes. The dose required for complete beta-receptor blockade is about 0.2 mg/kg. For serotonin syndrome, give 1 mg IV not to exceed 1 mg/min (children: 0.1 mg/kg per dose over 10 minutes; maximum, 1 mg per dose) every 2–5 minutes until a maximum of 5 mg. May repeat at 6- to 8-hour intervals.

B. Oral. Oral dosing may be initiated after the patient is stabilized; the dosage range is about 1–5 mg/kg/d in three or four divided doses for both children and adults. For serotonin syndrome, an adult dose of 20 mg every 8 hours has been used.

VII. **Formulations**

A. **Parenteral.** Propranolol hydrochloride (Generic), 1 mg/mL in 1-mL ampules, vials, and prefilled syringes.

B. **Oral.** Propranolol hydrochloride (Inderal and others), 60-, 80-, 120-, and 160-mg sustained-release capsules; 10-, 20-, 40-, 60-, and 80-mg tablets; 4- and 8-mg/mL in 500-mL oral solution, and 4.28 mg/mL in 120-mL alcohol-, paraben-, and sugar-free solution.

C. **Suggested minimum stocking levels** to treat a 100-kg adult for the first 8 hours and 24 hours: **propranolol hydrochloride,** *first 8 hours:* 6 mg or six vials (1 mg/mL, 1 mL each); *first 24 hours:* 20 mg or 20 vials (1 mg/mL, 1 mL each).

► PROTAMINE

Thomas E. Kearney, PharmD

I. **Pharmacology.** Protamine is a cationic protein obtained from fish sperm that rapidly binds to and inactivates heparin by forming a stable salt. The onset of action after intravenous administration is nearly immediate (30–60 seconds) and lasts up to 2 hours. It also partially neutralizes low-molecular-weight heparins (LMWHs) and can act as an anticoagulant by inhibiting thromboplastin.

II. **Indications**

A. Protamine is used for the reversal of the anticoagulant effect of heparin when an excessively large dose has been administered inadvertently. Protamine generally is not needed for the treatment of bleeding during standard heparin therapy because discontinuance of the heparin infusion is generally sufficient.

B. Protamine may be used for the reversal of regional anticoagulation in the hemodialysis circuit in cases in which anticoagulation of the patient is contraindicated (i.e., active GI or CNS bleeding).

C. Protamine may be used for the reversal of low–molecular-weight heparins (LMWHs). However, its effect may be partial and unpredictable and is generally reserved for cases with emergent and clinically significant bleeding.

III. **Contraindications**

A. **Black Box Warning.** Do not give protamine to patients with known sensitivity to the drug. Patients with diabetes who have used protamine insulin may be at the greatest risk for hypersensitivity reactions.

B. Protamine reconstituted with benzyl alcohol should not be used in neonates because of suspected toxicity from the alcohol.

IV. **Adverse effects**

A. **Black Box Warning.** Rapid intravenous administration and high doses are associated with hypotension, bradycardia, and anaphylactoid reactions. Have epinephrine (p 551), diphenhydramine (p 544), and cimetidine or another histamine$_2$ (H_2) blocker (p 532) ready. Reaction may be prevented by avoiding high infusion rates of more than 5 mg/min.

B. A rebound effect caused by heparin may occur within 8 hours of protamine administration.

C. Excess doses may lead to anticoagulation and the risk for bleeding.

D. **Use in pregnancy.** FDA Category C (indeterminate). A maternal hypersensitivity reaction or hypotension can result in placental ischemia. However, this does not preclude its acute, short-term use for a seriously symptomatic patient (p 498).

V. **Drug or laboratory interactions.** No known drug interactions other than the reversal of the effect of heparin.

VI. **Dosage and method of administration**

A. Administer protamine by slow intravenous injection, not to exceed 50 mg in a 10-minute period or 5 mg/min.

B. The dose of protamine depends on the total dose and the time since the administration of heparin.

1. If immediately after heparin administration, give 1–1.5 mg of protamine for each 100 units of heparin.
2. If 30–60 minutes after heparin administration, give only 0.5–0.75 mg of protamine for each 100 units of heparin.
3. If 60–120 minutes after heparin administration, give only 0.375–0.5 mg of protamine for each 100 units of heparin.
4. If more than 2 hours after heparin administration, give only 0.25–0.375 mg of protamine for each 100 units of heparin.
5. If heparin was being administered by constant infusion, give 25–50 mg of protamine.

C. If the patient is overdosed with an unknown quantity of heparin, give an empiric dose of 25–50 mg over 10 minutes (to minimize hypotension) and determine the activated partial thromboplastin time (aPTT) after 5–15 minutes and for up to 2–8 hours to determine the need for additional doses.

D. For an overdose of a low-molecular-weight heparin (LMWH)

1. **Dalteparin or tinzaparin.** Give 1 mg of protamine for every 100 anti–factor Xa international units of dalteparin and tinzaparin at a rate not to exceed 50 mg in a 10-minute period or 5 mg/min. If 8–12 hours has elapsed since administration of dalteparin or tinzaparin, then give only 0.5 mg of protamine for every 100 anti–factor Xa international units. Protamine administration may not be required if more than 12 hours has elapsed since administration of dalteparin or tinzaparin. If the aPTT remains prolonged 2–4 hours after the initial dose, then give an additional 0.5 mg of protamine for every 100 anti–factor Xa international units.
2. **Enoxaparin.** Give 1 mg of protamine for each 1 mg of enoxaparin at a rate not to exceed 50 mg in a 10-minute period or 5 mg/min. If 8–12 hours has elapsed since administration of enoxaparin, then give only 0.5 mg of protamine for each 1 mg of enoxaparin. Protamine administration may not be required if more than 12 hours has elapsed since administration of enoxaparin. If the aPTT remains prolonged 2–4 hours after the initial dose, then give an additional 0.5 mg of protamine for each 1 mg of enoxaparin.
3. If the LMWH overdose amount is unknown, consider an empiric dose of 25–50 mg given over 15 minutes. The ratios of anti–factor Xa to anti–factor IIa vary for LMWH products, and if they are high, as with an LMW heparinoid (e.g., danaparoid), protamine may be ineffective. Anti–factor Xa activity levels and aPTT values are usually not completely reversed, but they may be used to guide dosing (ideally measured 5–15 minutes after protamine administration). LMWHs have longer half-lives (4–6 hours) and accumulate with renal insufficiency; therefore, coagulopathies may persist, and protamine should be considered even several hours after the overdose.

VII. Formulations

A. Parenteral. Protamine sulfate, 10 mg/mL in 5- and 25-mL vials.

B. Suggested minimum stocking levels to treat a 100-kg adult for the first 8 hours and 24 hours: **protamine sulfate**, *first 8 hours:* 500 mg or two vials (10 mg/mL, 25 mL each); *first 24 hours:* 500 mg or two vials (10 mg/mL, 25 mL each).

▶ PRUSSIAN BLUE

Sandra A. Hayashi, PharmD

I. Pharmacology. Insoluble Prussian blue (ferric hexacyanoferrate) has been used to treat radioactive and nonradioactive cesium and thallium poisonings. Owing to the long half-lives of these isotopes, ingestion can pose significant long-term health risks. Insoluble Prussian blue binds thallium and cesium in the gastrointestinal tract as they undergo enterohepatic recirculation, enhancing fecal excretion. Proposed mechanisms of binding include chemical cation exchange, physical adsorption, and mechanical trapping within the crystal lattice structure. Insoluble Prussian blue is not absorbed across the intact GI wall.

II. Indications. Known or suspected internal contamination by:

A. Radioactive cesium (eg, ^{137}Cs) and nonradioactive cesium.

B. Radioactive thallium (eg, ^{201}Tl) and nonradioactive thallium.

III. Contraindications. There are no absolute contraindications. The efficacy of the agent relies on a functioning GI tract; thus, ileus may preclude its use and effectiveness.

IV. Adverse effects

A. Upset stomach and constipation.

B. May bind other elements, causing electrolyte or nutritional deficits, such as asymptomatic hypokalemia.

C. Does not treat the complications of radiation exposure.

D. Blue discoloration of feces (and teeth if capsules are opened).

E. Use in pregnancy. FDA Category C (indeterminate [p 498]). Because Prussian blue is not absorbed from the GI tract, effects on the fetus are not expected.

V. Drug or laboratory interactions

A. No major interactions.

B. May decrease absorption of tetracycline.

VI. Dosage and method of administration

A. Adults and adolescents. Usual dose is 3 g orally three times daily (9 g daily), although higher doses (>10 g daily) are often used for acute thallium poisoning (particularly if thallium is present in the GI tract). Doses may be decreased to 1–2 g three times daily when internal radioactivity is reduced and to improve patient tolerance.

B. Pediatrics (2–12 years): 1 g orally three times daily.

C. Capsules may be opened and mixed with food or water for those who have difficulty swallowing. However, this may cause blue discoloration of the mouth and the teeth.

D. Coingestion with food may increase effectiveness by stimulating bile secretion.

E. Treatment should continue for a minimum of 30 days. The duration of treatment should be guided by the level of contamination as measured by the amount of residual whole-body radioactivity.

VII. Formulations

A. Oral. Insoluble Prussian blue powder (Radiogardase®), 0.5 g in gelatin capsules packaged in amber bottles containing 30 capsules each.

B. Suggested minimum stocking level to treat a 100-kg adult for the first month is 540 capsules (18 bottles, 30 capsules each) based on a daily dose of 9 g. At this time, the minimum order is 25 bottles. Radiogardase cannot be sold directly to physicians but only with a prescription placed with McGuff Compounding Pharmacy at http://store.mcguff.com/products/5263.aspx or call 877-444-1133, fax 877-444-1155. Institutional and government agencies must begin order process by first contacting Heyltex at 281-395-7040 or lily@heyltex.com. Prussian blue is kept in the Strategic National Stockpile (SNS) at the Centers for Disease Control and prevention (CDC). The Radiation Emergency Assistance Center/Training Site (REAC/TS) can be contacted for information on obtaining Prussian blue and its recommended dosing by telephone at 1-865-576-3131(business hours) or 1-865-576-1005 (available 24 hours) or on the Internet at www.orau.gov/ reacts.

▶ PYRIDOXINE (VITAMIN B_6)

Thomas E. Kearney, PharmD

I. Pharmacology. Pyridoxine (vitamin B_6) is a water-soluble B-complex vitamin that acts as a cofactor in many enzymatic reactions. Overdose involving isoniazid or other hydrazines (eg, *Gyromitra* mushrooms, rocket propellant, or fuel-containing hydrazine, mono-, or di-methylhydrazine) may cause seizures by interfering with pyridoxine utilization in the brain, and pyridoxine given in high doses can control these seizures rapidly and may hasten consciousness. It can also correct the lactic acidosis secondary to isoniazid-induced impaired lactate metabolism. In ethylene glycol intoxication, pyridoxine may enhance metabolic conversion of the toxic metabolite glyoxylic acid to the nontoxic product glycine. Pyridoxine is well absorbed orally but usually is given intravenously for urgent uses. The biological half-life is about 15–20 days.

II. Indications

A. Acute management of seizures caused by intoxication with isoniazid (p 281), hydrazines, *Gyromitra* mushrooms (p 330), or possibly cycloserine. Pyridoxine may act synergistically with diazepam (p 516).

B. Adjunct to therapy for ethylene glycol intoxication (p 234).

C. May improve dyskinesias induced by levodopa.

III. Contraindications. Use caution in patients with known sensitivity to pyridoxine or parabens preservative.

IV. Adverse effects

A. Usually no adverse effects are noted from acute dosing of pyridoxine.

B. Chronic excessive doses may result in peripheral neuropathy.

C. Use of the 1-mL vials may cause mild CNS depression owing to the preservative if 50 or more vials (to deliver ≥5 g of pyridoxine) are administered (equivalent to ≥250 mg of chlorobutanol).

D. Preparations containing the preservative benzyl alcohol (eg, contained in some 1-mL and the 30-mL vials) have been associated with "gasping" syndrome in premature infants.

E. Use in pregnancy. FDA Category A (p 498). However, chronic excessive use in pregnancy has resulted in pyridoxine withdrawal seizures in neonates.

V. Drug or laboratory interactions. No adverse interactions are associated with acute dosing.

VI. Dosage and method of administration

A. Isoniazid poisoning. Give 1 g of pyridoxine intravenously for each gram of isoniazid known to have been ingested (as much as 52 g has been administered and tolerated). Dilute in 50 mL of dextrose or saline and give over 5 minutes (rate of 1 g/min). If the ingested amount is unknown, administer 4–5 g IV empirically and repeat every 5–20 minutes as needed.

B. Hydrazine and gyromitra mushroom poisoning. Give 25 mg/kg IV over 15–30 minutes for seizures; repeat as necessary and up to a maximum cumulative dose of 15–20 g daily has been suggested for mushroom poisoning.

C. Ethylene glycol poisoning. Give 50 mg IV or IM every 6 hours until intoxication is resolved.

D. Cycloserine poisoning. A dosage of 300 mg/d has been recommended.

VII. Formulations

A. Parenteral. Pyridoxine hydrochloride (various), 100 mg/mL (10% solution) in 1- and 30-mL vials (1-mL vial may contain the preservative chlorobutanol, and 30-mL vial contains 1.5% benzyl alcohol). ***Note:*** Only one US company, Legere Pharmaceuticals (Scottsdale, AZ; phone: 1-800-528-3144), manufactures and distributes the 3-g (30-mL) vials. See "Adverse effects" above regarding use of the 1-mL vials.

B. Suggested minimum stocking levels to treat a 100-kg adult for the first 8 hours and 24 hours: **pyridoxine hydrochloride**, *first 8 hours:* 9 g or three vials (100 mg/mL, 30 mL each or equivalent); *first 24 hours:* 24 g or eight vials (100 mg/mL, 30 mL each or equivalent).

▶ SILIBININ

Kent R. Olson, MD

I. **Pharmacology.** Extracts of the milk thistle plant (*Silybum marianum*) have been used since ancient times to treat a variety of hepatic and biliary disorders, including cholestasis, jaundice, cirrhosis, acute and chronic hepatitis, and primary malignancies, and to protect the liver against toxin-induced injury. The extract of the ripe seeds and leaves contains 70–80% **silymarin**, a flavanolignan mixture of which **silibinin** is the most biologically active constituent. The hypothesized mechanism of action is twofold: alteration of hepatocyte cell membrane permeability, preventing toxin penetration; and increased ribosomal protein synthesis, promoting hepatocyte regeneration.

Although the efficacy of silibinin has not been established in controlled studies in humans, it has been associated with reduced liver damage when administered intravenously in the treatment of amatoxin mushroom poisoning. Competitive inhibition of amatoxin entry via the membrane transport system for bile salts has been demonstrated. Silibinin also appears to inhibit tumor necrosis factor (TNF) release in the injured liver, thus slowing the process of amatoxin-induced apoptosis.

Silymarin also is reported to have antifibrotic, anti-inflammatory, and antioxidant activity and may have therapeutic efficacy in the treatment of prostate and skin cancer. There is preliminary evidence that milk thistle constituents may also protect against the nephrotoxic effects of drugs such as acetaminophen, cisplatin, and vincristine.

II. **Indications**

A. Intravenous silibinin is approved across Europe for the prevention and treatment of fulminant hepatic failure following ingestion of amatoxin-containing mushrooms (p 333). An FDA-sanctioned clinical trial has made the drug available in the United States as well.

B. Although this indication is unproven, silibinin may be effective as adjuvant therapy in cases of acute hepatic injury caused by acetaminophen toxicity and potentially other chemical- and drug-induced liver diseases.

III. **Contraindications.** None reported.

IV. **Adverse effects** are few and generally mild.

A. Nausea, diarrhea, abdominal fullness or pain, flatulence, and anorexia may occur in users of oral preparations.

B. Mild warmth and a flushing sensation are commonly reported during intravenous infusion.

C. Milk thistle is a member of the *Asteraceae* (daisy) family and can cause an allergic reaction in ragweed-sensitive individuals, including rash, urticaria, pruritus, and anaphylaxis.

D. **Use in pregnancy.** FDA Category B. Insufficient reliable information is available (p 498).

V. **Drug or laboratory interactions.** Although milk thistle has been shown to induce slight cytochrome P-450 enzyme inhibition in vitro, significant drug interactions with milk thistle extract have not been demonstrated in humans.

VI. **Dosage and method of administration**

A. Intravenous dosing for amatoxin mushroom poisoning is 20–50 mg/kg/d by continuous infusion or in four divided doses administered over 2 hours each.

B. Oral doses used in published studies have ranged from 280 to 800 mg/d of standardized silymarin. A typical dose used for chronic hepatitis is 420 mg/d in two or three oral doses.

VII. **Formulations**

A. **Oral.** In the United States, milk thistle extracts are available as over-the-counter dietary supplements (eg, Thisilyn). Oral formulations include Legalon (standardized to contain 70% silibinin) and Silipide (silibinin complexed with phosphatidylcholine, which has a higher oral bioavailability). Because silymarin is poorly water-soluble, milk thistle tea is not considered an effective preparation.

B. Parenteral. Intravenous silibinin can be obtained for the treatment of amatoxin mushroom poisoning as an FDA-sanctioned open Investigational New Drug (call toll-free 1-866-520-4412).

► SUCCIMER (DMSA)

Michael J. Kosnett, MD, MPH

I. Pharmacology

A. Succimer (*meso*-2,3-dimercaptosuccinic acid [DMSA]) is a chelating agent that is used in the treatment of intoxication from several heavy metals. A water-soluble analog of BAL (dimercaprol [p 514]), succimer enhances the urinary excretion of lead and mercury. Its effect on the elimination of the endogenous minerals calcium, iron, and magnesium is insignificant. Minor increases in zinc and copper excretion may occur. In an animal model, oral succimer was not associated with a significant increase in the GI absorption of lead or inorganic mercury (as mercuric chloride); the effect of oral succimer on the GI absorption of arsenic is not known.

B. After oral administration, peak blood concentrations occur in approximately 3 hours. Distribution is predominantly extracellular, and in the blood, succimer is extensively bound (>90%) to plasma proteins. Succimer is eliminated primarily in the urine, where 80–90% appears as mixed disulfides, mainly 2:1 or 1:1 cysteine–succimer adducts. Studies suggest that these adducts, rather than the parent drug, may be responsible for metal-chelating activity in vivo. Renal elimination of the metal chelates appears to be mediated in part by the multidrug resistance protein 2 (Mrp2). The elimination half-life of transformed succimer is approximately 2–4 hours. Renal clearance may be diminished in the setting of pediatric lead intoxication.

II. Indications

A. Succimer is approved for the treatment of lead intoxication, where it is associated with increased urinary excretion of the metal and concurrent reversal of metal-induced enzyme inhibition. At moderately elevated blood lead concentrations, oral succimer is comparable with parenteral calcium EDTA (p 548) in decreasing blood lead concentrations. The efficiency of succimer in eliminating lead from the blood and tissues may somewhat decline at very high blood concentrations of lead (eg, >100 mcg/dL). Although succimer treatment has been associated with subjective clinical improvement, controlled clinical trials demonstrating therapeutic efficacy have not been reported. A large, randomized, double-blind placebo-controlled trial of succimer in children with blood lead concentrations between 25 and 44 mcg/dL found no evidence of benefit in clinical outcome or long-term blood lead reduction.

B. Succimer is protective against the acute lethal and nephrotoxic effects of mercuric salts in animal models and increases urinary mercury excretion in animals and humans. It, therefore, may have clinical utility in the treatment of human poisoning by inorganic mercury. In a recent animal model of methylmercury exposure during pregnancy, succimer was effective in reducing the maternal and fetal mercury burden; however, unithiol (p 630) appeared to be somewhat more potent in that setting.

C. Succimer is protective against the acute lethal effects of arsenic in animal models and may have potential utility in acute human arsenic poisoning.

III. Contraindications. History of allergy to the drug. Because succimer and its transformation products undergo renal elimination, safety and efficacy in patients with severe renal insufficiency are uncertain. There is no available evidence that succimer increases the hemodialysis clearance of toxic metals in patients with anuria.

IV. Adverse effects

A. Gastrointestinal disturbances including anorexia, nausea, vomiting, and diarrhea are the most common side effects and occur in fewer than 10% of patients. There may be a mercaptan-like odor to the urine; this has no clinical significance.

B. Mild, reversible increases in liver transaminases have been observed in less than 5% of patients.

C. Rashes, some requiring discontinuation of treatment, may occur in fewer than 5% of patients. Isolated cases of mucocutaneous reactions have been reported.

D. Isolated cases of mild to moderate neutropenia have been reported.

E. Small increases (approximately two- to fivefold) in urinary excretion of zinc and copper have been observed.

F. When administered to juvenile rats *in the absence* of antecedent lead exposure or elevated blood lead levels, succimer was associated with persistent deficits in learning, attention, and arousal. The mechanism of this effect is uncertain but might involve detrimental succimer-induced changes in zinc and/or copper status during neurodevelopment.

G. Use in pregnancy. FDA Category C (indeterminate). Succimer has produced adverse fetal effects when administered to pregnant animals in amounts one to two orders of magnitude greater than recommended human doses. However, succimer has also diminished the adverse effects of several heavy metals in animal studies. Its effect on human pregnancy has not been determined (p 498).

V. Drug or laboratory interactions. No known interactions. Concurrent administration with other chelating agents has not been studied adequately.

VI. Dosage and method of administration (adults and children)

A. Lead poisoning. Availability in the United States is limited to an oral formulation (100-mg capsules) officially approved by the FDA for use in children with blood lead levels of 45 mcg/dL or higher. DMSA can also lower blood lead concentrations in adults. ***Note:*** Administration of DMSA should never be a substitute for removal from lead exposure. In adults, the federal OSHA lead standard requires removal from occupational lead exposure of any worker with a single blood lead concentration in excess of 60 mcg/dL or an average of three successive values in excess of 50 mcg/dL; however, recent data suggest that removal at lower blood lead levels may be warranted. ***Prophylactic chelation,*** defined as the routine use of chelation to prevent elevated blood lead concentrations or lower blood lead levels below the standard in asymptomatic workers, ***is not permitted.*** Consult the local or state health department or OSHA (see Table IV–3, p 652) for more detailed information.

1. Give 10 mg/kg (children: 350 mg/m^2) orally every 8 hours for 5 days and then give the same dose every 12 hours for 2 weeks.

2. An additional course of treatment may be considered on the basis of posttreatment blood lead levels and the persistence or recurrence of symptoms. Although blood lead levels may decline by more than 50% during treatment, patients with high body lead burdens may experience rebound to within 20% of pretreatment levels as bone stores equilibrate with tissue levels. Check blood lead levels 1 and 7–21 days after chelation to assess the extent of rebound and/or the possibility of reexposure.

3. Experience with oral succimer for severe lead intoxications (ie, lead encephalopathy) is limited. In such cases, consideration should be given to parenteral therapy with calcium EDTA (p 548). In resource limited settings where parenteral calcium EDTA was unavailable, oral succimer has been successfully administered to encephalopathic children via nasogastric tube.

B. **Mercury and arsenic poisoning**

1. Intoxication by inorganic mercury compounds and arsenic compounds may result in severe gastroenteritis and shock. In such circumstances, the capacity of the gut to absorb orally administered succimer may be impaired severely, and use of an available parenteral agent such as unithiol (p 630) or BAL (p 514) may be preferable.
2. Give 10 mg/kg (or 350 mg/m^2) orally every 8 hours for 5 days and then give the same dose every 12 hours for 2 weeks. Extending the duration of treatment in the presence of continuing symptoms or high levels of urinary metal excretion should be considered but is of undetermined value.

VII. **Formulations**

A. **Oral.** Succimer, *meso*-2,3-dimercaptosuccinic acid, DMSA (Chemet), 100-mg capsules in bottles of 100 capsules. A 200-mg capsule (Succicaptal) is available in Europe.

B. **Parenteral.** A parenteral form of DMSA (sodium 2,3-dimercaptosuccinate), infused at a dosage of 1–2 g/d, has been in use in the People's Republic of China but is not available in the United States.

C. **Suggested minimum stocking levels** to treat a 100-kg adult for the first 8 hours and 24 hours: **succimer,** *first 8 hours:* 1 g or 10 capsules (100 mg each); *first 24 hours:* 3 g or 30 capsules (100 mg each).

▶ TETANUS TOXOID AND IMMUNE GLOBULIN

Joshua B. Radke, MD

I. **Pharmacology.** Tetanus is caused by tetanospasmin, a protein toxin produced by *Clostridium tetani* (see p 432).

A. **Tetanus toxoid** uses modified tetanospasmin, which has been made nontoxic but still retains the ability to stimulate the formation of antitoxin. Tetanus toxoid provides active immunization to those with known, complete tetanus immunization histories as well as those with unknown or incomplete histories.

B. Human **tetanus immune globulin** (TIG) is an antitoxin that provides passive immunity by neutralizing circulating tetanospasmin and unbound toxin in a wound. It does not have an effect on toxin that has already bound to neural tissue. Tetanus antibody does not penetrate the blood–brain barrier. ***Note:*** Some international products may be equine based.

II. **Indications.** All wound injuries require consideration of tetanus prevention and treatment. This includes animal and insect bites and stings, injections from contaminated hypodermic needles, deep puncture wounds (including high-pressure, injection-type chemical exposures such as those from paint guns), burns, and crush wounds.

A. **Tetanus toxoid prophylaxis** (active immunization) is given as a primary series of three doses in childhood. The first and second doses are given 4–8 weeks apart, and the third dose is given 6–12 months after the second. A booster dose is required every 10 years.

1. **Unknown or incomplete history** of a previous primary series of three doses: tetanus toxoid is indicated for all wounds, including clean, minor wounds.
2. **Known complete histories** of a primary series of three doses: tetanus toxoid is indicated for clean, minor wounds if it has been longer than 10 years since the last dose and for all other wounds if it has been longer than 5 years since the last dose.

B. **Tetanus Immune Globulin (TIG)** (passive immunization) **is an antitoxin** indicated for persons with tetanus. TIG is also indicated as prophylaxis for wounds that are neither clean nor minor in persons who have unknown or incomplete histories of the primary three-dose series of tetanus toxoid.

III. Contraindications

A. Toxoid

1. History of a severe allergic reaction (acute respiratory distress and collapse) after a previous dose of tetanus toxoid.
2. History of encephalopathy within 72 hours of a previous dose of tetanus toxoid.
3. Precautions should be taken in individuals with histories of fever higher than 40.5°C (104.9°F) within 48 hours of a previous dose, collapse or a shock-like state within 48 hours of a previous dose, or seizures within 72 hours of a previous dose.

B. Antitoxin. The *human* tetanus immune globulin product is the only one available in the United Sates and no contraindications are listed by the manufacturer. *Equine* tetanus antitoxin (potentially available internationally) is contraindicated in persons who have had previous hypersensitivity or serum sickness reactions to other equine-derived products.

IV. Adverse effects of the toxoid

A. Local effects, including pain, erythema, and induration at the injection site. These effects are usually self-limiting and do not require therapy.

B. Exaggerated local (Arthus-like) reactions. These unusual reactions may present as extensive painful swelling from the shoulder to the elbow. They generally occur in individuals with preexisting high serum levels of tetanus antitoxin.

C. Severe systemic reactions such as generalized urticaria, anaphylaxis, and neurologic complications have been reported. A few cases of peripheral neuropathy and Guillain–Barré syndrome have also been reported.

D. **Use in pregnancy.** FDA Category C (indeterminate). Tetanus toxoid may be used during pregnancy. Pregnant patients not previously vaccinated should receive the three-dose primary series.

V. Adverse effects of tetanus immune globulin

A. Risk of transmissible agents. TIG is made from pooled human plasma and, therefore, carries the risk of containing infectious agents such as viral hepatitis, HIV, and the causative agent for Creutzfeldt–Jacob disease. Infections thought to be transmitted by this product should be reported to the manufacturer.

B. Hypersensitivity reactions. Angioedema, nephrotic syndrome, and anaphylactic shock have been reported, rarely. Epinephrine (1:1,000) should be readily available prior to administration. Use with caution in patients with isolated IgA deficiency or a history of systemic hypersensitivity to human immunoglobulins.

C. IM administration may cause bleeding in those with increased risk, such as thrombocytopenia, hemophilia, or in those receiving anticoagulant therapy.

D. Administration precautions: Not for IV administration. Do NOT administer TIG in the same syringe as tetanus toxoid.

E. **Use in pregnancy.** FDA Category C (intermediate). Use in pregnancy only when clearly needed.

VI. Drug or laboratory interactions. None.

VII. Dosage and method of administration

A. Tetanus toxoid

1. Adult Td consists of tetanus toxoid 5 Lf U/0.5 mL and diphtheria toxoid, adsorbed 2 Lf U/0.5 mL up to 12.5 Lf U/0.5 mL. A 0.5-mL dose is given intramuscularly. Adult Td is used for routine boosters and primary vaccination in persons 7 years of age and older. Three doses constitute a primary series of Td. The first two doses are separated by a minimum of 4 weeks, with the third dose given 6–12 months after the second. Boosters are given every 10 years thereafter.
2. In children younger than 7 years, primary tetanus immunization is with tetanus toxoid in combination with diphtheria toxoid and acellular pertussis (DTaP or TDaP). Pediatric DT (without pertussis) may also be used when there is a contraindication to pertussis vaccine. At least 4 weeks should separate the first and second and the second and third doses. A fourth dose should be

given no less than 6 months after the third dose. All doses are 0.5 mL given intramuscularly and usually contain tetanus toxoid 5 Lf U/0.5 mL.

B. Human tetanus immune globulin is given at 500 units intramuscularly, which has been found to be equally effective as larger doses (3,000–10,000 IU) that have been recommended previously. In countries where human tetanus immune globulin is not available, equine antitoxin is used and should be given in doses of 1,500–3,000 IU intramuscularly. The antitoxin is given in divided doses for both children and adults, with part of the dose infiltrated around the wound.

VIII. Formulations

A. Adult. Tetanus toxoid 5 Lf U/0.5 mL in combination with diphtheria toxoid, adsorbed 2 Lf U/0.5 mL, supplied in 0.5-mL single-dose vials; tetanus toxoid 5 Lf U/0.5 mL in combination with diphtheria toxoid, adsorbed 6.6–12.5 Lf U/0.5 mL, supplied in 5-mL multiple-dose vials.

B. Pediatric. Pediatric DT, 0.5-mL single-dose vials and 5-mL multiple-dose vials; DTaP, containing diphtheria toxoid 6.7 Lf U/0.5 mL, tetanus toxoid 5 Lf U/ 0.5 mL, and pertussis vaccine four protective units/0.5 mL.

C. Human tetanus immune globulin. HyperTET S/D (solvent/detergent treated). Supplied in single-dose vials containing 250 units.

D. Suggested minimum stocking level to treat a 100-kg adult for the first 8 hours and 24 hours is a single-dose vial of Td and immune globulin.

▶ THIAMINE (THIAMIN, VITAMIN B_1)

Thomas E. Kearney, PharmD

I. Pharmacology. Thiamine (vitamin B_1) is a water-soluble vitamin that acts as an essential cofactor for various pathways of carbohydrate metabolism. Thiamine also acts as a cofactor in the metabolism of glyoxylic acid (produced in ethylene glycol intoxication). Thiamine deficiency may result in beriberi and Wernicke–Korsakoff syndrome. Thiamine is absorbed rapidly after oral, intramuscular, or intravenous administration. However, parenteral administration is recommended for initial management of thiamine deficiency syndromes.

II. Indications

A. Empiric therapy to prevent and treat Wernicke–Korsakoff syndrome in alcoholic or malnourished patients. This includes any patient presenting with an altered mental status of unknown etiology. Thiamine should be given concurrently with glucose in such cases.

B. Adjunctive treatment in patients poisoned with ethylene glycol to possibly enhance the detoxification of glyoxylic acid.

III. Contraindications. Use caution in patients with known sensitivity to thiamine or preservatives.

IV. Adverse effects

A. Anaphylactoid reactions, vasodilation, hypotension, weakness, and angioedema after rapid intravenous injection. These may be attributable to the vehicle or contaminants of thiamine preparations in the past; rare reaction with new preparations.

B. Acute pulmonary edema in patients with beriberi owing to a sudden increase in vascular resistance.

C. Use in pregnancy. FDA Category A for doses up to the recommended daily allowance (RDA) and Category C for pharmacologic doses (p 498).

V. Drug or laboratory interactions. Theoretically, thiamine may enhance the effect of neuromuscular blockers, although the clinical significance is unclear.

VI. Dosage and method of administration. Parenteral, 100 mg (children: 10–50 mg) slowly IV (over 5 minutes) or IM; may repeat every 8 hours at doses of 5–100 mg. For Wernicke encephalopathy, follow with daily parenteral doses of 50–100 mg until the patient is taking a regular diet. ***Note:*** An alternate regimen for acute Wernicke–Korsakoff syndrome uses 500 mg IV three times a day for 2–3 days, then 250 mg daily for 5 days.

VII. Formulations

A. Parenteral. Thiamine hydrochloride (various), 100 mg/mL, in 2-mL multiple-dose vials (vials may contain chlorobutanol). Protect product from light.

B. Suggested minimum stocking levels to treat a 100-kg adult for the first 8 hours and 24 hours: **thiamine hydrochloride**, *first 8 hours:* 600 mg or three multiple-dose vials (100 mg/mL, 2 mL each); *first 24 hours:* 1,000 mg or five multiple-dose vials (100 mg/mL, 2 mL each).

▶ THIOSULFATE, SODIUM

Raymond Y. Ho, PharmD

I. Pharmacology. Sodium thiosulfate is a sulfur donor that promotes the conversion of cyanide to the less toxic thiocyanate by the sulfur transferase enzyme rhodanese. Unlike nitrites, thiosulfate is essentially nontoxic and may be given empirically in suspected cyanide poisoning. Animal studies suggest enhanced antidotal efficacy when hydroxocobalamin is used with thiosulfate. Sodium thiosulfate has poor oral bioavailability. Following IV injection, sodium thiosulfate is extensively distributed into the extracellular fluids and excreted unchanged in the urine, with a reported half-life of 0.65 hours.

II. Indications

A. May be given alone or in combination with nitrites (p 592) or hydroxocobalamin (p 563) to patients with acute cyanide poisoning; may also be used as empiric treatment of possible cyanide poisoning associated with smoke inhalation.

B. Prophylaxis during nitroprusside infusions (p 593).

C. Extravasation of mechlorethamine and cisplatin (infiltrate locally [p 114]).

D. Cisplatin overdose: sodium thiosulfate binds to free platinum to form a nontoxic thiosulfate–cisplatin complex, limiting damage to renal tubules.

E. Other reported uses: bromate salt ingestion (unproven); reduced calcium urolithiasis via formation of calcium thiosulfate, which is more soluble than other urinary calcium salts, and prophylaxis for cisplatin-induced nephrotoxicity.

III. Contraindications. No known contraindications.

IV. Adverse effects

A. Intravenous (IV) infusion may produce a burning sensation, muscle cramping and twitching, and nausea and vomiting.

B. Severe anion gap acidosis was reported following daily IV infusion of 25 g of sodium thiosulfate (>3 days) in a patient with nondialysis chronic kidney disease.

C. Use in pregnancy. FDA Category C (indeterminate). This does not preclude its acute, short-term use in a seriously symptomatic patient (p 498).

V. Drug or laboratory interactions. Thiosulfate falsely lowers measured cyanide concentrations in several methods. Sodium thiosulfate and hydroxocobalamin are chemically incompatible and should not be administered in the same IV line.

VI. Dosage and method of administration

A. For cyanide poisoning. Administer 12.5 g (50 mL of 25% solution) IV over 10 minutes or at 2.5–5 mL/min. The pediatric dose is 400 mg/kg (1.6 mL/kg of 25% solution) up to 50 mL. Half the initial dose may be given after 30–60 minutes if needed.

B. For prophylaxis during nitroprusside infusions. The addition of 10 mg of thiosulfate for each milligram of nitroprusside in the IV solution has been reported to be effective and physically compatible.

C. **For cisplatin overdose.** Administer (ideally within 1–2 hours of the overdose) 4 g/m^2 of sodium thiosulfate by IV bolus over 15 minutes, followed by an infusion of 12 g/m^2 over 6 hours. Although no optimal dosing regimen has been established, it is recommended to continue maintenance dosing until urinary platinum levels are below 1 mcg/mL.

VII. **Formulations**

A. **Parenteral.** As a component of the cyanide antidote kit (Nithiodote®), thiosulfate sodium, 25% solution, one 50-mL (12.5 g) vial per kit. Also available separately in vials containing 10% (100 mg/mL) in 10 mL or 25% (250 mg/mL) in 50 mL.

B. **Suggested minimum stocking levels** to treat a 100-kg adult for the first 8 hours and 24 hours: two Nithiodote® kits, containing two 12.5-g vials of sodium thiosulfate or the equivalent as a separate stock (which is a less expensive option). Suggested for hospitals to prepare for multiple patients: two cyanide antidote kits for small hospitals, six kits for major medical centers (one kit should be kept in the emergency department). ***Note:*** Consider stocking the hydroxocobalamin antidote kit (Cyanokit®) as an alternative antidote for cyanide poisoning.

► UNITHIOL (DMPS)

Michael J. Kosnett, MD, MPH

I. **Pharmacology.** Unithiol (DMPS; 2,3-dimercaptopropanol-sulfonic acid), a dimercapto chelating agent that is a water-soluble analog of BAL (p 514), is used in the treatment of poisoning by several heavy metals, principally mercury, arsenic, and lead. Available on the official formularies of Russia and former Soviet countries since 1958 and in Germany since 1976, unithiol has been legally available from compounding pharmacists in the United States since 1999. The drug can be administered orally and parenterally. Oral bioavailability is approximately 50%, with peak blood concentrations occurring in approximately 3.7 hours. It is bound extensively to plasma proteins, mainly albumin. More than 80% of an intravenous dose is excreted in the urine, 10% as unaltered unithiol, and 90% as transformed products, predominantly cyclic DMPS sulfides. The elimination half-life for total unithiol is approximately 20 hours. Unithiol and/or its in vivo biotransformation products form complexes with a variety of inorganic and organic metal compounds, increasing excretion of the metal in the urine and decreasing its concentration in various organs, particularly the kidneys. Renal elimination of the metal chelates appears to be mediated in part by the multidrug resistance protein 2 (Mrp2). Unlike BAL, unithiol does not redistribute mercury to the brain.

II. **Indications**

A. Unithiol has been used primarily in the treatment of intoxication by **mercury, arsenic**, and **lead**. In animal models, unithiol has averted or reduced the acute toxic effects of inorganic mercury salts and inorganic arsenic when administered promptly (minutes to hours) after exposure. Unithiol is associated with a reduction in tissue levels of mercury, arsenic, and lead in experimental animals, and it increases the excretion of those metals in humans. However, randomized, double-blind, placebo-controlled clinical trials demonstrating therapeutic efficacy in acute or chronic heavy metal poisoning have not been reported.

B. Animal studies and a few case reports suggest that unithiol may have utility in the treatment of poisoning by **bismuth** compounds. Animal studies suggest that unithiol may increase survival after acute exposure to **polonium 210;** however, redistribution to the kidneys may occur.

III. Contraindications

A. History of allergy to the drug.

B. Because renal excretion is the predominant route of elimination of unithiol and its metal complexes, caution is warranted in administering unithiol to patients with severe renal insufficiency. Published reports support the use of unithiol as an adjunct to high flux hemodialysis or hemodiafiltration in patients with anuric renal failure caused by mercury salts and bismuth.

IV. Adverse effects

A. The German manufacturer (Heyl) notes a low overall incidence (<4%) of adverse side effects.

B. Self-limited, reversible allergic dermatologic reactions such as exanthems and urticaria have been the most commonly reported adverse effect. Isolated cases of major allergic reactions, including erythema multiforme and Stevens–Johnson syndrome, have been reported.

C. Because rapid intravenous administration may be associated with vasodilation and transient hypotension, intravenous injections of unithiol should be administered slowly, over a 15- to 20-minute interval.

D. Unithiol increases the urinary excretion of copper and zinc, an effect that is not anticipated to be clinically significant in standard courses of treatment in patients without preexisting deficiency of these trace elements.

E. Use in pregnancy. Unithiol did not exhibit teratogenicity or other developmental toxicity in animal studies. Although protection against the adverse reproductive effects of selected toxic metals has been demonstrated in pregnant animals, there is insufficient clinical experience with the use of unithiol in human pregnancy.

V. Drug or laboratory interactions

A. Aqueous solutions of unithiol for intravenous injection should not be mixed with other drugs or minerals. Oral preparations should not be consumed simultaneously with mineral supplements.

B. Unithiol has been shown to form a complex with an arsenic metabolite, monomethylarsonous acid (MMA^{III}), which then is excreted in the urine. Laboratory techniques that use hydride reduction to measure urinary arsenic and its metabolites ("speciation") may not detect this complex. However, the complex will contribute to measurement of "total urinary arsenic."

VI. Dosage and method of administration. Unithiol may be administered by the oral, intramuscular, and intravenous routes. The intravenous route should be reserved for the treatment of severe acute intoxication by inorganic mercury salts or arsenic when compromised GI or cardiovascular status may interfere with rapid or efficient absorption from the GI tract. In animal models, oral unithiol did not increase the GI absorption of mercuric chloride.

A. Severe acute poisoning by inorganic mercury or arsenic. Administer 3–5 mg/kg every 4 hours by slow intravenous infusion over 20 minutes. If, after several days, the patient's GI and cardiovascular status has stabilized, consider changing to oral unithiol, 4–8 mg/kg every 6–8 hours.

B. Symptomatic poisoning by lead (without encephalopathy). Oral unithiol, 4–8 mg/kg orally every 6–8 hours, may be considered an alternative to succimer (p 624). ***Note:*** Parenteral therapy with EDTA (p 548) is preferable for the treatment of patients with severe lead intoxication (lead encephalopathy or lead colic) and for patients with extremely high blood lead concentrations (eg, blood lead >150 mcg/dL).

C. Mobilization or "chelation challenge" tests measuring an increase in urinary excretion of mercury and arsenic after a single dose of unithiol have been described, but their diagnostic or prognostic value has not been established.

VII. Formulations

A. In the United States, compounding pharmacists (including those in hospital inpatient pharmacies) may obtain bulk quantities of pharmaceutical-grade unithiol and dispense it as an injection solution for infusion (usually 50 mg/mL in sterile water). Capsules (typically in 100- or 300-mg sizes) may also be prepared in an oral dose form. ***Note:*** Bulk unithiol must be obtained outside the United States, and such supplies should have a certificate of analysis to ensure product purity.

B. Suggested minimum stocking levels to treat a 100-kg adult for the first 8 hours and 24 hours: **unithiol**, *first 8 hours:* 1 g; *first 24 hours:* 3 g.

► VASOPRESSIN

Ben Tsutaoka, PharmD

I. Pharmacology

A. Vasopressin is a peptide hormone that is synthesized in the hypothalamus. The primary stimuli for endogenous physiologic release are hyperosmolality, hypotension, and hypovolemia. It is used in the critical care setting for severe catecholamine-resistant vasodilatory shock, in which case, it acts as a potent vasoconstrictor. Conditions in which vasopressin has been used include septic shock, postcardiotomy shock, and hemorrhagic shock. There are insufficient and conflicting human and animal data to recommend its use routinely to manage shock from poisoning. Further data are needed to define its risks, benefits, and optimum dose. Increases in arterial pressure should be evident within 15 minutes. Its serum half-life is less than 10 minutes.

II. Indications

A. ***Note:*** Vasopressin should not be used as a first-line agent to treat hypotension. It is used as add-on therapy to treat severe vasodilator hypotension that is unresponsive or refractory to one or more adrenergic agents (eg, high-dose dopamine, epinephrine, norepinephrine, phenylephrine). There are limited case reports in the medical literature in which vasopressin was used for drug overdose.

B. As a means to reduce adrenergic agent requirements during the treatment of vasodilator hypotension.

III. Contraindications

A. Vasopressin infusion should be discontinued if there is a decrease in the cardiac index and/or stroke volume. ***Note:*** Serious consideration should be given to monitoring cardiac indexes invasively via a pulmonary artery catheter to titrate hemodynamic effects and dosing.

B. Use with extreme caution if there is evidence of decreased cardiac output despite adequate intravascular volume or evidence of cardiogenic shock.

C. Vasopressin should be used cautiously in treating a patient with an overdose of an agent that has myocardial depressant effects (eg, calcium channel blockers, beta-blockers).

IV. Adverse effects

A. Negative inotropic effect. Vasopressin may result in a decrease in the cardiac index. This may be attributed to an increase in systemic vascular resistance and afterload on a depressed myocardium or may be related in part to a compensatory decrease in the heart rate. Dobutamine and milrinone have been used in conjunction with vasopressin in attempts to attenuate this negative inotropic effect.

B. Ischemia (especially at doses >0.05 U/min).

1. Cardiac arrest has been reported at doses above 0.05 U/min.
2. Ischemic skin lesions of the distal extremities and trunk and lingual regions.
3. Mesenteric ischemia and hepatitis may occur.

C. Hyponatremia

D. Thrombocytopenia

E. **Use in pregnancy.** FDA Category C (p 498). There are no reports linking the use of vasopressin with congenital defects. Vasopressin and the related synthetic agents desmopressin and lypressin have been used during pregnancy to treat diabetes insipidus. Vasopressin and structurally related polypeptides may increase the frequency and amplitude of uterine contractions.

V. **Dosage and method of administration**

A. Intravenous infusion at 0.01–0.04 U/min. Vasopressin should be diluted with normal saline or 5% dextrose in water to a final concentration of 0.1–1 U/mL.

1. Doses of up to 0.07–0.1 U/min have been used for patients in septic shock or with postcardiotomy vasodilatory shock. However, doses higher than 0.04 U/min are associated with a greater incidence of adverse effects.
2. Administration through central venous access is recommended to minimize the risk of extravasation. Local skin necrosis has occurred when vasopressin was infused through a peripheral venous catheter.

B. Once an adequate blood pressure is achieved and stabilized, steps should be taken to reduce the doses of adrenergic agents and vasopressin gradually.

VI. **Formulations**

A. Vasopressin (Vasostrict®): 20 U/mL, 1-mL vial.

B. **Suggested minimum stocking levels** to treat a 100-kg adult for the first 8 hours and 24 hours: **vasopressin**, *first 8 hours*: 20 U or one vial (20 U/mL, 1 mL each); *first 24 hours*: 60 U or three vials (20 U/mL, 1 mL each).

► VITAMIN K_1 (PHYTONADIONE)

Thomas E. Kearney, PharmD

I. **Pharmacology.** Vitamin K_1 is an essential cofactor in the hepatic synthesis of coagulation factors II, VII, IX, and X. In adequate doses, vitamin K_1 reverses the inhibitory effects of coumarin and indanedione derivatives on the synthesis of these factors. ***Note:*** **Vitamin K_3 (menadione) is *not* effective** in reversing excessive anticoagulation caused by these agents. After parenteral vitamin K_1 administration, there is a 6- to 8-hour delay before vitamin K–dependent coagulation factors begin to achieve significant levels, and peak effects are not seen until 1–2 days after the initiation of therapy. The duration of effect is 5–10 days. The response to vitamin K_1 is variable, and the optimal dosage regimen is unknown; it is influenced by the potency and amount of the ingested anticoagulant, vitamin K pharmacokinetics, and the patient's hepatic biosynthetic capability.

II. **Indications**

A. Excessive anticoagulation caused by coumarin and indanedione derivatives, as evidenced by an elevated prothrombin time (p 459). Vitamin K_1 is ***not*** indicated for empiric treatment of anticoagulant ingestion, as most cases do not require treatment, and its use will delay the onset of an elevated prothrombin time as a marker of a toxic ingestion.

B. Vitamin K deficiency (eg, malnutrition, malabsorption, or hemorrhagic disease of the newborn) with coagulopathy.

C. Hypoprothrombinemia resulting from salicylate intoxication.

III. **Contraindications.** Do not use in patients with known hypersensitivity to vitamin K or preservatives.

IV. **Adverse effects**

A. **Black box warning.** Anaphylactoid reactions have been reported after intravenous administration and have been associated with fatalities. Although these are rare (incidence of 3 cases per 10,000 doses), intravenous use should be restricted to true emergencies; the patient must be monitored closely in an intensive care setting, and reducing the infusion rate may reduce the risk.

Severe reactions and fatalities have also been associated with intramuscular administration and resembled hypersensitivity reactions.

B. Intramuscular administration in patients receiving anticoagulants may cause large, painful hematomas. This can be avoided by using the oral or subcutaneous route.

C. Patients receiving anticoagulants for medical reasons (eg, deep vein thrombosis or prosthetic heart valves) may experience untoward effects from complete reversal of their anticoagulation status. Therapy in such patients should be based on the INR and presence or risk of bleeding.

D. Use in pregnancy. FDA Category C (indeterminate). Vitamin K_1 crosses the placenta readily. However, this does not preclude its acute, short-term use in a seriously symptomatic patient (p 498).

V. Drug or laboratory interactions. Empiric use after an acute anticoagulant overdose will delay (for up to several days) the onset of elevation of the prothrombin time, and this may give a false impression of insignificant ingestion in a case of serious "superwarfarin" overdose (p 459).

VI. Dosage and method of administration

A. Oral.

1. Reversal of therapeutic warfarin effect:
   - **a.** If INR less than 5 and no significant bleeding: hold warfarin dose, no vitamin K needed.
   - **b.** If INR 5–9 and no bleeding: hold warfarin dose and administer small titrated oral doses (1–2.5 mg) of vitamin K.
   - **c.** If INR exceeds 9 and no bleeding present, or only minor bleeding present regardless of INR: hold warfarin dose and administer 2.5–5 mg of oral vitamin K.
   - **d.** If serious hemorrhage is present (regardless of INR): hold warfarin dose and administer 10 mg of vitamin K orally or by slow IV infusion (see warning below). ***Note:*** For more rapid restoration of active clotting factors, use fresh frozen plasma or clotting factor replacement products (see p 534).
   - **e.** Adjunctive anticoagulation with heparin may be required until the desired prothrombin time is achieved.
2. Long-acting anticoagulant rodenticide poisoning. The usual dose of vitamin K_1 (***not*** menadione or vitamin K_3) is 10–50 mg two to four times a day in adults and 5–10 mg (or 0.4 mg/kg per dose) two to four times a day in children. Recheck the prothrombin time after 48 hours and increase the dose as needed. ***Note:*** Very high daily doses of 50–250 mg (typical daily dose is 100 mg) and up to 800 mg have been required in adults with brodifacoum poisoning; in addition, treatment for several weeks or months may be needed because of the long duration of effect of the "superwarfarin." Because the only available oral vitamin K_1 formulation is 5 mg, high-dose treatment may require patients to ingest up to 100 pills per day, and long-term compliance with the regimen is often problematic.

B. Parenteral injection is an alternative route of administration for patients with life-threatening or serious bleeding but is not likely to result in more rapid reversal of anticoagulant effects and is associated with potentially serious side effects. Subcutaneous administration is preferred over IM injection, although both can cause hematomas. The maximum volume is 5 mL or 50 mg per dose per injection site. The adult dose is 10–25 mg, and that for children is 1–5 mg; this may be repeated in 6–8 hours. Switch to oral therapy as soon as possible. Intravenous administration is used only rarely because of the risk for an anaphylactoid reaction. The usual dose is 10–25 mg (0.6 mg/kg in children younger than 12 years), depending on the severity of anticoagulation, diluted in preservative-free dextrose or sodium chloride solution. Give slowly at a rate not to exceed 1 mg/min or 5% of the total dose per minute, whichever is slower.

VII. Formulations. ***Note:*** Do ***not*** use menadione (vitamin K_3).

A. Parenteral. Phytonadione (AquaMEPHYTON and others), 2 mg/mL in 0.5-mL ampules and prefilled syringes, and 10 mg/mL in 1-mL ampules (ampules contain a fatty acid derivative and benzyl alcohol or propylene glycol).

B. Oral. Phytonadione (Mephyton), 5-mg tablets.

C. Suggested minimum stocking levels to treat a 100-kg adult for the first 8 hours and 24 hours: **phytonadione**, *first 8 hours:* 50 mg or 10 tablets (5 mg each) and five 1-mL (10 mg) ampules or the equivalent; *first 24 hours:* 100 mg or 20 tablets (5 mg each) and ten 1-mL (10 mg) ampules or the equivalent.

SECTION IV. Environmental and Occupational Toxicology

▶ EMERGENCY MEDICAL RESPONSE TO HAZARDOUS MATERIALS INCIDENTS

Kent R. Olson, MD and R. Steven Tharratt, MD, MPVM

With the constant threat of accidental releases of hazardous materials and the potential criminal use of chemical weapons, local emergency response providers must be prepared to handle victims who may be contaminated with chemical substances. Many local jurisdictions have developed hazardous materials (HazMat) teams; these usually are composed of fire, environmental, and paramedical personnel trained to identify hazardous situations quickly and take the lead in organizing a response. Health care providers such as ambulance personnel, nurses, physicians, and local hospital officials should participate in emergency response planning and drills with their local HazMat team before a chemical disaster occurs.

I. **General considerations.** The most important principles of successful medical management of a hazardous materials incident are the following:
   - A. Use extreme caution when dealing with unknown or unstable conditions.
   - B. Rapidly assess the potential hazard severity of the substances involved.
   - C. Determine the potential for secondary contamination of nearby personnel and facilities.
   - D. Perform any needed decontamination at the scene ***before*** victim transport, if possible.

II. **Organization.** Chemical incidents are managed under the Standardized Emergency Management System (SEMS). Integral to this system is the use of the **incident command system.** The incident commander or scene manager is usually the senior representative of the agency that has primary traffic investigative authority, but this authority may be delegated to a senior fire or health official. The first priorities of the incident commander are to secure the area, establish a command post, create hazard zones, and provide for the decontamination and immediate prehospital care of any victims. However, hospitals must be prepared to manage victims who leave the scene before teams arrive and may arrive at the emergency department unannounced, possibly contaminated, and needing medical attention.
   - A. **Hazard zones** (Figure IV–1) are determined by the nature of the spilled substance and the wind and geographic conditions. In general, the command post and support area are located upwind and uphill from the incident, with sufficient distance to allow rapid escape if conditions change.
     1. The **exclusion zone** (also known as the "hot" or "red" zone) is the area immediately adjacent to the chemical incident. This area may be extremely hazardous to persons without appropriate protective equipment. Only properly trained and equipped personnel should enter this zone, and they may require comprehensive decontamination when leaving the zone.
     2. The **contamination reduction zone** (also known as the "warm" or "yellow" zone) is where victims and rescuers are decontaminated before undergoing further medical assessment and prehospital care. Because of the limitations posed by protective equipment, patients in the exclusion zone and contamination reduction zone generally receive only rudimentary first aid and/or immediately life-saving interventions until they are decontaminated.
     3. The **support zone** (also known as the "cold" or "green" zone) is where the incident commander, support teams, media, medical treatment areas, and ambulances are situated. It is usually upwind, uphill, and a safe distance from the incident.

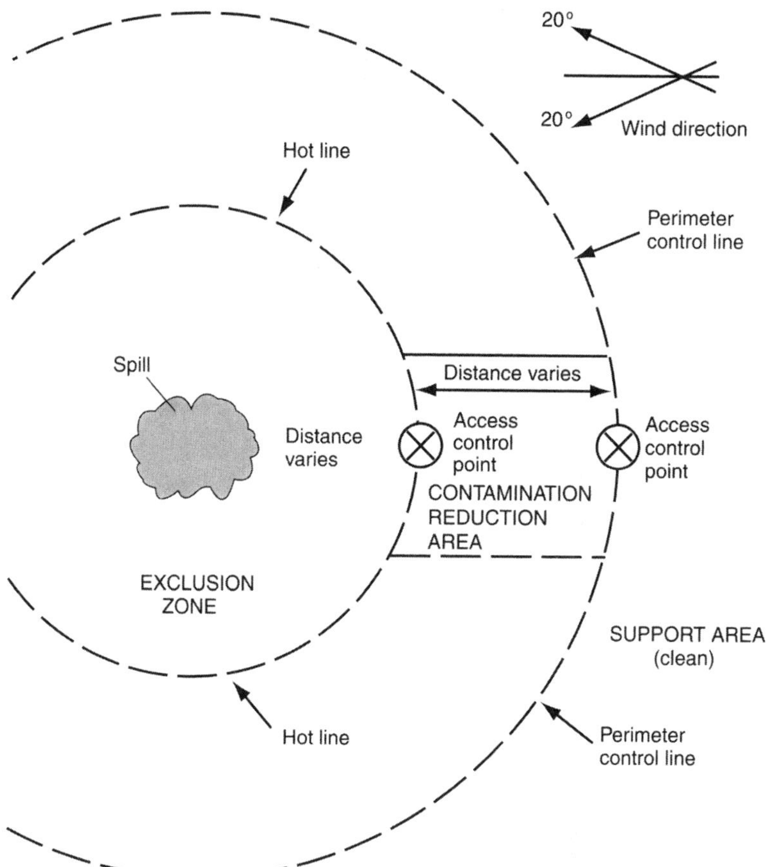

FIGURE IV–1. Control zones at a hazardous materials incident site.

B. Medical officer. A member of the HazMat team should already have been designated to be in charge of health and safety. This person is responsible, with help from the technical reference specialist, for determining the nature of the chemicals, the likely severity of their health effects, the need for specialized personal protective gear, the type and degree of decontamination required, and the supervision of triage and prehospital care. In addition, the medical officer, with the site safety officer, supervises the safety of response workers at the emergency site and monitors entry to and exit from the spill site. This person may also be in contact with receiving hospitals regarding the medical care and needs of the victims.

III. Assessment of hazard potential. Be prepared to recognize dangerous situations and respond appropriately. The potential for toxic or other types of injury depends on the chemicals involved, their toxicity, their chemical and physical properties, the conditions of exposure, and the circumstances surrounding their release. Be aware that the reactivity, flammability, explosiveness, or corrosiveness of a substance may be a source of greater hazard than its systemic toxicity.

Do not depend on your senses for safety, even though sensory input (eg, smell) may give clues to the nature of the hazard.

A. Identify the substances involved. Make inquiries and look for labels, warning placards, and shipping papers.

1. The **National Fire Protection Association (NFPA)** has developed a labeling system for describing chemical hazards that is widely used (Figure IV–2).
2. The **US Department of Transportation (DOT)** has developed a system of warning placards for vehicles carrying hazardous materials. The DOT placards usually bear a four-digit substance identification code and a single-digit hazard classification code (Figure IV–3). Identification of the substance from the four-digit code can be provided by the regional poison control center, CHEMTREC, or the DOT manual (see Item B below).
3. **Shipping papers,** which may include material safety data sheets (MSDSs), usually are carried by a driver or pilot or may be found in the truck cab or pilot's compartment.

B. Obtain toxicity information. Determine the acute health effects and obtain advice on general hazards, decontamination procedures, and the medical management of victims. Resources include the following:

1. **Regional poison control centers** (1-800-222-1222). The regional poison control center can provide information on immediate health effects, the need for decontamination or specialized protective gear, and specific treatment, including the use of antidotes. The regional center can also provide consultation with a medical toxicologist.
2. **CHEMTREC** (1-800-424-9300). Operated by the American Chemistry Council, this 24-hour hotline can provide information on the identity and hazardous properties of chemicals and, when appropriate, can put the caller in touch with industry representatives and medical toxicologists.

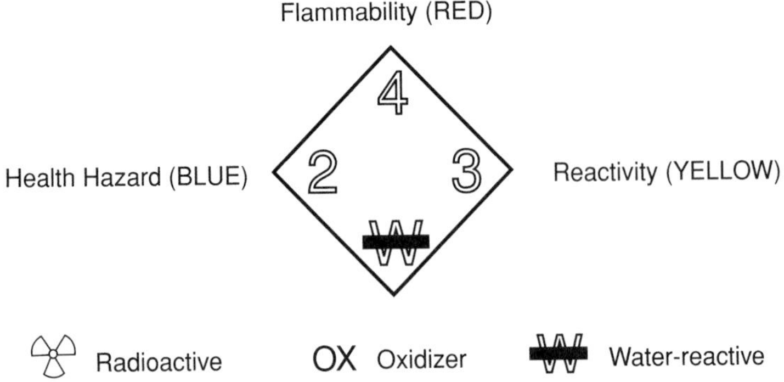

FIGURE IV–2. National Fire Protection Association (NFPA) identification of the hazards of materials (this page) and health hazard rating chart (next page). (Reprinted with permission from *NFPA 704-2017, System for the Identification of the Hazards of Materials for Emergency Response,* Copyright © 2016, National Fire Protection Association. This reprinted material is not the complete and official position of the NFPA on the referenced subject, which is represented solely by the standard in its entirety.) (*continued on next page*)

Degree of Hazard	Gas/Vapor: Inhalation LC_{50} (ppm-v)	Gas/Vapor: Saturated Vapor Concentration ($\times LC_{50}$ in ppm-v)	Dust/Mist Inhalation LC_{50} (mg/L)	Oral LD_{50} (mg/kg)	Dermal LD_{50} (mg/kg)	Skin/Eye Contact
4	0 to 1,000	10 to >10	0.00 to 0.5	0.00 to 5	0 to 40	—
3	1,001 to 3,000	1 to <10	0.51 to 2	5.01 to 50	40.1 to 200	Corrosive, irreversible eye injury Corrosive if pH ≤2 or ≥11.5
2	3,001 to 5,000	0.2 to <1	2.01 to 10	50.1 to 500	201 to 1,000	Severe irritation, reversible injury Sensitizers Lacrimators Frostbite from compressed liquefied gases
1	5,001 to 10,000	0 to <0.2	10.1 to 200	501 to 2,000	1,001 to 2,000	Slight to moderate eye irritation Mild irritation is borderline 0/1
0	>10,000	0 to <0.2	>200	>2,000	>2,000	Essentially nonirritating

FIGURE IV–2. (*Continued*) National Fire Protection Association (NFPA) health hazard rating chart.

EXAMPLE OF PLACARD AND PANEL WITH ID NUMBER

The Identification Number (ID No.) may be displayed on placards or on orange panels on tanks. Check the sides of the transport vehicle if the ID number is not displayed on the ends of the vehicle.

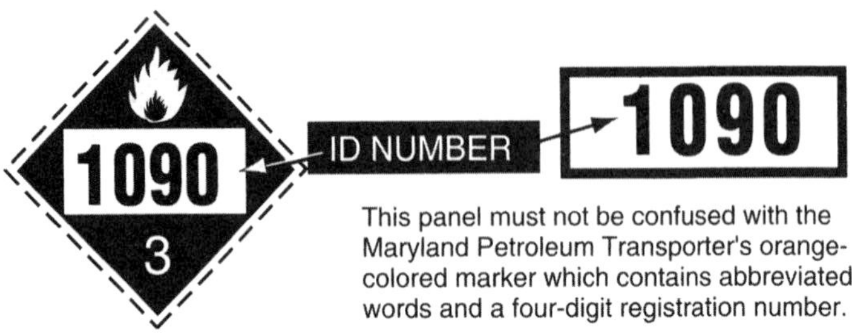

1090
3
ID NUMBER
1090
This panel must not be confused with the Maryland Petroleum Transporter's orange-colored marker which contains abbreviated words and a four-digit registration number.

FIGURE IV–3. Example of US Department of Transportation (DOT) vehicle warning placard and panel with DOT identification number.

3. See Table IV–4 (p 659) and specific chemicals covered in Section II of this manual.
4. A variety of texts, journals, and computerized information systems are available but are of uneven scope or depth. See the reference list at the end of this section.

C. **Recognize dangerous environments.** In general, environments likely to expose rescuers to the same conditions that caused grave injury to the victim(s) are not safe for unprotected entry. **These situations require trained and properly equipped rescue personnel.** Examples include the following:
1. Any indoor environment where the victim was rendered unconscious or otherwise disabled.
2. Environments causing acute onset of symptoms in rescuers, such as chest tightness, shortness of breath, eye or throat irritation, coughing, dizziness, headache, nausea, and loss of coordination.
3. Confined spaces such as large tanks or crawl spaces. (Their poor ventilation and small size can result in extremely high levels of airborne contaminants. In addition, such spaces permit only a slow or strenuous exit, which may become physically impossible for an intoxicated individual.)
4. Spills involving substances with poor warning properties or high vapor pressures, especially when they occur in an indoor or enclosed environment. Substances with poor warning properties can cause serious injury without any warning signs of exposure, such as smell and eye irritation. High vapor pressures increase the likelihood that dangerous air concentrations may be present. Also note that gases or vapors with a density greater than that of air may become concentrated in low-lying areas.

D. **Determine the potential for secondary contamination.** Although the threat of secondary contamination of emergency response personnel, equipment, and nearby facilities *may* be significant, it varies widely, depending on the chemical, its concentration, and whether basic decontamination has already been performed. Not all toxic substances carry a risk for secondary contamination, even though they may be extremely hazardous to rescuers in the hot zone. Exposures involving inhalation only and no external contamination generally do not pose a risk for secondary contamination.
1. Examples of substances with **no significant risk** for secondary contamination of personnel outside the hot zone are **gases**, such as carbon monoxide,

arsine, and chlorine, and **vapors,** such as those from xylene, toluene, and perchloroethylene.

2. Examples of substances that have **significant potential** for secondary contamination and require aggressive decontamination and protection of nearby personnel include potent organophosphorus insecticides, oily nitrogen-containing compounds, and highly radioactive compounds such as cesium and plutonium.
3. In many cases involving substances with a high potential for secondary contamination, this risk can be minimized by removing grossly contaminated clothing and thoroughly cleansing the body in the contamination reduction corridor, including washing with soap or shampoo. After these measures are followed, only rarely will the members of the medical team face significant, persistent personal threat to their health from an exposed victim.

IV. Personal protective equipment. Personal protective equipment includes chemical-resistant clothing and gloves and protective respiratory gear. The use of such equipment should be supervised by experts in industrial hygiene or others with appropriate training and experience. Particular care should be given to donning and removing protective equipment. Equipment that is incorrectly selected, improperly fitted, poorly maintained, or inappropriately used may provide a false sense of security and may fail, resulting in secondary contamination or serious injury.

A. Protective clothing may be as simple as a disposable apron or as sophisticated as a fully encapsulated chemical-resistant suit. However, no chemical-resistant clothing is completely impervious to all chemicals over the full range of exposure conditions. Each suit is rated for its resistance to specific chemicals, and many are also rated for chemical breakthrough time.

B. Protective respiratory gear may be a simple paper mask, a cartridge filter respirator, or a positive-pressure air-supplied respirator. Respirators must be properly fitted for each user.

1. **A paper mask** may provide partial protection against gross quantities of airborne dust particles but does not prevent exposure to gases, vapors, and fumes.
2. **Cartridge filter respirators** filter certain chemical gases and vapors out of the ambient air. They are used only when the toxic substance is known to be adsorbed by the filter, the airborne concentration is low, and there is adequate oxygen in the ambient air.
3. **Air-supplied respirators** provide an independent source of clean air. They may be fully self-contained units or masks supplied with air by a long hose. A **self-contained breathing apparatus** (SCBA) has a limited duration of air supply, from 5 to 30 minutes. Users must be fitted for their specific gear.

V. Victim management. Victim management includes rapid stabilization and removal from the exclusion zone, initial decontamination, delivery to emergency medical services personnel at the support zone perimeter, and medical assessment and treatment in the support area. Usually, only the HazMat team or other personnel with appropriate training and protective gear will be responsible for rescue from the hot zone, where skin and respiratory protection may be critical. Emergency medical personnel without specific training and appropriate equipment must not enter the hot zone unless it is determined to be safe by the incident commander and the medical officer.

A. Stabilization in the exclusion zone. If there is suspicion of trauma, the patient should be placed on a backboard, with a cervical collar applied if appropriate. Position the patient so that the airway remains open. Gross contamination may be brushed off the patient. No further medical intervention can be expected from rescuers who are wearing bulky suits, masks, and heavy gloves. Therefore, every effort should be made to get a seriously ill patient out of this area as quickly as possible. Victims who are ambulatory should be directed to walk to the contamination reduction area.

B. **Initial decontamination.** Gross decontamination may take place in the exclusion zone (eg, brushing off chemical powder and removing soaked clothing), but most decontamination occurs in the contamination reduction corridor before the victim is transferred to waiting emergency medical personnel in the support area. Do not delay critical treatment while decontaminating the victim unless the nature of the contaminant makes such treatment too dangerous. Consult a regional poison control center (1-800-222-1222) for specific advice on decontamination. See also Section I, p 50.

1. Remove contaminated clothing and flush exposed skin, hair, or eyes with copious plain water from a high-volume, low-pressure hose. For oily substances, additional washing with soap or shampoo may be required. Ambulatory, cooperative victims may be able to perform their own decontamination.
2. For eye exposures, remove contact lenses if present and irrigate eyes with plain water or, if available, normal saline dribbled from an intravenous bag. Continue irrigation until symptoms resolve or, if the contaminant is an acid or base, until the pH of the conjunctival sac is nearly normal (pH 6–8).
3. Double-bag and save all removed clothing and jewelry.
4. Collect runoff water if possible, but generally rapid flushing of exposed skin or eyes should not be delayed because of environmental concerns. Remember that protection of health takes precedence over environmental concerns in a hazardous materials incident.
5. In the majority of incidents, basic victim decontamination as outlined earlier will substantially reduce or eliminate the potential for secondary contamination of nearby personnel or equipment. Procedures for cleaning equipment are contaminant-specific and depend on the risk for chemical persistence as well as toxicity.

C. **Treatment in the support area.** Once the patient is decontaminated (if required) and released into the support area, triage, basic medical assessment, and treatment by emergency medical providers may begin. In the majority of incidents, once the victim has been removed from the hot zone and is stripped and flushed, there is little or no risk for secondary contamination of these providers, and sophisticated protective gear is not necessary. Simple surgical latex gloves, a plain apron, or disposable outer clothing is generally sufficient.

1. Maintain a patent airway and assist breathing if necessary (pp 1–7). Administer supplemental oxygen.
2. Provide supportive care for shock (p 15), arrhythmias (pp 10–15), coma (p 18), or seizures (p 23).
3. Treat with specific antidotes if appropriate and available.
4. Further skin, hair, or eye washing may be necessary.
5. Take notes on the probable or suspected level of exposure for each victim, the initial symptoms and signs, and the treatment provided. For victims exposed to chemicals with delayed toxic effects, this can be lifesaving.

VI. **Ambulance transport and hospital treatment.** For skin or inhalation exposures, no special precautions should be required if adequate decontamination has been carried out in the field before transport.

A. **Patients who have ingested toxic substances** may vomit en route; carry a large plastic bag–lined basin and extra towels to soak up and immediately isolate spillage. Vomitus may contain the original toxic material or even toxic gases created by the action of stomach acid on the substance (eg, hydrogen cyanide from ingested cyanide salts). When performing gastric lavage in the emergency department, isolate gastric washings if possible (eg, with a closed-wall suction container system).

B. For unpredictable situations in which **a contaminated victim arrives at the hospital before decontamination,** it is important to have a strategy ready that will minimize exposure of hospital personnel.

1. Ask the local HazMat team to set up a contamination reduction area outside the hospital emergency department entrance. However, keep in mind that all teams may already be committed and not available to assist.
2. Prepare in advance a hose with warm water at about 30°C (86°F), soap, and an old gurney for rapid decontamination ***outside*** the emergency department entrance. Have a child's inflatable pool or another container ready to collect water runoff, if possible. However, do not delay patient decontamination if water runoff cannot be contained easily.
3. Do not bring patients soaked with liquids into the emergency department until they have been stripped and flushed outside, as the liquids may emit gas vapors and cause illness among hospital staff.
4. For incidents involving radioactive materials or other highly contaminating substances that are not volatile, use the hospital's radiation accident protocol, which generally will include the following:
   a. Restricted access zones.
   b. Isolation of ventilation ducts leading out of the treatment room to prevent the spread of contamination throughout the hospital.
   c. Paper covering for floors and use of absorbent materials if liquids are involved.
   d. Protective clothing for hospital staff (gloves, paper masks, shoe covers, caps, and gowns).
   e. Double-bagging and saving all contaminated clothing and equipment.
   f. Monitoring to detect the extent and persistence of contamination (ie, using a radiation monitor for radiation incidents).
   g. Notifying appropriate local, state, and federal offices of the incident and obtaining advice on laboratory testing and decontamination of equipment.

VII. Summary. The emergency medical response to a hazardous materials incident requires prior training and planning to protect the health of response personnel and victims.

A. Response plans and training should be flexible. The level of hazard and the required actions vary greatly with the circumstances at the scene and the chemicals involved.

B. First responders should be able to do the following:

C. Recognize potentially hazardous situations.

D. Take steps to protect themselves from injury.

E. Obtain accurate information about the identity and toxicity of each chemical substance involved.

F. Use appropriate protective gear.

G. Perform victim decontamination before transport to a hospital.

H. Provide appropriate first aid and advanced supportive measures as needed.

I. Coordinate their actions with those of other responding agencies, such as the HazMat team, police and fire departments, and regional poison control centers.

USEFUL RESOURCES

Agency for Toxic Substances & Disease Registry (ATSDR): Managing Hazardous Materials Incidents (MHMIs). http://www.atsdr.cdc.gov/MHMI/index.asp (An excellent resource for planning as well as emergency care, including prehospital and hospital management and guidelines for triage and decontamination.) The ATSDR can also provide 24-hour assistance in emergencies involving hazardous substances in the environment at 1-770-488-7100.

Centers for Disease Control and Prevention: NIOSH Pocket Guide to Occupational Hazards. http://www.cdc.gov/niosh/npg (An excellent summary of workplace exposure limits and other useful information about the most common industrial chemicals.)

US Department of Transportation Pipeline and Hazardous Materials Safety Administration: Emergency Response Guidebook (ERG2008). http://phmsa.dot.gov/hazmat/library/erg

US National Library of Medicine: Wireless Information System for Emergency Responders (WISER). http://wiser.nlm.nih.gov (WISER is a system designed to assist first responders in hazardous material incidents. WISER provides a wide range of information on hazardous substances, including substance identification support, physical characteristics, human health information, and containment and suppression advice. It is freely available as a web-based tool, a downloadable freestanding version, or a mobile download for various mobile devices.)

▶ EVALUATION OF THE PATIENT WITH OCCUPATIONAL CHEMICAL EXPOSURE

Paul D. Blanc, MD, MSPH

This chapter highlights common toxicologic problems in the workplace. Occupationally related disease is encountered commonly in the outpatient setting. Estimates of the proportion of occupationally related medical problems in primary care practices range up to 15–20%, although this includes many patients with musculoskeletal complaints. However, approximately 5% of all symptomatic poison control center consultations are occupational in nature, suggesting a large number of work-related chemical exposures do occur.

I. General considerations

A. Occupational illness is rarely pathognomonic. The connection between illness and workplace factors is typically obscure unless a specific effort is made to link exposure to disease.

1. Massive or catastrophic events leading to the acute onset of symptoms, such as release of an irritant gas, are relatively uncommon but easily recognized.
2. For most workplace exposures, symptom onset is more often insidious, following a subacute or chronic pattern, as in heavy metal (e.g., lead) poisoning.
3. Long latency, often years between exposure and disease, makes linking cause and effect even more difficult—for example, in chronic lung disease or occupationally related cancer.

B. Occupational evaluation frequently includes legal and administrative components.

1. Occupational illness, even if suspected but not established, may be a reportable illness in certain states (eg, in California through its Doctor's First Report system).
2. Establishing quantifiable documentation of adverse effects at the time of exposure may be critical to future attribution of impairment (eg, spirometric evaluation soon after an irritant inhalant exposure).
3. Although workers' compensation is in theory a straightforward "no-fault" insurance system, in practice it often is arcane and adversarial. It is important to remember that the person being treated is the patient, not the employer or a referring attorney.

II. Components of the occupational exposure history

A. Job and job process

1. Ask specifics about the job. Do not rely on descriptions limited to a general occupation or trade, such as "machinist," "painter," "electronics worker," or "farmer."
2. Describe the industrial process and equipment used on the job. If power equipment is used, ascertain how it is powered to assess carbon monoxide exposure risk.
3. Determine whether the work process uses a closed system (eg, a sealed reaction vat) or an open system. Ascertain what other processes or workstations

are nearby. Work under a laboratory hood may be an effectively "closed" system, but not if the window is raised too far or if the airflow is not appropriately calibrated.

4. Find out who does maintenance and how often it is done.

B. Level of exposure

1. Ask whether dust, fumes, or mist can be seen in the air at the work site (even an outdoor work environment). If so, question whether coworkers or nearby objects can be seen clearly (very high levels actually obscure sight). A history of dust-laden sputum or nasal discharge at the end of the work shift is also a marker of heavy exposure.
2. Ask whether work surfaces are dusty or damp and whether the paint at the work site is peeling or discolored (eg, from a corrosive atmosphere).
3. Determine whether strong smells or tastes are present and, if so, whether they diminish over time, suggesting olfactory fatigue.
4. Find out whether there is any special ventilation system and where the fresh air intake is located (toxicants can be entrained and recirculated by a poorly placed air intake system).
5. Establish whether the person has direct skin contact with the materials worked with, especially solvents or other liquid chemicals.
6. Work in a confined space can be especially hazardous. Examples of such spaces include ship holds, storage tanks, and underground vaults.

C. Personal protective gear (p 641). Respiratory system and skin protection may be essential for certain workplace exposures. Just as important as the availability of equipment are proper selection, fit assessment, and use.

1. **Respiratory protection.** A disposable paper-type mask is inadequate for most exposures. A screw-in cartridge-type mask whose cartridges are rarely changed is also unlikely to be effective. For an air-supplied respirator with an air supply hose, ascertain the location of the air intake.
2. **Skin protection.** Gloves and other skin protection should be impervious to the chemical(s) used.

D. Temporal aspects of exposure

1. The most important question is whether there have been any changes in work processes, products used, or job duties that could be temporally associated with the onset of symptoms.
2. Patterns of recurring symptoms linked to the work schedule can be important—for example, if symptoms are different on the first day of the workweek, at the end of the first shift of the week, at the end of the workweek, or on days off or vacation days.

E. Other aspects of exposure

1. It is critical to assess whether anyone else from the workplace is also symptomatic and, if so, to identify that person's precise job duties.
2. Eating in work areas can result in exposure through ingestion; smoking on the job can lead to inhalation of native materials or toxic pyrolysis products of contaminated cigarettes.
3. Determine whether a uniform is provided and who launders it. For example, family lead poisoning can occur through work clothes brought home for laundering. After certain types of contamination (e.g., with pesticides), a uniform should be destroyed, not laundered, and reused.
4. Find out how large the work site is, because small operations are often the most poorly maintained. An active work safety and health committee suggests that better general protection is in place.

F. Common toxic materials of frequent concern that are appropriate to address in the occupational exposure history

1. **Two-part glues, paints, or coatings** that must be mixed just before use, or one-part variants of these, such as urethanes and epoxides. These reactive polymers are often irritants or sensitizers.

2. **Solvents or degreasers,** especially if the level of exposure by inhalation or through skin contact is high enough to cause dizziness, nausea, headache, or a sense of intoxication.
3. **Respirable dusts,** including friable insulation or heat-resistant materials, and sand or quartz dust, especially from grinding, drilling, or blasting.
4. **Combustion products or fumes** from fires, flame cutting, welding, and other high-temperature processes.

G. Identifying the specific chemical exposures involved may be difficult because the worker may not know or may not have been precisely informed about them. Even the manufacturer may be uncertain because components of the chemical mixture were obtained elsewhere or because exposure is due to undetermined process by-products. Finally, the exposure may have occurred long before. Aids to exposure identification include the following:

1. **Product labels.** Obtain product labels as a first step. However, the label alone is unlikely to provide sufficiently detailed information.
2. **Material safety data sheets.** Contact the manufacturer directly for a material safety data sheet (MSDS). These must be provided upon a physician's request in cases of suspected illness. ***Do not take no for an answer.*** You may need to supplement the MSDS information through direct discussion with a technical person working for the supplier because key information may not be provided (eg, an ingredient may not be specified because it is a small percentage of the product or treated as a "trade secret").
3. **Computerized databases.** Consult computerized databases, such as Poisindex, HSDB (Hazardous Substances Data Bank), Toxnet, TOMES (Toxicology Occupational Medicines and Environmental Sciences), NIOSHTIC (NIOSH Technical Information Center), and others, for further information. Regional poison control centers (1-800-222-1222) can be extremely useful.
4. **Department of Transportation identification placards.** In cases of transportation release, DOT identification placards may be available (p 640).
5. **Industrial exposure data.** Rarely, detailed industrial hygiene data may be available to delineate specific exposures and exposure levels in cases of ongoing, chronic exposure.
6. **Existing process exposure data.** Often, likely exposure can be inferred on the basis of known specific exposures strongly associated with certain work activities. Selected types of exposure are listed in Table IV–1.

III. **Organ-specific occupational toxidromes.** A list of the 10 leading work-related diseases and injuries has been developed by the National Institute for Occupational Safety and Health (NIOSH). This list, organized generally by organ system, is included in Table IV–2, along with additional disorders that were not on the original NIOSH list.

TABLE IV–1. SELECTED JOB PROCESSES AT HIGH RISK FOR SPECIFIC TOXIC EXPOSURES

Job Process	Exposure
Aerospace and other specialty metal work	Beryllium
Artificial nail application	Methacrylate
Artificial nail removal	Acetonitrile, nitroethane
Artificial leather making, fabric coating	Dimethylformamide
Auto body painting	Isocyanates
Battery recycling	Lead and cadmium fumes and dust
Carburetor cleaning (car repair)	Methylene chloride
Cement manufacture	Sulfur dioxide

(continued)

TABLE IV–1. SELECTED JOB PROCESSES AT HIGH RISK FOR SPECIFIC TOXIC EXPOSURES (CONTINUED)

Job Process	Exposure
Commercial refrigeration	Ammonia, sulfur dioxide
Concrete application	Chromic acid
Custodial work	Chlorine gas (hypochlorite + acid mixes)
Dry cleaning	Chlorinated hydrocarbon solvents
Epoxy glue and coatings use	Trimellitic anhydride
Explosives work	Nitrate oxidants
Fermentation operation	Carbon dioxide
Fire fighting	Carbon monoxide, cyanide, acrolein
Fumigation	Methyl bromide, methyl iodide, Vikane (sulfuryl fluoride), phosphine
Furniture stripping	Methylene chloride
Furniture and wood floor finishing	Isocyanates
Gas-shielded welding	Nitrogen dioxide
Gold refining	Mercury vapor, cyanide
Hospital sterilizer work	Ethylene oxide, glutaraldehyde
Indoor forklift or compressor operation	Carbon monoxide
Manure pit operation	Hydrogen sulfide
Metal blade specialty cutting	Tungsten carbide-cobalt (hard metal)
Metal degreasing	Chlorinated hydrocarbon solvents
Metal plating	Cyanide, acid mists
Microelectronics chip etching	Hydrofluoric acid
Microelectronic chip doping	Arsine gas, diborane gas
Paper pulp work	Chlorine, chlorine dioxide, ozone
Pool and hot tub disinfection	Chlorine, bromine
Pottery glazing and glassmaking	Lead dust
Radiator repair	Lead fumes
Rubber cement glue use	*n*-Hexane, other solvents
Rocket and jet fuel work	Hydrazine, monomethylhydrazine
Sandblasting, concrete finishing	Silica dust
Sewage work	Hydrogen sulfide
Silo work with fresh silage	Nitrogen dioxide
Sheet metal flame cutting or brazing	Cadmium fumes
Structural paint refurbishing	Lead fumes and dust
Superphosphate fertilizer manufacturing	Fluoride
Tobacco harvesting	Nicotine
Viscose production (rayon/cellophane)	Carbon disulfide
Water treatment or purification	Chlorine, ozone
Welding galvanized steel	Zinc oxide fumes
Welding solvent–contaminated metal	Phosgene

TABLE IV–2. LEADING WORK-RELATED DISEASES AND INJURIES AND THEIR RELEVANCE TO CLINICAL TOXICOLOGY

Work-Related Conditions	NIOSH[a]	Relevance	Examples of Relevant Conditions
Occupational lung disease	Yes	High	Irritant inhalation
Musculoskeletal	Yes	Low	Chemical-related Raynaud syndrome
Cancer	Yes	Moderate	Acute leukemia
Trauma	Yes	Low	High-pressure paint gun injury
Cardiovascular disease	Yes	Moderate	Carbon monoxide ischemia
Disorders of reproduction	Yes	Moderate	Spontaneous abortion
Neurotoxic disorders	Yes	High	Acetylcholinesterase inhibition
Noise-induced hearing loss	Yes	Low	Potential drug interactions
Dermatologic conditions	Yes	Moderate	Hydrofluoric acid burns
Psychological disorders	Yes	Moderate	Postexposure stress disorder
Hepatic injury	No	High	Chemical hepatitis
Renal disease	No	Moderate	Acute tubular necrosis
Hematologic conditions	No	High	Methemoglobinemia
Physical exposures	No	Moderate	Radiation sickness
Systemic illness	No	High	Cyanide toxicity

[a]NIOSH, National Institute for Occupational Safety and Health list of "10 leading work-related diseases and injuries."

A. Occupational lung diseases

1. In acute pulmonary injury from **inhaled irritants**, exposure is typically brief and intense; initial symptom onset occurs from within minutes to between 24 and 48 hours after exposure. The responses to irritant exposure, in order of increasing severity, are mucous membrane irritation, burning eyes and runny nose, tracheobronchitis, hoarseness, cough, laryngospasm, bronchospasm, and pulmonary edema progressing to acute respiratory distress syndrome (ARDS). Gases with lower water solubility (nitrogen dioxide, ozone, and phosgene) may produce little upper airway mucous membrane irritation. Injury from water-repellent fluoropolymer aerosol inhalation presents similarly to injury from the low-solubility gases. Any irritant (high or low solubility) can cause pulmonary edema and ARDS after sufficient exposure.
2. **Heavy metal** pneumonitis is clinically similar to irritant inhalation injury. As with low-solubility gases, upper airway mucous membrane irritation is minimal; thus, the exposure may have poor warning properties. Offending agents include cadmium, mercury, and, in limited industrial settings, nickel carbonyl. Other metal carbonyls (eg, iron pentacarbonyl) are rarely encountered.
3. **Febrile inhalational syndromes** are acute, self-limited, flulike syndromes that include the following: **metal fume fever** (caused by galvanized metal fumes); **polymer fume fever** after intermediate temperature thermal breakdown of certain fluoropolymers (a different syndrome from acute irritant injury from high temperature fluoropolymer breakdown or from water-repellent fluoropolymer injury); and **organic dust toxic syndrome** (ODTS; after heavy exposure to high levels of organic dust, such as occurs in shoveling wood chip mulch). In none of these syndromes is lung injury marked. The presence of hypoxemia or lung infiltrates suggests an alternative diagnosis (see Items 1 and 2 above).
4. **Work-related asthma** is a common occupational problem. Classic occupational asthma typically occurs after sensitization to either high–molecular-

weight chemicals (eg, inhaled foreign proteins) or small chemicals (the most common of which are urethane isocyanates such as **toluene diisocyanate** [TDI]) (p 280). After acute, high-level irritant inhalations of, for example, **chlorine** (p 191), a chronic irritant-induced asthma may persist (sometimes called reactive airways dysfunction syndrome [RADS]).

5. **Chronic fibrotic occupational lung diseases** include **asbestosis** (p 146), **silicosis, coal workers' pneumoconiosis,** and a few other, less common fibrotic lung diseases associated with occupational exposures to substances such as **beryllium,** hard metal **(cobalt-tungsten carbide)**, **indium tin oxide** (flat screen display manufacture) and short-length **synthetic textile fibers** (flock worker's lung). These conditions typically occur after years of exposure and have a long latency, although patients may present for evaluation after an acute exposure. Referral for follow-up surveillance is appropriate.
6. **Other occupational lung disorders. Hypersensitivity pneumonitis** (also called **allergic alveolitis**) includes a group of diseases most commonly caused by chronic exposure to organic materials, especially thermophilic bacteria or to bird-derived antigens. The most common of these is **farmer's lung.** Certain chemicals can also cause this disease (eg, isocyanates). Although the process is chronic, acute illness can occur in a sensitized host after heavy exposure to the offending agent. Other work-related lung syndromes include bronchiolitis obliterans from the flavorant diacetyl (eg, microwave popcorn worker's lung) and nitrogen dioxide (eg, silo filler's lung) and bronchiectasis following severe irritant inhalation injury.

B. **Musculoskeletal** conditions, including acute mechanical trauma, comprise the most common group of occupational medicine problems but rarely have direct toxicologic implications.
   1. **Raynaud syndrome** may be associated rarely with chemical exposure (eg, vinyl chloride monomer).
   2. **High-pressure injection injuries** (eg, from paint spray guns) are important not because of systemic toxicity resulting from absorption of an injected substance (eg, paint thinner) but because of extensive irritant-related tissue necrosis. Emergency surgical evaluation is mandatory.

C. **Occupational cancer** is a major public concern and often leads to referral for toxicologic evaluation. A variety of cancers have been associated with workplace exposure, some more strongly than others. Attributing a chemical cause to an individual case of cancer can be challenging. The process of attribution, however, tends to be far removed from the acute care setting, and clinical oncology management is not affected directly by such etiologic considerations.

D. **Cardiovascular disease**
   1. **Atherosclerotic** cardiovascular disease is associated with **carbon disulfide**. This chemical solvent is used in rayon manufacturing and in specialty applications and research laboratories. It is also a principal metabolite of **disulfiram**.
   2. **Carbon monoxide** (CO) at high levels can cause myocardial infarction in otherwise healthy individuals, and at lower levels it can aggravate ischemia in the face of established cardiovascular disease. Many jurisdictions automatically grant workers' compensation to firefighters or police officers with coronary artery disease, regarding it as a "stress-related" occupational disease in addition to possible CO effects in the former group.
   3. **Nitrate withdrawal–induced** coronary artery spasm has been reported among workers heavily exposed to nitrates during munitions manufacturing.
   4. **Hydrocarbon solvents,** especially chlorinated hydrocarbons, and chlorofluorocarbon propellants all enhance the sensitivity of the myocardium to catecholamine-induced dysrhythmias.

E. **Adverse reproductive outcomes** have been associated with or implicated in occupational exposures to **heavy metals** (eg, lead and organic mercury), hospital chemical exposures (including **anesthetic** and **sterilizing gases**), and **dibromochloropropane** (a soil fumigant now banned in the United States).

F. Occupational neurotoxins

1. Acute central nervous system (CNS) toxicity can occur with many pesticides (including both cholinesterase-inhibiting and chlorinated hydrocarbons). The CNS is also the target of **methyl bromide** (a structural fumigant [p 321]) as well as the related toxin methyl iodide. Cytotoxic and anoxic asphyxiant gases (e.g., carbon monoxide, cyanide, and hydrogen sulfide) all cause acute CNS injury, as can bulk asphyxiants (eg, carbon dioxide). **Hydrocarbon solvents** (p 266) are typically CNS depressants at high exposure levels.
2. **Chronic** CNS toxicity is the hallmark of heavy metals. These include inorganic forms (**arsenic, lead,** and **mercury**) and organic forms (tetraethyl lead, methyl mercury, and dimethylmercury). Chronic **manganese** (p 302) exposure can cause psychosis and parkinsonism. Other causes of parkinsonism include carbon disulfide and postanoxic injury (especially from **carbon monoxide**, p 182).
3. Established causes of **peripheral neuropathy** include lead, arsenic, carbon disulfide, *n*-hexane (magnified in combination with methyl ethyl ketone), 1-bromopropane, and certain organophosphates.

G. Occupational ototoxicity is common but is usually noise induced rather than chemically related. Pre-existing noise-induced hearing loss may magnify the impact of common ototoxic drugs and some chemicals.

H. Occupational skin disorders

1. Allergic and irritant contact dermatitis and urticaria and acute caustic chemical or acid injuries are the most common toxin-related skin problems. Systemic toxicity may occur but is not a common complicating factor.
2. **Hydrofluoric acid** burns present a specific set of management problems (p 269). Relevant occupations include not only those in the microelectronics industry but also maintenance or repair jobs in which hydrofluoric acid–containing rust removers are used.

I. Work-related psychological disorders include a heterogeneous mix of diagnoses. Among these, posttraumatic stress disorder (PTSD) and "mass psychogenic illness" can be extremely relevant to medical toxicology because the patients may believe that their symptoms have a chemical etiology. After reasonable toxicologic causes have been excluded, psychological diagnoses should be considered when nonspecific symptoms or multiple somatic complaints cannot be linked to abnormal signs or physiologic effects.

J. Occupational chemical hepatotoxins (see also p 42)

1. Causes of acute chemical hepatitis include exposure to industrial solvents such as **halogenated hydrocarbons** (methylene chloride, trichloroethylene, trichloroethane, and carbon tetrachloride, the latter only rarely encountered in modern industry), and nonhalogenated chemicals such as **dimethylformamide, dinitropropane,** and **dimethylacetamide.** The jet and rocket fuel components **hydrazine** and **monomethylhydrazine** are also potent nonhalogenated hepatotoxins.
2. Other hepatic responses that can be occupationally related include steatosis, cholestatic injury, hepatoportal sclerosis, and hepatic porphyria. The acute care provider should always consider a toxic chemical etiology in the differential diagnosis of liver disease.

K. Renal diseases

1. **Acute tubular necrosis** can follow high-level exposure to a number of toxins, although the more common exposure scenario is a suicide attempt by ingestion rather than workplace inhalation.
2. **Interstitial nephritis** is associated with chronic exposure to heavy metals, whereas hydrocarbon exposure has been associated epidemiologically with **glomerular nephritis,** particularly Goodpasture disease.

L. Hematologic toxicity

1. Industrial oxidants are an important potential cause of chemically induced **methemoglobinemia** (p 317), especially in the dyestuff and munitions industries.
2. **Bone marrow** is an important target organ for certain chemicals, such as **benzene** (p 154) and **methyl cellosolve.** Both can cause pancytopenia. Benzene exposure also causes leukemia in humans. **Lead** (p 286) causes anemia through interference with hemoglobin synthesis.
3. **Arsine gas** (p 144) is a potent cause of massive hemolysis. It is of industrial importance in microelectronics manufacturing.

M. Nonchemical physical exposures in the workplace are important because they can cause systemic effects that mimic chemical toxidromes. The most important example is **heat stress,** which is a major occupational health issue. Other relevant nonchemical, work-related types of physical exposure include **ionizing radiation, nonionizing radiation** (eg, ultraviolet, infrared, and microwave exposure), and **increased barometric pressure** (eg, among caisson workers). Except for extremes of exposure, the adverse effects of these physical factors generally are associated with chronic conditions.

N. Systemic poisons fit poorly into organ system categories but are clearly of major importance in occupational toxicology. Prime examples are the cytotoxic asphyxiants **hydrogen cyanide** (especially in metal plating and metal refining [p 208]), **hydrogen sulfide** (important as a natural by-product of organic material breakdown [p 271]), and **carbon monoxide** (principally encountered as a combustion by-product but also a metabolite of the solvent methylene chloride [p 323]). **Arsenic** (p 140) is a multiple-organ toxin with a myriad of effects. It has been used widely in agriculture and is an important metal smelting by-product. A systemic **disulfiram reaction** (p 226) can occur as a drug interaction with concomitant exposure to certain industrial chemicals. Toxicity from **dinitrophenol** (p 364), an industrial chemical that uncouples oxidative phosphorylation, is also best categorized as a systemic effect. **Pentachlorophenol** (p 364), a severely restricted wood preservative, acts similarly. Phosphine is a systemically toxic fumigant.

IV. Laboratory testing

A. Testing for specific occupational toxins has a limited but important role. Selected tests are listed in the descriptions of specific substances in Section II of this book. For significant irritant inhalation exposures, in addition to assessing oxygenation and chest radiographic status, early spirometric assessment is often important.

B. General laboratory testing for chronic exposure assessment should be driven by the potential organ toxicity delineated previously. Standard generic recommendations (eg, in NIOSH criteria documents) often include a complete blood cell count, electrolytes, tests of renal and liver function, and periodic chest radiographic and pulmonary function studies.

V. Treatment

A. Elimination or reduction of further exposure is a key treatment intervention in occupational toxicology. This includes prevention of exposure to coworkers. The **Occupational Safety and Health Administration (OSHA)** may be of assistance and should be notified immediately about an ongoing, potentially life-threatening workplace exposure situation. Contact information for regional OSHA offices is listed in Table IV–3. Workplace modification and control, especially the substitution of less hazardous materials, should always be the first line of defense. Worker-required personal protective equipment is, in general, less preferred as a preventive measure.

B. The medical treatment of occupational toxic illness should follow the general principles outlined earlier in this section and in Sections I and II of this book. In particular, the use of specific antidotes should be undertaken in consultation with a regional poison control center (1-800-222-1222) or other specialists. This is particularly true before chelation therapy is initiated for heavy metal poisoning.

TABLE IV–3. REGIONAL OFFICES OF THE OCCUPATIONAL SAFETY AND HEALTH ADMINISTRATION (OSHA)

Region	Regional Office	Phone Number	States Served
I	Boston	1-617-565-9860	Connecticut, Maine, Massachusetts, New Hampshire, Rhode Island, Vermont
II	New York City	1-212-337-2378	New York, New Jersey, Puerto Rico, Virgin Islands
III	Philadelphia	1-215-861-4900	Delaware, District of Columbia, Maryland, Pennsylvania, Virginia, West Virginia
IV	Atlanta	1-678-237-0400	Alabama, Florida, Georgia, Kentucky, Mississippi, North Carolina, South Carolina, Tennessee
V	Chicago	1-312-353-2220	Illinois, Indiana, Michigan, Minnesota, Ohio, Wisconsin
VI	Dallas	1-972-850-4145	Arkansas, Louisiana, New Mexico, Oklahoma, Texas
VII	Kansas City	1-816-283-8745	Iowa, Kansas, Missouri, Nebraska
VIII	Denver	1-720-264-6550	Colorado, Montana, North Dakota, South Dakota, Utah, Wyoming
IX	San Francisco	1-415-625-2547	Arizona, California, Hawaii, Nevada, Guam, American Samoa, Northern Mariana Islands
X	Seattle	1-206-757-6700	Alaska, Idaho, Oregon, Washington

▶ THE TOXIC HAZARDS OF INDUSTRIAL AND OCCUPATIONAL CHEMICALS

Timur S. Durrani, MD, MPH, MBA, Paul D. Blanc, MD, MSPH, Patricia Hess Hiatt, BS, and Kent R. Olson, MD[1]

Basic information on the toxicity of many of the most commonly encountered and toxicologically significant industrial chemicals is provided in Table IV–4. The table is intended to expedite the recognition of potentially hazardous exposure situations and therefore provides information such as vapor pressures, warning properties, physical appearance, occupational exposure standards and guidelines, and hazard classification codes, which may also be useful in the assessment of an exposure situation. Table IV–4 is divided into three sections: **health hazards, exposure guidelines,** and **comments.** To use the table correctly, it is important to understand the scope and limitations of the information it provides.

The chemicals included in Table IV–4 were selected on the basis of the following criteria: (1) toxic potential, (2) prevalence of use, (3) public health concern, and (4) availability of adequate toxicologic, regulatory, and physical and chemical property information. Several governmental and industrial lists of "hazardous chemicals" were used. Chemicals have been omitted in cases where little to no toxicologic information could be found, when there are no regulatory standards, or when chemicals have very limited use. Chemicals that were of specific interest, those with existing exposure recommendations, and those of frequent use (even if of low toxicity) generally were included.

I. **Health hazard information.** The health hazards section of Table IV–4 focuses primarily on the basic hazards associated with possible inhalation of or skin exposure to chemicals in a workplace. It is based predominantly on the extant occupational health literature. Much of our understanding of the potential effects of chemicals on human health is derived from occupational exposures, the levels of which are typically many times greater than those of environmental exposures.

[1]This chapter and Table IV–4 were originally conceived and created by Frank J. Mycroft, PhD.

Moreover, the information in Table IV–4 emphasizes *acute* health effects. Much more is known about the acute effects of chemicals on human health than about their chronic effects. The rapid onset of symptoms after exposure makes the causal association more readily apparent for acute health effects. Nonetheless, the table entries are also informed by nonoccupational human exposure data when relevant (eg, from outbreaks of consumer product exposures) and from experimental animal toxicology. The latter is critical to carcinogenesis assessment, a major chronic exposure endpoint in contradistinction to the acute exposure effects noted earlier.

A. The table is ***not*** a comprehensive source of the toxicology and medical information needed to manage a severely symptomatic or poisoned patient. Medical management information and advice for specific poisonings, where applicable, are found in Section I (see "Emergency Evaluation and Treatment," p 1, and "Decontamination," p 50) and Section II (see "Caustic and Corrosive Agents," p 186; "Gases, Irritant," p 255; and "Hydrocarbons," p 266).

B. Hydrocarbons, which are defined broadly as chemicals containing carbon and hydrogen, make up the majority of substances in Table IV–4. Hydrocarbons have a wide range of chemical structures and, not surprisingly, a variety of toxic effects. There are a few common features of hydrocarbon exposure, and the reader is directed to Section II, p 266, for information on general diagnosis and treatment. Some common features of hydrocarbon toxicity include the following:

1. **Skin.** Dermatitis caused by defatting or removal of oils in the skin is common, especially with prolonged contact. Some hydrocarbon agents also can cause frank chemical burns.
2. **Arrhythmias.** Many hydrocarbons, most notably fluorinated, chlorinated, and aromatic compounds, can sensitize the heart to the arrhythmogenic effects of epinephrine, resulting in premature ventricular contractions (PVCs), ventricular tachycardia, or fibrillation. Even simple aliphatic compounds such as butane can have this effect.
   - **a.** Because arrhythmias may not occur immediately, cardiac monitoring for 24 hours is recommended for all victims who have had significant hydrocarbon exposure (eg, associated with syncope or coma).
   - **b.** Ventricular arrhythmias preferably are treated with a beta-adrenergic blocker (eg, esmolol [p 552] or propranolol [p 617]). The use of epinephrine and other catecholamines should be avoided in the acutely hydrocarbon intoxicated patient, as these can precipitate arrhythmia.
3. **Pulmonary aspiration** of most hydrocarbons, especially those with relatively high volatility and low viscosity (eg, gasoline, kerosene, and naphtha), can cause severe chemical pneumonitis.

C. Carcinogens and Reproductive Hazards. To broaden the scope of the table, findings from human and animal studies relating to the carcinogenic or reproductive toxicity of a chemical are included when available. The **International Agency for Research on Cancer (IARC)** is the foremost authority in evaluating the carcinogenic potential of chemical agents for humans. The overall IARC evaluations are provided, when available, in the health hazards section of the table. The following IARC ratings are based primarily on human and animal data:

1. **IARC Group 1** substances are considered human carcinogens; generally, there is sufficient epidemiologic information to support a causal association between exposure and human cancer.
2. **IARC Group 2** compounds are suspected of being carcinogenic to humans, based on a combination of data from animal and human studies. IARC Group 2 is subdivided into two parts:
   - **a.** An **IARC 2A** rating indicates that a chemical is *probably* carcinogenic to humans. Most often, there is limited evidence of carcinogenicity in humans combined with sufficient evidence of carcinogenicity in animals.

b. **IARC 2B** indicates that a chemical is *possibly* carcinogenic to humans. This category may be used when there is limited evidence from epidemiologic studies and less than sufficient evidence for carcinogenicity in animals. It also may be used when there is inadequate evidence of carcinogenicity in humans and sufficient evidence in animals.

3. **IARC Group 3** substances cannot be classified in regard to their carcinogenic potential for humans because of inadequate data.
4. **IARC Group 4** substances are probably not carcinogenic to humans.
5. If a chemical is described in the table as carcinogenic but an IARC category is not given, IARC may not have classified the chemical at all or categorized it in Group 3, even though other sources (eg, the U.S. Environmental Protection Agency or the California Department of Public Health Hazard Evaluation System and Information Service [HESIS]) considers it carcinogenic.
6. Substances identified in the Table as reproductive toxicants are suspected to lead to adverse outcomes in human pregnancy based on clinical reports, epidemiologic investigation, or experimental animal data.

D. **Problems in assessing health hazards.** The nature and magnitude of the health hazards associated with occupational or environmental exposures to any chemical depend on its intrinsic toxicity and the conditions of exposure.

1. Characterization of these hazards is often difficult. Important considerations include the potency of the agent, route of exposure, level and temporal pattern of exposure, increased susceptibility (which may be genetic or due to other factors), overall health status, and lifestyle factors that may alter individual sensitivities (eg, alcohol consumption may cause "degreaser's flush" in workers exposed to trichloroethylene). Despite their value in estimating the likelihood and potential severity of an effect, quantitative measurements of the level of exposure associated with an adverse effect often are unavailable.
2. Hazard characterizations cannot address undiscovered or unappreciated health effects. The limited information available on the health effects of most chemicals makes this a major concern. For example, among the millions of compounds known to science, only about 100,000 are listed in the *Registry of the Toxic Effects of Chemical Substances* (RTECS) published by the National Institute for Occupational Safety and Health (NIOSH). Of these substances, fewer than 5,000 have any toxicity studies relating to their potential tumorigenic or reproductive effects in animals or humans. Because of these gaps, the absence of information does not imply the absence of hazard.
3. The predictive value of animal findings for humans is sometimes uncertain. For many effects, however, there is considerable concordance between test animals and humans.
4. The developmental toxicity information presented in Table IV–4 is not a sufficient basis upon which to make clinical judgments regarding whether a given exposure may affect a pregnancy adversely. For most chemicals known to have adverse effects on fetal development in test animals, there are insufficient data in humans. In general, so little is known about the effects of substances on fetal development that it is prudent to manage all chemical exposures conservatively. The information here is presented solely to identify those compounds for which available data further indicate the need to control exposures.

II. Exposure guidelines and National Fire Protection Association rankings

A. **Threshold limit values (TLVs)** are workplace exposure guidelines established by the American Conference of Governmental Industrial Hygienists (ACGIH), a professional nongovernmental organization. Although the ACGIH has no legally mandated regulatory authority, its recommendations are highly regarded and widely followed by the occupational health and safety community. The toxicologic basis for each TLV varies. A TLV may be based on such diverse effects as respiratory sensitization, sensory irritation, narcosis, or asphyxia, to list but a few adverse endpoints. The *Documentation of the Threshold Limit Values and Biological Exposure Indices*, which is published and regularly updated by the ACGIH and describes in detail the rationale for each value, should be consulted for specific information on the toxicologic significance of any particular TLV. Common units for a TLV are parts of a chemical per million parts of air **(ppm)** or milligrams of a chemical per cubic meter of air **(mg/m^3)**. **At standard temperature and pressure, TLV values in ppm can be converted to their equivalent concentrations in mg/m^3** by multiplying the TLV in ppm by the molecular weight (MW) in milligrams of the chemical and dividing the result by 22.4 (1 mole of gas displaces 22.4 L of air at standard temperature and pressure):

$$\text{mg/m}^3 = \frac{\text{ppm} \times \text{MW}}{22.4}$$

1. The **threshold limit value time-weighted average (TLV-TWA)** refers to airborne contaminants and is the time-weighted average concentration to which, per ACGIH findings, workers may be exposed repeatedly during a normal 8-hour workday and 40-hour workweek without an adverse effect. Unless otherwise indicated in Table IV–4, the values listed under the ACGIH TLV heading are the TLV-TWAs. Note that work days longer than 8 hours even below the TLV could nonetheless constitute excessive exposure.
2. The **threshold limit value–ceiling (TLV-C)** is the airborne concentration that should not be exceeded during any part of a working exposure. Ceiling guidelines often are set for rapidly acting agents for which an 8-hour time-weighted average exposure limit would be inappropriate. TLV-Cs are listed under the ACGIH TLV heading and are indicated by "**(C)**."
3. The **threshold limit value–short-term exposure limit (TLV-STEL)** is a time-weighted average exposure that should not be exceeded over any 15-minute period and no more than 4 times in an 8-hour workday. The TLV-STEL is set to avoid irritation, chronic adverse effects, impaired work performance, or injury.
4. Compounds for which **skin contact** is a significant route of exposure are designated with "**S**." This can refer to potential local corrosive effects or systemic toxicity due to skin absorption.
5. The ACGIH classifies some substances as **confirmed (A1) or suspected (A2) human carcinogens** or **confirmed animal carcinogens (A3)**. These designations are also provided in the table. The ACGIH does not consider A3 carcinogens likely to cause human cancer. This categorization may not conform with IARC designations.

B. **Occupational Safety and Health Administration (OSHA) regulations** are legally binding standards for exposure to airborne contaminants that are set and enforced by OSHA, an agency of the federal government.

1. The **permissible exposure limit (PEL)** set by OSHA is closely analogous to the ACGIH TLV-TWA. In fact, when OSHA was established in 1971, it formally adopted the 1969 ACGIH TLVs for nearly all of its PELs. In 1988, OSHA updated the majority of its PELs by adopting the 1986 TLVs. These revised PELs were printed in the 1990 edition of this manual. However, in early 1993, the 1988 PEL revisions were voided as a result of legal challenges and the earlier (1969) values were restored. These restored values cannot be assumed to protect worker health reliably.
2. Substances that are specifically **regulated as carcinogens** by OSHA are indicated by "**OSHA CA**" under the ACGIH TLV heading. For these carcinogens, additional regulations apply. The notation "**NIOSH CA**" in the TLV

column identifies the chemicals that the National Institute for Occupational Safety and Health (NIOSH) recommends be treated as potential human carcinogens.

3. Some states operate their own occupational health and safety programs in cooperation with OSHA. In these states, stricter standards may apply or the state may establish standards for a substance with no Federal OSHA PEL whatsoever. California, in particular, has several such standards—where relevant these are referred to in Table IV–4.
4. The NIOSH nonlegally binding corollary to the OSHA PEL is the **recommended exposure limit (REL)**. For NIOSH RELs, the time-weighted average is the concentration for up to a 10-hour workday (as opposed to 8 hours for OSHA) during a 40-hour work. For NIOSH, a short-term exposure limit is generally a 15-minute TWA exposure that should not be exceeded at any time during a workday (but can be specified as even shorter). A NIOSH ceiling value is a level recommended not be exceeded at any time. There are many compounds for which the NIOSH REL is lower than the OSHA PEL. NIOSH RELs are generally close to the ACGIH TLVs. Because the latter are included in Table IV–4, the former are presented only for selected compounds, in particular those where the NIOSH REL is ten times less permissive than the corresponding OSHA PEL or where there is no OSHA PEL at all. A NIOSH pocket guide table of 677 compounds can be accessed at http://www.cdc.gov/niosh/npg/pgintrod.html.

C. **Immediately dangerous to life or health (IDLH)** represents "a maximum concentration from which one could escape within 30 minutes without any escape-impairing symptoms or any irreversible health effects." The IDLH values originally were set jointly by OSHA and NIOSH for the purpose of respirator selection. They have been updated subsequently by NIOSH.

D. **Emergency Response Planning Guidelines (ERPGs)** have been developed by the American Industrial Hygiene Association (AIHA) for less than 150 specific substances. The values generally are based on limited human experience as well as available animal data and should be considered estimates only. Although these values may appear in the IDLH column, they have different meanings:
1. **ERPG-1** is "the maximum air concentration below which it is believed nearly all individuals could be exposed for up to 1 hour without experiencing other than mild transient adverse health effects or perceiving a clearly defined objectionable odor."
2. **ERPG-2** is "the maximum air concentration below which it is believed that nearly all individuals could be exposed for up to 1 hour without experiencing or developing irreversible or other serious health effects or symptoms which could impair their abilities to take protective action."
3. **ERPG-3** is "the maximum air concentration below which it is believed that nearly all individuals could be exposed for up to 1 hour without experiencing or developing life-threatening health effects."
4. The ERPGs were developed for purposes of emergency planning and response. They are not exposure guidelines and do not incorporate the safety factors normally used in establishing acceptable exposure limits. Reliance on the ERPGs for exposures lasting longer than 1 hour is not appropriately a safe practice.

E. **National Fire Protection Association (NFPA) codes** are part of the system created by the NFPA for identifying and ranking the potential fire hazards of materials. The system has three principal categories of hazard: **health (H), flammability (F),** and **reactivity (R).** Within each category, hazards are ranked from 4 (four), indicating a severe hazard, to 0 (zero), indicating no special hazard. The NFPA rankings for each substance are listed under their appropriate headings. The criteria for rankings within each category are found in Figure IV–2, p 639.

1. The NFPA health hazard rating is based on both the intrinsic toxicity of a chemical and the toxicities of its combustion or breakdown products. The overall ranking is determined by the greater source of health hazard under fire or other emergency conditions. Common hazards from the ordinary combustion of materials are not considered in these rankings. The NFPA health hazard rating may not provide appropriate toxicity guidance, especially for subacute or chronic adverse health effects.
2. This system is intended to provide basic information to firefighters and emergency response personnel. Its application to specific situations requires skill. Conditions at the scene, such as the amount of material involved and its rate of release, wind conditions, and the proximity to various populations and their health status, are as important as the intrinsic properties of a chemical in determining the magnitude of a hazard.

III. Comments section. The comments column of Table IV–4 provides supplementary information on the physical and chemical properties of substances that would be helpful in assessing their health hazards. Information such as physical state and appearance, vapor pressures, warning properties, and potential breakdown products is included. The comments section also includes, where applicable, a brief notation of common uses and exposure scenarios.

A. Information on the **physical state and appearance** of a compound may help in its identification and indicate whether dusts, mists, vapors, or gases are likely means of airborne exposure. ***Note:*** For many products, for example, pesticides, the appearance and some hazardous properties may vary with the formulation.

B. The **vapor pressure** of a substance helps determine its potential maximum air concentration and influences the degree of inhalation exposure or airborne contamination. Vapor pressures fluctuate greatly with temperature.

1. Substances with high vapor pressures tend to volatilize more quickly and can reach higher maximum air concentrations than substances with low vapor pressures. Some substances have such low vapor pressures that airborne contamination is a threat only if they are mechanically or otherwise dispersed, for example, as an aerosol.
2. A substance with a **saturated air concentration** below its TLV does not pose a significant *vapor* inhalation hazard (but this would be irrelevant to aerosol generation or skin exposure). Vapor pressure can be converted roughly to saturated air concentration expressed in parts per million by multiplying by a factor of 1,300. This is equivalent to dividing by 760 mm Hg and then multiplying the result by 1 million to adjust for the original unit of parts per million (a pressure of 1 atmosphere equals 760 mm Hg):

$$\text{ppm} = \frac{\text{vapor pressure (mm Hg)}}{760} \times 10^6$$

C. Warning properties such as odor and sensory irritation can be valuable indicators of exposure. However, because of olfactory fatigue and individual differences in odor thresholds, the sense of smell is often unreliable in detecting many compounds. There is no correlation between the quality of an odor and its toxicity. Pleasant-smelling compounds are not necessarily less toxic than foul-smelling ones.

1. The warning property assessments in the table are based on OSHA evaluations. For the purpose of this manual, chemicals described as having *good* warning properties can be detected by smell or irritation at levels below the TLV by most individuals. Chemicals described as having *adequate* warning properties can be detected at air levels near the TLV. Chemicals described as having *poor* warning properties can be detected only at levels significantly above the TLV or not at all.

2. Reported values for odor threshold in the literature vary greatly for many chemicals and are therefore frequently uncertain. These differences make assessments of warning qualities difficult.

D. Thermal breakdown products. Under fire conditions, many organic substances break down to other toxic substances. The amounts, kinds, and distribution of breakdown products vary with the fire conditions and are not easily modeled. Information on the likely thermal decomposition products is included because of their importance in the assessment of health hazards under fire conditions.

1. In general, incomplete combustion of *any* organic material will produce some carbon monoxide (p 182).
2. The partial combustion of compounds containing sulfur, nitrogen, or phosphorus atoms will also release their oxides (pp 341, 371, and 431).
3. Compounds with chlorine atoms will release some hydrogen chloride or chlorine (p 191) when exposed to high temperatures or fire; some chlorinated compounds may also generate phosgene (p 371).
4. Compounds containing the fluorine atom are similarly likely to break down to yield some hydrogen fluoride (p 269) or even more toxic fluorine-containing byproducts.
5. Some compounds (eg, polyurethane) that contain an unsaturated carbon-nitrogen bond will release cyanide (p 208) during decomposition.
6. Polychlorinated aromatic compounds may yield polychlorinated dibenzodioxins and polychlorinated dibenzofurans (p 224) when heated.
7. In addition, smoke from a chemical fire is likely to contain large amounts of the volatilized original chemical and still other well recognized (eg, acrolein) and poorly characterized products of partial breakdown.
8. The thermal breakdown product information in Table IV–4 is derived primarily from data found in the literature and the general considerations described immediately above. Aside from the NFPA codes, Table IV–4 does not cover the chemical reactivity or compatibility of substances.

IV. Summary. Table IV–4 provides basic information that describes the potential health hazards associated with exposure to several hundred chemicals. The table is not a comprehensive listing of all the possible health hazards for each chemical. The information compiled here comes from a wide variety of sources and focuses on the more likely or commonly reported health effects. Publications from NIOSH, OSHA, ACGIH, the California Hazard Evaluation System and Information Service, and NFPA; major textbooks in the fields of toxicology and occupational health; and major review articles are the primary sources of the information presented here. Table IV–4 is intended primarily to guide users in the quick qualitative assessment of common toxic hazards. Its application to specific situations requires skill. Contact a regional poison control center (1-800-222-1222) or medical toxicologist for expert assistance in managing specific emergency exposures.

TABLE IV–4. HEALTH HAZARD SUMMARIES FOR INDUSTRIAL AND OCCUPATIONAL CHEMICALS

IARC = Abbreviations and designations used in this table are defined as follows: International Agency for Research on Cancer overall classification (p 579): 1 = known human carcinogen; 2A = probable human carcinogen; 2B = possible human carcinogen; 3 = inadequate data available.
TLV = American Conference of Governmental Industrial Hygienists (ACGIH) threshold limit value 8-hour time-weighted average (TLV-TWA) air concentration (p 655); A1 = ACGIH-confirmed human carcinogen; A2 = ACGIH-suspected human carcinogen; A3 = ACGIH animal carcinogen.
ppm = parts of chemical per million parts of air.
mg/m^3 = milligrams of chemical per cubic meter of air.
mppcf = million particles of dust per cubic foot of air.
(C) = ceiling air concentration (TLV-C) that should not be exceeded at any time.
(STEL) = Short-term (15-minute) exposure limit.
S = skin absorption can be significant route of exposure.
SEN = potential for worker sensitization as a result of dermal contact or inhalation exposure.
NIOSH CA = Judged by the National Institute for Occupational Safety and Health to be a known or suspected human carcinogen (p 655).
OSHA CA = Regulated by the Occupational Safety & Health Administration as an occupational carcinogen (p 655).
IDLH = Immediately Dangerous to Life or Health air concentration (p 656).
LEL = For this substance, the IDLH value is set at 10% of the Lower Explosive Limit.
ERPG = Emergency Response Planning Guidelines air concentration values for a 1-hour period of exposure (p 656).
NFPA codes = National Fire Protection Association hazard classification codes (p 656):
0 (no hazard) <—> 4 (severe hazard)
H = health hazard
F = fire hazard
R = reactivity hazard
Ox = oxidizing agent
W = water-reactive substance

Health Hazard Summaries	ACGIH TLV	IDLH	NFPA Codes H F R	Comments
Acephate (AP, [CAS: 30560-19-1]): Widely available organophosphorus insecticide (p 353) considered to have low mammalian toxicity. Metabolized extensively to methamidophos, which is more toxic.				White or transparent solid, soluble in water with a strong odor similar to mercaptan. Vapor pressure is 1.7×10^{-6} mm Hg at 24°C.

(C), ceiling air concentration (TLV-C); S, skin absorption can be significant; SEN, potential sensitizer; STEL, short-term (15-minute) exposure level. A1, ACGIH-confirmed human carcinogen; A2, ACGIH-suspected human carcinogen; A3, ACGIH animal carcinogen. ERPG, Emergency Response Planning Guideline (see p 656 for an explanation of ERPG). IARC 1, known human carcinogen; IARC 2A, probable human carcinogen; IARC 2B, possible human carcinogen; IARC 3, inadequate data available. NFPA hazard codes: H, health; F, fire; R, reactivity; Ox, oxidizer; W, water-reactive; 0 (none) <—> 4 (severe).

(*continued*)

TABLE IV–4. HEALTH HAZARD SUMMARIES FOR INDUSTRIAL AND OCCUPATIONAL CHEMICALS (CONTINUED)

Health Hazard Summaries	ACGIH TLV	IDLH	NFPA Codes H F R	Comments
Acetaldehyde (CAS: 75-07-0): Corrosive; severe burns to eyes and skin may occur. Vapors strongly irritating to eyes and respiratory tract; evidence for adverse effects on fetal development in animals. A carcinogen in test animals (IARC 1).	25 ppm (C), A2 NIOSH CA	2,000 ppm ERPG-1: 10 ppm ERPG-2: 200 ppm ERPG-3: 1,000 ppm	2 4 2	Colorless liquid. Fruity odor and irritation are both adequate warning properties. Vapor pressure is 750 mm Hg at 20°C (68°F). Highly flammable. Carcinogenicity associated with consumption of alcoholic beverages.
Acetic acid (vinegar acid [CAS: 64-19-7]): Concentrated solutions are corrosive; severe burns to eyes and skin may occur. Vapors strongly irritating to eyes and respiratory tract.	10 ppm	50 ppm ERPG-1: 5 ppm ERPG-2: 35 ppm ERPG-3: 250 ppm	3 2 0	Colorless liquid. Pungent, vinegar-like odor and irritation both occur near the TLV and are adequate warning properties. Vapor pressure is 11 mm Hg at 20°C (68°F). Flammable.
Acetic anhydride (CAS: 108-24-7): Corrosive; severe burns to eyes and skin may result. Dermal sensitization has been reported. Vapors highly irritating to eyes and respiratory tract.	1 ppm	200 ppm ERPG-1: 0.5 ppm ERPG-2: 15 ppm ERPG-3: 100 ppm	3 2 1	Colorless liquid. Odor and irritation both occur below the TLV and are good warning properties. Vapor pressure is 4 mm Hg at 20°C (68°F). Flammable. Evolves heat upon contact with water.
Acetone (dimethyl ketone, 2-propanone [CAS: 67-64-1]): Vapors mildly irritating to eyes and respiratory tract. A CNS depressant at high levels. Eye irritation and headache are common symptoms of moderate overexposure.	250 ppm	2,500 ppm [LEL]	1 3 0	Colorless liquid with a sharp, aromatic odor. Eye irritation is an adequate warning property. Vapor pressure is 266 mm Hg at 25°C (77°F). Highly flammable.
Acetonitrile (methyl cyanide, cyanomethane, ethanenitrile [CAS: 75-05-8]): Vapors mildly irritating to eyes and respiratory tract. Inhibits several metabolic enzyme systems. Dermal absorption occurs. Metabolized to cyanide (p 208); fatalities have resulted. Symptoms include headache, nausea, vomiting, weakness, and stupor. Limited evidence for adverse effects on fetal development in test animals given large doses.	20 ppm, S	500 ppm	2 3 0	Colorless liquid. Ether-like odor, detectable at the TLV, is an adequate warning property. Vapor pressure is 73 mm Hg at 20°C (68°F). Flammable. Thermal breakdown products include oxides of nitrogen and cyanide. May be found in products for removing sculptured nails.

Acetophenone (phenyl methyl ketone [CAS: 98-86-2]): Direct contact irritating to eyes and skin. A CNS depressant at high levels.	10 ppm		2 2 0	Widely used in industry (eg, textile coatings).
Acetylene [CAS: 74-86-2]: Compressed gas used in welding and cutting of metals; previously used as a general anesthetic in the 1920s. An explosive hazard and simple asphyxiant.				Colorless gas with a faint to garlic-like odor. NIOSH recommended exposure limit (REL) 2,500 ppm (ceiling).
Acetylene tetrabromide (tetrabromoethane [CAS: 79-27-6]): Direct contact is irritating to eyes and skin. Vapors irritating to eyes and respiratory tract. Dermal absorption occurs. Highly hepatotoxic; liver injury can result from low-level exposures.	0.1 ppm (inhalable fraction and vapor)	8 ppm	3 0 1	Viscous, pale yellow liquid. Pungent, chloroform-like odor. Vapor pressure is less than 0.1 mm Hg at 20°C (68°F). Not combustible. Thermal breakdown products include hydrogen bromide and carbonyl bromide.
Acetylsalicyclic acid [CAS: 50-78-2] Skin and eye irritant. Systemic toxicity (see Salicylates, p 410).	5 mg/m^3			Odorless, colorless to white, crystalline powder.
Acrolein (acryaldehyde, 2-propenal [CAS: 107-02-8]): Highly corrosive; severe burns to eyes or skin may result. Vapors extremely irritating to eyes, skin, and respiratory tract; pulmonary edema has been reported. Permanent pulmonary function changes may result; see p 255 (IARC 3).	0.1 ppm (C), S	2 ppm ERPG-1: 0.05 ppm ERPG-2: 0.15 ppm ERPG-3: 1.5 ppm	4 3 3	Colorless to yellow liquid. Unpleasant odor. Eye irritation occurs at low levels and provides a good warning property. Formed in the pyrolysis of many substances. Vapor pressure is 214 mm Hg at 20°C (68°F). Highly flammable. Common combustion by-product in fire smoke.
Acrylamide (propenamide, acrylic amide [CAS: 79-06-1]): Concentrated solutions are slightly irritating. Well absorbed by all routes. A potent neurotoxin causing peripheral neuropathy. Contact dermatitis also reported. Testicular toxicity in test animals. A carcinogen in test animals (IARC 2A).	0.03 mg/m^3 (inhalable fraction and vapor), S, A3 NIOSH CA	60 mg/m^3	2 2 2	Colorless solid. Vapor pressure is 0.007 mm Hg at 20°C (68°F). Not flammable. Decomposes around 80°C (176°F). Breakdown products include oxides of nitrogen. Monomer used in the synthesis of polyacrylamide plastics.

(C), ceiling air concentration (TLV-C); S, skin absorption can be significant; SEN, potential sensitizer; STEL, short-term (15-minute) exposure level. A1, ACGIH-confirmed human carcinogen; A2, ACGIH-suspected human carcinogen; A3, ACGIH animal carcinogen. ERPG, Emergency Response Planning Guideline (see p 656 for an explanation of ERPG). IARC 1, known human carcinogen; IARC 2A, probable human carcinogen; IARC 2B, possible human carcinogen; IARC 3, inadequate data available. NFPA hazard codes: H, health; F, fire; R, reactivity; Ox, oxidizer; W, water-reactive; 0 (none) <—> 4 (severe).

(continued)

TABLE IV–4. HEALTH HAZARD SUMMARIES FOR INDUSTRIAL AND OCCUPATIONAL CHEMICALS (CONTINUED)

Health Hazard Summaries	ACGIH TLV	IDLH	NFPA Codes H F R	Comments
Acrylic acid (propenoic acid [CAS: 79-10-7]): Corrosive; severe burns may result. Vapors highly irritating to eyes, skin, and respiratory tract. Limited evidence of adverse effects on fetal development at high doses in test animals. Based on structural analogies, compounds containing the acrylate moiety may be carcinogens (IARC 3).	2 ppm, S	ERPG-1: 1 ppm ERPG-2: 50 ppm ERPG-3: 750 ppm	3 2 2	Colorless liquid with characteristic acrid odor. Vapor pressure is 31 mm Hg at 25°C (77°F). Flammable. Inhibitor added to prevent explosive self-polymerization. Odor threshold near 1 ppm.
Acrylonitrile (cyanoethylene, vinyl cyanide, propenenitrile [CAS: 107-13-1]): Direct contact can be strongly irritating to eyes and skin. Well absorbed by all routes. A CNS depressant at high levels. Metabolized to cyanide (p 208). Moderate acute overexposure will produce headache, weakness, nausea, and vomiting. Evidence of adverse effects on fetal development at high doses in animals. A carcinogen in test animals with limited epidemiologic evidence for carcinogenicity in humans (IARC 2B).	2 ppm, S, A3 OSHA CA NIOSH CA	85 ppm ERPG-1: 10 ppm ERPG-2: 35 ppm ERPG-3: 75 ppm	4 3 2	Colorless liquid with a mild odor. Odor threshold near 10 ppm. Vapor pressure is 83 mm Hg at 20°C (68°F). Flammable. Polymerizes rapidly. Thermal decomposition products include hydrogen cyanide and oxides of nitrogen. Used in the manufacture of ABS (acrylonitrile butadiene styrene) and SAN (styrene acrylonitrile) resins.
Alachlor (CAS: 15972-60-8): Not an eye irritant. Slightly irritating to the skin. A skin sensitizer.	1 mg/m^3, SEN, A3			Widely used as an herbicide. Colorless crystals. Vapor pressure is 0.000022 mm Hg at 25°C (77°F).
Aldicarb (CAS: 116-06-3): A potent carbamate-type cholinesterase inhibitor (p 353). Well absorbed dermally (IARC 3).				Widely used pesticide whose systemic absorption by fruits has caused human poisonings.
Aldrin (CAS: 309-00-2): Chlorinated insecticide (p 189). Minor skin irritant. Convulsant. Hepatotoxin. Well absorbed dermally. Limited evidence for carcinogenicity in test animals (IARC 3).	0.05 mg/m^3 (inhalable fraction and vapor), S, A3 NIOSH CA	25 mg/m^3		Tan to dark brown solid. A mild chemical odor. Vapor pressure is 0.000006 mm Hg at 20°C (68°F). Not flammable but breaks down, yielding hydrogen chloride gas. Most uses have been banned in the United States.

Allyl alcohol (2-propen-1-ol [CAS: 107-18-6]): Strongly irritating to eyes and skin; severe burns may result. Vapors highly irritating to eyes and respiratory tract. Systemic poisoning can result from dermal exposures. May cause liver and kidney injury.	0.5 ppm, S	20 ppm	4 3 1	Colorless liquid. Mustard-like odor and irritation occur near the TLV and serve as good warning properties. Vapor pressure is 17 mm Hg at 20°C (68°F). Flammable. Used in chemical synthesis and as a pesticide.
Allyl chloride (3-chloro-1-propene [CAS: 107-05-1]): Highly irritating to eyes and skin. Vapors highly irritating to eyes and respiratory tract. Well absorbed by the skin, producing both superficial and penetrating irritation and pain. Causes liver and kidney injury and neurotoxicity in test animals. Chronic exposures have been associated with reports of human peripheral neuropathy (IARC 3).	1 ppm, S, A3	250 ppm ERPG-1: 3 ppm ERPG-2: 40 ppm ERPG-3: 300 ppm	3 3 1	Colorless, yellow, or purple liquid. Pungent, disagreeable odor and irritation occur only at levels far above the TLV. Vapor pressure is 295 mm Hg at 20°C (68°F). Highly flammable. Breakdown products include hydrogen chloride and phosgene. Used as a chemical intermediate and in the synthesis of epichlorohydrin and glycerin.
Allyl glycidyl ether (AGE [CAS: 106-92-3]): Highly irritating to eyes and skin; severe burns may result. Vapors irritating to eyes and respiratory tract. Sensitization dermatitis has been reported. Hematopoietic and testicular toxicity occurs in test animals at modest doses. Well absorbed through the skin.	1 ppm	50 ppm		Colorless liquid. Unpleasant odor. Vapor pressure is 2 mm Hg at 20°C (68°F). Flammable.
Allyl propyl disulfide (onion oil [CAS: 2179-59-1]): Mucous membrane irritant and lacrimator.	0.5 ppm, SEN			Liquid with a pungent, irritating odor. A synthetic flavorant and food additive. Thermal breakdown products include sulfur oxide fumes.
alpha-Alumina (aluminum oxide [CAS: 1344-28-1]): Irritant dust with suspected fibrogenic potential; nanoparticles may have additional effects.	1 mg/m^3 (insoluble aluminum compounds, respirable)			"McIntyre's powder," predominantly aluminum oxide, was formerly administered intentionally as an inhalant to silica-exposed miners to prevent lung disease but was later discontinued for lack of efficacy.

(C), ceiling air concentration (TLV-C); S, skin absorption can be significant; SEN, potential sensitizer; STEL, short-term (15-minute) exposure level. A1, ACGIH-confirmed human carcinogen; A2, ACGIH-suspected human carcinogen; A3, ACGIH animal carcinogen. ERPG, Emergency Response Planning Guideline (see p 656 for an explanation of ERPG). IARC 1, known human carcinogen; IARC 2A, probable human carcinogen; IARC 2B, possible human carcinogen; IARC 3, inadequate data available. NFPA hazard codes: H, health; F, fire; R, reactivity; Ox, oxidizer; W, water-reactive; 0 (none) <—> 4 (severe).

(*continued*)

TABLE IV–4. HEALTH HAZARD SUMMARIES FOR INDUSTRIAL AND OCCUPATIONAL CHEMICALS (CONTINUED)

Health Hazard Summaries	ACGIH TLV	IDLH	NFPA Codes H F R	Comments
Aluminum metal (CAS: 7429-90-5): Dusts can cause mild eye and respiratory tract irritation. Long-term inhalation of large amounts of fine aluminum powders or fumes from aluminum ore (bauxite) has been associated with reports of pulmonary fibrosis (Shaver disease). Acute exposures in aluminum refining ("pot room") have been associated with asthma-like responses. Industrial processes used to produce aluminum have been associated with an increased incidence of cancer in workers. Nonoccupational exposure with renal insufficiency is associated with potential neurotoxicity.	1 mg/m^3 (metal and insoluble compounds, respirable)	031 (powder)		Oxidizes readily. Fine powders and flakes are flammable and explosive when mixed with air. Reacts with acids and caustic solutions to produce flammable hydrogen gas. Bauxite ore can contain trace beryllium.
Aluminum phosphide (CAS: 20859-73-8): Effects caused by phosphine gas that is produced on contact with moisture. Severe respiratory tract irritant. See "Phosphides," p 372.		442 W		Used as a structural fumigant (including in dwellings, silos, boxcars) as dry powder or pellet, similar to zinc phosphide. Bystander exposures can occur.
4-Aminodiphenyl (*p*-aminobiphenyl, *p*-phenylaniline [CAS: 92-67-1]): Potent bladder carcinogen in humans (IARC 1). Causes methemoglobinemia (p 317).	S, A1 OSHA CA NIOSH CA			Colorless crystals. Formerly used as a rubber antioxidant and as a dye intermediate. Present in cigarette smoke.
2-Aminopyridine (CAS: 504-29-0): Mild irritant. Potent CNS convulsant in humans. Very well absorbed by inhalation and skin contact. Signs and symptoms include headache, dizziness, nausea, elevated blood pressure, and convulsions.	0.5 ppm	5 ppm		Colorless solid with a distinctive odor and a very low vapor pressure at 20°C (68°F). Combustible. Much of the human experience is derived from its use as a pharmaceutical treatment in selected neurologic conditions.

Health Hazard Summaries	ACGIH TLV	IDLH	NFPA Codes H F R	Comments
Amitrole (3-amino-1,2,4-triazole [CAS: 61-82-5]): Mild irritant. Well absorbed by inhalation and skin contact. Overexposure can cause acute lung injury. Shows antithyroid activity in test animals. Evidence of adverse effects on fetal development in test animals at high doses. A carcinogen in test animals (IARC 3).	0.2 mg/m^3, A3 NIOSH CA			Used as an herbicide. Crystalline solid. Appearance and some hazardous properties vary with the formulation.
Ammonia (CAS: 7664-41-7): Corrosive; severe burns to eyes and skin result. Vapors highly irritating to eyes and respiratory tract; pulmonary edema has been reported. Severe responses are associated with anhydrous ammonia or with concentrated ammonia solutions (p 79).	25 ppm	300 ppm ERPG-1: 25 ppm ERPG-2: 150 ppm ERPG-3: 750 ppm	3 1 0	Colorless gas or aqueous solution. Pungent odor and irritation are good warning properties. Anhydrousammonia is flammable. Breakdown products include oxides of nitrogen. Although widely used in industry, concentrated forms are most frequently encountered in agriculture and from its use as a refrigerant.
Ammonium chloride a (CAS: 12125-02-9): Skin, eye, and respiratory tract irritant.	10 mg/m^3			Finely divided, odorless, white particulate. Decomposes on heating or burning, producing toxic and irritating fumes (nitrogen oxides, ammonia and hydrogen chloride). A large amount of fume may be generated in galvanizing operations.
***n*-Amyl acetate (CAS: 628-63-7):** Defats the skin, producing a dermatitis. Vapors mildly irritating to eyes and respiratory tract. A CNS depressant at very high levels. Reversible liver and kidney injury may occur at very high exposures.	50 ppm	1,000 ppm	1 3 0	Colorless liquid. Its banana-like odor, detectable below the TLV, is a good warning property. Vapor pressure is 4 mm Hg at 20°C (68°F). Flammable.
***sec*-Amyl acetate (alpha-methylbutyl acetate [CAS: 626-38-0]):** Defats the skin, producing a dermatitis. Vapors irritating to eyes and respiratory tract. A CNS depressant at very high levels. Reversible liver and kidney injury may occur at high-level exposures.	50 ppm	1,000 ppm	1 3 0	Colorless liquid. A fruity odor occurs below the TLV and is a good warning property. Vapor pressure is 7 mm Hg at 20°C (68°F). Flammable.

(C), ceiling air concentration (TLV-C); S, skin absorption can be significant; SEN, potential sensitizer; STEL, short-term (15-minute) exposure level. A1, ACGIH-confirmed human carcinogen; A2, ACGIH-suspected human carcinogen; A3, ACGIH animal carcinogen. ERPG, Emergency Response Planning Guideline (see p 656 for an explanation of ERPG). IARC 1, known human carcinogen; IARC 2A, probable human carcinogen; IARC 2B, possible human carcinogen; IARC 3, inadequate data available. NFPA hazard codes: H, health; F, fire; R, reactivity; Ox, oxidizer; W, water-reactive; 0 (none) <—> 4 (severe).

(*continued*)

TABLE IV–4. HEALTH HAZARD SUMMARIES FOR INDUSTRIAL AND OCCUPATIONAL CHEMICALS (CONTINUED)

Health Hazard Summaries	ACGIH TLV	IDLH	NFPA Codes H F R	Comments
Aniline (aminobenzene, phenylamine [CAS: 62-53-3]): Mildly irritating to eyes upon direct contact, with corneal injury possible. Potent inducer of methemoglobinemia (p 317). Well absorbed via inhalation and dermal routes. Limited evidence of carcinogenicity in test animals (IARC 3).	2 ppm, S, A3 NIOSH CA	100 ppm	2 2 0	Colorless to brown viscous liquid. Distinctive amine odor and mild eye irritation occur well below the TLV and are good warning properties. Vapor pressure is 0.6 mm Hg at 20°C (68°F). Combustible. Breakdown products include oxides of nitrogen.
***o*-Anisidine (*o*-methoxyaniline [CAS: 29191-52-4]):** Mild skin sensitizer causing dermatitis. Causes methemoglobinemia (p 317). Well absorbed through skin. Headaches and vertigo are signs of exposure. Possible liver and kidney injury. A carcinogen in test animals (IARC 2B).	0.5 mg/m^3, S, A3 NIOSH CA	50 mg/m^3	2 1 0	Colorless, red, or yellow liquid with the fishy odor of amines. Vapor pressure is less than 0.1 mm Hg at 20°C (68°F). Combustible. Primarily used in the dyestuffs industry.
Antimony and salts (antimony trichloride, antimony pentachloride [CAS: 7440-36-0]): Dusts and fumes irritating to eyes, skin, and respiratory tract. Toxicity through contamination with silica or arsenic may occur. **Antimony trioxide** (CAS: 1309-64-4) is carcinogenic in test animals, with limited evidence for carcinogenicity among antimony trioxide production workers (IARC 2B). See also p 112.	0.5 mg/m^3 (as Sb) A2 (antimony trioxide)	50 mg/m^3 (as Sb)		The metal is silver-white and has a very low vapor pressure. Some chloride salts release HCl upon contact with air.
ANTU (alpha-naphthylthiourea [CAS: 86-88-4]): Well absorbed by skin contact and inhalation. Pulmonary edema and liver injury may result from ingestion. Repeated exposures can injure the thyroid and adrenals, producing hypothyroidism. Possible trace contamination with alpha$_2$-naphthylamine, a human bladder carcinogen.	0.3 mg/m^3, S	100 mg/m^3		Colorless to gray solid powder. Odorless. A rodenticide. Breakdown products include oxides of nitrogen and sulfur dioxide.
Argon (CAS: 7440-37-1): Simple asphyxiant.				Inert gas that is colorless, odorless, and heavier than air. Bulk displacement of oxygen could occur in a confined space release.

Arsenic (CAS: 7440-38-2): Irritating to eyes and skin; hyperpigmentation, hyperkeratoses, and skin cancers have been described. A general cellular poison. May cause bone marrow suppression, peripheral neuropathy, and gastrointestinal, liver, and cardiac injury. Some arsenic compounds have adverse effects on fetal development in test animals. Exposure linked to skin, respiratory tract, and liver cancer in workers (IARC 1). See also p 140.	0.01 mg/m³ (as As), A1 OSHA CA NIOSH CA	5 mg/m³ (as As)		Elemental forms vary in appearance. Crystals are gray. Amorphous forms may be yellow or black. Vapor pressure is very low—about 1 mm Hg at 372°C (701°F).
Arsine (CAS: 7784-42-1): Extremely toxic hemolytic agent. Symptoms include abdominal pain, jaundice, hemoglobinuria, and renal failure. Low-level chronic exposures reported to cause anemia. See also p 144.	0.005 ppm NIOSH CA	3 ppm ERPG-2: 0.5 ppm ERPG-3: 1.5 ppm	4 4 2	Colorless gas with an unpleasant garlic-like odor. Flammable. Breakdown products include arsenic trioxide and arsenic fumes. Used in the semiconductor industry.
Asbestos (chrysotile, amosite, crocidolite, tremolite, anthophyllite): Effects of exposure include asbestosis (fibrosis of the lung), lung cancer, mesothelioma, and possible digestive tract cancer (IARC 1). Signs of toxicity are usually delayed at least 15–30 years. See also p 146.	0.1 fibers per cm³ (respirable fibers), A1 OSHA CA NIOSH CA			Exposure can occur through deconstruction and demolition work at prior asbestos use sites.
Asphalt fumes (CAS: 8052-42-4): Vapors and fumes irritating to eyes, skin, and respiratory tract. Skin contact can produce hyperpigmentation, dermatitis, or photosensitization. Some constituents are carcinogenic in test animals (IARC 2B).	0.5 mg/m³ (inhalable fraction) NIOSH CA			Smoke with an acrid odor. Asphalt is a complex mixture of parrafinic, aromatic, and heterocyclic hydrocarbons formed by the evaporation of lighter hydrocarbons from petroleum and the partial oxidation of the residue.
Atrazine (2-chloro-4-ethylamino-6-isoprylamino-s-triazine [CAS: 1912-24-9]): Skin and eye irritant. IARC 3.	2 mg/m³ (inhalable fraction)			Colorless crystals with a negligible vapor pressure. Slightly sensitive to light. The most heavily used triazine herbicide.

(C), ceiling air concentration (TLV-C); S, skin absorption can be significant; SEN, potential sensitizer; STEL, short-term (15-minute) exposure level. A1, ACGIH-confirmed human carcinogen; A2, ACGIH-suspected human carcinogen; A3, ACGIH animal carcinogen. ERPG, Emergency Response Planning Guideline (see p 656 for an explanation of ERPG). IARC 1, known human carcinogen; IARC 2A, probable human carcinogen; IARC 2B, possible human carcinogen; IARC 3, inadequate data available. NFPA hazard codes: H, health; F, fire; R, reactivity; Ox, oxidizer; W, water-reactive; 0 (none) <—> 4 (severe).

(continued)

TABLE IV–4. HEALTH HAZARD SUMMARIES FOR INDUSTRIAL AND OCCUPATIONAL CHEMICALS (CONTINUED)

Health Hazard Summaries	ACGIH TLV	IDLH	NFPA Codes H F R	Comments
Azinphos-methyl (Guthion [CAS: 86-50-0]): Low-potency organophosphate anticholinesterase insecticide (p 353). Requires metabolic activation.	0.2 mg/m^3 (inhalable fraction and vapor), S, SEN	10 mg/m^3		Brown, waxy solid with a negligible vapor pressure. Not combustible. Breakdown products include sulfur dioxide, oxides of nitrogen, and phosphoric acid.
Barium and soluble compounds (CAS: 7440-39-3): Powders irritating to eyes, skin, and respiratory tract. Although not typical of workplace exposures, ingestion of soluble barium salts (as opposed to the insoluble medical compounds used in radiography) is associated with muscle paralysis. See also p 152.	0.5 mg/m^3 (as Ba)	50 mg/m^3 (as Ba)		Most soluble barium compounds (eg, barium chloride, barium carbonate) are odorless white solids. Elemental barium spontaneously ignites on contact with air and reacts with water to form flammable hydrogen gas. Barium carbonate is a rodenticide; barium styphnate is an explosive propellant.
Benomyl (methyl 1-[butylcarbamoyl]-2-benzimidazolecarbamate, Benlate [CAS: 17804-35-2]): A carbamate cholinesterase inhibitor (p 353). Mildly irritating to eyes and skin. Of low systemic toxicity in test animals by all routes. Evidence of adverse effects on fetal development in test animals.	1 mg/m^3 (inhalable fraction), SEN, A3			White crystalline solid with a negligible vapor pressure at 20°C (68°F). Fungicide and miticide. Appearance and some hazardous properties vary with the formulation.
Benzene (CAS: 71-43-2): Vapors mildly irritating to eyes and respiratory tract. Well absorbed by all routes. A CNS depressant at high levels. Symptoms include headache, nausea, tremors, cardiac arrhythmias, and coma. Chronic exposure is causally associated with hematopoietic system depression, aplastic anemia, and leukemia (IARC 1). See also p 154.	0.5 ppm, S, A1 OSHA CA NIOSH CA	500 ppm ERPG-1: 50 ppm ERPG-2: 150 ppm ERPG-3: 1,000 ppm	1 3 0	Colorless liquid. Aromatic hydrocarbon odor near 50 ppm. Vapor pressure is 75 mm Hg at 20°C (68°F). Flammable. The generic term "benzine" is often used for gasoline or gasoline-like solvents and may not equate with benzene-containing materials.
Benzidine (*p*-diaminodiphenyl [CAS: 92-87-5]): Extremely well absorbed by inhalation and through skin. Causes bladder cancer in exposed workers (IARC 1).	S, A1 OSHA CA NIOSH CA			White or reddish solid crystals. Breakdown products include oxides of nitrogen. Found in dyestuffs, rubber industry, and analytic laboratories.

Benzoyl peroxide (CAS: 94-36-0): Dusts cause skin, eye, and respiratory tract irritation. A skin sensitizer. IARC 3.	5 mg/m^3	1,500 mg/m^3		White granules or crystalline solids with a very faint odor. Vapor pressure is negligible at 20°C (68°F). Strong oxidizer, reacting with combustible materials. Decomposes at 75°C (167°F). Unstable and explosive at high temperatures.
Benzyl chloride (alpha-chlorotoluene, [chloromethyl] benzene [CAS: 100-44-7]): Highly irritating to skin and eyes. A potent lacrimator. Vapors highly irritating to respiratory tract. Symptoms include weakness, headache, and irritability. May injure liver. Limited evidence for carcinogenicity and adverse effects on fetal development in test animals (IARC 2A).	1 ppm, A3	10 ppm ERPG-1: 1 ppm ERPG-2: 10 ppm ERPG-3: 50 ppm	3 2 1	Colorless liquid with a pungent odor near 1 ppm. Vapor pressure is 0·9 mm Hg at 20°C (68°F). Combustible. Breakdown products include phosgene and hydrogen chloride.
Beryllium (CAS: 7440-41-7): Very high acute exposure to dusts and fumes causes eye, skin, and respiratory tract irritation. However, more importantly, chronic low-level exposures to beryllium oxide dusts can produce an interstitial lung disease called berylliosis or chronic beryllium disease, which is a sarcoid-like condition that also can have extrapulmonary manifestations. A carcinogen in test animals. There is limited evidence of carcinogenicity in humans (IARC 1).	0.00005 ppm (inhalable fraction), S, SEN, A1 NIOSH CA	4 mg/m^3 (as Be) ERPG-2: 25 mcg/m^3 ERPG-3: 100 mcg/m^3	3 1 0	Silver-white metal or dusts. Reacts with some acids to produce flammable hydrogen gas. Exposures have occurred in nuclear and aerospace workers; may be present in any specialty metal alloy or metal ceramic manufacturing process; trace amounts naturally occur in bauxite, leading to exposure in aluminum smelting; dental technicians may also be exposed.
Biphenyl (diphenyl [CAS: 92-52-4]): Fumes mildly irritating to eyes. Chronic overexposures can cause bronchitis and liver injury. Peripheral neuropathy and CNS injury have also been reported.	0.2 ppm	100 mg/m^3	1 1 0	White crystals. Unusual but pleasant odor. Combustible. Previously used as antimold treatment for paper (eg, in wrapping citrus). An outbreak of parkinsonism has been reported in this context.

(C), ceiling air concentration (TLV-C); S, skin absorption can be significant; SEN, potential sensitizer; STEL, short-term (15-minute) exposure level. A1, ACGIH-confirmed human carcinogen; A2, ACGIH-suspected human carcinogen; A3, ACGIH animal carcinogen. ERPG, Emergency Response Planning Guideline (see p 656 for an explanation of ERPG). IARC 1, known human carcinogen; IARC 2A, probable human carcinogen; IARC 2B, possible human carcinogen; IARC 3, inadequate data available. NFPA hazard codes: H, health; F, fire; R, reactivity; Ox, oxidizer; W, water-reactive; 0 (none) <—> 4 (severe).

(*continued*)

TABLE IV–4. HEALTH HAZARD SUMMARIES FOR INDUSTRIAL AND OCCUPATIONAL CHEMICALS (CONTINUED)

Health Hazard Summaries	ACGIH TLV	IDLH	NFPA Codes H F R	Comments
Bisphenol A (BPA [CAS: 80-05-7]): Chronic exposure through food and environmental contamination may cause adverse reproductive and developmental effects, potentially as an "endocrine disruptor."	NIOSH CA			Widely used industrially as a starting material for carbonate plastics, in the formulation of epoxy resins, and as an additive to other plastics. Exposure occurs through migration of residual unreacted BPA.
Borates (anhydrous sodium tetraborate, borax [CAS: 1303-96-4]): Contact with dusts is highly irritating to eyes, skin, and respiratory tract. Contact with tissue moisture may cause thermal burns because hydration of borates generates heat. See also p 162.	2 mg/m^3 (inhalable fraction)			White or light gray solid crystals. Odorless.
Boron oxide (boric anhydride, boric oxide [CAS: 1303-86-2]): Contact with moisture generates boric acid (p 162). Direct eye or skin contact with dusts is irritating. Occupational inhalation exposure has caused respiratory tract irritation. Evidence for adverse effects on the testes in animals.	10 mg/m^3	2,000 mg/m^3		Colorless glassy granules, flakes, or powder. Odorless. Not combustible.
Boron tribromide (CAS: 10294-33-4): Corrosive; decomposed by tissue moisture to hydrogen bromide (p 166) and boric acid (p 162). Severe skin and eye burns may result from direct contact. Vapors highly irritating to eyes and respiratory tract.	1 ppm (C)		3 0 2 W	Colorless fuming liquid. Reacts with water, forming hydrogen bromide and boric acid. Vapor pressure is 40 mm Hg at 14°C (57°F).
Boron trifluoride (CAS: 7637-07-2): Corrosive; decomposed by tissue moisture to hydrogen fluoride (p 269) and boric acid (p 162). Severe skin and eye burns may result. Vapors highly irritating to eyes, skin, and respiratory tract.	1 ppm (C)	25 ppm ERPG-1: 2 mg/m^3 ERPG-2: 30 mg/m^3 ERPG-3: 100 mg/m^3	4 0 1	Colorless gas. Odor threshold near 2 mg/m^3. Dense, white, irritating fumes produced on contact with moist air. These fumes contain boric acid and hydrogen fluoride.

Bromine (CAS: 7726-95-6): Corrosive; severe skin and eye burns may result. Vapors highly irritating to eyes and respiratory tract; pulmonary edema may result. Measles-like eruptions may appear on the skin several hours after a severe exposure.	0.1 ppm	3 ppm ERPG-1: 0.1 ppm ERPG-2: 0.5 ppm ERPG 3: 5 ppm	3 0 0 Ox	Heavy red-brown fuming liquid. Odor and irritation thresholds are below the TLV and are adequate warning properties. Vapor pressure is 175 mm Hg at 20°C (68°F). Not combustible. Used as an alternative to chlorine in water purification (eg, hot tubs).
Bromine pentafluoride (CAS: 7789-30-2): Corrosive; severe skin and eye burns may result. Vapors extremely irritating to eyes and respiratory tract. Chronic overexposures caused severe liver and kidney injury in test animals.	0.1 ppm		4 0 3 W, Ox	Pale yellow liquid. Pungent odor. Not combustible. Highly reactive, igniting most organic materials and corroding many metals. Highly reactive with acids. Breakdown products include bromine and fluorine.
Bromoform (tribromomethane [CAS: 75-25-2]): Vapors highly irritating to eyes and respiratory tract. Well absorbed by inhalation and skin contact. CNS depressant. Liver and kidney injury may occur. Two preliminary tests indicate that it may be an animal carcinogen (IARC 3).	0.5 ppm, A3	850 ppm		Colorless to yellow liquid. Chloroform-like odor and irritation are adequate warning properties. Vapor pressure is 5 mm Hg at 20°C (68°F). Not combustible. Thermal breakdown products include hydrogen bromide and bromine.
1-Bromopropane (*n*-propyl bromide, 1-BP [CAS: 106-94-5]): Experimental reproductive and hepatotoxin. Human neurotoxin. A carcinogen in test animals (IARC 2B).	0.1 ppm, A3	46,000 ppm [LEL]		Vapor pressure is 111 mm Hg at 25°C (77°F). Used as alternative to ozone-depleting solvents in dry cleaning and spray adhesives. Documented neurotoxicity following occupational exposure in adhesive use.
1,3-Butadiene (CAS: 106-99-0): Vapors mildly irritating. A CNS depressant at very high levels. Evidence of adverse effects on reproductive organs and fetal development in test animals. A very potent carcinogen in test animals; evidence of carcinogenicity in exposed workers (IARC 1).	2 ppm, A2 OSHA CA NIOSH CA	20,000 ppm [LEL] ERPG-1: 10 ppm ERPG-2: 200 ppm ERPG-3: 5,000 ppm	2 4 2	Colorless gas. Mild aromatic odor is a good warning property. Readily polymerizes. Inhibitor added to prevent peroxide formation. Used in the formation of styrene-butadiene and ABS (acrylonitrile butadiene styrene) plastics.

(C), ceiling air concentration (TLV-C); S, skin absorption can be significant; SEN, potential sensitizer; STEL, short-term (15-minute) exposure level. A1, ACGIH-confirmed human carcinogen; A2, ACGIH-suspected human carcinogen; A3, ACGIH animal carcinogen. ERPG, Emergency Response Planning Guideline (see p 656 for an explanation of ERPG). IARC 1, known human carcinogen; IARC 2A, probable human carcinogen; IARC 2B, possible human carcinogen; IARC 3, inadequate data available. NFPA hazard codes: H, health; F, fire; R, reactivity; Ox, oxidizer; W, water-reactive; 0 (none) <—> 4 (severe).

(continued)

TABLE IV–4. HEALTH HAZARD SUMMARIES FOR INDUSTRIAL AND OCCUPATIONAL CHEMICALS (CONTINUED)

Health Hazard Summaries	ACGIH TLV	IDLH	NFPA Codes H F R	Comments
2-Butoxyethanol (ethylene glycol monobutyl ether, butyl cellosolve [CAS: 111-76-2]): Liquid very irritating to eyes and slightly irritating to skin. Vapors irritating to eyes and respiratory tract. Mild CNS depressant. A hemolytic agent in test animals. Well absorbed dermally. Liver and kidney toxicity in test animals. Reproductive toxicity much less than that of certain other glycol ethers, such as ethylene glycol monomethyl ether. See also p 234. IARC 3.	20 ppm, A3	700 ppm	3 2 0	Colorless liquid with a mild ether-like odor. Irritation occurs below the TLV and is a good warning property. Vapor pressure is 0.6 mm Hg at 20°C (68°F). Flammable.
***n*-Butyl acetate (CAS: 123-86-4):** Vapors irritating to eyes and respiratory tract. A CNS depressant at high levels. Limited evidence for adverse effects on fetal development in test animals.	150 ppm (proposed 50 ppm)	17,000 ppm [LEL] ERPG-1: 5 ppm ERPG-2: 200 ppm ERPG-3: 3,000 ppm	2 3 0	Colorless liquid. Fruity odor is a good warning property. Vapor pressure is 10 mm Hg at 20°C (68°F). Flammable.
***sec*-Butyl acetate (2-butanol acetate [CAS: 105-46-4]):** Vapors irritating to eyes and respiratory tract. A CNS depressant at high levels.	200 ppm (proposed 50 ppm)	1,700 ppm [LEL]	1 3 0	
***tert*-Butyl acetate (*tert*-butyl ester of acetic acid [CAS: 540-88-5]):** Vapors irritating to eyes and respiratory tract. A CNS depressant at high levels.	200 ppm (proposed 50 ppm)	1,500 ppm [LEL]		
***n*-Butyl acrylate (CAS: 141-32-2):** Highly irritating to skin and eyes; corneal necrosis may result. Vapors highly irritating to eyes and respiratory tract. Based on structural analogies, compounds containing the acrylate moiety may be carcinogens (IARC 3).	2 ppm, SEN	ERPG-1: 0.05 ppm ERPG-2: 25 ppm ERPG-3: 250 ppm	3 2 2	Colorless liquid. Odor threshold near 0.05 ppm. Vapor pressure is 3.2 mm Hg at 20°C (68°F). Flammable. Contains inhibitor to prevent polymerization.

***n*-Butyl alcohol (CAS: 71-36-3):** Irritating upon direct contact. Vapors mildly irritating to eyes and respiratory tract. A CNS depressant at very high levels. Chronic occupational overexposures associated with hearing loss and vestibular impairment.	20 ppm	1,400 ppm [LEL]	2 3 0	Colorless liquid. Strong odor and irritation occur below the TLV and are both good warning properties. Flammable.
***sec*-Butyl alcohol (CAS: 78-92-2):** Vapors mildly irritating to eyes and respiratory tract. A CNS depressant at high levels.	100 ppm	2,000 ppm	2 3 0	Colorless liquid. Pleasant odor occurs well below the TLV and is an adequate warning property. Vapor pressure is 13 mm Hg at 20°C (68°F). Flammable.
***tert*-Butyl alcohol (CAS: 75-65-0):** Vapors mildly irritating to eyes and respiratory tract. A CNS depressant at high levels.	100 ppm	1,600 ppm	2 3 0	Colorless liquid. Camphor-like odor and irritation occur slightly below the TLV and are good warning properties. Vapor pressure is 31 mm Hg at 20°C (68°F). Flammable.
***n*-Butylamine (CAS: 109-73-9):** Caustic alkali. Liquid highly irritating to eyes and skin upon direct contact; severe burns may result. Vapors highly irritating to eyes and respiratory tract. May cause histamine release.	5 ppm (C), S	300 ppm	3 3 0	Colorless liquid. Ammonia-like or fishlike odor occurs below the TLV and is an adequate warning property. Vapor pressure is about 82 mm Hg at 20°C (68°F). Flammable.
***tert*-Butyl chromate (CAS: 1189-85-1):** Liquid highly irritating to eyes and skin; severe burns may result. Vapors or mists irritating to eyes and respiratory tract. A liver and kidney toxin. By analogy to other Cr VI compounds, a possible carcinogen. No IARC evaluation. See p 196.	0.1 mg/m^3 (C) (as CrO_3), S NIOSH CA	15 mg/m^3 (as Cr VI)		Liquid. Reacts with moisture.
***n*-Butyl glycidyl ether (BGE, glycidylbutylether, 1,2-epoxy-3-butoxy propane [CAS: 2426-08-6]):** Liquid irritating to eyes and skin. Vapors irritating to the respiratory tract and cause GI distress. A CNS depressant. Causes sensitization dermatitis upon repeated exposures. Testicular atrophy and hematopoietic injury at modest doses in test animals.	3 ppm, S, SEN	250 ppm		Colorless liquid. Vapor pressure is 3 mm Hg at 20°C (68°F). Used in epoxy formulations.

(C), ceiling air concentration (TLV-C); S, skin absorption can be significant; SEN, potential sensitizer; STEL, short-term (15-minute) exposure level. A1, ACGIH-confirmed human carcinogen; A2, ACGIH-suspected human carcinogen; A3, ACGIH animal carcinogen. ERPG, Emergency Response Planning Guideline (see p 656 for an explanation of ERPG). IARC 1, known human carcinogen; IARC 2A, probable human carcinogen; IARC 2B, possible human carcinogen; IARC 3, inadequate data available. NFPA hazard codes: H, health; F, fire; R, reactivity; Ox, oxidizer; W, water-reactive; 0 (none) <—> 4 (severe).

(*continued*)

TABLE IV–4. HEALTH HAZARD SUMMARIES FOR INDUSTRIAL AND OCCUPATIONAL CHEMICALS (CONTINUED)

Health Hazard Summaries	ACGIH TLV	IDLH	NFPA Codes H F R	Comments
***n*-Butyl lactate (CAS: 138-22-7):** Vapors irritating to eyes and respiratory tract. Workers have complained of sleepiness, headache, coughing, nausea, and vomiting.	5 ppm		1 2 0	Colorless liquid. Vapor pressure is 0.4 mm Hg at 20°C (68°F). Combustible.
***n*-Butyl mercaptan (butanethiol [CAS: 109-79-5]):** Vapors mildly irritating to eyes and respiratory tract. Pulmonary edema occurred at high exposure levels in test animals. A CNS depressant at very high levels. Limited evidence for adverse effects on fetal development in test animals at high doses.	0.5 ppm	500 ppm	1 3 0	Colorless liquid. Strong, offensive, garlic-like odor. Vapor pressure is 35 mm Hg at 20°C (68°F). Flammable.
***o-sec*-Butylphenol (CAS: 89-72-5):** Irritating to skin upon direct, prolonged contact; burns have resulted. Vapors mildly irritating to eyes and respiratory tract.	5 ppm, S			A liquid.
***p-tert*-Butyltoluene (CAS: 98-51-1):** Mild skin irritant upon direct contact. Defatting agent causing dermatitis. Vapors irritating to eyes and respiratory tract. A CNS depressant. Limited evidence of adverse effects on fetal development in test animals at high doses.	1 ppm	100 ppm		Colorless liquid. Gasoline-like odor and irritation occur below the TLV and are both good warning properties. Vapor pressure is less than 1 mm Hg at 20°C (68°F). Combustible.
gamma-Butyrolactone (CAS: 96-48-0): Because of metabolism to gamma-hydroxybutyric acid (GHB), CNS and respiratory depression may occur (p 252). IARC 3.			1 2 0	Industrial solvent. Contained in some "acetone-free" nail polish removers (now restricted in United States because it is a GHB precursor). Vapor pressure 1.5 mm Hg at 20°C (68°F).

Cadmium and compounds (CAS 7440-43-9): Acute fumes and dust exposures can injure the respiratory tract; pulmonary edema can occur. Chronic exposures associated primarily with kidney injury and lung injury. Adverse effects on the testes and on fetal development in test animals. Cadmium and some of its compounds are carcinogenic in test animals. Limited direct evidence for carcinogenicity in humans (IARC 1). See also p 168.	0.01 mg/m^3 (total dust, as Cd), 0.002 mg/m^3 (respirable fraction, as Cd), A2 OSHA CA NIOSH CA	9 mg/m^3 (dust and fumes, as Cd)		Compounds vary in color. Give off fumes when heated or burned. Generally poor warning properties. Metal has a vapor pressure of about 1 mm Hg at 394°C (741°F) and reacts with acids to produce flammable hydrogen gas. "Silver solder" typically contains cadmium.
Calcium cyanamide (calcium carbimide, lime nitrogen [CAS: 156-62-7]): Dusts highly irritating to eyes, skin, and respiratory tract. Causes sensitization dermatitis. Systemic symptoms include nausea, fatigue, headache, chest pain, and shivering. A disulfiram-like interaction with alcohol (p 226),"cyanamide flush," may occur in exposed workers.	0.5 mg/m^3			Gray crystalline material. Reacts with water, generating ammonia and flammable acetylene. In addition to industrial exposure, used as a pharmaceutical alcohol aversive agent.
Calcium hydroxide (hydrated lime, caustic lime [CAS: 1305-62-0]): Corrosive (p 186); severe eye and skin burns may result. Dusts moderately irritating to eyes and respiratory tract.	5 mg/m^3			White, deliquescent crystalline powder. Odorless.
Calcium oxide (lime, quicklime, burnt lime [CAS: 1305-78-8]): Corrosive (p 186). Exothermic reactions with moisture. Highly irritating to eyes and skin upon direct contact. Dusts highly irritating to skin, eyes, and respiratory tract.	2 mg/m^3	25 mg/m^3	3 0 1	White or gray solid powder. Odorless. Hydration generates heat.

(C), ceiling air concentration (TLV-C); S, skin absorption can be significant; SEN, potential sensitizer; STEL, short-term (15-minute) exposure level. A1, ACGIH-confirmed human carcinogen; A2, ACGIH-suspected human carcinogen; A3, ACGIH animal carcinogen. ERPG, Emergency Response Planning Guideline (see p 656 for an explanation of ERPG). IARC 1, known human carcinogen; IARC 2A, probable human carcinogen; IARC 2B, possible human carcinogen; IARC 3, inadequate data available. NFPA hazard codes: H, health; F, fire; R, reactivity; Ox, oxidizer; W, water-reactive; 0 (none) <—> 4 (severe).

(*continued*)

TABLE IV–4. HEALTH HAZARD SUMMARIES FOR INDUSTRIAL AND OCCUPATIONAL CHEMICALS (CONTINUED)

Health Hazard Summaries	ACGIH TLV	IDLH	NFPA Codes H F R	Comments
Camphor, synthetic (CAS: 76-22-2): Irritating to eyes and skin upon direct contact. Vapors irritating to eyes and nose; may cause loss of sense of smell. A convulsant at doses typical of overdose ingestion rather than industrial exposure. See also p 176.	2 ppm	200 mg/m^3	2 2 0	Colorless, glassy solid. Sharp, obnoxious, aromatic odor near the TLV is an adequate warning property. Vapor pressure is 0.18 mm Hg at 20°C (68°F). Combustible.
Caprolactam (CAS: 105-60-2): Highly irritating to eyes and skin upon direct contact. Vapors, dusts, and fumes highly irritating to eyes and respiratory tract. Convulsant activity in test animals.	5 mg/m^3 (inhalable fraction and vapor)			White solid crystals. Unpleasant odor. Vapor pressure is 6 mm Hg at 120°C (248°F). Thermal breakdown products include oxides of nitrogen. Used in the production of Nylon 6; off-gassing of caprolactam from the polymerized product can be detected.
Captafol (Difolatan [CAS: 2425-06-1]): Dusts irritating to eyes, skin, and respiratory tract. A skin and respiratory tract sensitizer. May cause photoallergy dermatitis. Evidence for carcinogenicity in animal tests (IARC 2A).	0.1 mg/m^3, S NIOSH CA			White solid crystals. Distinctive, pungent odor. Fungicide. Thermal breakdown products include hydrogen chloride and oxides of nitrogen or sulfur.
Carbaryl (1-naphthyl *N*-methylcarbamate, sevin [CAS: 63-25-2]): A carbamate-type cholinesterase inhibitor (p 353). Evidence of adverse effects on fetal development in test animals at high doses (IARC 3).	0.5 mg/m^3 (inhalable fraction and vapor), S	100 mg/m^3		Colorless, white or gray solid. Odorless. Vapor pressure is 0.005 mm Hg at 20°C (68°F). Breakdown products include oxides of nitrogen and methylamine.
Carbofuran (2,3-dihydro-2,2'-dimethyl-7-benzofuranylmethyl-carbamate, Furadan [CAS: 1563-66-2]): A carbamate-type cholinesterase inhibitor (p 353). Not well absorbed by skin contact.	0.1 mg/m^3 (inhalable fraction and vapor)			White solid crystals. Odorless. Vapor pressure is 0.00005 mm Hg at 33°C (91°F). Thermal breakdown products include oxides of nitrogen.
Carbon black (CAS: 1333-86-4): Causes eye and respiratory irritation. A lung carcinogen in test animals (IARC 2B).	3 mg/m^3 (inhalable fraction), A3 NIOSH CA			Extremely fine powdery forms of elemental carbon; may have adsorbed polycyclic organic hydrocarbons.

Carbon dioxide (carbonic acid, dry ice [CAS: 124-38-9]): Acute asphyxiant and CNS depressant. Exposure to high levels can produce tachypnea, shortness of breath, headache and other neurologic symptoms and signs, including coma.	5,000 ppm	40,000 ppm		Colorless, odorless gas. Nonflammable. Heavier than air Exposure can occur through natural sources (geologic, including coal mines) and through man-made activities (industrial fermentation, dry ice sublimation). Enclosed space hazard.
Carbon disulfide (CAS: 75-15-0): Vapors mildly irritating to eyes and respiratory tract. A CNS depressant causing coma at high concentrations. Well absorbed by all routes. Acute symptoms include headache, dizziness, nervousness, and fatigue. Neuropathies, parkinsonian syndromes, and psychosis may occur. A liver and kidney toxin. An atherogenic agent causing stroke and heart disease. Adversely affects male and female reproductive systems in test animals and humans. Evidence for adverse effects on fetal development in test animals. See also p 181.	1 ppm, S	500 ppm ERPG-1: 1 ppm ERPG-2: 50 ppm ERPG-3: 500 ppm	3 4 0	Colorless to pale yellow liquid. Disagreeable odor occurs below the TLV and is a good warning property. Vapor pressure is 300 mm Hg at 20°C (68 F). Highly flammable. Major use is in viscose manufacture but is also used in chemical synthesis and as an industrial solvent. It was used in the past as an agricultural fumigant. It is one of the environmental breakdown products of the agricultural chemical metam sodium and is a metabolite of the pharmaceutical disulfiram.
Carbon monoxide (CAS: 630-08-0): Binds to hemoglobin, forming carboxyhemoglobin and causing cellular hypoxia. Persons with heart disease are more susceptible. Signs and symptoms include headache, dizziness, coma, and convulsions. Permanent CNS impairment and adverse effects on fetal development may occur after severe poisoning. See also p 182.	25 ppm	1,200 ppm ERPG-1: 200 ppm ERPG-2: 350 ppm ERPG-3: 500 ppm	2 4 0	Colorless, odorless gas. No warning properties. Important indoor sources of exposure include the indoor use of internal combustion engines, structural fires, and faulty space heaters. It is also an ambient air criteria pollutant regulated by the US Environmental Protection Agency. The solvent methlylene chloride and the antiseptic iodoform are both metabolized to carbon monoxide.
Carbon tetrabromide (tetrabromomethane [CAS: 558-13-4]): Highly irritating to eyes upon direct contact. Vapors highly irritating to eyes and respiratory tract. The liver and kidneys are also likely target organs.	0.1 ppm			White to yellow-brown solid. Vapor pressure is 40 mm Hg at 96°C (204°F). Nonflammable; thermal breakdown products may include hydrogen bromide and bromine.

(C), ceiling air concentration (TLV-C); S, skin absorption can be significant; SEN, potential sensitizer; STEL, short-term (15-minute) exposure level. A1, ACGIH-confirmed human carcinogen; A2, ACGIH-suspected human carcinogen; A3, ACGIH animal carcinogen. ERPG, Emergency Response Planning Guideline (see p 656 for an explanation of ERPG). IARC 1, known human carcinogen; IARC 2A, probable human carcinogen; IARC 2B, possible human carcinogen; IARC 3, inadequate data available. NFPA hazard codes: H, health; F, fire; R, reactivity; Ox, oxidizer; W, water-reactive; 0 (none) <—> 4 (severe).

(continued)

TABLE IV–4. HEALTH HAZARD SUMMARIES FOR INDUSTRIAL AND OCCUPATIONAL CHEMICALS (CONTINUED)

Health Hazard Summaries	ACGIH TLV	IDLH	NFPA Codes H F R	Comments
Carbon tetrachloride (tetrachloromethane [CAS 56-23-5]): Mildly irritating upon direct contact. A CNS depressant. May cause cardiac arrhythmias. Highly toxic to kidney and liver. Alcohol abuse increases risk for liver toxicity. A carcinogen in test animals (IARC 2B). See also p 184.	5 ppm, S, A2 NIOSH CA	200 ppm ERPG-1: 20 ppm ERPG-2: 100 ppm ERPG-3: 750 ppm	3 0 0	Colorless. Ether-like odor is a poor warning property (odor threshold is near 20 ppm). Vapor pressure is 91 mm Hg at 20°C (68°F). Not combustible. Breakdown products include hydrogen chloride, chlorine gas, and phosgene. Can contaminate antique fire extinguishers.
Carbonyl fluoride (COF_2 [CAS: 353-50-41]): Extremely irritating to eyes and respiratory tract; pulmonary edema may result. Toxicity results from its hydrolysis to hydrofluoric acid (p 269).	2 ppm			Colorless, odorless gas. Decomposes upon contact with water to produce hydrofluoric acid. Can be a combustion by-product of polyfluorocarbons.
Catechol (1,2-benzenediol, pyrocatechol [CAS: 120-80-9]): Highly irritating upon direct contact; severe eye and deep skin burns result. Well absorbed by skin. Systemic toxicity similar to that of phenol (p 368); however, catechol may be more likely to cause convulsions and hypertension. At high doses, renal and liver injury may occur. IARC 2B.	5 ppm, S, A3		3 1 0	Colorless solid crystals. Used in industrial chemical synthesis of pesticides and other organic chemicals.
Cerium (oxide or salt): Rare earth element. Fume and dust exposure associated with human interstitial lung disease.				Component of "rouge" used in glass polishing; fume from arc lamp use and specialty applications. Proposed diesel fuel additive.
Cesium hydroxide (cesium hydrate [CAS: 21351-79-1]): Corrosive (p 186). Highly irritating upon direct contact; severe burns may result. Dusts are irritating to eyes and respiratory tract.	2 mg/m^3			Colorless or yellow crystals that absorb moisture. Negligible vapor pressure.

Chloramine (monochloramine [CAS: 10599-90-3]): Vapors irritating to eyes and respiratory tract, can cause chemical pneumonitis (p 255). Liquid is a skin irritant. IARC 3. Closely related moieties include dichloramine and trichloramine (nitrogen trichloride).			Colorless or yellow liquid at 25°C, highly water-soluble. Often a mixture of mono-, di-, and trichloramines, produced when bleach and ammonia cleaners are combined or when urine comes in contact with chlorinated water. Small amounts off-gas from chlorinated public swimming pools. Occupational exposures include produce washing/packaging and water disinfection.
Chlordane (CAS: 57-74-9): Irritating to skin. A CNS convulsant. Skin absorption is rapid and has caused convulsions and death. Hepatotoxic. Evidence of carcinogenicity in test animals (IARC 2B). See also p 189.	0.5 mg/m^3, S, A3 NIOSH CA	100 mg/m^3	Viscous amber liquid. Formulations vary in appearance. A chlorine-like odor. Vapor pressure is 0.00001 mm Hg at 20°C (68°F). Not combustible. Thermal breakdown products include hydrogen chloride, phosgene, and chlorine gas. Pesticide use banned in the United States since 1976.
Chlorinated camphene (toxaphene [CAS: 8001-35-2]): Moderately irritating upon direct contact. A CNS convulsant. Acute symptoms include nausea, confusion, tremors, and convulsions. Well absorbed by skin. Potential liver and kidney injury. See also p 189.	0.5 mg/m^3, S, A3 NIOSH CA	200 mg/m^3	Waxy amber-colored solid. Formulations vary in appearance. Turpentine-like odor. Vapor pressure is about 0.3 mm Hg at 20°C (68°F). Pesticide use banned in the United States since 1990.
Chlorinated diphenyl oxide (CAS: 55720-99-5): Chloracne may result from even small exposures. A hepatotoxin in chronically exposed test animals. Signs and symptoms include gastrointestinal upset, jaundice, and fatigue. See also "Dioxins" (p 224).	0.5 mg/m^3	5 mg/m^3	Waxy solid or liquid. Vapor pressure is 0.00006 mm Hg at 20°C (68°F).

(C), ceiling air concentration (TLV-C); S, skin absorption can be significant; SEN, potential sensitizer; STEL, short-term (15-minute) exposure level. A1, ACGIH-confirmed human carcinogen; A2, ACGIH-suspected human carcinogen; A3, ACGIH animal carcinogen. ERPG, Emergency Response Planning Guideline (see p 656 for an explanation of ERPG). IARC 1, known human carcinogen; IARC 2A, probable human carcinogen; IARC 2B, possible human carcinogen; IARC 3, inadequate data available. NFPA hazard codes: H, health; F, fire; R, reactivity; Ox, oxidizer; W, water-reactive; 0 (none) <—> 4 (severe).

(*continued*)

TABLE IV–4. HEALTH HAZARD SUMMARIES FOR INDUSTRIAL AND OCCUPATIONAL CHEMICALS (CONTINUED)

Health Hazard Summaries	ACGIH TLV	IDLH	NFPA Codes H F R	Comments
Chlorine (CAS: 7782-50-5): Extremely irritating to eyes, skin, and respiratory tract; severe burns and pulmonary edema may occur. Symptoms include lacrimation, sore throat, headache, coughing, and wheezing. High concentrations may cause rapid tissue swelling and airway obstruction through laryngeal edema. See also p 191.	0.5 ppm	10 ppm ERPG-1: 1 ppm ERPG-2: 3 ppm ERPG-3: 20 ppm	4 0 0 Ox	Amber liquid or greenish-yellow gas. Irritating odor and irritation occur near the TLV and are both good warning properties. Can be formed when acid cleaners are mixed with hypochlorite bleach cleaners. Major releases can occur through transportation and water treatment mishaps and in industrial bleaching.
Chlorine dioxide (chlorine peroxide [CAS: 10049-04-4]): Extremely irritating to eyes and respiratory tract. Symptoms and signs are those of chlorine gas listed earlier (see also p 191), although chlorine dioxide is more potent.	0.1 ppm	5 ppm ERPG-2: 0.5 ppm ERPG-3: 3 ppm		Yellow-green or orange gas or liquid. Sharp odor at the TLV is a good warning property. Reacts with water to produce perchloric acid. Decomposes explosively in sunlight, with heat, or with shock to produce chlorine gas. Bleaching agent widely used in paper industry.
Chlorine trifluoride (chlorine fluoride [CAS: 7790-91-2]): Upon contact with moist tissues, hydrolyzes to chlorine (p 191), hydrogen fluoride (p 269), and chlorine dioxide. Extremely irritating to eyes, skin, and respiratory tract; severe burns or delayed pulmonary edema can result.	0.1 ppm (C)	20 ppm ERPG-1: 0.1 ppm ERPG-2: 1 ppm ERPG-3: 10 ppm	4 0 3 W, Ox	Greenish-yellow or colorless liquid or gas or white solid. Has a suffocating, sweet odor near 0.1 ppm. Not combustible. Water-reactive, yielding hydrogen fluoride and chlorine gas. Used as incendiary and rocket fuel additive.
Chloroacetaldehyde (CAS: 107-20-0): Extremely corrosive upon direct contact; severe burns will result. Vapors extremely irritating to eyes, skin, and respiratory tract.	1 ppm (C)	45 ppm		Colorless liquid with a pungent, irritating odor. Vapor pressure is 100 mm Hg at 20°C (68°F). Combustible. Readily polymerizes. Thermal breakdown products include phosgene and hydrogen chloride.
alpha-Chloroacetophenone (tear gas, chemical Mace [CAS: 532-27-4]): Extremely irritating to mucous membranes and respiratory tract. With extremely high inhalational exposures, lower respiratory injury is possible. A potent skin sensitizer. See also p 452.	0.05 ppm	15 mg/m^3	3 1 0	Sharp, irritating odor and irritation occur near the TLV and are adequate warning properties. Vapor pressure is 0.012 mm Hg at 20°C (68°F). Mace is a common crowd control agent.

Chlorobenzene (monochlorobenzene [CAS: 108-90-7]): Irritating; skin burns may result from prolonged contact. Vapors irritating to eyes and respiratory tract. A CNS depressant. May cause methemoglobinemia (p 317). Prolonged exposure to high levels has caused lung, liver, and kidney injury in test animals.	10 ppm, A3	1,000 ppm	3 3 0	Colorless liquid. Aromatic odor occurs below the TLV and is a good warning property. Vapor pressure is 8.8 mm Hg at 20°C (68°F). Flammable. Thermal breakdown products include hydrogen chloride and phosgene.
***o*-Chlorobenzylidene malononitrile (tear gas, OCBM, CS [CAS: 2698-41-1]):** Highly irritating on direct contact; severe burns may result. Aerosols and vapors very irritating to mucous membranes and upper respiratory tract. With extremely high inhalational exposures, lower respiratory injury is possible. Potent skin sensitizer. Symptoms include headache, nausea and vomiting, severe eye and nose irritation, excess salivation, and coughing. See also p 452.	0.05 ppm (C), S	2 mg/m^3 ERPG-1: 0.005 mg/m^3 ERPG-2: 0.1 mg/m^3 ERPG-3: 25 mg/m^3		White solid crystals. Pepper-like odor at 0.005 mg/m^3. Vapor pressure is much less than 1 mm Hg at 20°C (68°F). CS is a common crowd control agent.
Chlorobromomethane (bromochloromethane, Halon 1011 [CAS: 74-97-5]): Irritating upon direct contact. Vapors mildly irritating to eyes and respiratory tract. A CNS depressant. Disorientation, nausea, headache, seizures, and coma have been reported at high exposure. Chronic high doses caused liver and kidney injury in test animals.	200 ppm	2,000 ppm		Colorless to pale yellow liquid. Sweet, pleasant odor detectable far below the TLV. Vapor pressure is 117 mm Hg at 20°C (68°F). Thermal breakdown products include hydrogen chloride, hydrogen bromide, and phosgene.
Chlorodifluoromethane (Freon 22 [CAS: 75-45-6]): Irritating upon direct contact. Vapors mildly irritating to eyes and respiratory tract. A CNS depressant. High-level exposure may cause arrhythmias. There is evidence at high doses for adverse effects on fetal development in test animals (IARC 3). See also p 251.	1,000 ppm			Colorless, almost odorless gas. Nonflammable. Thermal breakdown products may include hydrogen fluoride. Widely used commercial refrigerant (eg, in seafood industry).

(C), ceiling air concentration (TLV-C); S, skin absorption can be significant; SEN, potential sensitizer; STEL, short-term (15-minute) exposure level. A1, ACGIH-confirmed human carcinogen; A2, ACGIH-suspected human carcinogen; A3, ACGIH animal carcinogen. ERPG, Emergency Response Planning Guideline (see p 656 for an explanation of ERPG). IARC 1, known human carcinogen; IARC 2A, probable human carcinogen; IARC 2B, possible human carcinogen; IARC 3, inadequate data available. NFPA hazard codes: H, health; F, fire; R, reactivity; Ox, oxidizer; W, water-reactive; 0 (none) <—> 4 (severe).

(continued)

TABLE IV–4. HEALTH HAZARD SUMMARIES FOR INDUSTRIAL AND OCCUPATIONAL CHEMICALS (CONTINUED)

Health Hazard Summaries	ACGIH TLV	IDLH	NFPA Codes H F R	Comments
Chloroform (trichloromethane [CAS: 67-66-3]): Mildly irritating upon direct contact; dermatitis may result from prolonged exposure. Vapors slightly irritating to eyes and respiratory tract. A CNS depressant. High levels (15,000–20,000 ppm) can cause coma and cardiac arrhythmias. Can produce liver and kidney damage. Limited evidence of adverse effects on fetal development in test animals. A carcinogen in test animals (IARC 2B). See also p 184.	10 ppm, A3 NIOSH CA	500 ppm ERPG-2: 50 ppm ERPG-3: 5,000 ppm	2 0 0	Colorless liquid. Pleasant, sweet odor. Not combustible. Vapor pressure is 160 mm Hg at 20°C (68°F). Thermal breakdown products include hydrogen chloride, phosgene, and chlorine gas.
Bis(chloromethyl) ether (BCME [CAS: 542-88-1]): A human lung carcinogen (IARC 1).	0.001 ppm, A1 OSHA CA NIOSH CA	ERPG-2: 0.1 ppm ERPG-3: 0.5 ppm	4 3 1	Colorless liquid with a suffocating odor. Vapor pressure is 100 mm Hg at 20°C (68°F). Used in the manufacture of ion-exchange resins. Can be formed when formaldehyde is mixed with hydrochloric acid.
Chloromethyl methyl ether (CMME, methyl chloromethyl ether [CAS: 107-30-2]): Vapors irritating to eyes and respiratory tract. Workers at increased risk for lung cancer, possibly owing to contamination of CMME with 1–7% BCME (IARC 1).	A2 OSHA CA NIOSH CA	ERPG-2: 1 ppm ERPG-3: 10 ppm	3 3 2	Combustible. Breakdown products include oxides of nitrogen and hydrogen chloride. Used in the manufacture of ion-exchange resins.
4-Chloro-2-methylphenoxyacetic acid (MCPA [CAS: 2698-38-6]): GI irritant with less toxicity than related phenoxherbicides 2,4-D and mecoprop (p 192).				White crystalline solid.
1-Chloro-1-nitropropane (CAS: 600-25-9): Based on animal studies, vapors highly irritating to eyes and respiratory tract and may cause pulmonary edema. High levels may cause injury to cardiac muscle, liver, and kidney.	2 ppm	100 ppm	3 2 3	Colorless liquid. Unpleasant odor and tearing occur near the TLV and are good warning properties. Vapor pressure is 5.8 mm Hg at 20°C (68°F). Used as a fungicide.

Chloropentafluoroethane (fluorocarbon 115 [CAS: 76-15-3]): Irritating upon direct contact. Vapors mildly irritating to eyes and respiratory tract. Produces coma and cardiac arrhythmias, but only at very high levels in test animals. See also p 251.	1,000 ppm			Colorless, odorless gas. Thermal breakdown products include hydrogen fluoride and hydrogen chloride.
Chloropicrin (trichloronitromethane [CAS: 76-06-2]): Extremely irritating upon direct contact; severe burns may result. Vapors extremely irritating to eyes, skin, and respiratory tract; delayed pulmonary edema has been reported. Kidney and liver injuries have been observed in test animals.	0.1 ppm	2 ppm ERPG-1: 0.075 ppm ERPG-2: 0.15 ppm ERPG-3: 1.5 ppm	4 0 3	Colorless, oily liquid. Sharp, penetrating odor and tearing occur near the TLV and are good warning properties. Vapor pressure is 20 mm Hg at 20°C (68°F). Breakdown products include oxides of nitrogen, phosgene, nitrosyl chloride, and chlorine gas. Used as a fumigant and also as an additive for its warning properties. Historically, used as a World War I chemical warfare agent.
beta-Chloroprene (2-chloro-1,3-butadiene [CAS: 126-99-8]): Irritating upon direct contact. Vapors irritating to eyes and respiratory tract. A CNS depressant at high levels. Liver and kidneys are major target organs. Limited evidence for adverse effects on fetal development and male reproduction in test animals. Equivocal evidence of carcinogenicity in test animals (IARC 2B).	10 ppm, S NIOSH CA	300 ppm	2 3 1	Colorless liquid with an ether-like odor. Vapor pressure is 179 mm Hg at 20°C (68°F). Highly flammable. Breakdown products include hydrogen chloride. Used in making neoprene.
***o*-Chlorotoluene (2-chloro-1-methylbenzene [CAS: 95-49-8]):** In test animals, direct contact produced skin and eye irritation; high vapor exposures resulted in tremors, convulsions, and coma. By analogy to toluene and chlorinated compounds, may cause cardiac arrhythmias.	50 ppm		2 2 0	Colorless liquid. Vapor pressure is 10 mm Hg at 43°C (109°F). Flammable.

(C), ceiling air concentration (TLV-C); S, skin absorption can be significant; SEN, potential sensitizer; STEL, short-term (15-minute) exposure level. A1, ACGIH-confirmed human carcinogen; A2, ACGIH-suspected human carcinogen; A3, ACGIH animal carcinogen. ERPG, Emergency Response Planning Guideline (see p 656 for an explanation of ERPG). IARC 1, known human carcinogen; IARC 2A, probable human carcinogen; IARC 2B, possible human carcinogen; IARC 3, inadequate data available. NFPA hazard codes: H, health; F, fire; R, reactivity; Ox, oxidizer; W, water-reactive; 0 (none) <—> 4 (severe).

(continued)

TABLE IV–4. HEALTH HAZARD SUMMARIES FOR INDUSTRIAL AND OCCUPATIONAL CHEMICALS (CONTINUED)

Health Hazard Summaries	ACGIH TLV	IDLH	NFPA Codes H F R	Comments
Chlorpyrifos (Dursban, 0,0-diethyl-0-[3,5,6-trichloro-2-pyridinyl] [CAS: 2921-88-2]): An organophosphate-type cholinesterase inhibitor (p 353). Peripheral neuropathy and dermatitis reported. Sodium 3,5,6-trichloropyridin-2-ol (STCP) is an important intermediate for synthesizing chlorpyrifos and has caused poisoning including chloracne and peripheral nerve damage.	0.1 mg/m^3, S (inhalable fraction and vapor)			White solid crystals. Vapor pressure is 0.00002 mm Hg at 25°C (77°F). Agricultural pesticide.
Chromic acid and chromates (chromium trioxide, sodium dichromate, potassium chromate): Highly irritating upon direct contact; severe eye and skin ulceration (chrome ulcers) may result. Dusts and mists highly irritating to eyes and respiratory tract. Skin and respiratory sensitization (asthma) may occur. Chromium trioxide is a teratogen in test animals. Certain hexavalent chromium compounds are carcinogenic in test animals and humans (IARC 1). Chromium III compounds and chromium metal are less strongly associated with cancer (IARC 3). See also p 196.	0.5 mg/m^3 (Cr III compounds), 0.05 mg/m^3, A1 (water-soluble Cr VI compounds), 0.01 mg/m^3, A1 (insoluble Cr IV compounds) NIOSH CA	15 mg/m^3 (Cr VI)	3 0 1 Ox (solid)	Soluble chromate compounds are water-reactive. Chromates are common components of cement in concrete fabrication. Hexavalent chromium exposure can occur in metal plating and in making and welding chrome containing (eg, stainless) steel. Selected yellow pigments and glazes can contain hexavalent chromium.
Chromium metal and insoluble chromium salts: Irritating upon direct contact with skin and eyes; dermatitis may result. Ferrochrome alloys possibly associated with pneumonoconiotic changes. See also p 196.	0.5 mg/m^3 (metal, as Cr), 0.01 mg/m^3, A1 (Cr VI compounds, as Cr) OSHA CA (Cr VI)	250 mg/m^3 (Cr II compounds) 25 mg/m^3 (Cr III compounds) 250 mg/m^3 (Cr metal)		Chromium metal, silver luster; copper chromite, greenish-blue solid. Odorless

Chromyl chloride (CAS: 14977-61-8): Hydrolyzes upon contact with moisture to produce chromic trioxide, HCl, chromic trichloride, and chlorine. Highly irritating upon direct contact; severe burns may result. Mists and vapors highly irritating to eyes and respiratory tract. Certain hexavalent chromium VI compounds are carcinogenic in test animals and humans. See also p 196.	0.025 ppm NIOSH CA			Dark red fuming liquid. Water-reactive, yielding hydrogen chloride, chlorine gas, chromic acid, and chromic chloride.
Coal tar pitch volatiles (particulate polycyclic aromatic hydrocarbons [CAS: 65996-93-2]): Irritating upon direct contact. Contact dermatitis, acne, hypermelanosis, and photosensitization may occur. Fumes irritating to eyes and respiratory tract. A carcinogen in test animals and humans (IARC 1).	0.2 mg/m^3, A1 NIOSH CA	80 mg/m^3		A complex mixture composed of a high percentage of polycyclic aromatic hydrocarbons. A smoky odor. Combustible. Creosote is an important source of exposure.
Cobalt and compounds: Irritating upon direct contact; dermatitis and skin sensitization may occur. Fumes and dusts irritate the respiratory tract; chronic interstitial pneumonitis and respiratory tract sensitization reported. Cardiotoxicity is associated with ingestion but has not been well documented with occupational exposures. Evidence of carcinogenicity in test animals (IARC 2B).	0.02 mg/m^3 (elemental and inorganic compounds, as Co), A3	20 mg/m^3 (as Co)		Elemental cobalt is a black or gray, odorless solid with a negligible vapor pressure. "Hard metal" used in specialty grinding and cutting is a tungsten carbide–cobalt amalgam and causes a specific (giant cell) pneumonitis pattern. Exposure through dysfunction of metal-on-metal cobalt-containing hip prostheses has occurred.
Cobalt hydrocarbonyl (CAS: 16842-03-8): In animal testing, overexposure produces symptoms similar to those of nickel carbonyl and iron pentacarbonyl. Effects include headache, nausea, vomiting, dizziness, fever, and pulmonary edema.	0.1 mg/m^3 (as Co)	ERPG-2: 0.9 mg/m^3 ERPG-3: 3 mg/m^3		Flammable gas.

(C), ceiling air concentration (TLV-C); S, skin absorption can be significant; SEN, potential sensitizer; STEL, short-term (15-minute) exposure level. A1, ACGIH-confirmed human carcinogen; A2, ACGIH-suspected human carcinogen; A3, ACGIH animal carcinogen. ERPG, Emergency Response Planning Guideline (see p 656 for an explanation of ERPG). IARC 1, known human carcinogen; IARC 2A, probable human carcinogen; IARC 2B, possible human carcinogen; IARC 3, inadequate data available. NFPA hazard codes: H, health; F, fire; R, reactivity; Ox, oxidizer; W, water-reactive; 0 (none) <—> 4 (severe).

(*continued*)

TABLE IV–4. HEALTH HAZARD SUMMARIES FOR INDUSTRIAL AND OCCUPATIONAL CHEMICALS (CONTINUED)

Health Hazard Summaries	ACGIH TLV	IDLH	NFPA Codes H F R	Comments
Copper fumes, dusts, and salts: Irritation upon direct contact varies with the compound. The salts are more irritating and can cause corneal ulceration. Allergic contact dermatitis is rare. Dusts and mists irritating to the respiratory tract; nasal ulceration has been described. Ingestion can cause severe gastroenteritis, hepatic injury, and hemolysis. See also p 206.	1 mg/m^3 (dusts and mists, as Cu), 0.2 mg/m^3 (fume)	100 mg/m^3 (as Cu)		Salts vary in color. Generally odorless. Agricultural pesticidal applications, especially as copper sulfate (blue vitriol)
Cotton dust: Chronic exposure causes a respiratory syndrome called byssinosis. Symptoms include cough and wheezing, which typically appear on the first day of the workweek and continue for a few days or all week, although they may subside within an hour after the affected individual leaves work. Can lead to irreversible obstructive airway disease. A flulike illness similar to metal fume fever (p 311) also occurs among cotton workers ("Monday morning fever").	0.1 mg/m^3 (thoracic fraction)	100 mg/m^3		Cotton textile manufacture is the principal source of exposure. "Card room" work (an early stage in cotton thread production) is the most significant source of exposure.
Creosote (coal tar creosote [CAS: 8001-58-9]): A primary irritant, photosensitizer, and corrosive. Direct eye contact can cause severe keratitis and corneal scarring. Prolonged skin contact can cause chemical acne, pigmentation changes, and severe penetrating burns. Exposure to the fumes or vapors causes irritation of mucous membranes and the respiratory tract. Systemic toxicity results from phenolic and cresolic constituents. Liver and kidney injury may occur with heavyexposure. A carcinogen in test animals. Some evidence for carcinogenicity in humans (IARC 2A). See also "Phenol and Related Compounds," p 368.	NIOSH CA		2 2 0	Oily, dark liquid. Appearance and some hazardous properties vary with the formulation. Sharp, penetrating, smoky odor. Combustible. Creosote is produced by the fractional distillation of coal tar but also can be derived from other fossil fuel sources. See entry on coal tar pitch volatiles. Plant-derived "creosote" is a different material that was used as a medicinal agent in the past and does not have the same carcinogenic potential.

Cresol (methylphenol, cresylic acid, hydroxymethylbenzene [CAS: 1319-77-3]): Corrosive. Skin and eye contact can cause severe burns. Exposure may be prolonged owing to local anesthetic action on skin. Well absorbed by all routes. Dermal absorption is a major route of systemic poisoning. Induces methemoglobinemia (p 317). CNS depressant. Symptoms include headache, nausea and vomiting, tinnitus, dizziness, weakness, and confusion. Severe lung, liver, and kidney injury may occur. See also "Phenol and Related Compounds," p 368.	20 mg/m^3 (inhalable fraction and vapor), S	250 ppm	3 2 0	Colorless, yellow, or pink liquid with a phenolic odor. Vapor pressure is 0.2 mm Hg at 20°C (68°F). Combustible.
Crotonaldehyde (2-butenal [CAS: 4170-30-3]): Highly irritating upon direct contact; severe burns may result. Vapors highly irritating to eyes and respiratory tract; delayed pulmonary edema may occur. Evidence for carcinogenicity in test animals (IARC 3).	0.3 ppm (C), S, A3	50 ppm ERPG-1: 0.2 ppm ERPG-2: 5 ppm ERPG-3: 15 ppm	4 3 2	Colorless to straw-colored liquid. Pungent, irritating odor occurs below the TLV and is an adequate warning property. A warning agent is added to fuel gases. Vapor pressure is 30 mm Hg at 20°C (68°F). Flammable. Polymerizes when heated.
Crufomate (4-*tert*-butyl-2-chlorophenyl *N*-methyl *O*-methylphosphoramidate [CAS: 299-86-5]): An organophosphate cholinesterase inhibitor (p 353).	5 mg/m^3			Crystals or yellow oil. Pungent odor. Flammable. Agricultural pesticide.
Cumene (isopropylbenzene [CAS: 98-82-8]): Mildly irritating upon direct contact. A CNS depressant at moderate levels. Well absorbed through skin. Adverse effects in fetal development in rats at high doses. IARC 2B.	50 ppm	900 ppm [LEL]	2 3 1	Colorless liquid. Sharp, aromatic odor below the TLV is a good warning property. Vapor pressure is 8 mm Hg at 20°C (68°F). Flammable.
Cyanamide (carbodiimide [CAS: 420-04-2]): Causes transient vasomotor flushing. Highly irritating and caustic to eyes and skin. Has a disulfiram-like interaction with alcohol, producing flushing, headache, and dyspnea (p 226).	2 mg/m^3		4 1 3	Combustible. Thermal breakdown products include oxides of nitrogen. Used as an agricultural chemical for plant growth regulation.

(C), ceiling air concentration (TLV-C); S, skin absorption can be significant; SEN, potential sensitizer; STEL, short-term (15-minute) exposure level. A1, ACGIH-confirmed human carcinogen; A2, ACGIH-suspected human carcinogen; A3, ACGIH animal carcinogen. ERPG, Emergency Response Planning Guideline (see p 656 for an explanation of ERPG). IARC 1, known human carcinogen; IARC 2A, probable human carcinogen; IARC 2B, possible human carcinogen; IARC 3, inadequate data available. NFPA hazard codes: H, health; F, fire; R, reactivity; Ox, oxidizer; W, water-reactive; 0 (none) <—> 4 (severe).

(*continued*)

TABLE IV–4. HEALTH HAZARD SUMMARIES FOR INDUSTRIAL AND OCCUPATIONAL CHEMICALS (CONTINUED)

Health Hazard Summaries	ACGIH TLV	IDLH	NFPA Codes H F R	Comments
Cyanide salts (sodium cyanide, potassium cyanide): Potent and rapidly fatal metabolic asphyxiants that inhibit cytochrome oxidase and stop cellular respiration. Well absorbed through skin; caustic action can promote dermal absorption. See also p 208.	5 mg/m^3 (C) (as cyanide), S	25 mg/m^3 (as cyanide)		Solids. Mild, almond-like odor. In presence of moisture or acids, hydrogen cyanide may be released. Odor is a poor indicator of exposure to hydrogen cyanide. May be generated in fires from the pyrolysis of such products as polyurethane and polyacrylonitrile. Cyanide salts are used in metal plating and metal pickling operations.
Cyanogen (dicyan, oxalonitrile [CAS: 460-19-5]): Hydrolyzes to release hydrogen cyanide and cyanic acid. Toxicity similar to that of hydrogen cyanide (p 208). Vapors irritating to eyes and respiratory tract.	10 ppm [proposed: 5 ppm (C)]		4 4 1	Colorless gas. Pungent, almond-like odor. Breaks down on contact with water to yield hydrogen cyanide and cyanate. Flammable.
Cyanogen chloride (CAS: 506-77-4): Vapors extremely irritating to eyes and respiratory tract; pulmonary edema may result. Cyanide interferes with cellular respiration (p 208).	0.3 ppm (C)	ERPG-2: 0.4 ppm ERPG-3: 4 ppm		Colorless liquid or gas with a pungent odor. Thermal breakdown products include hydrogen cyanide and hydrogen chloride. Formed by a reaction with hypochlorite in the treatment of cyanide-containing wastewater.
Cyclohexane (CAS: 110-82-7): Mildly irritating upon direct contact. Vapors irritating to eyes and respiratory tract. A CNS depressant at high levels. Chronically exposed test animals developed liver and kidney injury.	100 ppm	1,300 ppm [LEL]	1 3 0	Colorless liquid with a sweet, chloroform-like odor. Vapor pressure is 95 mm Hg at 20°C (68°F). Highly flammable. Organic solvent; principal industrial use in production of caprolactam.
Cyclohexanol (CAS: 108-93-0): Irritating upon direct contact. Vapors irritating to eyes and respiratory tract. Well absorbed by skin. A CNS depressant at high levels. Based on animal tests, it may injure the liver and kidneys at high doses.	50 ppm, S	400 ppm	1 2 0	Colorless, viscous liquid. Mild camphor-like odor. Irritation occurs near the TLV and is a good warning property. Vapor pressure is 1 mm Hg at 20°C (68°F). Combustible.

Cyclohexanone (CAS: 108-94-1): Irritating upon direct contact. Vapors irritate the eyes and respiratory tract. A CNS depressant at very high levels. Chronic, moderate doses caused slight liver injury in test animals. IARC 3.	20 ppm, S, A3	700 ppm	1 2 0	Clear to pale yellow liquid with peppermint-like odor. Vapor pressure is 2 mm Hg at 20°C (68°F). Flammable. A nylon industry chemical precursor.
Cyclohexene (1,2,3,4-tetrahydrobenzene [CAS: 110-83-8]): By structural analogy to cyclohexane, may cause respiratory tract irritation. A CNS depressant.	300 ppm	2,000 ppm	1 3 0	Colorless liquid with a sweet odor. Vapor pressure is 67 mm Hg at 20°C (68°F). Flammable. Readily forms peroxides and polymerizes.
Cyclohexylamine (aminocyclohexane [CAS: 108-91-8]): Corrosive and highly irritating upon direct contact. Vapors highly irritating to eyes and respiratory tract. Pharmacologically active, possessing sympathomimetic activity. Weak methemoglobin-forming activity (p 317). Very limited evidence for adverse effects on reproduction in test animals. Animal studies suggest brain, liver, and kidneys are target organs.	10 ppm		3 3 0	Liquid with an obnoxious, fishy odor. Flammable.
Cyclonite (RDX, trinitro-trimethylene-triamine, hexogen [CAS: 121-82-4]): Induces methemoglobinemia (p 317). Dermal and inhalation exposures affect the CNS with symptoms of confusion, headache, nausea, vomiting, multiple seizures, and coma.	0.5 mg/m^3, S			Explosive crystalline solid, principal ingredient in the plastic explosive C-4. Vapor pressure is negligible at 20°C (68°F). Thermal breakdown products include oxides of nitrogen. Exposure occurs among munitions workers and military personnel.
Cyclopentadiene [CAS: 542-92-7]): Mildly irritating upon direct contact. Vapors irritating to eyes and respiratory tract. A CNS depressant at high levels. Animal studies suggest some potential for kidney and liver injury at high doses.	75 ppm	750 ppm		Colorless liquid. Sweet, turpentine-like odor. Irritation occurs near the TLV and is a good warning property. Vapor pressure is high at 20°C (68°F). Flammable.

(C), ceiling air concentration (TLV-C); S, skin absorption can be significant; SEN, potential sensitizer; STEL, short-term (15-minute) exposure level. A1, ACGIH-confirmed human carcinogen; A2, ACGIH-suspected human carcinogen; A3, ACGIH animal carcinogen. ERPG, Emergency Response Planning Guideline (see p 656 for an explanation of ERPG). IARC 1, known human carcinogen; IARC 2A, probable human carcinogen; IARC 2B, possible human carcinogen; IARC 3, inadequate data available. NFPA hazard codes: H, health; F, fire; R, reactivity; Ox, oxidizer; W, water-reactive; 0 (none) <—> 4 (severe).

(continued)

TABLE IV–4. HEALTH HAZARD SUMMARIES FOR INDUSTRIAL AND OCCUPATIONAL CHEMICALS (CONTINUED)

Health Hazard Summaries	ACGIH TLV	IDLH	NFPA Codes H F R	Comments
Cyclopentane (CAS: 287-92-3]): Mildly irritating upon direct contact. Vapors irritating to eyes and respiratory tract. A CNS depressant at very high levels. Solvent mixtures containing cyclopentane have caused peripheral neuropathy, although this may have been related to *n*-hexane in combination.	600 ppm		1 3 0	Colorless liquid with a faint hydrocarbon odor. Vapor pressure is about 400 mm Hg at 31°C (88°F). Flammable.
Cyclotetramethylene-tetranitramine (HMX, octogen [CAS: 26914-41-0]): Dermally absorbed. Causes seizures in humans. Induces methemoglobinemia (p 317) in animals (human data limited).				White powder. Odorless. Explosive. Chemically related to RDX (hexahydro-1,3,5-trinitro-1,3,5-triazine). May be as potent a cause of seizures, but not as widely manufactured as RDX.
DDT (dichlorodiphenyltrichloroethane [CAS: 50-29-3]): Dusts irritating to eyes. Ingestion may cause tremor and convulsions. Chronic low-level exposure results in bioaccumulation. A carcinogen in test animals (IARC 2A). See also p 189.	1 mg/m^3, A3 NIOSH CA	500 mg/m^3		Colorless, white, or yellow solid crystals with a faint aromatic odor. Vapor pressure is 0.0000002 mm Hg at 20°C (68°F). Combustible. Banned for use in the United States in 1973.
Decaborane (CAS: 17702-41-9): A potent CNS toxin. Symptoms include headache, dizziness, nausea, loss of coordination, and fatigue. Symptoms may be delayed in onset for 1–2 days; convulsions occur in more severe poisonings. Systemic poisonings can result from dermal absorption. Animal studies suggest a potential for liver and kidney injury.	0.05 ppm, S	15 mg/m^3	3 2 2 W	Colorless solid crystals with a pungent odor. Vapor pressure is 0.05 mm Hg at 25°C (77°F). Combustible. Reacts with water to produce flammable hydrogen gas. Used as a rocket fuel additive and as a rubber vulcanization agent.
Demeton (Systox, mercaptophos [CAS: 8065-48-3]): An organophosphate-type cholinesterase inhibitor (p 353).	0.05 mg/m^3 (inhalable fraction and vapor), S	10 mg/m^3		A sulfur-like odor. A very low vapor pressure at 20°C (68°F). Thermal breakdown products include oxides of sulfur. Agricultural pesticide.

Substance	TLV	IDLH	NFPA	Comments
Diacetone alcohol (4-hydroxy-4-methyl-2 pentanone [CAS: 123-42-2]): Irritating upon direct contact. Vapors very irritating to eyes and respiratory tract. A CNS depressant at high levels. Possibly some hemolytic activity.	50 ppm	1,800 ppm [LEL]	1 2 0	Colorless liquid with an agreeable odor. Vapor pressure is 0.8 mm Hg at 20°C (68°F). Flammable.
Diacetyl (CAS: 625-34-3): Eye, skin, and respiratory irritant. Respiratory toxicity, producing bronchiolitis obliterans in occupationally exposed workers ("popcorn workers' lung").	0.01 ppm			Vapor pressure is 56.8 mm Hg at 25°C (77°F). Artificial butter flavoring agent. Removed from US microwavable popcorn but still in use industrially and as an additive to other products.
1,2-diacetylbenzene (1,2-DAB [CAS: 704-00-7]): Putative active metabolite of the organic solvent 1,2-diethylbenzene; forms blue-colored polymeric protein adducts and induces the formation of amyotrophic lateral sclerosis (ALS)-like giant, intraspinal neurofilamentous axonal swellings in an experimental animal model.				Yellow to light brown crystalline powder. The parent compound, 1,2-diethylbenzene, is used as an industrial solvent.
Diazinon (*O,O*-diethyl *O*-2-isopropyl-4-methyl-6-pyrimidinyl thiophosphate [CAS: 333-41-5]): An organophosphate-type cholinesterase inhibitor (p 353). Well absorbed dermally. Evidence of adverse reproductive effects in experimental testing. IARC 2A.	0.01 mg/m^3 (inhalable fraction and vapor), S			Commercial grades are yellow to brown liquids with a faint odor. Vapor pressure is 0.00014 mm Hg at 20°C (68°F). Thermal breakdown products include oxides of nitrogen and sulfur. Agricultural pesticide.
Diazomethane (azimethylene, diazirine [CAS: 334-88-3]): Extremely irritating to eyes and respiratory tract; pulmonary edema has been reported. Immediate symptoms include cough, chest pain, and respiratory distress. A potent methylating agent and respiratory sensitizer. IARC 3.	0.2 ppm, A2	2 ppm		Yellow gas with a musty odor. Air mixtures and compressed liquids can be explosive when heated or shocked. Used as a methylating agent in chemical synthesis.

(C), ceiling air concentration (TLV-C); S, skin absorption can be significant; SEN, potential sensitizer; STEL, short-term (15-minute) exposure level. A1, ACGIH-confirmed human carcinogen; A2, ACGIH-suspected human carcinogen; A3, ACGIH animal carcinogen. ERPG, Emergency Response Planning Guideline (see p 656 for an explanation of ERPG). IARC 1, known human carcinogen; IARC 2A, probable human carcinogen; IARC 2B, possible human carcinogen; IARC 3, inadequate data available. NFPA hazard codes: H, health; F, fire; R, reactivity; Ox, oxidizer; W, water-reactive; 0 (none) <—> 4 (severe).

(continued)

TABLE IV–4. HEALTH HAZARD SUMMARIES FOR INDUSTRIAL AND OCCUPATIONAL CHEMICALS (CONTINUED)

Health Hazard Summaries	ACGIH TLV	IDLH	NFPA Codes H F R	Comments
Diborane (boron hydride [CAS: 19287-45-7]): Extremely irritating to the respiratory tract; pulmonary edema may result. Repeated exposures have been associated with headache, fatigue, and dizziness; muscle weakness or tremors; and chills or fever. Animal studies suggest the liver and kidney are also target organs.	0.1 ppm	15 ppm ERPG-2: 1 ppm ERPG-3: 3 ppm	4 4 3 W	Colorless gas. Obnoxious, nauseatingly sweet odor. Highly flammable. Water-reactive; ignites spontaneously with moist air at room temperatures. A strong reducing agent. Breakdown products include boron oxide fumes. Used in microelectronics industry. Reacts violently with halogenated extinguishing agents.
1,2-Dibromo-3-chloropropane (DBCP [CAS: 96-12-8]): Irritant of eyes and respiratory tract. Has caused sterility (aspermia, oligospermia) in overexposed men. Well absorbed by skin contact and inhalation. A carcinogen in test animals (IARC 2B).	OSHA CA NIOSH CA			Brown liquid with a pungent odor. Combustible. Thermal breakdown products include hydrogen bromide and hydrogen chloride. Banned as a pesticide in the United States.
1,2-Dibromo-2,2-dichloroethyl dimethyl phosphate (naled, Dibrom [CAS: 300-76-5]): An organophosphate anticholinesterase agent (p 353). Highly irritating upon contact; eye injury is likely. Dermal sensitization can occur. Well absorbed dermally; localized muscular twitching results within minutes of contact.	0.1 mg/m^3 (inhalable fraction and vapor), S, SEN	200 mg/m^3		Has a pungent odor. Vapor pressure is 0.002 mm Hg at 20°C (68°F). Not combustible. Breaks down to dichlorvos. Thermal breakdown products include hydrogen bromide, hydrogen chloride, and phosphoric acid. Agricultural pesticide.
Dibutyl phosphate (di-*n*-butyl phosphate [CAS: 107-66-4]): A moderately strong acid likely to be irritating upon direct contact. Vapors and mists are irritating to the respiratory tract and have been associated with headache at low levels.	5 mg/m^3 (inhalable fraction and vapor), S	30 ppm		Colorless to brown liquid. Odorless. Vapor pressure is much less than 1 mm Hg at 20°C (68°F). Decomposes at 100°C (212°F) to produce phosphoric acid fumes.
Dibutyl phthalate (CAS: 84-74-2): Mildly irritating upon direct contact. Ingestion has produced nausea, dizziness, photophobia, and lacrimation but no permanent effects. Adverse effects on fetal development and male reproduction in test animals at very high doses.	5 mg/m^3	4,000 mg/m^3	2 1 0	Colorless, oily liquid with a faint aromatic odor. Vapor pressure is less than 0.01 mm Hg at 20°C (68°F). Combustible.

1, 2-Dichloroacetylene (CAS: 7572-29-4): Vapors extremely irritating to eyes and respiratory tract; pulmonary edema may result. CNS toxicity includes nausea and vomiting, headache, involvement of trigeminal nerve and facial muscles, and outbreaks of facial herpes. Limited evidence for carcinogenicity in test animals (IARC 3).	0.1 ppm (C), A3 NIOSH CA			Colorless liquid. Can be formed as a breakdown product of certain chlorinated organic compounds.
***o*-Dichlorobenzene (1,2-dichlorobenzene [CAS: 95-50-1]):** Irritating upon direct contact; skin blisters and hyperpigmentation may result from prolonged contact. Vapor also irritating to eyes and respiratory tract. Highly hepatotoxic in test animals. Evidence for adverse effects on male reproduction but limited evidence of carcinogenicity in test animals (IARC 3).	25 ppm	200 ppm	2 2 0	Colorless to pale yellow liquid. Aromatic odor and eye irritation occur well below the TLV and are adequate warning properties. Thermal breakdown products include hydrogen chloride and chlorine gas.
***p*-Dichlorobenzene (1,4-dichlorobenzene [CAS: 106-46-7]):** Irritating upon direct contact with the solid. Vapors irritating to eyes and respiratory tract. Systemic effects include headache, nausea, vomiting, and liver injury. The ortho isomer is more toxic to the liver. A carcinogen in test animals (IARC 2B).	10 ppm, A3 NIOSH CA	150 ppm	2 2 0	Colorless or white solid. Mothball odor and irritation occur near the TLV and are adequate warning properties. Vapor pressure is 0.4 mm Hg at 20°C (68°F). Combustible. Thermal breakdown products include hydrogen chloride. Used as a deodorizer and moth repellent. Industrially, used as a chemical intermediate for dyes and polyphenylene sulfide resin.
3,3'-Dichlorobenzidine (CAS: 91-94-1): Well absorbed by the dermal route. Animal studies suggest that severe eye injury and respiratory tract irritation may occur. A potent carcinogen in test animals (IARC 2B).	S, A3 OSHA CA NIOSH CA			Crystalline needles with a faint odor.

(C), ceiling air concentration (TLV-C); S, skin absorption can be significant; SEN, potential sensitizer; STEL, short-term (15-minute) exposure level. A1, ACGIH-confirmed human carcinogen; A2, ACGIH-suspected human carcinogen; A3, ACGIH animal carcinogen. ERPG, Emergency Response Planning Guideline (see p 656 for an explanation of ERPG). IARC 1, known human carcinogen; IARC 2A, probable human carcinogen; IARC 2B, possible human carcinogen; IARC 3, inadequate data available. NFPA hazard codes: H, health; F, fire; R, reactivity; Ox, oxidizer; W, water-reactive; 0 (none) <—> 4 (severe).

(*continued*)

TABLE IV–4. HEALTH HAZARD SUMMARIES FOR INDUSTRIAL AND OCCUPATIONAL CHEMICALS (CONTINUED)

Health Hazard Summaries	ACGIH TLV	IDLH	NFPA Codes H F R	Comments
Dichlorodifluoromethane (Freon 12, fluorocarbon 12 [CAS: 75-71-8]): Mild eye and respiratory tract irritant. Extremely high exposures (eg, 100,000 ppm) can cause coma and cardiac arrhythmias. See also p 251.	1,000 ppm	15,000 ppm		Colorless gas. Ether-like odor is a poor warning property. Vapor pressure is 5.7 mm Hg at 20°C (68°F). Not combustible. Decomposes slowly on contact with water or heat to produce hydrogen chloride, hydrogen fluoride, and phosgene.
1,3-Dichloro-5,5-dimethylhydantoin (Halane, Dactin [CAS: 118-52-5]): Releases hypochlorous acid and chlorine gas (p 191) on contact with moisture. Direct contact with the dust or concentrated solutions irritating to eyes, skin, and respiratory tract.	0.2 mg/m^3	5 mg/m^3		White solid with a chlorine-like odor. Odor and eye irritation occur below the TLV and are adequate warning properties. Not combustible. Thermal breakdown products include hydrogen chloride, phosgene, oxides of nitrogen, and chlorine gas.
1,1-Dichloroethane (ethylidene chloride [CAS: 75-34-3]): Mild eye and skin irritant. Vapors irritating to the respiratory tract. A CNS depressant at high levels. By analogy with its 1,2-isomer, may cause arrhythmias. Animal studies suggest some potential for kidney and liver injury.	100 ppm	3,000 ppm	1 3 0	Colorless, oily liquid. Chloroform-like odor occurs at the TLV. Vapor pressure is 182 mm Hg at 20°C (68°F). Flammable. Thermal breakdown products include vinyl chloride, hydrogen chloride, and phosgene.
1,2-Dichloroethane (ethylene dichloride [CAS: 107-06-2]): Irritating upon prolonged contact; burns may occur. Well absorbed dermally. Vapors irritating to eyes and respiratory tract. A CNS depressant at high levels; may be associated with chronic toxic encephalopathy. Can cause cardiac arrhythmias. Severe liver and kidney injury has been reported. A carcinogen in test animals (IARC 2B).	10 ppm NIOSH CA	50 ppm ERPG-1: 50 ppm ERPG-2: 200 ppm ERPG-3: 300 ppm	2 3 0	Odor threshold near 50 ppm. Flammable. Thermal breakdown products include hydrogen chloride and phosgene. A widely used industrial solvent.
1,1-Dichloroethylene (vinylidine chloride [CAS: 75-35-4]): Irritating upon direct contact. Vapors very irritating to eyes and respiratory tract. A CNS depressant. May cause cardiac arrhythmias. In test animals, damages the liver and kidneys. Limited evidence of carcinogenicity in test animals (IARC 3).	5 ppm NIOSH CA	ERPG-2: 500 ppm ERPG-3: 1,000 ppm	242	Colorless liquid. Sweet, ether-like or chloroform-like odor occurs below the TLV and is a good warning property. Polymerizes readily. Also used as a copolymer with vinyl chloride.

1,2-Dichloroethylene (1,2-dichloroethene, acetylene dichloride [CAS: 540-59-0]): Vapors mildly irritating to respiratory tract. A CNS depressant at high levels; once used as an anesthetic agent. May cause cardiac arrhythmias. Mildly hepatotoxic.	200 ppm	1,000 ppm	1 3 2	Colorless liquid with a slightly acrid, ether-like or chloroform-like odor. Vapor pressure is about 220 mm Hg at 20°C (68°F). Thermal breakdown products include hydrogen chloride and phosgene.
Dichloroethyl ether (bis[2-chloroethyl] ether, dichloroethyl oxide [CAS: 111-44-4]): Irritating upon direct contact; corneal injury may result. Vapors highly irritating to respiratory tract. A CNS depressant at high levels. Dermal absorption occurs. Animal studies suggest the liver and kidneys are also target organs at high exposures. Limited evidence for carcinogenicity in test animals (IARC 3).	5 ppm, S NIOSH CA	100 ppm	3 2 1	Colorless liquid. Obnoxious, chlorinated solvent odor occurs at the TLV and is a good warning property. Flammable. Breaks down on contact with water. Thermal breakdown products include hydrogen chloride.
Dichlorofluoromethane (fluorocarbon 21, Freon 21, Halon 112 [CAS: 75-43-4]): Animal studies suggest much greater hepatotoxicity than with most common chlorofluorocarbons. Causes CNS depression, respiratory irritation, and cardiac arrhythmias at very high air levels (eg, 100,000 ppm). Evidence for adverse effects on fetal development (preimplantation losses) in test animals at high levels. See also p 251.	10 ppm	5,000 ppm		Colorless liquid or gas with a faint ether-like odor. Thermal breakdown products include hydrogen chloride, hydrogen fluoride, and phosgene.
1,1-Dichloro-1-nitroethane [CAS: 594-72-9]): Based on animal studies, highly irritating upon direct contact. Vapors highly irritating to eyes, skin, and respiratory tract; pulmonary edema may result. In test animals, lethal doses also injured the liver, heart, and kidneys.	2 ppm	25 ppm	3 2 3	Colorless liquid. Obnoxious odor and tearing occur only at dangerous levels and are poor warning properties. Vapor pressure is 15 mm Hg at 20°C (68°F).

(C), ceiling air concentration (TLV-C); S, skin absorption can be significant; SEN, potential sensitizer; STEL, short-term (15-minute) exposure level. A1, ACGIH-confirmed human carcinogen; A2, ACGIH-suspected human carcinogen; A3, ACGIH animal carcinogen. ERPG, Emergency Response Planning Guideline (see p 656 for an explanation of ERPG). IARC 1, known human carcinogen; IARC 2A, probable human carcinogen; IARC 2B, possible human carcinogen; IARC 3, inadequate data available. NFPA hazard codes: H, health; F, fire; R, reactivity; Ox, oxidizer; W, water-reactive; 0 (none) <—> 4 (severe).

(continued)

TABLE IV–4. HEALTH HAZARD SUMMARIES FOR INDUSTRIAL AND OCCUPATIONAL CHEMICALS (CONTINUED)

Health Hazard Summaries	ACGIH TLV	IDLH	NFPA Codes H F R	Comments
2,4-Dichlorophenol [CAS: 120-83-2]: Extremely toxic, but the mechanism of action in human fatalities has not been determined.		ERPG-1: 0.2 ppm ERPG-2: 2 ppm ERPG-3: 20 ppm	3 1 0	Odor threshold near 0.2 ppm. Used as a chemical precursor in the manufacture of 2,4-dichlorophenoxyacetic acid (2,4-D). Exposure occurs through unintended releases in industrial settings.
2,4-Dichlorophenoxyacetic acid (2,4-D [CAS: 94-75-9]): Direct skin contact can produce a rash. Overexposed workers have manifested peripheral neuropathy. Severe rhabdomyolysis and minor liver and kidney injury may occur. Adverse effects on fetal development at high doses in test animals. There are weak epidemiologic associations of phenoxy herbicides with soft-tissue sarcomas. IARC 2B (chlorophenoxy herbicides). See also p 192.	10 mg/m^3, S	100 mg/m^3		White to yellow crystals. Appearance and some hazardous properties vary with the formulation. Odorless. Vapor pressure is negligible at 20°C (68°F). Thermal breakdown products include hydrogen chloride and phosgene. Used as an herbicide.
1,3-Dichloropropene (1,3-dichloropropylene, Telone [CAS: 542-75-6]): Based on animal studies, irritating upon direct contact. Well absorbed dermally. Vapors irritating to eyes and respiratory tract. In test animals, moderate doses caused severe injuries to the liver, pancreas, and kidneys. A carcinogen in test animals (IARC 2B).	1 ppm, S, A3 NIOSH CA	230		Colorless or straw-colored liquid. Sharp, chloroform-like odor. Polymerizes readily. Vapor pressure is 28 mm Hg at 25°C (77°F). Thermal breakdown products include hydrogen chloride and phosgene. A soil fumigant pesticide widely used in the United States
2,2-Dichloropropionic acid (CAS: 75-99-0): Corrosive upon direct contact with concentrate; severe burns may result. Vapors mildly irritating to eyes and respiratory tract.	5 mg/m^3 (inhalable fraction)			Colorless liquid. The sodium salt is a solid.

Dichlorotetrafluoroethane (fluorocarbon 114, Freon 114 [CAS: 76-14-2]): Vapors may sensitize the myocardium to arrhythmogenic effects of epinephrine at modestly high air levels (25,000 ppm). Other effects at higher levels (100,000–200,000 ppm) include respiratory irritation and CNS depression. See also p 251.	1,000 ppm	15,000 ppm		Colorless gas with a mild ether-like odor. Thermal breakdown products include hydrogen chloride, hydrogen fluoride, and phosgene.
Dichlorvos (DDVP, 2,2-dichlorovinyl diethyl phosphate [CAS: 62-73-7]): An organophosphate-type cholinesterase inhibitor (p 353). Peripheral neuropathy reported. Extremely well absorbed through skin. Evidence of carcinogenicity in test animals (IARC 2B).	0.1 mg/m^3 (inhalable fraction and vapor), S, SEN	100 mg/m^3	3 1 –	Colorless to amber liquid with a slight chemical odor. Vapor pressure is 0.032 mm Hg at 32°C (90°F). Pesticide in indoor "pest strips"; overexposure from misuse can occur.
Dicrotophos (dimethyl *cis*-2-dimethylcarbamoyl-1-methylvinyl phosphate, Bidrin [CAS: 141-66-2]): An organophosphate cholinesterase inhibitor (p 353). Dermal absorption occurs.	0.05 mg/m^3 (inhalable fraction and vapor), S			Brown liquid with a mild ester odor. Agricultural pesticide.
Dieldrin (CAS: 60-57-1): Minor skin irritant. Potent convulsant and hepatotoxin. Dermal absorption is a majorroute of systemic poisoning. Overexposures produce headache, dizziness, twitching, and convulsions. Limited evidence for adverse effects on fetal development and carcinogenicity in test animals (IARC 3). See also p 189.	0.1 mg/m^3 (inhalable fraction and vapor), S, A3 NIOSH CA	50 mg/m^3		Light brown solid flakes with a mild chemical odor. Appearance and some hazardous properties vary with the formulation. Vapor pressure is 0.0000002 mm Hg at 32°C (90°F). Not combustible. Agricultural pesticide.
Diesel exhaust: A respiratory irritant. May act as an adjuvant to immunologic sensitization. Animal and human epidemiologic studies provide evidence of pulmonary carcinogenicity (IARC 1).	100 mg/m^3 (inhalable fraction and vapor), S, A3 (uncombusted liquid) NIOSH CA			Diesel engines emit a complex mixture of gases, vapors, and respirable particulates, including many polycyclic aromatic and nitroaromatic hydrocarbons and oxides of nitrogen, sulfur, and carbon, including carbon monoxide.

(C), ceiling air concentration (TLV-C); S, skin absorption can be significant; SEN, potential sensitizer; STEL, short-term (15-minute) exposure level. A1, ACGIH-confirmed human carcinogen; A2, ACGIH-suspected human carcinogen; A3, ACGIH animal carcinogen. ERPG, Emergency Response Planning Guideline (see p 656 for an explanation of ERPG). IARC 1, known human carcinogen; IARC 2A, probable human carcinogen; IARC 2B, possible human carcinogen; IARC 3, inadequate data available. NFPA hazard codes: H, health; F, fire; R, reactivity; Ox, oxidizer; W, water-reactive; 0 (none) <—> 4 (severe).

(*continued*)

TABLE IV–4. HEALTH HAZARD SUMMARIES FOR INDUSTRIAL AND OCCUPATIONAL CHEMICALS (CONTINUED)

Health Hazard Summaries	ACGIH TLV	IDLH	NFPA Codes H F R	Comments
Diethylamine (CAS: 109-89-7): Corrosive. Highly irritating upon direct contact; severe burns may result. Vapors highly irritating to eyes and respiratory tract; pulmonary edema may occur. Subacute animal studies suggest liver and heart may be target organs.	5 ppm, S	200 ppm	3 3 0	Colorless liquid. Fishy, ammonia-like odor occurs below the TLV and is a good warning property. Vapor pressure is 195 mm Hg at 20°C (68°F). Highly flammable. Thermal breakdown products include oxides of nitrogen. Corrosion inhibitor with other industrial applications as well.
2-Diethylaminoethanol (*N,N*-diethylthanolamine, DEAE [CAS: 100-37-8]): Based on animal studies, highly irritating upon direct contact and a skin sensitizer. Vapors likely irritating to eyes, skin, and respiratory tract. Has been associated with irritant-induced asthma. Reports of nausea and vomiting after a momentary exposure to 100 ppm.	2 ppm, S	100 ppm	3 2 0	Colorless liquid. Weak to nauseating ammonia odor. Flammable. Thermal breakdown products include oxides of nitrogen. Corrosion inhibitor.
Diethylenetriamine (DETA [CAS: 111-40-0]): Corrosive; highly irritating upon direct contact; severe burns may result. Vapors highly irritating to eyes and respiratory tract. Dermal and respiratory sensitization can occur.	1 ppm, S		3 1 0	Viscous yellow liquid with an ammonia-like odor. Vapor pressure is 0.37 mm Hg at 20°C (68 F). Combustible. Thermal breakdown products include oxides of nitrogen.
Diethyl ketone (3-pentanone [CAS: 96-22-0]): Mildly irritating upon direct contact. Vapors mildly irritating to eyes and respiratory tract.	200 ppm		1 3 0	Colorless liquid with an acetone-like odor. Flammable.
Diethyl sulfate (CAS: 64-67-5): Strong eye and respiratory tract irritant. Sufficient evidence of carcinogenicity in test animals. Limited evidence (laryngeal cancers) in humans (IARC 2A).			3 1 1	An alkylating agent. Colorless oily liquid with a peppermint odor.

Difluorodibromomethane (dibromodifluoromethane, Freon 12B2 [CAS: 75-61-6]): Based on animal tests, vapors irritate the respiratory tract. A CNS depressant. By analogy to other freons, may cause cardiac arrhythmias. In test animals, high-level chronic exposures caused lung, liver, and CNS injury. See also p 251.	100 ppm	2,000 ppm		Heavy, volatile, colorless liquid with an obnoxious, distinctive odor. Vapor pressure is 620 mm Hg at 20°C (68°F). Not combustible. Thermal breakdown products include hydrogen bromide and hydrogen fluoride.
Diglycidyl ether (di[2,3-epoxypropyl]-ether, DGE [CAS: 2238-07-5]): Extremely irritating upon direct contact; severe burns result. Vapors highly irritating to eyes and respiratory tract; pulmonary edema may result. Testicular atrophy and adverse effects on the hematopoietic system at low doses in test animals. CNS depression also noted. An alkylating agent and a carcinogen in test animals. No IARC evaluation.	0.01 ppm NIOSH CA	10 ppm		Colorless liquid with a very irritating odor. Vapor pressure is 0.09 mm Hg at 25°C (77°F). Used in the epoxy industry.
Diisobutyl ketone (2,6-dimethyl-4-heptanone [CAS: 108-83-8]): Mildly irritating upon direct contact. Vapors mildly irritate eyes and respiratory tract. A CNS depressant at high levels.	25 ppm	500 ppm	1 2 0	Colorless liquid with a weak, ether-like odor. Vapor pressure is 1.7 mm Hg at 20°C (68°F).
Diisopropylamine (CAS: 108-18-9): Corrosive. Highly irritating upon direct contact; severe burns may result. Vapors very irritating to eyes and respiratory tract. Workers exposed to levels of 25–50 ppm have reported hazy vision, nausea, and headache.	5 ppm, S	200 ppm	3 3 0	Colorless liquid with an ammonia-like odor. Vapor pressure is 60 mm Hg at 20°C (68°F). Flammable. Thermal breakdown products include oxides of nitrogen.
Dimethoate (Phosphorodithiolate [CAS 60-51-5]): Organophosphate anticholinesterase agent. Suspect human teratogen.				White, crystalline solid with a camphor-like odor. Thermal breakdown to nitrogen, phosphorous, and sulfur oxides. Agricultural pesticide.

(C), ceiling air concentration (TLV-C); S, skin absorption can be significant; SEN, potential sensitizer; STEL, short-term (15-minute) exposure level. A1, ACGIH-confirmed human carcinogen; A2, ACGIH-suspected human carcinogen; A3, ACGIH animal carcinogen. ERPG, Emergency Response Planning Guideline (see p 656 for an explanation of ERPG). IARC 1, known human carcinogen; IARC 2A, probable human carcinogen; IARC 2B, possible human carcinogen; IARC 3, inadequate data available. NFPA hazard codes: H, health; F, fire; R, reactivity; Ox, oxidizer; W, water-reactive; 0 (none) <—> 4 (severe).

(continued)

TABLE IV–4. HEALTH HAZARD SUMMARIES FOR INDUSTRIAL AND OCCUPATIONAL CHEMICALS (CONTINUED)

Health Hazard Summaries	ACGIH TLV	IDLH	NFPA Codes H F R	Comments
Dimethyl acetamide (DMAC [CAS: 127-19-5]): Potent hepatotoxin similar to dimethylformamide (DMF). DMAC has also caused hallucinations. Inhalation and skin contact are major routes of absorption. Limited evidence for adverse effects on fetal development in test animals at high doses.	10 ppm, S	300 ppm	2 2 0	Colorless liquid with a weak ammonia-like odor. Vapor pressure is 1.5 mm Hg at 20°C (68°F). Combustible. Thermal breakdown products include oxides of nitrogen. Widely used industrial solvent, especially in film and fiber applications.
Dimethylamine (DMA [CAS: 124-40-3]): Corrosive upon direct contact; severe burns may result. Vapors extremely irritating to eyes and respiratory tract. Animal studies suggest liver is a target organ.	5 ppm, S	500 ppm ERPG-1: 0.6 ppm ERPG-2: 100 ppm ERPG-3: 350 ppm	3 4 0	Colorless liquid or gas. Fishy or ammonia-like odor far below TLV is a good warning property. Flammable. Thermal breakdown products include oxides of nitrogen.
Dimethylamine borane (DMAB [CAS: 74-94-2]): Eye, skin, and respiratory tract irritant. Absorbed through intact skin. Potent CNS and peripheral neurotoxin.			3 3 2	Vapor pressure is 266 mm Hg at 25°C (77°F). Used as reducing agent for nonelectric plating of semiconductors in the microelectronics industry.
4-Dimethylaminophenol (CAS: 619-60-3): Potent oxidizer used to induce methemoglobinemia in some countries outside the United States (especially Germany).				
***N,N*-Dimethylaniline (CAS: 121-69-7):** Causes methemoglobinemia (p 317). A CNS depressant. Well absorbed dermally. Limited evidence for carcinogenicity in test animals (IARC 3).	5 ppm, S	100 ppm	3 2 0	Straw-colored to brown liquid with an amine-like odor. Vapor pressure is less than 1 mm Hg at 20°C (68°F). Combustible. Thermal breakdown products include oxides of nitrogen.
Dimethylcarbamoyl chloride (CAS: 79-44-7): Rapidly hydrolyzed by moisture to dimethylamine, carbon dioxide, and hydrochloric acid. Expected to be extremely irritating upon direct contact or by inhalation. A carcinogen in test animals (IARC 2A).	0.005 ppm, S, A2 NIOSH CA			Liquid. Rapidly reacts with moisture to yield dimethylamine and hydrogen chloride.

***N,N*-Dimethylformamide (DMF [CAS: 68-12-2]):** Dermally well absorbed. Symptoms of overexposure include abdominal pain, nausea, and vomiting. Potent hepatotoxin in humans (liver enzyme elevations and fatty change). Interferes with ethanol to cause disulfiram-like reactions (p 226). Limited human evidence for testicular cancer (IARC 2A). Limited evidence for adverse effects on fetal development in animals.	10 ppm, S	500 ppm ERPG-1: 2 ppm ERPG-2: 100 ppm ERPG-3: 200 ppm	2 2 0	Colorless to pale yellow liquid. Faint ammonia-like odor is a poor warning property (odor threshold is near the TLV). Vapor pressure is 2.7 mm Hg at 20°C (68°F). Flammable. Thermal breakdown products include oxides of nitrogen. Multiple industrial applications as a solvent, in particular in coatings and artificial leather manufacturing.
1,1-Dimethylhydrazine (DMH, UDMH [CAS: 57-14-7]): Corrosive upon direct contact; severe burns may result. Vapors extremely irritating to eyes and respiratory tract; pulmonary edema may occur. Well absorbed through the skin. May cause methemoglobinemia (p 317); may cause hemolysis. A potent hepatotoxin; a carcinogen in test animals (IARC 2B).	0.01 ppm, S, A3 NIOSH CA	15 ppm	4 3 1	Colorless liquid with yellow fumes. Amine odor. Vapor pressure is 1.3 mm Hg at 20°C (68°F). Thermal breakdown products include oxides of nitrogen. Rocket fuel additive. "Aerozine 50" is a 50:50 mix of UDMH and hydrazine.
Dimethylmercury (mercury dimethyl [CAS: 593-74-8]): Extremely toxic liquid readily absorbed by inhalation or across intact skin; as little as 1–2 drops on a latex glove caused death in a research chemist. Neurotoxic effects include progressive ataxia, dysarthria, visual and auditory dysfunction, and coma. See also "Mercury," p 305.	(***Note:*** no TLV; OSHA PEL for alkyl mercury compounds in general: 0.01mg/m^3)			Colorless liquid with a weak, sweet odor. Density 3.2 g/ML Vapor pressure 50–82 mm Hg at 20°C (68°F). Permeable through latex, neoprene, and butyl rubber gloves. (OSHA recommends Silver Shield laminate gloves under outer gloves.)
Dimethyl sulfate (CAS: 77-78-1): Powerful vesicant action; hydrolyzes to sulfuric acid and methanol. Extremely irritating upon direct contact; severe burns have resulted. Vapors irritating to eyes and respiratory tract; delayed pulmonary edema may result. Skin absorption is rapid. Nervous system toxicity also manifested. A carcinogen in test animals (IARC 2A).	0.1 ppm, S, A3 NIOSH CA	7 ppm	4 2 1	Colorless, oily liquid. Very mild onion odor is barely perceptible and a poor warning property. Vapor pressure is 0.5 mm Hg at 20°C (68°F). Combustible. Thermal breakdown products include sulfur oxides. Methylating agent used in chemical synthesis.

(C), ceiling air concentration (TLV-C); S, skin absorption can be significant; SEN, potential sensitizer; STEL, short-term (15-minute) exposure level. A1, ACGIH-confirmed human carcinogen; A2, ACGIH-suspected human carcinogen; A3, ACGIH animal carcinogen. ERPG, Emergency Response Planning Guideline (see p 656 for an explanation of ERPG). IARC 1, known human carcinogen; IARC 2A, probable human carcinogen; IARC 2B, possible human carcinogen; IARC 3, inadequate data available. NFPA hazard codes: H, health; F, fire; R, reactivity; Ox, oxidizer; W, water-reactive; 0 (none) <—> 4 (severe).

(*continued*)

TABLE IV–4. HEALTH HAZARD SUMMARIES FOR INDUSTRIAL AND OCCUPATIONAL CHEMICALS (CONTINUED)

Health Hazard Summaries	ACGIH TLV	IDLH	NFPA Codes H F R	Comments
***N,N*-Dimethyl-*p*-toluidine (CAS: 99-97-8):** Oxidizing agent causing methemoglobinemia (p 317), presumably through its metabolite *p*-methylphenylhydroxylamine. A carcinogen in test animals (IARC 2B).				Used as a polymerization accelerator for ethyl methacrylate monomer. Exposure has occurred through artificial (sculpted) nail application.
Dinitrobenzene [CAS: 528-29-0 (ortho); 100-25-4 (para)]: May stain tissues yellow upon direct contact. Vapors are irritating to respiratory tract. Potent inducer of methemoglobinemia (p 317). Chronic exposures may result in anemia and liver damage. Injures testes in test animals. Very well absorbed through the skin.	0.15 ppm, S	50 mg/m^3	3 1 4 (ortho)	Pale yellow crystals. Explosive; detonated by heat or shock. Vapor pressure is much less than 1 mm Hg at 20°C (68°F). Thermal breakdown products include oxides of nitrogen. Munitions and other industrial applications.
Dinitro-*o*-cresol (2-methyl-4,6-dinitrophenol [CAS: 534-52-1]): Highly toxic; uncouples oxidative phosphorylation in mitochondria, increasing metabolic rate and leading to fatigue, sweating, rapid breathing, tachycardia, and fever. Liver and kidney injury may occur. Symptoms may last for days, as it is excreted very slowly. May induce methemoglobinemia (p 317). Poisonings may result from dermal exposure. Yellow-stained skin may mark exposure.	0.2 mg/m^3, S	5 mg/m^3		Yellow solid crystals. Odorless. Dust is explosive. Vapor pressure is 0.00005 mm Hg at 20°C (68°F). Thermal breakdown products include oxides of nitrogen.
2,4-Dinitrophenol (CAS: 25550-58-7): Potent uncoupler of oxidative phosphorylation. Initial findings include hypertension, fever, dyspnea, and tachypnea. May cause methemoglobinemia and harm liver and kidneys. May stain skin at point of contact. Limited evidence for adverse effects on fetal development. See also p 364.				Industrial chemical and pesticide. Abused as a chemical dietary supplement for weight loss and in body building. Fatal hyperthermia has been reported.

2,4-Dinitrotoluene (DNT [CAS: 25321-14-6]): May cause methemoglobinemia (p 317). Uncouples oxidative phosphorylation, leading to increased metabolic rate and hyperthermia, tachycardia, and fatigue. A hepatotoxin. May cause vasodilation; headache and drop in blood pressure are common. Cessation of exposure may precipitate angina pectoris in pharmacologically dependent workers. Well absorbed by all routes. May stain skin yellow. Injures testes in test animals and, possibly, exposed workers. A carcinogen in test animals.	0.2 mg/m^3, A3, S NIOSH CA	50 mg/m^3	3 1 3	Orange-yellow solid (pure) or oily liquid with a characteristic odor. Explosive. Thermal breakdown products include oxides of nitrogen. Vapor pressure is 1 mm Hg at 20°C (68°F). Exposure encountered in the munitions industry.
1,4-Dioxane (1,4-diethylene dioxide [CAS: 123-91-1]): Vapors irritating to eyes and respiratory tract. Inhalation or dermal exposures may cause gastrointestinal upset and liver and kidney injury. A carcinogen in test animals (IARC 2B).	20 ppm, S, A3 NIOSH CA	500 ppm	2 3 1	Colorless liquid. Mild ether-like odor occurs only at dangerous levels and is a poor warning property. Vapor pressure is 29 mm Hg at 20°C (68°F). Flammable. Industrial solvent and chemical additive stabilizer for chlorinated solvents.
Dioxathion (2,3-*p*-dioxanedithiol *S,S*-bis [*O,O*-diethyl phosphorodithioate] [CAS: 78-34-2]): An organophosphate-type cholinesterase inhibitor (p 353). Well absorbed dermally.	0.1 mg/m^3 (inhalable fraction and vapor), S			Amber liquid. Vapor pressure is negligible at 20°C (68°F). Thermal breakdown products include oxides of sulfur. Agricultural pesticide.
Dipropylene glycol methyl ether (DPGME [CAS: 34590-94-8]): Mildly irritating to eyes upon direct contact. A CNS depressant at very high levels.	100 ppm, S	600 ppm	2 2 0	Colorless liquid with a mild ether-like odor. Nasal irritation is a good warning property. Vapor pressure is 0.3 mm Hg at 20°C (68°F). Combustible.

(C), ceiling air concentration (TLV-C); S, skin absorption can be significant; SEN, potential sensitizer; STEL, short-term (15-minute) exposure level. A1, ACGIH-confirmed human carcinogen; A2, ACGIH-suspected human carcinogen; A3, ACGIH animal carcinogen. ERPG, Emergency Response Planning Guideline (see p 656 for an explanation of ERPG). IARC 1, known human carcinogen; IARC 2A, probable human carcinogen; IARC 2B, possible human carcinogen; IARC 3, inadequate data available. NFPA hazard codes: H, health; F, fire; R, reactivity; Ox, oxidizer; W, water-reactive; 0 (none) <—> 4 (severe).

(*continued*)

TABLE IV–4. HEALTH HAZARD SUMMARIES FOR INDUSTRIAL AND OCCUPATIONAL CHEMICALS (CONTINUED)

Health Hazard Summaries	ACGIH TLV	IDLH	NFPA Codes H F R	Comments
Diquat (1,1-ethylene-2,2'-dipyridinium dibromide, Reglone, Dextrone [CAS: 85-00-7]): Mucosal irritant; corrosive in high concentrations. Acute renal failure and liver injury may occur. Chronic feeding studies caused cataracts in test animals. Although pulmonary edema may occur, unlike with paraquat, pulmonary fibrosis has not been shown with human diquat exposures. See also p 361.	0.5 mg/m^3 (total dust, inhalable fraction), 0.1 mg/m^3 (respirable dust), S			Yellow solid crystals. Appearance and some hazardous properties vary with the formulation. Nonspecific contact herbicide.
Disulfiram (tetraethylthiuram disulfide, Antabuse [CAS: 97-77-8]): Inhibits aldehyde dehydrogenase, an enzyme involved in ethanol metabolism. Exposure to disulfiram and alcohol will produce flushing, headache, and hypotension. Disulfiram may also interact with other industrial solvents that share metabolic pathways with ethanol. Limited evidence for adverse effects on fetal development in test animals (IARC 3). See also p 226.	2 mg/m^3			Crystalline solid. Thermal breakdown products include oxides of sulfur. Metabolic pathways include carbon disulfide (p 181). Disulfiram and related compounds have been used in rubber industry vulcanization.
Disulfoton (*O,O*-diethyl-S-ethylmercapto-ethyl dithiophosphate [CAS: 298-04-4]): An organophosphate-type cholinesterase inhibitor (p 353). Dermally well absorbed.	0.05 mg/m^3 (inhalable fraction and vapor), S			Vapor pressure is 0.00018 mm Hg at 20°C (68°F). Thermal breakdown products include oxides of sulfur.
Divinylbenzene (DVB, diethylene benzene, vinylstyrene [CAS: 1321-74-0]): Mildly irritating upon direct contact. Vapors mildly irritating to eyes and respiratory tract. CNS depressant. May be metabolized to a neurotoxin 1,2-diacetylbenzene.	10 ppm		1 2 2	Pale yellow liquid. Combustible. Must contain inhibitor to prevent explosive polymerization.

Endosulfan (CAS: 115-29-7): Inhalation and skin absorption are major routes of exposure. Symptoms include nausea, confusion, excitement, twitching, and convulsions. Animal studies suggest liver and kidney injury from very high exposures. Limited evidence for adverse effects on male reproduction and fetal development in animal studies. See also p 189.	0.1 mg/m^3 (inhalable fraction and vapor), S			Chlorinated hydrocarbon insecticide. Tan, waxy solid with a mild sulfur dioxide odor. Thermal breakdown products include oxides of sulfur and hydrogen chloride.
Endrin (CAS: 72-20-8): Endrin is the stereoisomer of dieldrin, and its toxicity is very similar. Well absorbed through skin. Overexposure may produce headache, dizziness, nausea, confusion, twitching, and convulsions. Adverse effects on fetal development in test animals (IARC 3). See also p 189.	0.1 mg/m^3, S	2 mg/m^3		Colorless, white, or tan solid. A mild chemical odor and negligible vapor pressure of 0.0000002 mm Hg at 20°C (68°F). Not combustible. Thermal breakdown products include hydrogen chloride.
Environmental tobacco smoke: Passive smoking causes respiratory irritation and small reductions in lung function. It increases severity and frequency of asthmatic attacks in children. May cause coughing, phlegm production, chest discomfort, and reduced lung function in adults. Causes developmental toxicity in infants and children and reproductive toxicity in female adults. Epidemiologic studies show passive smoking causes lung cancer (IARC 1).				

(C), ceiling air concentration (TLV-C); S, skin absorption can be significant; SEN, potential sensitizer; STEL, short-term (15-minute) exposure level. A1, ACGIH-confirmed human carcinogen; A2, ACGIH-suspected human carcinogen; A3, ACGIH animal carcinogen. ERPG, Emergency Response Planning Guideline (see p 656 for an explanation of ERPG). IARC 1, known human carcinogen; IARC 2A, probable human carcinogen; IARC 2B, possible human carcinogen; IARC 3, inadequate data available. NFPA hazard codes: H, health; F, fire; R, reactivity; Ox, oxidizer; W, water-reactive; 0 (none) <—> 4 (severe).

(*continued*)

TABLE IV–4. HEALTH HAZARD SUMMARIES FOR INDUSTRIAL AND OCCUPATIONAL CHEMICALS (CONTINUED)

Health Hazard Summaries	ACGIH TLV	IDLH	NFPA Codes H F R	Comments
Epichlorohydrin (chloropropylene oxide [CAS: 106-89-8]): Extremely irritating upon direct contact; severe burns may result. Vapors highly irritating to eyes and respiratory tract; pulmonary edema has been reported. Other effects include nausea, vomiting, and abdominal pain. Sensitization has been reported (contact dermatitis). Animal studies suggest a potential for liver and kidney injury. High doses reduce fertility in test animals. A carcinogen in test animals (IARC 2A).	0.5 ppm, S, A3 NIOSH CA	75 ppm ERPG-1: 5 ppm ERPG-2: 20 ppm ERPG-3: 100 ppm	4 3 2	Colorless liquid. The irritating, chloroform-like odor is detectable only at extremely high exposures and is a poor warning property. Vapor pressure is 13 mm Hg at 20°C (68°F). Flammable. Thermal breakdown products include hydrogen chloride and phosgene. Used in epoxy manufacturing.
EPN (*O-ethyl O-p*-nitrophenyl phenylphosphonothioate [CAS: 210464–5]): An organophosphate-type cholinesterase inhibitor (p 353).	0.1 mg/m^3 (inhalable fraction), S	5 mg/m^3		Yellow solid or brown liquid. Vapor pressure is 0.0003 mm Hg at 100°C (212°F). Agricultural pesticide.
Ethanolamine (2-aminoethanol [CAS: 141-43-5]): Highly irritating upon direct contact; severe burns may result. Prolonged contact with skin is irritating. Animal studies suggest that at high levels, vapors are irritating to eyes and respiratory tract; liver and kidney injury may occur. Limited evidence for adverse effects on fetal development in animal studies.	3 ppm	30 ppm	3 2 0	Colorless liquid. A mild ammonia-like odor occurs at the TLV and is an adequate warning property. Vapor pressure is less than 1 mm Hg at 20°C (68°F). Combustible. Thermal breakdown products include oxides of nitrogen.
Ethion (phosphorodithioic acid [CAS: 563-12-2]): An organophosphate-type cholinesterase inhibitor (p 353). Well absorbed dermally.	0.05 mg/m^3 (inhalable fraction and vapor), S			Colorless, odorless liquid when pure. Technical products have an objectionable odor. Vapor pressure is 0.000002 mm Hg at 20°C (68°F). Thermal breakdown products include oxides of sulfur. Agricultural pesticide.

2-Ethoxyethanol (ethylene glycol monoethyl ether, EGEE, cellosolve [CAS: 110-80-5]): Mildly irritating on direct contact. Skin contact is a major route of absorption. Overexposures may reduce sperm counts in men. A potent teratogen in both rats and rabbits. Large doses cause lung, liver, testes, kidney, and spleen injury in test animals. See also p 234.	5 ppm, S	500 ppm	1 2 0	Colorless liquid. Very mild, sweet odor occurs only at very high levels and is a poor warning property. Vapor pressure is 4 mm Hg at 20°C (68°F).
2-Ethoxyethyl acetate (ethylene glycol monoethyl ether acetate, cellosolve acetate): Mildly irritating upon direct contact. May produce CNS depression and kidney injury. Skin contact is a major route of absorption. Metabolized to 2-ethoxyethanol. Adverse effects on fertility and fetal development in animals. See also p 234.	5 ppm, S	500 ppm	2 2 0	Colorless liquid. Mild ether-like odor occurs at the TLV and is a good warning property. Flammable.
Ethyl acetate (CAS: 141-78-6): Slightly irritating to eyes and skin. Vapors irritating to eyes and respiratory tract. A CNS depressant at very high levels. Metabolized to ethanol (p 231) and acetic acid, so may have some of the fetotoxic potential of ethanol.	400 ppm	2,000 ppm [LEL]	1 3 0	Colorless liquid. Fruity odor occurs at the TLV and is a good warning property. Vapor pressure is 76 mm Hg at 20°C (68°F). Flammable.
Ethyl acrylate (CAS: 140-88-5): Extremely irritating upon direct contact; severe burns may result. A skin sensitizer. Vapors highly irritating to eyes and respiratory tract. In animal tests, heart, liver, and kidney damage was observed at high doses. A carcinogen in test animals (IARC 2B).	5 ppm NIOSH CA	300 ppm ERPG-1: 0.01 ppm ERPG-2: 30 ppm ERPG-3: 300 ppm	2 3 2	Colorless liquid. Acrid odor occurs below the TLV and is a good warning property. Vapor pressure is 29.5 mm Hg at 20°C (68°F). Flammable. Contains an inhibitor to prevent dangerous self-polymerization.

(C), ceiling air concentration (TLV-C); S, skin absorption can be significant; SEN, potential sensitizer; STEL, short-term (15-minute) exposure level. A1, ACGIH-confirmed human carcinogen; A2, ACGIH-suspected human carcinogen; A3, ACGIH animal carcinogen. ERPG, Emergency Response Planning Guideline (see p 656 for an explanation of ERPG). IARC 1, known human carcinogen; IARC 2A, probable human carcinogen; IARC 2B, possible human carcinogen; IARC 3, inadequate data available. NFPA hazard codes: H, health; F, fire; R, reactivity; Ox, oxidizer; W, water-reactive; 0 (none) <—> 4 (severe).

(continued)

TABLE IV–4. HEALTH HAZARD SUMMARIES FOR INDUSTRIAL AND OCCUPATIONAL CHEMICALS (CONTINUED)

Health Hazard Summaries	ACGIH TLV	IDLH	NFPA Codes H F R	Comments
Ethyl alcohol (alcohol, grain alcohol, ethanol, EtOH [CAS: 64-17-5]): At high levels, vapors irritating to eyes and respiratory tract. A CNS depressant at high levels of exposure. Strong evidence for adverse effects on fetal development in test animals and humans with chronic ingestion (fetal alcohol syndrome). IARC 1. See also p 231.	1,000 ppm (STEL), A3	3,300 ppm [LEL] ERPG-1: 1,800 ppm ERPG-2: 3,300 ppm	0 3 0	Colorless liquid with a mild, sweet odor. Odor threshold near 1,800 ppm. Vapor pressure is 43 mm Hg at 20°C (68°F). Flammable.
Ethylamine (CAS: 75-04-7): Corrosive upon direct contact; severe burns may result. Vapors highly irritating to eyes, skin, and respiratory tract; delayed pulmonary edema may result. Animal studies suggest potential for liver and kidney injury at moderate doses.	5 ppm, S	600 ppm	3 4 0	Colorless liquid or gas with an ammonia-like odor. Highly flammable. Thermal breakdown products include oxides of nitrogen.
Ethyl amyl ketone (5-methyl-3-heptanone [CAS: 541-85-5]): Irritating to eyes upon direct contact. Vapors irritating to eyes and respiratory tract. A CNS depressant at high levels.	10 ppm	100 ppm		Colorless liquid with a strong, distinctive odor. Flammable.
Ethylbenzene (CAS: 100-41-4): Mildly irritating to eyes upon direct contact. May cause skin burns upon prolonged contact. Dermally well absorbed. Vapors irritating to eyes and respiratory tract. A CNS depressant at high levels of exposure. IARC 2B.	20 ppm, A3	800 ppm [LEL]	2 3 0	Colorless liquid. Aromatic odor and irritation occur at levels close to the TLV and are adequate warning properties. Vapor pressure is 7.1 mm Hg at 20°C (68°F). Flammable.
Ethyl bromide (CAS: 74-96-4): Irritating to skin upon direct contact. Irritating to respiratory tract. A CNS depressant at high levels and may cause cardiac arrhythmias. Former use as an anesthetic agent was discontinued because of fatal liver, kidney, and myocardial injury. Evidence for carcinogenicity in test animals (IARC 3).	5 ppm, S, A3	2,000 ppm	2 1 0	Colorless to yellow liquid. Ether-like odor detectable only at high, dangerous levels. Vapor pressure is 375 mm Hg at 20°C (68°F). Highly flammable. Thermal breakdown products include hydrogen bromide and bromine gas.

Ethyl butyl ketone (3-heptanone [CAS: 106-35-4]): Mildly irritating to eyes upon direct contact. Vapors irritating to eyes and respiratory tract. A CNS depressant at high levels.	50 ppm	1,000 ppm	2 2 0	Colorless liquid. Fruity odor is a good warning property. Vapor pressure is 4 mm Hg at 20°C (68°F). Flammable.
Ethyl chloride (CAS: 75-00-3): Mildly irritating to eyes and respiratory tract. A CNS depressant at high levels; has caused cardiac arrhythmias at anesthetic doses. Animal studies suggest the kidneys and liver are target organs at high doses. Structurally similar to the carcinogenic chloroethanes. IARC 3.	100 ppm, A3, S	3,800 ppm [LEL]	2 4 0	Colorless liquid or gas with a pungent, ether-like odor. Highly flammable. Thermal breakdown products include hydrogen chloride and phosgene.
Ethylene chlorohydrin (2-chloroethanol [CAS: 107-07-3]): Skin contact is extremely hazardous because it is not irritating and absorption is rapid. Vapors irritating to eyes and respiratory tract; pulmonary edema has been reported. Systemic effects include CNS depression, cardiomyopathy, shock, and liver and kidney damage.	1 ppm (C), S	7 ppm	4 2 0	Colorless liquid with a weak ether-like odor. Vapor pressure is 5 mm Hg at 20°C (68°F). Combustible. Thermal breakdown products include hydrogen chloride and phosgene. Industrial intermediate in chemical synthesis but can be created de novo during ethylene oxide sterilization of certain plastics.
Ethylenediamine (CAS: 107-15-3): Highly irritating upon direct contact; burns may result. Respiratory and dermal sensitization may occur. Vapors irritating to eyes and respiratory tract. Animal studies suggest potential for kidney injury at high doses.	10 ppm, S	1,000 ppm	3 2 0	Colorless viscous liquid or solid. Ammonia-like odor occurs at the PEL and may be an adequate warning property. Vapor pressure is 10 mm Hg at 20°C (68°F). Flammable. Thermal breakdown products include oxides of nitrogen. Widely used in industrial chemical and pharmaceutical synthesis.

(C), ceiling air concentration (TLV-C); S, skin absorption can be significant; SEN, potential sensitizer; STEL, short-term (15-minute) exposure level. A1, ACGIH-confirmed human carcinogen; A2, ACGIH-suspected human carcinogen; A3, ACGIH animal carcinogen. ERPG, Emergency Response Planning Guideline (see p 656 for an explanation of ERPG). IARC 1, known human carcinogen; IARC 2A, probable human carcinogen; IARC 2B, possible human carcinogen; IARC 3, inadequate data available. NFPA hazard codes: H, health; F, fire; R, reactivity; Ox, oxidizer; W, water-reactive; 0 (none) <—> 4 (severe).

(*continued*)

TABLE IV–4. HEALTH HAZARD SUMMARIES FOR INDUSTRIAL AND OCCUPATIONAL CHEMICALS (CONTINUED)

Health Hazard Summaries	ACGIH TLV	IDLH	NFPA Codes H F R	Comments
Ethylene dibromide (1,2-dibromoethane, EDB [CAS: 106-93-4]): Highly irritating upon direct contact; severe burns result. Highly toxic by all routes. Vapors highly irritating to eyes and respiratory tract. Severe liver and kidney injury may occur. A CNS depressant. Adverse effects on the testes in test animals and, possibly, humans. A carcinogen in test animals (IARC 2A).	S, A3 NIOSH CA	100 ppm	3 0 0	Colorless liquid or solid. Mild, sweet odor is a poor warning property. Vapor pressure is 11 mm Hg at 20°C (68°F). Not combustible. Thermal breakdown products include hydrogen bromide and bromine gas. Chemical intermediate used in organic synthesis. Formerly widely used as a pesticide but now banned in the United States except for limited fumigant applications.
Ethylene glycol (antifreeze [CAS: 107-21-1]): A CNS depressant. Metabolized to glycolic, oxalic and other acids; severe acidosis and renal failure may result. Precipitation of calcium oxalate crystals in tissues can cause extensive injury. Adversely affects fetal development in animal studies at very high doses. Not well absorbed dermally. See also p 234.	10 mg/m^3 (C) (aerosol only) 25 ppm (inhalable fraction and vapor)		2 1 0	Colorless viscous liquid. Odorless with a very low vapor pressure.
Ethylene glycol dinitrate (EGDN [CAS: 628-96-6]): Causes vasodilation similarly to other nitrate compounds. Headache, hypotension, flushing, palpitation, delirium, and CNS depression may occur. Well absorbed by all routes. Tolerance and dependence may develop to vasodilator effects; cessation after repeated exposures may cause angina pectoris. Can induce methemoglobinemia (p 317).	0.05 ppm, S	75 mg/m^3		Yellow oily liquid. Vapor pressure is 0.05 mm Hg at 20°C (68°F). Explosive. Historically, a munitions manufacturing chemical.

Ethyleneimine (aziridine [CAS: 151-56-4]): Strong caustic. Highly irritating upon direct contact; severe burns may result. Vapors irritating to eyes and respiratory tract; delayed-onset pulmonary edema may occur. Overexposures have resulted in nausea, vomiting, headache, and dizziness. Well absorbed dermally. Similar compounds are potent sensitizers. A carcinogen in animal studies (IARC 2B).	0.5 ppm, S, A3 OSHA CA NIOSH CA	100 ppm	4 3 3	Colorless liquid with an amine-like odor. Vapor pressure is 160 mm Hg at 20°C (68°F). Flammable. Contains inhibitor to prevent explosive self-polymerization. Explosive derivatives can be formed with exposure to silver. Aziridine-derived polyfunctional amines are widely used as hardeners and cross-linking agents in various reactive products.
Ethylene oxide (CAS: 75-21-8): Highly irritating upon direct contact. Vapors irritating to eyes and respiratory tract; delayed pulmonary edema has been reported. A CNS depressant at very high levels. Chronic overexposures can cause peripheral neuropathy and possible permanent CNS impairment. Adverse effects on fetal development and fertility in test animals and limited evidence in humans. A carcinogen in animal studies. Limited evidence of carcinogenicity in humans (IARC 1). See also p 238.	1 ppm, A2 OSHA CA NIOSH CA	800 ppm ERPG-2: 50 ppm ERPG-3: 500 ppm	3 4 3	Colorless. Highly flammable. Ether-like odor is a poor warning property. Important source of exposures has been instrument sterilization operations in health care industry.
Ethyl ether (diethyl ether, ether [CAS: 60-29-7]): Vapors irritating to eyes and respiratory tract. A CNS depressant and anesthetic agent; tolerance may develop to this effect. Overexposure produces nausea, headache, dizziness, anesthesia, and respiratory arrest. Evidence for adverse effects on fetal development in test animals.	400 ppm	1,900 ppm [LEL]	1 4 1	Colorless liquid. Ether-like odor occurs at low levels and is a good warning property. Vapor pressure is 439 mm Hg at 20°C (68°F). Highly flammable.

(C), ceiling air concentration (TLV-C); S, skin absorption can be significant; SEN, potential sensitizer; STEL, short-term (15-minute) exposure level. A1, ACGIH-confirmed human carcinogen; A2, ACGIH-suspected human carcinogen; A3, ACGIH animal carcinogen. ERPG, Emergency Response Planning Guideline (see p 656 for an explanation of ERPG). IARC 1, known human carcinogen; IARC 2A, probable human carcinogen; IARC 2B, possible human carcinogen; IARC 3, inadequate data available. NFPA hazard codes: H, health; F, fire; R, reactivity; Ox, oxidizer; W, water-reactive; 0 (none) <—> 4 (severe).

(*continued*)

TABLE IV–4. HEALTH HAZARD SUMMARIES FOR INDUSTRIAL AND OCCUPATIONAL CHEMICALS (CONTINUED)

Health Hazard Summaries	ACGIH TLV	IDLH	NFPA Codes H F R	Comments
Ethyl formate (CAS: 109-94-4): Slightly irritating to the skin upon direct contact. Vapors mildly irritating to eyes and upper respiratory tract. In test animals, very high levels caused rapid narcosis and pulmonary edema.	100 ppm (STEL)	1,500 ppm	2 3 0	Colorless liquid. Fruity odor and irritation occur near the TLV and are good warning properties. Vapor pressure is 194 mm Hg at 20°C (68°F). Highly flammable.
Ethyl methylacrylate monomer (CAS: 97-63-2): Irritant and sensitizing agent.			2 3 2	Precursor of ethyl methacrylate polymers. Flammable.
Ethyl mercaptan (ethanethiol [CAS: 75-08-1]): Vapors mildly irritating to eyes and respiratory tract. Respiratory paralysis and CNS depression at very high levels. Headache, nausea, and vomiting likely owing to strong odor.	0.5 ppm	500 ppm	2 4 1	Colorless liquid. Penetrating, offensive, mercaptan-like odor. Vapor pressure is 442 mm Hg at 20°C (68°F).
***N*-Ethylmorpholine (CAS: 100-74-3):** Irritating to eyes upon direct contact. Vapors irritating to eyes and respiratory tract. Workers exposed to levels near the TLV reported drowsiness and temporary visual disturbances, including corneal edema. Animal testing suggests potential for skin absorption.	5 ppm, S	100 ppm	2 3 0	Colorless liquid with ammonia-like odor. Vapor pressure is 5 mm Hg at 20°C (68°F). Flammable. Thermal breakdown products include oxides of nitrogen.
Ethyl silicate (tetraethyl orthosilicate, tetraethoxysilane [CAS: 78-10-4]): Irritating upon direct contact. Vapors irritating to eyes and respiratory tract. All human effects noted at vapor exposures above the odor threshold. In subchronic animal testing, high vapor levels produced liver, lung, and kidney damage and delayed-onset pulmonary edema.	10 ppm	700 ppm ERPG-1: 25 ppm ERPG-2: 100 ppm ERPG-3: 300 ppm	2 3 1	Colorless liquid. Faint alcohol-like odor and irritation are good warning properties. Vapor pressure is 2 mm Hg at 20°C (68°F). Flammable.

Etidronic acid (1-hydroxyethylidene 1,1-diphosphonic acid, HEDP [CAS: 2809-21-4]): Inadvertent ingestion in an industrial setting has caused renal failure.			A bisphosphonate used in detergents, corrosion inhibition in water cooling and boilers, cosmetics and medical treatment. It is available in powder and liquid forms. The liquid form is clear and colorless with a slight odor, and contains 58–62% of the active chemical substance.
Fenamiphos (ethyl 3-methyl-4-[methylthio]phenyl-[1-methylethyl]phosphoramide [CAS: 22224-92-6]): An organophosphate-type cholinesterase inhibitor (p 353). Well absorbed dermally.	0.05 mg/m^3 (inhalable fraction and vapor), S		Tan, waxy solid. Vapor pressure is 0.000001 mm Hg at 30°C (86°F). Agricultural pesticide.
Fensulfothion (*O,O*-diethyl *O*-[4-(methylsulfinyl) phenyl] phosphorothioate [CAS: 115-90-2]): An organophosphate-type cholinesterase inhibitor (p 353).	0.01 mg/m^3 (inhalable fraction and vapor), S		Brown liquid. Agricultural pesticide.
Fenthion (*O,O*-dimethyl *O*-[3-methyl-4-(methylthio) phenyl] phosphorothioate [CAS: 55-38-9]): An organophosphate-type cholinesterase inhibitor (p 353). Highly lipid-soluble; toxicity may be prolonged. Dermal absorption is rapid.	0.05 mg/m^3, S		Yellow to tan viscous liquid with a mild garlic-like odor. Vapor pressure is 0.00003 mm Hg at 20°C (68°F). Agricultural pesticide.
Ferbam (ferric dimethyldithiocarbamate [CAS: 14484-64-1]): Thiocarbamates do not act through cholinesterase inhibition. Dusts irritating upon direct contact; causes dermatitis in persons sensitized to sulfur. Dusts are mild respiratory tract irritants. Limited evidence for adverse effects on fetal development in test animals (IARC 3).	5 mg/m^3	800 mg/m^3	Odorless, black solid. Vapor pressure is negligible at 20°C (68°F). Thermal breakdown products include oxides of nitrogen and sulfur. Used as a fungicide.
Ferrovanadium dust (CAS: 12604-58-9): Mild irritant of eyes and respiratory tract.	1 mg/m^3	500 mg/m^3	Odorless, dark-colored powders.

(C), ceiling air concentration (TLV-C); S, skin absorption can be significant; SEN, potential sensitizer; STEL, short-term (15-minute) exposure level. A1, ACGIH-confirmed human carcinogen; A2, ACGIH-suspected human carcinogen; A3, ACGIH animal carcinogen. ERPG, Emergency Response Planning Guideline (see p 656 for an explanation of ERPG). IARC 1, known human carcinogen; IARC 2A, probable human carcinogen; IARC 2B, possible human carcinogen; IARC 3, inadequate data available. NFPA hazard codes: H, health; F, fire; R, reactivity; Ox, oxidizer; W, water-reactive; 0 (none) <—> 4 (severe).

(*continued*)

TABLE IV–4. HEALTH HAZARD SUMMARIES FOR INDUSTRIAL AND OCCUPATIONAL CHEMICALS (CONTINUED)

Health Hazard Summaries	ACGIH TLV	IDLH	NFPA Codes H F R	Comments
Fipronil (CAS: 120068-37-3): Phenylpyrazole insecticide; blocks GABA-gated chloride channels and can cause seizures. Mild irritant of eyes and respiratory tract.				Used to kill crickets, fire ants, fleas, ticks, termites, and roaches. Registered for use in more than 50 consumer products.
Fluoride dust (as fluoride): Irritating to eyes and respiratory tract. Workers exposed to levels 10 mg/m^3 experienced nasal irritation and bleeding. Lower-level exposures have produced nausea and eye and respiratory tract irritation. Chronic overexposures may result in skin rashes. Fluorosis, a bone disease associated with chronic high-level fluoride ingestion, is not associated with occupational dust inhalation. See also p 240.	2.5 mg/m^3 (as F)	250 mg/m^3 (as F)		Appearance varies with the compound. Sodium fluoride is a colorless to blue solid.
Fluorine (CAS: 7782-41-4): Rapidly reacts with moisture to form ozone and hydrofluoric acid. The gas is a severe eye, skin, and respiratory tract irritant; severe penetrating burns and pulmonary edema have resulted. Systemic hypocalcemia can occur with fluorine or hydrogen fluoride exposure. See also p 269.	1 ppm	25 ppm ERPG-1: 0.5 ppm ERPG-2: 5.0 ppm ERPG-3: 20 ppm	4 0 4 W	Pale yellow gas. Sharp odor is a poor warning property. Highly reactive; will ignite many oxidizable materials. Uses include rocket fuel oxidizer.
Fonofos (*O*-ethyl-*S*-phenyl ethylphosphonothiolothionate, Dyfonate [CAS: 944-22-9]): An organophosphate-type cholinesterase inhibitor (p 353). Highly toxic; oral toxicity in test animals ranged from 3 to 13 mg/kg for rats, and rabbits died after eye instillation.	0.1 mg/m^3 (inhalable fraction and vapor), S			Vapor pressure is 0.00021 mm Hg at 20°C (68°F). Thermal breakdown products include oxides of sulfur. Agricultural pesticide.

Formaldehyde (formic aldehyde, methanal, HCHO, formalin [CAS: 50-00-0]): Highly irritating to eyes upon direct contact; severe burns result. Irritating to skin; may cause sensitization dermatitis. Vapors highly irritating to eyes and respiratory tract. Sensitization may occur. A carcinogen in test animals (IARC 1). See also p 249.	0.3 ppm (C), SEN, A2 OSHA CA NIOSH CA	20 ppm ERPG-1: 1 ppm ERPG-2: 10 ppm ERPG-3: 40 ppm	3 2 0 (gas) 3 2 0 (formalin)	Colorless gas with a suffocating odor. Odor threshold near 1 ppm. Combustible. Formalin (15% methanol) solutions are flammable. Industrial chemical in wide use, including for urea-formaldehyde materials. Formaldehyde off-gassing can occur from formaldehyde-containing materials such as insulation and particle board.
Formamide (methanamide [CAS: 75-12-7]): In animal tests, mildly irritating upon direct contact. Adverse effects on fetal development in test animals at very high doses.	10 ppm, S		2 1 0	Clear, viscous liquid. Odorless. Vapor pressure is 2 mm Hg at 70°C (158°F). Combustible. Thermal breakdown products include oxides of nitrogen.
Formic acid (CAS: 64-18-6): Acid is corrosive; severe burns may result from contact of eyes and skin with concentrated acid. Vapors highly irritating to eyes and respiratory tract. Ingestion may produce severe metabolic acidosis. See "Methanol," p 314.	5 ppm	30 ppm ERPG-1: 3 ppm ERPG-2: 25 ppm ERPG-3: 250 ppm	3 2 0	Colorless liquid. Pungent odor and irritation occur near the TLV and are adequate warning properties. Vapor pressure is 30 mm Hg at 20°C (68°F). Combustible.
Furfural (bran oil [CAS: 98-01-1]): Highly irritating upon direct contact; burns may result. Vapors highly irritating to eyes and respiratory tract; pulmonary edema may result. Animal studies indicate the liver is a target organ. Hyperreflexia and convulsions occur at large doses in test animals. IARC 3.	2 ppm, S, A3	100 ppm ERPG-1: 2 ppm ERPG-2: 10 ppm ERPG-3:; 100 ppm	3 2 1	Colorless to light brown liquid. Almond-like odor occurs below the TLV and is a good warning property. Vapor pressure is 2 mm Hg at 20°C (68°F). Combustible. Thermal breakdown products include oxides of nitrogen.
Furfuryl alcohol (CAS: 98-00-0): Dermal absorption occurs. Vapors irritating to eyes and respiratory tract. A CNS depressant at high air levels.	10 ppm, S	75 ppm	3 2 1	Clear, colorless liquid. Upon exposure to light and air, color changes to red or brown. Vapor pressure is 0.53 mm Hg at 20°C (68°F). Combustible.
Gadolinium (CAS: 7440-54-2): Nephrogenic systemic sclerosis (fibrosis) in humans.				Used as a medical contrast agent in magnetic resonance imaging.

(C), ceiling air concentration (TLV-C); S, skin absorption can be significant; SEN, potential sensitizer; STEL, short-term (15-minute) exposure level. A1, ACGIH-confirmed human carcinogen; A2, ACGIH-suspected human carcinogen; A3, ACGIH animal carcinogen. ERPG, Emergency Response Planning Guideline (see p 656 for an explanation of ERPG). IARC 1, known human carcinogen; IARC 2A, probable human carcinogen; IARC 2B, possible human carcinogen; IARC 3, inadequate data available. NFPA hazard codes: H, health; F, fire; R, reactivity; Ox, oxidizer; W, water-reactive; 0 (none) <—> 4 (severe).

(*continued*)

TABLE IV–4. HEALTH HAZARD SUMMARIES FOR INDUSTRIAL AND OCCUPATIONAL CHEMICALS (CONTINUED)

Health Hazard Summaries	ACGIH TLV	IDLH	NFPA Codes H F R	Comments
Gasoline (CAS: 8006-61-9): Although exact composition varies, the acute toxicity of all gasoline mixes is similar. Vapors irritating to eyes and respiratory tract at high levels. A CNS depressant; symptoms include incoordination, dizziness, headaches, and nausea. Benzene (generally <1%) is one significant chronic health hazard. Other additives, such as ethylene dibromide and tetraethyl and tetramethyl lead, are present in low amounts and may be absorbed through the skin. Very limited evidence for carcinogenicity in test animals (IARC 2B). See also p 266.	300 ppm, A3 NIOSH CA	[LEL 14,000 ppm] ERPG-1: 200 ppm ERPG-2: 1,000 ppm ERPG-3: 4,000 ppm	1 3 0	Clear to amber liquid with a characteristic odor. Highly flammable. Gasoline is sometimes used inappropriately as a solvent. Substance abuse via inhalation has been reported.
Germanium tetrahydride (CAS: 7782-65-2): A hemolytic agent with effects similar to but less potent than those of arsine in animals. Symptoms include abdominal pain, hematuria, anemia, and jaundice.	0.2 ppm		4 4 3 W	Colorless gas. Highly flammable.
Glutaraldehyde (1,5-pentandial [CAS: 111-30-8]): The purity and therefore the toxicity of glutaraldehyde vary widely. Allergic dermatitis may occur. Highly irritating on contact; severe burns may result. Vapors highly irritating to eyes and respiratory tract; respiratory sensitization or irritant-induced asthma may occur. In animal studies, the liver is a target organ at high doses. See p 132.	0.05 ppm (C), SEN	ERPG-1: 0.2 ppm ERPG-2: 1 ppm ERPG-3: 5 ppm		Colorless solid crystals. Odor threshold near 0.2 ppm. Vapor pressure is 0.0152 mm Hg at 20°C (68°F). Can undergo hazardous self-polymerization. Commonly used as a sterilizing agent in medical settings, widely replacing ethylene oxide.
Glycidol (2,3-epoxy-1-propanol [CAS: 556-52-5]): Highly irritating to eyes on contact; burns may result. Moderately irritating to skin and respiratory tract. Evidence for carcinogenicity and testicular toxicity in test animals (IARC 2A).	2 ppm, A3	150 ppm		Colorless liquid. Vapor pressure is 0.9 mm Hg at 25°C (77°F) Combustible.

Glyphosate (CAS: 1071-83-6): Intentional self-poisoning has caused acute noncardiogenic pulmonary edema, renal failure; toxic effects may result from the surfactant component rather than from glyphosate itself. IARC 2A. See also p 257.				White or colorless solid. Odorless or slight amine odor; negligible vapor pressure. Stable to light and heat. Agricultural pesticide (herbicide).
Halothane (CAS: 151-67-7): Potential to cause hepatitis and may be teratogenic in occupationally exposed workers.	50 ppm			Clear, colorless liquid with a sweetish, pleasant odor; inhalation anesthetic
Hafnium (CAS: 7440-58-6): Based on animal studies, dusts are mildly irritating to eyes and skin. Liver injury may occur at very high doses.	0.5 mg/m^3	50 mg/m^3		The metal is a gray solid. Other compounds vary in appearance.
Heptachlor (CAS: 76-44-8): CNS convulsant. Skin absorption is rapid and has caused convulsions and death. Hepatotoxic. Stored in fatty tissues. Limited evidence for adverse effects on fetal development in test animals at high doses. A carcinogen in test animals (IARC 2B). See also p 189.	0.05 mg/m^3, S, A3 NIOSH CA	35 mg/m^3		White or light tan, waxy solid with a camphor-like odor. Vapor pressure is 0.0003 mm Hg at 20°C (68°F). Thermal breakdown products include hydrogen chloride. Not combustible. Pesticide use banned by EPA in 1988.
***n*-Heptane (CAS: 142-82-5):** Vapors only slightly irritating to eyes and respiratory tract. May cause euphoria, vertigo, CNS depression, and cardiac arrhythmias at high levels.	400 ppm	750 ppm	1 3 –	Colorless clear liquid. Mild gasoline-like odor occurs below the TLV and is a good warning property. Vapor pressure is 40 mm Hg at 20°C (68°F). Flammable. Industrial solvent also widely used in commercial consumer products.
Hexachlorobutadiene (CAS: 87-68-3): Based on animal studies, rapid dermal absorption is expected. The kidney is the major target organ but also hepatotoxic in animal studies. A carcinogen in test animals (nonetheless, IARC 3).	0.02 ppm, S, A3 NIOSH CA	ERPG-1: 1 ppm ERPG-2: 3 ppm ERPG-3: 10 ppm	3 1 0	Heavy, colorless liquid. Thermal breakdown products include hydrogen chloride and phosgene. Solvent and byproduct in industrial chemical synthesis.

(C), ceiling air concentration (TLV-C); S, skin absorption can be significant; SEN, potential sensitizer; STEL, short-term (15-minute) exposure level. A1, ACGIH-confirmed human carcinogen; A2, ACGIH-suspected human carcinogen; A3, ACGIH animal carcinogen. ERPG, Emergency Response Planning Guideline (see p 656 for an explanation of ERPG). IARC 1, known human carcinogen; IARC 2A, probable human carcinogen; IARC 2B, possible human carcinogen; IARC 3, inadequate data available. NFPA hazard codes: H, health; F, fire; R, reactivity; Ox, oxidizer; W, water-reactive; 0 (none) <—> 4 (severe).

(*continued*)

TABLE IV–4. HEALTH HAZARD SUMMARIES FOR INDUSTRIAL AND OCCUPATIONAL CHEMICALS (CONTINUED)

Health Hazard Summaries	ACGIH TLV	IDLH	NFPA Codes H F R	Comments
Hexachlorocyclopentadiene (CAS: 77-47-4): Vapors extremely irritating to eyes and respiratory tract; lacrimation and salivation. In animal studies, a potent kidney and liver toxin. At higher levels, the brain, heart, and adrenal glands were affected. Tremors occurred at high doses.	0.01 ppm			Yellow to amber liquid with a pungent odor. Vapor pressure is 0.08 mm Hg at 20°C (68°F). Not combustible.
Hexachloroethane (perchloroethane [CAS: 67-72-1]): Hot fumes irritating to eyes, skin, and mucous membranes. Based on animal studies, causes CNS depression and kidney and liver injury at high doses. Limited evidence of carcinogenicity in test animals (IARC 2B).	1 ppm, S, A3 NIOSH CA	300 ppm		White solid with a camphor-like odor. Vapor pressure is 0.22 mm Hg at 20°C (68°F). Not combustible. Thermal breakdown products include phosgene, chlorine gas, and hydrogen chloride.
Hexachloronaphthalene (Halowax 1014 [CAS: 1335-87-1]): Based on historical workplace experience, a potent toxin causing severe chloracne and severe, occasionally fatal liver injury. See p 224. Skin absorption can occur.	0.2 mg/m^3, S	2 mg/m^3		Light yellow solid with an aromatic odor. Vapor pressure is less than 1 mm Hg at 20°C (68°F). Not combustible.
Hexamethylphosphoramide (CAS: 680-31-9): Low-level exposures produced nasal cavity cancer in rats (IARC 2B). Adverse effects on the testes in test animals.	S, A3 NIOSH CA			Colorless liquid with an aromatic odor. Vapor pressure is 0.07 mm Hg at 20°C (68°F). Thermal breakdown products include oxides of nitrogen.
***n*-Hexane (normal hexane [CAS: 110-54-3]):** Vapors mildly irritating to eyes and respiratory tract. A CNS depressant at high levels, producing headache, dizziness, and gastrointestinal upset. Occupational overexposures have resulted in peripheral neuropathy. Methyl ethyl ketone potentiates this toxicity. Testicular toxicity in animal studies.	50 ppm, S	1,100 ppm [LEL]	– 3 0	Colorless, clear liquid with a mild gasoline odor. Vapor pressure is 124 mm Hg at 20°C (68°F). Highly flammable. Previously a widely used solvent, in particular in rubber cement–type glues.

Hexane isomers (other than *n*-hexane, isohexane, 2,3-demethylbutane): Vapors mildly irritating to eyes and respiratory tract. A CNS depressant at high levels, producing headache, dizziness, and gastrointestinal upset.	500 ppm			Colorless liquids with a mild petroleum odor. Vapor pressures are high at 20°C (68°F). Highly flammable.
***sec*-Hexyl acetate (1,3-dimethylbutyl acetate [CAS: 108-84-9]):** At low levels, vapors irritating to eyes and respiratory tract. Based on animal studies, a CNS depressant at high levels.	50 ppm	500 ppm	1 2 0	Colorless liquid. Unpleasant fruity odor and irritation are both good warning properties. Vapor pressure is 4 mm Hg at 20°C (68°F). Flammable.
Hexylene glycol (2-methyl-2,4-pentanediol [CAS: 107-41-5]): Irritating upon direct contact; vapors irritating to eyes and respiratory tract. A CNS depressant at very high doses in animal studies.	25 ppm (C)		2 1 0	Liquid with a faint sweet odor. Vapor pressure is 0.05 mm Hg at 20°C (68°F). Combustible.
Hydrazine (diamine [CAS: 302-01-2]): Corrosive upon direct contact; severe burns result. Vapors extremely irritating to eyes and respiratory tract; pulmonary edema may occur. Highly hepatotoxic. A convulsant and hemolytic agent. Kidneys are also target organs. Well absorbed by all routes. Limited human evidence of lung cancer (IARC 2A).	0.01 ppm, S, A3 NIOSH CA	50 ppm ERPG-1: 0.5 ppm ERPG-2: 5 ppm ERPG-3: 30 ppm	4 4 3 (vapors explosive)	Colorless, fuming, viscous liquid with an amine odor. Vapor pressure is 10 mm Hg at 20°C (68°F). Flammable. Thermal breakdown products include oxides of nitrogen. Used as a rocket fuel and in some military jet systems. Toxicity treated with pyridoxine (p 621).
Hydrogen bromide (HBr [CAS: 10035-10-6]): Direct contact with concentrated solutions may cause corrosive acid burns. Vapors highly irritating to eyes and respiratory tract; pulmonary edema may result.	2 ppm (C)	30 ppm	3 0 0	Colorless gas or pressurized liquid. Acrid odor and irritation occur near the TLV and are adequate warning properties. Not combustible.
Hydrogen chloride (hydrochloric acid, muriatic acid, HCl [CAS: 7647-01-0]): Direct contact with concentrated solutions may cause corrosive acid burns. Vapors highly irritating to eyes and respiratory tract; pulmonary edema has resulted. See p 255.	2 ppm (C)	50 ppm ERPG-1: 3 ppm ERPG-2: 20 ppm ERPG-3: 150 ppm	3 0 1	Colorless gas with a pungent, choking odor. Irritation occurs near the TLV and is a good warning property. Not combustible. Contact with water, including atmospheric humidity, leads to formation of hydrochloric acid.

(C), ceiling air concentration (TLV-C); S, skin absorption can be significant; SEN, potential sensitizer; STEL, short-term (15-minute) exposure level. A1, ACGIH-confirmed human carcinogen; A2, ACGIH-suspected human carcinogen; A3, ACGIH animal carcinogen. ERPG, Emergency Response Planning Guideline (see p 656 for an explanation of ERPG). IARC 1, known human carcinogen; IARC 2A, probable human carcinogen; IARC 2B, possible human carcinogen; IARC 3, inadequate data available. NFPA hazard codes: H, health; F, fire; R, reactivity; Ox, oxidizer; W, water-reactive; 0 (none) <—> 4 (severe).

(continued)

TABLE IV–4. HEALTH HAZARD SUMMARIES FOR INDUSTRIAL AND OCCUPATIONAL CHEMICALS (CONTINUED)

Health Hazard Summaries	ACGIH TLV	IDLH	NFPA Codes H F R	Comments
Hydrogen cyanide (hydrocyanic acid, prussic acid, HCN [CAS: 74 90–8]): A rapidly acting, potent metabolic asphyxiant that inhibits cytochrome oxidase and stops cellular respiration. See also p 208.	4.7 ppm (C), S	50 ppm ERPG-2: 10 ppm ERPG-3: 25 ppm	4 4 2 (vapors extremely toxic)	Colorless to pale blue liquid or colorless gas with a sweet, bitter almond smell that is an inadequate warning property, even for those sensitive to it. Vapor pressure is 620 mm Hg at 20°C (68°F). Cyanide salts will release HCN gas with exposure to acids or heat.
Hydrogen fluoride (hydrofluoric acid, HF [CAS: 7664-39-3]): Produces severe, penetrating burns to eyes, skin, and deeper tissues upon direct contact with solutions. Onset of pain and erythema may be delayed as much as 12–16 hours. As a gas, highly irritating to the eyes and respiratory tract; pulmonary edema has resulted. Severe hypocalcemia may occur with overexposure. See p 269.	0.5 ppm (C) (as F), S	30 ppm ERPG-1: 2 ppm ERPG-2: 20 ppm ERPG-3: 50 ppm	4 0 1	Colorless fuming liquid or gas. Irritation occurs at levels below the TLV and is an adequate warning property. Vapor pressure is 760 mm Hg at 20°C (68°F). Not combustible. Concentrated HF is used in the microelectronics industry. Over-the-counter rust-removing products may contain HF, but generally at lower concentrations (<10%).
Hydrogen peroxide (CAS: 7722-84-1): A strong oxidizing agent. Direct contact with concentrated solutions can produce severe eye damage and skin irritation, including erythema and vesicle formation. Vapors irritating to eyes, skin, mucous membranes, and respiratory tract. See also p 132. IARC 3.	1 ppm, A3	75 ppm ERPG-1: 10 ppm ERPG-2: 50 ppm ERPG-3: 100 ppm	2 0 3 Ox (≥60%) 2 0 1 Ox (40–60%)	Colorless liquid with a slightly sharp, distinctive odor. Vapor pressure is 5 mm Hg at 30°C (86°F). Because of instability, usually found in aqueous solutions (3% for home use, higher in some "health food" products and in industry). Not combustible but a very powerful oxidizing agent.
Hydrogen selenide (CAS: 7783-07-5): Vapors extremely irritating to eyes and respiratory tract. Systemic symptoms from low-level exposure include nausea and vomiting, fatigue, metallic taste in mouth, and a garlicky breath odor. Animal studies indicate hepatotoxicity.	0.05 ppm	1 ppm ERPG-2: 0.2 ppm ERPG-3: 2 ppm		Colorless gas. The strongly offensive odor and irritation occur only at levels far above the TLV and are poor warning properties. Flammable. Water-reactive.

Hydrogen sulfide (sewer gas [CAS: 7783-06-4]): Vapors irritating to eyes and respiratory tract. At higher levels, a potent, rapid systemic toxin causing cellular asphyxia and death. Systemic effects of low-level exposure include headache, cough, nausea, and vomiting. See also p 271.	1 ppm	100 ppm ERPG-1: 0.1 ppm ERPG-2: 30 ppm ERPG-3: 100 ppm	4 4 0	Colorless gas. Although the strong rotten egg odor can be detected at very low levels, olfactory fatigue occurs. Odor is therefore a poor warning property. Flammable. Produced by the decay of organic material, as may occur in sewers, manure pits, and fish processing. Fossil fuel production or storage also may generate the gas.
Hydroquinone (1,4-dihydroxybenzene [CAS: 123-31-9]): Highly irritating to eyes upon direct contact. Chronic occupational exposures may cause partial discoloration and opacification of the cornea. Systemic effects result from ingestion and include tinnitus, headache, dizziness, gastrointestinal upset, CNS excitation, and skin depigmentation. May cause methemoglobinemia (p 317). Limited evidence of carcinogenicity in test animals (IARC 3).	1 mg/m^3, SEN, A3	50 mg/m^3	2 1 0	White solid crystals. Vapor pressure is less than 0.001 mm Hg at 20°C (68°F). Combustible. Used in photographic development and as an industrial reducing agent; over-the-counter use as a skin depigmenting agent.
2-Hydroxypropyl acrylate (propylene glycol acrylate, HPA [CAS: 999-61-1]): Highly irritating upon direct contact; severe burns may result. Vapors highly irritating to eyes and respiratory tract. Based on structural analogies, compounds containing the acrylate moiety may be carcinogens. No IARC evaluation.	0.5 ppm, S, SEN		3 1 2	Combustible liquid.
Indene (CAS: 95-13-6): Polycyclic hydrocarbon. Repeated direct contact with the skin has produced dermatitis but no systemic effects. Vapors probably irritating to eyes and respiratory tract. Based on animal studies, high air levels may cause liver and kidney damage.	5 ppm			Colorless liquid. Used industrially in the manufacture of selected polymers.

(C), ceiling air concentration (TLV-C); S, skin absorption can be significant; SEN, potential sensitizer; STEL, short-term (15-minute) exposure level. A1, ACGIH-confirmed human carcinogen; A2, ACGIH-suspected human carcinogen; A3, ACGIH animal carcinogen. ERPG, Emergency Response Planning Guideline (see p 656 for an explanation of ERPG). IARC 1, known human carcinogen; IARC 2A, probable human carcinogen; IARC 2B, possible human carcinogen; IARC 3, inadequate data available. NFPA hazard codes: H, health; F, fire; R, reactivity; Ox, oxidizer; W, water-reactive; 0 (none) <—> 4 (severe).

(continued)

TABLE IV–4. HEALTH HAZARD SUMMARIES FOR INDUSTRIAL AND OCCUPATIONAL CHEMICALS (CONTINUED)

Health Hazard Summaries	ACGIH TLV	IDLH	NFPA Codes H F R	Comments
Indoxacarb (CAS: 173584-44-6): An oxadiazine insecticide that blocks neuronal voltage-dependent sodium channels. Intentional ingestion has resulted in methemoglobinemia (p 317) and acute kidney injury.				White powder with low water solubility. Vapor pressure is negligible. Used as broad spectrum insecticide in cotton, vegetables, and fruit; introduced as a new "reduced risk" pesticide to replace organophosphates.
Indium (CAS: 7440-74-6): Based on animal studies, the soluble salts are extremely irritating to eyes upon direct contact. Dusts irritating to eyes and respiratory tract. Linked to occupationally-related interstitial lung disease, including pulmonary fibrosis and alveolar proteinosis.	0.1 mg/m^3			Appearance varies with the compound. The elemental metal is a silver-white lustrous solid. Indium-tin oxide is a sintered metal combination used in flat screen displays.
Iodine (CAS: 7553-56-2): Extremely irritating upon direct contact; severe burns result. Vapors extremely irritating and corrosive to eyes and respiratory tract. Rarely, a skin sensitizer. Medicinal use of iodine-containing drugs has been associated with fetal goiter, a potentially life-threatening condition for a fetus or infant. Iodine causes adverse effects on fetal development in test animals. See also p 274.	0.01 ppm (inhalable fraction and vapor)	2 ppm ERPG-1: 0.1 ppm ERPG-2: 0.5 ppm ERPG-3: 5 ppm		Violet-colored solid crystals. Sharp, characteristic odor is a poor warning property. Vapor pressure is 0.3 mm Hg at 20°C (68°F). Not combustible.
Iron oxide fume (CAS: 1309-37-1): Fumes and dusts can produce a benign pneumoconiosis (siderosis) manifested by chest radiographic opacities. Fume is associated epidemiologically with infectious pneumonia.	5 mg/m^3 (respirable fraction)	2,500 mg/m^3 (as Fe)		Red-brown fume with a metallic taste. Vapor pressure is negligible at 20°C (68°F). Welders on mild steel are the principal exposure group.

Iron pentacarbonyl (iron carbonyl [CAS: 13463-40-6]): Acute toxicity resembles that of nickel carbonyl. Inhalation of vapors can cause lung and systemic injury without warning signs. Symptoms of overexposure include headache, nausea and vomiting, and dizziness. Symptoms of severe poisoning are fever, extreme weakness, and pulmonary edema; effects may be delayed for up to 36 hours.	0.1 ppm			Colorless to yellow viscous liquid. Vapor pressure is 40 mm Hg at 30.3°C (86.5°F). Highly flammable. Used in specialized chemical synthesis applications, including nanotubule formation.
Isoamyl acetate (banana oil, 3-methyl butyl acetate [CAS: 123-92-2]): May be irritating to skin upon prolonged contact. Vapors mildly irritating to eyes and respiratory tract. Symptoms in men exposed to 950 ppm for 0.5 hour included headache, weakness, dyspnea, and irritation of the nose and throat. A CNS depressant at high doses in test animals. Extrapyramidal syndrome (reversible) in one human case report.	50 ppm	1,000 ppm	1 3 0	Colorless liquid. Banana- or pearlike odor and irritation occur at low levels and are good warning properties. Vapor pressure is 4 mm Hg at 20°C (68°F). Flammable. Often used to test respirator fit, including in military recruits.
Isoamyl alcohol (3-methyl-1-butanol, isopentanol [CAS: 123-51-3]): Vapors irritating to eyes and respiratory tract. A CNS depressant at high levels.	100 ppm	500 ppm	1 2 0	Colorless liquid. Irritating alcohol-like odor and irritation are good warning properties. Vapor pressure is 2 mm Hg at 20°C (68°F). Flammable.
Isobutyl acetate (2-methylpropyl acetate [CAS: 110-19-0]): Vapors mildly irritating to eyes and respiratory tract. A CNS depressant at high levels.	50 ppm	1,300 ppm [LEL]	1 3 0	Colorless liquid. Pleasant fruity odor is a good warning property. Vapor pressure is 13 mm Hg at 20°C (68°F). Flammable.
Isobutyl alcohol (2-methyl-1 propanol [CAS: 78-83-1]): A CNS depressant at high levels.	50 ppm, A3	1,600 ppm	1 3 0	Colorless liquid. Mild characteristic odor is a good warning property. Vapor pressure is 9 mm Hg at 20°C (68°F). Flammable.

(C), ceiling air concentration (TLV-C); S, skin absorption can be significant; SEN, potential sensitizer; STEL, short-term (15-minute) exposure level. A1, ACGIH-confirmed human carcinogen; A2, ACGIH-suspected human carcinogen; A3, ACGIH animal carcinogen. ERPG, Emergency Response Planning Guideline (see p 656 for an explanation of ERPG). IARC 1, known human carcinogen; IARC 2A, probable human carcinogen; IARC 2B, possible human carcinogen; IARC 3, inadequate data available. NFPA hazard codes: H, health; F, fire; R, reactivity; Ox, oxidizer; W, water-reactive; 0 (none) <—> 4 (severe).

(*continued*)

TABLE IV–4. HEALTH HAZARD SUMMARIES FOR INDUSTRIAL AND OCCUPATIONAL CHEMICALS (CONTINUED)

Health Hazard Summaries	ACGIH TLV	IDLH	NFPA Codes H F R	Comments
Isophorone (trimethylcyclohexenone [CAS: 78-59-1]): Vapors irritating to eyes and respiratory tract. Workers exposed to 5–8 ppm experienced fatigue and malaise after 1 month. Higher exposures result in nausea, headache, dizziness, and a feeling of suffocation at 200–400 ppm. Limited evidence for adverse effects on fetal development in test animals.	5 ppm (C), A3	200 ppm	2 2 1	Colorless liquid with a camphor-like odor. Vapor pressure is 0.2 mm Hg at 20°C (68°F). Flammable.
Isophorone diisocyanate (CAS: 4098-71-9): Based on animal studies, extremely irritating upon direct contact; severe burns may result. By analogy with other isocyanates, vapors or mists likely to be potent respiratory sensitizers, causing asthma. See also p 280.	0.005 ppm		2 1 1 W	Colorless to pale yellow liquid. Vapor pressure is 0.0003 mm Hg at 20°C (68°F). Possible thermal breakdown products include oxides of nitrogen and hydrogen cyanide.
2-Isopropoxyethanol (isopropyl cellosolve, ethylene glycol monoisopropyl ether [CAS: 109-59-1]): Defatting agent causing dermatitis. May cause hemolysis.	25 ppm, S		3 2 1	Clear colorless liquid with a characteristic odor.
Isopropyl acetate (CAS: 108-21-4): Vapors irritating to the eyes and respiratory tract. A weak CNS depressant.	100 ppm	1,800 ppm	2 3 0	Colorless liquid. Fruity odor and irritation are good warning properties. Vapor pressure is 43 mm Hg at 20°C (68°F). Flammable.
Isopropyl alcohol (isopropanol, 2-propanol [CAS: 67-63-0]): Vapors produce mild eye and respiratory tract irritation. High exposures can produce CNS depression. See also p 282. IARC 3.	200 ppm	2,000 ppm [LEL]	1 3 0	Rubbing alcohol. Sharp odor and irritation are adequate warning properties. Vapor pressure is 33 mm Hg at 20°C (68°F). Flammable.
Isopropylamine (2-aminopropane [CAS: 75-31-0]): Corrosive upon direct contact; severe burns may result. Vapors highly irritating to the eyes and respiratory tract. Exposure to vapors can cause transient corneal edema.	5 ppm	750 ppm	3 4 0	Colorless liquid. Strong ammonia odor and irritation are good warning properties. Vapor pressure is 478 mm Hg at 20°C (68°F). Highly flammable. Thermal breakdown products include oxides of nitrogen.

Isopropyl ether (diisopropyl ether [CAS: 108-20-3]): A skin irritant upon prolonged contact with liquid. Vapors mildly irritating to the eyes and respiratory tract. A CNS depressant.	250 ppm	1,400 ppm [LEL]	2 3 1	Colorless liquid. Offensive and sharp ether-like odor and irritation are good warning properties. Vapor pressure is 119 mm Hg at 20°C (68°F). Highly flammable. Contact with air causes formation of explosive peroxides.
Isopropyl glycidyl ether (CAS: 4016-14-2): Irritating upon direct contact. Allergic dermatitis may occur. Vapors irritating to eyes and respiratory tract. In animals, a CNS depressant at high oral doses; chronic exposures produced liver injury. Some glycidyl ethers possess hematopoietic and testicular toxicity.	50 ppm	400 ppm		Flammable. Vapor pressure is 9.4 mm Hg at 25°C (77°F).
Kepone (chlordecone [CAS: 143-50-0]): Neurotoxin; overexposure causes slurred speech, memory impairment, incoordination, weakness, tremor, and convulsions. Causes infertility in males. Hepatotoxic. Well absorbed by all routes. A carcinogen in test animals (IARC 2B). See also p 189.	NIOSH CA			A solid. Banned pesticide, not manufactured in the United States since 1978.
Kerosene (CAS 8008-20-6; 64742-81-0): Mixture of medium-length aliphatic hydrocarbons (p 266). Reported to cause encephalopathy ("solvent syndrome") in those chronically exposed.	200 mg/m^3			Colorless to yellowish, oily liquid with a strong, characteristic odor; used in cooking and lighting fuels and jet fuel.
Ketene (ethenone [CAS: 463-51-4]): Vapors extremely irritating to the eyes and respiratory tract, leading to pulmonary edema. Toxicity similar to that of phosgene (p 371), of which it is the nonchlorinated analog. Human exposure data limited.	0.5 ppm	5 ppm		Colorless gas with a sharp odor. Acetylating agent. Water-reactive. Auto reacts to form the ketene dimer, which is also toxic.

(C), ceiling air concentration (TLV-C); S, skin absorption can be significant; SEN, potential sensitizer; STEL, short-term (15-minute) exposure level. A1, ACGIH-confirmed human carcinogen; A2, ACGIH-suspected human carcinogen; A3, ACGIH animal carcinogen. ERPG, Emergency Response Planning Guideline (see p 656 for an explanation of ERPG). IARC 1, known human carcinogen; IARC 2A, probable human carcinogen; IARC 2B, possible human carcinogen; IARC 3, inadequate data available. NFPA hazard codes: H, health; F, fire; R, reactivity; Ox, oxidizer; W, water-reactive; 0 (none) <—> 4 (severe).

(continued)

TABLE IV–4. HEALTH HAZARD SUMMARIES FOR INDUSTRIAL AND OCCUPATIONAL CHEMICALS (CONTINUED)

Health Hazard Summaries	ACGIH TLV	IDLH	NFPA Codes H F R	Comments
Lead (inorganic compounds, dusts, and fumes): Toxic to CNS and peripheral nerves, kidneys, and hematopoietic system. Toxicity may result from acute or chronic exposures. Inhalation and ingestion are the major routes of absorption. Symptoms and signs include abdominal pain, anemia, mood or personality changes, and peripheral neuropathy. Encephalopathy may develop with high blood levels. Adversely affects reproductive functions in men and women. Adverse effects on fetal development in test animals. Such inorganic lead compounds are carcinogenic in animal studies (IARC 2A). See also p 286.	0.05 mg/m^3, A3	100 mg/m^3 (as Pb)		The elemental metal is dark gray. Vapor pressure is low, about 2 mm Hg at 1,000°C (1,832°F). Major industrial sources include smelting, battery manufacture, radiator repair, and glass and ceramic processing. Construction and renovation work involving old leaded paint is another major source. Hobbyists and other unsalaried craft workers can also be exposed to lead (eg, stained glass window making). Environmental pollution (through contaminated water, air, and foodstuffs) is an important source of exposure and lead is found in some traditional (eg, Ayurvedic, Hispanic, Chinese) medicines.
Lead arsenate (CAS: 10102-48-4): Most common acute poisoning symptoms are caused by arsenic, with lead responsible for chronic toxicity. Symptoms include abdominal pain, headache, vomiting, diarrhea, nausea, itching, and lethargy. Suspected carcinogen. Liver and kidney damage may also occur. IARC 2A (inorganic lead). See "Lead," p 286, and "Arsenic," p 140.	(***Note:*** no TLV; OSHA PEL for inorganic lead compounds: 50 mcg/m^3)			White powder often dyed pink. Not combustible.
Lead chromate (chrome yellow [CAS: 7758-97-6]): Toxicity may result from both the chromium and the lead components. Lead chromate is a suspected human carcinogen owing to the carcinogenicity of hexavalent chromium (IARC 1) and inorganic lead compounds. See "Lead," p 286, and "Chromium," p 196.	0.05 mg/m^3 (as Pb), A2 0.012 mg/m^3 (as Cr), A2			Yellow pigment in powder or crystal form.

Lindane (gamma-hexachlorocyclohexane [CAS: 58-89-9]): A CNS stimulant and convulsant. Vapors irritating to the eyes and mucous membranes and produce severe headaches and nausea. Well absorbed by all routes. Animal feeding studies have resulted in lung, liver, and kidney damage. May injure bone marrow. Equivocal evidence of carcinogenicity in test animals. IARC 1. See also p 189.	0.5 mg/m^3, S, A3	50 mg/m^3		White crystalline substance with a musty odor if impure. Not combustible. Vapor is 0.0000094 mm Hg at 20°C (68°F). Use as a pesticide restricted by EPA to certified applicators. No longer licensed in the United States as a topical scabicide.
Lithium hydride (CAS: 7580-67-8): Strong vesicant and alkaline corrosive. Extremely irritating upon direct contact; severe burns result. Dusts extremely irritating to eyes and respiratory tract; pulmonary edema may develop. Symptoms of systemic toxicity include nausea, tremors, confusion, blurring of vision, and coma.	0.05 mg/m^3 (C)	0.5 mg/m^3 ERPG-1: 0.025 mg/m^3 ERPG-2: 0.1 mg/m^3 ERPG-3: 0.5 mg/m^3	3 2 2 W	Off-white, translucent solid powder that darkens on exposure. Odorless. Very water-reactive, yielding highly flammable hydrogen gas and caustic lithium hydroxide. Finely dispersed powder may ignite spontaneously.
LPG (liquefied petroleum gas [CAS: 68476-85-7]): A simple asphyxiant and possible CNS depressant. Flammability dangers greatly outweigh toxicity concerns. See also "Hydrocarbons," p 266.	1,000 ppm	2,000 ppm [LEL]		Colorless gas. An odorant usually is added because the pure product is odorless. Highly flammable.
Magnesium oxide fume (CAS: 1309-48-4): Slightly irritating to eyes and upper respiratory tract. There is little evidence to support magnesium oxide as a cause of metal fume fever (p 311).	10 mg/m^3 (inhalable fraction and vapor)	750 mg/m^3		White fume.
Malathion (*O,O*-dimethyl dithiophosphate of diethyl mercaptosuccinate [CAS: 121-75-5]): An organophosphate-type cholinesterase inhibitor (p 353). May cause skin sensitization. Absorbed dermally. IARC 2A.	1 mg/m^3 (inhalable fraction and vapor), S	250 mg/m^3		Colorless to brown liquid with mild skunklike odor. Vapor pressure is 0.00004 mm Hg at 20°C (68°F). Thermal breakdown products include oxides of sulfur and phosphorus. Agricultural pesticide.

(C), ceiling air concentration (TLV-C); S, skin absorption can be significant; SEN, potential sensitizer; STEL, short-term (15-minute) exposure level. A1, ACGIH-confirmed human carcinogen; A2, ACGIH-suspected human carcinogen; A3, ACGIH animal carcinogen. ERPG, Emergency Response Planning Guideline (see p 656 for an explanation of ERPG). IARC 1, known human carcinogen; IARC 2A, probable human carcinogen; IARC 2B, possible human carcinogen; IARC 3, inadequate data available. NFPA hazard codes: H, health; F, fire; R, reactivity; Ox, oxidizer; W, water-reactive; 0 (none) <—> 4 (severe).

(*continued*)

TABLE IV–4. HEALTH HAZARD SUMMARIES FOR INDUSTRIAL AND OCCUPATIONAL CHEMICALS (CONTINUED)

Health Hazard Summaries	ACGIH TLV	IDLH	NFPA Codes H F R	Comments
Maleic anhydride (2,5-furandione [CAS: 108-31-6]): Extremely irritating upon direct contact; severe burns may result. Vapors and mists extremely irritating to eyes, skin, and respiratory tract. A skin and respiratory tract sensitizer (asthma). IARC 3.	0.01 mg/m^3 (inhalable fraction and vapor), SEN	10 mg/m^3 ERPG-1: 0.2 ppm ERPG-2: 2 ppm ERPG-3: 20 ppm	3 1 1	Colorless to white solid. Strong, penetrating odor. Eye irritation occurs at the TLV and is an adequate warning property. Vapor pressure is 0.16 mm Hg at 20°C (68°F). Combustible.
Mancozeb (CAS: 1018-01-7): Manganese-containing dithiocarbmate fungicide. Based on animal testing and human experience, low acute toxicity. Produces dermatitis in some individuals.				Yellow powder. Odorless. Negligible vapor pressure. Decomposes at high temperature. A related manganese-containing herbicide, maneb, has been associated with parkinsonism.
Manganese compounds and fume (CAS: 7439-96-5): Chronic overexposure results in a CNS toxicity manifested as psychosis, which may be followed by a progressive toxicity manifested by parkinsonism (manganism). See also p 302.	0.02 mg/m^3 (elemental inhalable fraction, as Mn), 0.1 mg/m^3 (inorganic compounds, as Mn)	500 mg/m^3 (Mn compounds, as Mn)		Elemental metal is a gray, hard, brittle solid. Other compounds vary in appearance. Exposure occurs in mining and milling of the metal, in ferromanganese steel production, and through electric arc welding.
Manganese cyclopentadienyl tricarbonyl (MCT [CAS: 12079-65-1]): MCT is an organic manganese compound used as a gasoline antiknock additive. See "Manganese," p 302.	0.1 mg/m^3 (as elemental Mn), S			MCT is used in Canada but is still under EPA review in the United States. Ultrafine manganese is a combustion by-product.
Mecoprop (MCPP [CAS: 93-65-2]): See Chlorophenoxy Herbicides," p 192. IARC 2B (chlorophenoxy herbicides).				Colorless or white crystals and flakes. Agricultural pesticide (herbicide).
Melamine (CAS: 108-78-1): Eye and respiratory tract irritant. Animal tests and ingestion of contaminated pet food produce kidney damage and failure. Inadequate carcinogenicity data (IARC 3).				Colorless or white crystals and flakes. Sublimes. Decomposition produces cyanide and nitrogen oxides. In addition to occupational exposures, the lay public has been exposed through contaminated food.

Mercury (quicksilver [CAS: 7439-97-6]): Acute exposures to high vapor levels reported to cause toxic pneumonitis and pulmonary edema. Well absorbed by inhalation. Skin contact can produce irritation and sensitization dermatitis. Mercury salts but not metallic mercury are toxic primarily to the kidneys by acute ingestion. High acute or chronic overexposures can result in CNS toxicity (erythrism), chronic renal disease, brain injury, and peripheral neuropathy. Some inorganic mercury compounds have adverse effects on fetal development in test animals. See also p 305. IARC 3.	0.025 mg/m³ (inorganic and elemental), S	10 mg/m³ ERPG-2: 0.25 ppm ERPG-3: 0.5 ppm		Elemental metal is a dense, silvery liquid. Odorless. Vapor pressure is 0.0012 mm Hg at 20°C (68°F). Sources of exposure include small-scale gold refining or recycling operations by hobbyists and mercury-containing instruments. Vacuuming spilled mercury can lead to high airborne levels.
Mercury, alkyl compounds (methyl mercury, dimethylmercury, diethyl mercury, ethylmercuric chloride, phenylmercuric acetate): Well absorbed by all routes. Slow excretion may allow accumulation to occur. Readily crosses blood-brain barrier and placenta. Can cause kidney damage, organic brain disease, and peripheral neuropathy. Some compounds are extremely toxic. Methylmercury is teratogenic in humans. See also p 305.	0.01 mg/m³ (alkyl compounds, as Hg), S	2 mg/m³ (as Hg)		Colorless liquids or solids. Many alkyl compounds have a disagreeable odor. Inorganic mercury can be converted to alkyl mercury compounds in the environment. Can accumulate in food chain. Phenylmercuric acetate use as a fungicide was banned from indoor paints in 1990.
Mesityl oxide (4-methyl-3-penten-2-one [CAS: 141-79-7]): Causes dermatitis upon prolonged contact. Vapors very irritating to eyes and respiratory tract. Based on animal tests, a CNS depressant and injures kidney and liver at high levels.	15 ppm	1,400 ppm [LEL]	3 3 1	Colorless viscous liquid with a strong odor. Irritation is an adequate warning property. Vapor pressure is 8 mm Hg at 20°C (68°F). Flammable. Readily forms peroxides.

(C), ceiling air concentration (TLV-C); S, skin absorption can be significant; SEN, potential sensitizer; STEL, short-term (15-minute) exposure level. A1, ACGIH-confirmed human carcinogen; A2, ACGIH-suspected human carcinogen; A3, ACGIH animal carcinogen. ERPG, Emergency Response Planning Guideline (see p 656 for an explanation of ERPG). IARC 1, known human carcinogen; IARC 2A, probable human carcinogen; IARC 2B, possible human carcinogen; IARC 3, inadequate data available. NFPA hazard codes: H, health; F, fire; R, reactivity; Ox, oxidizer; W, water-reactive; 0 (none) <—> 4 (severe).

(*continued*)

TABLE IV–4. HEALTH HAZARD SUMMARIES FOR INDUSTRIAL AND OCCUPATIONAL CHEMICALS (CONTINUED)

Health Hazard Summaries	ACGIH TLV	IDLH	NFPA Codes H F R	Comments
Metam sodium (sodium methydithiocarbamate [CAS: 137-42-8]): Soil pesticide. Skin, eye, mucous membrane, and respiratory tract irritant. Reacts with water to yield methyl isothiocyanate, an irritant that has been associated with asthma. Carbon disulfide is also a breakdown product.				Olive green to light yellow liquid with fairly strong sulfur-like odor. Miscible in water. Boiling point 110°C. Vapor pressure 21 mm Hg at 25°C (77°F). Combustion may release oxides of sulfur and nitrogen.
Methacrylic acid (2-methylpropenoic acid [CAS: 79-41-4]): Corrosive upon direct contact; severe burns result. Vapors highly irritating to eyes and, possibly, respiratory tract. Based on structural analogies, compounds containing the acrylate moiety may be carcinogens. No IARC evaluation.	20 ppm		3 2 2	Liquid with an acrid, disagreeable odor. Vapor pressure is less than 0.1 mm Hg at 20°C (68°F). Combustible. Polymerizes above 15°C (59°F), emitting toxic gases.
Methamidophos (CAS: 10265-92-6): Irritating to the skin and eyes; can be absorbed dermally. Organophosphate-type cholinesterase inhibitor (p 353) that can also cause delayed peripheral neuropathy.				Colorless crystals with a mercaptan-like odor. Not water soluble; soluble in toluene, n-hexane, and 2-propanol. Oxidation produces toxic phosphorus oxides. Flammable and toxic phosphine gas produced in contact with strong reducing agents. Agricultural pesticide.
Methomyl (*S*-methyl-*N*-[(methylcarbamoyl)oxy] thioacetimidate, Lannate, Nudrin [CAS: 16752-77-5]): A carbamate-type cholinesterase inhibitor (p 353).	0.2 mg/m^3 (inhalable faction and vapors), S			A slight sulfur odor. Vapor pressure is 0.00005 mm Hg at 20°C (68°F). Thermal breakdown products include oxides of nitrogen and sulfur. Agricultural pesticide.
Methoxychlor (dimethoxy-DDT, 2,2-bis(*p*-methoxyphenol)-1,1,1-trichloroethane [CAS: 72-43-5]): Organochlorine (p 189). Convulsant at very high doses in test animals. Limited evidence for adverse effects on male reproduction and fetal development in test animals at high doses (IARC 3).	10 mg/m^3 NIOSH CA	5,000 mg/m^3		Colorless to tan solid with a mild fruity odor. Appearance and some hazardous properties vary with the formulation. Vapor pressure is very low at 20°C (68°F). Agricultural pesticide.

2-Methoxyethanol (ethylene glycol monomethyl ether, methyl cellosolve [CAS: 109-86-4]): Workplace overexposures have resulted in depression of the hematopoietic system and encephalopathy. Symptoms include disorientation, lethargy, and anorexia. Well absorbed dermally. Animal testing revealed testicular atrophy and teratogenicity at low doses. Overexposure associated with reduced sperm counts in workers. See also p 234.	0.1 ppm, S	200 ppm	1 2 1	Clear, colorless liquid with a faint odor. Vapor pressure is 6 mm Hg at 20°C (68°F). Flammable. Industrial solvent.
2-Methoxyethyl acetate (ethylene glycol monomethyl ether acetate, methyl cellosolve acetate [CAS: 110-49-6]): Mildly irritating to eyes upon direct contact. Dermally well absorbed. Vapors slightly irritating to the respiratory tract. A CNS depressant at high levels. Based on animal studies, may cause kidney damage, leukopenia, testicular atrophy, and birth defects. See also p 234.	0.1 ppm, S	200 ppm	2 2 0	Colorless liquid with a mild, pleasant odor. Flammable. Industrial solvent.
Methyl acetate (CAS: 79-20-9): Vapors moderately irritating to the eyes and respiratory tract. A CNS depressant at high levels. Hydrolyzed to methanol in the body with possible consequent toxicity similar to that of methanol (p 314).	200 ppm	3,100 ppm [LEL]	2 3 0	Colorless liquid with a pleasant, fruity odor that is a good warning property. Vapor pressure is 173 mm Hg at 20°C (68°F). Flammable.
Methyl acetylene (propyne [CAS: 74-99-7]): A CNS depressant and respiratory irritant at very high air concentrations in test animals.	1,000 ppm	1,700 ppm [LEL]	1 4 3	Colorless gas with sweet odor. Flammable.

(C), ceiling air concentration (TLV-C); S, skin absorption can be significant; SEN, potential sensitizer; STEL, short-term (15-minute) exposure level. A1, ACGIH-confirmed human carcinogen; A2, ACGIH-suspected human carcinogen; A3, ACGIH animal carcinogen. ERPG, Emergency Response Planning Guideline (see p 656 for an explanation of ERPG). IARC 1, known human carcinogen; IARC 2A, probable human carcinogen; IARC 2B, possible human carcinogen; IARC 3, inadequate data available. NFPA hazard codes: H, health; F, fire; R, reactivity; Ox, oxidizer; W, water-reactive; 0 (none) <—> 4 (severe).

(*continued*)

TABLE IV–4. HEALTH HAZARD SUMMARIES FOR INDUSTRIAL AND OCCUPATIONAL CHEMICALS (CONTINUED)

Health Hazard Summaries	ACGIH TLV	IDLH	NFPA Codes H F R	Comments
Methyl acrylate (2-propenoic acid methyl ester [CAS: 96-33-3]): Methacrylic acid. Highly irritating upon direct contact; severe burns may result. A sensitizer. Vapors highly irritating to the eyes and respiratory tract. Based on structural analogies, compounds containing the acrylate moiety may be carcinogens (IARC 3).	2 ppm, S, SEN	250 ppm	3 3 2	Colorless liquid with a sharp, fruity odor. Vapor pressure is 68.2 mm Hg at 20°C (68°F). Inhibitor included to prevent violent polymerization. Exposure can occur through artificial (sculpted) nail application.
Methylacrylonitrile (2-methyl-2-propenenitrile, methacrylonitrile, 2-cyanopropene [CAS: 126-98-7]): Mildly irritating upon direct contact. Well absorbed dermally. Metabolized to cyanide (p 208). In animal tests, acute inhalation at high levels caused death without signs of irritation, probably by a mechanism similar to that of acrylonitrile. Lower levels produced convulsions and loss of motor control.	1 ppm, S		4 3 2	Liquid. Vapor pressure is 40 mm Hg at 13°C (55°F). Industrial polymer.
Methylal (dimethoxymethane [CAS: 109-87-5]): Mildly irritating to eyes and respiratory tract. A CNS depressant at very high levels. Animal studies suggest a potential to injure heart, liver, kidneys, and lungs at very high air levels.	1,000 ppm	2,200 ppm [LEL]	1 3 1	Colorless liquid with pungent, chloroform-like odor. Highly flammable.
Methyl alcohol (methanol, wood alcohol [CAS: 67-56-1]): Mildly irritating to eyes and skin. Systemic toxicity may result from absorption by all routes. Toxic metabolites are formate and formaldehyde. A CNS depressant. Signs and symptoms include headache, nausea, abdominal pain, dizziness, shortness of breath, metabolic acidosis, and coma. Visual disturbances (optic neuropathy) range from blurred vision to blindness. See also p 314.	200 ppm, S	6,000 ppm ERPG-1: 200 ppm ERPG-2: 1,000 ppm ERPG-3: 5,000 ppm	1 3 0	Colorless liquid with a distinctive, sharp odor that is a poor warning property. Flammable. Found in windshield fluids and antifreezes.

Methylamine (CAS: 74-89-5): Corrosive. Vapors highly irritating to eyes, skin, and respiratory tract; severe burns and pulmonary edema may result.	5 ppm	100 ppm ERPG-1: 10 ppm ERPG-2: 100 ppm ERPG-3: 500 ppm	3 4 0	Colorless gas with a fishy or ammonia-like odor. Odor is a poor warning property owing to olfactory fatigue. Flammable. Used in a variety of organic synthesis applications, including methamphetamine production.
Methyl-*n*-amyl ketone (2-heptanone [CAS: 110-43-0]): Vapors are irritating to eyes and respiratory tract. A CNS depressant. Flammable.	50 ppm	800 ppm	1 2 0	Colorless or white liquid with a fruity odor. Vapor pressure is 2.6 mm Hg at 20°C (68°F).
***N*-Methylaniline (CAS: 100-61-8):** A potent inducer of methemoglobinemia (p 317). Well absorbed by all routes. Animal studies suggest potential for liver and kidney injury.	0.5 ppm, S			Yellow to light brown liquid with a weak ammonia-like odor. Vapor pressure is less than 1 mm Hg at 20°C (68°F). Thermal breakdown products include oxides of nitrogen.
Methyl bromide (bromomethane [CAS: 74-83-9]): Causes severe irritation and burns upon direct contact. Vapors irritating to the lung; pulmonary edema may result. The CNS, liver, and kidneys are major target organs; acute poisoning causes nausea, vomiting, delirium, and convulsions. Both inhalation and skin exposure may cause systemic toxicity. Chronic exposures associated with peripheral neuropathy in humans. Evidence for adverse effects on fetal development in test animals. Limited evidence of carcinogenicity in test animals (IARC 3). See also p 321 and entry for chloropicrin in this table.	1 ppm, S NIOSH CA	250 ppm ERPG-2: 50 ppm ERPG-3: 200 ppm	3 1 0	Colorless liquid or gas with a mild chloroform-like odor that is a poor warning property. Chloropicrin, a lacrimator, often is added as a warning agent. Methyl bromide has been widely used as a fumigant in agriculture and in structural pesticide control but is being phased out because of its ozone-depleting potential.
Methyl *n*-butyl ketone (MBK, 2-hexanone [CAS: 591-78-6]): Vapors irritating to eyes and respiratory tract at high levels. A CNS depressant at high doses. Causes peripheral neuropathy by a mechanism thought to be the same as that of *n*-hexane. Well absorbed by all routes. Causes testicular toxicity in animal studies.	5 ppm, S	1,600 ppm	2 3 0	Colorless liquid with an acetone-like odor. Vapor pressure is 3.8 mm Hg at 20°C (68°F). Flammable. NIOSH-recommended exposure limit is 1.0 ppm.

(C), ceiling air concentration (TLV-C); S, skin absorption can be significant; SEN, potential sensitizer; STEL, short-term (15-minute) exposure level. A1, ACGIH-confirmed human carcinogen; A2, ACGIH-suspected human carcinogen; A3, ACGIH animal carcinogen. ERPG, Emergency Response Planning Guideline (see p 656 for an explanation of ERPG). IARC 1, known human carcinogen; IARC 2A, probable human carcinogen; IARC 2B, possible human carcinogen; IARC 3, inadequate data available. NFPA hazard codes: H, health; F, fire; R, reactivity; Ox, oxidizer; W, water-reactive; 0 (none) <—> 4 (severe).

(*continued*)

TABLE IV–4. HEALTH HAZARD SUMMARIES FOR INDUSTRIAL AND OCCUPATIONAL CHEMICALS (CONTINUED)

Health Hazard Summaries	ACGIH TLV	IDLH	NFPA Codes H F R	Comments
Methyl chloride (chloromethane [CAS: 74-87-3]): Symptoms include headache, confusion, ataxia, convulsions, and coma. Liver, kidneys, and bone marrow are other target organs. Evidence for adverse effects on both the testes and fetal development	50 ppm, S NIOSH CA	2,000 ppm ERPG-1: 150 ppm ERPG-2: 1,000 ppm ERPG-3: 3,000 ppm	2 4 0	Colorless gas with a mild, sweet odor that is a poor warning property. Highly flammable. Industrial chemical also formerly used as an anesthetic and refrigerant.
Methyl-2-cyanoacrylate (CAS: 137-05-3): Vapors irritating to the eyes and upper respiratory tract. May act as a sensitizer (skin and lungs). A strong and fast-acting glue that can cause body parts to adhere to each other or surfaces. Direct contact with the eyes may result in mechanical injury if the immediate bonding of the eyelids is followed by forced separation.	0.2 ppm			Colorless viscous liquid. Commonly, this compound and related substances are known as "super glues."
Methylcyclohexane (CAS: 108-87-2): Irritating upon direct contact. Vapors irritating to eyes and respiratory tract. A CNS depressant at high levels. Based on animal studies, some liver and kidney injury may occur at chronic high doses.	400 ppm	1,200 ppm [LEL]	1 3 0	Colorless liquid with a faint benzene-like odor. Vapor pressure is 37 mm Hg at 20°C (68°F). Highly flammable.
***o*-Methylcyclohexanone (CAS: 583-60-8):** Based on animal studies, irritating upon direct contact. Dermal absorption occurs. Vapors irritating to eyes and respiratory tract. A CNS depressant at high levels.	50 ppm, S	600 ppm	2 2 0	Colorless liquid with mild peppermint odor. Irritation is a good warning property. Vapor pressure is about 1 mm Hg at 20°C (68°F). Flammable.
Methyl demeton (*O,O*-dimethyl 2-ethylmercaptoethyl thiophosphate [CAS: 8022-00-2]): An organophosphate-type cholinesterase inhibitor. See p 353.	0.5 mg/m^3, S			Colorless to pale yellow liquid with an unpleasant odor. Vapor pressure is 0.00036 mm Hg at 20°C (68°F). Thermal breakdown products include oxides of sulfur and phosphorus. Agricultural pesticide.
4,4'-Methylene-bis(2-chloroaniline) (MOCA [CAS: 101-14-4]): A human carcinogen (IARC 1). Dermal absorption occurs.	0.01 ppm, S, A2 NIOSH CA			Tan solid. Thermal breakdown products include oxides of nitrogen and hydrogen chloride.

Methylene bis (4-cyclohexylisocyanate, dmdi, 4-HMDI [CAS: 5124-30-1]): A strong irritant and skin and respiratory tract sensitizer (asthma).	0.005 ppm			White to pale yellow solid flakes. Odorless. Possible thermal breakdown products include oxides of nitrogen and hydrogen cyanide. Component of polyurethanes.
Methylene bisphenyl isocyanate (4,4-diphenylmethane diisocyanate, MDI [CAS: 101-68-8]): Irritating upon direct contact. Vapors and dusts highly irritating to eyes and respiratory tract. Potent respiratory tract sensitizer (asthma). IARC 3.	0.005 ppm	75 mg/m^3 ERPG-2: 5 mg/m^3 ERPG-3: 55 mg/m^3		White to pale yellow flakes. Odorless. Vapor pressure is 0.05 mm Hg at 20°C (68°F). Possible thermal breakdown products include oxides of nitrogen and hydrogen cyanide. Component of polyurethanes.
Methylene chloride (methylene dichloride, dichloromethane [CAS: 75-09-2]): Irritating upon prolonged direct contact. Dermal absorption occurs. Vapors irritating to eyes and respiratory tract. A CNS depressant. May cause cardiac arrhythmias. Liver and kidney injury at high concentrations. Converted to carbon monoxide in the body with resultant carboxyhemoglobin formation. A carcinogen in test animals (IARC 2A). See also p 323.	50 ppm, A3 OSHA CA NIOSH CA	2,300 ppm ERPG-1: 300 ppm ERPG-2: 750 ppm ERPG-3: 4,000 ppm	2 1 0	Heavy colorless liquid with a chloroform-like odor that is a poor warning property. Vapor pressure is 350 mm Hg at 20°C (68°F). Possible thermal breakdown products include phosgene and hydrogen chloride. Methylene chloride is a solvent with many industrial and commercial uses (eg, paint strippers, carburetor cleaners).
4,4-Methylene dianiline (4,4'-diaminodiphenylmethane [CAS: 101-77-9]): Vapors highly irritating to eyes and respiratory tract. Hepatotoxicity (cholestatic jaundice) observed in overexposed workers. Systemic toxicity may result from inhalation, ingestion, or skin contact. Methemoglobinemia (p 317), kidney injury, retinal injury, and evidence of carcinogenicity in animals (IARC 2B).	0.1 ppm, S, A3 OSHA CA NIOSH CA		2 1 0	Light brown solid crystals with a faint amine odor. Combustible. Thermal breakdown products include oxides of nitrogen. Used in synthesis of isocyanate and other polymer production. Historically, large scale exposure incident occurred from contaminated foodstuffs (Epping jaundice).

(C), ceiling air concentration (TLV-C); S, skin absorption can be significant; SEN, potential sensitizer; STEL, short-term (15-minute) exposure level. A1, ACGIH-confirmed human carcinogen; A2, ACGIH-suspected human carcinogen; A3, ACGIH animal carcinogen. ERPG, Emergency Response Planning Guideline (see p 656 for an explanation of ERPG). IARC 1, known human carcinogen; IARC 2A, probable human carcinogen; IARC 2B, possible human carcinogen; IARC 3, inadequate data available. NFPA hazard codes: H, health; F, fire; R, reactivity; Ox, oxidizer; W, water-reactive; 0 (none) <—> 4 (severe).

(*continued*)

TABLE IV–4. HEALTH HAZARD SUMMARIES FOR INDUSTRIAL AND OCCUPATIONAL CHEMICALS (CONTINUED)

Health Hazard Summaries	ACGIH TLV	IDLH	NFPA Codes H F R	Comments
Methylene iodide (iodoform [CAS: 75-47-8]): Severe liver toxin. Causes CNS impairment associated with elevated iodide levels. Metabolized to carbon monoxide. Elevated carboxyhemoglobin (COHb) noted following heavy acute ingestion. Iodide toxicity with chronic application to wounds and nonintact skin.	0.6 ppm	100 ppm		Colorless liquid. Acrid ether-like odor. Vapor pressure is 400 mm Hg at 25°C (77°F). Medical disinfectant.
Methyl ethyl ketone (2-butanone, MEK [CAS: 78-93-3]): Vapors irritating to eyes and respiratory tract. A CNS depressant at high levels. Limited evidence for adverse effects on fetal development in test animals. Potentiates neurotoxicity of methyl butyl ketone and *n*-hexane.	200 ppm	3,000 ppm	1 3 0	Colorless liquid with a mild acetone odor. Vapor pressure is 77 mm Hg at 20°C (68°F). Flammable.
Methyl ethyl ketone peroxide (CAS: 1338-23-4): Based on chemical reactivity, highly irritating upon direct contact; severe burns may result. Vapors or mists likely to be highly irritating to the eyes and respiratory tract. Corrosive if ingested. In animal tests, overexposure resulted in liver, kidney, and lung damage.	0.2 ppm (C)			Colorless liquid with a characteristic odor. Shock-sensitive. Breaks down above 50°C (122°F). Explodes upon rapid heating. May contain additives such as dimethyl phthalate, cyclohexanone peroxide, and diallylphthalate to add stability. Used as a hardener in manufacture of resins and plastics, including fiberglass.
Methyl formate (CAS: 107-31-3): Vapors highly irritating to eyes and respiratory tract. A CNS depressant at high levels. Exposure has been associated with visual disturbances, including temporary blindness.	50 ppm, S	4,500 ppm	2 4 0	Colorless liquid with a pleasant odor at high levels. Odor is a poor warning property. Vapor pressure is 476 mm Hg at 20°C (68°F). Highly flammable.

Methylhydrazine (monomethylhydrazine [CAS: 60-34-4]): Similar to hydrazine in its toxicity. Vapors likely to be highly irritating to the eyes and respiratory tract. Causes methemoglobinemia (p 317). Potent hemolysin. Highly hepatotoxic. Causes kidney injury. A convulsant. A carcinogen in test animals. No IARC evaluation.	0.01 ppm, S, A3 NIOSH CA	20 ppm	4 3 2	Colorless clear liquid. Vapor pressure is 36 mm Hg at 20°C (68°F). Flammable. Used as a rocket propellant like the related dimethyl hydrazine. Exposure to methylhydrazine can also occur from ingestion of false morel mushrooms (p 330).
Methyl iodide (iodomethane [CAS: 74-88-4]): An alkylating agent. Based on chemical properties, likely to be highly irritating upon direct contact; severe burns may result. Dermal absorption is likely. Vapors highly irritating to respiratory tract; pulmonary edema has resulted. Neurotoxic; signs and symptoms include nausea, vomiting, dizziness, slurred speech, visual disturbances, ataxia, tremor, irritability, convulsions, and coma. Delusions and hallucinations may persist following acute exposure. Severe hepatic injury may also occur. Limited evidence of carcinogenicity in test animals (IARC 3).	2 ppm, S NIOSH CA	100 ppm ERPG-1: 25 ppm ERPG-2: 50 ppm ERPG-3: 125 ppm		Colorless, yellow, red, or brown liquid. Not combustible. Vapor pressure is 375 mm Hg at 20°C (68°F). Thermal breakdown products include iodine and hydrogen iodide. Agricultural fumigant that was proposed as a replacement for methyl bromide, but withdrawn before widespread use.
Methyl isoamyl ketone (5-methyl-2-hexanone [CAS: 110-12-3]): By analogy to other aliphatic ketones, vapors are likely to be irritating to eyes and respiratory tract. Likely to be a CNS depressant.	20 ppm		1 3 0	Colorless liquid with a pleasant odor. Vapor pressure is 4.5 mm Hg at 20°C (68°F). Flammable.
Methyl isobutyl ketone (4-methyl-2-pentanone, hexone [CAS: 108-10-1]): Irritating to eyes upon direct contact. Vapors irritating to eyes and respiratory tract. Reported systemic symptoms in humans are weakness, dizziness, ataxia, nausea, vomiting, and headache. High-dose studies in animals suggest a potential for liver and kidney injury. IARC 2B.	20 ppm, A3	500 ppm	1 3 0	Colorless liquid with a mild odor. Vapor pressure is 7.5 mm Hg at 25°C (77°F). Flammable.

(C), ceiling air concentration (TLV-C); S, skin absorption can be significant; SEN, potential sensitizer; STEL, short-term (15-minute) exposure level. A1, ACGIH-confirmed human carcinogen; A2, ACGIH-suspected human carcinogen; A3, ACGIH animal carcinogen. ERPG, Emergency Response Planning Guideline (see p 656 for an explanation of ERPG). IARC 1, known human carcinogen; IARC 2A, probable human carcinogen; IARC 2B, possible human carcinogen; IARC 3, inadequate data available. NFPA hazard codes: H, health; F, fire; R, reactivity; Ox, oxidizer; W, water-reactive; 0 (none) <—> 4 (severe).

(continued)

TABLE IV–4. HEALTH HAZARD SUMMARIES FOR INDUSTRIAL AND OCCUPATIONAL CHEMICALS (CONTINUED)

Health Hazard Summaries	ACGIH TLV	IDLH	NFPA Codes H F R	Comments
Methyl isocyanate (MIC [CAS: 624-83-9]): Highly reactive; highly corrosive upon direct contact. Vapors extremely irritating to eyes, skin, and respiratory tract; severe burns and fatal pulmonary edema have resulted. A sensitizing agent. Toxicity is not related to cyanide. Evidence that severe poisonings have adverse effects on fetal development. See p 280.	0.02 ppm, S	3 ppm ERPG-1: 0.025 ppm ERPG-2: 0.25 ppm ERPG-3: 1.5 ppm	4 3 2 W	Colorless liquid with a sharp, disagreeable odor that is a poor warning property. Vapor pressure is 348 mm Hg at 20°C (68°F). Flammable. Reacts with water to release methylamine. Polymerizes upon heating. Thermal breakdown products include hydrogen cyanide and oxides of nitrogen. Used as a chemical intermediate in carbamate pesticide synthesis. MIC is not in urethanes.
Methyl mercaptan (CAS: 74-93-1): Causes delayed-onset pulmonary edema. CNS effects include narcosis and convulsions. Reported to have caused methemoglobinemia and hemolysis in a patient with G6PD deficiency.	0.5 ppm	150 ppm ERPG-1: 0.005 ppm ERPG-2: 25 ppm ERPG-3: 100 ppm	4 4 1	Colorless liquid with an offensive rotten egg odor. Odor and irritation are good warning properties.
Methyl methacrylate (CAS: 80-62-6): Irritating upon direct contact. Vapors irritating to the eyes, skin, and respiratory tract. A sensitizer (asthma and dermatitis). At very high levels may produce headache, nausea, vomiting, or dizziness. Possible peripheral nerve toxicity. Limited evidence for adverse effects on fetal development in animal tests. Limited evidence for carcinogenicity (IARC 3).	50 ppm, SEN	1,000 ppm	2 3 2	Colorless liquid with a pungent, acrid, fruity odor. Vapor pressure is 35 mm Hg at 20°C (68°F). Flammable. Contains inhibitors to prevent self-polymerization. Used in resin polymers, including medical applications.
Methyl parathion (*O,O*-dimethyl *O-p*-nitrophenylphosphorothioate [CAS: 298-00-01]): A highly potent organophosphate cholinesterase inhibitor (p 353). IARC 3.	0.02 mg/m^3 (inhalable fraction and vapor), S			Tan liquid with a strong garlic-like odor. Vapor pressure is 0.5 mm Hg at 20°C (68°F). Appearance may vary with formulation. Agricultural pesticide.
Methyl propyl ketone (2-pentanone [CAS: 107-87-9]): Vapors irritating to eyes and respiratory tract. Based on animal studies, a CNS depressant at high levels.	150 ppm (STEL)	1,500 ppm	2 3 0	Colorless liquid with a characteristic odor. Vapor pressure is 27 mm Hg at 20°C (68°F). Flammable.

Methyl silicate (tetramethoxy silane [CAS: 681-84-5]): Highly reactive; corrosive upon direct contact; severe burns and loss of vision may result. Vapors extremely irritating to eyes and respiratory tract; severe eye burns and pulmonary edema may result.	1 ppm	ERPG-2: 10 ppm ERPG-3: 20 ppm	4 3 2	Colorless crystals. Reacts with water, forming silicic acid and methanol.
alpha-Methylstyrene (CAS: 98-83-9): Slightly irritating upon direct contact. Vapors irritating to eyes and respiratory tract. A CNS depressant at high levels. IARC 2B.	10 ppm, A3	700 ppm	1 2 1	Colorless liquid with a characteristic odor. Irritation is an adequate warning property. Vapor pressure is 1.9 mm Hg at 20°C (68°F). Flammable.
Methyl *tert*-butyl ether (MTBE [CAS: 1634-04-4]): Vapors mildly irritating to eyes and respiratory tract. A CNS depressant; acute exposure at high levels can cause nausea, vomiting, dizziness, and sleepiness. Adverse effects on liver and kidney in test animals at high levels. Evidence for adverse effects on reproduction and carcinogenicity in test animals exposed to very high concentrations (IARC 3).	50 ppm, A3	[LEL: 1,600 ppm] ERPG-1: 50 ppm ERPG-2: 1,000 ppm ERPG-3: 5,000 ppm		A volatile colorless liquid at room temperature. Odor threshold near 50 ppm. Gasoline additive banned in several states. Vapor pressure is 248 mm Hg at 25°C (77°F).
Metribuzin (4-amino-6-[1,1-dimethylethyl]-3-[methylthio]-1,2,4-triazin-5[4H]-one [CAS: 21087-64-9]): Human data available reveal no irritation or sensitization after dermal exposure. In animal testing, was poorly absorbed through the skin and produced no direct skin or eye irritation. Repeated high doses caused CNS depression and liver and thyroid effects.	5 mg/m^3			Vapor pressure is 0.00001 mm Hg at 20°C (68°F). Thermal breakdown products include oxides of sulfur and nitrogen. Agricultural pesticide (herbicide).

(C), ceiling air concentration (TLV-C); S, skin absorption can be significant; SEN, potential sensitizer; STEL, short-term (15-minute) exposure level. A1, ACGIH-confirmed human carcinogen; A2, ACGIH-suspected human carcinogen; A3, ACGIH animal carcinogen. ERPG, Emergency Response Planning Guideline (see p 656 for an explanation of ERPG). IARC 1, known human carcinogen; IARC 2A, probable human carcinogen; IARC 2B, possible human carcinogen; IARC 3, inadequate data available. NFPA hazard codes: H, health; F, fire; R, reactivity; Ox, oxidizer; W, water-reactive; 0 (none) <—> 4 (severe).

(*continued*)

TABLE IV–4. HEALTH HAZARD SUMMARIES FOR INDUSTRIAL AND OCCUPATIONAL CHEMICALS (CONTINUED)

Health Hazard Summaries	ACGIH TLV	IDLH	NFPA Codes H F R	Comments
Mevinphos (2-carbomethoxy-1-methylvinyl dimethyl phosphate, phosdrin [CAS: 7786-34-7]): An organophosphate cholinesterase inhibitor (p 353). Well absorbed by all routes. With repeated exposures to low levels, can accumulate to produce symptoms.	0.01 mg/m^3 (inhalable fraction and vapor), S	4 ppm		Colorless or yellow liquid with a faint odor. Vapor pressure is 0.0022 mm Hg at 20°C (68°F). Combustible. Thermal breakdown products include phosphoric acid mist. Agricultural pesticide.
Mica (CAS: 12001-25-2): Dusts may cause pneumoconiosis upon chronic inhalation.	3 mg/m^3 (respirable fraction)	1,500 mg/m^3		Colorless solid flakes or sheets. Odorless. Vapor pressure is negligible at 20°C (68°F). Noncombustible.
Monocrotophos (dimethyl 2-methylcarbamoyl-1-methylvinyl phosphate [CAS: 6923-22-4]): An organophosphate-type cholinesterase inhibitor (p 353). Limited human data indicate it is well absorbed through the skin but is rapidly metabolized and excreted.	0.05 mg/m^3 (inhalable fraction and vapor), S			Reddish-brown solid with a mild odor. Agricultural pesticide.
Morpholine (tetrahydro-1,4-oxazine [CAS: 110-91-8]): Corrosive; extremely irritating upon direct contact; severe burns may result. Well absorbed dermally. Vapors irritating to eyes and respiratory tract. Exposure to vapors has caused transient corneal edema. May cause severe liver and kidney injury. Inadequate carcinogenicity data (IARC 3).	20 ppm, S	1,400 ppm [LEL]	3 3 1	Colorless liquid with mild ammonia-like odor. Vapor pressure is 7 mm Hg at 20°C (68°F). Flammable. Thermal breakdown products include oxides of nitrogen. Found in some consumer polish and wax products.
Monosodium methanearsonate (MSMA [CAS: 2163-80-6)]. Arsenical herbicide. Hepatoxin and auditory neurotoxin.				Light yellow liquid. Odorless.

Naphthalene (CAS: 91-20-3): Highly irritating to eyes upon direct contact. Vapors are irritating to eyes and may cause cataracts upon chronic exposure. Dermally well absorbed. May induce methemoglobinemia (p 317). Symptoms of overexposure include headache and nausea. Causes cataracts and retinal damage in animal studies. Suspected carcinogen (IARC 2B).	10 ppm, S, A3	250 ppm	2 2 0	White to brown solid. The mothball odor and respiratory tract irritation are good warning properties. Current mothball formulations in the United States do not contain naphthalene. Vapor pressure is 0.05 mm Hg at 20°C (68°F). Combustible. See also p 335.
beta-Naphthylamine (2-aminonaphthalene [CAS: 91-59-8]): Acute overexposures can cause methemoglobinemia (p 317) or acute hemorrhagic cystitis. Well absorbed through skin. Known human bladder carcinogen (IARC 1).	A1 OSHA CA NIOSH CA			White to reddish crystals. Vapor pressure is 1 mm Hg at 108°C (226°F). Combustible. Former rubber industry chemical.
Neonicitinoids: imidacloprid [CAS 13821-41-3], clothianidin [CAS 210880], dinotefuran [CAS 165252-80-0], nitenpyram [CAS 150824-47-8] and thiamethoxam [CAS 153719-23-4]: Agonists at postsynaptic nicotinic acetylcholine receptors. Poor permeability of the blood–brain barrier. Clinical effects of exposure may resemble nicotine (p 337) toxicity. Serious adverse effects such as respiratory failure, sedation, seizures, and rhabdomyolysis have been reported.				Agricultural pesticides. They are highly selective for the nicotinic receptors in insects compared with mammals.
Nickel carbonyl (nickel tetracarbonyl [CAS: 13463-39-3]): Inhalation of vapors can cause severe lung and systemic injury without irritant warning signs. Effects include headache, nausea, vomiting, fever, extreme weakness and ventilatory failure. Based on animal studies, liver and brain damage may occur. Adverse effects on fetal development in test animals. A carcinogen in test animals. No IARC evaluation.	0.05 ppm (as Ni), C, A3 NIOSH CA	2 ppm (as Ni)	4 3 3	Colorless liquid or gas. The musty odor is a poor warning property. Vapor pressure is 321 mm Hg at 20°C (68°F). Highly flammable. Exposures largely limited to nickel refining. Metal smelter byproduct.

(C), ceiling air concentration (TLV-C); S, skin absorption can be significant; SEN, potential sensitizer; STEL, short-term (15-minute) exposure level. A1, ACGIH-confirmed human carcinogen; A2, ACGIH-suspected human carcinogen; A3, ACGIH animal carcinogen. ERPG, Emergency Response Planning Guideline (see p 656 for an explanation of ERPG). IARC 1, known human carcinogen; IARC 2A, probable human carcinogen; IARC 2B, possible human carcinogen; IARC 3, inadequate data available. NFPA hazard codes: H, health; F, fire; R, reactivity; Ox, oxidizer; W, water-reactive; 0 (none) <—> 4 (severe).

(continued)

TABLE IV–4. HEALTH HAZARD SUMMARIES FOR INDUSTRIAL AND OCCUPATIONAL CHEMICALS (CONTINUED)

Health Hazard Summaries	ACGIH TLV	IDLH	NFPA Codes H F R	Comments
Nickel metal and soluble inorganic salts (nickel chloride, nickel sulfate, nickel nitrate, nickel oxide): May cause a severe sensitization dermatitis, "nickel itch," upon repeated contact. Fumes highly irritating to the respiratory tract. Some compounds have adverse effects on fetal development in test animals. Some compounds are human nasal and lung carcinogens (nickel compounds, IARC 1; nickel metal, IARC 2B).	1.5 mg/m^3 (elemental); 0.1 mg/m^3 (soluble compounds), as Ni; 0.2 mg/m^3, A1 (insoluble compounds), as Ni NIOSH CA	10 mg/m^3 (as Ni)		Gray metallic powder or green solids. All forms are odorless.
Nicotine (CAS: 54-11-5): A potent nicotinic cholinergic receptor agonist. Well absorbed by all routes of exposure. Symptoms include dizziness, confusion, weakness, nausea and vomiting, tachycardia and hypertension, tremors, convulsions, and muscle paralysis. Death from respiratory paralysis can be very rapid. Adverse effects on fetal development in animal studies. See also p 337.	0.5 mg/m^3, S	5 mg/m^3	3 1 0	Pale yellow to dark brown viscous liquid with a fishy or amine-like odor. Vapor pressure is 0.0425 mm Hg at 20°C (68°F). Combustible. Thermal breakdown products include oxides of nitrogen. Although generally thought of in context of tobacco use and abstinence products, nicotine is a widely used pesticide. Dermal exposure can occur in tobacco harvesters ("green tobacco illness").
Nitric acid (aqua fortis, engraver's acid [CAS: 7697-37-2]): Concentrated solutions corrosive to eyes and skin; very severe penetrating burns result. Vapors highly irritating to eyes and respiratory tract; acute lung injury has resulted. Chronic inhalation exposure can produce bronchitis and erosion of the teeth. See also "Gases, Irritant," p 255.	2 ppm	25 ppm ERPG-1: 1 ppm ERPG-2: 10 ppm ERPG-3: 78 ppm	3 0 0 Ox (~40%) 4 0 1 Ox (fuming)	Colorless, yellow, or red fuming liquid with an acrid, suffocating odor near 1 ppm. Vapor pressure is approximately 62 mm Hg at 25°C (77°F). Not combustible. Interaction with organic materials or selected metals can release nitrogen dioxide (p 341). Home exposures have occurred in hobbyists.

Nitric oxide (NO, nitrogen monoxide [CAS: 10102-43-9]): Nitric oxide slowly converts to nitrogen dioxide in air; eye and mucous membrane irritation and pulmonary edema are likely from nitrogen dioxide. Overexposures have been reported to result in acute and chronic obstructive airway disease. Based on animal studies, may cause methemoglobinemia (p 317). Binds to hemoglobin at the same site as oxygen, and this may contribute to the toxicity. See also p 341.	25 ppm	100 ppm		Colorless or brown gas. The sharp, sweet odor occurs below the TLV and is a good warning property.
***p*-Nitroaniline (CAS: 100-01-6):** Irritating to eyes upon direct contact; may injure cornea. Well absorbed by all routes. Over-exposure results in headache, weakness, respiratory distress, and methemoglobinemia (p 317). Liver damage may also occur.	3 mg/m^3, S	300 mg/m^3	3 1 2	Yellow solid with an ammonia-like odor that is a poor warning property. Vapor pressure is much less than 1 mm Hg at 20°C (68°F). Combustible. Thermal breakdown products include oxides of nitrogen.
Nitrobenzene (CAS: 98-95-3): Irritating upon direct contact; sensitization dermatitis may occur. Well absorbed by all routes. Causes methemoglobinemia (p 317). Symptoms include headache, cyanosis, weakness, and gastrointestinal upset. May injure liver. Injures testes in animals. Limited evidence for adverse effects on fetal development in animals (IARC 2B).	1 ppm, S, A3	200 ppm	3 2 1	Pale yellow to dark brown viscous liquid. Shoe polish–like odor is a good warning property. Vapor pressure is much less than 1 mm Hg at 20°C (68°F). Combustible. Thermal breakdown products include oxides of nitrogen. Used industrially in the manufacture of aniline.
***p*-Nitrochlorobenzene (CAS: 100-00-5):** Irritating upon direct contact; sensitization dermatitis may occur upon repeated exposures. Well absorbed by all routes. Causes methemoglobinemia (p 317). Symptoms include headache, cyanosis, weakness, and gastrointestinal upset. May cause liver and kidney injury.	0.1 ppm, S, A3 NIOSH CA	100 mg/m^3	2 1 3	Yellow solid with a sweet odor. Vapor pressure is 0.009 mm Hg at 25°C (77°F). Combustible. Thermal breakdown products include oxides of nitrogen and hydrogen chloride.

(C), ceiling air concentration (TLV-C); S, skin absorption can be significant; SEN, potential sensitizer; STEL, short-term (15-minute) exposure level. A1, ACGIH-confirmed human carcinogen; A2, ACGIH-suspected human carcinogen; A3, ACGIH animal carcinogen. ERPG, Emergency Response Planning Guideline (see p 656 for an explanation of ERPG). IARC 1, known human carcinogen; IARC 2A, probable human carcinogen; IARC 2B, possible human carcinogen; IARC 3, inadequate data available. NFPA hazard codes: H, health; F, fire; R, reactivity; Ox, oxidizer; W, water-reactive; 0 (none) <—> 4 (severe).

(*continued*)

TABLE IV–4. HEALTH HAZARD SUMMARIES FOR INDUSTRIAL AND OCCUPATIONAL CHEMICALS (CONTINUED)

Health Hazard Summaries	ACGIH TLV	IDLH	NFPA Codes H F R	Comments
4-Nitrodiphenyl (4-nitrobiphenyl [CAS: 92-93-3]): Extremely well absorbed through skin. Produces bladder cancer in dogs and rabbits. Metabolized to 4-aminodiphenyl, which is a potent carcinogen in humans. Inadequate carcinogenicity data for this chemical, however (IARC 3).	S, A2 OSHA CA NIOSH CA			White solid with a sweet odor. Thermal breakdown products include oxides of nitrogen.
Nitroethane (CAS: 79-24-3): Based on high-exposure studies in animals, vapors are irritating to the respiratory tract. A CNS depressant. Can cause methemoglobinemia (p 317). Causes liver injury at high levels of exposure in test animals. A structurally similar compound, 2-nitropropane, is a carcinogen. No IARC evaluation.	100 ppm	1,000 ppm	2 3 3 (explodes on heating)	Colorless viscous liquid with a fruity odor that is a poor warning property. Vapor pressure is 15.6 mm Hg at 20°C (68°F). Flammable. Thermal breakdown products include oxides of nitrogen. In addition to industrial applications, exposure has occurred use in consumer products (nail polish remover).
Nitrogen dioxide (CAS: 10102-44-0): Gases and vapors irritating to eyes and respiratory tract; fatal pulmonary edema has resulted. Initial symptoms include cough and dyspnea. Pulmonary edema may appear after a delay of several hours. The acute phase may be followed by a fatal secondary stage, with fever and chills, dyspnea, cyanosis, and delayed-onset bronchiolitis obliterans. See pp 255 and 341.	0.2 ppm	20 ppm ERPG-1: 1 ppm ERPG-2: 15 ppm ERPG-3: 30 ppm	3 0 0 Ox (oxides of N, NO_x)	Dark brown fuming liquid or gas. Pungent odor and irritation occur only slightly above the TLV and are adequate warning properties. Vapor pressure is 720 mm Hg at 20°C (68°F). Important exposures include the following: structural fires, silage (silo filling), gas-shielded (MIG [metal inert gas] or TIG [tungsten inert gas]) welding, and the interaction of nitric acid with other materials. The related **dinitrogen tetroxide [CAS: 10544-72-6]** is in equilibrium with nitrogen dioxide and is also highly toxic.
Nitrogen trifluoride (nitrogen fluoride [CAS: 7783-54-2]): Vapors may cause eye irritation. Based on animal studies, may cause methemoglobinemia (p 317) and liver and kidney damage.	10 ppm	1,000 ppm ERPG-2: 400 ppm ERPG-3: 800 ppm		Colorless gas with a moldy odor that is a poor warning property. Not combustible. Highly reactive and explosive under a number of conditions.

Health Hazard Summaries	ACGIH TLV	IDLH	NFPA Codes H F R	Comments
Nitroglycerin (glycerol trinitrate [CAS: 55-63-0]): Causes vasodilation, including vasodilation of coronary arteries. Headache and drop in blood pressure are common. Well absorbed by all routes. Tolerance to vasodilation can occur; cessation of exposure may precipitate angina pectoris in pharmacologically dependent workers. See also p 339.	0.05 ppm, S	75 mg/m^3	2 3 4	Pale yellow viscous liquid. Vapor pressure is 0.00026 mm Hg at 20°C (68°F). Highly explosive. Exposure can occur among munitions and pharmaceutical workers.
Nitromethane (CAS: 75-52-5): Based on high-dose animal studies, causes respiratory tract irritation, liver and kidney injury, and CNS depression with ataxia, weakness, convulsions, and, possibly, methemoglobinemia (p 317). Associated with an outbreak of human peripheral neuropathy. A suspected carcinogen (IARC 2B).	20 ppm, A3	750 ppm	2 3 4	Colorless liquid with a faint fruity odor that is a poor warning property. Vapor pressure is 27.8 mm Hg at 20°C (68°F). Thermal breakdown products include oxides of nitrogen. Used as an industrial chemical and as a fuel in model engines. Can interfere with some clinical assays for creatinine.
1-Nitropropane (CAS: 108-03-2): Vapors mildly irritating to eyes and respiratory tract. Liver and kidney injury may occur.	25 ppm	1,000 ppm	2 3 2 (may explode on heating)	Colorless liquid with a faint fruity odor that is a poor warning property. Vapor pressure is 27.8 mm Hg at 20°C (68°F). Flammable. Thermal breakdown products include oxides of nitrogen.
2-Nitropropane (CAS: 79-46-9): Mildly irritating, CNS depressant at high exposures. Highly hepatotoxic; fatalities have resulted. Renal toxicity also occurs. Well absorbed by all routes. Limited evidence for adverse effects on fetal development in test animals. A carcinogen in test animals (IARC 2B).	10 ppm, A3 NIOSH CA	100 ppm	2 3 2 (may explode on heating)	Colorless liquid. Vapor pressure is 12.9 mm Hg at 20°C (68°F). Flammable. Thermal breakdown products include oxides of nitrogen. A chemical solvent that has been used in commercial products.
***N*-Nitrosodimethylamine (dimethylnitrosamine [CAS: 62-75-9]):** Overexposed workers had severe liver damage. Based on animal studies, well absorbed by all routes. A potent animal carcinogen producing liver, kidney, and lung cancers (IARC 2A).	S, A3 OSHA CA NIOSH CA			Yellow viscous liquid. Combustible. Industrial intermediate in selected processes (eg, dimethyl hydrazine synthesis) and an environmental contaminant.

(C), ceiling air concentration (TLV-C); S, skin absorption can be significant; SEN, potential sensitizer; STEL, short-term (15-minute) exposure level. A1, ACGIH-confirmed human carcinogen; A2, ACGIH-suspected human carcinogen; A3, ACGIH animal carcinogen. ERPG, Emergency Response Planning Guideline (see p 656 for an explanation of ERPG). IARC 1, known human carcinogen; IARC 2A, probable human carcinogen; IARC 2B, possible human carcinogen; IARC 3, inadequate data available. NFPA hazard codes: H, health; F, fire; R, reactivity; Ox, oxidizer; W, water-reactive; 0 (none) <—> 4 (severe).

(*continued*)

TABLE IV–4. HEALTH HAZARD SUMMARIES FOR INDUSTRIAL AND OCCUPATIONAL CHEMICALS (CONTINUED)

Health Hazard Summaries	ACGIH TLV	IDLH	NFPA Codes H F R	Comments
Nitrotoluene (*o*-, *m*-, *p*-nitrotoluene [CAS: 99-08-1]): Weak inducer of methemoglobinemia (p 317). By analogy to structurally similar compounds, dermal absorption is likely. Inadequate carcinogenicity data (IARC 3).	2 ppm, S	200 ppm	3 1 1	*o*-Nitrotoluene and *m*-nitrotoluene, yellow liquid or solid; *p*-nitrotoluene, yellow solid. All isomers have a weak, aromatic odor. Vapor pressure is approximately 0.15 mm Hg at 20°C (68°F). Thermal breakdown products include oxides of nitrogen. Intermediate in synthesis of dyestuffs and explosives.
Nitrous oxide (CAS: 10024-97-2): A CNS depressant. Hematopoietic effects from chronic exposure include megaloblastic anemia. Substance abuse has resulted in neuropathy. May have an adverse effect on human fertility and fetal development. See also p 343.	50 ppm			Colorless gas. Sweet odor. Not combustible. Widely used as an anesthetic gas in dentistry, and a popular inhalant chemical of abuse.
Octachloronaphthalene (Halowax 1051 [CAS: 2234-13-1]): By analogy to other chlorinated naphthalenes, workers overexposed by inhalation or skin contact may experience chloracne and liver damage. For chloracne, see also "Dioxins," p 224.	0.1 mg/m^3, S	0.1 mg/m^3 (effective IDLH)		Pale yellow solid with an aromatic odor. Vapor pressure is less than 1 mm Hg at 20°C (68°F). Not combustible. Thermal breakdown products include hydrogen chloride.
Octane (CAS: 111-65-9): Vapors mildly irritating to eyes and respiratory tract. A CNS depressant at very high concentrations.	300 ppm	1,000 ppm [LEL]	1 3 0	Colorless liquid. Gasoline-like odor and irritation are good warning properties. Vapor pressure is 11 mm Hg at 20°C (68°F). Flammable.
Osmium tetroxide (osmic acid [CAS: 20816-12-0]): Corrosive upon direct contact; severe burns may result. Fumes are highly irritating to eyes and respiratory tract. Based on high-dose animal studies, bone marrow injury and kidney damage may occur.	0.0002 ppm (as Os)	1 mg/m^3 (as Os)		Colorless to pale yellow solid with a sharp and irritating odor like that of chlorine. Vapor pressure is 7 mm Hg at 20°C (68°F). Not combustible. Catalyst and laboratory reagent.

Oxalic acid (ethanedioic acid [CAS: 144-62-7]): A strong acid; corrosive to eyes and to skin upon direct contact (p 186). Fumes irritating to respiratory tract. Highly toxic upon ingestion; precipitation of calcium oxalate crystals can cause hypocalcemia and renal damage. See also p 360.	1 mg/m^3	500 mg/m^3	3 1 0	Colorless or white solid. Odorless. Vapor pressure is less than 0.001 mm Hg at 20°C (68°F).
Oxygen difluoride (oxygen fluoride, fluorine monoxide [CAS: 7783-41-7]): Extremely irritating to the eyes, skin, and respiratory tract. Effects similar to those of hydrofluoric acid (p 269). Based on animal studies, may also injure kidneys, internal genitalia, and other organs. Workers have experienced severe headaches after low-level exposures.	0.05 ppm (C)	0.5 ppm		Colorless gas with a strong and foul odor. Olfactory fatigue is common, so odor is a poor warning property. A strong oxidizing agent.
Ozone (triatomic oxygen [CAS: 10028-15-6]): Irritating to eyes and respiratory tract. Pulmonary edema has been reported. See also p 255.	0.05 ppm (heavy work), 0.08 ppm (moderate work), 0.1 ppm (light work), 0.2 ppm (≤2 h)	5 ppm		Colorless or bluish gas. Sharp, distinctive odor is an adequate warning property. A strong oxidizing agent. Gas-shielded and specialty welding are potential sources of exposure, in addition to water purification and industrial bleaching operations.
Paraquat (1,1-dimethyl-4,4'-bipyridinium dichloride [CAS: 4687-14-7]): Extremely irritating upon direct contact; severe corrosive burns may result. Well absorbed through skin. A potent toxin causing acute multiple-organ failure as well as progressive fatal pulmonary fibrosis after overexposure. See also p 361.	0.5 mg/m^3, 0.1 mg/m^3 (respirable fraction)	1 mg/m^3 (total dust), 0.1 mg/m^3 (respirable fraction)		Odorless white to yellow solid. Vapor pressure is negligible at 20°C (68°F). Not combustible. Thermal breakdown products include oxides of nitrogen and sulfur and hydrogen chloride. Although widely used as an agricultural herbicide, most deaths occur as a result of intentional ingestion.

(C), ceiling air concentration (TLV-C); S, skin absorption can be significant; SEN, potential sensitizer; STEL, short-term (15-minute) exposure level. A1, ACGIH-confirmed human carcinogen; A2, ACGIH-suspected human carcinogen; A3, ACGIH animal carcinogen. ERPG, Emergency Response Planning Guideline (see p 656 for an explanation of ERPG). IARC 1, known human carcinogen; IARC 2A, probable human carcinogen; IARC 2B, possible human carcinogen; IARC 3, inadequate data available. NFPA hazard codes: H, health; F, fire; R, reactivity; Ox, oxidizer; W, water-reactive; 0 (none) <—> 4 (severe).

(*continued*)

TABLE IV–4. HEALTH HAZARD SUMMARIES FOR INDUSTRIAL AND OCCUPATIONAL CHEMICALS (CONTINUED)

Health Hazard Summaries	ACGIH TLV	IDLH	NFPA Codes H F R	Comments
Parathion (*O,O*-diethyl *O-p*-nitrophenyl phosphorothioate [CAS: 56-38-2]): Highly potent organophosphate cholinesterase inhibitor (p 353). Systemic toxicity has resulted from inhalation, ingestion, and dermal exposures. Evidence for adverse effects on fetal development in test animals at high doses (IARC 2B).	0.05 mg/m^3 (inhalable fraction and vapor), S	10 mg/m^3		Yellow to dark brown liquid with garlic-like odor. Odor threshold of 0.04 ppm suggests it has good warning properties. Vapor pressure is 0.0004 mm Hg at 20°C (68°F). Thermal breakdown products include oxides of sulfur, nitrogen, and phosphorus. In the field, weathering/oxidation can convert parathion to paraoxon, an even more toxic organophosphate. Agricultural pesticide.
Pentaborane (CAS: 19624-22-7): Highly irritating upon direct contact; severe burns may result. Vapors irritating to the respiratory tract. A potent CNS toxin; symptoms include headache, nausea, weakness, confusion, hyperexcitability, tremors, seizures, and coma. Residual CNS effects may persist. Liver and kidney injury may also occur.	0.005 ppm	1 ppm	4 4 2	Colorless liquid. Vapor pressure is 171 mm Hg at 20°C (68°F). The pungent sour milk odor occurring only at air levels well above the TLV is a poor warning property. May ignite spontaneously. Reacts violently with halogenated extinguishing media. Thermal breakdown products include boron acids. Used as a dopant in the microelectronics industry
Pentachloronaphthalene (Halowax 1013 [CAS: 1321-64-8]): Chloracne results from prolonged skin contact or inhalation. May cause severe, potentially fatal liver injury or necrosis by all routes of exposure. For chloracne, see also "Dioxins," p 224.	0.5 mg/m^3, S	0.5 mg/m^3 (effective IDLH)		Pale yellow waxy solid with a pleasant aromatic odor. Odor threshold not known. Vapor pressure is less than 1 mm Hg at 20°C (68°F). Not combustible. Thermal breakdown products include hydrogen chloride fumes.
Pentachlorophenol (Penta, PCP [CAS: 87-86-5]): Irritating upon direct contact; burns may result. Vapors irritating to eyes and respiratory tract. A potent metabolic poison; uncouples oxidative phosphorylation. Well absorbed by all routes. Evidence for adverse effects on fetal development and carcinogenicity in test animals (IARC 2B). See also p 364. Case reports have associated PCP with bone marrow toxicity.	0.5 mg/m^3 (inhalable fraction and vapor), S, A3	2.5 mg/m^3	3 0 0	Eye and nose irritation occur slightly above the TLV and are good warning properties. Vapor pressure is 0.0002 mm Hg at 20°C (68°F). Not combustible. Thermal breakdown products include hydrogen chloride, chlorinated phenols, and octachlorodibenzodioxin. Has been widely used as a wood preservative. Trace dioxin contamination (p 224) can lead to chloracne.

Pentane (*n*-pentane [CAS: 109-66-0]): Vapors mildly irritating to eyes and respiratory tract. A CNS depressant at high levels.	1,000 ppm	1,500 ppm [LEL]	1 4 0	Colorless liquid with a gasoline-like odor that is an adequate warning property. Vapor pressure is 426 mm Hg at 20°C (68°F). Flammable.
Perfluoroallyl chloride (PFAC, [CAS: 79-47-0]). Severe inhalation irritant with human fatalities.				Colorless gas with a similar chemical structure to allyl chloride. Used in polymers and elastomers as a precursor to (chlorodifluoromethyl) trifluorooxirane.
Petroleum distillates (petroleum naphtha, petroleum ether): Vapors irritating to eyes and respiratory tract. A CNS depressant. If *n*-hexane, benzene, or other toxic contaminants are present, those hazards should be addressed. See also p 266.		1,100 ppm [LEL]	1 4 0 (petroleum ether)	Colorless liquid. Kerosene-like odor at levels below the TLV serves as a warning property. Highly flammable. Vapor pressure is about 40 mm Hg at 20°C (68°F).
Phenol (carbolic acid, hydroxybenzene [CAS: 108-95-2]): Corrosive acid and protein denaturant. Direct eye or skin contact causes severe tissue damage or blindness. Deep skin burns can occur without warning pain. Systemic toxicity by all routes; percutaneous absorption of vapor occurs. Vapors highly irritating to eyes and respiratory tract. Symptoms include nausea, vomiting, cardiac arrhythmias, circulatory collapse, convulsions, and coma. Toxic to liver and kidney. A tumor promoter; however, inadequate carcinogenicity data (IARC 3). See also p 368.	5 ppm, S	250 ppm ERPG-1: 10 ppm ERPG-2: 50 ppm ERPG-3: 200 ppm	4 2 0	Colorless to pink crystalline solid, or viscous liquid. Its odor has been described as distinct, acrid, and aromatic or as sweet and tarry. As the odor is detected at or below the TLV, it is a good warning property. Vapor pressure is 0.36 mm Hg at 20°C (68°F). Combustible.
Phenylenediamine (*p*-diaminobenzene, *p*-aminoaniline [CAS: 106-50-3]): Irritating upon direct contact. May cause skin and respiratory tract sensitization (asthma). Inflammatory reactions of larynx and pharynx have been noted often in exposed workers. Inadequate carcinogenicity data (IARC 3).	0.1 mg/m^3	25 mg/m^3	3 1 0	White to light purple or brown solid, depending on degree of oxidation. Combustible. Thermal breakdown products include oxides of nitrogen. Industrial chemical intermediate, but also present in some over-the-counter hair dyes.

(C), ceiling air concentration (TLV-C); S, skin absorption can be significant; SEN, potential sensitizer; STEL, short-term (15-minute) exposure level. A1, ACGIH-confirmed human carcinogen; A2, ACGIH-suspected human carcinogen; A3, ACGIH animal carcinogen. ERPG, Emergency Response Planning Guideline (see p 656 for an explanation of ERPG). IARC 1, known human carcinogen; IARC 2A, probable human carcinogen; IARC 2B, possible human carcinogen; IARC 3, inadequate data available. NFPA hazard codes: H, health; F, fire; R, reactivity; Ox, oxidizer; W, water-reactive; 0 (none) <—> 4 (severe).

(continued)

TABLE IV–4. HEALTH HAZARD SUMMARIES FOR INDUSTRIAL AND OCCUPATIONAL CHEMICALS (CONTINUED)

Health Hazard Summaries	ACGIH TLV	IDLH	NFPA Codes H F R	Comments
Phenyl ether (diphenyl ether [CAS: 101-84-8]): Mildly irritating upon prolonged direct contact. Vapors irritating to eyes and respiratory tract. Based on high-dose experiments in animals, liver and kidney damage may occur after ingestion.	1 ppm	100 ppm	1 1 0	Colorless liquid or solid. Mildly disagreeable odor detected below the TLV serves as a good warning property. Vapor pressure is 0.02 mm Hg at 25°C (77°F). Combustible.
Phenyl glycidyl ether (PGE, 1,2-epoxy-3-phenoxypropane [CAS: 122-60-1]): Irritating upon direct contact. A skin sensitizer. Based on animal studies, vapors are very irritating to eyes and respiratory tract. In high-dose animal studies, a CNS depressant producing injury to liver, kidneys, spleen, testes, thymus, and hematopoietic system. A carcinogen in test animals (IARC 2B).	0.1 ppm, S, SEN, A3 NIOSH CA	100 ppm		Colorless liquid with an unpleasant, sweet odor. Vapor pressure is 0.01 mm Hg at 20°C (68°F). Combustible. Readily forms peroxides.
Phenylhydrazine (CAS: 100-63-0): A strong base and corrosive upon direct contact. A potent skin sensitizer. Dermal absorption occurs. Vapors very irritating to eyes and respiratory tract. Causes hemolytic anemia in animals, with secondary kidney damage. Limited evidence of carcinogenicity in test animals. No IARC evaluation.	0.1 ppm, S, A3 NIOSH CA	15 ppm	3 2 0	Pale yellow crystals or oily liquid with a weakly aromatic odor. Darkens upon exposure to air and light. Vapor pressure is less than 0.1 mm Hg at 20°C (68°F). Combustible. Thermal breakdown products include oxides of nitrogen. Used industrially in dye synthesis.
Phenylphosphine (CAS: 638-21-1): In animals, subchronic inhalation at 2 ppm caused loss of appetite, diarrhea, tremor, hemolytic anemia, dermatitis, and irreversible testicular degeneration.	0.05 ppm (C)			Crystalline solid. Spontaneously combustible at high air concentrations.
Phorate (*O,O*-diethyl *S*-(ethylthio)methyl phosphorodithioate, Thimet, Timet [CAS: 298-02-2]): An organophosphate-type cholinesterase inhibitor (p 353). Well absorbed by all routes.	0.05 mg/m^3, (inhalable fraction and vapor), S			Clear liquid. Vapor pressure is 0.002 mm Hg at 20°C (68°F). Agricultural pesticide.

Phosgene (carbonyl chloride, $COCl_2$ [CAS: 75-44-5]): Extremely irritating to the lower respiratory tract. Exposure can be insidious because irritation and smell are inadequate as warning properties for pulmonary injury. Higher levels cause irritation of the eyes, skin, and mucous membranes. See also p 371.	0.1 ppm	2 ppm ERPG-2: 0.5 ppm ERPG-3: 1.5 ppm	4 0 1	Colorless gas. Sweet haylike odor at low concentrations; sharp and pungent odor at high concentrations. Dangerous concentrations may not be detected by odor. Chemical synthesis intermediate; can be a breakdown product of chlorinated solvents that are subjected to heat or ultraviolet light as well as a thermal breakdown product of other chlorinated organics.
Phosmet (imidan, phthalophos [CAS: 732-11-6]): Organophosphate cholinesterase inhibitor (p 353).				Thermal breakdown to nitrogen, phosphorus and sulfur oxides. Agricultural pesticide.
Phosphine (hydrogen phosphide [CAS: 7803-51-2]): Extremely irritating to the respiratory tract; fatal pulmonary edema has resulted. A multisystem poison. Symptoms in moderately overexposed workers included diarrhea, nausea, vomiting, cough, headache, and dizziness. See also p 372.	0.3 ppm	50 ppm ERPG-2: 0.5 ppm ERPG-3: 5 ppm	4 4 2	Colorless gas. A fishy or garlic-like odor detected well below the TLV is considered to be a good warning property. May ignite spontaneously on contact with air. A common fumigant, generated on site (eg, in grain storage and other enclosed spaces) by aluminum or zinc phosphide and atmospheric moisture.
Phosphoric acid (CAS: 7664-38-2): A strong corrosive acid; severe burns may result from direct contact. Mist or vapors irritating to eyes and respiratory tract.	1 mg/m^3	1,000 mg/m^3 ERPG-1: 3 mg/m^3 ERPG-2: 30 mg/m^3 ERPG-3: 150 mg/m^3	3 0 0	Colorless, syrupy, odorless liquid. Solidifies at temperatures below 20°C (68°F). Vapor pressure is 0.03 mm Hg at 20°C (68°F). Not combustible.
Phosphorus (yellow phosphorus, white phosphorus, P [CAS: 7723-14-0]): Severe, penetrating burns may result upon direct contact. Material may ignite upon contact with skin. Fumes irritating to eyes and respiratory tract; pulmonary edema may occur. Potent hepatotoxin. Systemic symptoms include abdominal pain, jaundice, and garlic odor on the breath. Historically, chronic poisoning caused jaw bone necrosis ("phossy jaw"). See also p 373.	0.1 mg/m^3 (yellow phosphorus)	5 mg/m^3	4 4 2	White to yellow, waxy or crystalline solid with acrid fumes. Flammable. Vapor pressure is 0.026 mm Hg at 20°C (68°F). Ignites spontaneously on contact with air. Thermal breakdown products include phosphoric acid fume. Historical exposures involved the match industry, which has long since substituted other forms of phosphorus. Current uses include munitions (including some fireworks) and pesticides.

(C), ceiling air concentration (TLV-C); S, skin absorption can be significant; SEN, potential sensitizer; STEL, short-term (15-minute) exposure level. A1, ACGIH-confirmed human carcinogen; A2, ACGIH-suspected human carcinogen; A3, ACGIH animal carcinogen. ERPG, Emergency Response Planning Guideline (see p 656 for an explanation of ERPG). IARC 1, known human carcinogen; IARC 2A, probable human carcinogen; IARC 2B, possible human carcinogen; IARC 3, inadequate data available. NFPA hazard codes: H, health; F, fire; R, reactivity; Ox, oxidizer; W, water-reactive; 0 (none) <—> 4 (severe).

(*continued*)

TABLE IV–4. HEALTH HAZARD SUMMARIES FOR INDUSTRIAL AND OCCUPATIONAL CHEMICALS (CONTINUED)

Health Hazard Summaries	ACGIH TLV	IDLH	NFPA Codes H F R	Comments
Phosphorus oxychloride (CAS: 10025-87-3): Reacts with moisture to release phosphoric and hydrochloric acids; highly corrosive upon direct contact. Fumes extremely irritating to eyes and respiratory tract; can cause acute lung injury. Systemic effects include headache, dizziness, and dyspnea. Kidney toxicity may occur.	0.1 ppm		4 0 2 W	Clear colorless to pale yellow, fuming liquid possessing a pungent odor. Vapor pressure is 40 mm Hg at 27.3°C (81°F). Not combustible.
Phosphorus pentachloride (CAS: 10026-13-8): Reacts with moisture to release phosphoric and hydrochloric acids; highly corrosive upon direct contact. Fumes extremely irritating to eyes and respiratory tract; can cause acute lung injury.	0.1 ppm	70 mg/m^3	3 0 2 W	Pale yellow solid with a hydrochloric acid–like odor. Not combustible.
Phosphorus pentasulfide (CAS: 1314-80-3): Rapidly reacts with moisture and moist tissues to form hydrogen sulfide (p 271) and phosphoric acid. Severe burns may result from prolonged contact with tissues. Dusts or fumes extremely irritating to eyes and respiratory tract. Systemic toxicology is caused predominantly by hydrogen sulfide.	1 mg/m^3	250 mg/m^3	2 1 2 W	Greenish-yellow solid with odor of rotten eggs. Olfactory fatigue reduces value of smell as a warning property. Thermal breakdown products include sulfur dioxide, hydrogen sulfide, phosphorus pentoxide, and phosphoric acid fumes. Ignites spontaneously in the presence of moisture. Industrial intermediate including in the production of selected pesticides.
Phosphorus trichloride (CAS: 7719-12-2): Reacts with moisture to release phosphoric and hydrochloric acids; highly corrosive upon direct contact. Fumes extremely irritating to eyes and respiratory tract; can cause acute lung injury.	0.2 ppm	25 ppm ERPG-1: 0.5 ppm ERPG-2: 3 ppm ERPG-3: 15 ppm	4 0 2 W	Fuming colorless to yellow liquid. Irritation provides a good warning property. Vapor pressure is 100 mm Hg at 20°C (68°F). Not combustible.
Phthalic anhydride (phthalic acid anhydride [CAS: 85-44-9]): Extremely irritating upon direct contact; chemical burns occur after prolonged contact. Dusts and vapors extremely irritating to respiratory tract. A potent skin and respiratory tract sensitizer (asthma).	1 ppm, SEN	60 mg/m^3	3 1 0	White crystalline solid with choking odor at very high air concentrations. Vapor pressure is 0.05 mm Hg at 20°C (68°F). Combustible. Thermal breakdown products include phthalic acid fumes.

Picloram (4-amino-3,5,6-trichloropicolinic acid [CAS: 1918-02-1]): Dusts mildly irritating to skin, eyes, and respiratory tract. Has low oral toxicity in test animals. Limited evidence of carcinogenicity in animals (IARC 3).	10 mg/m^3			White powder possessing a bleachlike odor. Vapor pressure is 0.0000006 mm Hg at 35°C (95°F). Thermal breakdown products include oxides of nitrogen and hydrogen chloride. Also used as an herbicide in combination with 2,4-D.
Picric acid (2,4,6-trinitrophenol [CAS: 88-89-1]): Irritating upon direct contact. Dust stains skin yellow and can cause sensitization dermatitis. Symptoms of low-level exposure are headache, dizziness, and gastrointestinal upset. May induce methemoglobinemia (p 317). Ingestion can cause hemolysis, nephritis, and hepatitis. Staining of the conjunctiva and aqueous humor can give vision a yellow hue. A weak uncoupler of oxidative phosphorylation.	0.1 mg/m^3	75 mg/m^3	3 4 4	Pale yellow crystalline solid or paste. Odorless. Vapor pressure is much less than 1 mm Hg at 20°C (68°F). Decomposes explosively above 120°C (248°F). May detonate when shocked. Contact with metals, ammonia, or calcium compounds can form salts that are much more sensitive to shock detonation. Exposure can occur in munitions manufacturing (historically a major source of exposure).
Pindone (Pival, 2-pivaloyl-1,3-indanedione (CAS: 83-26-1]): A vitamin K antagonist anticoagulant (p 459).	0.1 mg/m^3	100 mg/m^3		Bright yellow crystalline substance.
Piperazine dihydrochloride (CAS: 142-64-3): Irritating upon direct contact; burns may result. A moderate skin and respiratory sensitizer. Nausea, vomiting, and diarrhea are side effects of medicinal use. Overdose has caused confusion, lethargy, coma, and seizures.	0.03 ppm (inhalable fraction and vapors for piperazine salts), SEN			White crystalline solid with a mild fishy odor. This and other piperazine salts have been used as an antihelminthic (ascaricide), human use discontinued in the United States.
Piperidine (CAS: 110-89-4): Highly irritating upon direct contact; severe burns may result. Vapors irritating to eyes and respiratory tract. Neurotoxic. Small doses initially stimulate autonomic ganglia; larger doses depress them. A 30- to 60-mg/kg dose may produce symptoms in humans.			3 3 0	Flammable. Widely used industrial intermediate including in pharmaceutical synthesis.

(C), ceiling air concentration (TLV-C); S, skin absorption can be significant; SEN, potential sensitizer; STEL, short-term (15-minute) exposure level. A1, ACGIH-confirmed human carcinogen; A2, ACGIH-suspected human carcinogen; A3, ACGIH animal carcinogen. ERPG, Emergency Response Planning Guideline (see p 656 for an explanation of ERPG). IARC 1, known human carcinogen; IARC 2A, probable human carcinogen; IARC 2B, possible human carcinogen; IARC 3, inadequate data available. NFPA hazard codes: H, health; F, fire; R, reactivity; Ox, oxidizer; W, water-reactive; 0 (none) <—> 4 (severe).

(continued)

TABLE IV–4. HEALTH HAZARD SUMMARIES FOR INDUSTRIAL AND OCCUPATIONAL CHEMICALS (CONTINUED)

Health Hazard Summaries	ACGIH TLV	IDLH	NFPA Codes H F R	Comments
Platinum-soluble salts (sodium chloroplatinate, ammonium chloroplatinate, platinum tetrachloride): Sensitizers causing asthma and dermatitis. Metallic platinum does not share these effects. Soluble platinum compounds are also highly irritating to eyes, mucous membranes, and respiratory tract.	0.002 mg/m^3 (as Pt)		4 mg/m^3 (as Pt)	Appearance varies with the compound. Thermal breakdown products of some chloride salts include chlorine gas. Used as industrial catalysts and in specialized photographic applications.
Polychlorinated biphenyls (chlorodiphenyls, Aroclor 1242, PCBs; 42% chlorine, CAS:53469-21-9; 54% chlorine, CAS: 11097-69-1): Exposure to high concentrations is irritating to eyes, nose, and throat. Chronically overexposed workers have chloracne and liver injury. Reported symptoms are anorexia, gastrointestinal upset, and peripheral neuropathy. Some health effects may be caused by contaminants or thermal decomposition products. Adverse effects on fetal development and fertility in test animals. A carcinogen in test animals (IARC 2A). See also p 393.	1 mg/m^3 (42% chlorine), S NIOSH CA 0.5 mg/m^3 (54% chlorine), S, A3 NIOSH CA	5 mg/m^3 (42% or 54% chlorine)	2 1 0	42% chlorinated: a colorless to dark brown liquid with a slight hydrocarbon odor and a vapor pressure of 0.001 mm Hg at 20°C (68°F). 54% chlorinated: light yellow oily liquid with a slight hydrocarbon odor and a vapor pressure of 0.00006 mm Hg at 20°C (68°F). Thermal breakdown products include chlorinated dibenzofurans and chlorodibenzo dioxins. Although no longer used, old transformers may still contain PCBs.
Polytetrafluoroethylene decomposition products: Overexposures result in polymer fume fever, a disease with flulike symptoms that include chills, fever, and cough. See also p 648. **Perfluoroisobutylene (PFIB [CAS: 382-21-8]** has produced severe lung injury and death in occupational exposure acting similarly to, but approximately 10 times as potent as phosgene (p 371).	0.01 ppm (for PFIB)			Produced in the production (PFIB) and in pyrolysis of Teflon and related materials (PFIN, carbonyl fluoride and others).
Polyvinyl chloride decomposition products: Irritating to the respiratory tract.				Produced by the high-temperature partial breakdown of polyvinyl chloride plastics. Decomposition products include hydrochloric acid (p 255). Plasticizers and other additives and their breakdown products may also be released.

Portland cement (a mixture of mostly tricalcium silicate and dicalcium silicate with some alumina, calcium aluminate, and iron oxide): Alkaline irritant of the eyes, nose, and skin; corrosive burns may occur. Long-term heavy exposure has been associated with dermatitis and bronchitis.	1 mg/m^3 (with no asbestos and <1% crystalline silica)	5,000 mg/m^3		Gray powder. Odorless. Portland cement manufacture is typically is associated with sulfur dioxide exposure. Concrete is a combination of cement (typically with chromate as an additive) and aggregate (with sand as a potential source of silica exposure). May contain chromates (see p 196).
Potassium hydroxide (KOH [CAS: 1310-58-3]): A caustic alkali causing severe burns to tissues upon direct contact. Exposure to dust or mist causes eye, nose, and respiratory tract irritation.	2 mg/m^3 (C)		3 0 1	White solid that absorbs moisture. Vapor pressure is negligible at 20°C (68°F). Gives off heat and a corrosive mist when in contact with water.
Potassium permanganate (CAS: 7722-64-7): Powerful oxidizer. Contact with tissues produces necrosis, and ingestion is often fatal owing to multiple-organ failure. Eye contact produces severe damage. Exposure can cause manganese toxicity.	(proposed: 0.02 mg/m^3 [respirable fraction, as Mn])		3 0 3	Purple-gray crystals. Strong oxidizer. Contamination of potassium permanganate–treated illicit drugs has led to manganese toxicity following injection abuse.
Propane (CAS: 74-98-6): Simple asphyxiant. See also "Hydrocarbons," p 266.		2,100 ppm [LEL]	2 4 0	Highly flammable.
Propanil (CAS: 709-98-8). Chloracne and methemoglobinemia (p 317) reported in a study of workers in a pesticide plant producing propanil, the former likely from dioxin contamination (see p 224).				Colorless, white, or light brown odorless solid. Agricultural pesticide (herbicide).
Propargyl alcohol (2-propyn-1-ol [CAS: 107-19-7]): Irritating to skin upon direct contact. Dermally well absorbed. A CNS depressant. Causes liver and kidney injury in test animals.	1 ppm, S		4 3 3	Light to straw-colored liquid with a geranium-like odor. Vapor pressure is 11.6 mm Hg at 20°C (68°F). Flammable.

(C), ceiling air concentration (TLV-C); S, skin absorption can be significant; SEN, potential sensitizer; STEL, short-term (15-minute) exposure level. A1, ACGIH-confirmed human carcinogen; A2, ACGIH-suspected human carcinogen; A3, ACGIH animal carcinogen. ERPG, Emergency Response Planning Guideline (see p 656 for an explanation of ERPG). IARC 1, known human carcinogen; IARC 2A, probable human carcinogen; IARC 2B, possible human carcinogen; IARC 3, inadequate data available. NFPA hazard codes: H, health; F, fire; R, reactivity; Ox, oxidizer; W, water-reactive; 0 (none) <—> 4 (severe).

(continued)

TABLE IV–4. HEALTH HAZARD SUMMARIES FOR INDUSTRIAL AND OCCUPATIONAL CHEMICALS (CONTINUED)

Health Hazard Summaries	ACGIH TLV	IDLH	NFPA Codes H F R	Comments
Propionic acid (CAS: 79-09-4): Irritating to eyes and skin upon direct contact with concentrated solutions; burns may result. Vapors irritating to eyes, skin, and respiratory tract.	10 ppm		3 2 0	Colorless oily liquid with a pungent, somewhat rancid odor. Vapor pressure is 10 mm Hg at 39.7°C (103.5°F). Flammable.
Propoxur (*o*-isopropoxyphenyl-*N*-methylcarbamate, DDVP, Baygon [CAS: 114-26-1]): A carbamate anticholinesterase insecticide (p 353). Limited evidence for adverse effects on fetal development in test animals.	0.5 mg/m^3 (inhalable fraction and vapor), A3			White crystalline solid with a faint characteristic odor. Vapor pressure is 0.01 mm Hg at 120°C (248°F). Common insecticide found in many consumer pesticide formulations.
***n*-Propyl acetate (CAS: 109-60-4):** Vapors irritating to eyes and respiratory tract. Excessive inhalation may cause weakness, nausea, and chest tightness. Based on high-exposure studies in test animals, a CNS depressant.	200 ppm	1,700 ppm	1 3 0	Colorless liquid. Mild fruity odor and irritant properties provide good warning properties. Vapor pressure is 25 mm Hg at 20°C (68°F). Flammable.
Propyl alcohol (1-propanol [CAS: 71-23-8]): Vapors mildly irritating to eyes and respiratory tract. A CNS depressant. See also "Isopropyl Alcohol," p 282.	100 ppm	800 ppm	1 3 0	Colorless volatile liquid. Vapor pressure is 15 mm Hg at 20°C (68°F). Mild alcohol-like odor is an adequate warning property.
Propylene dichloride (1,2-dichloropropane [CAS: 78-87-5]): Vapors very irritating to eyes and respiratory tract. Causes CNS depression and severe liver and kidney damage at modest doses in animal studies. Testicular toxicity at high doses in test animals. IARC 1.	10 ppm, SEN NIOSH CA	400 ppm	2 3 0	Colorless liquid. Chloroform-like odor is considered an adequate warning property. Vapor pressure is 40 mm Hg at 20°C (68°F). Flammable. Thermal breakdown products include hydrogen chloride. Industrial chemical intermediate; no longer used as an agricultural nematocide in the United States.

Propylene glycol dinitrate (1,2-propylene glycol dinitrate, PGDN [CAS: 6423-43-4]): Chemically similar to nitroglycerin (see p 339). Mildly irritating upon direct contact. Dermal absorption occurs. May cause methemoglobinemia (p 317). Potential neurotoxic effects. Causes vasodilation, including vasodilation in coronary arteries and systemic hypotension. Headache common. Tolerance to vasodilation can occur; cessation of exposure may precipitate angina pectoris in pharmacologically dependent workers.	0.05 ppm, S			Colorless liquid with an unpleasant odor. Thermal breakdown products include oxides of nitrogen. Principal use as a torpedo fuel propellant (component of Otto Fuel II); military personnel comprise the primary at-risk group.
Propylene glycol monomethyl ether (1-methoxy-2-propanol [CAS: 107-98-2]): Vapors very irritating to the eyes and possibly the respiratory tract. A mild CNS depressant.	50 ppm		1 3 0	Colorless, flammable liquid.
Propylene imine (2-methylaziridine [CAS: 75-55-8]): Highly irritating upon direct contact; severe burns may result. Vapors highly irritating to eyes and respiratory tract. May also injure liver and kidneys. Well absorbed dermally. A carcinogen in test animals (IARC 2B).	0.2 ppm, S, A3 NIOSH CA	100 ppm		A fuming colorless liquid with a strong ammonia-like odor. Flammable. Thermal breakdown products include oxides of nitrogen. Alkylating agent used in polymer synthesis and other industrial applications.
Propylene oxide (2-epoxypropane [CAS: 75-56-9]): Highly irritating upon direct contact; severe burns result. Vapors highly irritating to eyes and respiratory tract. Based on high-dose animal studies, may cause CNS depression and peripheral neuropathy. A carcinogen in test animals (IARC 2B).	2 ppm, SEN, A3 NIOSH CA	400 ppm ERPG-1: 50 ppm ERPG-2: 250 ppm ERPG-3: 750 ppm	3 4 2	Colorless liquid. Its sweet, ether-like odor is considered to be an adequate warning property. Vapor pressure is 442 mm Hg at 20°C (68°F). Highly flammable. Polymerizes violently.

(C), ceiling air concentration (TLV-C); S, skin absorption can be significant; SEN, potential sensitizer; STEL, short-term (15-minute) exposure level. A1, ACGIH-confirmed human carcinogen; A2, ACGIH-suspected human carcinogen; A3, ACGIH animal carcinogen. ERPG, Emergency Response Planning Guideline (see p 656 for an explanation of ERPG). IARC 1, known human carcinogen; IARC 2A, probable human carcinogen; IARC 2B, possible human carcinogen; IARC 3, inadequate data available. NFPA hazard codes: H, health; F, fire; R, reactivity; Ox, oxidizer; W, water-reactive; 0 (none) <—> 4 (severe).

(continued)

TABLE IV–4. HEALTH HAZARD SUMMARIES FOR INDUSTRIAL AND OCCUPATIONAL CHEMICALS (CONTINUED)

Health Hazard Summaries	ACGIH TLV	IDLH	NFPA Codes H F R	Comments
***n*-Propyl nitrate (nitric acid *n*-propyl ester [CAS: 627-13-4]):** Vasodilator causing headaches and hypotension. Causes methemoglobinemia (p 317). See also "Nitrates and Nitrites," p 339.	25 ppm	500 ppm	2 3 3 Ox (may explode on heating)	Pale yellow liquid with an unpleasant sweet odor. Vapor pressure is 18 mm Hg at 20°C (68°F). Flammable. Thermal breakdown products include oxides of nitrogen.
Pyrethrum (pyrethrin I or II; cinerin I or II; jasmolin I or II): Dusts cause primary contact dermatitis and skin and respiratory tract sensitization (asthma). Of very low systemic toxicity. See also p 397.	5 mg/m^3	5,000 mg/m^3		Vapor pressure is negligible at 20°C (68°F). Combustible. Widely used insecticide including in consumer products.
Pyridine (CAS: 110-86-1): Irritating upon prolonged direct contact; occasional reports of skin sensitization. Vapors irritating to eyes and respiratory tract. A CNS depressant. Causes methemoglobinemia (p 317). Chronic ingestion of small amounts has caused fatal liver and kidney injury. Workers exposed to 6–12 ppm have experienced headache, dizziness, and gastrointestinal upset. Dermally well absorbed. Inadequate carcinogenicity data (IARC 3).	1 ppm, A3	1,000 ppm	3 3 0	Colorless or yellow liquid with a nauseating odor and a definite "taste" that serves as a good warning property. Vapor pressure is 18 mm Hg at 20°C (68°F). Flammable. Thermal breakdown products include oxides of nitrogen and cyanide. Large scale industrial chemical used in chemical synthesis, including pharmaceuticals.
Pyrogallol (1,2,3-trihydroxybenzene; pyrogallic acid [CAS: 87-66-1]): Highly irritating upon direct contact; severe burns may result. Potent reducing agent and general cellular poison. Causes methemoglobinemia (p 317). Attacks heart, lungs, liver, kidneys, red blood cells, bone marrow, and muscle. Causes sensitization dermatitis. Deaths have resulted from the topical application of salves containing pyrogallol.				White to gray odorless solid.

Quinone (1,4-cyclohexadienedione, *p*-benzoquinone [CAS: 106-51-4]): A severe irritant of the eyes and respiratory tract. May induce methemoglobinemia (p 317). Acute overexposure to dust or vapors can cause conjunctival irritation and discoloration, corneal edema, ulceration, and scarring. Chronic exposures can permanently reduce visual acuity. Skin contact can cause irritation, ulceration, and pigmentation changes. Inadequate carcinogenicity data (IARC 3).	0.1 ppm	100 mg/m^3	3 2 0	Pale yellow crystalline solid. The acrid odor is not a reliable warning property. Vapor pressure is 0.1 mm Hg at 20°C (68°F). Sublimes when heated.
Resorcinol (1,3-dihydroxybenzene [CAS: 108-46-3]): Corrosive acid and protein denaturant; extremely irritating upon direct contact; severe burns result. May cause methemoglobinemia (p 280). A sensitizer. Dermally well absorbed. See also "Phenol and Related Compounds," p 368. Inadequate carcinogenicity data (IARC 3).	10 ppm		3 1 0	White crystalline solid with a faint odor. May turn pink on contact with air. Vapor pressure is 1 mm Hg at 108°C (226°F). Combustible.
Rhodium (soluble salts): Respiratory irritant. Mild eye irritant. Acts as contact dermatitis allergen and as potential asthma-causing agent.	0.01 mg/m^3			Vapor pressure is less than 0.1 mm Hg at 25°C (77°F). Used in specialty metal (jewelry) plating and as a catalyst.
Ronnel (*O,O*-dimethyl-*O*-(2,4,5-trichlorophenyl) phosphorothioate, Fenchlorphos [CAS: 299-84-3]): One of the least toxic organophosphate anticholinesterase insecticides (p 353).	5 mg/m^3 (inhalable fraction and vapor)	300 mg/m^3		Vapor pressure is 0.0008 mm Hg at 20°C (68°F). Not combustible. Unstable above 149°C (300°F); harmful gases such as sulfur dioxide, dimethyl sulfide, and trichlorophenol may be released. Agricultural pesticide.

(C), ceiling air concentration (TLV-C); S, skin absorption can be significant; SEN, potential sensitizer; STEL, short-term (15-minute) exposure level. A1, ACGIH-confirmed human carcinogen; A2, ACGIH-suspected human carcinogen; A3, ACGIH animal carcinogen. ERPG, Emergency Response Planning Guideline (see p 656 for an explanation of ERPG). IARC 1, known human carcinogen; IARC 2A, probable human carcinogen; IARC 2B, possible human carcinogen; IARC 3, inadequate data available. NFPA hazard codes: H, health; F, fire; R, reactivity; Ox, oxidizer; W, water-reactive; 0 (none) <—> 4 (severe).

(*continued*)

TABLE IV–4. HEALTH HAZARD SUMMARIES FOR INDUSTRIAL AND OCCUPATIONAL CHEMICALS (CONTINUED)

Health Hazard Summaries	ACGIH TLV	IDLH	NFPA Codes H F R	Comments
Rotenone (tubatoxin, cube root, derris root, derrin [CAS: 83-79-4]): Irritating upon direct contact. Dusts irritate the respiratory tract. A metabolic poison; depresses cellular respiration and inhibits mitotic spindle formation. Ingestion of large doses numbs oral mucosa and causes nausea and vomiting, muscle tremors, and convulsions. Chronic exposure caused liver and kidney damage in animal studies. Limited evidence for adverse effects on fetal development in animals at high doses.	5 mg/m^3	2,500 mg/m^3		White to red crystalline solid. Vapor pressure is negligible at 20°C (68°F). A natural pesticide extracted from plants such as cube, derris, and timbo. Odorless. Decomposes upon contact with air or light. Unstable to alkali.
Sarin (GB [CAS: 107-44-8]): Extremely toxic chemical warfare nerve agent (p 452) by all routes of contact. Readily absorbed via respiratory tract and skin and eyes. A potent cholinesterase inhibitor with rapid onset of symptoms. Vapors highly irritating.				Clear, colorless liquid. Odorless. Most volatile of nerve agents. Vapor pressure is 2.1 mm Hg at 20°C (68°F). Not flammable. Chemical warfare agent.
Selenium and inorganic compounds (as selenium): Fumes, dusts, and vapors irritating to eyes, skin, and respiratory tract; pulmonary edema may occur. Many compounds are well absorbed dermally. A general cellular poison. Chronic intoxication causes depression, nervousness, dermatitis, gastrointestinal upset, metallic taste in mouth and garlicky odor of breath, excessive caries, and loss of fingernails or hair. The liver and kidneys are also target organs. Some selenium compounds have been found to cause birth defects and cancers in test animals; inadequate carcinogenicity data, however (IARC 3). See also p 416.	0. 2 mg/m^3 (as Se)	1 mg/m^3 (as Se)		Elemental selenium is a black, gray, or red crystalline or amorphous solid and is odorless. Used as bluing agent in weapons maintenance. Selenium shampoos can cause elevated hair levels on hair heavy metals screens. Can be an important environmental contaminant.

Selenium dioxide (selenium oxide [CAS: 7446-08-4]): Strong vesicant; severe burns result from direct contact. Converted to selenious acid in the presence of moisture. Well absorbed dermally. Fumes and dusts very irritating to eyes and respiratory tract. See also p 416.			White solid. Reacts with water to form selenious acid.
Selenium hexafluoride (CAS: 7783-79-1): Vesicant. Reacts with moisture to form selenium acids and hydrofluoric acid; severe HF burns may result from direct contact (p 269). Fumes highly irritating to eyes and respiratory tract; pulmonary edema and lung injury may result.	0.05 ppm	2 ppm	Colorless gas. Not combustible.
Selenium oxychloride (CAS: 7791-23-3): Strong vesicant. Direct contact can cause severe burns. Dermally well absorbed. Fumes extremely irritating to eyes and respiratory tract; delayed pulmonary edema and lung injury may result.			Colorless to yellow liquid. Hydrogen chloride and selenious acid fumes produced on contact with moisture.
Silica, amorphous (diatomaceous earth, precipitated and gel silica): Possesses little or no potential to cause silicosis. Most sources of amorphous silica contain quartz (see entry for crystalline silica, below). If greater than 1% quartz is present, the quartz hazard must be addressed. When diatomaceous earth is strongly heated (calcined) with limestone, it becomes crystalline and can cause silicosis. Amorphous silica has been associated with lung fibrosis, but the role of crystalline silica contamination remains controversial. For silicates, as opposed to silica (below), there are inadequate carcinogenicity data (IARC 3).		3,000 mg/m^3	White to gray powders. Odorless with a negligible vapor pressure. The TLV for dusts is 10 mg/m^3 if no asbestos and less than 1% quartz are present.

(C), ceiling air concentration (TLV-C); S, skin absorption can be significant; SEN, potential sensitizer; STEL, short-term (15-minute) exposure level. A1, ACGIH-confirmed human carcinogen; A2, ACGIH-suspected human carcinogen; A3, ACGIH animal carcinogen. ERPG, Emergency Response Planning Guideline (see p 656 for an explanation of ERPG). IARC 1, known human carcinogen; IARC 2A, probable human carcinogen; IARC 2B, possible human carcinogen; IARC 3, inadequate data available. NFPA hazard codes: H, health; F, fire; R, reactivity; Ox, oxidizer; W, water-reactive; 0 (none) <—> 4 (severe).

(*continued*)

TABLE IV–4. HEALTH HAZARD SUMMARIES FOR INDUSTRIAL AND OCCUPATIONAL CHEMICALS (CONTINUED)

Health Hazard Summaries	ACGIH TLV	IDLH	NFPA Codes H F R	Comments
Silica, crystalline (quartz, fused amorphous silica, cristobolite, tridymite, tripoli [CAS: 14464-46-1]): Inhalation of dusts causes silicosis, a progressive, fibrotic scarring of the lungs. Individuals with silicosis are much more susceptible to tuberculosis. Crystalline silica is a human carcinogen (IARC 1).	0.025 mg/m^3 (respirable fraction), A2 NIOSH CA	25 mg/m^3 (cristobolite, tridymite), 50 mg/m^3 (quartz, tripoli)		Colorless, odorless solid with a negligible vapor pressure. A component of many mineral dusts. Exposure can occur in a variety of occupational settings, including sand blasting, secondary concrete work, stone cutting (including synthetic materials containing silica), and mining and quarrying.
Silicon (CAS: 7440-21-3): A nuisance dust that does not cause pulmonary fibrosis. Parenteral exposure has been associated with systemic toxicity.				Gray to black, lustrous, needle-like crystals. Vapor pressure is negligible at 20°C (68°F).
Silicon tetrachloride (tetrachlorosilane [CAS: 10026-04-7]): Generates hydrochloric acid vapor upon contact with moisture; severe burns may result. Extremely irritating to eyes and respiratory tract; pulmonary edema and lung injury may result.		ERPG-1: 0.75 ppm ERPG-2: 5 ppm ERPG-3: 37 ppm	3 0 2 W	Odor threshold near 0.75 ppm. Not combustible.
Silver (CAS: 7440-22-4): Silver compounds cause argyria, a blue-gray discoloration of tissues, which may be generalized throughout the viscera or localized to the conjunctivae, nasal septum, and gums. Some silver salts are corrosive upon direct contact with tissues.	0.01 mg/m^3 (soluble compounds, as Ag), 0.1 mg/m^3 (metal)	10 mg/m^3 (Ag compounds, as Ag)		Compounds vary in appearance. Silver nitrate is a strong oxidizer. Heavy systemic exposure is typically through intentional chronic ingestion as an alternative self-treatment rather than occupational inhalation.
Sodium azide (hydrazoic acid, sodium salt, NaN_3 [CAS: 26628-22-8]): Potent cellular toxin; inhibits cytochrome oxidase. Eye irritation, bronchitis, headache, hypotension, and collapse have been reported in overexposed workers. See also p 147.	0.29 mg/m^3 (C) (as sodium azide), 0.11 ppm (C) (as hydrazoic acid vapor)			White, odorless, crystalline solid. Present in some motor vehicle air bag systems.

Sodium bisulfide (NaSH [CAS: 16721-80-5]): Decomposes in the presence of water to form hydrogen sulfide (p 271) and sodium hydroxide (p 186). Highly corrosive and irritating to eyes, skin, and respiratory tract.				White crystalline substance with a slight odor of sulfur dioxide.
Sodium bisulfite (sodium hydrogen sulfite, $NaHSO_3$ [CAS: 7631-90-5]): Irritating to eyes, skin, and respiratory tract. Hypersensitivity reactions (angioedema, bronchospasm, or anaphylaxis) may occur.	5 mg/m^3			White crystalline solid with a slight sulfur dioxide odor and disagreeable taste. Widely used as a food and chemical preservative.
Sodium fluoroacetate (compound 1080 [CAS: 62-74-8]): A highly toxic metabolic poison. Metabolized to fluorocitrate, which prevents the oxidation of acetate in the Krebs cycle. Human lethal oral dose ranges from 2 to 10 mg/kg. See also p 242.	0.05 mg/m^3, S	2.5 mg/m^3		Fluffy white solid or a fine white powder. Sometimes dyed black. Hygroscopic. Odorless. Vapor pressure is negligible at 20°C (68°F). Not combustible. Thermal breakdown products include hydrogen fluoride. Has been used as a rodenticide.
Sodium hydroxide (NaOH [CAS: 1310-73-2]): A caustic alkali; may cause severe burns. Fumes or mists are highly irritating to eyes, skin, and respiratory tract. See also p 186.	2 mg/m^3 (C)	10 mg/m^3 ERPG-1: 0.5 mg/m^3 ERPG-2: 5 mg/m^3 ERPG-3: 50 mg/m^3	3 0 1	White solid that absorbs moisture. Odorless. Emits great amount of heat upon solution in water. Soda lye is an aqueous solution.
Sodium metabisulfite (sodium pyrosulfite [CAS: 7681-57-4]): Very irritating to eyes and skin upon direct contact. Dusts irritating to eyes and respiratory tract; pulmonary edema may result. Hypersensitivity reactions may occur.	5 mg/m^3			White powder or crystalline material with a slight odor of sulfur dioxide. Reacts to form sulfur dioxide in the presence of moisture.
Soman (GD [96-64-0]): Extremely toxic chemical warfare nerve agent (p 452) by all routes of contact. Readily absorbed via respiratory tract and skin and eyes. A potent cholinesterase inhibitor with rapid onset of symptoms. Vapors highly irritating.				Clear, colorless liquid. Slight camphor-like odor that is not an adequate indication of exposure. Vapor pressure is 0.4 mm Hg at 25°C (77°F).

(C), ceiling air concentration (TLV-C); S, skin absorption can be significant; SEN, potential sensitizer; STEL, short-term (15-minute) exposure level. A1, ACGIH-confirmed human carcinogen; A2, ACGIH-suspected human carcinogen; A3, ACGIH animal carcinogen. ERPG, Emergency Response Planning Guideline (see p 656 for an explanation of ERPG). IARC 1, known human carcinogen; IARC 2A, probable human carcinogen; IARC 2B, possible human carcinogen; IARC 3, inadequate data available. NFPA hazard codes: H, health; F, fire; R, reactivity; Ox, oxidizer; W, water-reactive; 0 (none) <—> 4 (severe).

(continued)

TABLE IV–4. HEALTH HAZARD SUMMARIES FOR INDUSTRIAL AND OCCUPATIONAL CHEMICALS (CONTINUED)

Health Hazard Summaries	ACGIH TLV	IDLH	NFPA Codes H F R	Comments
Stibine (antimony hydride [CAS: 7803-52-3]): A potent hemolytic agent similar to arsine. Gases irritating to the lung; pulmonary edema may occur. Liver and kidneys are secondary target organs. See also p 112.	0.1 ppm	5 ppm ERPG-2: 0.5 ppm ERPG-3: 1.5 ppm	4 4 2	Colorless gas. Odor similar to that of hydrogen sulfide but may not be a reliable warning property. Formed when acid solutions of antimony are treated with zinc or strong reducing agents. Used in the microelectronics industry.
Stoddard solvent (mineral spirits, a mixture of aliphatic and aromatic hydrocarbons [CAS: 8052-41-3]): Dermal absorption can occur. Vapors irritating to eyes and respiratory tract. A CNS depressant. Chronic overexposures associated with headache, fatigue, bone marrow hypoplasia, and jaundice. May contain a small amount of benzene. See also "Hydrocarbons," p 266.	100 ppm	20,000 mg/m^3	1 2 0	Colorless liquid. Kerosene-like odor and irritation are good warning properties. Vapor pressure is approximately 2 mm Hg at 20°C (68°F). Flammable.
Strychnine (CAS: 57-24-9): Neurotoxin binds to inhibitory, postsynaptic glycine receptors, which results in excessive motor neuron activity associated with convulsions and muscular hyperrigidity leading to respiratory impairment or paralysis. See also p 429.	0.15 mg/m^3	3 mg/m^3		White solid. Odorless. Vapor pressure is negligible at 20°C (68°F). Thermal breakdown products include oxides of nitrogen. Commonly used as a rodenticide (gopher bait).
Styrene monomer (vinylbenzene [CAS: 100-42-5]): Irritating upon direct contact. Dermal absorption occurs. Vapors irritating to respiratory tract. A CNS depressant. Symptoms include headache, nausea, dizziness, and fatigue. Cases of peripheral neuropathy have been reported. Neurotoxic in animal studies. Limited evidence for adverse effects on fetal development. Possible carcinogen (IARC 2B).	20 ppm	700 ppm ERPG-1: 50 ppm ERPG-2: 250 ppm ERPG-3: 1,000 ppm	2 3 2	Colorless viscous liquid. Sweet aromatic odor at low concentrations is an adequate warning property. Odor at high levels is acrid. Vapor pressure is 4.5 mm Hg at 20°C (68°F). Flammable. Inhibitor must be included to avoid explosive polymerization. Used in SBR (styrene butadiene rubber), ABS (acrylonitrile butadiene styrene), and SAN (styrene acrylonitrile) polymers.
Subtilisins (proteolytic enzymes of *Bacillus subtilis* [CAS: 1395-21-7]): Primary skin and respiratory tract irritants. Potent sensitizers causing asthma.	0.06 mcg/m^3 (C)			Light-colored powder. Occupational asthma was associated with introduction into detergent in a powder formulation.

Sulfur dioxide (CAS: 7446-09-5): Forms sulfurous acid upon contact with moisture. Strongly irritating to eyes and skin; burns may result. Extremely irritating to the respiratory tract; irritation of the upper airways has caused obstruction of the upper airways and pulmonary edema. Persons with asthma are of documented increased sensitivity to the bronchoconstrictive effects of sulfur dioxide air pollution. Inadequate carcinogenicity data (IARC 3). See also p 431.	0.25 ppm (STEL)	100 ppm ERPG-1: 0.3 ppm ERPG-2: 3 ppm ERPG-3: 15 ppm	3 0 0 (liquefied)	Colorless gas. Pungent, suffocating odor with a "taste" and irritative effects that are good warning properties. Criteria air pollutant. Fossil fuel burning is a major environmental source. Byproduct of smelting and other industrial processes. Prior use as a refrigerant with potential exposure from antique refrigerators.
Sulfur hexafluoride (CAS: 2551-62-4): Considered to be essentially a nontoxic gas. Asphyxiation by the displacement of air is suggested as the greatest hazard.	1,000 ppm			Odorless, colorless dense gas. May be contaminated with other fluorides of sulfur, including the highly toxic sulfur pentafluoride, which release HF or oxyfluorides on contact with moisture.
Sulfuric acid (oil of vitriol, H_2SO_4 [CAS: 7664-93-9]): Highly corrosive (p 186) upon direct contact; severe burns may result. Breakdown may release sulfur dioxide (p 431). Exposure to the mist can irritate the eyes, skin, and respiratory tract.	0.2 mg/m^3 (thoracic fraction), A2 (strong acid mists)	15 mg/m^3 ERPG-1: 2 mg/m^3 ERPG-2: 10 mg/m^3 ERPG-3: 120 mg/m^3	3 0 2 W	Colorless to dark brown heavy, oily liquid. Odorless. Eye irritation may be an adequate warning property. A strong oxidizer. Addition of water creates strong exothermic reaction. Vapor pressure is less than 0.001 mm Hg at 20°C (68°F).
Sulfur monochloride (CAS: 10025-67-9): Forms hydrochloric acid and sulfur dioxide (p 431) upon contact with water; direct contact can cause burns. Vapors highly irritating to the eyes, skin, and respiratory tract.	1 ppm (C)	5 ppm	3 1 1	Fuming, amber to red oily liquid with a pungent, irritating, sickening odor. Eye irritation is a good warning property. Vapor pressure is 6.8 mm Hg at 20°C (68°F). Combustible. Breakdown products include hydrogen sulfide, hydrogen chloride, and sulfur dioxide.
Sulfur pentafluoride (disulfur decafluoride [CAS: 5714-22-7]): Vapors are extremely irritating to the respiratory tract, and acute lung injury may occur; causes pulmonary edema at low levels (0.5 ppm) in test animals.	0.01 ppm (C)	1 ppm		Colorless liquid or vapor with a sulfur dioxide–like odor. Vapor pressure is 561 mm Hg at 20°C (68°F). Not combustible. Thermal breakdown products include sulfur dioxide and hydrogen fluoride.

(C), ceiling air concentration (TLV-C); S, skin absorption can be significant; SEN, potential sensitizer; STEL, short-term (15-minute) exposure level. A1, ACGIH-confirmed human carcinogen; A2, ACGIH-suspected human carcinogen; A3, ACGIH animal carcinogen. ERPG, Emergency Response Planning Guideline (see p 656 for an explanation of ERPG). IARC 1, known human carcinogen; IARC 2A, probable human carcinogen; IARC 2B, possible human carcinogen; IARC 3, inadequate data available. NFPA hazard codes: H, health; F, fire; R, reactivity; Ox, oxidizer; W, water-reactive; 0 (none) <—> 4 (severe).

(*continued*)

TABLE IV–4. HEALTH HAZARD SUMMARIES FOR INDUSTRIAL AND OCCUPATIONAL CHEMICALS (CONTINUED)

Health Hazard Summaries	ACGIH TLV	IDLH	NFPA Codes H F R	Comments
Sulfur tetrafluoride (SF_4 [CAS: 7783-60-0]): Readily hydrolyzed by moisture to form sulfur dioxide (p 431) and hydrogen fluoride (p 269). Extremely irritating to the respiratory tract; pulmonary edema and lung injury may occur. Vapors also highly irritating to eyes and skin.	0.1 ppm (C)			Colorless gas. Reacts with moisture to form sulfur dioxide and hydrogen fluoride.
Sulfuryl fluoride (Vikane, SO_2F_2 [CAS: 2699-79-8]): Irritating to eyes and respiratory tract; fatal pulmonary edema has resulted. Acute high exposure causes tremors and convulsions in test animals. Chronic exposures may cause kidney and liver injury and elevated fluoride. See also p 269.	5 ppm	200 ppm		Colorless, odorless gas with no warning properties. Chloropicrin, a lacrimator, often is added to provide a warning property. Thermal breakdown products include sulfur dioxide and hydrogen fluoride. A widely used structural pesticide fumigant, and poisoning can occur from inappropriate early reentry.
Sulprofos (*O*-ethyl *O*-[4-(methylthio)phenyl] *S*-propylphosphorodithioate [CAS: 35400-43-2]): An organophosphate anticholinesterase insecticide (p 353).	0.1 mg/m^3 (inhalable fraction and vapor), S			Tan-colored liquid with a characteristic sulfide odor. Agricultural pesticide.
Tabun (GA [CAS: 77-81-6]): Extremely toxic chemical warfare nerve agent (p 452) by all routes of contact. Readily absorbed via respiratory tract and skin and eyes. A potent cholinesterase inhibitor with rapid onset of symptoms. Vapors are highly irritating.				Clear, colorless liquid. Slight fruity odor that is not an adequate indication of exposure. Vapor pressure is 0.037 mm Hg at 20°C (68°F).
Talc, containing no asbestos fibers or crystalline silica (CAS: 14807-96-6): A tissue irritant. Pulmonary inhalation may cause pneumonitis; parenteral injection can also cause lung disease. Inadequate carcinogenicity data (IARC 3).	2 mg/m^3 (respirable fraction, with no asbestos fibers and $<1\%$ crystalline silica)	1,000 mg/m^3		Used in many industries and in cosmetics.

Tantalum compounds (as Ta): Of low acute toxicity. Dusts mildly irritating to the lungs.		2,500 mg/m^3 (metal and oxide dusts, as Ta)		Metal is a gray-black solid, platinum-white if polished. Odorless. Tantalum pentoxide is a colorless solid. Used in aerospace and other specialty alloys.
Tellurium and compounds (as Te): Reports of sleepiness, nausea, metallic taste, and garlicky odor on breath and perspiration associated with workplace exposures. Neuropathy has been noted in high-dose studies. Hydrogen telluride causes pulmonary irritation and hemolysis; however, its ready decomposition reduces likelihood of a toxic exposure. Some tellurium compounds are fetotoxic or teratogenic in test animals.	0.1 mg/m^3 (as Te)	25 mg/m^3 (as Te)		Metallic tellurium is a solid with a silver-white or grayish luster. Used in specialty alloys and in the semiconductor industry.
Tellurium hexafluoride (CAS: 7783-80-4): Slowly hydrolyzes to release hydrofluoric acid (p 269) and telluric acid. Extremely irritating to the eyes and respiratory tract; pulmonary edema may occur. Has caused headaches, dyspnea, and garlicky odor on the breath of overexposed workers.	0.02 ppm	1 ppm		Colorless gas. Offensive odor. Not combustible. Thermal breakdown products include hydrogen fluoride.
Temephos (Abate, *O,O,O′,O′*-tetramethyl *O,O*-thiodi-*p*-phenylene phosphorothioate [CAS: 3383-96-8]): Primary irritant of eyes, skin, and respiratory tract; a moderately toxic organophosphate-type cholinesterase inhibitor (p 353). Well absorbed by all routes.	1 mg/m^3 (inhalable fraction and vapor), S			Colorless or white crystals; liquid above 87° F. Not water soluble; soluble in toluene, ether, and hexane. Very low vapor pressure. Agricultural pesticide.
Terphenyls (diphenyl benzenes, triphenyls [CAS: 26140-60-3]): Irritating upon direct contact. Vapors and mists irritating to respiratory tract; pulmonary edema has occurred at very high levels in test animals. Animal studies also suggest a slight potential for liver and kidney injury.	5 mg/m^3 (C)	500 mg/m^3	1 1 0	White to light yellow crystalline solids. Irritation is a possible warning property. Vapor pressure is very low at 20°C (68°F). Combustible. Commercial grades are mixtures of *o*-, *m*-, and *p*-isomers.

(C), ceiling air concentration (TLV-C); S, skin absorption can be significant; SEN, potential sensitizer; STEL, short-term (15-minute) exposure level. A1, ACGIH-confirmed human carcinogen; A2, ACGIH-suspected human carcinogen; A3, ACGIH animal carcinogen. ERPG, Emergency Response Planning Guideline (see p 656 for an explanation of ERPG). IARC 1, known human carcinogen; IARC 2A, probable human carcinogen; IARC 2B, possible human carcinogen; IARC 3, inadequate data available. NFPA hazard codes: H, health; F, fire; R, reactivity; Ox, oxidizer; W, water-reactive; 0 (none) <—> 4 (severe).

(*continued*)

TABLE IV–4. HEALTH HAZARD SUMMARIES FOR INDUSTRIAL AND OCCUPATIONAL CHEMICALS (CONTINUED)

Health Hazard Summaries	ACGIH TLV	IDLH	NFPA Codes H F R	Comments
2,3,7,8-Tetrachlorodibenzo-*p*-dioxin (TCDD [CAS 1746-01-6]): A potent form of acne (chloracne) is a specific marker of exposure. Human carcinogen (IARC 1). See also "Dioxins," p 224.	NIOSH CA			White crystalline solid. A toxic contaminant of numerous chlorinated herbicides, including 2,4,5-T and 2,4-D.
1,1,1,2-Tetrachloro-2,2-difluoroethane (halocarbon 112a; refrigerant 112a [CAS: 76-11-9]): Of low acute toxicity. Very high air levels irritating to the eyes and respiratory tract. A CNS depressant at high levels. By anology to other freons, may cause cardiac arrhythmias. High-dose studies in animals suggest possible kidney and liver in jury. See also p 251.	100 ppm	2,000 ppm		Colorless liquid or solid with a slight ether-like odor. Vapor pressure is 40 mm Hg at 20°C (68°F). Not combustible. Thermal breakdown products include hydrogen chloride and hydrogen fluoride.
1,1,2,2-Tetrachloro-1,2-difluoroethane (halocarbon 112; refrigerant 112 [CAS: 76-12-0]): Of low acute toxicity. Once used as an antihelminthic. Very high air levels cause CNS depression. Vapors mildly irritating. By analogy to other freons, may cause cardiac arrhythmias. See also p 251.	50 ppm	2,000 ppm		Colorless liquid or solid with a slight ether-like odor. Odor is of unknown value as a warning property. Vapor pressure is 40 mm Hg at 20°C (68°F). Not combustible. Thermal breakdown products include hydrogen chloride and hydrogen fluoride.
1,1,2,2-Tetrachloroethane (acetylene tetrachloride [CAS: 79-34-5]): Dermal absorption may cause systemic toxicity. Vapors irritating to the eyes and respiratory tract. A CNS depressant. By analogy to other (p 439) chlorinated ethane derivatives, may cause cardiac arrhythmias. May cause hepatic or renal injury. Inadequate evidence of carcinogenicity in test animals (IARC 2B).	1 ppm, S, A3 NIOSH CA	100 ppm		Colorless to light yellow liquid. Sweet, suffocating, chloroform-like odor is a good warning property. Vapor pressure is 8 mm Hg at 20°C (68°F). Not combustible. Thermal breakdown products include hydrogen chloride and phosgene. Prior heavy use as a solvent in the United States.

Tetrachloroethylene (perchloroethylene, PERC [CAS: 127-18-4]): Irritating upon prolonged contact; mild burns may result. Vapors irritating to eyes and respiratory tract. A CNS depressant. By analogy to trichloroethylene and other chlorinated solvents, may cause arrhythmias. May cause liver and kidney injury. Chronic overexposure may cause short-term memory loss and personality changes. Limited evidence of adverse effects on male reproductive function and fetal development in test animals. Evidence for carcinogenicity in test animals (IARC 2A). See also p 439.	25 ppm, A3 NIOSH CA	150 ppm ERPG-1: 100 ppm ERPG-2: 200 ppm ERPG-3: 1,000 ppm		Colorless liquid. Chloroform-like or ether-like odor and eye irritation are adequate warning properties. Vapor pressure is 14 mm Hg at 20°C (68°F). Not combustible. Thermal breakdown products include phosgene and hydrochloric acid. Used in the dry cleaning industry.
Tetrachloronaphthalene (Halowax [CAS: 1335-88-2]): Causes chloracne and jaundice. Stored in body fat. Dermal absorption occurs. For chloracne, see also "Dioxins," p 224.	2 mg/m^3	50 mg/m^3 (effective IDLH)		White to light yellow solid. Aromatic odor of unknown value as a warning property. Vapor pressure is less than 1 mm Hg at 20°C (68°F). Thermal breakdown products include hydrogen chloride and phosgene.
Tetraethyl dithionopyrophosphate (TEDP, sulfotepp [CAS: 3689-24-5]): An organophosphate anticholinesterase insecticide (p 353). Well absorbed dermally.	0.1 mg/m^3 (inhalable fraction and vapor), S	10 mg/m^3		Yellow liquid with garlic odor. Not combustible. Thermal breakdown products include sulfur dioxide and phosphoric acid mist. Agricultural pesticide.
Tetraethyl lead (CAS: 78-00-2): A potent CNS toxin. Dermally well absorbed. Can cause psychosis, mania, convulsions, and coma. Reports of reduced sperm counts and impotence in overexposed workers. See also "Lead," p 286.	0.1 mg/m^3 (as Pb), S	40 mg/m^3 (as Pb)	3 2 3 W	Colorless liquid. May be dyed blue, red, or orange. Slight musty odor of unknown value as a warning property. Vapor pressure is 0.2 mm Hg at 20°C (68°F). Combustible. Decomposes in light. As a gasoline additive, largely phased out; heavy exposure has occurred historically through inappropriate use of gasoline as a solvent and in substance abuse.

(C), ceiling air concentration (TLV-C); S, skin absorption can be significant; SEN, potential sensitizer; STEL, short-term (15-minute) exposure level. A1, ACGIH-confirmed human carcinogen; A2, ACGIH-suspected human carcinogen; A3, ACGIH animal carcinogen. ERPG, Emergency Response Planning Guideline (see p 656 for an explanation of ERPG). IARC 1, known human carcinogen; IARC 2A, probable human carcinogen; IARC 2B, possible human carcinogen; IARC 3, inadequate data available. NFPA hazard codes: H, health; F, fire; R, reactivity; Ox, oxidizer; W, water-reactive; 0 (none) <—> 4 (severe).

(*continued*)

TABLE IV–4. HEALTH HAZARD SUMMARIES FOR INDUSTRIAL AND OCCUPATIONAL CHEMICALS (CONTINUED)

Health Hazard Summaries	ACGIH TLV	IDLH	NFPA Codes H F R	Comments
Tetraethyl pyrophosphate (TEPP [CAS: 107-49-3]): A potent organophosphate cholinesterase inhibitor (p 353). Rapidly absorbed through skin.	0.01 mg/m^3 (inhalable fraction and vapor), S	5 mg/m^3		Colorless to amber liquid with a faint fruity odor. Slowly hydrolyzed in water. Vapor pressure is 1 mm Hg at 140°C (284°F). Not combustible. Thermal breakdown products include phosphoric acid mist.
Tetrahydrofuran (THF, diethylene oxide [CAS: 109-99-9]): Mildly irritating upon direct contact. Vapors mildly irritating to eyes and respiratory tract. A CNS depressant at high levels. A liver and kidney toxin at high doses in test animals.	50 ppm, S, A3	20,000 ppm [LEL] ERPG-1: 100 ppm ERPG-2: 500 ppm ERPG-3: 5,000 ppm	2 3 1	Colorless liquid. The ether-like odor is detectable well below the TLV and provides a good warning property. Flammable. Vapor pressure is 145 mm Hg at 20°C (68°F).
Tetrahydrothiophene (THT [CAS: 110-01-0]): Eye and respiratory tract irritant. Case report association with severe airway obstruction.			1 3 0	Pale yellow or clear liquid with pungent, objectionable odor. Odorant additive to gas. Vapor pressure is 18 mm Hg at 25°C (77°F). Highly flammable. Used as an odorant (eg, added to natural gas).
Tetramethyl lead (CAS: 75-74-1): A potent CNS toxin thought to be similar to tetraethyl lead. See also “lead,” p 286.	0.15 mg/m^3 (as Pb), S	40 mg/m^3 (as Pb)	2 3 3 W	Colorless liquid. May be dyed red, orange, or blue. Slight musty odor is of unknown value as a warning property. Vapor pressure is 22 mm Hg at 20°C (68°F).
Tetramethyl succinonitrile (TMSN [CAS: 3333-52-6]): A potent neurotoxin. Headaches, nausea, dizziness, convulsions, and coma have occurred in overexposed workers.	0.5 ppm, S	5 ppm		Colorless, odorless solid. Thermal breakdown products include oxides of nitrogen.
Tetramethylammonium hydroxide (TMAH [CAS: 75-59-2): A corrosive substance that can cause injury to the skin, eyes, and respiratory tract. Exposure has resulted in human fatalities.				A very strong base that forms corrosive alkaline solutions. Used in semiconductor manufacturing.

Tetranitromethane (CAS: 509-14-8): Highly irritating upon direct contact; mild burns may result. Vapors extremely irritating to eyes and respiratory tract; pulmonary edema has been reported. May cause methemoglobinemia (p 317). Liver, kidney, and CNS injury in test animals at high doses. Overexposure associated with headaches, fatigue, dyspnea. See also "Nitrates and Nitrites," p 339. A carcinogen in animal tests (IARC 2B).	0.005 ppm, A3	4 ppm	Colorless to light yellow liquid or solid with a pungent, acrid odor. Irritative effects are a good warning property. Vapor pressure is 8.4 mm Hg at 20°C (68°F). Not combustible. A weak explosive and oxidizer. Highly explosive in the presence of impurities.
Tetryl (nitramine, 2,4,6-trinitrophenylmethylnitramine [CAS: 479-45-8]): Causes skin sensitization with dermatitis. Dusts extremely irritating to the eyes and respiratory tract. Stains tissues bright yellow. May injure the liver and kidneys. Overexposures also associated with malaise, headache, nausea, and vomiting.	1.5 mg/m^3	750 mg/m^3	White to yellow solid. Odorless. A strong oxidizer. Vapor pressure is much less than 1 mm Hg at 20°C (68°F). Explosive used in detonators and primers.
Thallium (CAS: 7440-28-0) and soluble compounds (thallium sulfate, thallium acetate, thallium nitrate): A potent toxin causing diverse chronic effects, including psychosis, peripheral neuropathy, optic neuritis, alopecia, abdominal pain, irritability, and weight loss. Liver and kidney injury may occur. Ingestion causes severe hemorrhagic gastroenteritis. Absorption possible by all routes. See also p 433.	0.02 mg/m^3 (inhalable fraction, as Tl), S	15 mg/m^3 (as Tl)	Appearance varies with the compound. The elemental form is a bluish-white ductile heavy metal with a negligible vapor pressure. Thallium has been used as a rodenticide.
Thioglycolic acid (mercaptoacetic acid [CAS: 68-11-1]): Skin or eye contact with concentrated acid causes severe burns. Vapors irritating to eyes and respiratory tract.	1 ppm, S		Colorless liquid. Unpleasant mercaptan-like odor. Vapor pressure is 10 mm Hg at 18°C (64°F). Found in some cold wave and depilatory formulations.

(C), ceiling air concentration (TLV-C); S, skin absorption can be significant; SEN, potential sensitizer; STEL, short-term (15-minute) exposure level. A1, ACGIH-confirmed human carcinogen; A2, ACGIH-suspected human carcinogen; A3, ACGIH animal carcinogen. ERPG, Emergency Response Planning Guideline (see p 656 for an explanation of ERPG). IARC 1, known human carcinogen; IARC 2A, probable human carcinogen; IARC 2B, possible human carcinogen; IARC 3, inadequate data available. NFPA hazard codes: H, health; F, fire; R, reactivity; Ox, oxidizer; W, water-reactive; 0 (none) <—> 4 (severe).

(*continued*)

TABLE IV–4. HEALTH HAZARD SUMMARIES FOR INDUSTRIAL AND OCCUPATIONAL CHEMICALS (CONTINUED)

Health Hazard Summaries	ACGIH TLV	IDLH	NFPA Codes H F R	Comments
Thiram (tetramethylthiuram disulfide [CAS: 137-26-8]): Dusts mildly irritating to eyes, skin, and respiratory tract. A moderate allergen and a potent skin sensitizer. Has disulfiram-like effects in exposed persons who consume alcohol (p 226). An experimental goitrogen. Adverse effects on fetal development in test animals at very high doses. Inadequate carcinogenicity data (IARC 3).	0.05 mg/m^3, SEN	100 mg/m^3		White to yellow powder with a characteristic odor. May be dyed blue. Vapor pressure is negligible at 20°C (68°F). Thermal breakdown products include sulfur dioxide and carbon disulfide (p 181). Used in rubber manufacture (vulcanization) and as a fungicide.
Tilmicosin phosphate (Micotil 300 [CAS: 137330-13-3]): Severe allergen and acute human cardiotoxin.				Yellow to amber liquid. Veterinary antibiotic. Has been used for intentional self-poisoning. Exposure can occur through syringe mishap leading to auto-injection.
Tin, metal and inorganic compounds: Dusts irritating to the eyes, nose, throat, and skin. Prolonged inhalation may cause chest radiographic abnormalities. Some compounds react with water to form acids (tin tetrachloride, stannous chloride, and stannous sulfate) or bases (sodium and potassium stannate).	2 mg/m^3 (as Sn)	100 mg/m^3 (as Sn)		Metallic tin is odorless with a dull, silvery color.
Tin, organic compounds: Highly irritating upon direct contact; burns may result. Dusts, fumes, or vapors highly irritating to the eyes and respiratory tract. Triethyltin is a potent neurotoxin; triphenyltin acetate is highly hepatotoxic. Trialkyltins are the most toxic, followed in order by the dialkyltins and monoalkyltins. Within each of these classes, the ethyltin compounds are the most toxic. All are well absorbed dermally.	0.1 mg/m^3, S (as Sn)	25 mg/m^3 (as Sn)		There are many kinds of organotin compounds: mono-, di-, tri-, and tetra-alkyltin and -aryltin compounds exist. Combustible. Organic tin compounds are used in some polymers and paints (as a mildewcide).
Titanium dioxide (CAS: 13463-67-7): A mild pulmonary irritant. IARC 2B.	10 mg/m^3 NIOSH CA	5,000 mg/m^3		White odorless powder. Rutile is a common crystalline form. Vapor pressure is negligible.

Tolidine (*o*-tolidine, 3,3'-dimethylbenzidine [CAS: 119-93-7]): A carcinogen in test animals (IARC 2B).	S, A3 NIOSH CA			White to reddish solid. Oxides of nitrogen are among thermal breakdown products. Nanoparticle preparations have widespread applications including consumer products.
Toluene (toluol, methylbenzene [CAS: 108-88-3]): Vapors mildly irritating to eyes and respiratory tract. A CNS depressant; may cause brain, kidney, and muscle damage with frequent intentional abuse. May cause cardiac arrhythmias. Liver and kidney injury with heavy exposures. Abusive sniffing during pregnancy associated with birth defects. Inadequate carcinogenicity data (IARC 3). See also p 437.	20 ppm, S	500 ppm ERPG-1: 50 ppm ERPG-2: 300 ppm ERPG-3: 1,000 ppm	2 3 0	Colorless liquid. Aromatic, benzene-like odor detectable at very low levels. Irritation serves as a good warning property. Vapor pressure is 22 mm Hg at 20°C (68°F). Flammable. Common industrial solvent also found in many consumer products (eg, adhesives, strippers).
Toluene-2,4-diisocyanate (TDI [CAS: 584-84-9]): A potent respiratory tract sensitizer (asthma) and potent irritant of the eyes, skin, and respiratory tract. Pulmonary edema has resulted with higher exposures. A carcinogen in test animals (IARC 2B). See also p 280.	[proposed: 0.001 ppm (inhalable fraction and vapor), S, SEN], A3 NIOSH CA	2.5 ppm ERPG-1: 0.01 ppm ERPG-2: 0.15 ppm ERPG-3: 0.6 ppm	3 1 2	Colorless needles or a liquid with a sharp, pungent odor near 0.01 ppm. Vapor pressure is approximately 0.04 mm Hg at 20°C (68°F). Combustible. Starting material for polyurethane; exposure to TDI may occur during polymerization including in field applications.
***o*-Toluidine (2-methylaniline [CAS: 95-53-4]):** A corrosive alkali; can cause severe burns. May cause methemoglobinemia (p 317). Dermal absorption occurs. A human carcinogen (IARC 1).	2 ppm, S, A3 NIOSH CA	50 ppm	3 2 0	Colorless to pale yellow liquid. The weak aromatic odor is thought to be a good warning property. Vapor pressure is less than 1 mm Hg at 20°C (68°F).
***m*-Toluidine (3-methylaniline [CAS: 108-44-1]):** A corrosive alkali; can cause severe burns. May cause methemoglobinemia (p 317). Dermal absorption occurs.	2 ppm, S			Pale yellow liquid. Vapor pressure is less than 1 mm Hg at 20°C (68°F).
***p*-Toluidine (4-methylaniline [CAS: 106-49-0]):** A corrosive alkali; can cause severe burns. May cause methemoglobinemia (p 317). Dermal absorption occurs. A carcinogen in test animals.	2 ppm, S, A3 NIOSH CA		3 2 0	White solid. Vapor pressure is 1 mm Hg at 20°C (68°F).

(C), ceiling air concentration (TLV-C); S, skin absorption can be significant; SEN, potential sensitizer; STEL, short-term (15-minute) exposure level. A1, ACGIH-confirmed human carcinogen; A2, ACGIH-suspected human carcinogen; A3, ACGIH animal carcinogen. ERPG, Emergency Response Planning Guideline (see p 656 for an explanation of ERPG). IARC 1, known human carcinogen; IARC 2A, probable human carcinogen; IARC 2B, possible human carcinogen; IARC 3, inadequate data available. NFPA hazard codes: H, health; F, fire; R, reactivity; Ox, oxidizer; W, water-reactive; 0 (none) <—> 4 (severe).

(*continued*)

TABLE IV–4. HEALTH HAZARD SUMMARIES FOR INDUSTRIAL AND OCCUPATIONAL CHEMICALS (CONTINUED)

Health Hazard Summaries	ACGIH TLV	IDLH	NFPA Codes H F R	Comments
Tributyl phosphate (CAS: 126-73-8): Highly irritating upon direct contact; causes severe eye injury and skin irritation. Vapors or mists irritating to the eyes and respiratory tract; high exposure in test animals caused pulmonary edema. Weak anticholinesterase activity. Headache and nausea are reported.	5 mg/m^3 (inhalable fraction and vapor), A3	30 ppm	3 1 0	Colorless to pale yellow liquid. Odorless. Vapor pressure is very low at 20°C (68°F). Combustible. Thermal breakdown products include phosphoric acid fume.
Trichloroacetic acid (CAS: 76-03-9): A strong acid. A protein denaturant. Corrosive to eyes and skin upon direct contact. Insufficient data for carcinogenicity (IARC 2B).	0.5 ppm, A3			Deliquescent crystalline solid. Vapor pressure is 1 mm Hg at 51°C (128.3°F). Thermal breakdown products include hydrochloric acid and phosgene.
1,2,4-Trichlorobenzene (CAS: 120-82-1): Prolonged or repeated contact can cause skin and eye irritation. Vapors irritating to the eyes, skin, and respiratory tract. High-dose animal exposures injure the liver, kidneys, lungs, and CNS. Does not cause chloracne.	5 ppm (C)		2 1 0	A colorless liquid with an unpleasant, mothball-like odor. Vapor pressure is 1 mm Hg at 38.4°C (101.1°F). Combustible. Thermal breakdown products include hydrogen chloride and phosgene.
1,1,1-Trichloroethane (methyl chloroform, TCA [CAS: 71-55-6]): Vapors mildly irritating to eyes and respiratory tract. A CNS depressant. May cause cardiac arrhythmias. Some dermal absorption occurs. Liver and kidney injury may occur. See also p 439. IARC 3.	350 ppm	700 ppm ERPG-1: 350 ppm ERPG-2: 700 ppm ERPG-3: 3,500 ppm	2 1 0	Colorless liquid. Odor threshold near 350 ppm. Vapor pressure is 100 mm Hg at 20°C (68°F). Not combustible. Thermal breakdown products include hydrogen chloride and phosgene. Widely used chlorinated solvent.
1,1,2-Trichloroethane (CAS: 79-00-5): Dermal absorption may occur. Vapors mildly irritating to eyes and respiratory tract. A CNS depressant. May cause cardiac arrhythmias. Causes liver and kidney injury in test animals. Limited evidence for carcinogenicity in test animals (IARC 3). See also p 439.	10 ppm, S, A3 NIOSH CA	100 ppm	2 1 0	Colorless liquid. Sweet, chloroform-like odor is of unknown value as a warning property. Vapor pressure is 19 mm Hg at 20°C (68°F). Not combustible. Thermal breakdown products include phosgene and hydrochloric acid.

Trichloroethylene (trichloroethene, TCE [CAS: 79-01-6]): Dermal absorption may occur. Vapors mildly irritating to eyes and respiratory tract. A CNS depressant. May cause cardiac arrhythmias. May cause cranial and peripheral neuropathy and liver damage. Has a disulfiram-like effect, "degreasers' flush" (p 226). Reported to cause liver and lung cancers in mice (IARC 1). See also p 439.	10 ppm, A2 NIOSH CA	1,000 ppm ERPG-1: 100 ppm ERPG-2: 500 ppm ERPG-3: 5,000 ppm	2 1 0	Colorless liquid. Sweet chloroform-like odor near 100 ppm. Vapor pressure is 58 mm Hg at 20°C (68°F). Not combustible at room temperature. Decomposition products include hydrogen chloride and phosgene. Widely used chlorinated solvent.
Trichlorofluoromethane (Freon 11 [CAS: 75-69-4]): Vapors mildly irritating to eyes and respiratory tract. A CNS depressant. May cause cardiac arrhythmias. See also p 251.	1,000 ppm (C)	2,000 ppm		Colorless liquid or gas at room temperature. Vapor pressure is 690 mm Hg at 20°C (68°F). Not combustible. Thermal breakdown products include hydrogen chloride and hydrogen fluoride.
Trichloronaphthalene (Halowax [CAS: 1321-65-9]): Causes chloracne. A hepatotoxin at low doses, causing jaundice. Stored in body fat. Systemic toxicity may occur after dermal exposure. For chloracne, see also "Dioxins," p 224.	5 mg/m^3, S	20 mg/m^3 (effective IDLH)		Colorless to pale yellow solid with an aromatic odor of uncertain value as a warning property. Vapor pressure is less than 1 mm Hg at 20°C (68°F). Flammable. Decomposition products include phosgene and hydrogen chloride.
2,4,5-Trichlorophenoxyacetic acid (2,4,5-T [CAS: 93-76-5]): Moderately irritating to eyes, skin, and respiratory tract. Ingestion can cause gastroenteritis and injury to the CNS, muscle, kidney, and liver. A weak uncoupler of oxidative phosphorylation. Polychlorinated dibenzodioxin (dioxin) compounds are contaminants (p 224). There are reports of sarcomas occurring in applicators. Adverse effects on fetal development in test animals.	10 mg/m^3	250 mg/m^3		Colorless to tan solid. Appearance and some hazardous properties vary with the formulation. Odorless. Vapor pressure is negligible at 20°C (68°F). Not combustible. Thermal breakdown products include hydrogen chloride and dioxins. An herbicide once widely used as a defoliant and in Vietnam ("Agent Orange").

(C), ceiling air concentration (TLV-C); S, skin absorption can be significant; SEN, potential sensitizer; STEL, short-term (15-minute) exposure level. A1, ACGIH-confirmed human carcinogen; A2, ACGIH-suspected human carcinogen; A3, ACGIH animal carcinogen. ERPG, Emergency Response Planning Guideline (see p 656 for an explanation of ERPG). IARC 1, known human carcinogen; IARC 2A, probable human carcinogen; IARC 2B, possible human carcinogen; IARC 3, inadequate data available. NFPA hazard codes: H, health; F, fire; R, reactivity; Ox, oxidizer; W, water-reactive; 0 (none) <—> 4 (severe).

(*continued*)

TABLE IV–4. HEALTH HAZARD SUMMARIES FOR INDUSTRIAL AND OCCUPATIONAL CHEMICALS (CONTINUED)

Health Hazard Summaries	ACGIH TLV	IDLH	NFPA Codes H F R	Comments
1,1,2-Trichloro-1,2,2-trifluoroethane (Freon 113 [CAS: 76-13-1]): Vapors mildly irritating to eyes and mucous membranes. Very high air levels cause CNS depression and may injure the liver. May cause cardiac arrhythmias at air concentrations as low as 2,000 ppm in test animals. See also p 251.	1,000 ppm	2,000 ppm		Colorless liquid. Sweet, chloroform-like odor occurs only at very high concentrations and is a poor warning property. Vapor pressure is 284 mm Hg at 20°C (68°F). Not combustible. Thermal breakdown products include hydrogen chloride, hydrogen fluoride, and phosgene.
Triethylamine (CAS: 121-44-8): An alkaline corrosive; highly irritating to eyes and skin; severe burns may occur. Vapors very irritating to eyes and respiratory tract; pulmonary edema may occur. High doses in animals cause heart, liver, and kidney injury. CNS stimulation possibly resulting from inhibition of monoamine oxidase.	0.5 ppm, S	200 ppm	3 3 0	Colorless liquid with a fishy, ammonia-like odor of unknown value as a warning property. Vapor pressure is 54 mm Hg at 20°C (68°F). Flammable. Industrial chemical but also used as an insect "anesthetic" in research and other applications.
Trifluorobromomethane (Halon 1301; Freon 13B1 [CAS: 75-63-8]): Extremely high air levels (150,000–200,000 ppm) can cause CNS depression and cardiac arrhythmias. See also p 251.	1,000 ppm	40,000 ppm		Colorless gas with a weak ether-like odor at high levels and poor warning properties. Not combustible.
Trifluoromethane (Freon 23 [CAS: 75-46-7]): Vapors mildly irritating to the eyes and mucous membranes. Very high air levels cause CNS depression and cardiac arrhythmias. See also p 251.				Not combustible. Thermal breakdown products include hydrogen fluoride (p 269).
Trimellitic anhydride (TMAN [CAS: 552-30-7]): Dusts and vapors extremely irritating to eyes, nose, throat, skin, and respiratory tract. Potent respiratory sensitizer (asthma). Can also cause diffuse lung hemorrhage (and subsequent pulmonary hemosiderosis).	0.0005 mg/m^3 (inhalable fraction and vapor), S, SEN			Colorless solid. Hydrolyzes to trimellitic acid in aqueous solutions. Vapor pressure is 0.000004 mm Hg at 25°C (77°F). TMAN is an important component of certain epoxy formulations.

Trimethylamine (CAS: 75-50-3): An alkaline corrosive; highly irritating upon direct contact; severe burns may occur. Vapors very irritating to respiratory tract.	5 ppm	ERPG-1: 0.1 ppm ERPG-2: 100 ppm ERPG-3: 500 ppm	3 4 0	Highly flammable gas with a pungent, fishy, ammonia-like odor near 0.1 ppm. May be used as a warning agent in natural gas.
Trimethyl phosphite (phosphorous acid trimethylester [CAS: 121-45-9]): Very irritating upon direct contact; severe burns may result. Vapors highly irritating to respiratory tract. Cataracts have developed in test animals exposed to high air levels. Evidence for adverse effects on fetal development in test animals.	2 ppm		1 3 1	Colorless liquid with a characteristic strong, fishy, or ammonia-like odor. Hydrolyzed in water. Vapor pressure is 24 mm Hg at 25°C (77°F). Combustible.
Trinitrotoluene (2,4,6-trinitrotoluene, TNT [CAS: 118-96-7]): Irritating upon direct contact. Stains tissues yellow. Causes sensitization dermatitis. Vapors irritating to respiratory tract. May cause liver injury, methemoglobinemia (p 317). Occupational overexposure associated with cataracts. Causes vasodilation, including vasodilation in coronary arteries. Headache and drop in blood pressure are common. Well absorbed by all routes. Tolerance to vasodilation can occur; cessation of exposure may precipitate angina pectoris in pharmacologically dependent workers. See also "Nitrates and Nitrites," p 339. Inadequate carcinogenicity data (IARC 3).	0.1 mg/m^3, S	500 mg/m^3		White to light yellow crystalline solid. Odorless. Vapor pressure is 0.05 mm Hg at 85°C (185°F). Explosive upon heating or shock. Exposure can occur among munitions workers.
Triorthocresyl phosphate (TOCP [CAS: 78-30-8]): Inhibits acetylcholinesterase (p 353). Potent neurotoxin causing delayed, partially reversible peripheral neuropathy by all routes.	[proposed: 0.02 mg/m^3 (inhalable fraction and vapor)], S	40 mg/m^3	1 1 0	Colorless viscous liquid. Odorless. Not combustible. Although an anticholinesterase inhibitor, it is widely used as a chemical additive and in chemical synthesis. Exposure has occurred through contaminated foodstuffs.

(C), ceiling air concentration (TLV-C); S, skin absorption can be significant; SEN, potential sensitizer; STEL, short-term (15-minute) exposure level. A1, ACGIH-confirmed human carcinogen; A2, ACGIH-suspected human carcinogen; A3, ACGIH animal carcinogen. ERPG, Emergency Response Planning Guideline (see p 656 for an explanation of ERPG). IARC 1, known human carcinogen; IARC 2A, probable human carcinogen; IARC 2B, possible human carcinogen; IARC 3, inadequate data available. NFPA hazard codes: H, health; F, fire; R, reactivity; Ox, oxidizer; W, water-reactive; 0 (none) <—> 4 (severe).

(continued)

TABLE IV–4. HEALTH HAZARD SUMMARIES FOR INDUSTRIAL AND OCCUPATIONAL CHEMICALS (CONTINUED)

Health Hazard Summaries	ACGIH TLV	IDLH	NFPA Codes H F R	Comments
Triphenyl phosphate (CAS: 115-86-6): Weak anticholinesterase activity in humans (p 353). Delayed neuropathy reported in test animals.	3 mg/m^3	1,000 mg/m^3	1 1 0	Colorless solid. Faint phenolic odor. Not combustible. Thermal breakdown products include phosphoric acid fumes.
Tungsten and compounds: Few reports of human toxicity. Some salts may release acid upon contact with moisture. Chronic exposure to tungsten carbide–cobalt amalgams in the hard metals industry may be associated with fibrotic lung disease.	5 mg/m^3 (insoluble compounds) 1 mg/m^3 (soluble compounds)			Elemental tungsten is a gray, hard, brittle metal. Finely divided powders are flammable. Hard metal is used in specialty saw blades and in diamond cutting, among other applications.
Turpentine (CAS: 8006-64-2): Irritating to eyes upon direct contact. Dermal sensitizer. Dermal absorption occurs. Vapors irritating to respiratory tract. A CNS depressant at high air levels. See also "Hydrocarbons," p 266.	20 ppm, SEN	800 ppm	2 3 0	Colorless to pale yellow liquid with a characteristic paintlike odor that serves as a good warning property. Vapor pressure is 5 mm Hg at 20°C (68°F). Flammable.
Uranium compounds: Many salts are irritating to the respiratory tract; soluble salts are potent kidney toxins. Uranium is a weakly radioactive element (alpha emitter); decays to the radionuclide thorium 230. Uranium has the potential to cause radiation injury to the lungs, tracheobronchial lymph nodes, bone marrow, and skin.	0.2 mg/m^3 (soluble and insoluble compounds, as U), A1 NIOSH CA	10 mg/m^3		Dense, silver-white, lustrous metal. Finely divided powders are pyrophoric. Radioactive (see p 401). Depleted uranium-containing weaponry has been investigated as a potential source of exposure (eg, through retained shrapnel).
Valeraldehyde (pentanal [CAS: 110-62-3]): Very irritating to eyes and skin; severe burns may result. Vapors highly irritating to the eyes and respiratory tract.	50 ppm		1 3 0	Colorless liquid with a fruity odor. Flammable.

Compound				
Vanadium pentoxide (CAS: 1314-62-1): Dusts or fumes highly irritating to eyes, skin, and respiratory tract. Acute overexposures have been associated with persistent bronchitis and asthma-like responses ("boilermakers' asthma"). Sensitization dermatitis reported. Low-level exposure may cause a greenish discoloration of the tongue, metallic taste, and cough. IARC 2B.	0.05 mg/m^3 (inhalable fraction), A3	35 mg/m^3 (as V)		Yellow-orange to rust-brown crystalline powder or dark gray flakes. Odorless. Not combustible.
Vinyl acetate (CAS: 108-05-4): Highly irritating upon direct contact; severe skin and eye burns may result. Vapors irritating to the eyes and respiratory tract. Mild CNS depressant at high levels. Limited evidence for adverse effects on male reproduction in test animals at high doses. IARC 2B.	10 ppm, A3	ERPG-1: 5 ppm ERPG-2: 75 ppm ERPG-3: 500 ppm	2 3 2	Volatile liquid with a pleasant fruity odor at low levels. Vapor pressure is 115 mm Hg at 25°C (77°F). Flammable. Polymerizes readily. Must contain inhibitor to prevent auto-polymerization.
Vinyl bromide (CAS: 593-60-2): At high air levels, an eye and respiratory tract irritant and CNS depressant; a kidney and liver toxin. Animal carcinogen (IARC 2A).	0.5 ppm, A2 NIOSH CA		2 4 1	Colorless, highly flammable gas with a distinctive odor.
Vinyl chloride (CAS: 75-01-4): An eye and respiratory tract irritant at high air levels. Degeneration of distal phalanges with "acro-osteolysis," Raynaud disease, and scleroderma has been associated with heavy workplace overexposures. A CNS depressant at high levels, formerly used as an anesthetic. May cause cardiac arrhythmias. Causes angiosarcoma of the liver in humans (IARC 1).	1 ppm, A1 OSHA CA NIOSH CA	[LEL: 36,000 ppm] ERPG-1: 500 ppm ERPG-2: 5,000 ppm ERPG-3: 20,000 ppm	2 4 2	Colorless, highly flammable gas with a sweet ether-like odor. Polymerizes readily. Current potential exposure is limited to vinyl chloride synthesis and polymerization to PVC.

(C), ceiling air concentration (TLV-C); S, skin absorption can be significant; SEN, potential sensitizer; STEL, short-term (15-minute) exposure level. A1, ACGIH-confirmed human carcinogen; A2, ACGIH-suspected human carcinogen; A3, ACGIH animal carcinogen. ERPG, Emergency Response Planning Guideline (see p 656 for an explanation of ERPG). IARC 1, known human carcinogen; IARC 2A, probable human carcinogen; IARC 2B, possible human carcinogen; IARC 3, inadequate data available. NFPA hazard codes: H, health; F, fire; R, reactivity; Ox, oxidizer; W, water-reactive; 0 (none) <—> 4 (severe).

(continued)

TABLE IV–4. HEALTH HAZARD SUMMARIES FOR INDUSTRIAL AND OCCUPATIONAL CHEMICALS (CONTINUED)

Health Hazard Summaries	ACGIH TLV	IDLH	NFPA Codes H F R	Comments
Vinyl cyclohexene dioxide (vinylhexane dioxide [CAS: 106-87-6]): Moderately irritating upon direct contact; severe burns may result. Vapors highly irritating to eyes and respiratory tract. Testicular atrophy, leukemia, and necrosis of the thymus in test animals. Topical application causes skin cancer in animal studies (IARC 2B).	0.1 ppm, S, A3 NIOSH CA			Colorless liquid. Vapor pressure is 0.1 mm Hg at 20°C (68°F).
Vinyl toluene (methylstyrene [CAS: 25013-15-4]): Vapors irritating to eyes and respiratory tract. A CNS depressant at high levels. Hepatic, renal, and hematologic toxicities observed at high doses in test animals. Limited evidence for adverse effects on the developing fetus at high doses. Inadequate carcinogenicity data (IARC 3).	50 ppm	400 ppm	2 2 2	Colorless liquid. Strong, unpleasant odor is considered to be an adequate warning property. Vapor pressure is 1.1 mm Hg at 20°C (68°F). Flammable. Inhibitor added to prevent explosive auto-polymerization.
VM&P naphtha (varnish makers' and printers' naphtha; ligroin [CAS: 8032-32-4]): Vapors irritating to eyes and respiratory tract. A CNS depressant at high levels. May contain a small amount of benzene. See also "Hydrocarbons," p 266.			1 3 0	Colorless volatile liquid. Common solvent.
VX (CAS 50782-69-9): Extremely toxic chemical warfare nerve agent (p 452) by all routes of contact. Readily absorbed via respiratory tract and skin and eyes. A potent cholinesterase inhibitor with rapid onset of symptoms. Vapors highly irritating.			4 1 1	Colorless or amber liquid. Least volatile of the chemical nerve agents: vapor pressure is 0.007 mm Hg at 25°C (77°F). Odor is not an adequate warning of exposure. Flammability unknown.
Warfarin (CAS: 81-81-2): An anticoagulant by ingestion. Medicinal doses associated with adverse effects on fetal development in test animals and humans. See also p 459.	0.1 mg/m^3 (inhalable fraction and vapors)	100 mg/m^3		Colorless crystalline substance. Odorless. Used as a rodenticide and pharmaceutical anticoagulant. Exposure is typically from inadvertent or deliberate ingestion rather than through workplace contamination.

Xylene (mixture of *o*-, *m*-, and *p*-dimethylbenzenes [CAS: 1330-20-7]): Vapors irritating to eyes and respiratory tract. A CNS depressant. By analogy to toluene and benzene, may cause cardiac arrhythmias. May injure kidneys. Limited evidence for adverse effects on fetal development in test animals at very high doses. Inadequate carcinogenicity data (IARC 3). See also p 437.	100 ppm	900 ppm	2 3 0	Colorless liquid or solid. Weak, somewhat sweet aromatic odor. Irritant effects are adequate warning properties. Vapor pressure is approximately 8 mm Hg at 20°C (68°F). Flammable.
Xylidine (dimethylaniline [CAS: 1300-73-8]): May cause methemoglobinemia (p 317). Dermal absorption may occur. Liver and kidney damage seen in test animals.	0.5 ppm (inhalable fraction and vapor), S, A3	50 ppm	3 1 0	Pale yellow to brown liquid. Weak, aromatic amine odor is an adequate warning property. Vapor pressure is less than 1 mm Hg at 20°C (68°F). Combustible. Thermal breakdown products include oxides of nitrogen. Used in chemical synthesis including in the dye industry.
Yttrium and compounds (yttrium metal, yttrium nitrate hexahydrate, yttrium chloride, yttrium oxide): Dusts may be irritating to the eyes and respiratory tract.	1 mg/m^3 (as Y)	500 mg/m^3 (as Y)		Appearance varies with compound.
Zinc chloride (CAS: 7646-85-7): Caustic and highly irritating upon direct contact; severe burns may result. Ulceration of exposed skin from exposure to fumes has been reported. Fumes extremely irritating to respiratory tract; pulmonary edema has resulted.	1 mg/m^3 (fume)	50 mg/m^3		White powder or colorless crystals that absorb moisture. The fume is white and has an acrid odor. Exposure is principally through smoke bombs.
Zinc chromates (basic zinc chromate, $ZnCrO_4$; zinc potassium chromate, $KZn_2(CrO_4)$; zinc yellow): Contains hexavalent chromium, which is associated with lung cancer in workers. See also p 196.	0.01 mg/m^3 (as Cr), A1			Basic zinc chromate is a yellow pigment; dichromates are orange.

(C), ceiling air concentration (TLV-C); S, skin absorption can be significant; SEN, potential sensitizer; STEL, short-term (15-minute) exposure level. A1, ACGIH-confirmed human carcinogen; A2, ACGIH-suspected human carcinogen; A3, ACGIH animal carcinogen. ERPG, Emergency Response Planning Guideline (see p 656 for an explanation of ERPG). IARC 1, known human carcinogen; IARC 2A, probable human carcinogen; IARC 2B, possible human carcinogen; IARC 3, inadequate data available. NFPA hazard codes: H, health; F, fire; R, reactivity; Ox, oxidizer; W, water-reactive; 0 (none) <—> 4 (severe).

(*continued*)

TABLE IV–4. HEALTH HAZARD SUMMARIES FOR INDUSTRIAL AND OCCUPATIONAL CHEMICALS (CONTINUED)

Health Hazard Summaries	ACGIH TLV	IDLH	NFPA Codes H F R	Comments
Zinc oxide (CAS: 1314-13-2): Fumes irritating to the respiratory tract. Causes metal fume fever (p 311). Symptoms include headache, fever, chills, and muscle aches.	2 mg/m^3 (respirable fraction)	500 mg/m^3		A white or yellowish-white powder. Fumes of zinc oxide are formed when elemental zinc is heated above its melting point. Principal exposure is through brass foundries or welding on galvanized steel.
Zirconium compounds (zirconium oxide, ZrO_2; zirconium oxychloride, ZrOCl; zirconium tetrachloride, $ZrCl_4$): Zirconium compounds are generally of low toxicity. Some compounds are irritating; zirconium tetrachloride releases HCl upon contact with moisture. Granulomata caused by the use of deodorants containing zirconium have been observed. Dermal sensitization has not been reported.	5 mg/m^3 (as Zr)	50 mg/m^3 (as Zr)		The elemental form is a bluish-black powder or a grayish-white, lustrous metal. The finely divided powder can be flammable.

(C), ceiling air concentration (TLV-C); S, skin absorption can be significant; SEN, potential sensitizer; STEL, short-term (15-minute) exposure level. A1, ACGIH-confirmed human carcinogen; A2, ACGIH-suspected human carcinogen; A3, ACGIH animal carcinogen. ERPG, Emergency Response Planning Guideline (see p 656 for an explanation of ERPG). IARC 1, known human carcinogen; IARC 2A, probable human carcinogen; IARC 2B, possible human carcinogen; IARC 3, inadequate data available. NFPA hazard codes: H, health; F, fire; R, reactivity; Ox, oxidizer; W, water-reactive; 0 (none) <—> 4 (severe).

Index

NOTE: A *t* following a page number indicates tabular material and an *f* following a page number indicates an illustration. Both proprietary and generic product names are listed in the index. When a proprietary name is used, the reader is encouraged to review the full reference under the generic name for complete information on the product.